WL 385 SHO 2013

Oxford Textbook of

Epilepsy and Epileptic Seizures

Oxford Textbook of
Epilepsy and Epileptic Seizures

Edited by

Simon Shorvon
UCL Institute of Neurology, University College London, London, UK

Renzo Guerrini
Pediatric Neurology Unit and Laboratories,
Children's Hospital A. Meyer – University of Florence, Firenze, Italy

Mark Cook
University of Melbourne, St Vincent's Hospital, Fitzroy, Victoria, Australia

Samden D. Lhatoo
Epilepsy Center, University Hospitals - Case Medical Center and Case Western Reserve University School of Medicine, Cleveland, Ohio, USA

Series Editor

Christopher Kennard

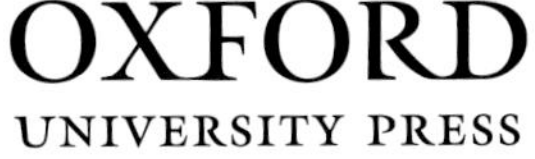

OXFORD
UNIVERSITY PRESS

Great Clarendon Street, Oxford, OX2 6DP,
United Kingdom

Oxford University Press is a department of the University of Oxford.
It furthers the University's objective of excellence in research, scholarship, and education by publishing worldwide. Oxford is a registered trade mark of Oxford University Press in the UK and in certain other countries

© Oxford University Press 2013

The moral rights of the authors have been asserted

Impression: 1

All rights reserved. No part of this publication may be reproduced, stored in a retrieval system, or transmitted, in any form or by any means, without the prior permission in writing of Oxford University Press, or as expressly permitted by law, by licence or under terms agreed with the appropriate reprographics rights organization. Enquiries concerning reproduction outside the scope of the above should be sent to the Rights department, Oxford University Press, at the address above

You must not circulate this work in any other form
and you must impose this same condition on any acquirer

British Library Cataloguing in publication data
Data available

ISBN 978-0-19-965904-3

Printed in China by
C&C Offset Printing Co. Ltd

Oxford University Press makes no representation, express or implied, that the drug dosages in this book are correct. Readers must therefore always check the product information and clinical procedures with the most up-to-date published product information and data sheets provided by the manufacturers and the most recent codes of conduct and safety regulations. The authors and the publishers do not accept responsibility or legal liability for any errors in the text or for the misuse or misapplication of material in this work. Except where otherwise stated, drug dosages and recommendations are for the non-pregnant adult who is not breast feeding.

Links to third party websites are provided by Oxford in good faith and for information only. Oxford disclaims any responsibility for the materials contained in any third party website referenced in this work.

Contents

List of Contributors

Shahram Amina, MD Epilepsy Center, University Hospitals Case Medical Center and Case Western Reserve University School of Medicine, Cleveland, Ohio, USA

Florin Amzica Associate Professor of Stomatology, Faculty of Dentistry, University of Montreal, Quebec, Canada

Richard Appleton Consultant Paediatric Neurologist, The Roald Dahl EEG Unit, Paediatric Neurosciences Foundation, Alder Hey Children's Hospital, Liverpool, UK

Sallie Baxendale Department of Clinical & Experimental Epilepsy, Institute of Neurology, UCL, London, UK

Jessie Bendavid Psychological Sciences, The University of Melbourne, Victoria, Australia

Adriana C. Bermeo Rush University Medical Center, Department of Neurological Sciences, Chicago, IL, USA

Tom Berney Institute of Health & Society (Child & Adolescent Psychiatry), Sir James Spence Institute, Royal Victoria Infirmary, Newcastle upon Tyne, UK

Ingmar Blümcke Department of Neuropathology, University Hospital Erlangen, Erlangen, Germany

Paul A.J.M. Boon Reference Center for Refractory Epilepsy, Department of Neurology & Institute for Neuroscience, Ghent University Hospital, Gent, Belgium

Trevor T.-J. Chong Department of Medicine, University of Melbourne, St Vincent's Hospital, Fitzroy, Victoria, Australia

Mark Cook University of Melbourne, St Vincent's Hospital, Fitzroy, Victoria, Australia

John J. Craig Department of Neurology, Belfast Health and Social Care Trust, Belfast, UK

B. Keith Day Department of Neurology, Washington University in St. Louis, St. Louis, MO, USA

Shoumitro Deb Imperial College London, Computational, Cognitive, and Clinical Neuroimaging Laboratory Hammersmith Hospital, London, UK

Ding Ding Institute of Neurology, Fu Dan University, Shanghai, China

Wendyl D'Souza Department of Medicine, St Vincent's Hospital Melbourne, The University of Melbourne, Fitzroy, Victoria, Australia

Lawrence Eisenman Department of Neurology, Washington University in St. Louis, St. Louis, MO, USA

Zachary Grinspan Division of Child Neurology, Weill Cornell Medical College, New York, NY, USA

Renzo Guerrini Pediatric Neurology Unit and Laboratories, Children's Hospital A. Meyer – University of Florence, Firenze, Italy

R. Edward Hogan Department of Neurology, Washington University in St. Louis, St. Louis, MO, USA

Ann Jacoby University of Liverpool, Department of Public Health and Policy, Institute of Psychology, Health and Society, Liverpool, UK

Michael R. Johnson Centre for Neuroscience, Imperial College Healthcare, Charing Cross Hospital, London, UK

Kitti Kaiboriboon Epilepsy Center, University Hospitals Case Medical Center and Case Western Reserve University School of Medicine, Cleveland, Ohio, USA

Samden D. Lhatoo Epilepsy Center, University Hospitals - Case Medical Center and Case Western Reserve University School of Medicine, Cleveland, Ohio, USA

Shichuo Li China Association Against Epilepsy, Beijing, China

Katia Lin Neurology Unit, Department of Internal Medicine University Hospital, Federal University of Santa Catarina, Florianopolis, SC, Brazil

Simon V. Liubinas Departments of Neurosurgery and Neurology, The Royal Melbourne Hospital, Parkville, Victoria, Australia

Hans O. Lüders Epilepsy Center, University Hospitals Case Medical Center and Case Western Reserve University School of Medicine, Cleveland, Ohio, USA

Kristina Malmgren Institute of Neuroscience and Physiology, Sahlgrenska Acedemy at Gothenburg University, Göteborg, Sweden

Carla Marini Pediatric Neurology Unit and Laboratories, Children's Hospital A. Meyer-University of Florence, Florence, Italy

Andrew P. Morokoff Departments of Surgery and Medicine, The Royal Melbourne Hospital, The University of Melbourne, Parkville, Victoria, Australia

Marco Mula Department of Clinical & Experimental Medicine, Amedeo Avogadro University, Division of Neurology, University Hospital Maggiore della Carità, Novara, Italy

J.M.K. Murthy The Institute of Neurological Sciences, CARE Hospital, Hyderabad, India

Aidan Neligan UCL Institute of Neurology, University College London, London, UK

Marina Nikanorova Danish Epilepsy Centre, Dianalund, Denmark

Terence J. O'Brien Departments of Surgery and Medicine, The Royal Melbourne Hospital, The University of Melbourne, Parkville, Victoria, Australia

Morris Odell Victorian Institute of Forensic Medicine Department of Forensic Medicine, Monash University, Victoria, Australia

Elena Parrini Pediatric Neurology Unit and Laboratories,, Children's Hospital A. Meyer – University of Florence, Firenze, Italy

Philip N. Patsalos UCL Institute of Neurology, University College London, London, UK

Elia Pestana Knight Case Western Reserve University, Division of Pediatric Epilepsy, Rainbow Babies and Children's Hospital, Cleveland, OH, USA

Bettina Pfausler Neurological Intensive Care Unit, Department of Neurology, University Hospital Innsbruck, Innsbruck, Austria

Ashalatha Radhakrishnan R. Madhavan Nayar Centre for Comprehensive Epilepsy Care, Sree Chitra Tirunal Institute for Medical Sciences and Technology, Thiruvananthapuram, Kerala, India

Markus Reuber Academic Neurology Unit, University of Sheffield, Sheffield, UK

Andrea O. Rossetti Department of Neurosciences, Service de Neurologie, Lausanne, Switzerland

Erich Schmutzhard Neurological Intensive Care Unit, Department of Neurology, University Hospital Innsbruck, Innsbruck, Austria

Stephan U. Schuele Northwestern University Comprehensive Epilepsy Center, Department of Neurology, Northwestern Memorial Hospital, Chicago, IL, USA

Jerry J. Shih Director, Comprehensive Epilepsy Program, Mayo Clinic Florida, Associate Professor of Neurology, Mayo Clinic College of Medicine

Shlomo Shinnar Comprehensive Epilepsy Management Center, Montefiore Medical Center, Albert Einstein College of Medicine, Bronx, NY, USA

Simon Shorvon UCL Institute of Neurology, University College London, London, UK

Gagandeep Singh Professor and Head Department of Neurology, Dayanand Medical College, Ludhiana, 141 001, Punjab, IndiaHonary Senior Research FellowDepartment of Clinical & Experimental Epilepsy, Institute of Neurology, Queen Square, London, UK

Ingrid E.B. Tuxhorn Case Western Reserve University, Division of Pediatric Epilepsy, Rainbow Babies and Children's Hospital, Cleveland, OH, USA

Kristl E. Vonck Reference Center for Refractory Epilepsy, Department of Neurology & Institute for Neuroscience, Ghent University Hospital, Gent, Belgium

Sarah J. Wilson Psychological Sciences, The University of Melbourne, Victoria, Australia, Comprehensive Epilepsy Program, Austin Health, Melbourne, Australia

Peter Wolf Danish Epilepsy Centre, Dianalund, Denmark

Jianzhong Wu Beijing Neurosurgical Institute, Beijing, China

List of Abbreviations

5-HT	serotonin
AED	antiepileptic drug
ACRM	American Congress of Rehabilitation Medicine
ACTH	adrenocorticotropic hormone
ADA	acute drug administration
ADNFLE	autosomal dominant nocturnal frontal lobe epilepsy
ADTLE	autosomal dominant temporal lobe epilepsy
AMACR	alpha-methylacyl-CoA racemase
AMPA	alpha-amino-3-hydroxyl-5-methyl-4-isoxazole-propionate
AMT	alpha-methyl-L-tryptophan
AN	anterior nucleus
AVM	arteriovenous malformation
BECTS	benign epilepsy of childhood with centrotemporal spikes
BFNC	benign familial neonatal convulsion
BFNIS	benign familial neonatal-infantile seizures
BFNS	benign familial neonatal seizures
BFPP	bilateral frontoparietal polymicrogyria
BIRD	brief ictal rhythmic electrographic discharge
BOLD	blood-oxygen level dependent
BPP	bilateral perisylvian polymicrogyria
Ca^{2+}	calcium
CAE	childhood absence epilepsy
CBZ	carbamazepine
CFR	case fatality rate
CGH	comparative genomic hybridization
CI	confidence interval
CK	creatine kinase
Cl^-	chloride
CM	centromedian
CNS	central nervous system
CNV	copy number variant
CPSE	complex partial status epilepticus
CRH	corticotropin-releasing hormone
CS	cortical stimulation
CSF	cerebrospinal fluid
CSH	carotid sinus hypersensitivity
CT	computed tomography
CVD	cerebrovascular disease
CYP	cytochrome P450
DALY	disability-adjusted life year
DAS	dialysis-associated seizures
DBS	deep brain stimulation
DDS	dialysis disequilibrium syndrome
DMPA	depot medroxyprogesterone acetate
DNET	dysembryoplastic neuroepithelial tumour
DTI	diffusion tensor imaging
EAAT	excitatory amino acid transporter
ECG	electrocardiography
ECoG	electrocortigogram
EDS	excessive daytime sleepiness
EE	epileptic encephalopathy
EEG	electroencephalogram
EIEE	early infantile epileptic encephalopathy
EME	early myoclonic epilepsy
EMG	electromyography
EPO	erythropoietin
EPSP	excitatory postsynaptic potential
ESES	electrical status epilepticus during sleep
ESI	electroencephalogram source imaging
ESM	ethosuximide
ESRD	end-stage renal disease
FCD	focal cortical dysplasia
FDA	Food and Drug Administration
FDG	fluro-2-deoxy-D-glucose
FER	facial emotion recognition
FLAIR	fluid attenuated inversion recovery
FLE	frontal lobe epilepsy
fMRI	functional magnetic resonance imaging
FS	febrile seizure
GABA	gamma-aminobutyric acid
GCD	granule cell dispersion
GCSE	generalized convulsive status epilepticus
GEFS+	generalized epilepsy with febrile seizure plus
GTCS	generalized tonic–clonic seizure
GVG	vigabatrin
H&E	haematoxylin and eosin
H^+	hydrogen
HD	haemodialysis
HFO	high-frequency oscillation
HIE	hypoxic-ischaemic encephalopathy

HP	hypothalamic–pituitary
HRF	haemodynamic response function
HS	hippocampal sclerosis
HSE	herpes simplex encephalitis
HSV-1	herpes simplex virus type-1
HUS	haemolytic uraemic syndrome
HWE	hot-water epilepsy
ICD-10	International Statistical Classification of Diseases and Related Health Problems, 10th revision
ICOE	idiopathic childhood occipital epilepsy
ICU	intensive care unit
IDD	interictal dysphoric disorder
IED	interictal epileptiform discharge
IGE	idiopathic generalized epilepsy
IHD	ischaemic heart disease
ILAE	International League Against Epilepsy
IPOLE	idiopathic photosensitive occipital lobe epilepsy
IPSP	inhibitory postsynaptic potential
IQ	intelligence quotient
IS	infantile spasms
ISSX	X-linked infantile spasms syndrome
JAE	juvenile absence epilepsy
JME	juvenile myoclonic epilepsy
K^+	potassium
LD	learning disability
LGS	Lennox–Gastaut syndrome
LIS	lissencephaly
LTG	lamotrigine
MCD	malformation of cortical development
MCM	major congenital malformation
MEG	magnetoencephalography
MERRF	myoclonus epilepsy with ragged red fibres
MHT	multiple hippocampal transection
MMIGS	multimodality image-guided surgery
MPRAGE	magnetization-prepared rapid acquisition with gradient echo
MRI	magnetic resonance imaging
MRS	magnetic resonance spectroscopy
MSI	magnetic source imaging
MST	multiple subpial transection
MTLE	mesial temporal lobe epilepsy
NAA	N-acetylaspartate
NALD	neonatal adrenoleucodystrophy
NCL	neuronal ceroid-lipofuscinosis
NES	non-epileptic seizures
NFLE	nocturnal frontal lobe epilepsy
NICE	National Institute for Health and Clinical Excellence
NMDA	N-methyl-D-aspartate
NREM	non-rapid eye movement
OR	odds ratio
pCO_2	partial pressure of carbon dioxide
PCOS	polycystic ovarian syndrome
PD	peritoneal dialysis
PDS	paroxysmal depolarizing shift
PEHO	progressive encephalopathy with oedema, hypsarrhythmia, and optic atrophy
PET	positron emission tomography
PHT	phenytoin
PMG	polymicrogyria
PMR	proportional mortality ratio
PNES	psychogenic non-epileptic seizure
PNH	periventricular nodular heterotopia
pO_2	partial pressure of oxygen
PRE	primary reading epilepsy
PRES	posterior reversible encephalopathy syndrome
PRIS	propofol infusion syndrome
PSW	polyspike wave
QOL	quality of life
RCDP	rhizomelic chondrodysplasia punctata
REM	rapid eye movement
RNS	responsive neurostimulator system
RR	relative risk
SBH	subcortical band heterotopia
SE	status epilepticus
SIGN	Scottish Intercollegiate Guidelines Network
SISCOM	subtraction ictal SPECT coregistered to MRI
SLE	systemic lupus erythematosus
SMA	supplementary motor area
SMEI	severe myoclonic epilepsy of infancy
SMR	standardized mortality ratio
SPC	Summary of Product Characteristics
SPECT	single-positron emission computed tomography
SpGR	spoiled gradient recalled
SSRI	selective serotonin reuptake inhibitor
SUDEP	sudden unexpected death in epilepsy
SW	spike wave
SWI	susceptibility-weighted image
TCI	tricyclic antidepressant drug
TEA	transient epileptic amnesia
TGA	transient global amnesia
TIA	transient ischaemic attack
TLE	temporal lobe epilepsy
TLOC	transient loss of consciousness
TLS	temporal lobe sclerosis
TPM	topiramate
TRH	thyrotropin-releasing hormone
TSC	tuberous sclerosis complex
UGT	uridine diphosphate glucuronyltransferase
VBM	voxel-based morphometry
VEM	video electroencephalography monitoring
VGLUT	vesicular glutamate transporter
VLCFA	very long chain fatty acid
VNS	vagus nerve stimulation
VPA	valproate
WoG	week of gestation
XLAG	X-linked lissencephaly with absent corpus callosum and ambiguous genitalia
XLMR	X-linked mental retardation

CHAPTER 1

Neurophysiology of Epilepsy

Florin Amzica

The epileptic syndrome encompasses a complex pathological reality with numerous and various aetiological origins. Each of these induces as many structural and functional alterations at the cellular and molecular level. Despite this rich diversity that eventually triggers epileptic or epileptic-like paroxysms, the electrical discharges, and ensuing behavioural correlates, during seizures share a surprisingly reduced variety of patterns, suggesting some common underlying mechanisms.

Both experimental and clinical evidence show that several types of epileptic seizures preferentially occur during slow-wave sleep. This is the case of absence (petit mal) seizures with spike-wave (SW) complexes at 2–4 Hz that appear during drowsiness or light sleep in children (1) and behaving monkeys (2), and in association with sleep spindles in stage 2 of human sleep (3). The Lennox–Gastaut syndrome (4–6), which is accompanied by SW and polyspike-wave (PSW) complexes that recur at relatively lower frequencies (generally 1.5–2.5 Hz) and are associated with episodes of fast runs (10–15 Hz), is also prevalently activated during slow-wave sleep (5, 7).

The behaviour of neurons during paroxysmal discharges has been extensively studied. However, for reasons that will become clear in this chapter, the understanding of the neurophysiological mechanisms of epilepsies has not progressed as much as one would have expected from the bulk of means that were invested in the sole study of neurons. Some pioneering studies have repeatedly acknowledged the abnormal activity of glial cells during epileptic events (8–11), and only few recent studies have addressed the interaction between neurons and glia. Therefore I will emphasize the contribution of glial cells to the triggering of the seizures and to the oscillating process accompanying them especially because the neuronal activity is modulated by several ionic species (mainly potassium (K^+), calcium (Ca^{2+}), and hydrogen (H^+)) of the extracellular space.

The analysis of the mechanisms underlying the occurrence of nocturnal SW seizures has to take into consideration the precipitating factors acting before and throughout the paroxysmal episode, as well as the (minimal) critical structures required to generate SW discharges. Interestingly, the same elements that rule and promote the behaviour of complex neuron, glia, and extracellular space loops during slow-wave sleep may also contribute to the triggering of pathological states such as seizures. The transition from normal (sleep) to abnormal (paroxysms) states may rely on a multitude of factors ranging from genetic causes (12) to imbalances of ionic concentrations (13) or the abnormal recruitment of cellular aggregates (14–16). As a precipitating factor, one may also consider the irregularity of respiration during the initial stages of sleep (17). Most of the time seizures result from a combination of factors. However, a basal condition that is already present in all sleeping patients is the presence of coherent oscillations during slow-wave sleep. Thus I will start with a brief survey of the mechanisms underlying slow sleep oscillations.

Mechanisms of slow sleep oscillations

The slow-wave sleep is dominated by a coherent cortical activity that imposes a slow (less than but close to 1 Hz) oscillation to both neurons (18) and glial cells (19) belonging to cortical networks (Fig. 1.1A). At the neuronal level, the slow oscillation is made of alternating steady depolarizations and hyperpolarizations. The depolarizing phase is made of synaptic events (excitatory as well as inhibitory) and intrinsic membrane currents (18). In parallel with the neuronal depolarization phase, glial cells are also depolarized, but at a slower pace that reflects the variation of extracellular K^+ concentration (20). The persistent neuronal depolarization is associated with a progressive depletion of extracellular Ca^{2+} (Fig. 1.1B) (21), which in turn initiates a disfacilitation process (22, 21) leading to the onset of the persistent hyperpolarizing phase of the slow oscillation.

During the hyperpolarizing phase, no neurons are active, their membrane potential reaching values much more hyperpolarized than the threshold for action potential generation. In parallel, glial cells slowly repolarize, as the extracellular K^+ concentrations return to control values (20). Extracellular Ca^{2+} is restored through ionic pumps and reaches concentrations compatible with efficient synaptic transmission (Fig. 1.1B) (21).

Several lines of evidence support the idea that the slow oscillation is generated within cortical networks. First, the slow oscillation survives in the cortex after extensive thalamic lesions and in preparations with high brainstem transactions (23). Second, the slow oscillation is absent from the thalamus of decorticated

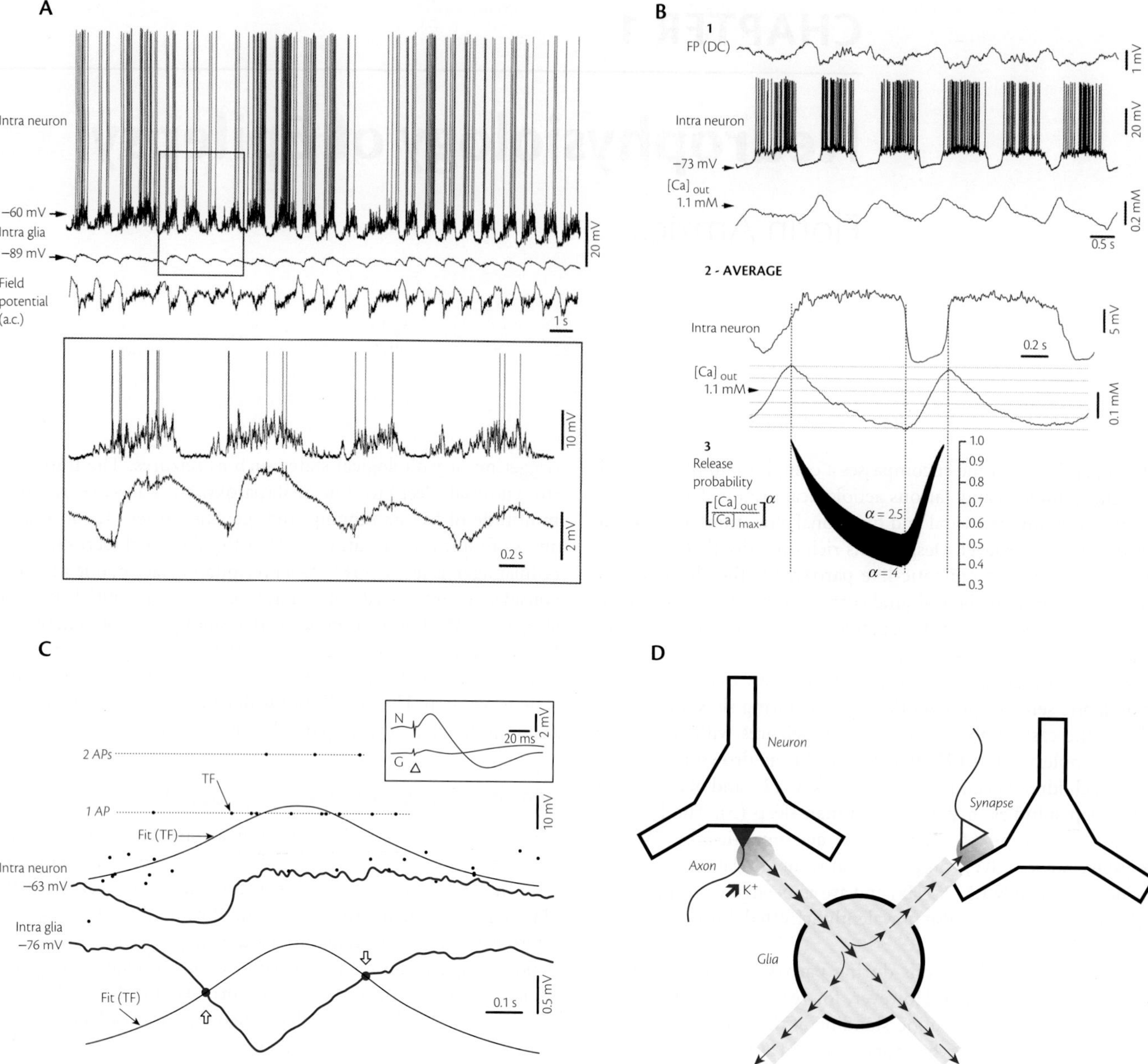

Fig. 1.1 Mechanisms of genesis of the slow (<1 Hz) sleep oscillation. A) Recordings from cortical areas 5 (neuron and depth field potential) and 7 (glia), displaying periodic depolarizations of the neuronal membrane, made of synaptic potentials and triggering somatic action potentials. Depolarizations are followed by hyperpolarizations with reduced synaptic noise. In synchrony with the onset of the neuronal depolarization, the glia depolarizes. The end of the depolarization coincides with the onset of the neuronal hyperpolarization. Note that the amplitude of the glial depolarization increases as the slow oscillation in the neuron becomes more rhythmic and of higher amplitude (*top right*; see also detail in box). In this and the following figures, polarities always are depicted with positivity upward. B) Relationships between intracellular membrane potential, extracellular Ca^{2+} ($(Ca)_{out}$) and estimated synaptic release probability. B1) Alternating neuronal depolarizations and hyperpolarization corresponding to negative and positive field potential waves, respectively. $(Ca)_{out}$ dropped by about 0.25 mM during the depolarizing phase reaching a minimum just before the onset of the hyperpolarization. Then, $(Ca)_{out}$ rose back until the beginning of the next cycle. B2) Thirty oscillatory cycles were averaged (neuronal spikes clipped) after being extracted around the onset of the neuronal depolarization. The vertical dotted lines tentatively indicate the boundaries of the two phases of the slow oscillation. B3) The transmitter release probability is contained within the black area between the estimations with $\alpha = 2.5$ (90) and $\alpha = 4$ (91) exponents. The release probability dropped to around 50% before the onset of the hyperpolarizing phase. C) Neuronal excitability during the oscillatory cycle of the slow oscillation. The *thick traces* represent the wave-triggered averages of a neuron–glia pair recorded intracellularly. The *dots* constitute the excitability curve and correspond to the maximum of the voltage values reached by the synaptic response elicited with a cortical volley. Artificial levels were attributed when the synaptic potential was crowned by 1 or 2 action potentials (*dotted horizontal lines* for *1AP* and *2APs*). The *thin curve* (*fit*) is for the Lorentzian fit of the excitability score. In the glial trace, the fitting curve is replicated in order to suggest the relative points of intersection with the intraglial potential (*open arrows*). Maximum neuronal excitability is achieved during the trough of the glial oscillation. The *inset* provides the shape of the intracellular responses evoked by the cortical shock (*triangle*) in the neuron (*N*) and glia (*G*). The former display and EPSP–IPSP sequence, while the latter contain a very slight initial depolarization (~0.3 mV). D) Schematic functioning of the spatial buffering during the slow oscillation. During the depolarizing phase of the slow oscillation, small and local increases of extracellular K^+ (*circle*) may occur in the proximity of the axon hillock. The neighbouring glial cells take up the K^+ and redistribute it at sites where the values of extracellular K^+ are normal. These locations may be close to a synapse, in which case the synaptic efficiency may be modulated, or close to a neuronal membrane such to modify the excitability of that membrane. Modified from: A (19), B (21), C (28), and D (20).

animals (24), while it is expressed by thalamic reticular and thalamocortical cells in intact animals (25). Moreover, the slow oscillation has been recently replicated in cortical slices (26). Thus, the slow oscillation is generated within cortical neurons.

The mechanisms underlying this oscillatory behaviour are partly elucidated at the neuronal level. It was shown that the slow oscillations were expressed by various cortical areas (18) and by virtually all types of neurons (27). The slow oscillation is marked by a variable neuronal responsiveness that is maximal during the first third of the depolarizing phase and progressively decays during the rest of the depolarizing phase (Fig. 1.1C) (28). Having demonstrated that the slow oscillation is synchronized between all cortical areas (29), we have sought for the mechanisms underlying this coherent behaviour and found that, beyond the essential role played by synaptic intracortical projections (30), glial cells, through local K^+ spatial buffering (31–33) and Ca^{2+}-dependent neurotransmitter release (34), might modulate the neuronal excitability and activity, respectively (Fig. 1.1D) (20). The presence of a large current sink in cortical layer III during the depolarizing phase (35) further strengthened the contribution of intracortical linkages to the propagation of the slow oscillation. Thus, the slow oscillation relies on widespread cortical networks.

The long-lasting hyperpolarization of the neuronal membrane often de-inactivates additional excitatory currents of the low-threshold Ca^{2+} spike type, which in turn will have a greater impact on the synchronization of the network. It has been therefore proposed that the slow oscillation acts as a precursor of nocturnal SW seizures (14, 16).

Electroencephalographic correlates of the slow oscillation

The synchronous nature of the slow oscillation has a direct impact on the electroencephalogram (EEG). Therefore the slow oscillation is detectable in the gross brain activity of the sleeping brain. First, the slow oscillation is expressed in the local field potentials reflecting the membrane currents generated by neurons and, possibly, glial cells. Since the depolarizing phase of the slow oscillation reflects the excitation of all neurons, the corresponding extracellular field potential consists of a negative deflection (27). The shape of this negative potential has been found similar to the one of the K-complex (36, 35). Besides disclosing the cellular bases of the K-complex, our studies have also established that this EEG event has a periodic and spontaneous recurrence (with the exception of occasional, sensory evoked K-complexes), and is generated in all sleep stages.

The hyperpolarizing phase of the slow oscillation corresponds to a round wave that has a negative polarity in the cortical depth (27) when measured with alternating current (AC) amplifiers (i.e. after removal of direct current (DC) and very slow components). Although AC recordings are the rule in routine EEG, it should be kept in mind that the procedure is altering the real shape of field potential and EEG waves by introducing some artificial components, like the negative wave during the hyperpolarizing phase of the slow oscillation. In fact, being the result of network disfacilitation, the field expression of the hyperpolarizing phase marks a return to resting extracellular potential (see comparison between DC and AC recordings in figure 3 from reference 37).

Transformation of the slow oscillation into SW seizures

The smooth transition from the physiological (slow oscillation) to the pathological (SW sequences) pattern suggests that the slow and the paroxysmal oscillations share common mechanisms. The electroencephalographic SW is made at the neuronal level by a paroxysmal depolarizing shift (PDS). The PDS is a giant excitatory postsynaptic potential (EPSP) (38–41) that also contains inhibitory postsynaptic potential (IPSPs) (42). Occasionally, the PDSs and their EEG counterparts, the 'spikes', are superimposed by faster oscillations at about 10–15 Hz that produce corresponding indentations on the EEG 'spike' with a polyspike shape (Fig. 1.2). This pattern of seizure is a quite typical signature for those occurring in the Lennox–Gastaut syndrome (5) and their frequency appears as a resonating phenomenon within the cortical network (43).

The wave component of the SW complex is not due to active inhibition because, as demonstrated with multiple intracellular recordings, virtually all neurons (local inhibitory interneurons included) are silent during this phase of the oscillation. In addition, the firing rate tends to diminish towards the end of the PDS due to the inactivation of action potentials. Therefore, the activity of local-circuit inhibitory cells tends to weaken towards the end of the PDS and undergoes the general disfacilitation affecting all neurons belonging to the cortical network. The somatic input resistance is lowest at the beginning of the PDS and continuous to increase up to the next PDS, assuming its largest value during the hyperpolarization (44). This behaviour would not be consistent with the possibility that gamma-aminobutyric acid (GABA)ergic currents induce the arrest of firing. The disfacilitation could be promoted, as in the case of the slow oscillation, by reduced synaptic efficacy consequent to depletion of extracellular Ca^{2+} ions (28). This reduced synaptic efficacy corroborates the relative refractoriness of cortically elicited PDSs (45).

Among the ions with a significant impact on the neuronal excitability, K^+ and Ca^{2+} were repeatedly investigated. The more synchronized the network, the higher the amplitude of its oscillations, with more K^+ being expelled in the extracellular space during action potentials and other currents. During SW seizures, the extracellular concentration of K^+ increases from resting values around 3–3.5 mM to pathological levels around 9–12 mM (46–50). An increase in the extracellular K^+ concentration has proved to favour SW seizures (13, 46, 51). Extracellular K^+ is regulated by glial cells uptake (32, 52, 53,) followed by spatial buffering through gap junctions connecting the glial syncytium (54, 55). The latter phenomenon evens out K^+ but may also contribute to the general depolarization of the neuronal membrane potential (Fig. 1.3) by positively shifting the Nernst equilibrium potential.

Cortical seizures developing in a circumscribed focus generate a local increase in extracellular K^+, which is then spatially buffered through the syncytium of glial cells at more distant locations. The neuronal population of the latter would thus become the target of synchronous synaptic bombardment from the seizure focus and would act in an environment with increased K^+ concentration. Hence, synchronization of neuronal activity, the striking feature of sleep activities, creates favourable premises for seizure genesis. The protective mechanism against this seems to rely on the ability of glial cells to regulate the extracellular K^+ concentration through

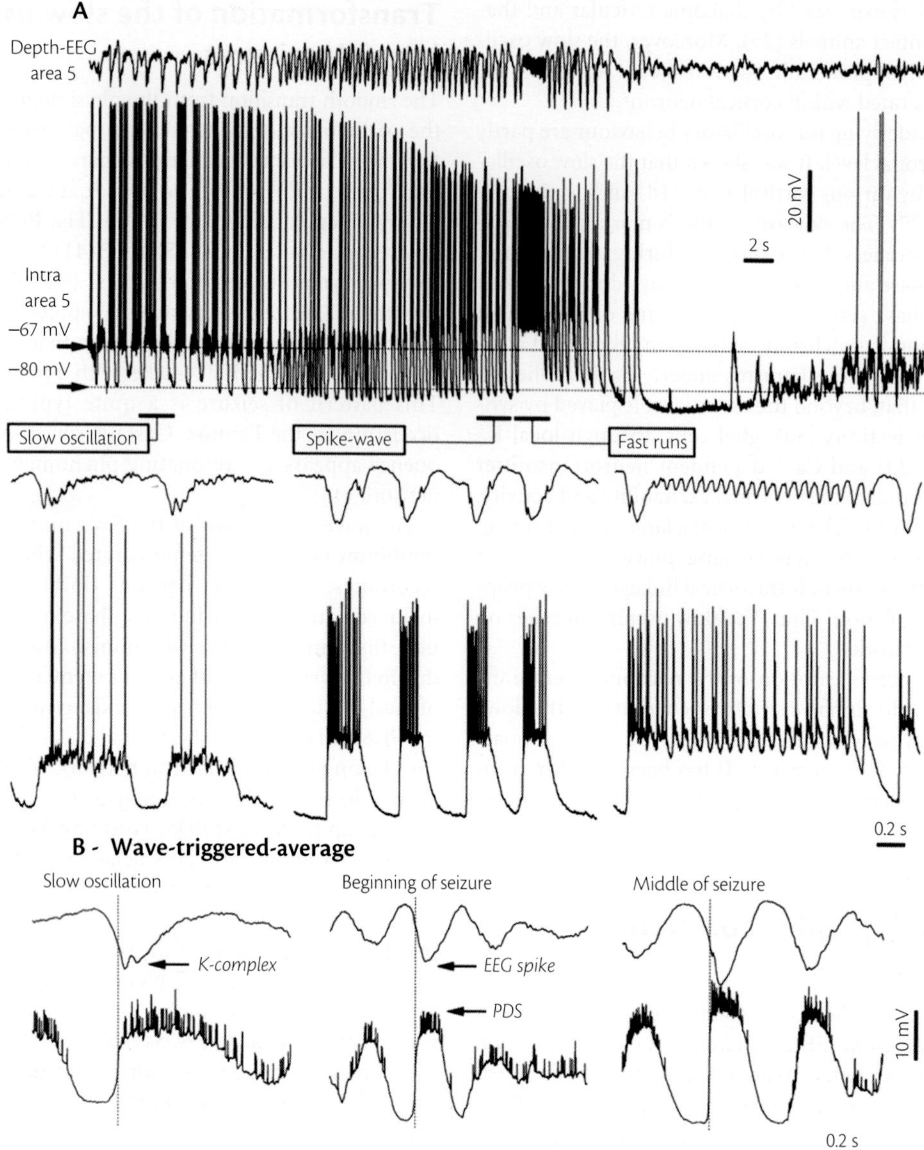

Fig. 1.2 Spontaneously occurring seizure, developing without discontinuity from slow sleep-like oscillation. Intracellular recording from regular-spiking area 5 neuron together with depth-EEG from the vicinity in area 5 in a cat under ketamine-xylazine anaesthesia. A) Smooth transition from slow oscillation to complex seizure consisting of SW complexes at ~2 Hz and fast runs at ~15 Hz. The seizure lasted for ~25 s. Epochs of slow oscillation preceding the seizure, SW complexes, and fast runs are indicated and expanded below. Note postictal depression (hyperpolarization) in the intracellularly recorded neuron (~6 s), associated with suppression of EEG slow oscillation (compare to left part of trace). B) Wave-triggered-average during the slow oscillation, at the beginning of seizure and during the middle part of seizure. Averaged activity was triggered by the steepest part of the depolarizing component in cortical neuron (dotted lines), during the three epochs. The depth-negative field component of the slow oscillation (associated with cell's depolarization) is termed *K-complex*. During the seizure, the depolarizing component reaches the level of a paroxysmal depolarizing shift (*PDS*), associated with an *EEG spike*. Modified from (16).

uptake, since impaired glial uptake of K^+ may cause epileptiform activity in the hippocampus (56).

Variations of the glial membrane potentials during sleep SW seizures

It has been well known for a long time that epileptic seizures are accompanied by significant increases in the extracellular K^+ concentration (46–48) and persistent depolarization of glial cells (8– 10). Simultaneous intracellular recordings of pairs of neurons and glia, together with extracellular ionic concentrations (mainly K^+ and Ca^{2+}) and the intracortical field activity during SW seizures (19, 20, 37) have allowed us to establish a pattern of correlation between these functional entities. Thus, it appeared that glial cells also express phasic depolarizations in relation to interictal and ictal PDSs (Fig. 1.3).

The estimate of neuronal and glial depolarizations during the phasic events building up the SW cycles led to high correlative values (>84%) (28). Since the neuronal phasic depolarizations are made of entry of Na^+ and Ca^{2+} and exit of chloride (Cl^-) and K^+, while the glial ones mostly reflect entry of K^+ (and possibly Ca^{2+}), the increased correlation between the depolarizations of the two

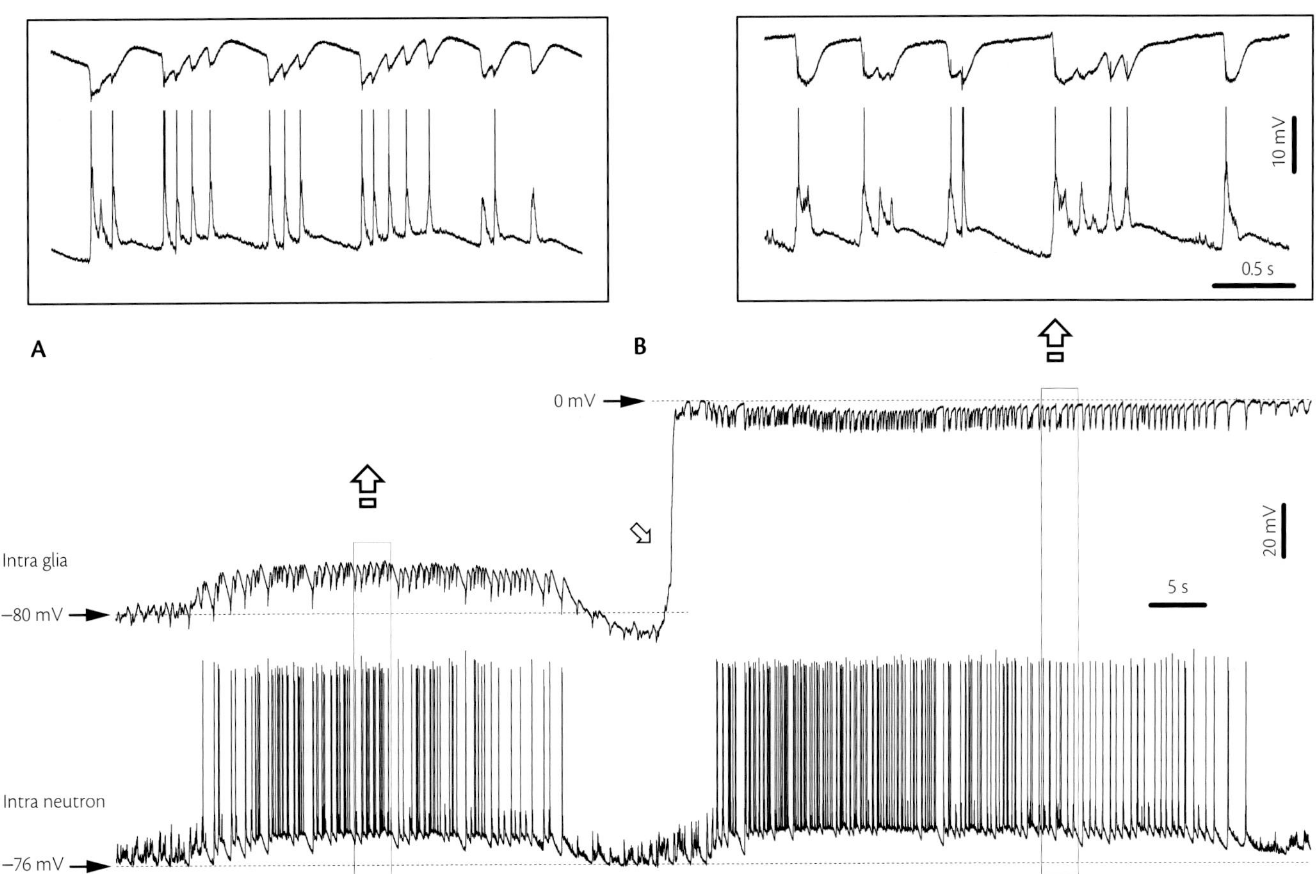

Fig. 1.3 Neuron–glia interaction during SW seizures. Continuous recording containing a double neuron–glia impalement (A), and neuron-field recording (B) in cortical association area 7. The two electrodes are separated by <1 mm. The transition from A to B is marked by the withdrawal of the pipette from the glia (*oblique open arrowhead*). Epochs within the squares are expanded above the respective panels. Modified from (37).

cell types suggests that the ionic activity of Na^+ and Ca^{2+} is proportional to that of K^+ and/or that the neuronal phasic depolarizations depend on the amount of extracellular K^+. Alternatively, it could be that SW seizures are accompanied by a more active glial uptake of extracellular K^+.

Measurements of membrane capacitance of both cortical glia and neurons during control sleep periods and SW seizures developing from the slow sleep oscillations suggests that the glial cells (not the neurons) undergo swelling and/or increased communication through gap junctions during paroxysmal discharges (Fig. 1.4) (19). The swelling of glial cells corroborates with previous experiments demonstrating shrinkage of the extracellular space during periods of increased extracellular K^+ (57). Therefore, in both cases, ephaptic transmission through the cortex might be favoured during SW discharges, as previously observed in the hippocampus (58) and could account, at least in part, for the increased synchronization recorded during epileptic seizures (14).

Correlates of paroxysmal glial activities with extracellular ionic (K^+ and/or Ca^{2+}) concentrations

Compared with the slow sleep oscillation, SW seizures appear as hypersynchronous phenomena. The progressive reduction of time lags between the activities of pairs of neurons in parallel with the development of the seizure might suggest increased synaptic coupling (14, 59). On the other hand, numerous studies have demonstrated that the extracellular Ca^{2+} concentrations decrease during SW seizures (Fig. 1.5A) (20, 60–63). Knowing that synaptic efficacy critically depends on extracellular Ca^{2+} levels (64), and assuming that the observed depletion is due to postsynaptic Ca^{2+} entry, these data challenge the classical view of the synaptic synchronization during SW seizures. Although Ca^{2+} uptake may also occur at the presynaptic level (65, 66), several lines of evidence suggest the preponderance of the postsynaptic uptake (67–71). This phenomenon alone could produce a steady decoupling of the neuronal networks during seizures.

Nevertheless, ictal extracellular Ca^{2+} levels display phasic variations in relation to rhythmic occurring PDSs (Fig. 1.5B) (20). A locally increased extracellular Ca^{2+} concentration coincides with the onset of a PDS and, although the overall variations have relatively low amplitude (~0.1 mM), they might explain the relative increased network excitability at the onset of a PDS (see figure 10 in reference 28). These data seem to confirm a previous report (45) in which the ability of the seizure-prone neocortical network to respond to electrical stimuli with interictal PDSs depended on the time lag between the end of the previous spontaneous PDS and the moment at which the stimulus was presented (Fig. 1.5C).

Intraglial as well as extracellular K^+ recordings during SW discharges show, in parallel with the Ca^{2+} depletion, a progressive

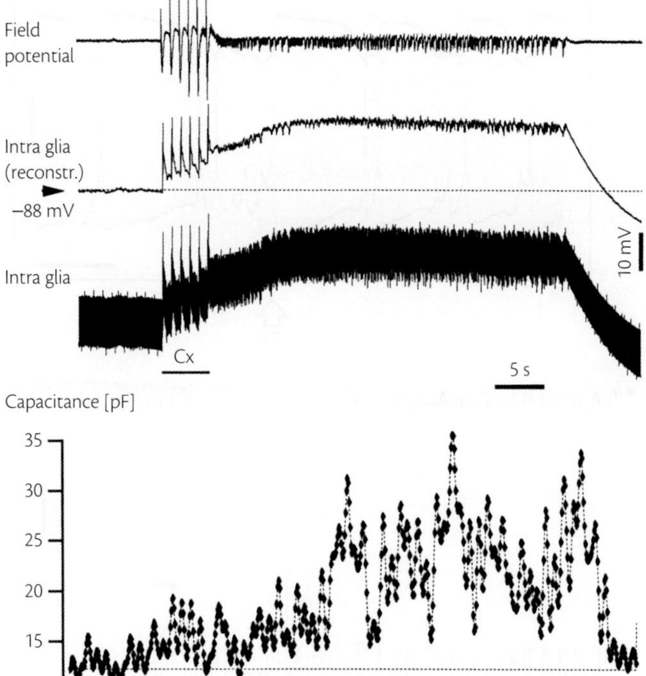

Fig. 1.4 Glial capacitance measurements during SW seizures elicited by electrical stimulation. The seizure was evoked by six trains of cortical stimuli at 1 Hz (every train contains 10 stimuli at 100 Hz). The second trace (*reconstr.*) represents the glial membrane potential after artificially eliminating the hyperpolarizing pulses (third trace) applied in order to calculate the membrane capacitance from the charging curve of the membrane. The capacitance increase reflects swelling and/or enhanced gap junction communication. Modified from (19).

depolarization and, respectively, an increase in extracellular K^+. Ca^{2+} and K^+ dynamics are clearly different (Fig. 1.5D). The epileptic tissue benefits from an enhanced gap junction communication (19, 72, 73), thus supporting the hypothesis that large cortical territories may be synchronized during SW seizures by means of K^+ waves travelling through a functional gap junction syncytium. This observation gains more weight in the presence of depleted extracellular Ca^{2+} at levels that are incompatible with synaptic functionality. Indeed, simultaneous extracellular K^+ concentrations at cortical sites separated by more than 2 mm, together with an intracellular recording close to one of the K^+ electrodes (Fig. 1.6A) have shown that, at some distance from a presumed epileptic focus, the estimated intracellular K^+ concentration increases faster than the K^+ concentration of its extracellular environment (20). These data suggest that the propagation of the epileptic activity in the cortex may use spatial buffering through the glial syncytium rather than the simple diffusion through the extracellular space.

This hypothesis gains corroborative support from the fact that isoflurane and other volatile anaesthetics, known to block gap junctions communication (74), are widely used to prevent status epilepticus (75, 76). Thus, in the absence of an efficient synaptic pathway to synchronize networks of neurons, the alternative pathway using the spatial buffering of K^+ appears as a compensatory mechanism contributing to the spreading of the seizures and to the synchronization of large cortical territories (Fig. 1.6B). Two ions could be involved in this process. First, glial cells take up Ca^{2+} through voltage-dependent channels (77), further contributing to the extracellular depletion of this ion. The subsequent increase of the intraglial Ca^{2+}, together with the increase resulting from the glutamate-mediated neuronal activity (78), may result in glutamate release from glia (79–81) and excitation of the neighbouring neurons. Such an effect may be enhanced by the increased excitability of axons resulting from the extracellular Ca^{2+} depletion (82).

It appears, therefore, that the tight homeostasis of the extracellular potassium plays a pivotal role in keeping the normal brain oscillations from evolving into paroxysmal ones. Glial cells normally fulfil this function. However, once the potassium regulation is compromised, the same cells also participate in the propagation/generalization of the ictal activities. Several studies have drawn the attention to the fact that glial dysfunction is intimately associated with the genesis of epileptic behaviour. Among others, the opening of the blood–brain barrier and the ensuing extravasation of blood proteins entrain a cascade of events beginning with astrocytic activation (83), downregulation of inward-rectifying potassium (Kir 4.1) channels in astrocytes, and impaired interstitial potassium buffering, ultimately leading to the genesis of epileptogenic foci (84).

Are nocturnal SW seizures generated in the cortex or in the thalamus?

The site of genesis of SW seizures has been hotly debated during the past decades. The hypothesis that SW seizures are generated within thalamic networks stemmed from old studies in which, however, no self-sustained activity outlasted SW-like cortical responses to medial thalamic stimulation (85). This hypothesis was replaced by the more reasonable idea that sleep spindles develop into SW seizures because of an enhanced excitability of neocortical neurons (86). Marcus and Watson (87) and Steriade (2) had emphasized the leading role of the cortex. More recently, intracellular studies in our laboratory have demonstrated that the cortically generated slow oscillation is the seed for paroxysmal developments such as SW seizures (14, 15, 59). Moreover, the thalamus of decorticated cats was unable to trigger seizures even after systemic or local injection of bicuculline (88). In contrast, local microinjections of bicuculline in the cortex of athalamic cats produced widespread synchronous seizures (88). It was thus concluded that the minimal substrate for the generation of such SW seizures is the neocortex, although the active participation of some thalamocortical cells was not precluded.

The minor role played by the thalamus in the genesis of such SW seizures is in agreement with recordings from a majority (at least 60%) of thalamic neurons in intact animals showing a tonic hyperpolarization, superimposed by phasic IPSPs, during seizures (Fig. 1.7) (15, 89). The behaviour of such thalamocortical cells further precludes their active implication in reinforcing the oscillations during seizures. It was suggested that the tonic hyperpolarization was induced by the corticofugal projections of GABAergic thalamic reticular neurons that faithfully follow cortical PDSs. A minority of thalamocortical cells was, however, discharging spike-bursts or spike-trains at 2–4 Hz, in phase with the depolarizing components of the cortical seizure. Therefore, during paroxysmal attacks the thalamic activity undergoes the antagonist influence of the steady excitatory cortex and inhibitory thalamic reticular neurons. This balance may evolve during the seizure itself,

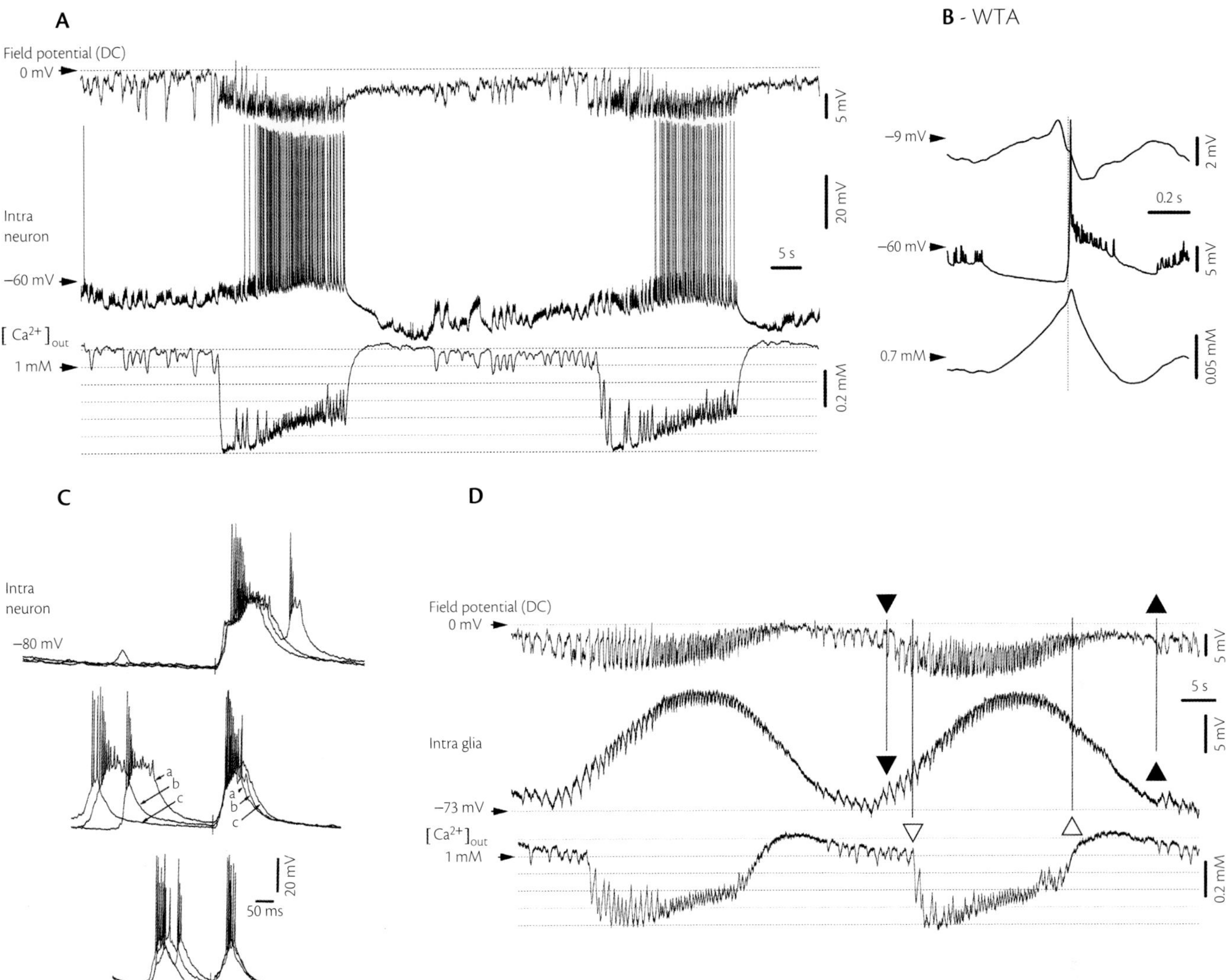

Fig. 1.5 A) Decrease of extracellular Ca^{2+} concentrations ($(Ca^{2+})_{out}$) during SW seizures. Simultaneous intracellular recording of a neuron in the suprasylvian gyrus and of neighbouring DC field potentials and $(Ca^{2+})_{out}$. SW seizures are accompanied by a persistent drop of ~0.6 mM of the extracellular Ca^{2+} concentration and by phasic oscillations of the $(Ca^{2+})_{out}$ during the SW complexes B) The wave-triggered averages (n = 40) were aligned with the maximum slope of the neuronal depolarization (*vertical dotted line*), and depict the relationship between the neuronal paroxysmal depolarization, the field potential and the Ca^{2+} concentration. Extracellular Ca^{2+} increases during the hyperpolarizing phase foregoing the onset of the ictal discharge, and decreases during the subsequent neuronal depolarization.
C) Relative refractoriness of cortically-elicited PDSs. Intracellular recording of a neuron in area 7. Three PDSs elicited by cortical stimuli to area 5 were superimposed and aligned; see stimuli artefacts from top to bottom. The amplitude and duration of cortically-evoked PDS depended on their 'time-distance' from the preceding (spontaneously occurring) PDSs: PDSs decreased both in duration and amplitude as the stimulus was closer to the spontaneous PDS. D) Relationship between $(Ca^{2+})_{out}$ and glial activities during recurrent SW seizures. Intraglial, DC field potentials, and Ca^{2+} concentrations were measured at short distance (<1 mm) in the suprasylvian gyrus. During seizures, the glial steady depolarization and presumably the $(K^{+})_{out}$, had a different time course from the $(Ca^{2+})_{out}$: the onset of the seizure was simultaneous in glia and field potential (black arrowheads oriented downward) and before the Ca^{2+} started to decrease (empty arrowhead downward). The end of the seizure was marked first by a rapid return of Ca^{2+} to normal values (empty arrowhead upward), followed by a much slower return of the glia and field potential to control potentials (black arrowhead upward). Modified from: (A), (B), and (D) (20), and (C) (45).

as suggested by the progression of the overall synchronization in corticothalamic networks, which becomes stronger as the seizure develops and more territories are recruited (59).

Conclusions

The developing of SW seizures is far from exclusively being a neuronal phenomenon. From the data presented here, we believe that glial cells and the extracellular environment, mainly through the traffic of ions, have an active role in modulating the neuronal behaviour. In the absence of reliable neuron-to-neuron synaptic transmission, alternative pathways may be used by the extraneuronal partners. Further investigation of the blood–brain barrier and the implication of its transporters may bring new insights as to their contribution to paroxysmal discharges. From this perspective, intractability may well be the reflection of our limited knowledge of the ensemble of mechanisms underlying epileptic syndromes.

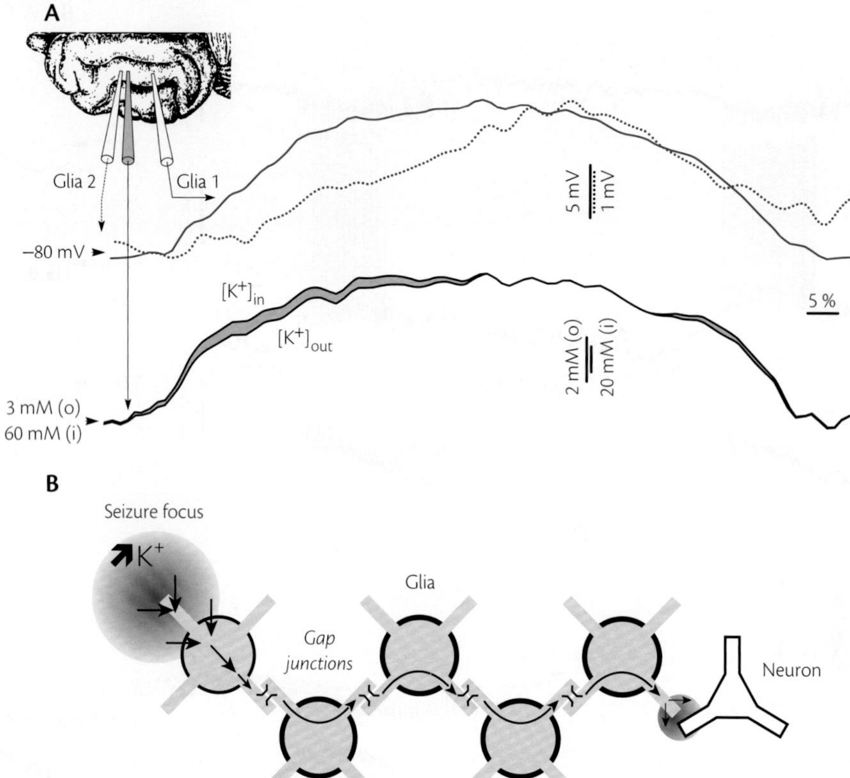

Fig. 1.6 Propagation of K^+ waves during SW seizures. A) Dual intraglial recording together with the $(K^+)_{out}$. The disposition of the recording electrodes in the suprasylvian gyrus is shown in the inset. The traces represent the average of 20 normalized seizure envelopes. The *upper* superimposition contains the intracellular seizures in the pair of glial cells expanded at their maximum amplitude (see different voltage calibrations—*continuous line* for *cell 1* and *dotted line* for *cell 2*, also corresponding to the envelope traces). From the higher amplitude of the signal, it may be inferred that *cell 1* is closer to a presumed seizure focus. The *lower* panel displays the intra- and extracellular K^+ concentrations superimposed and expanded at their maximum amplitude. The $(K^+)_{in}$ was calculated from the Nernst equilibrium potential in relation with the $(K^+)_{out}$ and the intracellular trace that was recorded closely to the K^+ microelectrode (2). Toward the beginning of the seizure, the estimated $(K^+)_{in}$ rose faster than the $(K^+)_{out}$ (*grey area* between the two traces). B) Schematic functioning of the spatial buffering during SW seizures. Important increases in the $(K^+)_{out}$ may not be buffered at short distances, in which case the internalized K^+ may travel through the glial syncytium and is externalized at a location with lower $(K^+)_{out}$ values, where it would modulate the activity of nearby neurons. Modified from (20).

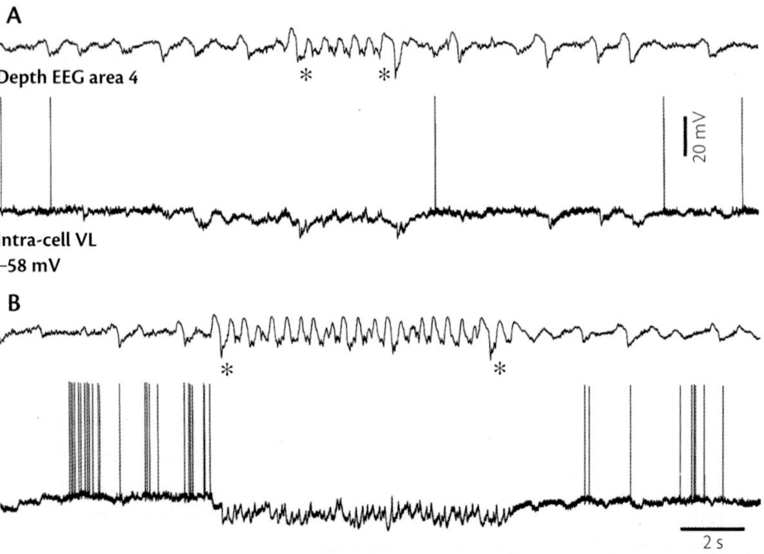

Fig. 1.7 Hyperpolarization of a thalamocortical neuron during cortical SW seizures. Cat under ketamine-xylazine anesthesia. Intracellular recording from a thalamocortical neuron in the ventrolateral (VL) nucleus, together with depth-EEG from cortical area 4. Development from embryonic SW activity (A, between asterisks) to longer-lasting seizures with SW complexes at about 2.5 Hz (B, between asterisks). Modified from (15).

References

1. Sato S, Dreifuss FE, Penry JK. The effect of sleep on spike-wave discharges in absence seizures. *Neurology* 1973: 23:1335–45.
2. Steriade M. Interneuronal epileptic discharges related to spike-and-wave cortical seizures in behaving monkeys. *Electroencephalogr Clin Neurophysiol* 1974; 37:247–63.
3. Kellaway P. Sleep and epilepsy. *Epilepsia* 1985; 26(Suppl 1):S15–S30.
4. Gastaut H, Roger J, Soulayrol R, Saint-Jean M, Tassinari CA, Regis H, *et al.* Epileptic encephalopathy of children with diffuse slow spikes and waves (alias 'petit mal variant') or Lennox syndrome. *Ann Pediatr (Paris)* 1966; 13:489–99.
5. Niedermeyer E. Abnormal EEG patterns (epileptic and paroxysmal). In: Niedermeyer E, Lopes da Silva F (eds) *Abnormal EEG patterns (epileptic and paroxysmal)*, pp.235–60. Baltimore, MD: Williams & Wilkins, 1999.
6. Velasco M, Diaz-de-Leon AE, Brito F, Velasco AL, Velasco F. Sleep-epilepsy interactions in patients with intractable generalized tonic seizures and depth electrodes in the centro median thalamic nucleus. *Arch Med Res* 1995; 26(Spec No):S117–25.
7. Halasz P. Runs of rapid spikes in sleep: a characteristic EEG expression of generalized malignant epileptic encephalopathies. A conceptual review with new pharmacological data. *Epilepsy Res Suppl*1991; 2:49–71.
8. Dichter MA, Herman CJ, Selzer M. Silent cells during interictal discharges and seizures in hippocampal penicillin foci. Evidence for the role of extracellular K^+ in the transition from the interictal state to seizures. *Brain Res* 1972; 48:173–83.
9. Grossman RG, Hampton T. Depolarization of cortical glial cells during electrocortical activity. *Brain Res* 1968; 11:316–24.
10. Sypert GW, Ward AA, Jr. Unidentified neuroglia potentials during propagated seizures in neocortex. *Exp Neurol* 1971; 33:239–55.
11. Somjen GG. Influence of potassium and neuroglia in the generation of seizures and their treatment. *Adv Neurol* 1980; 27:155–67.
12. Scheffer IE, Bhatia KP, Lopes-Cendes I, Fish DR, Marsden CD, Andermann F, *et al.* Autosomal dominant frontal epilepsy misdiagnosed as sleep disorder. *Lancet* 1994; 343:515–17.
13. Zuckermann EC, Glaser GH. Hippocampal epileptic activity induced by localized ventricular perfusion with high-potassium cerebrospinal fluid. *Exp Neurol* 1968; 20:87–110.
14. Steriade M, Amzica F. Dynamic coupling among neocortical neurons during evoked and spontaneous spike-wave seizure activity. *J Neurophysiol* 1994; 72:2051–69.
15. Steriade M, Contreras D. Relations between cortical and thalamic cellular events during transition from sleep patterns to paroxysmal activity. *J Neurosci* 1995; 15:623–42.
16. Steriade M, Amzica F, Neckelmann D, Timofeev I. Spike-wave complexes and fast components of cortically generated seizures. II. Extra- and intracellular patterns. *J Neurophysiol* 1998; 80:1456–79.
17. Krieger J. Respiratory physiology: breathing in normal subjects. In: Kryger MH, Roth T, Dement W (eds) *Respiratory physiology: breathing in normal subjects*, pp.229–41. Philadelphia, PA: Saunders, 2000.
18. Steriade M, Nunez A, Amzica F. A novel slow (< 1 Hz) oscillation of neocortical neurons in vivo: depolarizing and hyperpolarizing components. *J Neurosci* 1993; 13:3252–65.
19. Amzica F, Neckelmann D. Membrane capacitance of cortical neurons and glia during sleep oscillations and spike-wave seizures. *J Neurophysiol* 1999; 82:2731–46.
20. Amzica F, Massimini M, Manfridi A. Spatial buffering during slow and paroxysmal sleep oscillations in cortical networks of glial cells in vivo. *J Neurosci* 2002; 22:1042–53.
21. Massimini M, Amzica F. Extracellular calcium fluctuations and intracellular potentials in the cortex during the slow sleep oscillation. *J Neurophysiol* 2001; 85:1346–50.
22. Contreras D, Timofeev I, Steriade M. Mechanisms of long-lasting hyperpolarizations underlying slow sleep oscillations in cat corticothalamic networks. *J Physiol* 1996; 494:251–64.
23. Steriade M, Nuñez A, Amzica F. Intracellular analysis of relations between the slow (<1 Hz) neocortical oscillation and other sleep rhythms of the electroencephalogram. *J Neurosci* 1993; 13:3266–83.
24. Timofeev I, Steriade M. Low-frequency rhythms in the thalamus of intact-cortex and decorticated cats. *J Neurophysiol* 1996; 76:4152–68.
25. Steriade M, Contreras D, Curró Dossi R, Nuñez A. The slow (<1 Hz) oscillation in reticular thalamic and thalamocortical neurons: scenario of sleep rhythm generation in interacting thalamic and neocortical networks. *J Neurosci* 1993; 13:3284–99.
26. Sanchez-Vives MV, McCormick DA. Cellular and network mechanisms of rhythmic recurrent activity in neocortex. *Nature Neurosci* 2000; 3:1027–34.
27. Contreras D, Steriade M. Cellular basis of EEG slow rhythms: a study of dynamic corticothalamic relationships. *J Neurosci* 1995; 15:604–22.
28. Amzica F, Massimini M. Glial and neuronal interactions during slow wave and paroxysmal activities in the neocortex. *Cereb Cortex* 2002; 12:1101–13.
29. Amzica F, Steriade M. Short- and long-range neuronal synchronization of the slow (< 1 Hz) cortical oscillation. *J Neurophysiol* 1995; 73:20–38.
30. Amzica F, Steriade M. Disconnection of intracortical synaptic linkages disrupts synchronization of a slow oscillation. *J Neurosci* 1995; 15:4658–77.
31. Orkand RK, Nicholls JG, Kuffler SW. Effect of nerve impulses on the membrane potential of glial cells in the central nervous system of amphibia. *J Neurophysiol* 1966; 29:788–806.
32. Walz W. Role of glial cells in the regulation of the brain ion microenvironment. *Prog Neurobiol* 1989; 33:309–33.
33. Newman EA. Glial cell regulation of extracellular potassium. In: Kettenmann H, Ransom BR (eds) *Glial cell regulation of extracellular potassium*, pp.717–31. New York: Oxford University Press, 1995.
34. Araque A, Li N, Doyle RT, Haydon PG. SNARE protein-dependent glutamate release from astrocytes. *J Neurosci* 2000; 20:666–73.
35. Amzica F, Steriade M. Cellular substrates and laminar profile of sleep K-complex. *Neuroscience* 1998; 82:671–86.
36. Amzica F, Steriade M. The K-complex: its slow (<1 Hz) rhythmicity and relation to delta waves. *Neurology* 1997; 49:952–9.
37. Amzica F, Steriade M. Neuronal and glial membrane potentials during sleep and paroxysmal oscillations in the neocortex. *J Neurosci* 2000; 20:6648–65.
38. Matsumoto H, Ajmone-Marsan C. Cortical cellular phenomena in experimental epilepsy: interictal manifestations. *Exp Neurol* 1964; 9:286–304.
39. Matsumoto H, Ajmone-Marsan C. Cortical cellular phenomena in experimental epilepsy: ictal manifestations. *Exp Neurol* 1964; 9:305–26.
40. Ayala GF, Dichter M, Gumnit RJ, Matsumoto H, Spencer WA. Genesis of epileptic interictal spikes. New knowledge of cortical feedback systems suggests a neurophysiological explanation of brief paroxysms. *Brain Res* 1973; 52:1–17.
41. Johnston D, Brown TH. Giant synaptic potential hypothesis for epileptiform activity. *Science* 1981; 211:294–7.
42. Steriade M, Timofeev I, Grenier F. Inhibitory components of cortical spike-wave seizures in vivo. *Soc Neurosci Abstr* 1998; 24:2143.
43. Amzica F, Steriade M. Spontaneous and artificial activation of neocortical seizures. *J Neurophysiol* 1999; 82:3123–38.
44. Neckelmann D, Amzica F, Steriade M. Changes in neuronal conductance during different components of cortically generated spike-wave seizures. *Neuroscience* 2000; 96:475–85.
45. Steriade M, Amzica F. An intracellular study of excitability in the seizure-prone neocortex in vivo. *J Neurophysiol* 1999; 82:3108–22.
46. Fertziger AP, Ranck JB, Jr . Potassium accumulation in interstitial space during epileptiform seizures. *Exp Neurol* 1970; 26:571–85.

47. Futamachi KJ, Mutani R, Prince DA. Potassium activity in rabbit cortex. *Brain Res* 1974; 75:5–25.
48. Moody WJ, Futamachi KJ, Prince DA. Extracellular potassium activity during epileptogenesis. *Exp Neurol* 1974; 42:248–63.
49. Sypert GW, Ward AA Jr. Changes in extracellular potassium activity during neocortical propagated seizures. *Exp Neurol* 1974; 45:19–41.
50. Somjen GG. Extracellular potassium in the mammalian central nervous system. *Prog Biophys Mol Biol* 1979; 42:135–90.
51. McBain CJ, Traynelis SF, Dingledine R. High potassium induced synchronous bursts and electrographic seizures. In: Schwartzkroin PA (ed) *Epilepsy: Models, Mechanisms and Concepts*, pp.437–61. Cambridge: Cambridge University Press, 1993.
52. Ballanyi K, Grafe P, Ten Bruggencate G. Ion activities and potassium uptake mechanisms of glial cells in guinea-pig olfactory cortex slices. *J Physiol (Lond)* 1987; 382:159–74.
53. Kettenmann H. K^+ and Cl^- uptake by cultured oligodendrocytes. *Can J Physiol Pharmacol* 1987; 65:1033–7.
54. Kettenmann H, Ransom BR. Electrical coupling between astrocytes and between oligodendrocytes studied in mammalian cell cultures. *Glia* 1988; 1:64–73.
55. Nicholson C. Extracellular space as the pathway for neuron-glial cell interaction. In: Kettenmann H, Ransom BR (eds) *Neuroglia*, pp.387–97. New York: Oxford University Press, 1995.
56. Janigro D, Gasparini S, D'Ambrosio R, McKhann G II, DiFrancesco D. Reduction of K^+ uptake in glia prevents long-term depression maintenance and causes epileptiform activity. *J Neurosci* 1997; 17:2813–24.
57. Dietzel I, Heinemann U, Hofmeier G, Lux HD. Transient changes in the size of the extracellular space in the sensorimotor cortex of cats in relation to stimulus-induced changes in potassium concentration. *Exp Brain Res* 1980; 40:432–9.
58. Taylor CP, Dudek FE. Synchronization without active chemical synapses during hippocampal afterdischarges. *J Neurophysiol* 1984; 52:143–55.
59. Neckelmann D, Amzica F, Steriade M. Spike-wave complexes and fast components of cortically generated seizures. III. Synchronizing mechanisms. *J Neurophysiol* 1998; 80:1480–94.
60. Heinemann U, Lux HD, Gutnick MJ. Extracellular free calcium and potassium during paroxysmal activity in the cerebral cortex of the cat. *Exp Brain Res* 1977; 27:237–43.
61. Somjen GG. Stimulus-evoked and seizure-related responses of extracellular calcium activity in spinal cord compared to those in cerebral cortex. *J Neurophysiol* 1980; 44:617–32.
62. Pumain R, Kurcewicz I, Louvel J . Fast extracellular calcium transients: involvement in epileptic processes. *Science* 1983; 222:177–9.
63. Hablitz JJ, Heinemann U. Extracellular K^+ and Ca^{2+} changes during epileptiform discharges in the immature rat neocortex. *Brain Res* 1987; 433:299–303.
64. King RD, Wiest MC, Montague PR. Extracellular calcium depletion as a mechanism of short-term synaptic depression. *J Neurophysiol* 2001; 85:1952–9.
65. Alici K, Heinemann U. Effects of low glucose levels on changes in $(Ca^{2+})o$ induced by stimulation of Schaffer collaterals under conditions of blocked chemical synaptic transmission in rat hippocampal slices. *Neurosci Lett* 1995; 185:5–8.
66. Igelmund P, Zhao YQ, Heinemann U. Effects of T-type, L-type, N-type, P-type, and Q-type calcium channel blockers on stimulus-induced pre- and postsynaptic calcium fluxes in rat hippocampal slices. *Exp Brain Res* 1996; 109:22–32.
67. Heinemann U, Pumain R. Effects of tetrodotoxin on changes in extracellular free calcium induced by repetitive electrical stimulation and iontophoretic application of excitatory amino acids in the sensorimotor cortex of cats. *Neurosci Lett* 1981; 21:87–91.
68. Bollmann JH, Helmchen F, Borst JG, Sakmann B. Postsynaptic Ca^{2+} influx mediated by three different pathways during synaptic transmission at a calyx-type synapse. *J Neurosci* 1998; 18:10409–19.
69. Borst JG, Sakmann B. Depletion of calcium in the synaptic cleft of a calyx-type synapse in the rat brainstem. *J Physiol (Lond)* 1999; 521:123–33.
70. Rusakov DA, Kullmann DM, Stewart MG. Hippocampal synapses: do they talk to their neighbours? *Trends Neurosci* 1999; 22:382–8.
71. King RD, Wiest MC, Montague PR, Eagleman DM. Do extracellular Ca^{2+} signals carry information through neural tissue? *Trends Neurosci* 2000; 23:12–13.
72. Lee SH, Magge S, Spencer DD, Sontheimer H, Cornell-Bell AH. Human epileptic astrocytes exhibit increased gap junction coupling. *Glia* 1995; 15:195–202.
73. Bordey A, Lyons SA, Hablitz JJ, Sontheimer H. Electrophysiological characteristics of reactive astrocytes in experimental cortical dysplasia. *J Neurophysiol* 2001; 85:1719–31.
74. Mantz J, Cordier J, Giaume C. Effects of general anesthetics on intercellular communications mediated by gap junctions between astrocytes in primary culture. *Anesthesiology* 1993; 78:892–901.
75. Kofke WA, Snider MT, Young RS, Ramer JC. Prolonged low flow isoflurane anesthesia for status epilepticus. *Anesthesiology* 1985; 62:653–6.
76. Kofke WA, Young RS, Davis P, Woelfel SK, Gray L, Johnson D, *et al.* Isoflurane for refractory status epilepticus: a clinical series. *Anesthesiology* 1989; 71:653–9.
77. MacVicar BA. Voltage-dependent calcium channels in glial cells. *Science* 1984; 226:1345–7.
78. Cornell-Bell AH, Finkbeiner SM, Cooper MS, Smith SJ. Glutamate induces calcium waves in cultured astrocytes: long-range glial signaling. *Science* 1990; 247:470–3.
79. Parpura V, Basarsky TA, Liu F, Jeftinija K, Jeftinija S, Haydon PG. Glutamate-mediated astrocyte-neuron signalling. *Nature* 1994; 369:744–7.
80. Pasti L, Volterra A, Pozzan T, Carmignoto G. Intracellular calcium oscillations in astrocytes: a highly plastic, bidirectional form of communication between neurons and astrocytes in situ. *J Neurosci* 1997; 17:7817–30.
81. Bezzi P, Carmignoto G, Pasti L, Vesce S, Rossi D, Rizzini BL, *et al.* Prostaglandins stimulate calcium-dependent glutamate release in astrocytes. *Nature* 1998; 391:281–5.
82. Hille B. *Ion Channels of Excitable Membranes.* Sunderland, MA: Sinauer, 1991.
83. Seiffert E, Dreier JP, Ivens S, Bechmann I, Tomkins O, Heinemann U, *et al.* Lasting blood-brain barrier disruption induces epileptic focus in the rat somatosensory cortex. *J Neurosci* 2004; 24:7829–36.
84. Ivens S, Kaufer D, Flores LP, Bechmann I, Zumsteg D, Tomkins O, *et al.* TGF-beta receptor-mediated albumin uptake into astrocytes is involved in neocortical epileptogenesis. *Brain* 2007; 130:535–47.
85. Jasper HH, Droogleever-Fortuyn J . Experimental studies on the functional anatomy of petit-mal epilepsy. *Res Publ Assoc Nerv Ment Dis* 1949; 26:272–98.
86. Gloor P, Fariello RG. Generalized epilepsy: some of its cellular mechanisms differ from those of focal epilepsy. *Trends Neurosci* 1988; 11:63–8.
87. Marcus EM, Watson CW. Symmetrical epileptogenic foci in monkey cerebral cortex. *Arch Neurol* 1968; 19:99–116.
88. Steriade M, Contreras D. Spike-wave complexes and fast components of cortically generated seizures. I. Role of neocortex and thalamus. *J Neurophysiol* 1998; 80:1439–55.
89. Pinault D, Leresche N, Charpier S, Deniau JM, Marescaux C, Vergnes M, *et al* . Intracellular recordings in thalamic neurones during spontaneous spike and wave discharges in rats with absence epilepsy. *J Physiol (Lond)* 1998; 509:449–56.
90. Mintz IM, Sabatini BL, Regehr WG. Calcium control of transmitter release at a cerebellar synapse. *Neuron* 1995; 15:675–88.
91. Qian J, Colmers WF, Saggau P. Inhibition of synaptic transmission by neuropeptide Y in rat hippocampal area CA1: modulation of presynaptic Ca^{2+} entry. *J Neurosci* 1997; 17:8169–77.

CHAPTER 2

Neurogenetics of Epilepsy

Renzo Guerrini and Elena Parrini

Epilepsy can be caused by genetic or acquired factors, although, often, both contribute to its determinism. Epilepsies of unknown cause are classically divided into two main aetiological categories: 'presumed symptomatic' epilepsies are those whose cause is suspected to be induced by a pathology that is below the limit of detection of the available diagnostic tests; 'idiopathic' epilepsies are instead thought to be caused by a genetic predisposition. Symptomatic epilepsies are caused by an obvious brain abnormality, which can in turn be genetically determined or by external factors acting prenatally or after birth. Defining as 'symptomatic' a genetically determined epilepsy is easy, for example, in front of a neuronal migration disorder, or a neurocutaneous disease such as tuberous sclerosis or a syndromic form of mental retardation. The same applies to many forms of progressive myoclonus epilepsy, whose clinical expression is relatively homogeneous in relation to the genetically determined degenerative or metabolic causes. The task is much more complex when the genetic cause is hidden and will only be recognizable or hypothesizable later during the course, when a given electroclinical pattern or syndrome will become obvious. This is, for example, the case of several early-onset epileptic encephalopathies such as those caused by alterations of the *CDKL5*, *STXBP1*, or *ARX* genes. For this reason, the category of 'genetic epilepsy' which has recently been proposed is controversial and, perhaps, somewhat uncertain as what is presumed to be symptomatic today, may become genetic after a molecular screening, or remain as such if screening is unavailable.

Genetic research in epilepsy represents an area of great interest for both clinical purposes and for understanding of the mechanisms underlying epilepsy. In the past, genetic studies on families and twins contributed to the definition of genetic epilepsy, and especially to the evaluation of the risk of familial occurrence. After the first report in 1988 of the chromosomal mapping of juvenile myoclonic epilepsy (1), several additional loci were demonstrated to be implicated in syndromic epilepsies. In 1995, the first mutation in the gene coding for the nicotinic acetylcholine receptor was identified in a family with autosomal dominant nocturnal frontal lobe epilepsy (2). The subsequent identification of new epilepsy genes has greatly improved our understanding of the pathophysiological mechanisms underlying epilepsy and has favoured research into experimental models and new therapeutic strategies. A targeted molecular diagnosis is now available for different forms of epilepsy. However, ethical problems may arise especially in asymptomatic mutation carriers or in individuals and families in which although mutations of specific genes have been identified, severity of the associated phenotype is unpredictable.

Genetic epilepsy syndromes without structural brain abnormalities

About 30% of all epilepsies are idiopathic (3). The idiopathic epilepsies are characterized by age-related onset, normal neurological and cognitive development, and absence of brain damage. The study of electroencephalogram (EEG) anomalies while awake and during sleep is useful for characterizing the different forms. An underlying genetic defect has been identified for some forms with Mendelian inheritance. Most idiopathic epilepsies, however, do not follow a simple Mendelian pattern of inheritance. Even in families where involvement of a single gene is suspected, a high degree of complexity can actually be present. The phenotypic variability in some families has been ascribed to genetic modifiers (polymorphisms) or environmental factors that influence phenotypic expression (4).

The genetic alterations identified so far are responsible for rare forms of idiopathic epilepsies with a dominant pattern of inheritance, which occur with repeated seizures in the neonatal or early infantile period, and with febrile, generalized, or partial seizures that persist into adulthood. These forms are observed in a limited number of patients, but they are of great interest as they are caused by alterations in genes that encode voltage-gated ion channel subunits or receptor subunits. The identified mutations are located in the neuronal nicotinic acetylcholine receptor in familial forms of frontal epilepsy, the K^+ channels in benign familial neonatal seizures, the Na^+ channels in a particular form of generalized epilepsy with febrile seizures, and the gamma aminobutyric acid (GABA) receptor in a variant of juvenile myoclonic epilepsy (5). For the most common forms of idiopathic epilepsy, however, the molecular bases have not yet been defined; it is possible that different mutations can cause similar phenotypes in different families or in patients from different geographical areas (Table 2.1).

Table 2.1 Epilepsy syndromes with known genetic basis

Epilepsy syndromes	Type of seizures	Gene	Protein	Locus	OMIM
Generalized epilepsy with febrile seizures plus (GEFS+)	Febrile and afebrile, complex partial, generalized tonic–clonic, absences, myoclonic	*SCN1A*	Sodium channel, neuronal type 1, α subunit	2q24.3	*182389
		SCN1B	Sodium channel, neuronal type 1, β subunit	19q13.1	*600235
		GABRG2	Gamma-aminobutyric acid receptor, γ-2	5q31.1–q33.1	*137164
Severe myoclonic epilepsy of infancy (SMEI)	Febrile, partial, absences, myoclonic, generalized tonic–clonic	*SCN1A*	Sodium channel, neuronal type 1, α subunit	2q24.3	*182389
Benign familial neonatal seizures (BFNS)	Multifocal neonatal convulsions, generalized tonic–clonic	*KCNQ2*	Potassium channel, voltage-gated, KQT-like subfamily, member 2	20q13.3	*602235
		KCNQ3	Potassium channel, voltage-gated, KQT-like subfamily, member 3	8q24	*602232
Benign familial neonatal/infantile seizures (BFNIS)	Multifocal neonatal convulsions, generalized tonic–clonic	*SCN2A*	Sodium channel, voltage-gated, type 2, α subunit	2q23–q24.3	*182390
Benign familial infantile seizures (BFIS) with familial hemiplegic migraine	Multifocal neonatal convulsions, generalized tonic–clonic, hemiplegic migraine	*ATP1A2*	ATPase, Na^+/K^+ Transporting, α-2 polypeptide	1q21–q23	*182340
Autosomal dominant nocturnal frontal lobe epilepsy (ADNLFE)	Partial nocturnal motor seizures with hyperkinetic or tonic manifestations	*CHRNA4*	Cholinergic receptor, neuronal nicotinic, α polypeptide 4	20q13.2–q13.3	*118504
		CHRNB2	Cholinergic receptor, neuronal nicotinic, β polypeptide 2	1q21	*118507
		CHRNA2	Cholinergic receptor, neuronal nicotinic, α polypeptide 2	8p21	*118502
Autosomal dominant temporal lobe epilepsy (ADTLE)	Partial seizures with auditory or visual hallucinations	*LGI1*	Leucine-rich, glioma-inactivated 1	10q24	*604619
Childhood absence epilepsy (CAE)	Absences, tonic–clonic	*GABRG2*	Gamma-aminobutyric acid receptor, γ-2	5q31.1–q33.1	*137164
		CLCN2	Chloride channel 2	3q26	*600570
Juvenile myoclonic epilepsy (JME)	Myoclonic, tonic–clonic	*GABRA1*	Gamma-aminobutyric acid receptor, α-1	5q34–q35	*137160
Juvenile myoclonic epilepsy (JME)	Myoclonic, tonic–clonic	*EFHC1*	EF-hand domain (C-terminal)-containing protein 1	6p12.2	*608815
Infantile spasms, West syndrome	Infantile spasms, hypsarrhythmia	*ARX*	Gene homeobox aristaless related	Xq22.13	*300382
Early infantile epileptic encephalopathy	Myoclonic, infantile spasms	*CDKL5*	Cyclin-dependent kinase 5	Xp22X	*300203
Epilepsy and mental retardation restricted to females	Febrile, partial, absences, myoclonic, generalized tonic–clonic	*PCDH19*	Protocadherin 19	Xq22	*300460
Epileptic encephalopathy (Ohtahara syndrome)	Tonic, infantile spasms	*STXBP1*	Syntaxin binding protein 1	9q34.1	*602926

Severe myoclonic epilepsy of infancy or Dravet syndrome

Dravet syndrome starts at about 6 months of age in previously healthy infants, typically with prolonged generalized or hemiclonic febrile seizures. Between 1 and 4 years, other types of seizures appear, including myoclonic, partial, and absence seizures. Hyperthermia, such as fever or a warm bath, often precipitates seizures (6). Development in the first year of life is normal but subsequently slows and may regress. The EEG may be normal until age 2 years when generalized spike wave activity is seen; approximately 10% of patients are photosensitive. The magnetic resonance imaging (MRI) scan is either normal or shows non-specific features (7, 8).

Dravet syndrome is related to *SCN1A* mutations in at least 85% of cases. The majority of patients exhibiting mutations of this gene carry *de novo* mutations (90%); about 40% of these mutations are truncation and 40% are missense mutations. 10% of patients who are negative on sequence-based mutational analysis, have copy number variations including exonic deletions or duplications that can involve several exons or the whole gene (9, 10). Some rare patients have a mutation in the *GABRG2* gene (11). Germline mosaicism may result in siblings with Dravet syndrome born from an unaffected or mildly unaffected parent carrying a low level of mosaicism for the mutation (12, 13).

SCN1A mutations are also commonly found in the borderline variant of severe myoclonic epilepsy of infancy (SMEB), whose separation from Dravet syndrome may be arbitrary (14). Mutations are less commonly found in patients that have been categorized within different subgroups exhibiting various elements of Dravet syndrome (15–17).

Generalized epilepsy with febrile seizures plus

Generalized epilepsy with febrile seizures plus (GEFS+) is a familial epilepsy syndrome, diagnosed on the basis of at least two individuals with GEFS+ phenotypes in a family. The GEFS+ spectrum denotes the phenotypic heterogeneity observed in families including febrile seizures (FS) and febrile seizures plus (FS+). Overlap with classical idiopathic generalized epilepsy (IGE) is also seen. The course and response to antiepileptic drugs may be considerably variable within the same family: in some patients FS are rare, or disappear after a few years, while in other individuals within the same family, epilepsy is severe and drug resistant. GEFS+ was originally recognized because of remarkable large autosomal dominant pedigrees with 60–70% penetrance. It is likely that most cases, however, occur in small families or are sporadic (18).

Mutations in genes that encode alpha and beta subunits of the voltage-gated Na^+ channel (*SCN1A* and *SCN1B*) have been associated with GEFS + (19, 20). Missense mutations in *SCN1A* are the commonest identified molecular abnormalities and are found in about 10% of families (21). In some families, mutations in the gene encoding the gamma 2 subunit of the $GABA_A$ receptor (*GABRG2*) have been identified (22, 23). The phenotypic variability observed in GEFS + could be linked to the combined action of mutations in different genes.

The neuronal sodium (Na^+) channels consist of two subunits: alpha and beta (Fig. 2.1). *In vitro* functional studies have shown that mutations in the gene that encode the alpha 1 subunit determine a persistent depolarization of the Na^+ current resulting in neuronal hyperexcitability (24). The expression of many *SCN1A* mutations in human embryonic kidney cells or *Xenopus* oocytes has revealed both gain- and loss-of-function mechanisms. However, loss-of function seems to be the predominant mechanism of action causing FS and GEFS+, which is in agreement with genetic and functional studies in Dravet syndrome (25). Two recently published mouse models for SCN1A, in which loss of function mutations were introduced into the endogenous mouse gene, exhibited spontaneous seizures and reduced sodium currents with decreased sodium-channel expression selectively affecting inhibitory interneurons (26, 27). These findings suggest that Dravet syndrome, and maybe the other *SCN1A*-linked seizure disorders, are caused by a decreased excitability of GABAergic interneurons owing to *SCN1A* haploinsufficiency (26, 27). GABA receptors were long suspected to be involved in epileptogenesis. Functional expression of some *GABRG2* mutations, identified in patients with GEFS+, revealed a pronounced loss-of-function by altered gating or defective trafficking and reduced surface expression as a common pathogenic mechanism (25). Hence, these mutations reduce the main mechanism for neuronal inhibition in the brain, which can explain the occurrence of seizures.

Benign epilepsies of the first year of life

Benign epilepsies of the first year of life represent a group of syndromes that are defined as 'benign' because their clinical manifestations, which occur in otherwise asymptomatic babies, regress and eventually disappear spontaneously. These forms are quite rare and are transmitted with an autosomal dominant pattern of inheritance. Molecular diagnosis, where possible, is important in order to avoid unnecessary invasive testing and support genetic counselling. The clinical manifestations of these forms of epilepsy are rather similar, while age of onset is variable.

Benign familial neonatal seizures

Benign familial neonatal seizures (BFNS) are characterized by clusters of seizures that appear from the first days of life up to the 3rd month, and disappear spontaneously after weeks to months. Seizures have a focal onset, often with hemitonic or hemiclonic symptoms or with apnoeic spells, or can clinically appear as generalized. Interictal EEG is usually normal. The rare available ictal EEGs show focal and generalized discharges. The risk of seizures recurring later in life is about 15% (28). Although psychomotor development is usually normal, an increasing number of cases with learning disability have recently been described (29). BFNS are autosomal dominantly inherited with a penetrance of 85%. Most patients have mutations in the gene encoding the K^+ channel voltage-dependent, KQT-like subtype member (*KCNQ2*), and deletions/duplications involving one or more exons of *KCNQ2* (30–32). A small proportion of families carry mutations in the associated gene voltage-dependent K^+ channel, KQT-like subtype, member 3 (*KCNQ3*) (33). *KCNQ2* and *KCNQ3* form a heteromeric K^+ channel, which determines the M-current, influencing the membrane potential at rest (34). Co-expression of the heteromeric wild-type and mutant KCNQ2/3 channels usually revealed a reduction of about 20–30% in the resulting potassium current, which is apparently sufficient to cause BFNS (35). Although the reduction of the potassium current can cause epileptic seizures by a subthreshold membrane depolarization, which increases neuronal firing, it is not fully understood why seizures preferentially occur in neonates (36). It is possible that the neonatal brain be more

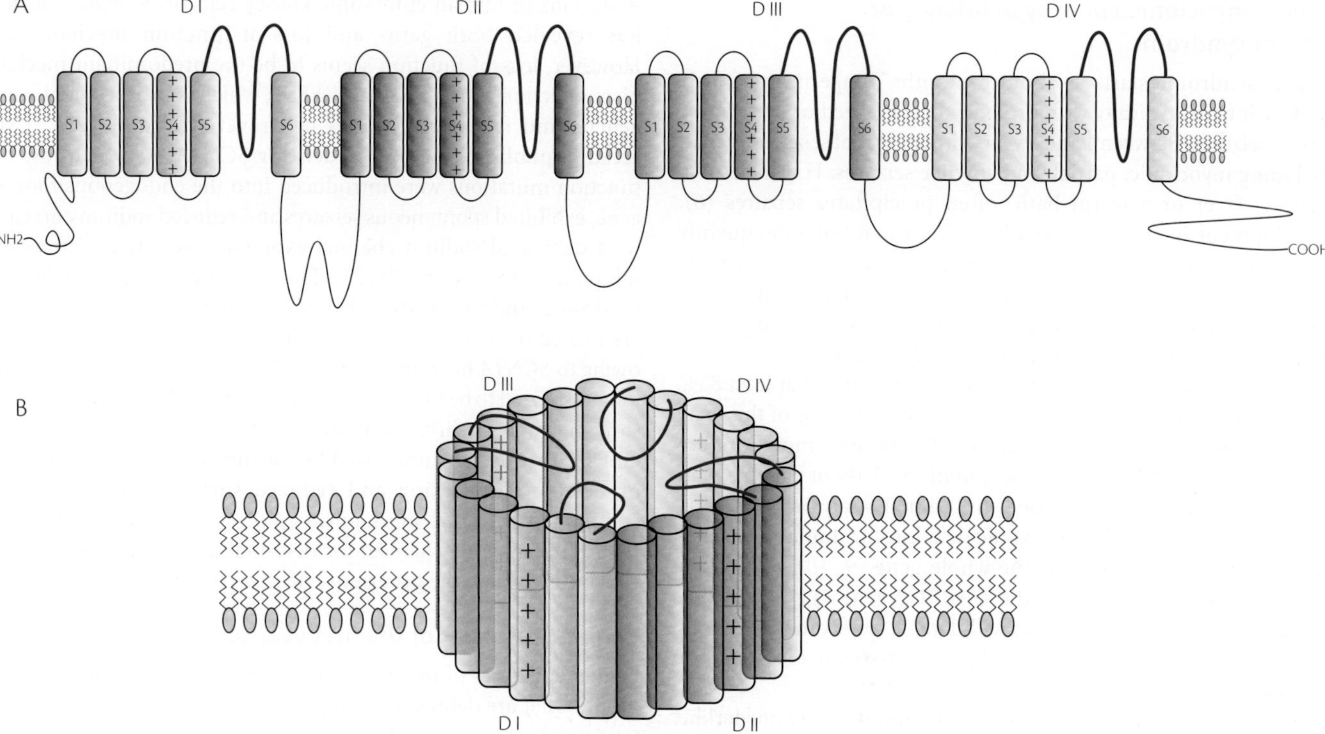

Fig. 2.1 A) Scheme of the structure of the linearized voltage-gated sodium channel α-subunit. The α-subunit consists of four repeated domains (DI–DIV), each of which is in turn composed of 6 α-helix transmembrane segments (S1–S6). Segment S4 is the voltage sensor. The S5 and S6 segments and the linkers form the pore that acts as ion selectivity filter. β-subunits, not represented here, modulate the kinetic and the voltage-dependence of the channel. B) Three-dimensional configuration of the sodium channel.

vulnerable to changes, even small, of neuronal excitability. An alternative is that KCNQ2 and KCNQ3 channels, when mutated, are replaced by other K^+ channels that become functional after the first months of life.

Benign familial neonatal-infantile seizures

Benign familial neonatal-infantile seizures (BFNIS) are characterized by seizures similar to those observed in children with BFNS. However, age at onset of seizures ranges from the neonatal period to infancy in different family members, with a mean onset age of 3 months. Remission occurs by 12 months with a very low risk of later seizures (37, 38). Mutations in *SCN2A* have been identified in most families with BFNS (39).

Benign familial infantile seizures

Benign familial infantile seizures (BFIS) are characterized by seizures similar to those observed in BNFS with an onset at around 6 months (40). Linkage studies have identified two loci for this type of epilepsy, one in the pericentromeric region of chromosome 16 and another on chromosome 19 (41, 42). However, the disease gene has not yet been identified. Some families also have paroxysmal dyskinesia beginning in later childhood (infantile convulsions and choreoathetosis) (41). Long-term prognosis for seizure remission is excellent. Several families with mutations in the *ATP1A2* gene have benign infantile seizures in conjunction with hemiplegic migraine (43). Rare families with mutations in *SCN2A* or *KCNQ2* have also been described in which only infantile seizures occur (44, 45).

Autosomal dominant nocturnal frontal lobe epilepsy

Autosomal dominant nocturnal frontal lobe epilepsy (ADNFLE) includes frequent brief seizures that occur from childhood, with hyperkinetic or tonic manifestations, typically in clusters at night (46). Ictal video-EEG studies have revealed partial seizures originating from the frontal lobe but also from parts of the insula and temporal lobe suggesting a defect of a broader network (47, 48). Penetrance is estimated at approximately 70–80%. A mutation was identified in the gene *CHRNA4* encoding the a4-subunit of a neuronal nicotinic acetylcholine receptor as the first ion channel mutation found in an inherited form of epilepsy (2). Altogether, six mutations in *CHRNA4*, three in *CHRNB2*, which encodes the beta2-subunit of neuronal nicotinic acetylcholine receptor, and one in *CHRNA2*, encoding the neuronal nicotinic acetylcholine receptor alpha2-subunit, have been reported so far (25, 49–52). These receptors are heteropentamers consisting of various combinations of subunits. The alpha4-beta2 combination is the most represented in the thalamus and cerebral cortex (Fig. 2.2). All the identified mutations reside in the pore-forming M2 transmembrane segments. The exact pathomechanism is not fully understood, but an increased acetylcholine sensitivity could be the main common gating defect of the mutations.

Autosomal dominant temporal lobe epilepsy

Autosomal dominant temporal lobe epilepsy (ADTLE) is a form of autosomal dominant partial epilepsy associated to auditory symptoms. The first clinical manifestations, usually occurring during

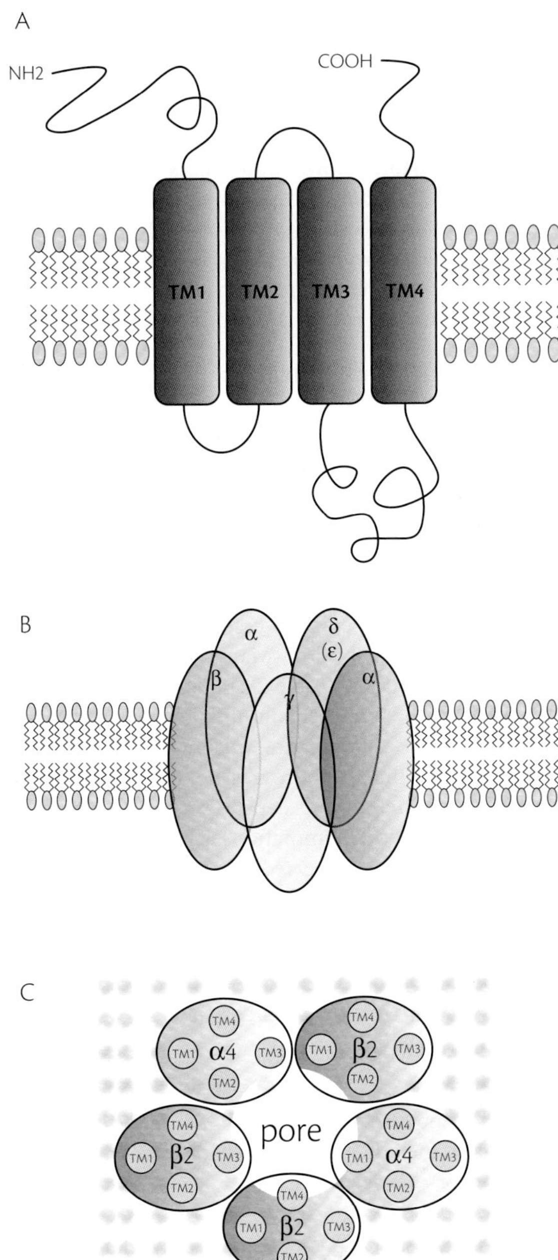

Fig. 2.2 A) General structure of a single subunit of the nicotinic receptor. B) Nicotinic receptors are formed by five subunits (pentamers), symmetrically arranged to delimit a pore through which cations flow, with Na^+ and Ca^{2+} incoming, and K^+ outgoing. Nine different types of α-subunits and four different types of β-subunits are known. Isoforms for subunits δ, ε, and γ are not yet known. Numerous receptor subtypes that have specific anatomical locations (e.g. muscle or neuronal) are generated by multiple combinations of different types of these subunits. In the central nervous system, the pentameric structures of the receptor are composed of α-subunit homodimers or of α-subunits/β-subunits combinations. C) Top view of the structure of a neuronal nicotinic receptor composed by two α4-subunits (CHRNA4) and three β2-subunits (CHRNB2). Abnormalities in this receptor, caused by mutations of its subunits, cause nocturnal frontal lobe epilepsy.

childhood or adolescence, are auditory hallucinations, sometimes accompanied by vision or olfactory manifestations, or dizziness (53, 54). Mutations in the *LGI1* gene (leucine-rich, glioma-inactivated 1) have been associated with ADTLE in several families (55, 56). The *LGI1* pathogenetic mechanism remains to be clarified. Functional inactivation of one allele leads to ADTLE, whereas silencing of both alleles has been observed in several high-grade gliomas (57). The LGI1 protein harbours a domain consisting of a sevenfold repeat of 44 amino acids, the EAR (epilepsy-associated repeat) domain (58). This domain is common to MASS1, a large G-protein coupled receptor, mutated in the Frings murine model of audiogenic epilepsy (59).

Febrile seizures

FS are classified as a nosological entity distinct from epilepsy. FS affect 2–4% of children between the ages of 3 months and 6 years (60). The differential diagnosis includes seizures with fever in a child with epilepsy, seizures with central nervous system infection, or an acute metabolic disturbance (60). A positive family history is one of the few known risk factors for febrile seizures, with recurrence risk ratios of 3–5 in first-degree relatives (61). About 3–6% of children with FS will have epilepsy later in life, including idiopathic generalized epilepsy and temporal lobe epilepsy with hippocampal sclerosis that might be related to prolonged FS (62). Segregation analysis of a population-based sample showed that most FS have polygenic inheritance, although a small proportion have autosomal-dominant inheritance (63). Using large, multigeneration families with presumed autosomal dominant inheritance, four loci for FS have been identified (FEB1–FEB4) but no gene defect has yet been identified (64).

Single gene severe epilepsies and epileptic encephalopathies

Some types of severe epilepsies have a genetic basis. Patients often have severe epilepsy with early onset and infantile spasms, delayed neurological and cognitive development, and behavioural problems. Some examples of genes in which, in recent years, mutations have been identified in patients with particular forms of severe epilepsy are discussed in this section.

PCDH19 (protocadherin 19)

PCDH19 mutations have been associated to epilepsy and mental retardation limited to females (EFMR) (65), an X-linked disorder surprisingly affecting only females and sparing transmitting males, but also often appearing *de novo* (66). It is characterized by a variable clinical presentation, including slow development from birth, normal early development followed by regression starting at seizure onset, and normal development without regression (65, 67). The epilepsy spectrum associated with *PCDH19* mutations is in turn variable and includes mild focal epilepsy starting in infancy or epilepsy with recurrent episodes of focal or generalized seizures in series or status epilepticus triggered by fever (66). Protocadherin 19 is part of the protocadherin delta-2 subclass of the cadherin superfamily. Protocadherin members are expressed predominantly in the nervous system, where they have a role in establishing neuronal connections and in signal transduction at synaptic membranes (65). Males which are hemizygous for *PCDH19* mutations have normal cognitive level and no epilepsy. Cellular interference has been proposed to explain the discrepancy between the clinical manifestations of heterozygous females and hemizygous males (68). This model suggests that if an individual has two populations of protocadherin cells (mutated and non-mutated) then a pathological phenotype occurs. A normal female or a transmitting male have only one protocadherin population of cells, protocadherin-wildtype or protocadherin-mutant cells, respectively, then they do not present a pathological phenotype. The development of genetically modified animal models will allow this puzzling disease mechanism to be better explored.

ARX (aristaless-related homeobox)

The *ARX* gene, on chromosome Xp22, is a transcription factor that belongs to a family of paired class homeobox genes, and plays an important role in embryogenesis, especially in the development of the central nervous system (69). To date, *ARX* mutations have been identified in about 10 different clinical conditions, with or without brain malformations (70–72). Malformation phenotypes, including X-linked lissencephaly with abnormal genitalia (XLAG), XLAG with severe hydrocephalus, and Proud syndrome (agenesis of the corpus callosum with abnormal genitalia), are associated with protein truncation mutations and missense mutations in the homeobox (70, 73). Non-malformation phenotypes are associated with missense mutations outside of the homeobox or expansion of the second polyA tract and include X-linked infantile spasms (ISS)/West syndrome, Partington syndrome (mental retardation with mild distal dystonia), and non-specific X-linked mental retardation (XLMR) (70, 73). Expansions in the first polyA tract cause X-linked infantile spasms (ISSX)/West syndrome (tonic spasms with clustering, severe psychomotor delay and hypsarrhythmia on the EEG) (74, 75), a severe epileptic-dyskinetic encephalopathy (71), tonic seizures and dystonia without infantile spasms (76), and Ohtahara syndrome (77).

CDKL5 (cyclin-dependent, kinase-like 5)

Mutations in the X-linked gene *CDKL5* cause early onset intractable seizures, severe developmental delay and, often, subsequent appearance of Rett syndrome (RTT)–like features (78). The phenotypic spectrum associated with *CDKL5* mutations also includes X-linked infantile spasms syndrome (ISSX) (79), a form of myoclonic encephalopathy (80), and severe encephalopathy with refractory seizures (81). Mutations in *CDKL5* are mainly found in females, suggesting gestational lethality in males (82). Parental germline mosaicism has been reported (83). In affected females, a seemingly normal early development, followed by onset of intractable seizures between the first days and 4th month of life are early key diagnostic criteria. Severe developmental delay with regression become apparent after seizures onset. Seizures are usually manifested as infantile spasms, or prolonged tonic seizures followed by spasms and myoclonus, with a peculiar electroclinical pattern (84) variably associated with, migrating focal seizures during the course. Overall, 16.3% of girls with early-onset intractable epilepsy, with or without infantile spasms, exhibit either mutations or genomic deletions involving *CDKL5* (85).

STXBP1 (syntaxin binding protein 1)

Mutations in the *STXBP1* gene have been associated with Ohtahara syndrome or early infantile epileptic encephalopathy (EIEE), characterized by early onset of tonic spasms, seizure intractability, a characteristic suppression-burst pattern on the EEG and poor outcome with severe psychomotor retardation (86, 87). *STXBP1* mutations have also been found in some children with infantile spasms (88, 89). The transition from EIEE to West syndrome occurs in 75% of individuals with EIEE (86, 87). STXBP1 protein plays an essential role in synaptic vesicle release and secretion of neurotransmitters (90). The Ohtahara syndrome–infantile spasms spectrum can also be caused by polyalanine expansions of the *ARX* gene (71, 77). Available information suggests a mutation rate of about 6% for *ARX* in boys with isolated or X-linked infantile spasms and no brain lesions (71) and up to 37% for *STXBP1* in infants with Ohtahara syndrome (90). However, larger series are needed to fully elucidate the phenotypic spectrum and better understand the causative role of this gene in epilepsy.

Progressive myoclonus epilepsies

These genetically heterogeneous disorders (Table 2.2) share clinical features that include action myoclonus, myoclonic jerks that are segmental and arrhythmic, appearing both at rest and as stimulus sensitive manifestations, epileptic seizures, predominantly generalized tonic–clonic. Progressive mental deterioration, cerebellar and extrapyramidal signs are also present in a variable proportion of patients (91, 92). Progressive myoclonus epilepsies (PMEs) represent less than 1% of all epilepsy cases and have a variable geographic and ethnic distribution. Many gene defects underlying PMEs have been identified (Table 2.3) but in a considerable proportion of patients the cause remains unknown. Most PMEs result from the intracellular accumulation of abnormal deposit material (93). The age onset, the rapid progression of the symptoms, and the prognosis are different and depend on the specific aetiology and on the type of causative mutations. The diagnostic approach varies in relation to the suspected form (Table 2.4). While the Unverricht–Lundborg disease, although disabling, can reach a degree of stabilization, all other forms progress relentlessly, leading to severe disability or death in matter of years.

Idiopathic generalized epilepsies with complex inheritance

Mode of inheritance

The idiopathic generalized epilepsies (IGEs) represent 20–30% of all epilepsies and include a group of syndromes characterized by

Table 2.2 Clinical classification of progressive myoclonic epilepsies

PMEs type	Age of onset
Unverricht–Lundborg disease (ULD)	7–16 years
Lafora disease (LD)	6–19 years
Neuronal ceroid-lipofuscinoses (NCLs):	
◆ Infantile (Haltia–Santavuori)	6 months–2 years
◆ Late infantile (Jansky–Bielschowsky)	1–4 years
◆ Intermediate (Lake or Cavanagh)	5–8 years
◆ Juvenile (Spielmeyer–Vogt)	4–14 years
◆ Adult (Kufs)	15–50 years
Myoclonic epilepsy with ragged-red fibres (MERRF)	3–65 years
Sialidosis:	8–15 years
◆ Type 1	
◆ Galactosialidosis (type 2)	
Dentato-rubro-pallido-luysian atrophy (DRPLA)	Childhood
Gaucher disease (type III)	Variable

Table 2.3 Molecular genetics of progressive myoclonic epilepsies

PMEs type	Pattern of inheritance	Locus	Gene
Unverricht–Lundborg disease (ULD)	AR	21q22.3	*CSTB*
Lafora disease (LD)	AR	6q 24.3 6p22.3	*EPM2A* *NHLRC1*
Neuronal ceroid-lipofuscinoses (NCLs):			
Infantile	AR	1p34.2	*PPT1*
Late infantile	AR	11p15.4	*TPP1*
Finnish variant	AR	13q22.3	*CLN5*
Gipsy variant	AR	15q23	*CLN6*
Turkish variant	AR	4q28.2	*MFSD8*
Juvenile	AR	16p12.1	*CLN3*
Juvenile variant	AR	8p23.3	*CLN8*
Juvenile variant	AR	–	*CLN9*
Adult	AR	15q23	*CLN4*
Congenital	AD AR	20q13.33 11p15.5	*DNAJC5* *CTSD*
Myoclonic epilepsy with ragged-red fibres (MERRF)	Mitochondrial	Mt DNA	$tRNA^{Lys}$
Sialidosis:			
Type I	AR	6p21.33	*NEU1*
Galactosialidosis	AR	20q13.12	*CTSA*
Gaucher disease, type III	AR	1q22	*GBA*
Dentato-rubro-pallido-luysian atrophy (DRPLA)	AD	12p13.31	*ATN1*

AD, autosomal dominant; AR, autosomal recessive; Mt, mitochondrial.

absence seizures, myoclonus, and generalized tonic–clonic seizures. There is a partial overlap in age of onset, type, and frequency of seizures, prognosis, and response to treatment. Among these disorders there are several subsyndromes, including childhood absence epilepsy (CAE), juvenile absence epilepsy (JAE), juvenile myoclonic epilepsy (JME), and epilepsy with generalized tonic–clonic seizures alone. Generalized spike-wave activity and normal background are observed in the EEG. Among epilepsies with complex inheritance, IGEs seem very suitable for genetic studies because they are common, have a relatively well-defined phenotype and occur in familial clusters. Close relatives of IGE probands have 4–10% risk of developing epilepsy (94). Higher risk is seen in siblings and offspring, and is lower in second-degree relatives. In contrast to monogenic inheritance, polygenic inheritance leads to a more rapid decrease of the risk in relatives as the distance from the affected individuals increases (95). Twin studies have shown higher concordance for IGE in monozygotic than in dizygotic twins (0.76 versus 0.33), which is consistent with polygenic inheritance (96). IGEs have a genetic aetiology with complex inheritance. It has been suggested that they might result from the interaction of two or more genes (97). However a high degree of complexity is operating as large-scale exome sequencing of ion channels reveals that rare missense variation in known Mendelian disease genes are equally prevalent in healthy individuals and in those with idiopathic generalized epilepsy, revealing that even deleterious ion channel mutations confer an uncertain risk to an individual depending on the other variants with which they are combined (98).

Table 2.4 Diagnostic tools for progressive myoclonic epilepsies

PMEs type	Methods	Marker
Unverricht–Lundborg disease (ULD)	Molecular biology	*CSTB*
Lafora disease (LD)	Axillar biopsy Molecular biology	Lafora bodies *EPM2A* and *NHLRC1*
Neuronal ceroid-lipofuscinoses (NCLs)	Biopsy Molecular biology	Storage lipopigment in lysosomes *PPT1, TPP1, CLN3, CLN4, CLN5, CLN6, CLN8, CLN9, MFSD8, DNAJC5, CTSD*
Myoclonic epilepsy with ragged-red fibres (MERRF)	Muscle biopsy Molecular biology	Ragged-red fibres A8344G substitution (90%) (mitochondrial DNA)
Sialidosis	Urine Lymphocytes, fibroblasts Molecular biology	↑Urinary oligosaccharides α-N-acetyl neuroaminidase deficit *NEU1*
Galactosialidosis	Urine, leukocytes, and fibroblasts Molecular biology	β-galactosidase deficit *CTSA*
Gaucher disease, type III	Lymphocytes, fibroblasts Molecular biology	β-glucocerebrosidase deficit *GBA*
Dentato-rubro-pallido-luysian atrophy (DRPLA)	Molecular biology	*ATN1*

Molecular basis

Although several chromosomal loci for different forms of IGEs have been identified, they have not often been replicated. Linkage studies on a large number of families with IGE led to the identification of several susceptibility loci (18q, 2q, 3q, and 14q) (99, 100). In rare families pathogenic mutations in single genes have been reported. Mutations in the *GABRG2* gene were identified in families with febrile seizures and childhood absence epilepsy (22, 23), a mutation in the *GABRA1* gene was identified in a family with dominantly inherited juvenile myoclonic epilepsy (101). Mutations in *CLCN2* have been identified in families with heterogeneous IGE phenotypes, including CAE (102). Rare variants in *CACNA1H* have been identified in CAE and other generalized epilepsy phenotypes (103, 104). Finally, the study of variants has provided some evidence that *GABRD* (105), *ME2* (106), *BRD2* (107), and *NEDD4L* (108) are susceptibility genes for IGE.

Symptomatic epilepsy

Epilepsies are defined symptomatic when an external cause can be identified. Often, these epilepsies persist over time and are resistant to drug treatment. Advances in diagnostics, especially the use of brain MRI, has brought to attention how often structural brain anomalies, even discrete, are the cause of epilepsy. Developmental abnormalities of the cerebral cortex are a frequent cause of epilepsy. They occur as isolated manifestations or may be one expression of neurocutaneous diseases, vascular malformations, structural abnormalities associated with chromosomal disorders (Down syndrome, Angelman and Prader–Willi syndromes, Ring 20 syndrome, Wolff–Hirschhorn syndrome and many pathogenic copy number variations), mitochondrial encephalomyopathies, the organic acidurias, and the peroxisomal diseases. All these disorders have usually an early onset. However, even a relatively late onset of seizures (2nd to 3rd decade of life) may occur when a discrete developmental abnormality of the brain is the cause of seizures.

Malformations of the cerebral cortex

It has been estimated that at least 40% of children with drug-resistant epilepsy have a malformation of the cerebral cortex (109). These malformations consist of an abnormal distribution, organization, or sometimes differentiation of the neuronal components (110). Several cortical malformations associated with epilepsy are caused by alterations that occur during embryonic development, especially during the migration of neurons to form the cerebral cortex in its definitive shape. In recent years, several genes have been identified that, when mutated, cause abnormalities of cortical development. In the following sections, the most frequent cortical malformations associated with epilepsy (lissencephaly, periventricular heterotopia, and polymicrogyria) and those whose disease genes have been identified will be presented (Table 2.5).

Lissencephaly and subcortical band heterotopia

Lissencephaly (LIS) and subcortical band heterotopia (SBH) are malformations resulting from anomalies in cortical neuronal migration. LIS is characterized by absent (agyria) or decreased (pachygyria) convolutions, producing cortical thickening and a smooth cerebral surface (111). SBH is a related disorder in which bands of grey matter are interposed in the white matter between the cortex and the lateral ventricles (110).

Classical LIS is rare, with a prevalence of about 12 per million births. Patients with severe LIS have early developmental delay, early diffuse hypotonia, later spastic quadriplegia, and eventual severe or profound mental retardation. Seizures occur in over 90% of LIS children (112), with onset before 6 months in about 75% of cases. About 80% of children have infantile spasms, although EEG does not show typical hypsarrhythmia. Most LIS children subsequently have multiple seizure types. Epilepsy is present in almost all patients with SBH and is intractable in about 65% of them. About 50% of patients with epilepsy have focal seizures, and the remaining 50% have generalized epilepsy, often within the spectrum of Lennox–Gastaut syndrome (109).

Two major genes have been associated with classical LIS and SBH. The *LIS1* gene is responsible for the autosomal form of LIS (113), while the *doublecortin* gene (*DCX*) is X-linked (114, 115). Although either gene can result in either LIS or SBH, most cases of classical LIS are due to deletions or mutations of *LIS1* (116), whereas most cases of SBH are due to mutations of *DCX* (117). *LIS1*-related *LIS* is more severe in the posterior brain regions (p>a gradient) (Fig. 2.3A), whereas *DCX*-related LIS is more severe in the anterior brain (a>p gradient) (Fig. 2.3B). About 60% of patients with p>a isolated lissencephaly (ILS) carry genomic alterations or mutations involving *LIS1* (116). Most mutations (84%) are truncating (118). Small genomic deletions and duplications of *LIS1* occur in almost 50% of patients (116). A simplified gyral pattern in the posterior brain, with underlying SBH, has been associated with mosaic mutations of *LIS1* (119). Miller–Dieker syndrome (MDS) is caused by deletion of *LIS1* and contiguous genes and features severe p>a LIS (Fig. 2.3C), accompanied by distinct dysmorphic facial features and additional malformations. Most *DCX* mutations cause a>p SBH/pachygyria. Mutations of *DCX* have been found in all reported pedigrees and in 80% of sporadic females and 25% of sporadic males with SBH (117). Genomic deletions of *DCX* are a rare cause of SBH or X-linked lissencephaly in patients who are mutation negative after Sanger sequencing of *DCX* (Fig. 2.3D) (120). Maternal germline or mosaic *DCX* mutations may occur in about 10% of cases of either SBH or X-linked LIS (121).

Three rarer forms of LIS-pachygyria have been identified in recent years. One form, X-linked LIS with absent corpus callosum and ambiguous genitalia (XLAG), results from mutations of the *ARX* gene. XLAG is a severe condition that is only observed in boys. Female carriers have normal brain MRI scan or partial to complete agenesis of the corpus callosum, with normal cognition to mild retardation (73) (Fig. 2.3, E and F). A second form, due to mutations of the *TUBA1A* gene, exhibits characteristics that partially overlap with the LIS-SBH spectrum but is often accompanied by cerebellar hypoplasia (Fig. 2.3G) (122). A third, recessive form, results from homozygous mutations of the *RELN* gene and is characterized by moderate lissencephaly, severe cerebellar hypoplasia, dysmorphic facial features, developmental delay and epilepsy (123).

Periventricular nodular heterotopia

Periventricular nodular heterotopia (PNH) consists of nodules of grey matter located along the lateral ventricles with a total failure of migration of a subset of neurons (110); it ranges from isolated, single, to confluent bilateral nodules (Fig. 2.3H). Many patients

Table 2.5 Genes and chromosomal loci associated with cortical malformations

Cortical malformations	Pattern of inheritance	Gene	Locus	OMIM
Malformations from abnormal proliferation				
Tuberous sclerosis	AD	*TSC1*	9q34.13	* 605284
Tuberous sclerosis	AD	*TSC2*	16p13.3	* 191092
Malformations from abnormal migration				
Lissencephaly (LIS)				
Miller–Dieker syndrome (MDS)	AD	*LIS1+YWHAE*	17p13.3	*601545
Isolated lissencephaly sequence (ILS) or subcortical band heterotopia (SBH)	AD	*LIS1*	17p13.3	*601545
ILS or SBH	X-linked	*DCX*	Xq22.3–q23	*300121
ILS or SBH	AD	*TUBA1A*	12q12–q14	*602529
X-linked lissencephaly with abnormal genitalia (XLAG)	X-linked	*ARX*	Xp22.13	*300382
LIS with cerebellar hypoplasia (LCH)	AR	*RELN*	7q22	*600514
LCH group B	AR	*VLDLR*	9p24.2	
Periventricular nodular heterotopia (PNH)				
Classical bilateral PNH	X-linked	*FLNA*	Xq28	*300017
Ehlers–Danlos syndrome and PNH	X-linked	*FLNA*	Xq28	*300017
Facial dysmorphisms, severe constipation and PNH	X-linked	*FLNA*	Xq28	*300017
Fragile-X syndrome and PNH	X-linked	*FMR1*	Xq27.3	*309550
PNH with limb abnormalities (limb reduction abnormality or syndactyly)	X-linked	...	Xq28	
Williams syndrome and PNH	AD	...	7q11.23	
PH	AD	...	5p15.1	
PH	AD	...	5p15.33	
Agenesis of the corpus callosum, polymicrogyria and PNH	AD	...	6q26–qter	
PH	AD		4p15	
PH	AD	...	5q14.3–q15	
Agenesis of the corpus callosum and PNH	AD	...	1p36.22–pter	
Microcephaly and PNH	AR	*ARFGEF2*	20q13.13	*605371
Donnai–Barrow syndrome and PNH	AR	*LRP2*	2q24–q31	*600073
Cobblestone cortical malformations				
Fukuyama congenital muscular dystrophy or Walker–Warburg syndrome (WWS)	AR	*FKTN*	9q31.2	*607440
Muscle–eye–brain disease (MEB) or WWS	AR	*FKRP*	19q13.32	*606596
MEB	AR	*LARGE*	22q12.3	*603590
MEB	AR	*POMGnT1*	1p34.1	*606822
MEB or WWS	AR	*POMT1*	9q34.13	*607423
MEB or WWS	AR	*POMT2*	14q24.3	*607439
CEDNIK syndrome	AR	*SNAP29*	22q11.2	*604202
Malformations from abnormal cortical organization				
Polymicrogyria (PMG)				
Bilateral frontoparietal PMG	AR	*GPR56*	16q13	*604110
Asymmetric PMG	AD	*TUBB2B*	6p25.2	*612850
PMG and rolandic seizures, oromotor dyspraxia	X-linked	*SRPX2*	Xq21.33–q23	*300642
PMG and Agenesis of the corpus callosum (ACC), microcephaly	AD	*TBR2*	3p21.3–p21.2	*604615
PMG and aniridia	AD	*PAX6*	11p13	*607108
PMG	AD	...	1p36.3–pter	
PMG and microcephaly	AD	...	1q44–qter	
PMG and facial dysmorphisms	AD	...	2p16.1–p23	
PMG and microcephaly, hydrocephalus	AD		4q21–q22	
PMG	AD	...	21q2	
PMG and DiGeorge syndrome	AD	...	22q11.2	
PMG and Warburg Micro syndrome	AR	RAB3GAP1	2q21.3	*602536
PMG and Goldberg–Shprintzen syndrome	AR	KIAA1279	10q21.3	*609367

AD, autosomal dominant; AR, autosomal recessive.

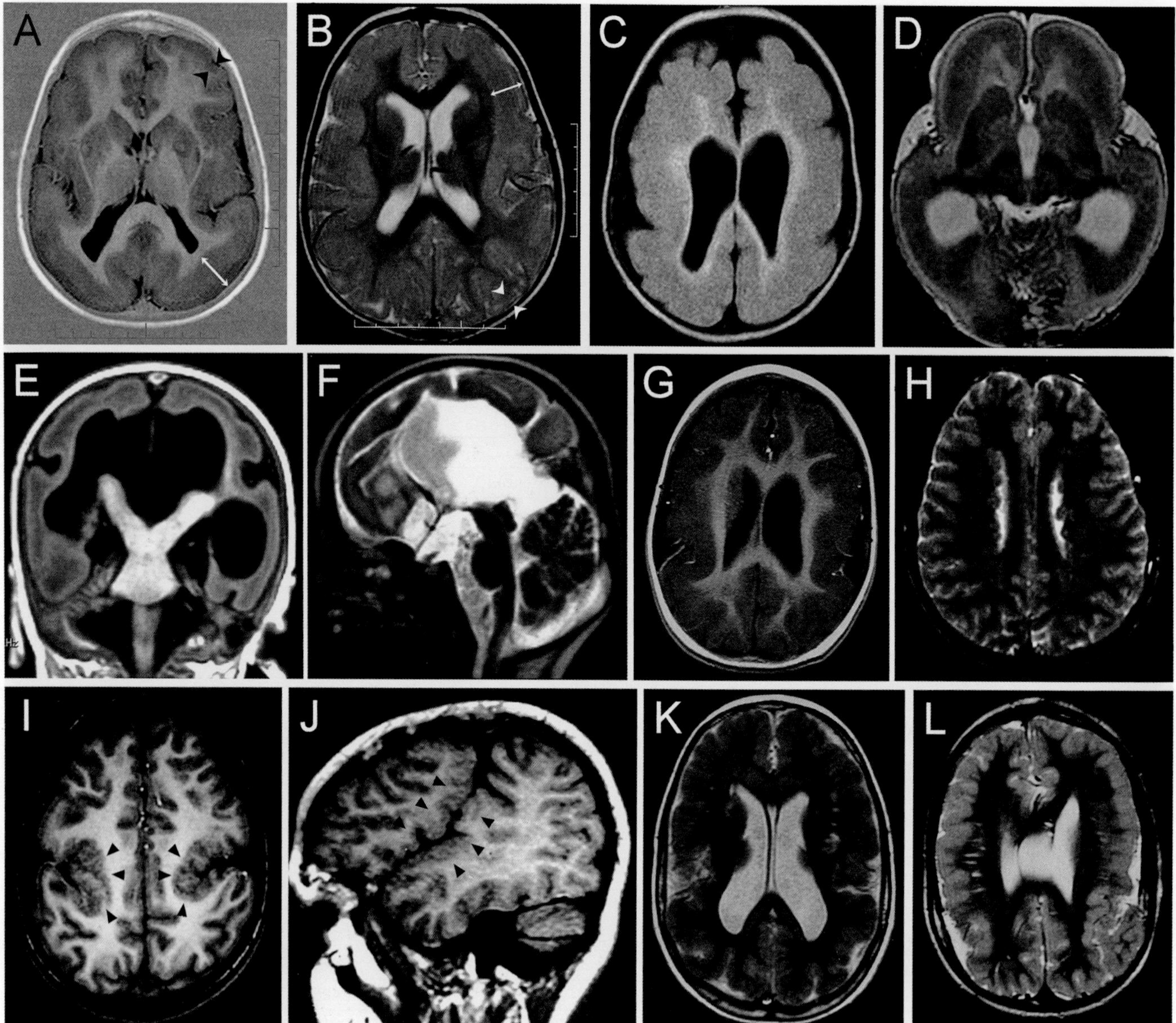

Fig. 2.3 Brain MRI of patients with different malformations of the cerebral cortex. A) Axial section. Classical lissencephaly in a boy with *LIS1* mutation. B) Axial section. Lissencephaly in a girl with *DCX* mutation. C) Axial section. Lissencephaly in a patient with Miller–Dieker syndrome. D) Axial section. Severe diffuse lissencephaly with relatively small frontal lobes in a boy with *DCX* mutation. E) and F) Coronal section and sagittal section of a boy with X-linked lissencephaly, complete corpus callosum agenesis, and ambiguous genitalia due to an *ARX* mutation. G) Axial section. Thickened cortex with simplified gyral pattern in a girl with a *TUBA1A* gene mutation. H) Axial section. Classical bilateral periventricular nodular heterotopia in a woman with a *FLNA* mutation. I) and J) belong to the same patient. I) Axial section. Bilateral perisylvian polymicrogyria. The sylvian fissures are open and the perisylvian cortex is thickened and irregular (black arrows). J) Sagittal section. Note the abnormally vertical orientation of the sylvian fissure, which appears to be fused with the rolandic fissure. K) Axial section. Bilateral frontoparietal polymicrogyria in a girl with a *GPR56* mutation and Lennox–Gastaut syndrome. L) Axial section. Polymicrogyria in a patient with *TUBB2B* mutation. The cortical mantle is diffusely polymicrogyric, with prominent infoldings in the posterior aspect of the abnormally oriented sylvian fissures, more on the left.

have epilepsy, with normal or borderline cognitive level. However, a wide spectrum of clinical presentations and associated features is possible, with a loose correlation between size of PNH, structural abnormality of the cortex, and clinical severity (124). PNH occurs most frequently in women as an X-linked trait (125) defined as 'classical bilateral PNH', associated with high rates of prenatal lethality in male fetuses, and 50% recurrence risk in the female offspring. Almost 100% of families and 26% of sporadic patients, harbour mutations of the *FLNA* gene (124), which also cause coagulopathy and cardiovascular abnormalities in some patients. Only a few living male patients with PNH owing to *FLNA* mutations have been reported (126, 127). Mild missense mutations or mosaic mutations account for survival of affected males, who can, in turn, pass their genetic defect to their daughters. A rare recessive form of PNH owing to mutations of the *ARFGEF2* gene was described in two consanguineous pedigrees in which affected children had microcephaly, severe delay, and early-onset seizures (128). PNH has been described in association with known genetic syndromes and a number of copy number variants (CNVs) in patients with variably impaired cognitive skills (129) (Table 2.5).

Polymicrogyria

The term 'polymicrogyria' (PMG) defines an excessive number of abnormally small gyri that produce an irregular cortical surface with lumpy aspect (110). PMG can be localized to a single gyrus, involve a portion of one hemisphere, be bilateral and asymmetrical, bilateral and symmetrical, or diffuse. The imaging appearance of PMG varies with the patient's age. In newborns and young infants, the malformed cortex is very thin with multiple, very small undulations. After myelination, PMG appears as thickened cortex with irregular cortex–white matter junction (130). Polymicrogyria is associated with a wide number of patterns and syndromes and with mutations in several genes (Table 2.5). Various PMG syndromes have been described, which have been designated according to their lobar topography (130). Bilateral perisylvian polymicrogyria (BPP) (Fig. 2.3I, J) is the most frequent form. It is associated with mild to moderate mental retardation, epilepsy, and impaired oromotor skills. Most cases are sporadic but genetic heterogeneity is apparent (130, 131). A missense mutation in the Xq22 gene *SRPX2* was found in an affected male (131). However, *SRPX2* does not account for X-linked pedigrees. BPP, frequently asymmetric and with a striking predisposition for the right hemisphere, has also been reported in association with 22q11.2 deletion (132). Bilateral frontoparietal polymicrogyria (BFPP) (Fig. 2.3K) has been reported in families with recessive pedigrees and has been associated with mutations of the *GPR56* gene (133). The imaging characteristics of BFPP resemble those of the cobblestone malformative spectrum (muscle-eye-brain disease and Fukuyama congenital muscular dystrophy) (130). Mutations of the *TUBB2B* gene have been associated with asymmetric polymicrogyria (134) but genotype–phenotype correlations need to be clarified (Fig. 2.3L). Different types of PMG as part of complex syndromes have been associated with several different pathogenic CNVs (Table 2.5) (135).

Metabolic disorders

Epilepsy is part of the clinical spectrum of a large number of inherited metabolic disorders (136, 137), often within the context of a complex neurological syndrome. Sometimes epilepsy is a prominent, or presenting, symptom, and, in a minority of patients can be cured by an appropriate dietary supplementation or regimen. Pyridoxine-dependent seizures, a recessive disorder due to mutations of the *antiquitin* (*ALDH7A1*) gene, respond dramatically to the intravenous injection of pyridoxine and recur within a few days if maintenance therapy is discontinued. The disorder is caused by a defect of alpha-amino adipic semialdehyde (α-AASA) dehydrogenase (antiquitin) in the cerebral lysine degradation pathway (138). The possibility of dosing specific metabolites such as α-AASA (139) and of mutation analysis has meant that pyridoxine withdrawal is no longer needed to establish the diagnosis. Epilepsy related to glucose transporter type 1 deficiency syndrome (GLUT1-DS) provides a paradigmatic example of how once the core phenotypic spectrum of a genetically determined inherited neurometabolic disorder has been defined, availability of biological and molecular markers allows progressive delineation of the syndrome spectrum. The cause of GLUT1-DS is heterozygous mutations of the *SLC2A1* gene encoding GLUT1, the molecule that transports glucose across the blood–brain barrier (140). Hypoglycorrachia is a key diagnostic laboratory feature. Clinical features classically comprise a combination of infantile-onset seizures, complex movement disorders, ataxia, cognitive impairment, and, in some children, microcephaly (141). Generalized spike-and-wave discharges and a combination of absence, myoclonic, and tonic–clonic seizures have been reported (142). A syndrome of paroxysmal exercise-induced dyskinesia and epilepsy (143) and recently an IGE phenotype (144) and more specifically early-onset absence epilepsy (145) and myoclonic-astatic epilepsy have been associated to *SLC2A1* mutations (146).

Chromosomal abnormalities

Chromosomal abnormalities are relatively common genetically determined conditions that increase the risk of epilepsy. Epilepsy has been associated with over 400 different chromosomal imbalances (147, 148). Among patients with epilepsy and intellectual disability, about 6% have chromosomal abnormalities, but this figure climbs to 50% if multiple congenital abnormalities are also present (147). The use of such current techniques as high-resolution chromosome banding, fluorescent *in situ* hybridization (FISH), comparative genomic hybridization (array CGH), and multiplex ligand-dependent probe amplification (MLPA) would certainly increase these detection rates. However, the likelihood of developing seizures varies greatly among the different chromosomal disorders. Chromosomal abnormalities almost constantly result from rearrangements or deletions/duplications that affect the function of more than one gene. As a consequence, even when the chromosomal imbalance can only be detected using techniques with the highest resolution, such as array CGH, affected patients have a combination of clinical features and only exceptionally have isolated epilepsy. Most often cognitive impairment and dysmorphic features, even subtle, co-occur with epilepsy. The ring chromosome 20 syndrome represents the most striking example in which a highly specific epilepsy phenotype can be, at least in some patients, the only expression of the chromosomal disorder.

Most pathogenic CNVs detected by array-CGH are rare or unique, making it difficult to collect a sufficient number of patients to identify characteristic features of epilepsy for each chromosomal syndrome. However, at the research level on the causes of epilepsy, the association between cryptic deletions/duplications and epilepsy is improving our ability to clone new critical genes, translating in turn in improved diagnosis. For example, heterozygous missense mutations in *STXBP1* in patients with infantile epileptic encephalopathy with suppression bursts (Ohtahara syndrome) were found after a *de novo* 2.0-Mb microdeletion at 9q33.3–q34.11 in an affected girl prompted analysis of candidate genes mapping to the deleted region in patients with similar phenotypes (90).

Array CGH has greatly improved the diagnostic yield of chromosomal imbalances, allowing the identification of new syndromes caused by imbalances as small as a few dozen kilobases (149). However, little information is available on genome-wide cytogenetic array screening in patients specifically selected for epilepsy. Engels et al. (150) analysed 60 patients with mental retardation combined with congenital anomalies, 25% of whom also had epilepsy. Novel imbalances were found in six patients (10%), two of whom had epilepsy. Kim et al. (151) reported various CNVs in patients with idiopathic generalized or partial epilepsies and FS. A study investigating the impact of these five microdeletions on the genetic risk for common IGE syndromes, using high-density single nucleotide polymorphism arrays, in a large cohort, found significant associations with microdeletions at 15q11.2 and 16p13.11 (152).

Genetic counselling

Genetic testing can be offered for single-gene or Mendelian epilepsy syndromes, or epilepsy-associated disorders, if the gene has been identified. If not, empirical counselling can be offered, based on the type of epilepsy, mode of inheritance, and penetrance. Although we can now carry out preclinical and prenatal diagnosis in many cases, the severity and prognosis of the epilepsy in specific individuals, particularly in those with idiopathic epilepsies, is difficult to predict. However, in symptomatic monogenic epilepsies, such as the progressive myoclonus epilepsies, phakomatoses, and malformations of cortical development, carrier detection, prenatal diagnosis, and presymptomatic testing may lead to prevention. Unfortunately, no curative treatment has emerged from any genetic finding in epilepsy to date (with the possible exception of the ketogenic diet in *GLUT1* deficiency syndrome), nor have the many pharmacogenomic studies in epilepsy yielded any widely applicable treatment advances. This is a disappointing lack of progress, reflecting as it does on the complex nature of epilepsy and its treatment. Counselling needs to consider these issues.

Future perspectives

The next steps include identifying additional genes both in monogenic epilepsies and epilepsies with complex inheritance, genotype–phenotype correlations, and functional studies of the abnormal proteins. These studies may have practical applications for diagnosis, genetic counselling, and possible treatment. Most of the epilepsy syndromes listed in this chapter are characterized by marked clinical and genetic heterogeneity. This may be explained by pleiotropic expression of a single-gene mutation, modifying genes, or by several genes producing a similar phenotype, at times because they affect the same developmental or metabolic pathway. It is hoped that a constantly updated database will be established for all the known gene mutations and polymorphisms and their clinical correlates, so that genotype–phenotype correlations can be determined. This is the objective of the Human Variome project (153). For example, over 600 mutations in *SCN1A* associated with Dravet syndrome have now been identified and the severity of the related phenotype can be predicted early, with reasonable accuracy for those recurrent mutations in which sufficient numbers of clinical observations are available.

References

1. Greenberg DA, Delgado-Escueta AV, Widelitz H, Sparkes RS, Treiman L, Maldonado HM, *et al.* Juvenile myoclonic epilepsy (JME) may be linked to the BF and HLA loci on human chromosome 6. *Am J Med Genet* 1988; 31:185–92.
2. Steinlein OK, Mulley JC, Propping P, Wallace RH, Phillips HA, Sutherland GR, *et al.* A missense mutation in the neuronal nicotinic acetylcholine receptor alpha 4 subunit is associated with autosomal dominant nocturnal frontal lobe epilepsy. *Nat Genet* 1995; 11:201–3.
3. Heron SE, Scheffer IE, Berkovic SF, Dibbens LM, Mulley JC. Channelopathies in idiopathic epilepsy. *Neurotherapeutics* 2007; 4:295–304.
4. Martin MS, Tang B, Papale LA, Yu FH, Catterall WA, Escayg A . The voltage-gated sodium channel Scn8a is a genetic modifier of severe myoclonic epilepsy of infancy. *Hum Mol Genet* 2007; 16:2892–9.
5. Gourfinkel-An I, Baulac S, Nabbout R, Ruberg M, Baulac M, Brice A, *et al.* Monogenic idiopathic epilepsies. *Lancet Neurol* 2004; 3:209–18.
6. Guerrini R, Dravet CH. Severe epileptic encephalopathies of infancy. In: Engel J, Pedley TA (eds) *Epilepsy*, pp.2285–302. Philadelphia, PA: Lippincott-Raven, 1997.
7. Guerrini R, Striano P, Catarino C, Sisodiya SM. Neuroimaging and neuropathology of Dravet syndrome. *Epilepsia* 2011; 52:30–4.
8. Catarino CB, Liu JY, Liagkouras I, Gibbons VS, Labrum RW, Ellis R, *et al.* Dravet syndrome as epileptic encephalopathy: evidence from long-term course and neuropathology. *Brain* 2011; 134:2982–3010.
9. Suls A, Claeys KG, Goossens D, Harding B, Van Luijk R, Scheers S, *et al.* Microdeletions involving the SCN1A gene may be common in SCN1A-mutation-negative SMEI patients. *Hum Mutat* 2006; 27:914–20.
10. Marini C, Scheffer IE, Nabbout R, Mei D, Cox K, Dibbens LM, *et al.* SCN1A duplications and deletions detected in Dravet syndrome: implications for molecular diagnosis. *Epilepsia* 2009; 50:1670–8.
11. Macdonald RL, Kang JQ. Molecular pathology of genetic epilepsies associated with GABAA receptor subunit mutations. *Epilepsy Curr* 2009; 9:18–23.
12. Depienne C, Arzimanoglou A, Trouillard O, Fedirko E, Baulac S, Saint-Martin C, *et al.* Parental mosaicism can cause recurrent transmission of SCN1A mutations associated with severe myoclonic epilepsy of infancy. *Hum Mutat* 2006; 27:389.
13. Marini C, Mei D, Helen CJ, Guerrini R. Mosaic SCN1A mutation in familial severe myoclonic epilepsy of infancy. *Epilepsia* 2006; 47:1737–40.
14. Guerrini R, Oguni H. Borderline Dravet syndrome: a useful diagnostic category? *Epilepsia* 2011; 52:10–12.
15. Fujiwara T, Sugawara T, Mazaki-Miyazaki E, Takahashi Y, Fukushima K, Watanabe M, *et al.* Mutations of sodium channel alpha subunit type 1 (SCN1A) in intractable childhood epilepsies with frequent generalized tonic-clonic seizures. *Brain* 2006; 126:531–46.
16. Wallace RH, Scheffer IE, Barnett S, Richards M, Dibbens L, Desai RR, *et al.* Neuronal sodium-channel alpha1-subunit mutations in generalized epilepsy with febrile seizures plus. *Am J Hum Genet* 2001; 68:859–65.
17. Harkin LA, McMahon JM, Iona X, Dibbens L, Pelekanos JT, Zuberi SM, *et al.* The spectrum of SCN1A-related infantile epileptic encephalopathies. *Brain* 2007; 130:843–52.
18. Scheffer IE, Berkovic SF. Generalized epilepsy with febrile seizures plus: a genetic disorder with heterogeneous clinical phenotypes. *Brain* 1997; 120:479–90.
19. Wallace RH, Wang DW, Singh R, Scheffer IE, George AL Jr, Phillips HA, *et al.* Febrile seizures and generalized epilepsy associated with a mutation in the Na+channel beta1 subunit gene SCN1B. *Nat Genet* 1998; 19:366–70.
20. Escayg A, MacDonald BT, Meisler MH, Baulac S, Huberfeld G, An-Gourfinkel I, *et al.* Mutations of SCN1A, encoding a neuronal sodium channel, in two families with GEFS+2. *Nat Genet* 2000; 24:343–5.
21. Marini C, Mei D, Temudo T, Ferrari AR, Buti D, Dravet C, *et al.* Idiopathic epilepsies with seizures precipitated by fever and SCN1A abnormalities. *Epilepsia* 2007; 48:1678–85.
22. Wallace RH, Marini C, Petrou S, Harkin LA, Bowser DN, Panchal RG, *et al.* Mutant GABA(A) receptor gamma2-subunit in childhood absence epilepsy and febrile seizures. *Nat Genet* 2001; 28:49–52.
23. Baulac S, Huberfeld G, Gourfinkel-An I, Mitropoulou G, Beranger A, Prud'homme JF, *et al.* First genetic evidence of GABA(A) receptor dysfunction in epilepsy: a mutation in the gamma2-subunit gene. *Nat Genet* 2001; 28:46–8.
24. Mantegazza M, Rusconi R, Scalmani P, Avanzini G, Franceschetti S. Epileptogenic ion channel mutations: from bedside to bench and, hopefully, back again. *Epilepsy Res* 2010; 92:1–29.
25. Lerche H, Weber YG, Jurkat-Rott K, Lehmann-Horn F. Ion channel defects in idiopathic epilepsies. *Curr Pharm* 2005; 11:2737–52.

26. Yu FH, Mantegazza M, Westenbroek RE, Robbins CA, Kalume F, Burton KA, *et al.* Reduced sodium current in GABAergic interneurons in a mouse model of severe myoclonic epilepsy in infancy. *Nat Neurosci* 2006; 9:1142–9.
27. Ogiwara I, Miyamoto H, Morita N, Atapour N, Mazaki E, Inoue I, *et al.* Na(v)1.1 localizes to axons of parvalbumin-positive inhibitory interneurons: a circuit basis for epileptic seizures in mice carrying an Scn1a gene mutation. *J Neurosci* 2007; 27:5903–14.
28. Plouin P, Anderson VE. Benign familial and non-familial neonatal seizures. In: Roger J, Bureau M, Dravet C, Genton P, Tassinari CA, Wolf P (eds) *Epileptic syndromes in infancy*, childhood and adolescence, pp. 89–113. Mountrouge: John Libbey Eurotext Ltd, 2005.
29. Steinlein OK, Conrad C, Weidner B. Benign familial neonatal convulsions: always benign? *Epilepsy Res* 2007; 73:245–9.
30. Biervert C, Schroeder BC, Kubisch C, Berkovic SF, Propping P, Jentsch TJ, *et al.* A potassium channel mutation in neonatal human epilepsy. *Science* 1998; 279:403–6.
31. Singh NA, Charlier C, Stauffer D, DuPont BR, Leach RJ, Melis R, *et al.* A novel potassium channel gene, KCNQ2, is mutated in an inherited epilepsy of newborns. *Nat Genet* 1998; 18:25–9.
32. Heron SE, Cox K, Grinton BE, Zuberi SM, Kivity S, Afawi Z, *et al.* Deletions or duplications in KCNQ2 can cause benign familial neonatal seizures. *J Med Genet* 2007; 44:791–6.
33. Singh NA, Westenskow P, Charlier C, Pappas C, Leslie J, Dillon J, *et al.* KCNQ2 and KCNQ3 potassium channel genes in benign familial neonatal convulsions:expansion of the functional and mutation spectrum. *Brain* 2003; 126:2726–37.
34. Delmas P, Brown DA. Pathways modulating neural KCNQ/M (Kv7) potassium channels. *Nat Rev Neurosci* 2005; 6:850–62.
35. Schroeder BC, Kubisch C, Stein V, Jentsch TJ. Moderate loss of function of cyclic-AMP-modulated KCNQ2/KCNQ3 K^+ channels causes epilepsy. *Nature* 1998; 396:687–90.
36. Weber YG, Lerche H. Genetic mechanisms in idiopathic epilepsies. *Dev Med Child Neurol* 2008; 50:648–54.
37. Heron SE, Crossland KM, Andermann E, Phillips HA, Hall AJ, Bleasel A, *et al.* Sodium-channel defects in benign familial neonatal-infantile seizures. *Lancet* 2002; 360:851–2.
38. Berkovic SF, Heron SE, Giordano L, Marini C, Guerrini R, Kaplan RE, *et al.* Benign familial neonatal infantile seizures: characterization of a new sodium channelopathy. *Ann Neurol* 2004; 55:550–7.
39. Herlenius E, Heron SE, Grinton BE, Keay D, Scheffer IE, Mulley JC, *et al.* SCN2A mutations and benign familial neonatal-infantile seizures: the phenotypicspectrum. *Epilepsia* 2007; 48:1138–42.
40. Vigevano F. Benign familial infantile seizures. *Brain Dev* 2005; 27:172–7.
41. Szepetowski P, Rochette J, Berquin P, Piussan C, Lathrop GM, Monaco AP. Familial infantile convulsions and paroxysmal choreoathetosis: a new neurological syndrome linked to the pericentromeric region of human chromosome 16. *Am J Hum Genet* 1997; 61:889–98.
42. Guipponi M, Rivier F, Vigevano F, Gastaldi M, Echenne B, Motte J, *et al.* Linkage mapping of benign familial infantile convulsions (BFIC) to chromosome 19q. *Hum Mol Genet* 1997; 6:473–7.
43. Vanmolko KR, Kors EE, Hottenga JJ, Terwindt GM, Haan J, Hoefnagels WA, *et al.* Novel mutations in the Na^+, K^+-ATPase pump gene ATP1A2 associated with familial hemiplegic migraine and benign familial infantile convulsions. *Ann Neurol* 2003; 54:360–6.
44. Zhou X, Ma A, Liu X, Huang C, Zhang Y, Shi R, *et al.* Infantile seizures and other epileptic phenotypes in a Chinese family with a missense mutation of KCNQ2. *Eur J Pediatr* 2006; 165:691–5.
45. Striano P, Bordo L, Lispi ML, Specchio N, Minetti C, Vigevano F, *et al.* A novel SCN2A mutation in family with benign familial infantile seizures. *Epilepsia* 2006; 47:218–20.
46. Scheffer IE, Bhatia KP, Lopes-Cendes I, Fish DR, Marsden CD, Andermann E, *et al.* Autosomal dominant nocturnal frontal lobe epilepsy: a distinctive clinical disorder. *Brain* 1995; 118:61–73.
47. Picard F, Baulac S, Kahane P, Hirsch E, Sebastianelli R, Thomas P, *et al.* Dominant partial epilepsies. A clinical, electrophysiological and genetic study of 19 European families. *Brain* 2000; 123:1247–62.
48. Ryvlin P, Minotti L, Demarquay G, Hirsch E, Arzimanoglou A, Hoffman D, *et al.* Nocturnal hypermotor seizures, suggesting frontal lobe epilepsy, can originate in the insula. *Epilepsia* 2006; 47:755–65.
49. Steinlein OK. Genetic mechanisms that underlie epilepsy. *Nat Rev Neurosci* 2004; 5:443–8.
50. Aridon P, Marini C, Di Resta C, Brilli E, De Fusco M, Politi F, *et al.* Increased sensitivity of the neuronal nicotinic receptor alpha 2 subunit causes familial epilepsy with nocturnal wandering and ictal fear. *Am J Hum Genet* 2006; 79:342–50.
51. Chen Y, Wu L, Fang Y, He Z, Peng B, Shen Y, *et al.* A novel mutation of the nicotinic acetylcholine receptor gene CHRNA4 in sporadic nocturnal frontal lobe epilepsy. *Epilepsy Res* 2009; 83:152–6.
52. Liu H, Lu C, Li Z, Zhou S, Zhou S, Li X, Ji L, *et al.* The identification of a novel mutation of nicotinic acetylcholine receptor gene CHRNB2 in a Chinese patient: Its possible implication in non-familial nocturnal frontal lobe epilepsy. *Epilepsy Res* 2011; 95:94–9.
53. Ottman R, Risch N, Hauser WA, Pedley TA, Lee JH, Barker-Cummings C, *et al.* Localization of a gene for partial epilepsy to chromosome 10q. *Nat Genet* 1995; 10:56–60.
54. Michelucci R, Poza JJ, Sofia V, de Feo MR, Binelli S, Bisulli F, *et al.* Autosomal dominant lateral temporal epilepsy: clinical spectrum, new epitempin mutations, and genetic heterogeneity in seven European families. *Epilepsia* 2003; 44:1289–97.
55. Kalachikov S, Evgrafov O, Ross B, Winawer M, Barker-Cummings C, Martinelli Boneschi F, *et al.* Mutations in LGI1 cause autosomal-dominant partial epilepsy with auditory features. *Nat Genet* 2002; 30:335–41.
56. Ottman R, Winawer MR, Kalachikov S, Barker-Cummings C, Gilliam TC, Pedley TA, *et al.* LGI1 mutations in autosomal dominant partial epilepsy with auditory features. *Neurology* 2004; 62:1120–6.
57. Chernova OB, Somerville RP, Cowell JK. A novel gene, LGI1, from 10q24 is rearranged and down-regulated in malignant brain tumors. *Oncogene* 1998; 17:2873–81.
58. Scheel H, Tomiuk S, Hofmann K. A common protein interaction domain links two recently identified epilepsy genes. *Hum Mol Genet* 2002; 11:1757–62.
59. Skradski SL, Clark AM, Jiang H, White HS, Fu YH, Ptácek LJ. A novel gene causing a mendelian audiogenic mouse epilepsy. *Neuron* 2001; 31:537–44.
60. Sadleir LG, Scheffer IE. Febrile seizures. *Br Med J* 2007; 334:307–11.
61. Hauser WA, Annegers JF, Anderson VE, Kurland LT. The risk of seizure disorders among relatives of children with febrile convulsions. *Neurology* 1985; 35:1268–73.
62. Maher J, McLachlan RS. Febrile convulsions. Is seizure duration the most important predictor of temporal lobe epilepsy? *Brain* 1995; 118:1521–8.
63. Johnson WG, Kugler SL, Stenroos ES, Meulener MC, Rangwalla I, Johnson TW, *et al.* Pedigree analysis in families with febrile seizures. *Am J Med Genet* 1996; 61:345–52.
64. Baulac S, Gourfinkel-An I, Nabbout R, Huberfeld G, Serratosa J, Leguern E, *et al.* Fever, genes, and epilepsy. *Lancet Neurol* 2004; 3:421–30.
65. Dibbens LM, Tarpey PS, Hynes K, Bayly MA, Scheffer IE, Smith R, *et al.* X-linked protocadherin 19 mutations cause female-limited epilepsy and cognitive impairment. *Nat Genet* 2008; 40:776–81.
66. Marini C, Mei D, Parmeggiani L, Norci V, Calado E, Ferrari A, *et al.* Protocadherin 19 mutations in girls with infantile onset epilepsy. *Neurology* 2010; 75:646–53.

67. Deprez L, Jansen A, De Jonghe P. Genetics of epilepsy syndromes starting in the first year of life. *Neurology* 2009; 72:273–81.
68. Depienne C, Bouteiller D, Keren B, Cheuret E, Poirier K, Trouillard O, *et al.* Sporadic infantile epileptic encephalopathy caused by mutations in PCDH19 resembles Dravet syndrome but mainly affects females. *PLoS Genet* 2009; 5:e1000381.
69. Ohira R, Zhang YH, Guo, Dipple K, Shih SL, Doerr J, *et al.* Human ARX gene: Genomic characterization and expression. *Mol Genet Metab* 2002; 77:179–88.
70. Gécz J, Cloosterman D, Partington M. ARX: A gene for all seasons. *Curr Opin Genet Dev* 2006; 16:308–16.
71. Guerrini R, Moro F, Kato M, Barkovich AJ, Shiihara T, McShane MA, *et al.* Expansion of the first PolyA tract of ARX causes infantile spasms and status dystonicus. *Neurology* 2007; 69:427–33.
72. Marsh E, Fulp C, Gomez E, Nasrallah I, Minarcik J, Sudi J, *et al.* Targeted loss of Arx results in a developmental epilepsy mouse model and recapitulates the human phenotype in heterozygous females. *Brain* 2009; 132:1563–76.
73. Kato M, Das S, Petras K, Kitamura K, Morohashi K, Abuelo DN, *et al.* Mutations of ARX are associated with striking pleiotropy and consistent genotype–phenotype correlation. *Hum Mutat* 2004; 23:147–59.
74. Stromme P, Mangelsdorf ME, Scheffer IE, Gecz J. Infantile spasms, dystonia, and other X-linked phenotypes caused by mutations in Aristaless related homeobox gene, ARX. *Brain Dev* 2002; 24:266–8.
75. Wallerstein R, Sugalski R, CohnL, Jawetz R, Friez M. Expansion of the ARX spectrum. *Clin Neurol Neurosurg* 2008; 110:631–4.
76. Shinozaki Y, Osawa M, Sakuma H, Komaki H, Nakagawa E, Sugai K, *et al.* Expansion of the first polyalanine tract of the ARX gene in a boy presenting with generalized dystonia in the absence of infantile spasms. *Brain Dev* 2008; 31:469–72.
77. Kato M, Saitoh S, Kamei A, Shiraishi H, Ueda Y, Akasaka M, *et al.* A longer polyalanine expansion mutation in the ARX gene causes early infantile epileptic encephalopathy with suppression-burst pattern (Ohtahara syndrome). *Am J Hum Genet* 2007; 81:361–6.
78. Mari F, Azimonti S, Bertani I, Bolognese F, Colombo E, Caselli R, *et al.* CDKL5 belongs to the same molecular pathway of MeCP2 and it is responsible for the early-onset seizure variant of Rett syndrome. *Hum Mol Genet* 2005; 14:1935–46.
79. Kalscheuer VM, Tao J, Donnelly A, Hollway G, Schwinger E, Kübart S, *et al.* Disruption of the serine/threonine kinase 9 gene causes severe X-linked infantilespasms and mental retardation. *Am J Hum Genet* 2003; 72:1401–11.
80. Buoni S, Zannolli R, Colamaria V, Macucci F, di Bartolo RM, Corbini L, *et al.* Myoclonic encephalopathy in the CDKL5 gene mutation. *Clin Neurophysiol* 2006; 117:223–7.
81. Archer HL, Evans J, Edwards S, Spalletta A, Bottitta M, Calabrese G, *et al.* CDKL5 mutations cause infantile spasms, early onset seizures, and severe mental retardation in female patients. *J Med Genet* 2006; 43:729–34.
82. Elia M, Falco M, Ferri R, *et al.* CDKL5 mutations in boys with severe encephalo pathy early-onset intractable epilepsy. *Neurology* 2008; 71:997–9.
83. Weaving LS, Christodoulou J, Williamson SL, Friend KL, McKenzie OL, Archer H, *et al.* Mutations of CDKL5 cause a severe neurodevelopmental disorder with infantile spasms and mental retardation. *Am J Hum Genet* 2004; 75:1079–93.
84. Melani F, Mei D, Pisano T, Savasta S, Franzoni E, Ferrari AR, *et al.* CDKL5 gene-related epileptic encephalopathy: electroclinical findings in the first year of life. *Dev Med Child Neurol* 2011; 53:54–60.
85. Mei D, Marini C, Novara F, Bernardina BD, Granata T, Fontana E, *et al.* Xp22.3 genomic deletions involving the CDKL5 gene in girls with early onset epileptic encephalopathy. *Epilepsia* 2010; 51:647–54.
86. Djukic A, Lado FA, Shinnar S, Moshe SL. Are early myoclonic encephalopathy (EME) and the Ohtahara syndrome (EIEE) independent of each other? *Epilepsy Res* 2006; 70:S68–76.
87. Ohtahara S, Yamatogi Y. Ohtahara syndrome: with special reference to its developmental aspects for differentiating from early myoclonic encephalopathy. *Epilepsy Res* 2006; 70:S58–67.
88. Mignot C, Moutard ML, Trouillard O, Gourfinkel-An I, Jacquette A, Arveiler B, *et al.* STXBP1-related encephalopathy presenting as infantile spasms and generalized tremor in three patients. *Epilepsia* 2011; 52:1820–7.
89. Milh M, Villeneuve N, Chouchane M, Kaminska A, Laroche C, Barthez MA, *et al.* Epileptic and nonepileptic features in patients with early onset epileptic encephalopathy and STXBP1 mutations. *Epilepsia* 2011; 52:1828–34.
90. Saitsu H, Kato M, Mizuguchi T, Hamada K, Osaka H, Tohyama J, *et al.* De novo mutations in the gene encoding STXBP1 (MUNC18–1) cause early infantile epileptic encephalopathy. *Nat Genet* 2008; 40:782–8.
91. Berkovic SF, Andermann F, Carpenter S, Wolfe LS. Progressive myoclonus epilepsies: specific causes and diagnosis. *N Engl J Med* 1986; 315:296–305.
92. Genton P, Malafosse A, Moulard B, Rogel-Ortiz FJ, Dravet C, Bureau M, *et al.* Progressive myoclonus epilepsies. Roger J, Bureau M, Dravet C, Genton P, Tassinari CA, Wolf P (eds) *Epileptic syndromes in infancy*, childhood and adolescence (3rd edn), pp. 89–113. London: John Libbey, 2002.
93. Delgado-Escueta AV, Ganesh S, Yamakawa K. Advances in the genetics of progressive myoclonus epilepsy. *Am J Med Genet* 2001; 106:129–38.
94. Annegers JF, Hauser WA, Anderson VE, Kurland LT. The risk of seizure disorders among relatives of patients with childhood onset epilepsy. *Neurology* 1982; 32:174–79.
95. Risch N. Linkage strategies for genetically complex traits. (1) Multilocus models. *Am J Hum Genet* 1990; 46:222–8.
96. Berkovic SF, Howell RA, Hay DA, Hopper JL. Epilepsies in twins: genetics of the major epilepsy syndromes. *Ann Neurol* 1998; 43:435–45.
97. Berkovic SF, Scheffer IE. Genetics of the epilepsies. *Epilepsia* 2001; 42:16–23.
98. Klassen T, Davis C, Goldman A, Burgess D, Chen T, Wheeler D, *et al.* Exome sequencing of ion channel genes reveals complex profiles confounding personal risk assessment in epilepsy. *Cell* 2011; 145:1036–48.
99. Sander T, Schulz H, Saar K, Gennaro E, Riggio MC, Bianchi A, *et al.* Genome search for susceptibility loci of common generalized epilepsies. *Hum Mol Genet* 2000; 9:1465–72.
100. Durner M, Keddache MA, Tomasini L, Shinnar S, Resor SR, Cohen J, *et al.* Genome scan of idiopathic generalized epilepsy: evidence for major susceptibility gene and modifying genes influencing the seizure type. *Ann Neurol* 2001; 49:328–35.
101. Cossette P, Liu L, Brisebois K, Dong H, Lortie A, Vanasse M, *et al.* Mutation of GABRA1 in an autosomal dominant form of juvenile myoclonic epilepsy. *Nat Genet* 2002; 31:184–9.
102. D'Agostino D, Bertelli M, Gallo S, Cecchin S, Albiero E, Garofalo PG, *et al.* Mutations and polymorphisms of the CLCN2 gene in idiopathic epilepsy. *Neurology* 2004; 63:1500–2.
103. Chen Y, Lu J, Pan H, Wu H, Xu K, Liu X, *et al.* Association between genetic variation of CACNA1H and childhood absence epilepsy. *Ann Neurol* 2003; 54:239–43.
104. Heron SE, Phillips HA, Mulley JC, Mazarib A, Neufeld MY, Berkovic SF, *et al.* Genetic variation of CACNA1H in idiopathic generalized epilepsy. *Ann Neurol* 2004; 55:595–6.
105. Dibbens LM, Feng HJ, Richards MC, Harkin LA, Hodgson BL, Scott D, *et al.* GABRD encoding a protein for extra- or peri-synaptic GABAA receptors is a susceptibility locus for generalized epilepsies. *Hum Mol Genet* 2004; 13:1315–19.
106. Greenberg DA, Cayanis E, Strug L, Marathe S, Durner M, Pal DK, *et al.* Malic enzyme 2 may underlie susceptibility to adolescent-onset idiopathic generalized epilepsy. *Am J Hum Genet* 2003; 76:139–46.

107. Pal DK, Evgrafov OV, Tabares P,Zhang F, Durner M, Greenberg DA. BRD2 (RING3) is a probable major susceptibility gene for common juvenile myoclonic epilepsy. *Am J Hum Genet* 2003; 73:261–70.
108. Dibbens LM, Ekberg J, Taylor I, Hodgson BL, Conroy SJ, Lensink IL, *et al.* NEDD4-2 as a potential candidate susceptibility gene for epileptic photosensitivity. *Genes Brain Behav* 2007; 6:750–5.
109. Guerrini R, Carrozzo R. Epilepsy and genetic malformations of the cerebral cortex. *Am J Med Genet* 2001; 106:160–73.
110. Barkovich AJ, Kuzniecky RI, Jackson GD, Guerrini R, Dobyns WB. A developmental and genetic classification for malformations of cortical development. *Neurology* 2005; 65:1873–87.
111. Friede RL. *Developmental neuropathology.* New York: Springer-Verlag, 1989.
112. Guerrini R, Filippi T. Neuronal migration disorders, genetics, and epileptogenesis. *J Child Neurol* 2005; 20:287–99.
113. Reiner O, Carrozzo R, Shen Y, Wehnert M, Faustinella F, Dobyns WB, *et al.* Isolation of a Miller–Dieker lissencephaly gene containing G protein beta-subunit-like repeats. *Nature* 1993; 364:717–21.
114. des Portes V, Francis Pinard JM, Desguerre I, Moutard ML, Snoeck I, *et al.* doublecortin is the major gene causing X-linked subcortical laminar heterotopia (SCLH). *Hum Mol Genet* 1998; 7:1063–70.
115. Gleeson JG, Allen KM, Fox JW, Lamperti ED, Berkovic S, Scheffer I, *et al.* Doublecortin, a brain-specific gene mutated in human X-linked lissencephaly and double cortex syndrome, encodes a putative signaling protein. *Cell* 1998; 92:63–72.
116. Mei D, Lewis R, Parrini, Lazarou LP, Marini C, Pilz DT, *et al.* High frequency of genomic deletions and duplication in the LIS1 gene in lissencephaly: implications for molecular diagnosis. *J Med Genet* 2008; 45:355–61.
117. Matsumoto N, Leventer RJ, Kuc JA, Mewborn SK, Dudlicek LL, Ramocki MB, *et al.* Mutation analysis of the DCX gene and genotype/phenotype correlation in subcortical band heterotopia. *Eur J Hum Genet* 2001; 9:5–12.
118. Cardoso C, Leventer RJ, Dowling JJ, Ward HL, Chung J, Petras KS, *et al.* Clinical and molecular basis of classical lissencephaly: mutations in the LIS1 gene (PAFAH1B1). *Hum Mutat* 2002; 19:4–15.
119. Sicca F, Kelemen A, Genton, Das S, Mei D, Moro F, *et al.* Mosaic mutations of the LIS1 gene cause subcortical band heterotopia. *Neurology* 2003; 61:1042–6.
120. Mei, D., Parrini, E., Pasqualetti, M, Tortorella G, Franzoni E, Giussani U, *et al.* Multiplex ligation-dependent probe amplification detects DCX gene deletions in band heterotopia. *Neurology* 2007; 68:446–50.
121. Gleeson JG, Minnerath S, Kuzniecky RI, Dobyns WB, Young ID, Ross ME, *et al.* Somatic and germline mosaic mutations in the doublecortin gene are associated with variable phenotypes. *Am J Hum Genet* 2000; 67:574–81.
122. Poirier K, Keays DA, Francis, Saillour Y, Bahi N, Manouvrier S, *et al.* Large spectrum of lissencephaly and pachygyria phenotypes resulting fromde novomissensemutations in tubulin alpha 1A (TUBA1A). *Hum Mutat* 2007; 28:1055–64.
123. Hong SE, Shugart YY, Huang DT, Shahwan SA, Grant PE, Hourihane JO, *et al.* Autosomal recessive lissencephaly with cerebellar hypoplasia is associated with human RELN mutations. *Nat Genet* 2000; 26:93–6.
124. Parrini E, Ramazzotti A, Dobyns WB, Guerrini R. Periventricular heterotopia: phenotypic heterogeneity and correlation with Filamin A mutations. *Brain* 2006; 129:1892–906.
125. Sheen VL, Dixon PH, Fox JW, Hong SE, Kinton L, Sisodiya SM, *et al.* Mutations in the X-linked filamin 1 gene cause periventricular nodular heterotopia in males as well as in females. *Hum Mol Genet* 2001; 10:1775–83.
126. Guerrini R, Mei D, Sisodiya S, Sicca F, Harding B, Takahashi Y, *et al.* Germline and mosaic mutations of FLN1 in men with periventricular heterotopia. *Neurology* 2004; 63:51–6.
127. Parrini E, Rivas IL, Toral JF, Pucatti D, Giglio S, Mei D, *et al.* In-frame deletion in FLNA causing familial periventricular heterotopia with skeletal dysplasia in males. *Am J Med Genet A* 2011; 155A:1140–6.
128. Sheen VL, Ganesh VS, Topcu M, Sebire G, Bodell A, Hill RS, *et al.* Mutations in ARFGEF2 implicate vesicle trafficking in neural progenitor proliferation and migration in the human cerebral cortex. *Nat Genet* 2004; 36:69–76.
129. Guerrini R, Parrini E. Neuronal migration disorders. *Neurobiol Dis* 2010; 38:154–66.
130. Guerrini R, Dobyns W, Barkovich A. Abnormal development of the human cerebral cortex: genetics, functional consequences and treatment options. *Trends Neurosci* 2008; 31:154–62.
131. Roll P, Rudolf G, Pereira S, Scheffer IE, Massacrier A, Valenti MP, *et al.* SRPX2 mutations in disorders of language cortex and cognition. *Hum Mol Genet* 2006; 15:1195–207.
132. Robin NH, Taylor CJ, McDonald-McGinn DM, Zackai EH, Bingham P, Collins KJ, *et al.* Polymicrogyria and deletion 22q11.2 syndrome: window to the etiology of a common cortical malformation. *Am J Med Genet A* 2006; 140:2416–25.
133. Piao X, Hill RS, Bodell A, Chang BS, Basel-Vanagaite L, Straussberg R, *et al.* G protein-coupled receptor-dependent development of human frontal cortex. *Science* 2004; 303:2033–6.
134. Jaglin XH, Poirier K, Saillour Y, Buhler E, Tian G, Bahi-Buisson N, *et al.* Mutations in the beta-tubulin gene TUBB2B result in asymmetrical polymicrogyria. *Nat Genet* 2009; 41:746–52.
135. Dobyns WB, Mirzaa G, Christian SL, Petras K, Roseberry J, Clark GD, *et al.* Consistent chromosome abnormalities identify novel polymicrogyria loci in 1p36.3, 2p16.1-p23.1, 4q21.21-q22.1, 6q26-q27, and 21q2. *Am J Med Genet A* 2008; 146:1637–54.
136. Kolodny EH, Sathe S. Lysosomal disorders and Menkes syndrome. In: Shorvon SD, Andermann F, Guerrini R (eds) *The Causes of Epilepsy: Common and Uncommon Causes in Adults and Children*, pp. 206–11. New York: Cambridge University Press, 2011.
137. Donati MA, Gasperini S, Guerrini R. Organic acid, amino acids and peroxisomal disorders. In: Shorvon SD, Andermann F, Guerrini R (eds) *The Causes of Epilepsy: Common and Uncommon Causes in Adults and Children*, pp. 216–30. New York: Cambridge University Press, 2011.
138. Plecko B, Paul K, Paschke E, Stoeckler-Ipsiroglu S, Struys E, Jakobs C, *et al.* Biochemical and molecular characterization of 18 patients with pyridoxine-dependent epilepsy and mutations of the antiquitin (ALDH7A1) gene. *Hum Mutat* 2007; 28:19–26.
139. Sadilkova K, Gospe SM Jr, Hahn SH. Simultaneous determination of alpha-aminoadipic semialdehyde, piperideine-6-carboxylate and pipecolic acid by LC-MS/MS for pyridoxine-dependent seizures and folinic acid-responsive seizures. *J Neurosci Methods* 2009; 184:136–41.
140. Seidner G, Alvarez MG, Yeh JI, O'Driscoll KR, Klepper J, Stump TS, *et al.* GLUT-1 deficiency syndrome caused by haploinsufficiency of the blood–brain barrier hexose carrier. *Nat Genet* 1998; 18:188–91.
141. De Vivo DC, Trifiletti RR, Jacobson RI, Ronen GM, Behmand RA, Harik SI. Defective glucose transport across the blood–brain barrier as a cause of persistent hypoglycorrhachia, seizures, and developmental delay. *N Engl J Med* 1991; 325:703–9.
142. Leary LD, Wang D, Nordli DR Jr, Engelstad K, De Vivo DC. Seizure characterization and electroencephalographic features in Glut-1 deficiency syndrome. *Epilepsia* 2003; 44:701–7.
143. Suls A, Dedeken P, Goffin K, Van Esch H, Dupont P, Cassiman D, *et al.* Paroxysmal exercise-induced dyskinesia and epilepsy is due to mutations in SLC2A1, encoding the glucose transporter GLUT1. *Brain* 2008; 131:1831–44.
144. Roulet-Perez E, Ballhausen D, Bonafé L, Cronel-Ohayon S, Maeder-Ingvar M. Glut-1 deficiency syndrome masquerading as idiopathic generalize epilepsy. *Epilepsia* 2008; 49:1955–8.
145. Suls A, Mullen SA, Weber YG, Verhaert K, Ceulemans B, Guerrini R, *et al.* Early-onset absence epilepsy caused by mutations in the glucose transporter GLUT1. *Ann Neurol* 2009; 66:415–19.
146. Mullen SA, Marini C, Suls A, Mei D, Della Giustina E, Buti D, *et al.* Glucose transporter 1 deficiency as a treatable cause of myoclonic astatic epilepsy. *Arch Neurol* 2011; 68:1152–5.

147. Singh R, McKinlay Gardner RJ, Crossland KM, Scheffer IE, Berkovic SF. Chromosomal abnormalities and epilepsy: a review for clinicians and gene hunters. *Epilepsia* 2002; 43:127–40.
148. Guerrini R, Battaglia A, Carrozzo R, Gobbi G, Parrini E, Pramparo T, *et al.* Chromosomal abnormalities. In: Engel J Jr., Pedley TA (eds) *Epilepsy: A Comprehensive Textbook* (2nd edn), pp. 2589–601. Philadelphia, PA: Lippincott Williams and Wilkins, 2008.
149. Ledbetter DH. Cytogenetic technology: genotype and phenotype. *N Engl J Med* 2008; 359:1728–30.
150. Engels H, Brockschmidt A, Hoischen A, Landwehr C, Bosse K, Walldorf C, *et al.* DNA microarray analysis identifies candidate regions and genes in unexplained mental retardation. *Neurology* 2007; 68:721–2.
151. Kim HS, Yim SV, Jung KH, Zheng LT, Kim YH, Lee KH, *et al.* Altered DNA copy number in patients with different seizure disorder type: by array-CGH. *Brain Devel* 2007; 29:639–43.
152. de Kovel CG, Trucks H, Helbig I, Mefford HC, Baker C, Leu C, *et al.* Recurrent microdeletions at 15q11.2 and 16p13.11 predispose to idiopathic generalized epilepsies. *Brain* 2010; 133:23–32.
153. Cotton RG, Auerbach AD, Axton M, Barash CI, Berkovic SF, Brookes AJ, *et al.* GENETICS: the Human Variome Project. *Science* 2008; 322:861–2.

CHAPTER 3

Neurochemistry of Epilepsy

B. Keith Day, Lawrence Eisenman, and
R. Edward Hogan

Introduction

Epileptic seizures emerge from complex biochemical processes in the human brain. Physicians and scientists engaged in the study of this disease process have gained significant knowledge about the neurochemical basis for epilepsy. The earliest studies at the turn of the 20th century focused attention and subsequent theories on changes in chemicals detected in the urine, serum, and cerebrospinal fluid, many of which we today recognize as non-specific associated biochemical changes (1). However, with advances in studies of the human brain on cellular and molecular levels and the evolution of the pharmacology of epilepsy, the early idea that excitatory and inhibitory influences in the brain existed in balance that could be tipped toward excitation or away from inhibition to produce seizures was supported in numerous types of epilepsies and seizure-related conditions. With this simple yet elegant view in mind, studies advancing our knowledge of the neurochemistry of epilepsy continue to aid our understanding of the pathophysiology of epileptic disorders as well as our approach to their diagnosis and treatment.

The focus of this chapter will be on synaptic neurotransmission and its role in epilepsy. The main excitatory and inhibitory neurochemicals in the human brain are glutamate and gamma-aminobutyric acid (GABA), respectively, which have gained wide acceptance as the major neurochemical influences in epilepsy. However, other neurotransmitters such as aspartate and glycine remain chemicals of interest as excitatory and inhibitory amino acids. Also, the roles of acetylcholine, serotonin, and the catecholamines (dopamine and noradrenaline) in epilepsy have been studied. We will review the basic chemistry of neurotransmission for the major neurotransmitters glutamate and GABA to provide a substrate for further discussion. Next, we briefly consider the contribution of selective neuronal circuits to seizure generation. Animal models of seizures and epilepsy have been a critical source of knowledge of the neurochemistry of epilepsy, and we briefly review relevant data from several such models with a focus on microdialysis experiments. We turn back to human studies, again focusing on microdialysis experiments. We also review magnetic resonance spectroscopy and the emerging technology of microelectrode arrays as newer methods that are complementary to microdialysis. We then address potential contributions of the other neurotransmitter systems noted earlier. Having reviewed the neurochemistry of the neurotransmitter systems, we next turn to the neurochemistry of antiepileptic drugs (AEDs). Finally, we conclude with a review of a clinical trial of a drug specifically designed to modulate the GABA system that highlights some of the complexities of applying our knowledge of neurochemistry to patient care.

GABA

GABA is the major inhibitory molecule in the mammalian brain. GABA was recognized as a neurochemical in 1950 and as the amino acid in the inhibitory nerves of crustaceans by 1963 (2). It was later accepted as satisfying criteria as a neurotransmitter in the mammalian brain in 1973 (3). The idea that reduction of GABAergic inhibition results in epilepsy while its potentiation is antiepileptic became known as the GABA hypothesis of epilepsy and continues to withstand experimental scrutiny (4, 5). As discussed in more detail later, its role in epilepsy became viewed as so important that designer drugs (including vigabatrin, tiagabine, and gabapentin) were created in hopes of mimicking the effects of GABA.

GABA is biochemically synthesized in presynaptic terminals with the removal of a carboxyl group from the alpha carbon of L-glutamate by the enzyme glutamic acid decarboxylase (GAD) (6). Depolarization of GABA-producing presynaptic terminals leads to voltage-gated calcium channel activation. Calcium entering the terminals facilitates vesicular docking and release of GABA into the extracellular space at the synaptic cleft where it is able to interact with two recognized receptor types, $GABA_A$ and $GABA_B$. $GABA_A$ receptors are ligand-gated ion channels. When GABA binds $GABA_A$ receptors in the adult brain, a conformational change in the shape of the receptor allows chloride to flow along its concentration gradient into the postsynaptic cell increasing the negative membrane potential and hyperpolarizing the cell. $GABA_B$ receptors are metabotropic receptors that are coupled to G-proteins which activate adenylate cyclase leading to changes in cyclic adenosine monophosphate (cAMP) signalling to alter the conductance of a potassium channel. This, in turn, releases potassium from within the cell leading again to hyperpolarization. Both GABA receptor types make it more difficult for excitatory influences to depolarize the cell body to the point of creating new action potentials. GABA is actively removed from the extracellular space by

GABA transporters (GAT-1 through GAT-4). GAT is present on perisynaptic glia and the presynaptic cell. Coupled to the uptake of one GABA molecule is the influx of two sodium ions and one chloride ion (7, 8). The reversal of GATs may serve as a non-synaptic mechanism for GABA receptor activation as well (9).

Glutamate

Glutamate is the major excitatory neurotransmitter in the mammalian brain. It is also one of the 20 amino acids used to synthesize proteins in humans and is readily available through dietary consumption of L-glutamic acid salts (such as monosodium glutamate) and protein. However, most intracellular glutamate originates from glucose through glycolysis and the Krebs cycle. The Krebs cycle intermediate α-ketoglutarate is converted to glutamate through transamination. Because of its ubiquitous nature in the body and very high concentrations in the central nervous system, its role as a neurotransmitter was doubted for many decades. However, by the mid to late 1970s, investigators were demonstrating biochemical pathways of glutamate synthesis, specialized uptake by glia, and pharmacological antagonism of neuronal excitation by compounds which prevented glutamate binding (10–13).

Depolarization at glutamatergic presynaptic terminals leads to vesicular release of glutamate at the synaptic cleft where it can act on multiple receptor types, both ionotropic and metabotropic. Ligand-gated ion channels activated by glutamate include alpha-amino-3-hydroxyl-5-methyl-4-isoxazole-propionate (AMPA), N-methyl-D-aspartate (NMDA), and kainate receptors. AMPA receptors permit sodium to rapidly enter the postsynaptic cell accompanied by a smaller efflux of intracellular potassium, with the net result being depolarization. Kainate receptors act very similarly to AMPA receptors although the duration of the open ion channel is shorter. Kainate receptors are also found presynaptically on some GABAergic terminals facilitating the release of GABA and, thus, can have an inhibitory effect at times. NMDA receptors require glycine as a co-ligand for activation and also have divalent magnesium ions blockading the channels. The depolarization of the cell membrane by AMPA activation leads to expulsion of magnesium ions, so that movement of sodium and potassium can occur. Although there is also a small calcium conductance through AMPA and kainate receptors, NMDA receptors are the main glutamate ionotropic receptors that allow the passage of calcium into the cell. The overall result is depolarization of the postsynaptic cell (14).

Metabotropic glutamate receptors are G-protein coupled receptors that can be divided into three groups: Group I (mGluR1 and 5), Group II (mGluR2 and 3), and Group III (mGluR4, 6, 7, and 8). Group I receptors activate phospholipase C via G_q proteins leading to phospholipid-related cell signalling through inositol 1,4,5-triphosphate (IP3) and diacyl glycerol (DAG), the latter of which can increase protein kinase C activity. Though they can be found presynaptically, Group I receptors are primarily postsynaptic. Experimentally, Group I receptor activation is both excitatory and inhibitory with capacity to modulate sodium, potassium, and voltage-gated calcium channels, inhibit glutamate release, and enhance NMDA receptor activity. Group II and III receptors coupled to G_0 proteins inhibit adenylate cyclase activity and decrease cAMP concentrations. These receptors are primarily presynaptic and inhibit further release of glutamate. Postsynaptic ligand-bound Group II and III receptors do not directly change the membrane potential but reduce the activities of other excitatory and inhibitory ion channels. Overall, in addition to an important role in positive feedback inhibiting further glutamate release, mGluRs modulate the postsynaptic cell's response to both excitatory and inhibitory influences (14, 15).

Glutamate is actively removed from the extracellular space by glial and postsynaptic neuronal uptake through five subtypes of excitatory amino acid transporters (EAATs) each with a predominant neuroanatomical distribution: EAAT1 (cerebellar glia), EAAT2 (forebrain glia), EAAT3 (cortical neurons), EAAT4 (cerebellar Purkinje neurons), and EAAT5 (retina) (16, 17). Glutamate is not taken back up into the presynaptic terminal, so to replenish vesicles, the glutamate must be shuttled back to the original cell. This is accomplished through the glutamate-glutamine cycle in which glial intracellular glutamate is converted to glutamine by glutamine synthetase. Glutamine is released by the glia and taken up by the presynaptic cell where it is converted back to glutamate by the enzyme glutaminase. Glutamate is actively transported along with protons into vesicles by the vesicular glutamate transporters (VGLUTs). Whereas EAATs will transport aspartate, VGLUTs will not (16). Reversal of glutamate uptake may also contribute to extracellular release with both potential physiological and pathologically effects (18).

GABA, glutamate, and epileptic circuitry

GABA and glutamate neurotransmission are integral components of how seizures emerge, spread, and recur, and modulation of their effects is one of the mechanisms by which many of our current AEDs prevent and abort seizures. In localization-related epilepsy, prolonged depolarization of neurons in the seizure focus leads to firing of multiple sodium-dependent action potentials, a phenomenon referred to as the paroxysmal depolarization shift (PDS). The PDS is also commonly referred to as the intracellular correlate of the epileptiform discharges seen with electroencephalographic recordings. The PDS is typically followed by GABA-mediated hyperpolarization. If GABAergic inhibition fails, the bursting behaviour of the PDS may precipitate continuous high-frequency neuronal firing which can propagate locally, spread through longer circuits to affect larger brain regions, or generalize to the entire brain (19). A typical seizure will end when the affected brain repolarizes, and the postictal state is characterized by hyperpolarization. In generalized epilepsies, where many or all brain areas begin firing abnormally simultaneously, the normal oscillatory rhythms of the thalamocortical loops are dysfunctional. The thalamic nucleus reticularis controls GABAergic thalamic relay neurons via T-type calcium channels. The thalamic relay neurons influence the activity of glutamatergic pyramidal cortical neurons (20, 21). Seizure creation results from an imbalance in excitatory and inhibitory influences within these focal and generalized networks with glutamate and GABA playing dominant roles.

The hippocampus within the temporal lobe is a region of extraordinary importance in epilepsy research and clinical practice. Temporal lobe epilepsy (TLE) represents about 40% of adult onset epilepsies. The hippocampus has been extensively studied microstructurally dating back to the initial studies of Ramón Y Cajal in the late 1800s, and with more advanced techniques, we now also understand much of the neurochemistry complementing the neuroanatomy. The major circuit within the hippocampus is the trisynaptic pathway. Glutamatergic projections from the entorhinal cortex perforate across a fold of the spiral hippocampal structure to synapse on the dendrites of the granule cells of the dentate gyrus creating the perforant pathway. Glutamatergic projections from the granule cells project to the CA3 region. These axons are called mossy fibres due to their microstructural appearance. The third type of synapse of the pathway arises from glutamatergic projections from CA3 to CA1 pyramidal neurons called Schaffer collaterals. There are also recurrent pathways including dentate gyrus and CA1 to entorhinal cortex which are excitatory. Inhibitory control of this feedforward positive loop is provided by GABAergic interneurons found in the hilum (22). Finally, there is also subcortical modulation of the system along the septohippocampal pathway which broadly projects cholinergic connections throughout the hippocampus and well as specific GABAergic projections onto the GABA interneurons which would disinhibit the trisynaptic loop (23). More recently, glutamatergic projections have also been identified in the septohippocampal pathway with a lesser known role (24).

The pathological structural correlate of mesial temporal lobe epilepsy (MTLE) is mesial temporal sclerosis (MTS). MTS is the most common postsurgical histopathological finding from patients with refractory epilepsy who undergo epilepsy surgery (25, 26). It was first grossly recognized in the early 1800s followed by extensive study by Sommer in 1880 (27). MTS became widely recognized as a common correlate of temporal lobe epilepsy in the 1970s (28) and was histopathologically defined in a modern sense in the 1980s (29, 30). MTS has the same pathological findings as the very closely related Ammon's horn sclerosis but extends into other neighbouring regions including the entorhinal cortex and amygdala. Pathologically there is significant segmental neuronal loss accompanied by astrogliosis. Specifically, this damage is at minimum observed in Sommer's sector made up of the CA1 and presubiculum. Grossly, the tissue appears shrunken and hardened which can be appreciated with brain magnetic resonance imaging (MRI) and the corresponding metabolic dysfunction can be observed with positron emission tomography and single-positron emission computed tomography (31, 32). Additional histopathological changes in MTLE include loss of hilar mossy cells, hilar somatostatin-containing GABAergic interneurons, and CA1 pyramidal neurons with associated dispersion of the granule cell layer and aberrant sprouting from the granule cells, spared GABAergic interneurons, and remaining CA1 pyramidal neurons (26). The resulting alterations in glutamate and GABA transmission are widely assumed to contribute to the pathophysiology of MTLE and remain areas of intense study.

A lesser known epileptic region in which glutamate and GABA are important is the area tempestas, a structure in the forebrain's deep prepiriform cortex. It has been identified as a particularly epileptogenic region with connections to the temporal lobes. Initial studies showed that injections directly into this region with chemicals such as kainate, glutamate, aspartate, and NMDA as well as bicuculline produce seizures. At the same time, treatment with the NMDA receptor antagonist 2-amino-phosphonoheptanoic acid (2APH) or the $GABA_A$ agonist muscimol was found to prevent seizures (33, 34). Further studies attempted to elucidate specific neurotransmitter-receptor pathways through which seizures could propagate from the area tempestas into temporal regions. They found that GABA inhibition was sufficiently antiepileptic throughout the system, while NMDA receptor activation is needed to initiate seizures in the area tempestas and non-NMDA receptors (AMPA and KA) are required for the seizures to spread into temporal regions (35).

Lessons from animal models of epilepsy

In 1989, R.S. Fisher (36) published a review which described over 50 different animal models of epilepsy, several of which are still used today. Many of the neuroactive chemicals that were found to produce seizures have both historical relevance and academic importance in epilepsy. For example, penicillin was found to induce seizures during neurosurgical procedures when it was applied directly to the cortex for antibiotic prophylaxis. Later, while conducting intracellular recordings of cat neocortex following focal penicillin administration, the PDS was first described (37, 38). The chemical pentylenetetrazol (PTZ) was so reliable that it was used in British mental hospitals to provoke seizures to treat psychiatric illness until 1939 when it was supplanted by electroconvulsive therapy. For a time, it was also thought of as the prototypical epilepsy-invoking agent because of its ability to induce spike-wave or polyspike discharges on EEG. It even became an industry standard in AED screening; the ability to prevent PTZ-provoked seizures was associated with a higher chance of preventing primary generalized seizures, especially absence seizures. Much later, PTZ was found to work in part through the $GABA_A$ receptor although the exact mechanism by which it provokes seizures remains unclear. In fact, with the exception of the bromides and phenobarbital, every AED used today was first studied using animal models of epilepsy (36). Of special note, use of the maximal electroshock model to screen barbiturate derivatives led to the discovery of phenytoin in the late 1930s (39).

Fortunately, interest in developing animal models of epilepsy over decades has provided further insight into the role of GABA in epilepsy. In addition to PTZ, there are numerous additional GABA antagonists that have been shown to be effective in producing recurrent seizures in animals, including bemegride ($GABA_A$ antagonist), picrotoxin (non-competitive $GABA_A$ antagonist that acts by blocking the ion channel itself and not the receptor binding site), and bicuculline (competitive $GABA_A$ antagonist). In 1974, Meldrum et al. (40) showed that allylglycine, which inhibits glutamate decarboxylase (GAD) and prevents GABA synthesis, caused prolonged status epilepticus in monkeys. Treiman (41) outlined multiple GABAergic mechanisms found in animal models of epilepsy including alterations in GABA levels, receptor binding, and uptake as well as the antiepileptic properties of drugs which enhance GABA neurotransmission.

The animal models also support a significant role for glutamate in epilepsy. Most animal models of complex partial seizures utilize enhanced excitation either through genetic manipulation, kindling, or the administration of excitatory chemicals. Both glutamate and its structural analogue kainate, first discovered in red algae in 1953 (42), were known to be potent excitotoxins. Kainate became one of the most widely used neuroactive chemicals to induce seizures in animals starting in the late 1970s and 1980s (43). These animals also show structural changes in the brain which are very similar to human MTS. Studies show that mice genetically designed to be deficient in glutamate uptake are susceptible to seizures (44). Those strains without the ability to post-transcriptionally edit glutamate receptor subunits (Q/R GluR-B subunit), causing poorly regulated

AMPA-related calcium influx, are useful models of temporal lobe epilepsy. Kindling to the point of status epilepticus is associated with elevated glutamate levels as well as increased NMDA receptor number and activity and other glutamate receptor changes (26, 45).

Microdialysis: animal studies

In the last few decades, investigators have developed techniques to measure extracellular levels of neurochemicals in animal models of epilepsy, resected human tissue, and patients with epilepsy, both ictally and interictally. To date, microdialysis, in which a small probe with a dialysis membrane at its tip is inserted into a brain region of interest, has been the most widely used of these technologies. Fluid can run through the probe in a contained loop, allowing chemicals to pass from the extracellular space across the membrane into the fluid for sampling, or in some cases, chemicals can be directly applied in the area of the probe for experimental purposes. Measurements of the chemicals of interest are typically performed off-line using highly sensitive techniques, such as high-performance liquid chromatography (HPLC). Because multiple samples can be taken serially, the time course of chemical changes in the brain can be studied (46).

Experience with using intracerebral microdialysis to study epileptic and non-epileptic brain regions in animal models of epilepsy revealed the significant roles of neuroactive amino acids in the brain, especially glutamate and GABA. Zhang et al. (47) studied amino acid changes in the ventral hippocampus before and during kindling using electrical stimulation of the deep prepiriform cortex which showed that both glutamate and glycine increased during kindling, with elevated basal glutamate levels for up to 30 days thereafter. Millan et al. (48) examined amino acid levels in the hippocampus in rats finding significant increases in aspartate and glutamate after kindling. They also found if pilocarpine was used to induce seizures in kindled animals, both glutamate and aspartate concentrations rose prior to the onset of seizures. This effect of kindling has been shown by others as well (49). In 2001, a study using the rat kainate model of partial epilepsy showed decreased protein and messenger RNA levels for the main rodent glutamate transporters GLAST and GLT-1 as well as changes in potassium-evoked neurotransmitter release (increased glutamate, decreased GABA) interictally in freely-moving animals which they interpreted as a result of impaired glutamate uptake (50). In a rat model of absence epilepsy, which likely involves pathophysiological changes in GABAergic regulation of the glutamatergic thalamocortical loops, $GABA_B$ antagonists are highly anticonvulsant. Using *in vivo* microdialysis, investigators were able to measure an increased basal level of GABA in this animal model, although treatment with $GABA_B$ antagonist baclofen or GAT inhibitor tiagabine did not significantly change GABA levels (51). Lacking, minimal, or conflicting microdialysis neuroactive amino acid findings in animal models of epilepsy, as demonstrated in this study, are unfortunately common (52–56).

Several investigators have attempted to reconcile the conflicting results by conducting their own potentially definitive studies. Wilson et al. (57) posited that prior studies showing little to no change in neuroactive amino acids might be because the investigators had not allowed enough time for pathophysiological changes to occur in the animal models of chronic epilepsy. Their study was unique insofar as they compared measurements of hippocampal amino acid changes sampled using microdialysis between the rat kainate model of chronic partial epilepsy and twelve patients with TLE. At least 90 days elapsed between intrahippocampal kainate injections and microdialysis sampling in the rat group. For both groups, they used electrographic monitoring and sampled microdialysate every 30 minutes interictally and every 5 minutes for an hour at the time of a seizure. Ictally in the patients, there was a significant elevation of hippocampal glutamate, aspartate, GABA, and taurine, while during seizures in the rat hippocampus, all of these were elevated except taurine. More recently, Meurs et al. (58) published the results of their own microdialysis studies of three animal models of acute epilepsy using intrahippocampal reverse dialysis to apply pilocarpine (cholinergic muscarine agonist), picrotoxin ($GABA_A$ antagonist), and a Group I metabotropic glutamate antagonist, all of which had previously been shown to provoke seizures. During seizures, both glutamate and GABA were significantly increased in all three models, especially glutamate following picrotoxin administration.

Microdialysis: human studies

In contrast to findings in animal models, intracerebral microdialysis studies of epileptic patients are more consistent. Prior to extracellular studies of resected human epileptic and non-epileptic tissue, whole tissue studies showed evidence of increased glutamate levels and increased glutamate receptor binding. This was coupled with decreased GABA binding without changes in whole tissue levels or number of hippocampal GABAergic synapses despite clear loss of some of the hilar GABAergic interneurons (59). In 1981, Perry and Hansen (60) studied the amino acid composition of resected epileptic foci from 35 patients and found no change in total GABA or aspartate concentrations but a significant increase in glutamate, including levels greater than two standard deviations above the mean in six patients, and postulated a possible aetiological role for glutamate in epilepsy. However, the ability to measure extracellular amino acids in real time while monitoring patients having seizures was a breakthrough in understanding the neurochemistry of epilepsy. In 1992, Ronne-Engstrom et al. (61) reported amino acid levels from seven patients undergoing epilepsy surgery in whom they collected samples via intraoperative *in vivo* microdialysis capturing five spontaneous and five electrically-induced seizures. Compared to basal levels measured before seizures, aspartate, glycine, glutamate, and serine were significantly elevated during the seizures. GABA levels were not analysed.

Shortly thereafter During and Spencer (62) reported changes in glutamate and GABA in six patients who had bilaterally implanted hippocampal microdialysis probes. In the period prior to their epilepsy surgeries, they were electrographically and behaviourally monitored for seizures. They found that increased extracellular glutamate preceded seizure onset by over a minute and during this period there was also relatively lower extracellular GABA. During seizures, glutamate levels increased significantly bilaterally and persisted much longer on the side of seizure onset. GABA also rose to a lesser degree, and interestingly was significantly higher on the contralateral side. This work was followed in 1995 by an investigation focused on GABA. Previous work showed diminished GABA inhibition in the human epileptic hippocampus, despite relatively preserved GABAergic interneurons and receptors. They compared potassium- and glutamate-evoked GABA release in the bilateral hippocampi and found increased potassium-evoked release and diminished glutamate-evoked release on the epileptogenic side. Unlike potassium-evoked release, glutamate-evoked release was calcium-independent (i.e. non-synaptic), and they speculated that the high concentrations of glutamate causing depolarization might reverse the sodium-dependent GATs. In parallel studies in amygdala-kindled rat hippocampus, they reported a 48% reduction in GAT, suggesting that decreased extracellular GABA might be related to decreased GAT density (63).

Since these landmark studies, investigators have continued to study additional aspects of glutamate and GABA in human epileptogenic brain. Starting in 2003, O'Connor's group published a series of papers highlighting increased glutamate, aspartate, and GABA intraoperatively in spontaneously epileptiform human hippocampus (64). In 2005, the metabolism of glutamate was examined by Cavus et al. (65) using microdialysis and depth electrodes interictally in 38 patients with both TLE and cortical epilepsy. In the epileptogenic hippocampus, they measured elevated basal glutamate and high lactate as well as poor glucose utilization and a low glutamine-to-glutamate ratio raising the possibility of impaired glutamate uptake and glutamate-glutamine cycling in association with inefficient regional energy use. In epileptogenic cortex, glutamate was only marginally increased which might indicate a different regional pathophysiology. In 2008, related groups published multiple papers on the epileptogenic hippocampus, linking higher glutamate levels with diminished tissue volumes, energy impairment, and hyperexcitability and correlating GABA levels with neurometabolism (66–68). Of particular note, Eid et al. (69) reviewed the previous data and advanced the concept of the 'glutamate hypothesis' in MTLE tying together the importance of astrogliosis in MTS with the special role that astrocytes play in extracellular glutamate regulation. Astrocytes control extracellular glutamate levels through rapid uptake and the glutamate-glutamine cycle, but they noted a 35–40% decrease in glutamine synthetase (GS) and approximately 40% decrease in activity of glutamine synthetase in MTLE and proposed that astrocytic glutamate release through uptake reversal may play a significant role in its pathophysiology.

Magnetic resonance spectroscopy: human studies

Nuclear magnetic resonance spectroscopy (MRS) is an attractive tool for both clinical and investigational use in epilepsy given its ready availability at most academic medical centres, safety, and non-invasive nature. MRS measures the resonance frequencies of naturally occurring radioisotopes, such as ^{1}H, ^{31}P, and ^{13}C, to identify and quantitate a broad number of neurochemicals. These include N-acetyl aspartate (NAA, primarily neuronal), creatine- and choline-containing compounds (primarily glial), and lactate, which in combination can provide evidence of neuronal damage and energy deficiency. Other neurochemicals of special interest in epilepsy which can be measured include GABA, glutamate, and glutamine (59, 70) which allows MRS to provide complementary data to that obtained using microdialysis. MRS is limited primarily insofar as it provides a measurement of a total level and cannot differentiate between intra- and extracellular pools. GABA was first detected with ^{1}H MRS in 1984, whereas glutamate was detected initially in 1985 but required an 8.5 Tesla magnet. Currently ^{13}C MRS can detect glutamate at much lower field strengths (71). The best use of MRS in epilepsy is not yet clear. Studies over the last two decades have investigated metabolic and energy abnormalities in generalized epilepsies, Rasmussen's encephalitis, and temporal lobe epilepsy (72–75), as well as lateralization of seizure onset when MRI was inconclusive (76, 77). Clearly, applications for researching the role of GABA have been the most prolific to date, including predicting poorer seizure control in one study (78). However, the primary use has been investigation of GABA levels as they relate to the mechanisms of action of multiple AEDs (79–81). There are also MRS studies of glutamate and the glutamate-glutamine cycle in temporal lobe epilepsy (66, 82).

Microelectrode arrays: animal studies and clinical potential

A major limitation of whole tissue levels, MRS, and even microdialysis is temporal resolution. Whole tissue and MRS provide interictal snapshots of chemical profiles. The vast majority of microdialysis-based techniques cannot sample more quickly than every few minutes because higher flow rates would disrupt tissue and confound measurements. A typical seizure lasts less than one minute, and the kinetics of the neurochemical changes that occur during a seizure are likely to occur over the time course of seconds to minutes, especially with respect to extracellular neurochemicals with high affinity uptake systems like glutamate and GABA. One intriguing approach to address this problem is the use of implantable microelectrode arrays which can provide second-by-second electrochemical detection of extracellular neurochemicals. Using an enzyme coating coupled with voltammetric techniques for identifying specific neurochemicals, Dr Greg Gerhardt's group has refined a platinum-based, glutamate oxidase-coated microeletrode array capable of measuring basal and stimulated release of glutamate in anesthetized and awake mice, rats, and monkeys (83–87). In animal studies, potassium-evoked release of glutamate has very fast kinetics and is completely cleared back to baseline within seconds (88). Efforts are ongoing to complete refinements of a combined depth electrode and glutamate-sensitive microelectrode array for human use. The details of potential microelectrode-based epilepsy therapy were published in 2008 (89).

Other neurotransmitters and epilepsy

There are studies of other neurotransmitters in epilepsy. As neuroactive amino acids, both aspartate and glycine show variable changes during seizures as previously detailed. The excitatory neurochemical aspartate is a pervasive non-essential amino acid which may be co-released with glutamate. Its importance as a neurotransmitter is questionable considering that, other than NMDA receptors which bind glutamate more tightly than aspartate, there are no currently identified aspartate receptors. Aspartate can be removed from the extracellular space by glutamate transporters, but is not packaged into vesicles by VGLUTs. On the other hand, the inhibitory neurotransmitter glycine exerts its effects through specific glycine receptors which are chloride ion channels, like $GABA_A$ receptors, although GABA cannot activate them. The glycine receptor is found predominantly in the brainstem and spinal cord and plays a role in motor reflex circuits and nociception as well as the rare neurological disorder hyperekplexia, or startle disease (90).

However, glycine receptors are also present in hippocampal neurons where activation by extrasynaptic glycine may provide tonic inhibition (91). The NMDA receptor also has a glycine binding site giving glycine a role in excitation as well. To date, there are no studies reporting significant pathophysiologic roles in epilepsy for either aspartate or glycine although glycine encephalopathy (nonketotic hyperglycinemia), an inborn error of glycine metabolism, is associated with refractory seizures (92).

Dopamine, on the other hand, seems to have a complex role in subcortical modulation of epileptogenic circuits (93). Alterations in dopamine pathways occur in ring chromosome 20 epilepsy, temporal lobe epilepsy, juvenile myoclonic epilepsy, and autosomal dominant nocturnal frontal lobe epilepsy (ADNFLE) (94). The thalamocortical pathways which underlie generalized epilepsies are regulated by GABAergic projections from the thalamus; however, oscillatory pathways within the basal ganglia also have projections which modulate the thalamocortical loops. This includes the dopaminergic nigrostriatal pathway originating in the substantia nigra. Based on this, many investigators have proposed that basal ganglia dysfunction has a significant role in the pathophysiology of some epilepsies (95, 96). Also of potential interest is the dopaminergic mesocorticolimbic pathway from the ventral tegmental area to the frontal cortex which might help explain both motor and behavioural symptoms seen in epilepsy. These findings have yet to inspire any significant pursuit of dopaminergic drugs as antiepileptic agents. Nonetheless, further definition of the role of dopamine, especially in specific epileptic syndromes, remains an intriguing area of active research.

Acetylcholine was the first identified neurotransmitter, largely due to its prominence in the parasympathetic nervous system and neuromuscular junction. Its discovery earned Dale and Loewi the Nobel Prize in Physiology or Medicine in 1936. As a result, early studies of the neurochemical basis for epilepsy focused on acetylcholine, even prompting Foster in 1946 to conjecture that 'the physiological cause of epilepsy may be defined as abnormalities of acetylcholine metabolism' (97). However a major role for acetylcholine in epilepsy remained controversial for decades. Obvious support stemmed from findings that either direct intrahippocampal or systemic treatment with muscarinic cholinergic agonists such as pilocarpine could provoke status epilepticus followed by chronic seizures in rodents (98–100). Anatomically in humans, cholinergic projections to the hippocampus arise from cells in the medial septum and the diagonal band of Broca along the septohippocampal pathway which also carries GABAergic and glutamatergic projections (24). This pathway regulates hippocampal theta rhythms most prominent during wakefulness and REM sleep, which are periods of decreased seizure likelihood in patients with epilepsy. This antiepileptic role is also further supported by the fact that the cholinergic agonist carbachol induces hippocampal theta and protects against epileptogenesis in rodent models of chronic epilepsy (101). The major cholinergic pathways in the brain begin in the basal nucleus of Meynert in the forebrain and project diffusely throughout the cortex with a significant role in arousal. Some of these projections also terminate in the thalamic reticular nucleus, where acetylcholine has a modulatory effect on the thalamocortical loops (102). Separately, the neuronal nicotinic acetylcholine receptor mutations CHRNA4 (α4 subunit) and CHRNB2 (β subunit) are implicated in ADNFLE types 1 and type 3, respectively. The CHRNA4 mutation, in fact, was the first demonstration that a heritable ion channel mutation can cause epilepsy (103, 104). Overall, acetylcholine has a significant modulatory role in multiple types of epilepsy as well as an etiological role in one type. However, beyond the potential benefits of future gene therapy for ADNFLE, cholinergic modulation has not shown efficacy in treating seizures, and its importance as target for further AED development remains unclear.

Support for serotonin's contribution to epilepsy has been growing since the mid 1980s. Serotonergic projections originate in the midbrain raphe nuclei and make diffuse connections throughout the brain, including most well-known epileptic brain regions including the cortex, hippocampus, and thalamus. Bagdy has summarized several key points (105). In animal models of epilepsy, increased serotonergic activity tends to be antiepileptic whereas decreased activity is proconvulsant. Furthermore, provoked or genetic mouse models of epilepsy with knockout for 5-HT_{1A} or 5-HT_{2C} receptors tend to have more seizures. There is some evidence of changes in serotonin neurotransmission in resected tumours and epileptogenic tissue. Among the multitude of serotonin receptors, the 5-HT_{2C} receptor appears to be of particular importance in epilepsy. Some currently used antiepileptic medications including valproic acid, lamotrigine, carbamazepine, phenytoin, and zonisamide, when administered experimentally in animals, are associated with increased extracellular serotonin levels. Altogether, there is some sentiment that serotonin should be more closely investigated for possible AED development.

Lastly, noradrenaline also has support as an antiepileptic neurotransmitter. Of the multiple noradrenergic brainstem nuclei, it is the most rostral pontine nucleus, the locus coeruleus (LC), which appears to have a role in epilepsy. The LC projects along two small ascending pathways, the dorsal bundle and the rostral limb of the dorsal periventricular pathway, before extensively branching to innervate the entire cerebrum. There are also descending projections to the cerebellum, medulla, and spinal cord. Evidence for the anticonvulsant properties of noradrenaline stem from pharmacologic agonism of its receptors and from lesional studies of the LC in which seizure magnitude and associated pathological destruction was heightened in both genetic and acquired animal models of epilepsy. Furthermore, when animal models of epilepsy are also exposed to common AEDs, including valproic acid, carbamazepine, phenytoin, and phenobarbital, increased levels of noradrenaline can be measured in some brain regions. In addition, noradrenaline is associated with the efficacy of vagal nerve stimulation (VNS), a treatment for refractory partial epilepsy thought to exert its effects through stimulation of the nucleus of the solitary tract and other neighbouring brainstem nuclei that modulate the subcortical gating of epileptic circuits. In 1998, Krahl et al. (106) showed that bilateral LC lesions eliminated the seizure-suppressing ability of VNS. Finally, several other neurotransmitters are co-released with noradrenaline including galanin, neuropeptide Y, and adenosine which may also be contributory (107).

The neurochemical basis of antiepileptic drugs

Given our modern understanding of the contributions of multiple neurotransmitter systems that drive inhibition and excitation of the epileptic circuits, one might expect that the neurobiology has driven the drug designs. At times, this has been true; however, the drug development evolved with our understanding of the biology such that most of the current AEDs which we use today were not borne out of newly identified molecular targets. For example, bromide salts were found to be effective antiseizure treatments in 1853, used for well over 50 years in humans, and are still used in veterinary medicine today. However, after discovery of safer agents, like phenobarbital in 1912 and phenytoin in 1937, their use in humans ceased (108). The proposed GABAergic mechanism of action was not reported until the 1980s (109), highlighting that rational drug design is often challenging because our observations outpace our understanding. A later chapter will detail the AEDs, but because the neurochemical basis of epilepsy offers us significant insight into the use of medications, a brief discussion is merited.

The major mechanisms by which AEDs exert their effects can be subdivided into three categories as described by Rogawski and Loscher (104): (1) modulation of voltage-gated ion channels including sodium and calcium, (2) enhancement of synaptic inhibition, and (3) inhibition of synaptic excitation. The first category includes what clinicians often refer to as the sodium channel blockers, which includes the voltage-gated fast and the persistent sodium currents. Modulation affects neuronal ability to respond to depolarization with generation of an action potential. Relevant AEDs include phenytoin, carbamazepine, oxcarbazepine, lamotrigine, zonisamide, and lacosamide (110) as well as rufinamide, felbamate, valproic acid, and topiramate. This effect on action potentials reduces downstream synaptic transmission, with evidence that glutamate release may be more affected than other neurotransmitters, such as GABA (111, 112). Sodium channel blockers tend to be effective against partial and generalized tonic–clonic seizures. The voltage-gated calcium channel blockers include the high voltage-activated (HVA) (L-, R-, P/Q-, and N-types) and the low voltage-activated (LVA) (T-type). HVA calcium channels are primarily involved in presynaptic neurotransmitter release, while LVA calcium channels regulate bursting and oscillations such as previously described in the thalamus. Probably the most recognizable of the AEDs that primarily affect calcium channels is ethosuximide which blocks T-type channels and disrupts the hypersynchronized thalamocortical loops responsible for absence epilepsy. Other AEDs which interact with T-type channels include zonisamide and possibly valproic acid, while the AEDs which have HVA calcium channel activity include lamotrigine, felbamate, topiramate, gabapentin, and phenobarbital. Levetiracetam at clinically relevant doses reportedly also inhibits HVA (N-type) calcium channels (113, 114). More recently, voltage-gated potassium channels were recognized as another potential target for AEDs. In particular, the KCNQ/Kv7 activating drug retigabine has shown significant promise in clinical trials (115).

Potentiation of GABA systems has been the major AED mechanism since effective treatments became recognized. Despite that excitatory synapses in epileptic regions often significantly outnumber inhibitory ones, the ability of GABA to inhibit feedforward positive loops is critically important and a potent strategy for seizure treatment. Both benzodiazepines and phenobarbital accentuate the effects of GABA at the $GABA_A$ receptor through different mechanisms. Valproic acid increases both GABA synthesis and turnover. The first example of rational drug design focused on GABA and produced three agents in use today. Gabapentin, a lipophilic 3-cyclohexyl analogue of GABA, was synthesized in an attempt to create a GABA agonist, but it does not activate GABA receptors, and, in fact, the most likely mechanism of action is via binding the $\alpha2\delta$ subunit of voltage-gated calcium channels (117). However, there is also some evidence that gabapentin modulates GABA systems including increasing GABA synthesis and turnover as well as possibly inhibiting or reversing GABA transport. The second agent vigabatrin was found to be an irreversible inhibitor of GABA transaminase, the enzyme which breaks down GABA. Without GABA catabolism, GABA levels increase, possibly by way of reversal of GAT. Approximately 10 years following its introduction on the market, reports of visual field loss because of retinal side effects limited enthusiasm for continued use, especially in the US, although it is still used in many other countries around the world, though almost exclusively for the treatment of infantile spasms. Finally, tiagabine is a GAT inhibitor which also effectively increases GABA levels (116). Rounding out the story, both felbamate and topiramate have some effects on $GABA_A$ receptors, and though the main mechanism of action of levetiracetam is likely related to binding to the synaptic vesicular protein SV2A which may inhibit calcium-dependent vesicular release (117), levetiracetam reportedly also reverses an exogenous allosteric modulator of $GABA_A$ receptors (118).

Finally, glutamate receptors are also molecular targets for AED development. In animal models, antagonism of AMPA and NMDA is effective, but clinical trials have been disappointing due to significant side effects. The NMDA receptor blocker ketamine is sometimes beneficial in the treatment of refractory status epilepticus. Furthermore, felbamate may somewhat selectively block NMDA receptors containing the NR2B subunit which is largely restricted in its CNS distribution to the forebrain, perhaps explaining why its side effect profile is better. Phenobarbital also blocks AMPA receptors, and topiramate antagonizes both AMPA and kainate receptors. Recall that kainate may be an especially intriguing target for blockade as it causes both postsynaptic excitation and presynaptically inhibits GABA release. Most recently, the first-in-class, highly selective, non-competitive AMPA receptor blocker peramapanel (investigation compound E2007) is currently being evaluated for clinical use.

Clinical complexities of the neurochemistry of epilepsy

The development of multiple antiepileptic medications with different mechanisms of action has led to the concept of 'rational polypharmacy' for the treatment of refractory epilepsy. The idea is that combining medications with different mechanisms of action may produce synergistic effects that improve efficacy. Unfortunately, there is surprisingly little clinical data to guide treatment (119) and despite our ever increasing understanding of the neurochemistry of epilepsy, it is still necessary to assess combinations of medications with different proposed mechanisms of action in clinical trials in patients with epilepsy. One trial, designed as a 'first add-on' study, compared effects of tiagabine to phenytoin and carbamazepine, using a parallel design. Because the study allowed comparison of drugs with different proposed mechanisms and highlights the complexities of 'rational polypharmacy', the study will be presented in detail.

Patients with complex partial seizures with or without secondary generalization, which were not satisfactorily controlled on phenytoin or carbamazepine monotherapy, were randomized to either a tiagabine or carbamazepine/phenytoin add-on treatment group. Efficacy determinations were based on seizure frequency. The add-on AED was titrated to effect or unacceptable adverse effects to permit patients to find the best tolerated and effective dose and provide a fair comparison between the study drugs (120).

Eight tests of mental abilities and three of mood and adjustment were administered prior to assignment of add-on treatment and after up to 16 weeks of add-on treatment. Overall, add-on tiagabine showed few or no differences in comparison with add-on carbamazepine and add-on phenytoin (121). Slightly more side effects were reported with the addition of either phenytoin or carbamazepine compared to addition of tiagabine. Measuring the median seizure reduction of the two 'combined' groups, which compared the average of the add-on carbamazepine and add-on phenytoin groups with the average of the tiagabine add-on groups, showed a statistically significant difference in favour of the carbamazepine/phenytoin groups which was attributed to the carbamazepine add-on to phenytoin group (122, 123).

This well-designed study showed better tolerability with add-on tiagabine, few differences in effects on cognitive ability, mood, and adjustment between the groups, and better efficacy with add-on carbamazepine/phenytoin. The concept of 'rational polypharmacy' was not supported by this trial since add-on therapy with tiagabine (GABAergic mechanism) was less effective than add-on therapy with carbamazepine/phenytoin. Improved efficacy in the carbamazepine add-on group may well reflect mechanisms of action of carbamazepine beyond sodium channel modulation (124), differential efficacy between carbamazepine, phenytoin, and tiagabine, an effect of the trial design or some combination of factors. One other unexplained outcome is the observation that the addition of carbamazepine to phenytoin was apparently superior to the addition of phenytoin to carbamazepine. The findings illustrate that interactions of medications with different proposed mechanisms of action are difficult to predict in the absence of testing in clinical trials, and highlight the need for additional studies.

Conclusions

The dedicated efforts of several generations of investigators have greatly expanded our understanding of the neurochemistry of epilepsy. Epilepsy results from an imbalance between excitation mediated by glutamatergic transmission and inhibition mediated by GABAergic transmission. While previous efforts have resulted in the development of multiple medications for the effective treatment of epilepsy, a significant minority of patients continue to have seizures despite treatment with antiepileptic medications.

Many questions remain unanswered. For example, there is uncertainty about the roles of the other transmitter systems in the pathophysiology of epilepsy, as well as the mechanisms of action of our current antiepileptic medications. The inherent complexity of the neurochemistry of the brain provides challenges for understanding, but also opportunities for identification of additional therapeutic targets for treatment. Past successes in understanding of the neurochemistry of epilepsy and associated development of antiepileptic medications provides a roadmap for the future, providing insights for additional clinical trials to leverage our knowledge of neurochemistry and provide optimal treatment to all epilepsy patients.

References

1. Van Rijn C, Meinardi H. Neurochemistry and epileptology. *Epilepsia* 2009; 50(Suppl 3):17–29.
2. Kravitz EA, Kuffler SW, Potter DD. Gamma-aminobutyric acid and other blocking compounds in crustacea. Iii. Their relative concentrations in separated motor and inhibitory axons. *J Neurophysiol* 1963; 26:739–51.
3. Otsuka M. Gamma-aminobutyric acid and some other neurotransmitter candidates in the nervous system. In: Acheson GH, Bloom FE (eds) *Pharmacology and the Future of Man: Proceedings of the Fifth International Congress on Pharmacology*, pp. 186–201. Basel: S. Karger, 1973.
4. De Deyn PP, Marescau B, MacDonald RL. Epilepsy and the GABA-hypothesis a brief review and some examples. *Acta Neurol Belg* 1990; 90(2):65–81.
5. Jones EA, Yurdaydin C, Basile AS. The GABA hypothesis—state of the art. *Adv Exp Med Biol* 1994; 368:89–101.
6. Bloom FE. Neurotransmission and the central nervous system. In: Molinoff PB, Ruddon RW (eds) *Goodman and Gilman's the pharmacological basis of therapeutics* (9th edn), pp. 267–93. New York: McGraw-Hill, 1996.
7. Lu CC, Hilgemann DW. GAT1 (GABA:Na+:Cl−) cotransport function. Kinetic studies in giant Xenopus oocyte membrane patches. *J Gen Physiol* 1999; 114(3):445–57.
8. Mathern GW, Mendoza D, Lozada A, Pretorius JK, Dehnes Y, Danbolt NC, *et al.* Hippocampal GABA and glutamate transporter immunoreactivity in patients with temporal lobe epilepsy. *Neurology* 1999; 52(3):453–72.
9. Wu Y, Wang W, Diez-Sampedro A, Richerson GB. Nonvesicular inhibitory neurotransmission via reversal of the GABA transporter GAT-1. *Neuron* 2007; 56(5):851–65.
10. Hamberger A, Chiang GH, Sandoval E, Cotman CW. Glutamate as a CNS transmitter. II. Regulation of synthesis in the releasable pool. *Brain Res* 1979; 168(3):531–41.
11. Hamberger AC, Chiang GH, Nylen ES, Scheff SW, Cotman CW. Glutamate as a CNS transmitter. I. Evaluation of glucose and glutamine as precursors for the synthesis of preferentially released glutamate. *Brain Res* 1979; 168(3):513–30.
12. Henn FA, Goldstein MN, Hamberger A. Uptake of the neurotransmitter candidate glutamate by glia. *Nature* 1974; 249(458):663–4.
13. Sandoval ME, Cotman CW. Evaluation of glutamate as a neurotransmitter of cerebellar parallel fibers. *Neuroscience* 1978; 3(2):199–206.
14. Meldrum BS. Glutamate as a neurotransmitter in the brain: review of physiology and pathology. *J Nutr* 2000; 130(4S Suppl):1007S–15S.
15. Ferraguti F, Shigemoto R. Metabotropic glutamate receptors. *Cell Tissue Res* 2006; 326(2):483–504.
16. Danbolt NC. Glutamate uptake. *Prog Neurobiol* 2001; 65(1):1–105.
17. O'Kane RL, Martinez-Lopez I, DeJoseph MR, Vina JR, Hawkins RA. Na(+)-dependent glutamate transporters (EAAT1, EAAT2, and EAAT3) of the blood-brain barrier. A mechanism for glutamate removal. *J Biol Chem* 1999; 274(45):31891–5.
18. Szatkowski M, Barbour B, Attwell D. Non-vesicular release of glutamate from glial cells by reversed electrogenic glutamate uptake. *Nature* 1990; 348(6300):443–6.
19. Bradford HF. Glutamate, GABA and epilepsy. *Prog Neurobiol* 1995; 47(6):477–511.
20. Blumenfeld H, McCormick DA. Corticothalamic inputs control the pattern of activity generated in thalamocortical networks. *J Neurosci* 2000; 20(13):5153–62.
21. Crunelli V, Leresche N. Childhood absence epilepsy: genes, channels, neurons and networks. *Nat Rev Neurosci* 2002; 3(5): 371–82.

22. Swaiman KF, Ashwal S, Ferriero DM. *Neurophysiology of epilepsy. Pediatric neurology: principles and practice* (4th edn). Philadelphia, PA: Mosby, 2006.
23. Freund TF, Antal M. GABA-containing neurons in the septum control inhibitory interneurons in the hippocampus. *Nature* 1988; 336(6195):170–3.
24. Colom LV, Castaneda MT, Reyna T, Hernandez S, Garrido-Sanabria E. Characterization of medial septal glutamatergic neurons and their projection to the hippocampus. *Synapse* 2005; 58(3):151–64.
25. Bronen RA, Fulbright RK, Spencer DD, Spencer SS, Kim JH, Lange RC, *et al.* Refractory epilepsy: comparison of MR imaging, CT, and histopathologic findings in 117 patients. *Radiology* 1996; 201(1): 97–105.
26. Dalby NO, Mody I. The process of epileptogenesis: a pathophysiological approach. *Curr Opin Neurol* 2001; 14(2):187–92.
27. Sommer W. Erkrankung des Ammonshorns als aetiologisches Moment der Epilepsie. *Arch Psychiatr Nervenkr* 1880; 10:631–75.
28. Falconer MA. Mesial temporal (Ammon's horn) sclerosis as a common cause of epilepsy. Aetiology, treatment, and prevention. *Lancet* 1974; 2(7883):767–70.
29. Williamson PD, French JA, Thadani VM, Kim JH, Novelly RA, Spencer SS, *et al.* Characteristics of medial temporal lobe epilepsy: II. Interictal and ictal scalp electroencephalography, neuropsychological testing, neuroimaging, surgical results, and pathology. *Ann Neurol* 1993; 34(6):781–7.
30. Babb TL, Brown WJ. Pathological findings in epilepsy. In: Engel J (ed) *Surgical treatment of the epilepsies*, pp. 511–40. New York: Raven; 1987.
31. Hogan RE. Mesial temporal sclerosis: clinicopathological correlations. *Arch Neurol* 2001; 58(9):1484–6.
32. Wolf H, Blumcke I. Pathologic findings in mesial temporal sclerosis. In: Kotagal P (ed) *The Epilepsies: Etiologies and Prevention*, pp. 133–9. San Diego, CA: Academic Press, Inc.; 1999.
33. Piredda S, Gale K. A crucial epileptogenic site in the deep prepiriform cortex. *Nature* 1985; 317(6038):623–5.
34. Piredda S, Gale K. Anticonvulsant action of 2-amino-7-phosphonoheptanoic acid and muscimol in the deep prepiriform cortex. *Eur J Pharmacol* 1986; 120(1):115–18.
35. Halonen T, Tortorella A, Zrebeet H, Gale K. Posterior piriform and perirhinal cortex relay seizures evoked from the area tempestas: role of excitatory and inhibitory amino acid receptors. *Brain Res* 1994; 652(1):145–8.
36. Fisher RS. Animal models of the epilepsies. *Brain Res Brain Res Rev* 1989; 14(3):245–78.
37. Matsumoto H, Ajmonemarsan C. Cellular mechanisms in experimental epileptic seizures. *Science* 1964; 144:193–4.
38. Prince DA. The depolarization shift in 'epileptic' neurons. *Exp Neurol* 1968; 21(4):467–85.
39. Merritt HH, Putnam TJ. Landmark article Sept 17, 1938: Sodium diphenyl hydantoinate in the treatment of convulsive disorders. By H. Houston Merritt and Tracy J. Putnam. *JAMA* 1984; 251(8):1062–7.
40. Meldrum BS, Horton RW, Brierley JB. Epileptic brain damage in adolescent baboons following seizures induced by allylglycine. *Brain* 1974; 97(2):407–18.
41. Treiman DM. GABAergic mechanisms in epilepsy. *Epilepsia* 2001; 42(Suppl 3):8–12.
42. Murakami S, Takemoto T, Shimizu Z. The effective principle of Digenea simplex Aq I. Separation of the effective fraction by liquid chromatography. *J Pharm Soc Japan* 1953; 73:1026–8.
43. Schwarcz R, Zaczek R, Coyle JT. Microinjection of kainic acid into the rat hippocampus. *Eur J Pharmacol* 1978; 50(3):209–20.
44. Meldrum BS, Akbar MT, Chapman AG. Glutamate receptors and transporters in genetic and acquired models of epilepsy. *Epilepsy Res* 1999; 36(2–3):189–204.
45. Chapman AG. Glutamate receptors in epilepsy. *Prog Brain Res* 1998; 116:371–83.
46. Khan SH, Shuaib A. The technique of intracerebral microdialysis. *Methods* 2001; 23(1):3–9.
47. Zhang WQ, Hudson PM, Sobotka TJ, Hong JS, Tilson HA. Extracellular concentrations of amino acid transmitters in ventral hippocampus during and after the development of kindling. *Brain Res* 1991; 540(1–2):315–8.
48. Millan MH, Chapman AG, Meldrum BS. Extracellular amino acid levels in hippocampus during pilocarpine-induced seizures. *Epilepsy Res* 1993; 14(2):139–48.
49. Meldrum BS. The role of glutamate in epilepsy and other CNS disorders. *Neurology* 1994; 44(11 Suppl 8):S14–23.
50. Ueda Y, Doi T, Tokumaru J, Yokoyama H, Nakajima A, Mitsuyama Y, *et al.* Collapse of extracellular glutamate regulation during epileptogenesis: down-regulation and functional failure of glutamate transporter function in rats with chronic seizures induced by kainic acid. *J Neurochem* 2001; 76(3):892–900.
51. Richards DA, Lemos T, Whitton PS, Bowery NG. Extracellular GABA in the ventrolateral thalamus of rats exhibiting spontaneous absence epilepsy: a microdialysis study. *J Neurochem* 1995; 65(4):1674–80.
52. Bruhn T, Cobo M, Berg M, Diemer NH. Limbic seizure-induced changes in extracellular amino acid levels in the hippocampal formation: a microdialysis study of freely moving rats. *Acta Neurol Scand* 1992; 86(5):455–61.
53. Lehmann A. Alterations in hippocampal extracellular amino acids and purine catabolites during limbic seizures induced by folate injections into the rabbit amygdala. *Neuroscience*. 1987; 22(2):573–8.
54. Millan MH, Obrenovitch TP, Sarna GS, Lok SY, Symon L, Meldrum BS. Changes in rat brain extracellular glutamate concentration during seizures induced by systemic picrotoxin or focal bicuculline injection: an in vivo dialysis study with on-line enzymatic detection. *Epilepsy Res* 1991; 9(2):86–91.
55. Ueda Y, Tsuru N. Bilateral seizure-related changes of extracellular glutamate concentration in hippocampi during development of amygdaloid kindling. *Epilepsy Res* 1994; 18(1):85–8.
56. Wade JV, Samson FE, Nelson SR, Pazdernik TL. Changes in extracellular amino acids during soman- and kainic acid-induced seizures. *J Neurochem* 1987; 49(2):645–50.
57. Wilson CL, Maidment NT, Shomer MH, Behnke EJ, Ackerson L, Fried I, *et al.* Comparison of seizure related amino acid release in human epileptic hippocampus versus a chronic, kainate rat model of hippocampal epilepsy. *Epilepsy Res* 1996; 26(1):245–54.
58. Meurs A, Clinckers R, Ebinger G, Michotte Y, Smolders I. Seizure activity and changes in hippocampal extracellular glutamate, GABA, dopamine and serotonin. *Epilepsy Res* 2008; 78(1):50–9.
59. Sherwin AL. Neuroactive amino acids in focally epileptic human brain: a review. *Neurochem Res* 1999; 24(11):1387–95.
60. Perry TL, Hansen S. Amino acid abnormalities in epileptogenic foci. *Neurology* 1981; 31(7):872–6.
61. Ronne-Engstrom E, Hillered L, Flink R, Spannare B, Ungerstedt U, Carlson H. Intracerebral microdialysis of extracellular amino acids in the human epileptic focus. *J Cereb Blood Flow Metab* 1992; 12(5):873–6.
62. During MJ, Spencer DD. Extracellular hippocampal glutamate and spontaneous seizure in the conscious human brain. *Lancet* 1993; 341(8861):1607–10.
63. During MJ, Ryder KM, Spencer DD. Hippocampal GABA transporter function in temporal-lobe epilepsy. *Nature* 1995; 376(6536):174–7.
64. Thomas PM, Phillips JP, Delanty N, O'Connor WT. Elevated extracellular levels of glutamate, aspartate and gamma-aminobutyric acid within the intraoperative, spontaneously epileptiform human hippocampus. *Epilepsy Res* 2003; 54(1):73–9.
65. Cavus I, Kasoff WS, Cassaday MP, Jacob R, Gueorguieva R, Sherwin RS, *et al.* Extracellular metabolites in the cortex and hippocampus of epileptic patients. *Ann Neurol* 2005; 57(2):226–35.

66. Cavus I, Pan JW, Hetherington HP, Abi-Saab W, Zaveri HP, Vives KP, *et al.* Decreased hippocampal volume on MRI is associated with increased extracellular glutamate in epilepsy patients. *Epilepsia* 2008; 49(8):1358–66.
67. Pan JW, Cavus I, Kim J, Hetherington HP, Spencer DD. Hippocampal extracellular GABA correlates with metabolism in human epilepsy. *Metab Brain Dis* 2008; 23(4):457–68.
68. Pan JW, Williamson A, Cavus I, Hetherington HP, Zaveri H, Petroff OA, *et al.* Neurometabolism in human epilepsy. *Epilepsia* 2008; 49(Suppl 3):31–41.
69. Eid T, Williamson A, Lee TS, Petroff OA, de Lanerolle NC. Glutamate and astrocytes—key players in human mesial temporal lobe epilepsy? *Epilepsia* 2008; 49(Suppl 2):42–52.
70. Duncan JS. Magnetic resonance spectroscopy. *Epilepsia* 1996; 37(7):598–605.
71. Petroff OA, Mattson RH, Rothman DL. Proton MRS: GABA and glutamate. *Adv Neurol* 2000; 83:261–71.
72. Hajek M, Dezortova M, Komarek V. 1H MR spectroscopy in patients with mesial temporal epilepsy. *Magma* 1998; 7(2):95–114.
73. Helms G, Ciumas C, Kyaga S, Savic I. Increased thalamus levels of glutamate and glutamine (Glx) in patients with idiopathic generalised epilepsy. *J Neurol Neurosurg Psychiatry* 2006; 77(4):489–94.
74. Lin K, Carrete H, Jr., Lin J, Peruchi MM, de Araujo Filho GM, Guaranha MS, *et al.* Magnetic resonance spectroscopy reveals an epileptic network in juvenile myoclonic epilepsy. *Epilepsia* 2009; 50(5):1191–200.
75. Wellard RM, Briellmann RS, Wilson JC, Kalnins RM, Anderson DP, Federico P, *et al.* Longitudinal study of MRS metabolites in Rasmussen encephalitis. *Brain* 2004; 127(Pt 6):1302–12.
76. Doelken MT, Stefan H, Pauli E, Stadlbauer A, Struffert T, Engelhorn T, *et al.* (1)H-MRS profile in MRI positive- versus MRI negative patients with temporal lobe epilepsy. *Seizure* 2008; 17(6):490–7.
77. Hammen T, Kerling F, Schwarz M, Stadlbauer A, Ganslandt O, Keck B, *et al.* Identifying the affected hemisphere by (1)H-MR spectroscopy in patients with temporal lobe epilepsy and no pathological findings in high resolution MRI. *Eur J Neurol* 2006; 13(5):482–90.
78. Briellmann RS, Mark Wellard R, Masterton RA, Abbott DF, Berkovic SF, Jackson GD. Hippocampal sclerosis: MR prediction of seizure intractability. *Epilepsia* 2007; 48(2):315–23.
79. Errante LD, Williamson A, Spencer DD, Petroff OA. Gabapentin and vigabatrin increase GABA in the human neocortical slice. *Epilepsy Res* 2002; 49(3):203–10.
80. Garcia M, Huppertz HJ, Ziyeh S, Buechert M, Schumacher M, Mader I. Valproate-induced metabolic changes in patients with epilepsy: assessment with H-MRS. *Epilepsia* 2009; 50(3):486–92.
81. Kuzniecky R, Ho S, Pan J, Martin R, Gilliam F, Faught E, *et al.* Modulation of cerebral GABA by topiramate, lamotrigine, and gabapentin in healthy adults. *Neurology* 2002; 58(3):368–72.
82. Spencer SS. Neural networks in human epilepsy: evidence of and implications for treatment. *Epilepsia* 2002; 43(3):219–27.
83. Day BK, Pomerleau F, Burmeister JJ, Huettl P, Gerhardt GA. Microelectrode array studies of basal and potassium-evoked release of L-glutamate in the anesthetized rat brain. *J Neurochem* 2006; 96(6):1626–35.
84. Hascup KN, Hascup ER, Pomerleau F, Huettl P, Gerhardt GA. Second-by-second measures of L-glutamate in the prefrontal cortex and striatum of freely moving mice. *J Pharmacol Exp Ther* 2008; 324(2):725–31.
85. Quintero JE, Day BK, Zhang Z, Grondin R, Stephens ML, Huettl P, *et al.* Amperometric measures of age-related changes in glutamate regulation in the cortex of rhesus monkeys. *Exp Neurol* 2007; 208(2):238–46.
86. Rutherford EC, Pomerleau F, Huettl P, Stromberg I, Gerhardt GA. Chronic second-by-second measures of L-glutamate in the central nervous system of freely moving rats. *J Neurochem* 2007; 102(3): 712–22.
87. Stephens ML, Pomerleau F, Huettl P, Gerhardt GA, Zhang Z. Real-time glutamate measurements in the putamen of awake rhesus monkeys using an enzyme-based human microelectrode array prototype. *J Neurosci Methods* 2010; 185(2):264–72.
88. Hascup KN, Rutherford EC, Quintero JE, Day BK, Nickell JR, Pomerleau F, *et al.* Second-by-second measures of L-glutamate and other neurotransmitters using enzyme-based microelectrode arrays. In: Michael AC, Borland LM (eds) *Electrochemical Methods for Neuroscience*, pp. 407–50. Boca Raton, FL: CRC Press, 2007.
89. Stephens ML, Spencer DD, Cavus I, Hsiao MC, Song D, Courellis SH, *et al.* Microelectrode-based epilepsy therapy: A hybrid neural prosthesis incorporating seizure prediction and intervention with biomemetic maintenance of normal hippocampal function. In: Soltesz I, Staley K (eds) *Computational Neuroscience in Epilepsy*. London: Academic Press, 2008.
90. Lynch JW. Molecular structure and function of the glycine receptor chloride channel. *Physiol Rev* 2004; 84(4):1051–95.
91. Xu TL, Gong N. Glycine and glycine receptor signaling in hippocampal neurons: diversity, function and regulation. *Prog Neurobiol* 2010; 91(4):349–61.
92. Applegarth DA, Toone JR. Glycine encephalopathy (nonketotic hyperglycinemia): comments and speculations. *Am J Med Genet A* 2006; 140(2):186–8.
93. Starr MS. The role of dopamine in epilepsy. *Synapse* 1996; 22(2): 159–94.
94. Haut SR, Albin RL. Dopamine and epilepsy: hints of complex subcortical roles. *Neurology* 2008; 71(11):784–5.
95. Bouilleret V, Semah F, Biraben A, Taussig D, Chassoux F, Syrota A, *et al.* Involvement of the basal ganglia in refractory epilepsy: an 18F-fluoro-L-DOPA PET study using 2 methods of analysis. *J Nucl Med* 2005; 46(3):540–7.
96. Bouilleret V, Semah F, Chassoux F, Mantzaridez M, Biraben A, Trebossen R, *et al.* Basal ganglia involvement in temporal lobe epilepsy: a functional and morphologic study. *Neurology* 2008; 70(3):177–84.
97. Lennox WG. The literature for 1945. *Epilepsia* 1946; 3:131–43.
98. Olney JW, de Gubareff T, Labruyere J. Seizure-related brain damage induced by cholinergic agents. *Nature* 1983; 301(5900):520–2.
99. Turski WA, Cavalheiro EA, Schwarz M, Czuczwar SJ, Kleinrok Z, Turski L. Limbic seizures produced by pilocarpine in rats: behavioural, electroencephalographic and neuropathological study. *Behav Brain Res* 1983; 9(3):315–35.
100. Vezzani A. Pilocarpine-induced seizures revisited: what does the model mimic? *Epilepsy Curr* 2009; 9(5):146–8.
101. Colom LV. Septal networks: relevance to theta rhythm, epilepsy and Alzheimer's disease. *J Neurochem* 2006; 96(3):609–23.
102. Berdiev RK, van Luijtelaar G. Cholinergic stimulation of the nucleus basalis of Meynert and reticular thalamic nucleus affects spike-and-wave discharges in WAG/Rij rats. *Neurosci Lett* 2009; 463(3):249–53.
103. Bertrand D. Neuronal Nicotinic Acetylcholine Receptors and Epilepsy. *Epilepsy Curr* 2002; 2(6):191–3.
104. Rogawski MA, Loscher W. The neurobiology of antiepileptic drugs. *Nat Rev Neurosci* 2004; 5(7):553–64.
105. Bagdy G, Kecskemeti V, Riba P, Jakus R. Serotonin and epilepsy. *J Neurochem* 2007; 100(4):857–73.
106. Krahl SE, Clark KB, Smith DC, Browning RA. Locus coeruleus lesions suppress the seizure-attenuating effects of vagus nerve stimulation. *Epilepsia* 1998; 39(7):709–14.
107. Giorgi FS, Pizzanelli C, Biagioni F, Murri L, Fornai F. The role of norepinephrine in epilepsy: from the bench to the bedside. *Neurosci Biobehav Rev* 2004; 28(5):507–24.
108. Ryan M, Baumann RJ. Use and monitoring of bromides in epilepsy treatment. *Pediatr Neurol* 1999; 21(2):523–8.

109. Balcar VJ, Erdo SL, Joo F, Kasa P, Wolff JR. Neurochemistry of GABAergic system in cerebral cortex chronically exposed to bromide in vivo. *J Neurochem* 1987; 48(1):167–9.
110. Beydoun A, D'Souza J, Hebert D, Doty P. Lacosamide: pharmacology, mechanisms of action and pooled efficacy and safety data in partial-onset seizures. *Expert Rev Neurother* 2009; 9(1):33–42.
111. Leach MJ, Marden CM, Miller AA. Pharmacological studies on lamotrigine, a novel potential antiepileptic drug: II. Neurochemical studies on the mechanism of action. *Epilepsia* 1986; 27(5):490–7.
112. Prakriya M, Mennerick S. Selective depression of low-release probability excitatory synapses by sodium channel blockers. *Neuron* 2000; 26(3):671–82.
113. Lukyanetz EA, Shkryl VM, Kostyuk PG. Selective blockade of N-type calcium channels by levetiracetam. *Epilepsia* 2002; 43(1):9–18.
114. Niespodziany I, Klitgaard H, Margineanu DG. Levetiracetam inhibits the high-voltage-activated Ca(2+) current in pyramidal neurones of rat hippocampal slices. *Neurosci Lett* 2001; 306(1–2):5–8.
115. Czuczwar P, Wojtak A, Cioczek-Czuczwar A, Parada-Turska J, Maciejewski R, Czuczwar SJ. Retigabine: the newer potential antiepileptic drug. *Pharmacol Rep* 2010; 62(2):211–19.
116. Fink-Jensen A, Suzdak PD, Swedberg MD, Judge ME, Hansen L, Nielsen PG. The gamma-aminobutyric acid (GABA) uptake inhibitor, tiagabine, increases extracellular brain levels of GABA in awake rats. *Eur J Pharmacol* 1992; 220(2–3):197–201.
117. Lynch BA, Lambeng N, Nocka K, Kensel-Hammes P, Bajjalieh SM, Matagne A, *et al.* The synaptic vesicle protein SV2A is the binding site for the antiepileptic drug levetiracetam. *Proc Natl Acad Sci U S A* 2004; 101(26):9861–6.
118. Rigo JM, Hans G, Nguyen L, Rocher V, Belachew S, Malgrange B, *et al.* The anti-epileptic drug levetiracetam reverses the inhibition by negative allosteric modulators of neuronal GABA- and glycine-gated currents. *Br J Pharmacol* 2002; 136(5):659–72.
119. Brodie MJ, Sills GJ. Combining antiepileptic drugs-Rational polytherapy? *Seizure* 2011; 20(5):369–75.
120. Sommerville KW. *Special issue: Gabitril (tiagabine HCl) receives FDA approval. Abbott Investigator Update*, pp. 1–6. Abbott Park, IL: Abbott Laboratories; 1997.
121. Dodrill CB, Arnett JL, Deaton R, Lenz GT, Sommerville KW. Tiagabine versus phenytoin and carbamazepine as add-on therapies: effects on abilities, adjustment, and mood. *Epilepsy Res* 2000; 42(2–3):123–32.
122. Sommerville KW. *Tiagabine (Gabitril): Best tolerated add-on to carbamazepine or phenytoin. Abbott Investigator Update*, pp. 1–6. Abbott Park, IL: Abbott Laboratories; 1998.
123. Sommerville KW. *Special issue: tiagabine (Gabitril) as first add-on (Study M92-825) Part II* ~ The final analysis. Abbott Investigator Update, pp. 1–6. Abbott Park, IL: Abbott Laboratories; 1998.
124. Ambrosio AF, Soares-Da-Silva P, Carvalho CM, Carvalho AP. Mechanisms of action of carbamazepine and its derivatives, oxcarbazepine, BIA 2-093, and BIA 2-024. *Neurochem Res* 2002; 27(1–2):121–30.

CHAPTER 4

Developmental Neurobiology, Neuroanatomy, and Neuropathology of Epilepsy

Ingmar Blümcke

Introduction

Histopathological brain abnormalities can be recognized in 93% of patients suffering from intractable focal seizures and submitted to epilepsy surgery treatment (Table 4.1). These numbers are similar to those obtained from earlier postmortem studies in primary and secondary generalized seizure disorders (1). In our hands, hippocampal sclerosis (synonyms: Ammon's horn sclerosis, mesial temporal sclerosis), long-term epilepsy associated glio-neuronal tumours (gangliogliomas, dysembryoplastic neuroepithelial tumours), and malformations of cortical development (e.g. focal cortical dysplasia, polymicrogyria) were most frequently encountered. Other lesions comprise vascular malformations (cavernomas, arteriovenous malformations), glial scars (ischaemic or traumatic brain injuries) or brain inflammation (Rasmussen encephalitis). In a small proportion (7%), thorough and systematic histomorphological analysis cannot identify a specific anatomical alteration.

The history of neuropathological studies in brains of patients with intractable epilepsy is, however, often characterized by a controversial debate concerning the primacy of structural abnormalities in seizure genesis. In this regard, only an interdisciplinary approach will be successful in identifying the 'epileptogenic potential' of distinct morphological alterations and should include clinical faculty as well as basic sciences. In this chapter, I will focus on our recent advance in classifying the morphological spectrum of focal cortical dysplasias (FCDs) and hippocampal sclerosis (HS). As both lesions are likely to result from insults compromising brain development and/or early postnatal maturation, anatomical data of neocortical and hippocampal development will also be included to comprehensively review and better understand the complex and

Table 4.1 Surgical specimens collected by the European Epilepsy Brain Bank

Entity	Var.	Number	Age OP	Hemisphere	Gender	Onset	Duration
HS		1591	34.6	659 L/611 R	786 M/805 F	11.5	23.3
DUAL		218	24.8	78 L/112 R	127 M/91 F	9.7	14.6
LEAT		1236	28.5	407 L/397 R	638 M/565 F	16.5	12.8
	GG	570	25.4	184 L/158 R	285 M/263 F	12.7	13.5
	DNT	189	26.3	59 L/68 R	105 M/84 F	15.2	12.3
Dysplasia		577	18.5	228 L/242 R	299 M/276 F	5.6	12.4
	FCD I	66	11.5	35 L/26 R	16 M/33 F	3.5	7.2
	FCD II	216	18.4	76 L/96 R	112 M/104 F	4.1	14.1
Vascular		271	36.4	91 L/108 R	157 M/114 F	23.5	13.4
Scars		239	25.2	92 L/91 R	147 M/90 F	10.3	14.8
Encephalitis		73	22.0	26 L/29 R	43 M/29 F	13.9	9.4
No lesion		307	29.2	117 L/58 R	161 M/146 F	12.7	16.1

All data were obtained from the European Epilepsy Brain Bank. Histopathological evaluation and clinical histories are as following: Var.: frequent variants of specific entities are highlighted; HS: hippocampal sclerosis; DUAL: dual pathologies; LEAT: long-term epilepsy associated tumours; GG: ganglioglioma; DNT: dysembryoplastic neuroepithelial tumour; FCD: focal cortical dysplasia; Age OP = age of patients at surgery (in years); Hemisphere: L (left), R (right); Gender: F = female, M = male; Onset = age at onset of spontaneous seizure activity (in years); Duration = duration of seizure disorder before surgical treatment (in years).

often diverse lesion patterns to be recognized. It will be a future task to deduce specific prognostic or predictive values from these pathology patterns and whether they will be helpful for diagnostic and treatment purposes in these difficult-to-treat epileptic disorders.

Neocortical pathology in focal epilepsies

Malformations of cortical development (MCDs) are increasingly recognized in patients suffering from intractable focal epilepsies (2). The histopathological spectrum of MCDs is large, ranging from prominent to only minute changes. Whereas schizencephalic brain lesions, hemimegalencephaly, polymicrogyria, nodular or band heterotopia can be reliably diagnosed *in vivo*, FCDs often escape imaging techniques (magnetic resonance imaging (MRI)) and may vary considerably in their size and localization (3). Hence, I will particularly focus on the peculiar histopathological aspects of FCD, either appearing as an isolated lesion within the cerebral hemisphere, or in conjunction with another principal lesion, i.e. HS, glio-neuronal tumour, or glial scarring.

The term 'focal cortical dysplasia (FCD)' was coined in 1971 by David Taylor and colleagues to describe localized malformative brain lesions in a series of 10 patients with drug-resistant epilepsy (4). Meanwhile, the term has also been applied to refer to a wide range of derangements of cortical anatomy and numerous classifications of these structural abnormalities have been proposed. Hence, the histopathological, clinical, and neuroradiological classification of these lesions remains difficult or even controversial. The most widely recognized classification system was published by Palmini et al. in 2004 (5). It was the report of an international working group, hence only a small contribution and recognition of neuropathology data was included. Unfortunately, this classification has not yielded a reliable prediction of proposed FCD variants and postsurgical seizure control (6). This applies in particular to so-called Type I FCDs. A recently published neuropathological study showed that inter- and intraobserver reproducibility of FCD Type I cases were in the range of only 50% when using the Palmini system (7). A Task Force of the International League Against Epilepsy (ILAE) was addressing this clinically important issue and redefined clinicopathological FCD subtypes (8, 9). The new 'ILAE FCD classification system 2011' (Table 4.2) also takes into account insights from experimental neurodevelopmental studies, i.e. sustained plasticity and neurogenesis in the postnatal brain, which is compromised by various pathogenic conditions. Similarly, the 'dysmature cerebral developmental hypothesis' suggested that there is partial failure in later phases of cortical development that might explain the distinctive histopathology of FCD and that local interactions of dysmature cells with normal postnatal neurons promote seizures (10).

Focal cortical dysplasia Type Ia

The ILAE classification system introduced this new FCD subtype, because it is likely representing a specific clinicopathological entity (11, 12). Patients are young and have early seizure onset, severe psycho-motor retardation, and mild hemispheric hypoplasia without magnetic resonance visibility of any other lesion (12, 13). Drug resistance is frequent and surgical resection procedures achieve seizure control in only 50% of affected children (14). However, brain surgery can be helpful as palliative strategy to reduce seizure burden, thereby accelerating developmental delay. Neuropathological hallmarks include abnormal cortical layering affecting both radial migration and maturation of neurons (Fig. 4.1G, H). This aberrant pattern resembles those neurodevelopmental minicolumns described by the 'radial unit lineage model' (15). Furthermore, cortical thickness is often decreased and recent MRI data confirmed a significantly smaller hemisphere ipsilateral to the ictal onset (12). In addition, neuronal cell density tended to be increased and neuronal body area decreased, which might point towards immaturity of the neuronal cells of these lesions. These findings are consistent with the recently introduced concept of postmigrational FCD (16). However, to date, there are no molecular-biological or genetic data available to clarify or even suggest the underlying pathomechanism in this difficult-to-treat-epileptic disorder. Recent studies addressed aberrant expression of layer-specific markers in FCD variants (17). Indeed, cortical tissue obtained from patients that would be classified to the new FCD Type Ia was characterized by abnormal expression of transcription factors *Tbr1* and *Otx1* in layer 2 and *Map1B* was abnormally expressed in vertical microcolumns. In addition, immature cell types (expressing *Otx1*, *Pax6*, and *Tbr2*) were also noted, suggesting activation of progenitor cell populations or a persisting immature phenotype. These data suggest that abundant vertical microcolumnar arrangements may result from severely compromised cortical maturation, in which neuroblasts that migrated along the radial glial scaffold into the cortex cannot equally distribute within their appropriate cortical layers.

To better understand this intriguing histomorphological phenotype, I will briefly review moving aspects of human cortical developmental referring mainly to the seminal work of Pasko Rakic and Vernon Mountcastle on the columnar organization of the human brain.

Table 4.2 ILAE consensus classification system for FCD

Isolated FCD Type I (Fig. 4.1)	FCD Ia: abnormal radial (vertical) cortical lamination	FCD Ib: abnormal tangential (horizontal) cortical lamination	FCD Ic: abnormal radial and tangential cortical lamination	
Isolated FCD Type II (Fig. 4.2)	FCD IIa: with dysmorphic neurons		FCD IIb: with dysmorphic neurons and balloon cells	
Associated FCD Type III (Fig. 4.3)	FCD IIIa: cortical lamination abnormalities in the temporal lobe associated with HS	FCD IIIb: cortical lamination abnormalities adjacent to a glial or glio-neuronal tumour	FCD IIIc: cortical lamination abnormalities adjacent to vascular malformation	FCD IIId: cortical lamination abnormalities adjacent to any other lesion acquired during early life

The three-tiered ILAE classification system of FCD distinguishes isolated forms (FCD Type I and II) from those associated with another principal lesion, i.e. hippocampal sclerosis (FCD Type IIIa), tumours (FCD Type IIIb), vascular malformations (FCD Type IIIc), or lesions acquired during early life (i.e. traumatic injury, ischemic injury or encephalitis, FCD Type IIId).

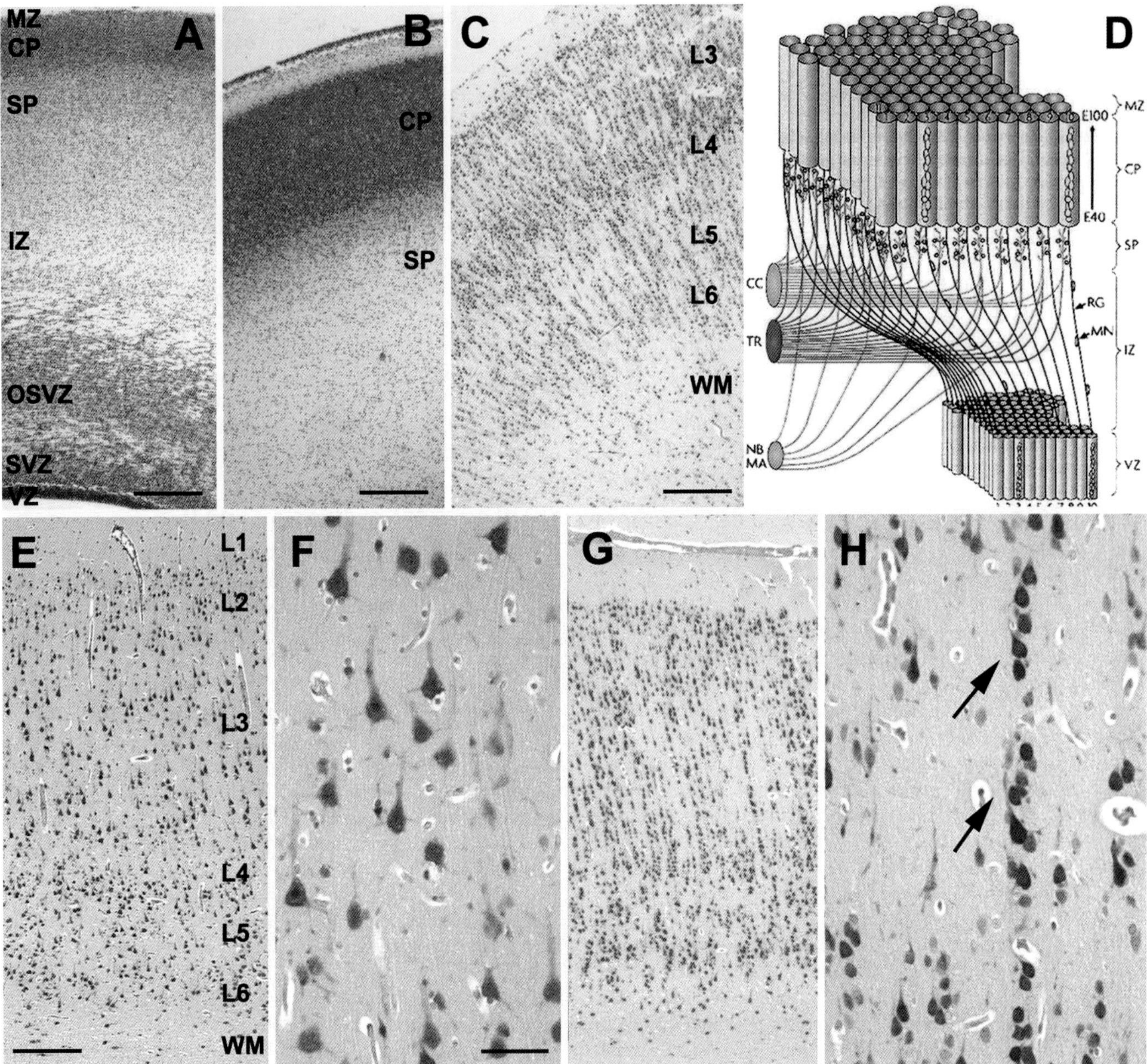

Fig. 4.1 (See also Colour plate 1.) FCD Type Ia compared to normal development and anatomy of the human neocortex. A) The developing human neocortex reviewed at 17th week of gestation (WoG). Cortical neurons (stained purple by thionine) arise from radial glial cells, the epithelial stem cells that line the ventricle. Radial glial cells in the ventricular zone (VZ) generate intermediate progenitor cells that migrate into the subventricular zone (SVZ). The outer subventricular zone (OSVZ) is massively expanding at this time period and most likely contribute to the evolutionary advance underlying cortical size and complexity in human brain (21). CP, cortical plate; IZ, intermediate zone; MZ, marginal zone; SP, subcortical plate (also see (D)). B) Expansion of the cortical plate at 19th WoG. Migrating neurons follow an inside-out pattern forming different pyramidal cell layers. C) The hexalaminar cortical architecture is fully developed in the premature brain (35th WoG), with prominent radial (vertical) columnar arrangements still being visible (4 µm thin paraffin sections were used for all preparations shown here). Note the similarity with a surgical specimens obtained from a 15-year-old child with epilepsy and FCD Type Ia (G–H). D) This well-recognized model of radial neuronal migration that underlies cortical organization is based on (20). The cohorts of neurons generated in the VZ traverse IZ and SP, containing 'waiting' afferents from several sources (cortico-cortical connections (CC), thalamic radiation (TR), nucleus basalis (NB), monoamine subcortical centers (MA)), and finally pass through the earlier generated deep layers before setting in at the interface between the cortical plate (CP) and marginal zone (MZ). MN, migrating neurons; RG, radial glial cell. E–F) Adult human temporal neocortex (NeuN immunohistochemistry). Scale bar in E = 200 µm (applies also to G); in F = 50 µm (applies also to (H)). G–H) Fifteen-year-old child with drug-resistant epilepsy and severe psycho-motor retardation. Seizure onset was recorded from only one hemisphere and histopathological analysis revealed persistent vertical microcolumns in the temporal and occipital lobe specimen. Note that neurons are also significantly smaller (arrow in (H)), compared to controls shown in (F). NeuN immunohistochemistry.

Columnar organization of the neocortex

The six-layered human neocortex is a convoluted ribbon with a surface area of approximately 2600 mm^2, and 3–4 mm thickness. It contains up to 28×10^9 neurons and a similar amount of glial cells (18). The earliest event in the formation of the neocortex is the generation of a horizontal layer called the preplate, composed of a superficial sublayer of the earliest corticopetal nerve fibres, and the earliest generated neurons. These are the Cajal–Retzius cells and a lower layer of cells that will become the subplate. Subsequent waves of migrating neurons form the cortical plate in an inside to outside temporal sequence creating future layers VI–II of the mature neocortex (19). This general pattern of migration and cortical plate formation has been observed in a number of mammalian species, and is particularly pronounced in primates. The cortical plate is inserted into the preplate, splitting it into an outermost marginal zone, the future layer I, and a lower, thick, and partially transient band called the subplate (Fig. 4.1A). Neurons migrating to the neocortex move along radial glial fibres that form palisades linking the neural epithelium and the developing cortical plate (20). The time of generation of a neuron determines its final laminar (vertical) position in the mature cortex. It is probable that humans acquire their full complement of neocortical neurons during the 2nd trimester.

The basic unit of the mature neocortex is the 'minicolumn', a narrow chain of neurons extending vertically across the cellular layers II–VI, perpendicular to the pial surface (18). Each minicolumn in primates contains 80–100 neurons, except for the striate cortex where the number is 2.5 times larger. Minicolumns contain all the major cortical neural cell phenotypes, interconnected in the vertical dimension. The minicolumn is produced by the iterative division of a small cluster of progenitor cells in the neuroepithelium or is derived from neurogenic radial glia in the intermediate zone (21, 22). A cortical column is a complex processing and distributing unit that links a number of inputs to a number of outputs via overlapping internal processing chains. Cortical efferent neurons with different extrinsic targets are partially segregated; those of layers II/III project to other cortical areas, those of layers V/VI to subcortical structures. The most widely studied columnar organization is that of the visual cortex (23), confirming preferential input to neighbouring 'ocular dominance columns' by stimuli delivered to one or the other eye.

There are two broad classes of cortical neurons that differ in their mode of migration, morphology, and functional characteristics. They also originate from different embryonic areas. Projection neurons (glutamatergic excitatory) extend axons to distant targets and are generated from progenitors of the neocortical germinal zone (located in the dorsolateral wall of the telencephalon). Inhibitory interneurons (gamma-aminobutyric acid (GABA)ergic) are those that make local connections and are primarily generated from progenitors in the ganglionic eminence, the primordium of the future basal ganglia, located in the ventral forebrain. The cells generated in the ganglionic eminence follow a long tangential migratory route to reach the cortical plate and form the majority of non-pyramidal neurons (i.e. cortical interneurons). While neocortical cells born in the ventricular zone utilize radial glia as scaffold to migrate to the developing cortical plate, tangentially migrating neurons move in close association with axons of the corticofugal fibre system (24). All these neurons will be located in distinct layers at the end of corticogenesis, and a growing body of evidence suggests that most essential features of cortical neurons, and differences between them, are programmed genetically during development. The gene expression profiles that define neuronal properties are broadly controlled by transcription factors, which activate or repress the transcription of a multitude of downstream genes.

Focal cortical dysplasia Type Ib and Ic

The 2011 ILAE classification of FCD further specifies cortical lamination abnormalities that affect horizontal layering (FCD Ib) or both vertical and horizontal layering (FCD Ic). As for all new FCD Type I variants, they should occur as an isolated feature and not be associated with any other structural brain lesion (described later in the chapter). To the best of my knowledge, FCD Type Ib or Ic are very rare and there is still no systematic analysis available characterizing clinically phenotypes, aetiology, or pathogenesis.

Focal cortical dysplasia Type II

It becomes evident from the aforementioned anatomical and developmental data that any (genetic or environmental) insult during early time windows and involving one or more of the leading neurodevelopmental processes of corticogenesis, will determine cortical malformation and thus predispose the affected brain to enhanced seizure susceptibility. The most prominent and better studied example is that of FCD Type II (Fig. 4.2), which is characterized as cortical malformation with an almost complete disruption of lamination (with the exception of layer 1). In addition, distinct cytological abnormalities are present, which differentiate nowadays FCD Type IIa (dysmorphic neurons without balloon cells) from FCD Type IIb (dysmorphic neurons and balloon cells). Dysmorphic neurons were likely to be first described by Crome (25). They are morphologically the same in both Type II variants and microscopically characterized by severe abnormalities. Neuronal cell diameters and cell nucleus diameter are significantly enlarged, Nissl substance is aggregated and displaced towards the cell membrane, and phosphorylated and non-phosphorylated neurofilament isoforms accumulate in their cytoplasm (Fig. 4.2). In the centre of the lesion, dysmorphic neurons cluster in large aggregates. They are distributed throughout the cortical thickness and dislocate also into the white matter. However, distant from the core of the main lesion, isolated dysmorphic neurons can also be observed. In addition, multiple FCD Type II lesions have been recognized and individually contribute to seizure generation (26). Balloon cells are the distinguishing hallmark of FCD Type IIb. They present with a large cell body and opalescent glassy eosinophilic cytoplasm (using haematoxylin and eosin (H&E) stain), which lacks Nissl substance. Multiple nuclei are often present. Balloon cells can occur at any cortical location (including layer 1) and are often found in the underlying white matter. Balloon cells commonly accumulate intermediate filaments vimentin and nestin, which can be used as histopathological markers (27, 28). Balloon cells have gross histomorphological similarities with giant cells, and can be observed in cortical tubers from patients with tuberous sclerosis complex (TSC). The TSC1/TSC2 signalling pathway (including insulin growth factor receptor and mTOR) is, therefore, a promising candidate pathomechanism for FCD Type II (29, 30).

Determination of characteristic molecular genetic alterations for specific FCD variants will further advance our clinicopathological classification system and help to identify molecular pathways with potential therapeutic relevance. As a matter of fact, the mTOR inhibitor rapamycin, and its derivative everolimus, have recently been shown beneficial for tumour reduction in TSC patients and likely translate also into drug treatment of epilepsies (31).

As children and adolescents frequently develop drug resistance and surgical resection offers complete seizure control in up to 80% of all patients (6), high-resolution imaging is an important tool for clinical management of patients with FCD Type II. Indeed, most FCD Type IIb lesions can be detected by presurgical MRI. They usually present with a 'transmantle sign' in FLAIR (fluid attenuated inversion recovery) sequences (28, 32). In contrast, FCD Type IIa lesions are less clearly visible by structural MRI but may be detectable using specialized post-processing protocols (9). In addition, a distinctive pattern of repetitive, high amplitude, fast spikes, followed by high amplitude slow waves, interspersed with relatively flat periods can be detected in FCD Type IIb. During drowsiness and slow sleep, fast spikes become more prominent, increase in frequency and tend to spread into contiguous non-lesional areas (33). During REM sleep, there is a marked decrease in these electrical abnormalities.

Focal cortical dysplasia type III

This entity is newly introduced into the ILAE FCD classification system and refers to a compilation of cortical abnormalities associated with and adjacent to another principal lesion (Fig. 4.3). A most prominent example refers to FCD Type IIIa encountered in mesial temporal lobe epilepsy (MTLE) patients with hippocampal sclerosis (formerly classified mostly as FCD Type Ia in Palmini's system (5)). This diagnosis was probably very much fostered by abnormal anterior temporal lobe white matter signal changes detectable by MRI as well as from ictogenic EEG patterns evolving independent from hippocampal location. Yet, not all patients showed histomorphologically confirmed and approved FCDs. Thom et al. suggested, that one easy to recognize FCD Type IIIa variant should be termed 'temporal lobe sclerosis' (TLS), as its pathogenesis is reactive rather than malformative (34). This hypothesis is supported by recent findings from Garbelli et al. using high-resolution 7T MRI in the temporal lobe in HS patients (35). They suggest the origin of abnormal white matter intensities (accompanied by anterior temporal lobe atrophy) in MTLE-HS patterns to derive from punctate myelin loss being of reactive/degenerative nature rather than malformative. The very similar postoperative seizure control in patients with a principal lesion, compared to those without any associated FCD, further argue against an independent origin and pathogenesis (14). However, a total of four subtypes have been proposed by the new ILAE classification system (Table 4.2): FCD Type IIIa, when associated with hippocampal sclerosis; FCD Type IIIb, when associated with tumours; FCD Type IIIc, when associated with vascular malformations; and FCD Type IIId when associated with any other principal lesion acquired during early life. Early head injury, bleeding, or inflammation are amongst the most frequent causes for FCD Type IIId. The new FCD category has not yet been clinically well described, although many patients were included in cohorts of previously published Palmini FCD Type I series (6).

The hippocampal formation

The anatomy of the human hippocampus has a long and controversial history since its first description by Julius Caesar Arantius in 1587, who was a pupil of the famous Italian anatomist Andreas Vesalius (36). Arantius compared the anatomical elevations within the inferior horn of the lateral ventricles with that of a seahorse (genus *Hippocampus*), with the animal's head pointing either to the third ventricle or the anterior part of the temporal lobe. This controversy was further promoted by another term introduced by de Garengoet in 1742. He compared the mesial view of the hippocampus with the Ammon's horn adopted from the Egyptian god Ammun Kneph (36, 37). It is the pyramidal cell layer of the various hippocampal subregions that is microscopically recognized as cornu ammonis (CA areas) these days and, indeed, also resembles a ram's horn (Fig. 4.4). The anatomical classification of hippocampal subfields is no less contradictory with many classification systems available. This may also result from differences between rodent and human hippocampus. The classification introduced by Lorente de No in 1934 is mostly used, designating four hippocampal sectors, namely CA1 to CA4 (38). The transition areas between CA1 and subiculum or between the CA3–CA4 regions remain, however, difficult to clarify using routine staining techniques.

The hippocampus is a main constituent of the allocortex (39). It is situated in the mesial temporal lobe and occupies the floor of the inferior horn of the lateral ventricle from the level of the corpus amygdaloideum up to the splenium of the corpus callosum. Three major parts can be distinguished: the dentate gyrus (or fascia dentata), the cornu ammonis, and the subiculum. The dentate gyrus consists of three laminae: the molecular layer, the granular layer, and an ill-defined plexiform layer. Small nerve cells usually referred to as 'granule cells' dominate in the dentate gyrus. The perikarya of granule cells assemble tightly together and form a clear-cut band. The basal tip of the soma shows a distinct axon hillock from which a relatively thick axon is generated which enters the cornu ammonis and forms synaptic contacts with the pyramids of the 3rd and the 4th sector (mossy fibre system). The apical dendrites ramify within the molecular layer and received topographically restricted efferents from the collateral hippocampus and ipsilateral tractus perforans. The granule cell layer is functionally regarded as 'gate keeper' of the hippocampus, as it receives the majority of axonal input. A helpful and interactive overview of the parahippocampal–hippocampal network is presented in van Strien et al. (40).

Hippocampal neuropathology in MTLE

The human hippocampus is particularly prone to generate seizures and to perpetuate chronic focal temporal lobe epilepsies (TLEs). The end stage of the disease often results in a pathomorphological pattern recognized as hippocampal sclerosis (HS; synonym Ammon's horn sclerosis, Table 4.1). In HS patients, diagnostic MRI protocols (T2, FLAIR) prove severe atrophy of the affected hippocampus and histopathological examination of surgical resections identifies segmental neuronal cell loss in the pyramidal cell layer of the cornu ammonis, most dramatically affecting CA1 and CA4 (41, 42). In a large series of 3311 patients suffering from TLE, HS can be identified in 48%. Within our entire cohort of 4512 epilepsy patients undergoing surgical resection for various aetiologies, HS was recognized in 35.2%, with 5% presenting as dual pathology,

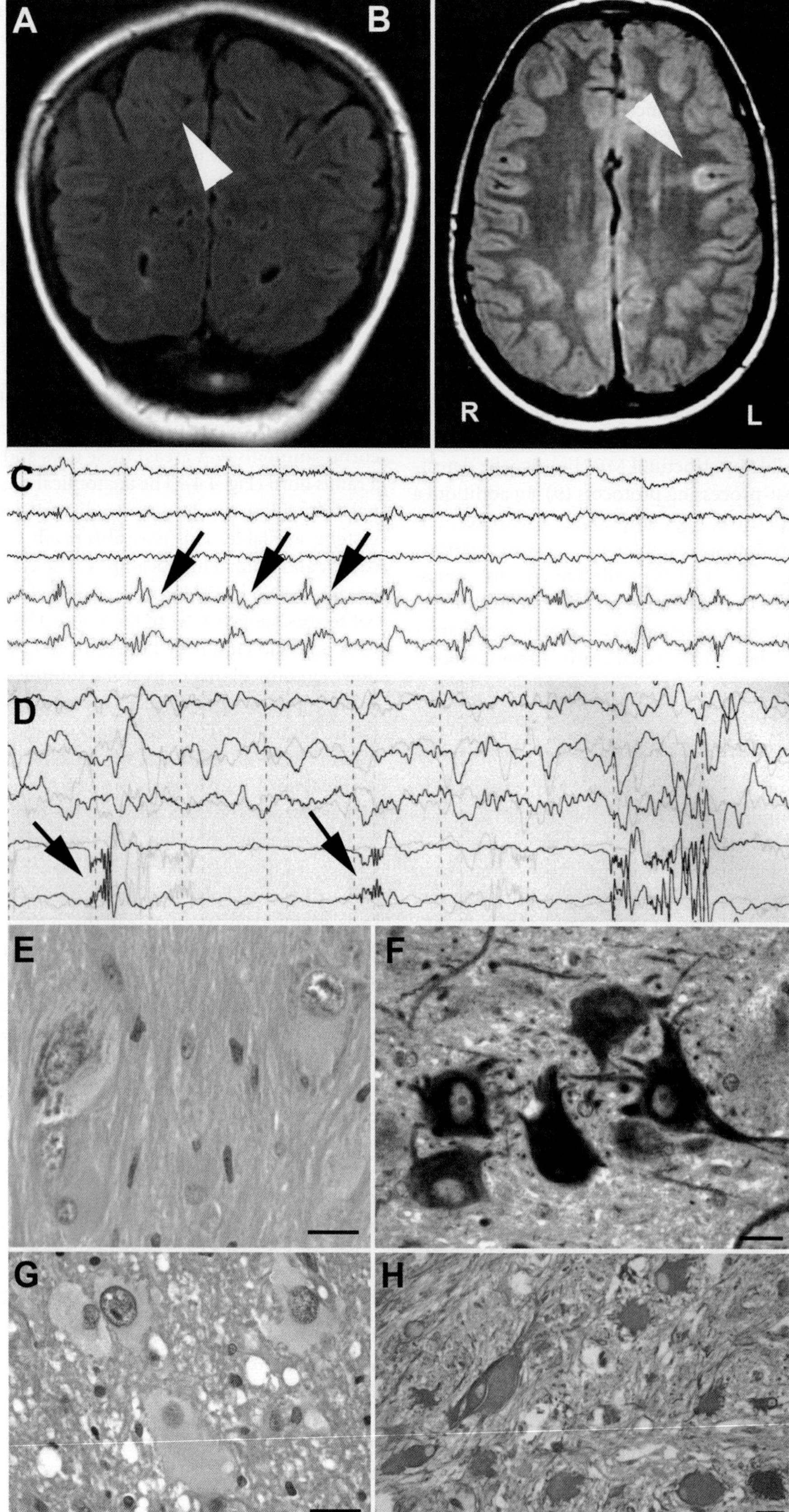

Fig. 4.2 (See also Colour plate 2.) Clinicopathological findings in FCD Type II. A) FCD Type IIa in an 18-year-old female patient with refractory seizures from age 5 years, that would start with sensory disturbance in the left foot. Coronal T2 FLAIR did not reveal definitely abnormal signal intensities, which is often reported for FCD Type IIa. Indeed, histopathological inspection showed characteristic hallmarks of FCD Type IIa (see (E) and (F)) in surgical specimen obtained from the indicated brain region (arrowhead). MRI figure kindly provided by Dr Duncan (London, UK). B) Proton density imaging reveals a hyperintense signal change in the left frontal lobe of the patient with drug-resistant seizures, tapering from the depth of the gyrus towards the ventricle ('transmantle sign', arrowhead). C) Interictal EEG recording from the scalp surface of the patient shown in (B). Arrows point to characteristic 'brushes', which can be often recognized in patients with FCD Type IIB. D) The peculiar electrographic pattern ('brushes') becomes more evident when recording is obtained from depth electrodes implanted into the lesion (patient with histopathologically confirmed FCD Type IIB). (C) and (D) were kindly provided by Dr Spreafico (Milan, Italy). E–F) Dysmorphic neurons revealed by HE (E), or neurofilament immunostaining (SMI311 (F)) are typical findings in FCD Type IIa and IIb. G–H) Balloon cells revealed by HE (H), or vimentin immunostaining (H) can be seen only in FCD Type IIb. Scale bars in (E)–(H) = 20 μm.

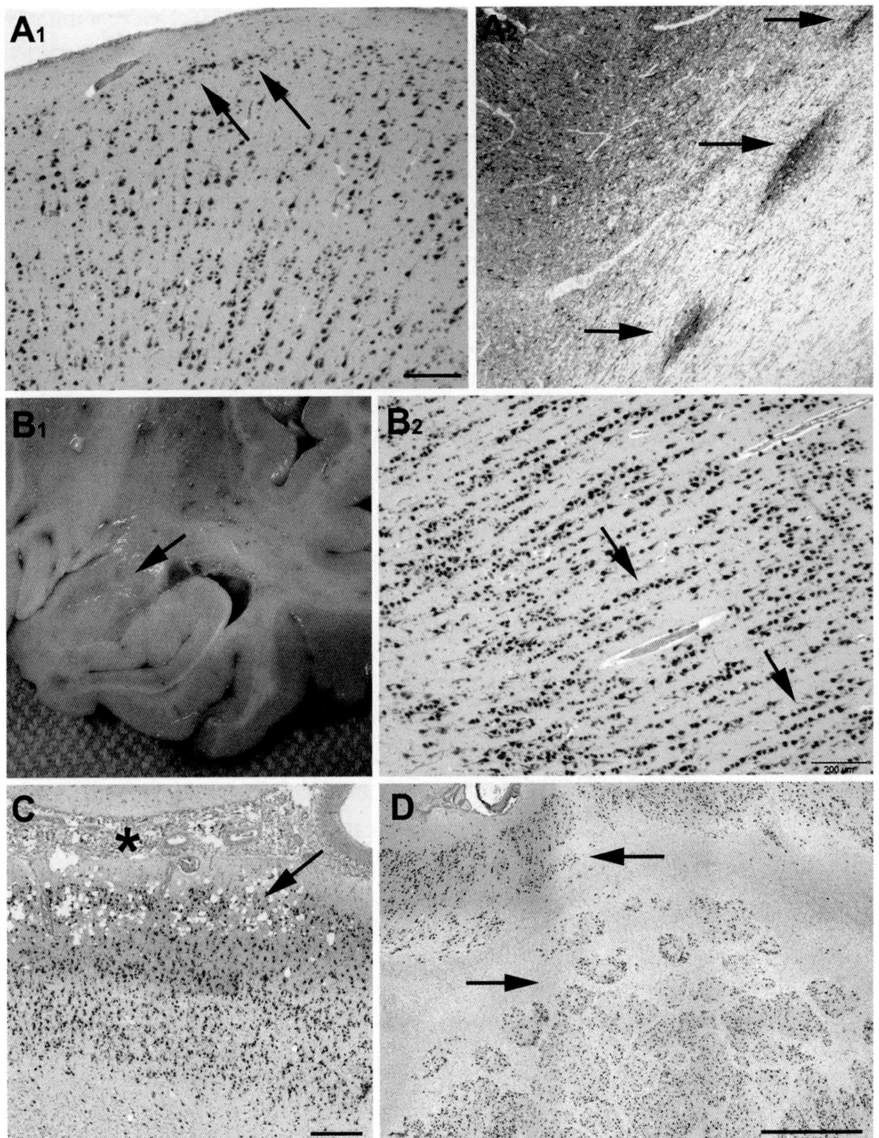

Fig. 4.3 (See also Colour plate 3.) Associated FCDs Type III. A1) This abnormal pattern of superficial cortical lamination (arrows) was associated with hippocampal sclerosis in an MTLE patient and should be diagnosed as FCD Type IIIa. It is similar to that described by Thom et al. as temporal lobe sclerosis (34). Scale bar = 200 μm (applies also to (A2) and (B2)). Another characteristic FCD Type IIIa pattern is that of heterotopic 'lentiform' neuronal islets in the white matter of the temporal lobe in MTLE-HS patients (A2). B1) Dysembryoplastic neuroepithelial tumour of the right mesial temporal lobe. Courtesy of Dr Macaulay (Halifax, Canada). B2) Persisting vertical microcolumns can be observed in the vicinity of long-term epilepsy associated tumours and should be diagnosed as FCD Type IIIb. C) Leptomeningeal vascular malformations (asterisk) usually associate with abnormal lamination in adjacent neocortex (FCD Type IIIc) marked by an arrow. D) These massive cortical lamination abnormalities were registered adjacent to a glial scar (acquired by perinatal head trauma) and classify as FCD Type IIId. Such lesions can be progressive in nature and were first described by Marin-Padilla et al. in 2002 (93).

i.e. in combination with tumours or scars. Although the pathogenesis of HS remains to be identified, clinical histories follow a characteristic schedule in most patients. Approximately 50% of patients suffered from an 'initial precipitating injury' before the age of 4 years (41). In this cohort, complex febrile seizures are the most frequently noted events. Birth trauma, head injury, or meningitis were other early childhood lesions observed in TLE patients. The mean age at onset of spontaneous complex partial seizures is 11.5 years (43). As a matter of fact, structural, molecular, or functional analysis can usually not be obtained at this early and clinically silent period and the diagnosis of HS is verified after a long period of unsuccessful antiepileptic medication. The mean age at the time of surgery is 34.6 years with a history of epileptic seizures for 23.3 years. As in most other series reported so far, both genders were equally affected and a family history of TLE was very rare indicating that hereditary factors do not play a major role in HS associated TLE.

HS is characterized at the histopathological level by segmental pyramidal cell loss in CA1 (Sommer's sector), CA3, and CA4, whereas CA2 pyramidal and dentate gyrus granule cells are more seizure resistant (44). Notwithstanding, several interneuronal cell populations are also affected, i.e. neuropeptide Y- and somatostatin-immunoreactive interneurons and/or mossy cells in the CA4 sector (45, 46). Neuronal cell loss is invariably associated with reactive astrogliosis, which results in stiffening of the tissue and established the traditional term of 'Ammon's horn sclerosis' (44). An intriguing question relates to the mechanisms of selective neuronal vulnerability between these morphologically similar neuronal cell populations. This topic is a matter of ongoing studies and will not be further discussed. Major pathomechanisms include, besides many others, abnormal neuronal circuitries (aberrant mossy fibre sprouting) (47), and molecular rearrangement/plasticity of ion channel and neurotransmitter receptor expression (29, 48).

Clinical studies assume MTLE as a heterogenic entity with different aetiologies and clinical histories (49–51). Hence, neuropathological investigations describe different patterns of neuronal cell loss within hippocampal subfields and adjacent temporal lobe structures (46, 52, 53). An intriguing issue is, therefore, to identify determining factors on hippocampal pathology patterns. A reliable neuropathological classification system will be helpful to separate distinct pathological subgroups and to better predict postsurgical seizure control. We have recently proposed a clinicopathological classification system for hippocampal cell loss in MTLE patients (54). Five distinct patterns were recognized (Table 4.3), which associated with specific clinical histories or a probability for postsurgical seizure control (54, 55).

The largest group of HS cases presents with a classical or severe pattern of segmental neuronal cell loss affecting CA1, CA3, and CA4 (Table 4.3; Fig. 4.4). There are, however, considerable similarities between HS Type 1a (classical pattern) and 1b (severe pattern). It is the degree of CA3 and CA2 pyramidal cell loss which makes the difference. This distinction is reasonably similar to Wyler scores W3 and W4 (52). Correlation with clinical data pointed to an early age of preceding events (<3 years) as important predictor of classical and severe hippocampal pathology pattern.

Two atypical variants are characterized either by severe neuronal loss restricted to sector CA1 (HS Type 2) or to CA4 (HS Type 3). In HS Type 2, preceding events were documented at a later age (mean 6 years), whereas in HS Type 3 and normal appearing hippocampus (no HS) the first event appeared beyond the age of 13 and 16 years, respectively.

The proposed HS classification system allows some prediction of postsurgical outcome (54, 55). The most favourable outcome was achieved in patients presenting with HS Type 1a and HS Type 1b (> 83% seizure freedom), whereas only half of patients with atypical HS patterns (Type 2 and Type 3) became seizure free. However, this classification system will need further confirmation in independent patient cohorts to assess its interobserver reliability. Meanwhile, Thom and colleagues published another HS classification system describing similar cell loss patterns (56). Differences with respect to postsurgical outcome need, however, clarification.

Despite electrophysiological evidence for mesial temporal lobe generation of seizures, a cohort of approximately 20% of MTLE cases do not show microscopical features of neuronal cell loss (54) and cell density measurements were not significantly different from age-matched autopsy controls (10% difference in neuronal cell densities, either up or down, are obtained already by standard deviation from human control values!). We designated this group as 'no hippocampal sclerosis (no HS)'. This observation has been frequently reported in neuropathological surveys of similar HS series (41, 42). The epileptogenic pathomechanisms of hippocampal seizure generation remains to be further determined, but is suggested to be similar to kindling in animal TLE models.

Table 4.3 Neuropathological grading scale of hippocampal sclerosis

	Pattern of neuronal loss[a] and gliosis (complete samples)				
DG[b]	0–2	1–2	0–2	0–2	0–1
CA4	1–2	2	0	1–2	0
CA3	0–1	2	0	0–1	0
CA2	0–1	1–2	0	0	0
CA1	2	2	1–2	0	0
Class	Type 1a[c]	Type 1b[c]	Type 2[c]	Type 3[c]	No HS[c]

Semiquantitative microscopic examination based on formalin-fixed, paraffin-embedded surgical specimen (4–7 μm section thickness), H&E, CV/LFB, NeuN (recommended), and GFAP stainings. Grading scale is defined as following: 0 = no obvious neuronal loss or gliosis only; 1 = neuronal loss or gliosis (GFAP) but moderate or patchy; 2 = severe neuronal loss (majority of neurons) and fibrillary gliosis.

[a] Please note limitations of visual inspection as first visible sign of cell loss is usually 30–40% cell loss (H&E stains, shown by quantified neuronal density measurements). Quantitative methods will be more reliable for scoring.

[b] Granule cell layer is normal (score = 0), dispersed (score 1; can be focal), or shows severe granule cell loss (score 2; can be focal).

[c] If surgical specimen is anatomically well-preserved (en bloc resection recommended).

Dentate gyrus pathology in TLE patients

It remains an intriguing observation, that dentate granule cell loss significantly associates with deficient memory acquisition and recall in TLE patients (57–59). Indeed, the population of dentate granule cells is pathologically affected in the majority of HS patients. Lesional patterns in this anatomical distinct compartment range from granule cell dispersion (GCD), which occurs in almost 50% of patients (59) to severe cell loss in HS Type 1a and 1b (Fig. 4.4). Neuropathological criteria for granule cell alterations include increased granule cell lamination above 10 layers with smaller perikarya and larger intercellular gaps, as well as ectopic cluster and bilamination into the molecular layer. Since grading scales for granule cell pathology are not yet internationally standardized, clinicopathological studies yielded complementary but also controversial results (59–63).

Our current understanding of these intriguing pathology patterns were much influenced from developmental neurobiology studies of the dentate gyrus and its propensity to generate neurons throughout life. Assembly of the granule cell layer follows different migration streams building first its internal limb (Fig. 4.4A), from which newly generated granule cells progressively expand into lateral direction, thus forming the external limb (64). Most intriguingly, the neurogenic capacity of the dentate gyrus maintains throughout life, also in human brain (65). Within the adult mammalian hippocampus, multipotent precursor cells have been characterized in the dentate gyrus, residing directly below the granule cell layer (66). These cells proliferate upon diverse functional and molecular stimuli, generate migratory neuroblasts, and further differentiate into granule cells upon migration into the dentate gyrus (67, 68). Migratory guidance is provided by a scaffold of radial glial cells within the dentate gyrus as well as from Reelin molecules secreted by Cajal–Retzius cells (69–71). Newborn granule cells

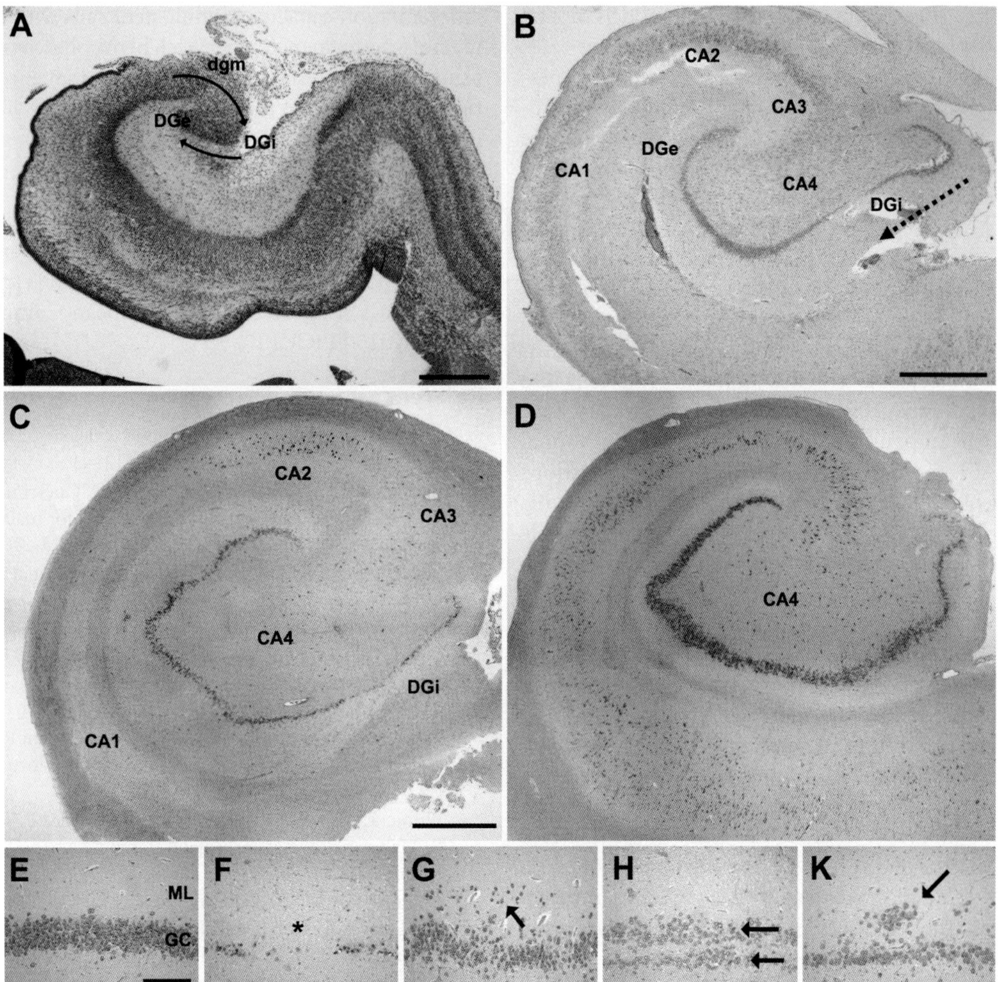

Fig. 4.4 (See also Colour plate 4.) Microscopic anatomy of the developing human hippocampus and in MTLE patients with hippocampal sclerosis. A) Human hippocampal development at 17th WoG. Scale bar = 500 µm. The figure should also illustrate the particular development of the dentate gyrus, which retains its neurogenic propensity throughout life. The dentate gyrus matrix is bending through the dentate notch and form the internal limb (DGi). From here, newly generated granule cells were continuously integrated and form the external limb (DGe) (64). B) Human hippocampus at birth (42nd WoG). Scale bar = 1 mm (applies also to (C) and (D)). All hippocampal sectors were clearly visible (CA1–4). The term 'hilus' should be restricted to the rodent hippocampus, and is not defined by Lorente de No (38). The same applies for the term 'endfolium', which is not a proper anatomical terminology for this region. The dashed line should indicate that the DGi is likely the portion of the DG maintaining its neurogenic capacity throughout life. C) Severe hippocampal sclerosis (HS Type 1b, Table 4.3) in an adult patient with febrile seizures at age 3 years and onset of spontaneous recurrent and drug-resistant seizures since his 14th year of life. NeuN immunohistochemistry with haematoxylin counterstaining (4 µm thin paraffin embedded section; applies to all images shown here). Note that restricted cell loss in DGi, compared to the mid portion or DG3 area. Experimental data has shown that this patterns correlates with the patient's ability to store and recall memory with this isolated hippocampus/hemisphere (Wada-testing; (58)). D) A patient with limbic encephalitis and late onset of her MTLE. The surgical specimen showed restricted cell loss within the CA4 region. This rare pattern is classified as atypical HS (Type 3, Table 4.3). E) Normal appearance of the human dentate gyrus with densely packed granule cells and sharp borders to subgranular and molecular layers (10× magnification, bar = 100µm, refers also to (F)–(K)). F) Granule cell pathology with significant granule cell loss indicated by thinning of dentate gyrus and cell free gaps (asterisk). G) Granule cell dispersion with spreading of granule cells into the molecular layer (arrow): H) Bilaminar architecture of the granule cell layer (arrows). K) granule cell dispersion with spreading of granule cell clusters into the molecular layer (arrow), as described by (62). GC, granule cell layer; ML, molecular layer.

functionally integrate into the trisynaptic hippocampal pathway (72–74), expand dendrites into the molecular layer and axonal collaterals into the CA3 region (mossy fibres), where they form synaptic connections on large excrescences of pyramidal neurons within stratum lucidum (75). The time period from proliferation to functional integration has been estimated in the range of 4 weeks in adult rodents, although maturation of newborn neurons extends over several months (74). In the mouse, axons reach the CA3 region about 2 weeks after neurogenesis (76). In adult rats, the number of newborn hippocampal neurons per day has been estimated to approximate 9000 or 250,000 per month, respectively (77), while cell proliferation in humans is likely to be much lower (78). The number of new and functionally integrated neurons is, however, challenged by apoptosis and most newborn cells die within 1–2 weeks after their birth (79).

The obvious association between HS and GCD leads to the hypothesis, that newly built granule cells aberrantly integrate into the dentate gyrus and disturb the trisynaptic hippocampal pathway, thereby increasing seizure susceptibility (80). Recurrent mossy fibre sprouting (mossy fibres are axonal projections of granule cells) has long been recognized in animal models of TLE (81) as well as in surgical human hippocampal specimens (82). Indeed, seizure-induced granule cell neurogenesis and/or dispersion may then represent a major pathomechanism underlying hippocampal seizure activity (80). Further studies on this intriguing topic challenged this assumption. Irradiation of hippocampal precursor cells did not abolish mossy fibre sprouting after experimental induction of status epilepticus (83), and fostered the discussion on the relevance of neurogenesis to architectural abnormalities within the epileptogenic hippocampus and to the aetiology of TLEs (84). However, newborn granule cells not only anatomically and functionally integrate into the granule cell layer (as destined) or ectopically into the molecular layer (GCD) but also ectopically into CA4 (85). Ectopic granule cells at the CA4/CA3 boundary have been first identified and functionally characterized in animal models for TLE (86). Using immunohistochemical preparations for *Prox-1*, a homeobox gene specifically expressed in postmitotic dentate granule cells (68), a significant number of ectopic granule cells can now be reliably recognized in rat models as well as human surgical specimens (85). These findings are compatible with the notion that aberrant anatomical organization of the epileptic hippocampus contribute to increased seizure susceptibility and that neurogenesis is critically involved in this process. The majority of findings points to a predominately young age of seizure-induced neurogenesis, which contributes to aberrant network integration and seizure progression. The decreased propensity of neurogenesis in chronic TLE stages, whether reflecting a depletion or exhaustion of the precursor cell pool (87), would rather result in the well-recognized cell loss patterns and severe cognitive deterioration (57). This hypothesis is in good agreement with a recently proposed pathogenic model on the 'two faces' of seizure-related neurogenesis in human TLE (84).

The hippocampus serves a major role in all aspects of conscious, declarative memory, i.e. semantic memory for facts and concepts, episodic memory, and spatial memory (88). Notwithstanding, bilateral damage of both hippocampi induces profound anterograde amnesia in humans. (89). Neuropsychological lesion studies, functional imaging in humans, as well as experimental animal models linked memory function particularly with the dentate gyrus (90). Thus, standardized cognitive evaluation programmes in epilepsy patients submitted to surgical treatment offer the unique opportunity to study such higher brain function in humans. Evidence has already been achieved pointing to the impact of dentate granule cell neurogenesis on learning and behaviour in rodents (91, 92). We have studied this issue in human hippocampus obtained from epilepsy surgery. Comparing memory performance (tested by amobarbital anaesthesia (Wada test) in patients subsequently submitted to surgical resection of either the left or right hippocampus) with the extent of hippocampal cell loss within the internal limb identified granule cell density as most significant predictor accounting for 78% of the total memory capacity in an individual patient (57). It 'suggestively' points to neurogenesis as neurobiological substrate of memory acquisition (rather than seizure aetiology) and that a run-down of the neurogenic propensity in chronic seizure disorders compromises higher cognitive brain function. Indeed, we experimentally confirmed this hypothesis when isolating, proliferating, and differentiating adult human stem cells from the dentate gyrus of TLE patients with HS (58). There was a highly significant correlation between the proliferation and differentiation capacity of adult stem cells with the same patient's memory performance, when each hemisphere was tested separately using the Wada test. Our results suggest that encoding new memories is also related to the regenerative capacity of the hippocampus in the human brain.

Acknowledgements

The author is grateful to Drs Angelika Mühlebner (Wien/Erlangen) and Roland Coras (Milan/Erlangen) for their critical comments. The work is supported by the European Community (LSH-CT-2006-037315 EPICURE).

References

1. Meencke HJ. Pathology of childhood epilepsies. *Cleve Clin J Med* 1989; 56(Suppl Pt 1):S111–20; discussion S121–3.
2. Barkovich AJ, Kuzniecky RI, Jackson GD, Guerrini R, Dobyns WB. A developmental and genetic classification for malformations of cortical development. *Neurology* 2005; 65:1873–87.
3. Guerrini R, Dobyns WB, Barkovich AJ. Abnormal development of the human cerebral cortex: genetics, functional consequences and treatment options. *Trends Neurosci* 2008; 31:154–62.
4. Taylor DC, Falconer MA, Bruton CJ, Corsellis JA. Focal dysplasia of the cerebral cortex in epilepsy. *J Neurol Neurosurg Psychiatry* 1971; 34:369–87.
5. Palmini A, Najm I, Avanzini G, Babb T, Guerrini R, Foldvary-Schaefer N, *et al.* Terminology and classification of the cortical dysplasias. *Neurology* 2004; 62:S2–8.
6. Blumcke I, Vinters HV, Armstrong D, Aronica E, Thom M, Spreafico R. Malformations of cortical development and epilepsies. *Epileptic Disord* 2009; 11:181–93.
7. Chamberlain WA, Cohen ML, KAGyure, Kleinschmidt-DeMasters BK, Perry A, Powell SZ, *et al.* Interobserver and intraobserver reproducibility in focal cortical dysplasia (malformations of cortical development). *Epilepsia* 2009; 50:2593–8.
8. Blumcke I, Spreafico R. An international consensus classification for focal cortical dysplasias. *Lancet Neurol* 2011; 10:26–7.
9. Blümcke I, Thom M, Aronica E, Armstrong DD, Vinters HV, Palmini A, *et al.* The clinico-pathological spectrum of Focal Cortical Dysplasias: a consensus classification proposed by an ad hoc Task Force of the ILAE Diagnostic Methods Commission. *Epilepsia* 2011; 52:158–74.
10. Cepeda C, Andre VM, Levine MS, Salanion N, Miyata H, Vinters HV, *et al.* Epileptogenesis in pediatric cortical dysplasia: The dysmature cerebral developmental hypothesis. *Epilepsy Behav* 2006; 9:219–35.
11. Hildebrandt M, Pieper T, Winkler P, Kolodziejczyk D, Holthausen H, Blumcke I. Neuropathological spectrum of cortical dysplasia in children with severe focal epilepsies. *Acta Neuropathol* 2005; 110:1–11.
12. Blumcke I, Pieper T, Pauli E, Hildebrandt M, Kudernatsch M, Winkler P, *et al.* A distinct variant of focal cortical dysplasia type I characterised by magnetic resonance imaging and neuropathological examination in children with severe epilepsies. *Epileptic Disord* 2010; 12:172–80.
13. Krsek P, Pieper T, Karlmeier A, Hildebrandt M, Kolodziejczyk D, Winkler P, *et al.* Different presurgical characteristics and seizure outcomes in children with focal cortical dysplasia type I or II. *Epilepsia* 2009; 50:125–37.
14. Tassi L, Garbelli R, Colombo N, Bramerio M, Lo Russo G, Deleo F, *et al.* Type I focal cortical dysplasia: surgical outcome is related to histopathology. *Epileptic Disord* 2010; 12:181–91.
15. Rakic P, Ayoub AE, Breunig JJ, Dominguez MH. Decision by division: making cortical maps. *Trends Neurosci* 2009; 32:291–301.
16. Spreafico R. Are some focal cortical dysplasias post-migratory cortical malformaitons? *Epileptic Disord* 2010; 12:169–71.
17. Hadjivassiliou G, Martinian L, Squier W, Blumcke I, Aronica E, Sisodiya SM, *et al.* The application of cortical layer markers in the

evaluation of cortical dysplasias in epilepsy. *Acta Neuropathol* 2010; 120:517–28.

18. Mountcastle VB. The columnar organization of the neocortex. *Brain* 1997; 120(Pt 4):701–22.
19. Angevine JB, Jr, Sidman RL. Autoradiographic study of cell migration during histogenesis of cerebral cortex in the mouse. *Nature* 1961; 192:766–8.
20. Rakic P. Specification of cerebral cortical areas. *Science* 1988; 241:170–6.
21. Hansen DV, Lui JH, Parker PR, Kriegstein AR. Neurogenic radial glia in the outer subventricular zone of human neocortex. *Nature* 2010; 464:554–61.
22. Rakic P. Evolution of the neocortex: a perspective from developmental biology. *Nat Rev Neurosci* 2009; 10:724–35.
23. Hubel DH, Wiesel TN, Stryker MP. Orientation columns in macaque monkey visual cortex demonstrated by the 2-deoxyglucose autoradiographic technique. *Nature* 1977; 269:328–30.
24. Nadarajah B, Parnavelas JG. Modes of neuronal migration in the developing cerebral cortex. *Nat Rev Neurosci* 2002; 3:423–32.
25. Crome L. Infantile cerebral gliosis with giant nerve cells. *J Neurol Neurosurg Psychiatry* 1957; 20:117–24.
26. Fauser S, Sisodiya SM, Martinian L, Thom M, Gumbinger C, Huppertz HJ, *et al.* Multi-focal occurrence of cortical dysplasia in epilepsy patients. *Brain* 2009; 132:2079–90.
27. Garbelli R, Munari C, De Biasi S, Vitellaro-Zuccarello L, Galli C, Bramerio M, *et al.* Taylor's cortical dysplasia: a confocal and ultrastructural immunohistochemical study. *Brain Pathol* 1999; 9:445–61.
28. Urbach H, Scheffler B, Heinrichsmeier T, von Oertzen J, Kral T, Wellmer J, *et al.* Focal cortical dysplasia of Taylor's balloon cell type: a clinicopathological entity with characteristic neuroimaging and histopathological features, and favorable postsurgical outcome. *Epilepsia* 2002; 43:33–40.
29. Becker AJ, Urbach H, Scheffler B, Baden T, Normann S, Lahl R, *et al.* Focal cortical dysplasia of Taylor's balloon cell type: Mutational analysis of the TSC1 gene indicates a pathogenic relationship to tuberous sclerosis. *Ann Neurol* 2002; 52:29–37.
30. Baybis M, Yu J, Lee A, Golden JA, Weiner H, McKhann G, 2nd, *et al.* mTOR cascade activation distinguishes tubers from focal cortical dysplasia. *Ann Neurol* 2004; 56:478–87.
31. Krueger DA, Care MM, Holland K, Agricola K, Tudor C, Mangeshkar P, *et al.* Everolimus for subependymal giant-cell astrocytomas in tuberous sclerosis. *N Engl J Med* 2010; 363: 1801–11.
32. Barkovich AJ, Kuzniecky RI, Bollen AW, Grant PE. Focal transmantle dysplasia: a specific malformation of cortical development. *Neurology* 1997; 49:1148–52.
33. Nobili L, Cardinale F, Magliola U, Cicolin A, Didato G, Bramerio M, *et al.* Taylor's focal cortical dysplasia increases the risk of sleep-related epilepsy. *Epilepsia* 2009; 50:2599–604.
34. Thom M, Eriksson S, Martinian L, Caboclo LO, McEvoy AW, Duncan JS, *et al.* Temporal lobe sclerosis associated with hippocampal sclerosis in temporal lobe epilepsy: Neuropathological features. *J Neuropathol Exp Neurol* 2009; 68:928–38.
35. Garbelli R, Zucca I, Milesi G, Mastropietro A, D'Incerti L, Tassi L, *et al.* Combined 7-T MRI and histopathologic study of normal and dysplastic samples from patients with TLE. *Neurology* 2011; 76:1177–85.
36. Lewis FT. The significance of the term hippocampus. *J Comp Neurol* 1923; 35:213–30.
37. Walther C. Hippocampal terminology: concepts, misconceptions, origins. *Endeavour* 2002; 26:41–4.
38. Lorente de Nó R. Studies on the structure of the cerebral cortex. II: Continuatiuon of the study of the Ammonic system. *J Psychol Neurol* 1934; 46:113–77.
39. Braak H. Architectonics of the human telencephalic cortex. In: Barlow HB, Bizzi E, Florey E, Grüsser OJ, van der Loos H (eds) *Studies of Brain Function*, Vol. 4, pp. 1–147. Berlin: Springer. 1980.
40. van Strien NM, Cappaert NL, Witter MP. The anatomy of memory: an interactive overview of the parahippocampal-hippocampal network. *Nat Rev Neurosci* 2009; 10:272–82.
41. Blumcke I, Thom M, Wiestler OD. Ammon's horn sclerosis: a maldevelopmental disorder associated with temporal lobe epilepsy. *Brain Pathol* 2002; 12:199–211.
42. Thom M, Zhou J, Martinian L, Sisodiya S. Quantitative post-mortem study of the hippocampus in chronic epilepsy: seizures do not inevitably cause neuronal loss. *Brain* 2005; 128:1344–57.
43. Blumcke I. Neuropathology of focal epilepsies: a critical review. *Epilepsy Behav* 2009; 15:34–9.
44. Sommer W. Die Erkrankung des Ammonshorns als aetiologisches Moment der Epilepsie. *Arch Psychiat Nervenkr* 1880; 308:631–75.
45. Blumcke I, Suter B, Behle K, Kuhn R, Schramm J, Elger CE, *et al.* Loss of hilar mossy cells in Ammon's horn sclerosis. *Epilepsia* 2000; 41:S174–80.
46. de Lanerolle NC, Kim JH, Williamson A, Spencer SS, Zaveri HP, Eid T, *et al.* A retrospective analysis of hippocampal pathology in human temporal lobe epilepsy: evidence for distinctive patient subcategories. *Epilepsia* 2003; 44:677–87.
47. Sutula TP, Cascino G, Cavazos J, Parada I, Ramirez L. Mossy fiber synaptic reorganization in the epileptic human temporal lobe. *Ann Neurol* 1989; 26:321–30.
48. Bernard C, Anderson A, Becker A, Poolos NP, Beck H, Johnston D. Acquired dendritic channelopathy in temporal lobe epilepsy. *Science* 2004; 305:532–5.
49. Janszky J, Janszky I, Schulz R, Hoppe M, Behne F, Pannek HW, *et al.* Temporal lobe epilepsy with hippocampal sclerosis: predictors for long-term surgical outcome. *Brain* 2005; 128:395–404.
50. Mathern GW, Babb TL, Vickrey BG, Melendez M, Pretorius JK. The clinical-pathogenic mechanisms of hippocampal neuron loss and surgical outcomes in temporal lobe epilepsy. *Brain* 1995; 118(Pt 1):105–18.
51. Wieser HG. ILAE Commission Report. Mesial temporal lobe epilepsy with hippocampal sclerosis. *Epilepsia* 2004; 45:695–714.
52. Wyler AR, Dohan FC, Schweitzer JB, Berry AD. A grading system for mesial temporal pathology (hippocampal sclerosis) from anterior temporal lobectomy. *J Epilepsy* 1992; 5:220–5.
53. Mathern GW, Pretorius JK, Babb TL. Quantified patterns of mossy fiber sprouting and neuron densities in hippocampal and lesional seizures. *J Neurosurg* 1995; 82:211–19.
54. Blumcke I, Pauli E, Clusmann H, Schramm J, Becker A, Elger C, *et al.* A new clinico-pathological classification system for mesial temporal sclerosis. *Acta Neuropathol* 2007; 113:235–44.
55. Stefan H, Hildebrandt M, Kerling F, Kasper BS, Hammen T, Dorfler A, *et al.* Clinical prediction of postoperative seizure control: structural, functional findings and disease histories. *J Neurol Neurosurg Psychiatry* 2009; 80:196–200.
56. Thom M, Liagkouras I, Elliot KJ, Martinian L, Harkness W, McEvoy A, *et al.* Reliability of patterns of hippocampal sclerosis as predictors of postsurgical outcome. *Epilepsia* 2010; 51:1801–8.
57. Pauli E, Hildebrandt M, Romstock J, Stefan H, Blumcke I. Deficient memory acquisition in temporal lobe epilepsy is predicted by hippocampal granule cell loss. *Neurology* 2006; 67:1383–9.
58. Coras R, Siebzehnrubl FA, Pauli E, Huttner HB, Njunting M, Kobow K, *et al.* Low proliferation and differentiation capacities of adult hippocampal stem cells correlate with memory dysfunction in humans. *Brain* 2010; 133:3359–72.
59. Blumcke I, Kistner I, Clusmann H, Schramm J, Becker AJ, Elger CE, *et al.* Towards a clinico-pathological classification of granule cell dispersion in human mesial temporal lobe epilepsies. *Acta Neuropathol* 2009; 117:535–44.

60. Mathern GW, Kuhlman PA, Mendoza D, Pretorius JK. Human fascia dentata anatomy and hippocampal neuron densities differ depending on the epileptic syndrome and age at first seizure. *J Neuropathol Exp Neurol* 1997; 56:199–212.
61. Thom M, Martinian L, Williams G, Stoeber K, Sisodiya SM. Cell proliferation and granule cell dispersion in human hippocampal sclerosis. *J Neuropathol Exp Neurol* 2005; 64:194–201.
62. Houser CR. Granule cell dispersion in the dentate gyrus of humans with temporal lobe epilepsy. *Brain Res* 1990; 535:195–204.
63. Sagar HJ, Oxbury JM. Hippocampal neuron loss in temporal lobe epilepsy: correlation with early childhood convulsions. *Ann Neurol* 1987; 22:334–40.
64. Altman J, Bayer SA. Migration and distribution of two populations of hippocampal granule cell precursors during the perinatal and postnatal periods. *J Comp Neurol* 1990; 301:365–81.
65. Eriksson PS, Perfilieva E, Bjork-Eriksson T, Alborn AM, Nordborg C, Peterson DA, *et al.* Neurogenesis in the adult human hippocampus. *Nat Med* 1998; 4:1313–17.
66. Gage FH. Mammalian neural stem cells. *Science* 2000; 287:1433–8.
67. Seri B, Garcia-Verdugo JM, Collado-Morente L, McEwen BS, Alvarez-Buylla A. Cell types, lineage, and architecture of the germinal zone in the adult dentate gyrus. *J Comp Neurol* 2004; 478:359–78.
68. Pleasure SJ, Collins AE, Lowenstein DH. Unique expression patterns of cell fate molecules delineate sequential stages of dentate gyrus development. *J Neurosci* 2000; 20:6095–105.
69. Frotscher M, Haas CA, Forster E. Reelin controls granule cell migration in the dentate gyrus by acting on the radial glial scaffold. *Cereb Cortex* 2003; 13:634–40.
70. Kim HM, Qu T, Kriho V, Lacor P, Smalheiser N, Pappas GD, *et al.* Reelin function in neural stem cell biology. *Proc Natl Acad Sci U S A* 2002; 99:4020–5.
71. Zhao S, Chai X, Forster E, Frotscher M. Reelin is a positional signal for the lamination of dentate granule cells. *Development* 2004; 131:5117–25.
72. Ge S, Goh EL, Sailor KA, Kitabatake Y, Ming GL, Song H. GABA regulates synaptic integration of newly generated neurons in the adult brain. *Nature* 2006; 439:589–93.
73. Ramirez-Amaya V, Marrone DF, Gage FH, Worley PF, Barnes CA. Integration of new neurons into functional neural networks. *J Neurosci* 2006; 26:12237–41.
74. van Praag H, Schinder AF, Christie BR, Toni N, Palmer TD, Gage FH. Functional neurogenesis in the adult hippocampus. *Nature* 2002; 415:1030–4.
75. Hastings NB, Gould E. Rapid extension of axons into the CA3 region by adult-generated granule cells. *J Comp Neurol* 1999; 413:146–54.
76. Zhao S, Chai X, Bock HH, Brunne B, Forster E, Frotscher M. Rescue of the reeler phenotype in the dentate gyrus by wild-type coculture is mediated by lipoprotein receptors for Reelin and Disabled 1. *J Comp Neurol* 2006; 495:1–9.
77. Cameron HA, McKay RD. Adult neurogenesis produces a large pool of new granule cells in the dentate gyrus. *J Comp Neurol* 2001; 435: 406–17.
78. Del Bigio MR. Proliferative status of cells in adult human dentate gyrus. *Microsc Res Tech* 1999; 45:353–8.
79. Gould E, Reeves AJ, Fallah M, Tanapat P, Gross CG, Fuchs E. Hippocampal neurogenesis in adult Old World primates. *Proc Natl Acad Sci U S A* 1999; 96:5263–7.
80. Parent JM, Yu TW, Leibowitz RT, Geschwind DH, Sloviter RS, Lowenstein DH. Dentate granule cell neurogenesis is increased by seizures and contributes to aberrant network reorganization in the adult rat hippocampus. *J Neurosci* 1997; 17:3727–38.
81. Tauck DL, Nadler JV. Evidence of mossy fiber sprouting in hippocampal formation of kainic acid-treated rats. *J Neurosci* 1985; 5:1016–22.
82. Sutula T, Cascino G, Cavazos J, Parada I, Ramirez L. Mossy fiber synaptic reorganization in the epileptic human temporal lobe. *Ann Neurol* 1989; 26:321–30.
83. Parent JM, Tada E, Fike JR, Lowenstein DH. Inhibition of dentate granule cell neurogenesis with brain irradiation does not prevent seizure-induced mossy fiber synaptic reorganization in the rat. *J Neurosci* 1999; 19:4508–19.
84. Scharfman HE, Gray WP. Relevance of seizure-induced neurogenesis in animal models of epilepsy to the etiology of temporal lobe epilepsy. *Epilepsia* 2007; 48(Suppl 2):33–41.
85. Parent JM, Elliott RC, Pleasure SJ, Barbaro NM, Lowenstein DH. Aberrant seizure-induced neurogenesis in experimental temporal lobe epilepsy. *Ann Neurol* 2006; 59:81–91.
86. Scharfman HE, Goodman JH, Sollas AL. Granule-like neurons at the hilar/CA3 border after status epilepticus and their synchrony with area CA3 pyramidal cells: functional implications of seizure-induced neurogenesis. *J Neurosci* 2000; 20:6144–58.
87. Blumcke I, Schewe JC, Normann S, Brustle O, Schramm J, Elger CE, *et al.* Increase of nestin-immunoreactive neural precursor cells in the dentate gyrus of pediatric patients with early-onset temporal lobe epilepsy. *Hippocampus* 2001; 11:311–21.
88. Squire LR, Stark CE, Clark RE. The Medial Temporal Lobe. *Annu Rev Neurosci* 2004; 27:279–306.
89. Scoville WB, Milner B. Loss of recent memory after bilateral hippocampal lesions. *J Neurol Neurosurg Psychiatry* 1957; 20:11–21.
90. Kesner RP, Lee I, Gilbert P. A behavioral assessment of hippocampal function based on a subregional analysis. *Rev Neurosci* 2004; 15: 333–51.
91. Leuner B, Mendolia-Loffredo S, Kozorovitskiy Y, Samburg D, Gould E, Shors TJ. Learning enhances the survival of new neurons beyond the time when the hippocampus is required for memory. *J Neurosci* 2004; 24:7477–81.
92. Shors TJ, Miesegaes G, Beylin A, Zhao M, Rydel T, Gould E. Neurogenesis in the adult is involved in the formation of trace memories. *Nature* 2001; 410:372–6.
93. Marin-Padilla M, Parisi JE, Armstrong DL, Sargent SK, Kaplan JA. Shaken infant syndrome: developmental neuropathology, progressive cortical dysplasia, and epilepsy. *Acta Neuropathol (Berl)* 2002; 103: 321–32.

CHAPTER 5

Definitions and Epidemiology of Epilepsy

Shichuo Li, Ding Ding, and Jianzhong Wu

Worldwide, an estimated 50 million people have epilepsy and around 85% of people with epilepsy live in developing countries. There are two million new cases occurring in the world every year. Up to 70% of people with epilepsy could lead normal lives if properly treated, but for an overwhelming majority of patients this is not the case (1). Overall, epilepsy contributed more than seven million disability-adjusted life years (DALYs) (0.5%) to the global burden of disease in 2000 (2). Among neurological disorders, more than half of the burden in DALYs is contributed by cerebrovascular disease. Epilepsy contributed approximately 8% of the burden, following Alzheimer and other dementias (12%) and migraine (8.3%). It is apparent that close to 90% of the worldwide burden of epilepsy is to be found in developing regions, with more than half occurring in the 39% of the global population living in countries with the highest levels of premature mortality and lowest levels of income (3).

Definitions of epilepsy and epileptic seizures

In 2005, the International League Against Epilepsy (ILAE) proposed a conceptual definition for clinicians diagnosing epilepsy: 'a disorder characterized by an enduring predisposition to generate epileptic seizures and by neurobiologic, cognitive, psychological and social consequences of this condition. The definition requires the occurrence of at least one epileptic seizure' (4). Evidence of recurrence may be the only information available to most epidemiological studies with which to identify the presence of an 'enduring predisposition to seizures'. Therefore, epilepsy is defined in practice as 'two or more unprovoked seizures occurring at least 24 hours apart' for the purpose of conducting most population-based studies of epilepsy epidemiology (5). This operational approach has the additional advantage of permitting comparison of epidemiological studies across time periods.

Active epilepsy indicates a person who is either currently being treated for epilepsy or whose most recent seizure has occurred within a time interval usually defined as the past 2 or 5 years (6). In low- and middle-income countries, active epilepsy may be defined over a 1-year period, due to problems in recalling dates beyond that period (7–11).

Epileptic seizure is defined in principle as 'a transient occurrence of signs and/or symptoms due to abnormal excessive or synchronous neuronal activity in the brain' (4). Operationally, these signs or symptoms include sudden and transitory abnormal phenomena such as alterations of consciousness, or involuntary motor, sensory, autonomic, or psychic events, perceived by the patient or an observer. Epileptic seizures, even if recurrent, are not always synonymous with epilepsy per se. Traditionally, and based on strong epidemiological data supporting the distinctions, certain conditions under which seizures occur are generally not considered to be epilepsy proper, although they are still considered within a broader spectrum of seizure-related disorders: (1) solitary unprovoked epileptic seizures, or a single cluster occurring within a 24-hour period or as a single episode of status epilepticus (SE); (2) febrile seizures or neonatal seizures (occurring in infants less than 28 days of age); (3) seizures 'in close temporal association with an acute systemic, metabolic or toxic insult or in association with an acute central nervous system (CNS) insult (infection, stroke, cranial trauma, intracerebral hemorrhage, or acute alcohol intoxication or withdrawal)', i.e. seizures not necessarily due to an established and 'enduring alteration in the brain'. Seizures due to such acute and transient conditions have also been described as *provoked* or *acute symptomatic* epileptic seizures. In these cases, the interval between the insult and the seizure—which can be used to separate acute symptomatic from unprovoked seizures—may vary according to the underlying clinical condition (6).

Aetiology

According to ILAE commission reports, aetiology is partitioned into three categories:

Remote symptomatic refers to epilepsy that occurs in association with an antecedent condition that has been demonstrated to increase the risk of developing epilepsy. Antecedent factors include history of stroke, brain malformation, cerebral palsy, history of bacterial meningitis or viral encephalitis, certain chromosomal and genetic disorders, and tumors. Epilepsy in the context of a progressive condition (e.g. neurodegenerative disease or an aggressive tumor) is often considered a subgroup within the category of remote symptomatic.

Idiopathic refers to a group of well-characterized disorders whose initial onset is concentrated during infancy, childhood, and adolescence. The intent of the term is to reflect a presumed genetic aetiology in which the primary and often the sole manifestation is seizures.

Cryptogenic is meant to be viewed neutrally and to designate that the nature of the underlying cause is as yet unknown; it may have a fundamental genetic defect at its core or it may be the consequence of a separate as yet unrecognized disorder.

The range of aetiologies for the development of epilepsy varies with age and geographic location. Congenital, developmental, and genetic conditions are mostly associated with the development of epilepsy in childhood, adolescence, and early adulthood. Head trauma, CNS infections, and tumors may occur at any age and may lead to the development of epilepsy, although tumors are more likely over the age of 40. Cerebrovascular disease (CVD) is the most common risk factor for epilepsy in people over the age of 60 years. Endemic infections are associated with epilepsy in certain environments, particularly in resource-poor countries, and these include malaria, neurocysticercosis, paragonomiasis, and toxocariasis (4, 12–18). The presence of a family history of epilepsy seems to enhance other risk factors and this may suggest that the aetiology of epilepsy is multifactorial (19–22). Based on community-based studies, proportions of presumed identified causes of epilepsy are as follows: CVD 11–21%; trauma 2–6%; tumors 4–7%; infection 0–3%, and idiopathic 54–65% (23–25).

It is evident that the successful detection of an aetiological factor depends upon the extent of investigation and unless this is standardized and specified in any study, evaluation of the results is problematic (26). The use of the terms idiopathic epilepsy and cryptogenic epilepsy is a particular source of confusion. Thus, new terminology and concepts advanced by the ILAE divide the causes of epilepsy into categories of structural/metabolic, genetic, and unknown, corresponding roughly to the former categories of remote symptomatic, idiopathic, and cryptogenic. The concepts and terminology were updated to keep them relevant in the context of increasing advances in genomics and neuroimaging and improved understanding of epilepsy (27).

Epidemiology

Epidemiology is the study of the dynamics of a medical condition in terms of its distribution, determinants, and natural history in a population. It consists of three domains: descriptive, analytical, and experimental epidemiology. Descriptive epidemiology concerns the vital statistics of a condition and is usually observational, with no designed control group. Analytical epidemiology attempts to establish associations and determinants of a condition, often by comparing individuals with the condition or risk factors for it with those without, for example, in cohort and case–control studies. Studies under conditions that allow an investigator to control relevant factors constitute experimental epidemiology (28). The epidemiology of epilepsy is largely based on descriptive and analytical studies, as very little experimental work has been carried out for a number of reasons, including logistical and ethical considerations (26).

The first landmark epidemiological study of epilepsy was conducted in 1959 by Leonard T. Kurland and colleagues who reported population-based data from Rochester, Minnesota, USA, over a 10-year period (29). Early epidemiological studies that followed from Kurland's work contributed substantially to our current understanding of epilepsy. Additional studies exploring the Rochester longitudinal population-based data sets provided an evidence base of the occurrence and prognosis of epilepsy that contributed to advances in the treatment and management of seizures.

Diagnostic accuracy and case ascertainment

Major problems in epilepsy epidemiology are diagnostic accuracy and case ascertainment (30, 31). Epileptic seizures are pleomorphic, although usually stereotyped for a given individual. Unlike most neurological disorders, the majorities of patients with epilepsy do not have permanent physical signs and can be diagnosed only by taking a history or by the chance observation of a seizure. Diagnosis of epilepsy is essentially a discretionary judgement that may vary depending on the skill and experience of the diagnostician and the quality of witness information available. Electroencephalography is useful in classifying epilepsy, but is of limited help in making the diagnosis. In practice, both false positive and false negative diagnoses are common. Even if the diagnosis of epilepsy is accurate, case ascertainment poses a variety of problems. Some patients with seizures may never seek medical attention because they ignore or misinterpret the symptoms, or indeed may be unaware of them. Some patients conceal or deny their seizure history because of barriers of traditional prejudice, especially in less developed regions. It is likely, therefore, that epidemiological studies of epilepsy often miss patients unless sensitive screening techniques are included (26).

The incidence and prevalence of epilepsy

The common standard measures of the frequency of epilepsy in a population are incidence rate and prevalence rate:

Incidence rate is the frequency with which new cases occur in a population. It is expressed as a frequency per standard population (e.g. 100,000) per time period (usually per year). *Incidence density* is also useful for estimating the incidence in dynamic populations, when the denominator is the sum of the person-year of the at-risk population. Incidence is informative about the rate of new cases regardless of the prognosis or cause of the disorder. For aetiological and prognostic investigations, incidence-based studies are superior to prevalence-based studies (6). The overall incidence of epilepsy is generally taken to be around 50 per 100,000 population per year (range 40–70 per 100,000 population per year) while the incidence of epilepsy in resource-poor countries is generally higher in the range of 100–190 cases per 100,000 population per year (32–37). It has been shown that people from a socioeconomically deprived background are at higher risk of developing epilepsy (38). In industrialized countries, there is evidence of a decrease in the incidence in children and a simultaneous increase in the elderly over the last three decades (39, 40).

Table 5.1 presents findings from incidence studies of epilepsy worldwide. In North America, age-adjusted incidence of epilepsy ranged from 16 per 100,000 person-years (41) to 51 per 100,000 person-years (24). The only incidence study that could be age-adjusted in South America, conducted in rural Chile, reported the highest age-adjusted incidence in the world (111 per 100,000 person-years) (42). Age- adjusted incidence of epilepsy in European studies ranged from 26 per 100,000 person-years in Norway (43) to 47 per 100,000 person years in England (33). Only one incidence study that could be age-adjusted was conducted in India in Asia, this reported an age-adjusted incidence of 35 per

100,000 person-years (44). In Africa, studies reported age-adjusted incidence of epilepsy of 51 per 100,000 in Tanzania (12) and 43 per 100,000 in Ethiopia (45).

Point prevalence is the proportion of individuals in the population who are affected by a health condition at a single point in time, usually designated as a specific day. It is useful for indicating the degree of disease burden in a population. With epilepsy, the point prevalence of *active epilepsy* is typically considered of most interest (6). A plethora of studies has been made of the prevalence of epilepsy in many different settings and it has usually been found to be 4–10 per 1000 persons (26). Most large-scale studies of populations in resource-poor countries have reported prevalence rates for active epilepsy of 6–10 per 1,000; many of these studies have, however, reported different rates for urban and rural areas, usually with higher rates in the latter (11, 30, 31, 46, 47). The differences seem unlikely to be artefactual or attributable to differential case ascertainment between regions as many of these studies used identical methods, study design, and diagnostic confirmation in each area.

Table 5.2 presents age-adjusted prevalence of epilepsy in studies that used door-to-door survey methodology worldwide. In the North American studies, the prevalence was 5.0 in New York (48) and 7.1 per 1000 (49) in Mississippi. In Central and South America, the overall prevalence ranged from 3.7 per 1000 in Argentina (50) to 22.2 per 1000 in Ecuador (51). Real differences in prevalence may be related to the presence of endemic conditions such as neurocysticercosis or malaria, the medical infrastructure in place, including availability of preventive regional health programmes, and accessible local medical care. A region which has eradicated the porcine tapeworm, has established effective malaria prevention strategies, or has established immunization programmes, can reduce or minimize risk factors associated with epilepsy (52). In Europe, prevalence was low, 2.7 per 1000 and 3.3 per 1000, respectively in each study conducted in Italy (53, 54), when compared to a prevalence of 7.0 per 1000 in the study conducted in the European region of Turkey (55). In contrast to the majority of studies conducted in Asia, the prevalence of 10.2 per 1000 in Asian Turkey (56)

Table 5.1 Incidence of epilepsy in population based studies of all ages worldwide

Region	Publication year (reference)	Gender	Population	Number of cases	Incidence (per 100,000 population)	
					Crude	Age-adjusted to 2000 US standard population
North America						
Rochester, MN 1935–44	1993 (24)	M > F	245,969	94	38	41
Rochester, MN 1945–54	1993 (24)	M > F	282,452	142	50	49
Rochester, MN 1955–64	1993 (24)	M > F	384,881	187	45	44
Rochester, MN 1965–74	1993 (24)	M > F	516,903	182	35	36
Rochester, MN 1975–84	1993 (24)	M > F	573,152	275	48	51
Texas	1999 (117)	M > F	601,448	197	33	28
New York	2008 (41)	M > F	279,677	82	15	16
Central and South America						
Chile	1992 (42)	M > F	90,596	102	113	111
Europe						
England	1966 (118)	–	497,707	141	29	28
Norway	1974 (43)	M > F	213,116	70	33	26
Italy	1983 (119)	M > F	697,000	230	33	33
Faroes	1986 (120)	M > F	452,584	194	43	37
Iceland	1996 (121)	M > F	90,237	42	47	43
England	2000 (33)	–	100,230	46	46	47
Netherlands	2002 (34)	M > F	316,828	94	30	29
Iceland	2005 (122)	M > F	882,151	290	33	31
Asia						
India	1998 (44)	M > F	64,963	32	49	35
Africa						
Tanzania	1992 (12)	–	165,684	122	73	51
Ethiopia	1997 (45)	M > F	215,901	139	64	43

From Banerjee et al. (52).

Table 5.2 Age-adjusted prevalence of epilepsy in studies that used door-to-door survey methodology worldwide

Region	Publication year (reference number)	Gender	Population	Number of cases	Prevalence (per 1000 population)	
					Crude	Age-adjusted to 2000 US standard population
North America						
Mississippi	1986 (49)	M > F	23,597	160	6.8	7.1
New York	2007 (48)[a]	M < F	208,301	42	5.2	5.0
Central and South America						
Ecuador	1985 (51)	M < F	1113	19	17.1	22.2
Ecuador	1992 (46)	M < F	72,121	575	8.0	9.1
Ecuador	1997 (123)	M > F	221	5[b]	22.6	11.4
Bolivia	1999 (124)	M < F	10,124	112	11.1	14.0
Honduras	2005 (125)	M < F	6473	100	15.4	16.0
Argentina	2007 (50)	M < F	17,049	64	3.8	3.7
Europe						
Italy	1996 (53)	M < F	9956	27	2.7	2.7
Italy	2001 (54)	M > F	24,496	81	3.3	3.3
Turkey	2002 (55)	M > F	2817	17	6.0	7.0
Asia						
China	1985 (61)	M > F	63,195	289	4.6	4.4
India 1988	1988 (58)	M > F	63,645	157	2.5	2.2
India	1988 (59)	M > F	14,010	50	3.6	3.6
Pakistan	1997 (57)	M < F	24,130	241	9.9	9.8
Turkey[c]	1997 (57)	M > F	11,497	81	7.0	6.6
Turkey[c]	1999 (56)	M > F	4803	49	10.2	10.2
India 2000	2000 (60)	M > F	238,102	1,175	4.9	4.4
Saudi Arabia	2001 (126)	M > F	23,700	155	6.5	5.1
Africa						
Nigeria	1982 (127)	M < F	903	33	37	41.0
Nigeria	1987 (128)	M < F	18,954	101	5.3	4.9
Nigeria	1989 (8)	M < F	2925	18	6.2	4.7
Ethiopia	1990 (129)	M > F	60,820	316	5.2	5.4
Tanzania	1992 (12)	M < F	18,183	185	10.2	12.5
Tunisia	1993 (130)	M > F	35,370	141	4.0	3.9
Kenya	1994 (131)	M > F	7450 (5+)	30	4.0	3.7
Uganda	1996 (132)	M < F	4743	61	12.9	9.2
Zambia	2004 (10)	M > F	55,000	799	14.5	13.2
Tanzania	2005 (133)	M > F	4905	42	8.6	6.8
Pacific Islands						
Guam	1968 (134)	–	6967	16	2.3	2.7

[a] This study was done using random-digit dial methodology in the Northern Manhattan community. A follow-up interview was administered to those who screened positive for epilepsy over the telephone.

Epileptologists reviewed all information from interviews to determine whether each potential case was actually a case.

[b] All 5 cases were between 7–14 years of age.

[c] These studies were conducted in a region of Turkey that is geographically part of Asia. However, the population may be more comparable to the western region of Turkey, which is part of Europe.

From Banerjee et al. (52).

was higher than that reported in studies conducted in Pakistan, India, and China, where prevalence ranged from 2.2–4.4 per 1000 (57–61).

Lifetime prevalence is the risk of having a non-febrile epileptic seizure at some point in an average lifetime. In both industrialized and resource-poor countries, up to 5% of a population will experience non-febrile seizures at some point in life (30, 31). From the difference between lifetime prevalence and the point prevalence of active epilepsy it is apparent that most patients developing epilepsy will either cease to have seizures or die (62). It is likely that in most patients the condition remits. Epilepsy, however, is associated with increased mortality particularly, but not exclusively, in symptomatic cases (63–65). Patients with chronic epilepsy are most at risk but the impact of mortality on the prevalence of epilepsy and the extent to which the difference in lifetime and point prevalence rates is due to mortality has not yet been fully appraised.

Mortality

Different measures are used to estimate mortality, depending upon the study design and available information on deaths. The measures include mortality rate, case fatality, standardized mortality ratio, and proportionate mortality.

Mortality rate is the number of deaths that occur in the defined population divided by the person-years at risk in that population, and can be an indirect estimator of severity (66). People with epilepsy have a mortality rate 2–3 times higher than that of the general population (67). Mortality rate from epilepsy shows a small peak in early life, which possibly reflects the mortality of those children with severe hypoxic-ischaemic encephalopathy, brain malformations, and inherited metabolic disorders. The risk then falls to a minimum around the age of 10 years. It rises again in late adolescence and early adulthood before levelling off throughout most of adult life. There is a late peak of epilepsy-related mortality in old age, presumably secondary to CVD (68).

Mortality is best expressed as the *standardized mortality ratio* (SMR), the ratio of the observed number of deaths in an epilepsy population to that expected based on the age- and sex-specific mortality rates in a reference population, in a given time. The *proportional mortality ratio* (PMR), the proportion of deaths due to a particular cause in a cohort of patients in a given period, can be used to compare the relative contribution of various causes to the overall mortality in the population. *Case fatality rate* (CFR), the number of deaths caused by a disease divided by the number of diagnosed cases of the disease, can also be used to describe the severity of mortality (5, 69).

In large cohort studies of patients over 15 years, SMRs ranging from 2.1–5.1 were reported (63, 70–73). The majority of deaths in people whose seizures start in childhood occur in adulthood. Prospective studies in which children with large sample size were followed for 15 to more than 30 years reported higher SMRs of 8.8–13.2 (74–77). For patients with epilepsy, population-based studies demonstrate PMRs of 12–39% for CVD, 12–37% for ischaemic heart disease (IHD), 18–40% for neoplasia (including brain tumours), 9–15% for brain tumours, 8–18% for pneumonia, 0–7% for suicides, 0–12% for accidents, 0–4% for sudden unexpected death in epilepsy (SUDEP), 0–10% for seizure-related causes (including SE), and 5–30% for other causes (63, 78–83).

Death in people with epilepsy can be classified into three groups: epilepsy-related deaths, deaths related to the underlying cause of the epilepsy, and deaths that are unrelated to the epilepsy or its underlying aetiology (Table 5.3) (84). The PMRs for epilepsy-related conditions range from 1–45% (63, 76, 78, 80, 82, 84).

SUDEP is defined as a sudden, unexpected, witnessed or unwitnessed, non-traumatic, and non-drowning death in patients with epilepsy, with or without evidence of seizure and excluding documented SE, in which postmortem examination does not reveal a toxicological or anatomical cause of death (85). The reported incidence of SUDEP has ranged from 0.35–9.3 per 1000 person-years depending on the different study population and methodologies employed (86). The incidence of death for young adults with intractable epilepsy is many times that of the general population, with a peak between the ages of 20–40 years (87).

SE accounts for between 0.5–10% of all deaths in epilepsy, with a SMR of 2.8 (95% confidence interval (CI) 2.1–3.5) (88). The CFR from SE was reported as 7.6–22% for short-term mortality (within 30 days of SE) (89–93) and 43% for long-term mortality (30 days after SE to 10 years) (88).

People with epilepsy may sustain a fatal accident either during a seizure or as a consequence of a seizure. Accidental deaths related to epilepsy are commonly due to drowning, traffic accidents, trauma, falls, burns, or aspiration. Based on attendance records of 4 accident and emergency departments, the risk of injury as a result of a seizure was estimated to be 29.5 per 100,000 per year (94).

Table 5.3 Causes of death in epilepsy

Unrelated deaths
Neoplasms outside the central nervous system
Ischaemic heart disease
Pneumonia
Others
Related to underlying disease
Brain tumours
Cerebrovascular disease
Cerebral infection—abscesses and encephalitis
Inherited disorders, e.g. Batten disease
Epilepsy-related deaths
Suicides
Treatment-related deaths
Idiosyncratic drug reactions
Medication adverse effects
Seizure-related deaths
Status epilepticus
Trauma, burns, drowning
Asphyxiation, aspiration
Aspiration pneumonia after a seizure
Sudden unexpected death in epilepsy

From Nashef and Shorvon (84).

Accident-related deaths in people with epilepsy comprise 1.2–6.5% of all deaths in community-based studies (63, 74, 82) and 7.3–42% in selected population studies with SMRs ranging from 2.4–5.6 (67, 71, 95–101). People with epilepsy have an increased risk of drowning with SMR of 5.4–96.9 that varied depending on the study population (102). Studies performed during the 1970s and 1980s demonstrated that the suicide PMRs range from 0–20% and the SMRs from 1–5.8 (103–105).

Common non-epileptic causes of death cited in mortality studies include neoplasia, CVD, IHD, and pneumonia. Reports have noted increased SMR for malignant neoplasia of the lung, pancreas, hepatobiliary system, breast, and lymphoid and haematopoietic tissue (89). Cancer accounts for 16–29% of deaths with reported SMRs ranging from 3.4–5.4 (70, 96, 98); although in one study, hospitalized patients with epilepsy appeared to be at much higher risk, with a reported SMR of 29.9 (71). The SMR for neoplasia remains at 1.4–2.5 even when CNS tumours are excluded (63, 71, 72, 78, 96). The SMR for all cancers in an institutional cohort with more severe epilepsy (SMR 1.42; 95% CI 1.18–1.69) was higher than that for the milder cases in a community-based population (SMR 0.93; 95% CI 0.84–1.03). The SMR for brain and CNS neoplasms was significantly elevated in the group with milder epilepsy (106).

Prognosis of epilepsy

Remission of treated epilepsy

Given that in developed countries antiepileptic medication is usually commenced after two unprovoked seizures, prognostic studies from Western countries are essentially those of treated epilepsy. A landmark study of the natural history of treated epilepsy was a community-based project carried out in Rochester, Minnesota, USA. The probability of being in remission for 5 years at 20 years after diagnosis (terminal remission) was 75% (107). The National General Practice Study of Epilepsy (NGPSE) conducted in the UK reported that, when patients with acute symptomatic seizures and those who had only one seizure were excluded, 60% had achieved a 5-year remission by 9 years of follow up (108, 109). Other modern large-scale studies that include only newly diagnosed patients followed for long periods also tend to suggest a remission rate of 60–90% (110). At a conservative estimate, at least 60% of newly diagnosed patients will enter long-term remission on treatment initiation, and approximately 50% of these patients will remain in remission after antiepileptic medication withdrawal. A long-term study of newly diagnosed patients in Glasgow, Scotland demonstrated that, among the 470 patients who had never previously received antiepileptic drug (AED) treatment, 64% entered terminal remission of at least 1 year, including 47% of patients who became and remained seizure-free on the first drug, 13% on the second drug, but only 4% on the third drug or a combination of two drugs. Thus, response to the first AED was the most powerful predictor of prognosis (111).

Spontaneous remission and untreated epilepsy

Evidence from studies from resource-poor countries where a significant treatment gap exists suggests that many patients may enter spontaneous remission with no AED treatment (112). The similar prevalence rates in resource-poor and developed nations may reflect the occurrence of spontaneous remission of many of the untreated cases. In the late 1980s, 49% of 643 patients who lived in northern Ecuador and who had never received AED treatment were seizure free for at least 12 months (112). A recent study from rural Bolivia reported 43.7% of untreated epilepsy cases were seizure free for more than 5 years when the cohort was revisited after 10 years (113). Besides developing countries, spontaneous remission of epilepsy has also been observed in developed countries. In a Finnish study, it was found that 42% of 33 untreated epilepsy patients entered a 2-year remission within 10 years after onset (114).

Prognosis of intractable epilepsy

Only 5–10% of all incidence cases of epilepsy ultimately result in truly intractable disease. These cases probably account for half the prevalence cases of epilepsy. Approximately 60% of patients with intractable epilepsy can be expected to suffer from partial seizures. Studies suggest that failure to control seizures with the first or second AED implies that the probability of subsequent seizure control with further AEDs is only about 4% (110). Recent studies reported that approximately 5% per year of patients with intractable epilepsy were seizure free for 12 months following medication changes. This finding highlights the fact that, irrespective of the number of previous AEDs, there is still a small possibility of inducing meaningful seizure remission in the population (115, 116).

References

1. Shorvon SD, Farmer PJ. Epilepsy in developing countries: a review of epidemiological, sociocultural, and treatment aspects. *Epilepsia* 1988: 29(Suppl. 1):36–54.
2. Leonardi M, Ustun B. The global burden of epilepsy. *Epilepsia* 2002: 43(Suppl. 6):21–5.
3. World Health Organization. Neurological disorders a public health approach. In: *Neurological Disorders: Public Health Challenges*, pp. 41– 111. Geneva: World Health Organization, 2006.
4. Fisher R, van Emde Boas W, Blume W, Elger C, Genton P, Lee P, *et al.* Epileptic seizures and epilepsy: definitions proposed by ILAE and IBE. *Epilepsia* 2005; 46(4):470–2.
5. Commission on Epidemiology and Prognosis of the International League Against Epilepsy. Guidelines for epidemiologic studies on epilepsy. *Epilepsia* 1993; 34:592–6.
6. Guidelines for epidemiologic studies on epilepsy. Commission on Epidemiology and Prognosis, International League Against Epilepsy. *Epilepsia* 2011; 34:592–6.
7. Mung'ala-Odera V, Meehan R, Njuguna P, Mturi N, Alcock K, Carter JA, *et al.* Validity and reliability of the 'Ten Questions' questionnaire for detecting moderate to severe neurological impairment in children aged 6–9 years in rural Kenya. *Neuroepidemiology* 2004; 23:67–72.
8. Longe AC, Osuntokun BO. Prevalence of neurological disorders in Udo, a rural community in southern Nigeria. *Trop Geogr Med* 1989; 41:36– 40.
9. Edwards T, Scott AG, Munyoki G, Odera VM, Chengo E, Bauni E, *et al.* Active convulsive epilepsy in a rural district of Kenya: a study of prevalence and possible risk factors. *Lancet Neurol* 2008; 7:50–6.
10. Birbeck GL, Kalichi EM. Epilepsy prevalence in rural Zambia: a door-to-door survey. *Trop Med Int Health* 2004; 9:92–5.
11. Wang WZ, Wu JZ, Wang DS, Dai XY, Yang B, Wang TP, *et al.* The prevalence and treatment gap in epilepsy in China: An ILAE/IBE/WHO study. *Neurology* 2003; 60:1544–5.
12. Rwiza HT, Kilonzo GP, Haule J, Matuja WB, Mteza I, Mbena P, *et al.* Prevalence and incidence of epilepsy in Ulanga, a rural Tanzanian district: a community-based study. *Epilepsia* 1992; 33:1051–6.
13. Commission on Tropical Diseases of the International League Against Epilepsy. Relationship between epilepsy and tropical diseases. *Epilepsia* 1994; 35:89–93.

14. Molyneux ME. Impact of malaria on the brain and its prevention. *Lancet* 2000; 355:671–2.
15. Bergen DC. Preventable neurological diseases worldwide. *Neuroepidemiology* 1998; 17:67–73.
16. Waruiru CM, Newton CR, Forster D, New L, Winstanley P, Mwangi I, *et al.* Epileptic seizures and malaria in Kenyan children. *Trans R Soc Trop Med Hyg* 1996; 90:152–5.
17. Pal DK, Carpio A, Sander JW. Neurocysticercosis and epilepsy in developing countries. *J Neurol Neurosurg Psychiatry* 2000; 68:137–43.
18. Nicoletti A, Bartoloni A, Reggio A, Bartalesi F, Roselli M, Sofia V, *et al.* Epilepsy, cysticercosis, and toxocariasis: a population-based case-control study in rural Bolivia. *Neurology* 2002; 58:1256–61.
19. Anderson VE, Hauser WA, Rich SS. Genetic heterogeneity and epidemiology of the epilepsies. *Adv Neurol* 1999; 79:59–73.
20. Johnson MR, Sander JW. The clinical impact of epilepsy genetics. *J Neurol Neurosurg Psychiatry* 2001; 70:428–30.
21. Berkovic SF, Scheffer IE. Genetics of the epilepsies. *Epilepsia* 2001; 42(Suppl 5):16–23.
22. Anderson E, Berkovic S, Dulac O, Gardiner M, Jain S, Laue Friis M, *et al.* ILAE genetics commission conference report: molecular analysis of complex genetic epilepsies. *Epilepsia* 2002; 43:1262–7.
23. Sander JW, Hart YM, Johnson AL, Shorvon SD. National General Practice Study of Epilepsy: newly diagnosed epileptic seizures in a general population. *Lancet* 1990; 336:1267–71.
24. Hauser WA, Annegers JF, Kurland LT. Incidence of epilepsy and unprovoked seizures in Rochester, Minnesota: 1935–1984. *Epilepsia* 1993; 34:453–68.
25. Forsgran L, Bucht G, Eriksson S, Bergmark L. Incidence and clinical characterization of unprovoked seizures in adults: a prospective population-based study. *Epilepsia* 1996; 37:224–9.
26. Sander JW. The epidemiology of epilepsy revisited. *Current Opinion in Neurology* 2003; 16:165–70.
27. Revised terminology and concepts for organization of the epilepsies: Report of the Commission on Classification and Terminology. *Epilepsia*, 2010; 51(4):676–85.
28. Jallon P. Epilepsy and epileptic disorders, an epidemiological marker? Contributions of descriptive epidemiology. *Epileptic Disord* 2002; 4:1–13.
29. Kurland LT. The incidence and prevalence of convulsive disorders in a small urban community. *Epilepsia* 1959; 1:143–61.
30. Sander JW, Shorvon SD. Epidemiology of the epilepsies. *J Neurol Neurosurg Psychiatry* 1996; 61:433–43.
31. Bell GS, Sander JW. The epidemiology of epilepsy: the size of the problem. *Seizure* 2001; 10:306–14.
32. Zarrelli MM, Beghi E, Rocca WA, Hauser WA. Incidence of epileptic syndromes in Rochester, Minnesota: 1980–1984. *Epilepsia* 1999; 40:1708–14.
33. MacDonald BK, Cockerell OC, Sander JW, Shorvon SD. The incidence and lifetime prevalence of neurological disorders in a prospective community-based study in the UK. *Brain* 2000; 123:665–76.
34. Kotsopoulos IA, Merode T, Kessels FG, de Krom MC, Knottnerus JA. Systematic review and metaanalysis of incidence studies of epilepsy and unprovoked seizures. *Epilepsia* 2002; 43:1402–9.
35. Heaney DC, MacDonald BK, Everitt A, Stevenson S, Leonardi GS, Wilkinson P, *et al.* Socioeconomic variation in incidence of epilepsy: prospective community based study in south east England. *BMJ* 2002; 325:1013–16.
36. Gaitatzis A, Purcell B, Carroll K, Sander JW, Majeed A. Differences in the use of health services among people with and without epilepsy in the United Kingdom: socio-economic and disease-specific determinants. *Epilepsy Res* 2002; 50:233–41.
37. Lindsten H, Stenlund H, Edlund C, Forsgren L. Socioeconomic prognosis after a newly diagnosed unprovoked epileptic seizure in adults: a population-based case-control study. *Epilepsia* 2002; 43:1239–50.
38. Heaney DC, Bell GS, Sander JW. The socioeconomic, cultural, and emotional implications of starting or withholding treatment in a patient with a first seizure. *Epilepsia* 2008; 49(S1):35–9.
39. ILAE Commission of Epidemiology and Prognosis. The epidemiology of the epilepsies: future directions. *Epilepsia* 1997; 38:614–18.
40. Everitt AD, Sander JW. Incidence of epilepsy is now higher in elderly people than children. *BMJ* 1998; 316:780.
41. Benn EK, Hauser WA, Shih T, Leary L, Bagiella E, Dayan P, *et al.* Estimating the incidence of first unprovoked seizure and newly diagnosed epilepsy in the low-income urban community of Northern Manhattan, New York City. *Epilepsia* 2008; 49(8):1431–9.
42. Lavados J, Germain L, Morales A, Campero M, Lavados P. A descriptive study of epilepsy in the district of El Salvador, Chile, 1984–1988. *Acta Neurol Scand* 1992; 85(4):249–56.
43. De Graaf AS. Epidemiological aspects of epilepsy in northern Norway. *Epilepsia* 1974; 15(3):291–9.
44. Mani KS, Rangan G, Srinivas HV, Kalyanasundaram S, Narendran S, Reddy AK. The Yelandur study: a community-based approach to epilepsy in rural South India—epidemiological aspects. *Seizure* 1998; 7(4):281–8.
45. Tekle-Haimanot R, Forsgren L, Ekstedt J. Incidence of epilepsy in rural central Ethiopia. *Epilepsia* 1997; 38(5):541–6.
46. Placencia M, Shorvon SD, Paredes V, Bimos C, Sander JW, Suarez J, *et al.* Epileptic seizures in an Andean region of Ecuador: incidence and prevalence and regional variation. *Brain* 1992; 115:771–82.
47. Aziz H, Ali SM, Frances P, Khan MI, Hasan KZ.Epilepsy in Pakistan: a population-based epidemiologic study. *Epilepsia* 1994; 35:950–8.
48. Kelvin EA, Hesdorffer DC, Bagiella E, Andrews H, Pedley TA, Shih TT, *et al.* Prevalence of self-reported epilepsy in a multiracial and multiethnic community in New York City. *Epilepsy Res* 2007; 77(2– 3):141–50.
49. Haerer AF, Anderson DW, Schoenberg BS. Prevalence and clinical features of epilepsy in a biracial United States population. *Epilepsia* 1986; 27(1):66–75.
50. Melcon MO, Kochen S, Vergara RH. Prevalence and clinical features of epilepsy in Argentina. A community-based study. *Neuroepidemiology* 2007; 28(1):8–15.
51. Cruz ME, Schoenberg BS, Ruales J, Barberis P, Proano J, Bossano F, *et al.* Pilot study to detect neurologic disease in Ecuador among a population with a high prevalence of endemic goiter. *Neuroepidemiology* 1985; 4(2):108–16.
52. Banerjee PN, Filippi D, Hauser WA. The descriptive epidemiology of epilepsy-a review. *Epilepsy Res* 2009; 85(1):31–45.
53. Reggio A, Failla G, Patti F, Nicoletti A, Grigoletto F, Meneghini F, *et al.* Prevalence of epilepsy. A door-to-door survey in the Sicilian community of Riposto. *Ital J Neurol Sci* 1996; 17(2):147–51.
54. Rocca WA, Savettieri G, Anderson DW, Meneghini F, Grigoletto F, Morgante L, *et al.* Door-to-door prevalence survey of epilepsy in three Sicilian municipalities. *Neuroepidemiology* 2001; 20(4):237–41.
55. Onal AE, Tumerdem Y, Ozturk MK, Gurses C, Baykan B, Gokyigit A, *et al.* Epilepsy prevalence in a rural area in Istanbul. *Seizure* 2002; 11(6):397–401.
56. Karaagac N, Yeni SN, Senocak M, Bozluolcay M, Savrun FK, Ozdemir H, *et al.* Prevalence of epilepsy in Silivri, a rural area of Turkey. *Epilepsia* 1999; 40(5):637–42.
57. Aziz H, Guvener A, Akhtar SW, Hasan KZ. Comparative epidemiology of epilepsy in Pakistan and Turkey: population-based studies using identical protocols. *Epilepsia* 1997; 38(6):716–22.
58. Koul R, Razdan S, Motta A. Prevalence and pattern of epilepsy (Lath/Mirgi/Laran) in rural Kashmir, India. *Epilepsia* 1988; 29(2):116–22.
59. Bharucha NE, Bharucha EP, Bharucha AE, Bhise AV, Schoenberg BS. Prevalence of epilepsy in the Parsi community of Bombay. *Epilepsia* 1988; 29(2):111–15.

60. Radhakrishnan K, Pandian JD, Santhoshkumar T, Thomas SV, Deetha TD, Sarma PS, *et al.* Prevalence, knowledge, attitude, and practice of epilepsy in Kerala, South India. *Epilepsia* 2000; 41(8):1027–35.
61. Li SC, Schoenberg BS, Wang CC, Cheng XM, Zhou SS, Bolis CL. Epidemiology of epilepsy in urban areas of the People's Republic of China. *Epilepsia* 1985; 26(5):391–4.
62. Sander JW. Some aspects of prognosis in the epilepsies: a review. *Epilepsia* 1993; 34:1007–16.
63. Lhatoo SD, Johnson AL, Goodridge DM, MacDonald BK, Sander JW, Shorvon SD. Mortality in epilepsy in the first 11 to 14 years after diagnosis: multivariate analysis of a long-term, prospective, population-based cohort. *Ann Neurol* 2001; 49:336–44.
64. Shackleton DP, Westendorp RG, Kasteleijn-Nolst Trenite DG, de Craen AJ, Vandenbroucke JP. Survival of patients with epilepsy: an estimate of the mortality risk. *Epilepsia* 2002; 43:445–50.
65. Morgan CL, Kerr MP. Epilepsy and mortality: a record linkage study in a U.K. population. *Epilepsia* 2002; 43:1251–5.
66. Logroscino G, Hesdorffer DC. Methodologic issues in studies of mortality following epilepsy: measures, types of studies, sources of cases, cohort effects, and competing risks. *Epilepsia* 2005; 46: S3–7.
67. Gaitatzis A, Sander JW. The mortality of epilepsy revisited. *Epileptic Disord* 2004; 6:3–13.
68. O'Callaghan FJK, Osborne JP, Martyn CN. Epilepsy related mortality. *Arch Dis Child* 2004; 89:705–7.
69. Tomson T. Mortality in epilepsy. *J Neurol* 2000; 247:15–21.
70. Lindsten H, Nystrom L, Forsgren L. Mortality risk in an adult cohort with a newly diagnosed unprovoked epileptic seizure: a population-based study. *Epilepsia* 2000; 41:1469–73.
71. Nilsson L, Tomson T, Farahmand BY, Diwan V, Persson PG. Cause-specific mortality in epilepsy: a cohort study of more than 9,000 patients once hospitalized for epilepsy. *Epilepsia* 1997; 38:1062–8.
72. Shackleton DP, Westendorp RG, Trenite DG, Vandenbroucke JP. Mortality in patients with epilepsy: 40 years of follow-up in a Dutch cohort study. *J Neurol Nerosurg Psychiatry* 1999; 66:636–40.
73. Nashef L, Fish DR, Sander JW, Shorvon SD. Incidence of sudden unexpected death in an adult outpatient cohort with epilepsy at a tertiary referral centre. *J Neurol Nerosurg Psychiatry* 1995; 58:462–4.
74. Sillanpää M, Jalava M, Kaleva O, Shinnar S. Long-term prognosis of seizures with onset in childhood. *N Engl J Med* 1998; 338:1715–22.
75. Kurtz Z, Tookey P, Ross E. Epilepsy in young people: 23 year follow-up of the British national child development study. *BMJ* 1998; 316:339–42.
76. Harvey AS, Nolan T, Carlin JB. Community-based study of mortality in children with epilepsy. *Epilepsia* 1993; 34:597–603.
77. Camfield CS, Camfield PR, Veugelers PJ. Death in children with epilepsy: a population-based study. *Lancet* 2002; 359:1891–5.
78. Hauser WA, Annegers JF, Elveback LR. Mortality in patients with epilepsy. *Epilepsia* 1980; 21:399–412.
79. Cockerell OC, Johnson AL, Sander JW, Hart YM, Goodridge DM, Shorvon SD. Mortality from epilepsy: results from a prospective population-based study. *Lancet* 1994; 344:918–21.
80. Loiseau J, Picot MC, Loiseau P. Short-term mortality after a first epileptic seizure: a population-based study. *Epilepsia* 1999; 40:1388–92.
81. Ding D, Wang W, Wu J, Ma G, Dai X, Yang B, *et al.* Premature mortality in people with epilepsy in rural China: a prospective study. *Lancet Neurol* 2006:823–7.
82. Zielinski JJ. Epilepsy and mortality rate and cause of death. *Epilepsia* 1974; 15:191–201.
83. Annegers JF, Hauser WA, Shirts SB. Heart disease mortality and morbidity in patients with epilepsy. *Epilepsia* 1984; 25:699–704.
84. Nashef L, Shorvon SD. Mortality in epilepsy. *Epilepsia* 1997; 38:1059–61.
85. Nashef L. Sudden unexplained death in epilepsy: terminology and definitions. *Epilepsia* 1997; 38: S6–8.
86. Jehi L, Najm IM. Sudden unexpected death in epilepsy: impact, mechanisms, and prevention. *Cleve Clin Med* 2008; 75(S2):66–70.
87. Hitiris N, Suratman S, Kelly K, Stephen LJ, Sills GJ, Brodie MJ. Sudden unexpected death epilepsy: A search for risk factors. *Epilepsy Behav* 2007; 10:138–41.
88. Logroscino G, Hesdorffer DC, Cascino GD, Annegers JF, Bagiella E, Hauser WA. Long-term mortality after a first episode of status epilepticus. *Neurology* 2002; 58:537–41.
89. DeLorenzo RJ, Hauser WA, Towne AR, Boggs JG, Pellock JM, Penberthy L, *et al.* A prospective, population-based epidemiologic study of status epilepticus in Richmond, Virginia. *Neurology* 1996; 46:1029–235.
90. Waterhouse EJ, Garnett LK, Towne AR, Morton LD, Barnes T, Ko D, *et al.* Prospective population-based study of intermittent and continuous convusive status epilepticus in Richmond, Virginia. *Epilepsia* 1999; 40:752–8.
91. Knake S, Rosenow F, Vescovi M, Oertel WH, Mueller HH, Wirbatz A, *et al.* Incidence of status epilepticus in adults in Germany: a prospective, population-based study. *Epilepsia* 2001; 42:714–18.
92. Logroscino G, Hesdorffer DC, Cascino GD, Annegers JF, Hauser WA. Short-term mortality after a first episode of status epilepticus. *Epilepsia* 1997; 38:1344–9.
93. Coeytaux A, Jallon P, Galobardes B, Morabia A. Incidence of status epilepticus in French-speaking Switzerland (EPISTAR). *Neurology* 2000; 55:693–7.
94. Kirby S, Sadler RM. Injury and death as a result of seizures. *Epilepsia* 1995; 36:25–8.
95. Rafnsson V, Olafsson E, Hauser WA, Gudmundsson G. Cause-specific mortality in adults with unprovoked seizures. A population-based incidence cohort study. *Neuroepidemiology* 2001; 20: 232–6.
96. White SJ, McLean AE, Howland C. Anticonvulsant drugs and cancer. A cohort study in patients with severe epilepsy. *Lancet* 1979; 2:458–61.
97. Krumholz A, Sung GY, Fisher RS, Barry E, Bergey GK, Grattan LM. Complex partial status epilepticus accompanied by serious morbidity and mortality. *Neurology* 1995; 45:1499–504.
98. Shackleton DP, Westendorp RG, Kasteleijn-Nolst Trenite DG, de Craen AJ, Vandenbroucke JP. Survival of patients with epilepsy: an estimate of the mortality risk. *Epilepsia* 2002; 43:445–50.
99. Hashimoto K, Fukushima Y, Saito F, Wada K. Mortality and cause of death in patients with epilepsy over 16 years of age. *Jpn J Psychiatry Neurol* 1989; 43:546–7.
100. Henriksen B, Juul-Jensen P, Lund M. The mortality of epilepsy. In: Brackenridge RDC (ed) *Proceedings of the International Congress of Life Assurance Medicine*, pp. 139–48. London: Pitman, 1970.
101. Livanainen M, Lehtinen J. Causes of death in institutionalized epileptics. *Epilepsia* 1979; 20:485–91.
102. Bell GS, Gaitatzis A, Bell CL, Johnson AL, Sander JW. Drowning in people with epilepsy: how great is the risk? *Neurology* 2008; 71:578–82.
103. Barraclough BM. The suicide rate of epilepsy. *Acta Psychiatr Scand* 1987; 76:339–45.
104. Nilsson L, Ahlbom A, Farahmand BY, Asberg M, Tomson T. Risk factors for suicide in epilepsy: a case control study. *Epilepsia* 2002; 43:644–51.
105. Christensen J, Vestergaard M, Mortensen PB, Sidenius P, Agerbo E. Epilepsy and risk of suicide: a population-based case-control study. *Lancet Neurol* 2007; 6:693–8.
106. Singh G, Fletcher O, Bell GS, McLean AE, Sander JW. Cancer mortality amongst people with epilepsy: a study of two cohorts with severe and presumed milder epilepsy. *Epilepsy Res* 2009; 83:190–7.
107. Shafer SQ, Hauser WA, Annegers JF, Klass DW. EEG and other early predictors of epilepsy remission: a community study. *Epilepsia* 1988; 29:590–60.
108. Cockerell OC, Johnson AL, Sander JW, Hart YM, Shorvon SD. Remission of epilepsy: results from the National General Practice Study of Epilepsy. *Lancet* 1995; 346:140–4.

109. Cockerell OC, Johnson AL, Sander JW, Shorvon SD. Prognosis of epilepsy: a review and further analysis of the first nine years of the British National General Practice Study of Epilepsy, a prospective population-based study. *Epilepsia* 1997; 38:31–46.
110. Kwan P, Sander JW. The natural history of epilepsy: an epidemiological view. *J Neurol Neurosurg Psychiatry* 2004; 75:1376–81.
111. Kwan P, Brodie MJ. Early identification of refractory epilepsy. *N Engl J Med* 2000; 342:314–19.
112. Placencia M, Sander JW, Roman M, Madera A, Crespo F, Cascante S, *et al.* The characteristics of epilepsy in a largely untreated population in rural Ecuador. *J Neurol Neurosurg Psychiatry* 1994; 57:320–5.
113. Nicoletti A, Sofia V, Vitale G, Bonelli SI, Bejarano V, Bartalesi F, *et al.* Natural history and mortality of chronic epilepsy in an untreated population of rural Bolivia: a follow-up after 10 years. *Epilepsia* 2009; 50:2199–206.
114. Keranen T, Riekkinen PJ. Remission of seizures in untreated epilepsy. *BMJ* 1993; 307:483.
115. Luciano AL, Shorvon SD. Results of treatment changes in patients with apparently drug-resistant chronic epilepsy. *Ann Neurol* 2007; 62:375–81.
116. Callaghan BC, Anand K, Hesdorffer D, Hauser WA, French JA. Likelihood of seizure remission in an adult population with refractory epilepsy. *Ann Neurol* 2007; 62:382–9.
117. Annegers JF, Dubinsky S, Coan SP, Newmark ME, Roht L. The incidence of epilepsy and unprovoked seizures in multiethnic, urban health maintenance organizations. *Epilepsia* 1999; 40(4):502–6.
118. Brewis, M. *Neurological disease in an English city*. Copenhagen: Munksgaard, 1966.
119. Granieri E, Rosati G, Tola R, Pavoni M, Paolino E, Pinna L, Mon*et al.* A descriptive study of epilepsy in the district of Copparo, Italy, 1964–1978. *Epilepsia* 1983; 24(4):502–14.
120. Joensen P. Prevalence, incidence, and classification of epilepsy in the Faroes. *Acta Neurol Scand* 1986; 74 (2):150–5.
121. Olafsson E, Hauser WA, Ludvigsson P, Gudmundsson G. Incidence of epilepsy in rural Iceland: a population-based study. *Epilepsia* 1996; 37(10):951–5.
122. Olafsson E, Ludvigsson P, Gudmundsson G, Hesdorffer D, Kjartansson O, Hauser WA. Incidence of unprovoked seizures and epilepsy in Iceland and assessment of the epilepsy syndrome classification: a prospective study. *Lancet Neurol* 2005; 4(10):627–34.
123. Basch EM, Cruz ME, Tapia D, Cruz A. Prevalence of epilepsy in a migrant population near Quito, Ecuador. *Neuroepidemiology* 1997; 16(2):94–8.
124. Nicoletti A, Reggio A, Bartoloni A, Failla G, Sofia V, Bartalesi F, *et al.* Prevalence of epilepsy in rural Bolivia: a door-to-door survey. *Neurology* 1999; 53(9):2064–9.
125. Medina MT, Duron RM, Martinez L, Osorio JR, Estrada AL, Zuniga C, *et al.* Prevalence, incidence, and etiology of epilepsies in rural Honduras: the Salama Study. *Epilepsia* 2005; 46(1):124–31.
126. Al Rajeh S, Awada A, Bademosi O, Ogunniyi A. The prevalence of epilepsy and other seizure disorders in an Arab population: a community-based study. *Seizure* 2001; 10(6):410–14.
127. Osuntokun BO, Schoenberg BS, Nottidge VA. Research protocol for measuring the prevalence of neurologic disorders in developing countries: results of a pilot study in Nigeria. *Neuroepidemiology* 1982; 1:143–53.
128. Osuntokun BO, Adeuja AO, Nottidge VA, Bademosi O, Olumide A, Ige O, *et al.* Prevalence of the epilepsies in Nigerian Africans: a community-based study. *Epilepsia* 1987; 28(3):272–9.
129. Tekle-Haimanot R, Forsgren L, Abebe M, Gebre-Mariam A, Heijbel J, Holmgren G, *et al.* Clinical and electroencephalographic characteristics of epilepsy in rural Ethiopia: a community-based study. *Epilepsy Res* 1990; 7(3):230–9.
130. Attia-Romdhane N, Mrabet A, Ben Hamida M. Prevalence of epilepsy in Kelibia, Tunisia. *Epilepsia* 1993; 34(6):1028–32.
131. Snow RW, Williams RE, Rogers JE, Mung'ala VO, Peshu N. The prevalence of epilepsy among a rural Kenyan population. Its association with premature mortality. *Trop Geogr Med* 1994; 46(3):175–9.
132. Kaiser C, Kipp W, Asaba G, Mugisa C, Kabagambe G, Rating D, *et al.* The prevalence of epilepsy follows the distribution of onchocerciasis in a west Ugandan focus. *Bull World Health Organ* 1996; 74(4):361–7.
133. Dent W, Helbok R, Matuja WB, Scheunemann S, Schmutzhard E. Prevalence of active epilepsy in a rural area in South Tanzania: a door-to-door survey. *Epilepsia* 2005; 46(12):1963–9.
134. Mathai KV, Dunn DP, Kurland LT, Reeder FA. Convulsive disorders in the Mariana Islands. *Epilepsia* 1968; 9(2):77–85.

CHAPTER 6

The Causes of Epilepsy

Simon Shorvon

In any individual, the occurrence of seizures is often the result of both genetic and acquired influences and provoking factors. Despite this multifactorial nature of causation, cases can be classified according to the predominant cause (or presumed cause) into four categories (1):

1. Idiopathic epilepsy. Defined as: epilepsy of predominately genetic origin and in which there is no gross neuroanatomical or neuropathological abnormality. There are a small number of rare epilepsies which are caused by a single gene. More common are epilepsies with presumed polygenic or complex inheritance but the nature of the genetic mechanisms has remained elusive. Most 'idiopathic generalized epilepsies' and most 'benign epilepsies of childhood' fall into this category. The term idiopathic is preferred as the production of the epilepsy is a complex mix of likely genetic and non-genetic mechanisms, and includes epigenetic and epistatic mechanisms, with chance and environmental influences operating over time as the brain develops.
2. Symptomatic epilepsy. Defined as: epilepsy, of an acquired or genetic cause, associated with neuroanatomical or neuropathological abnormalities indicative of an underlying disease or condition. This category includes both (a) acquired conditions and also (b) developmental and congenital disorders where these are associated with cerebral pathological changes, whether genetic or acquired (or indeed cryptogenic) in origin.
3. Provoked epilepsy. Defined as: epilepsy in which a specific systemic or environmental factor is the predominant cause of the seizures and in which there are no gross causative neuroanatomical or neuropathological changes.

   Some 'provoked epilepsies' will have a genetic basis and some an acquired basis. The reflex epilepsies are included in this category (which are usually genetic) as well as the epilepsies with a marked seizure precipitant.
4. Cryptogenic epilepsy. Defined as: epilepsy of presumed symptomatic nature in which the cause has not been identified. The number of such cases is diminishing, but currently this is still an important category, accounting for at least 40% of adult-onset cases of epilepsy.

It is important to note that these categories do not map easily to focal/generalized groupings, and some symptomatic epilepsies are generalized and some idiopathic epilepsies are focal. Furthermore, both generalized and focal seizures may be 'provoked', and provoked seizures can be either genetic or acquired. It is also noteworthy that the meaning of 'aetiology' now refers to the 'underlying cause' where in the past it referred often to the mechanisms of epileptogenesis (1). Both approaches would be valid, and it is likely that many downstream causes converge on a final common pathway of epileptogenesis. This is a poorly researched area. It is also clear that the mechanisms underpinning idiopathic, symptomatic, and provoked epilepsy are quite distinct. Bearing these issues in mind, a list of aetiologies divided into the four categories is presented in Table 6.1.

It must be emphasized that there are obviously cases where categorization is, to a significant extent, arbitrary, especially where the genetic or symptomatic influences are 'presumed' rather than identified.

Idiopathic epilepsy

As Hippocrates realized, 2000 years ago, inheritance is very important as a cause of epilepsy. In the 19th century too, epilepsy was considered a largely inherited disorder, often as one symptom of the 'neurological trait'. With the recent discoveries of molecular genetics and the unravelling of the human genome, genetics is again the focus of much interest (2).

Pure epilepsies as a result of single-gene disorders

'Pure epilepsy' (i.e. a condition with seizures as the only predominant symptom) resulting from a single-gene defect is very rare, and some have been described in single families only. Fifteen genes so far have been identified. Interestingly, almost all of the genes identified are genes that code for ion channels (see Chapter 11, Table 11.9). It is notable that mutations in the same gene can cause different epilepsy syndromes (phenotypic heterogeneity) and the same syndrome can be caused by mutations in different genes (genotypic heterogeneity) and clearly even in these single-gene disorders, there are more complex polygenic or environmental influences (3, 4).

Table 6.1 An aetiological classification of epilepsy

Main category	Subcategory	Subcategory	Examples[a]
Idiopathic epilepsy	Pure epilepsies due to single gene disorders		Benign familial neonatal convulsions; autosomal dominant nocturnal frontal lobe epilepsy; generalized epilepsy with febrile seizures plus; severe myoclonic epilepsy of childhood (and others)
	Pure epilepsies with complex inheritance		Idiopathic generalized epilepsy (and its subtypes); benign partial epilepsies of childhood (various subtypes)
Symptomatic epilepsy	Predominately genetic or developmental causation	Childhood epilepsy syndromes	West syndrome; Lennox–Gastaut syndrome
		Progressive myoclonic epilepsies	Unverricht–Lundborg disease; dentato-rubro-pallido-luysian atrophy; Lafora body disease; mitochondrial cytopathy; neuronal ceroid lipofuscinosis; myoclonus renal failure syndrome
		Neurocutaneous syndromes	Tuberose sclerosis, neurofibromatosis, Sturge–Weber syndrome
		Other single-gene disorders	Angelman syndrome; lysosomal disorders; neuroacanthocytosis; organic acidurias; porphyria; pyridoxine-dependent epilepsy; Rett syndrome; urea cycle disorders; Wilson disease
		Disorders of chromosome function	Down syndrome; fragile X syndrome; 4p-syndrome; ring chromosome 20
		Developmental anomalies of cerebral structure	Hemimegalencephaly; focal cortical dysplasia; agyria-pachygyria-band spectrum; agenesis of corpus callosum; polymicrogyria; schizencephaly; periventricular nodular heterotopia; microcephaly
	Predominately acquired causation	Hippocampal sclerosis	
		Perinatal and infantile causes	Neonatal seizures (various causes); cerebral palsy; post-vaccination
		Cerebral trauma	Open head injury; closed head injury; neurosurgery; non-accidental head injury in infants
		Cerebral tumour	Glioma; ganglioglioma and hamatoma; DNET; hypothalamic hamartoma; meningioma; secondary tumours
		Cerebral infection	Viral meningitis and encephalitis; bacterial meningitis and abscess; malaria; neurocysticercosis, tuberculosis; HIV
		Cerebrovascular disorders	Cerebral haemorrhage; cerebral infarction; arteriovenous malformation; cavernous haemangioma
		Cerebral immunological disorders	Rasmussen encephalitis; SLE and collagen vascular disorders; inflammatory disorders
		Degenerative diseases, and other neurological conditions	Alzheimer disease and other dementing disorders; multiple sclerosis and demyelinating disorders; hydrocephalus; arachnoid cyst and porencephaly
Provoked epilepsy		Provoking factors	Fever; menstrual cycle and catamenial epilepsy sleep–wake cycle; metabolic and endocrine-induced seizures; drug-induced seizures; alcohol- and toxin-induced seizures
		Reflex epilepsies	Photosensitive epilepsies; startle-induced epilepsies; reading epilepsy; auditory-induced epilepsy; eating epilepsy; hot-water epilepsy
Cryptogenic epilepsies[b]			

[a] These examples are not comprehensive, and in every category there are other causes (usually lumped together in a final section chapter).
[b] By definition, the causes of the cryptogenic epilepsies are 'unknown'. However, these are an important category, accounting for at least 40% of epilepsies encountered in adult practice and a lesser proportion in paediatric practice.
(Derived from reference 1.)

Pure epilepsies with complex (presumed polygenic) inheritance

Pure epilepsies with complex inheritance are much more frequent than the single-gene epilepsies. These conditions are divided into the idiopathic generalized epilepsies (IGEs) and the benign partial epilepsies of childhood. Both have been the subject of intensive genetic study, but to date no common susceptibility genes have been identified and the genetic mechanisms are obscure (5).

Idiopathic generalized epilepsy

IGE (also known as primary generalized epilepsy) is a very common condition, accounting for up to 20% of all cases of epilepsy, which probably has a genetic basis, although the genetic mechanisms and causes have not been elucidated. The condition is often subdivided into subgroups (Table 6.2), although the basis for this is arguable and certainly overlap between syndromes occurs (6). The commonest variant is juvenile myoclonic epilepsy (JME) which may account for 10% of all epilepsies. The core clinical features are shared to a greater or lesser extent by these syndromes (at least those with onset in later childhood or early adult life) and are shown in Table 6.2.

Benign partial epilepsy

The most common condition in this category, accounting for up to 15% of all epilepsies, is benign partial epilepsy with centrotemporal spikes (BECTS; also known as rolandic epilepsy or benign epilepsy with rolandic spikes) (7, 8). The core clinical features are shown in Table 6.3. Other benign partial syndromes include childhood epilepsy with occipital paroxysms (benign occipital epilepsy; Gastaut type—idiopathic childhood occipital epilepsy) and early-onset benign occipital epilepsy (synonym: Panayiotopoulos syndrome).

Symptomatic epilepsy of predominantly genetic or congenital causation

Childhood epilepsy syndromes

These have multiple causes and are included in this section for convenience as, although some causes are acquired, the majority are genetic or developmental in origin.

West syndrome

West syndrome is a severe epileptic encephalopathy, with an incidence of 1–2 per 4000 live births (9). It is defined by the occurrence of infantile spasms with an electroencephalographic (EEG) pattern of hypsarrhythmia. Ninety per cent of cases develop in the first years of life and the peak age of onset is 4–6 months. A wide variety of conditions have been reported to cause this encephalopathy (Table 6.4).

Table 6.2 Subgroups and core clinical features of idiopathic generalized epilepsy

Subgroups
◆ Epilepsy with myoclonic absences
◆ Childhood absence epilepsy (petit mal; pyknolepsy)
◆ Juvenile absence epilepsy
◆ Juvenile myoclonic epilepsy (impulsive petit mal)
◆ Epilepsy with grand mal seizures on awakening
◆ Absence epilepsy with peri-oral myoclonia
Core clinical features
◆ Onset in childhood or early adult life
◆ Positive family history in some cases
◆ Generalized seizure types—myoclonus, generalized absence (petit mal), and generalized tonic–clonic seizures
◆ A diurnal pattern of seizure recurrence, with seizures especially on waking and during sleep
◆ Normal intellect and low comorbidity
◆ Absence of identifiable underlying structural aetiology
◆ Normal EEG background
◆ Paroxysms of generalized EEG discharges, either 3 Hz spike and wave or polyspike bursts, often exacerbated by over-breathing and photosensitivity
◆ Excellent response to therapy with sodium valproate

Table 6.3 Benign epilepsy with centrotemporal spikes

- 15% of all childhood epilepsy
- Age of onset 5–10 years
- Simple partial seizures with frequent secondary generalization
- Partial seizures involve the face, oropharynx, and upper limb.
- Typically, spasm or clonic jerking of one side of the face, speech arrest, gutteral sounds
- Seizures infrequent—50% of cases have 5 seizures or less
- Seizures typically during sleep
- No other neurological features; normal intelligence
- Some cases have a positive family history
- EEG shows typical centrotemporal spikes
- Excellent response to antiepileptic drugs
- Excellent prognosis with remission by mid-teenage years

NB There are transitional cases which show some features of the benign and more severe childhood syndromes. Some cases of BECTS show features of the Landau–Kleffner syndrome and electrical status epilepticus during sleep (ESES). Some also consider febrile seizures, Panayiotopoulos syndrome and BECTS to be manifestations of a continuum (the benign childhood seizure susceptibility syndrome).

Lennox–Gastaut syndrome

Lennox–Gastaut syndrome is a term used to describe the severe epilepsies of childhood in which multiple types of epileptic seizure occur and are associated with slow (2–3 Hz) spike-wave discharges on the EEG (10). The most characteristic seizure type in this syndrome is the tonic seizure, and this is usually associated with atypical absence, myoclonic, tonic–clonic seizures, and later complex partial seizures. Learning disability is always present and is often severe. The syndrome accounts for up to 5% of all childhood epilepsies. The age of onset is usually 1–7 years. Whether this is a specific syndrome, or simply a reflection of severe epilepsy in childhood associated with learning disability is unclear. There are also overlap cases with other epilepsy syndromes, and Lennox–Gastaut syndrome can evolve from West syndrome or neonatal convulsions. There are a number of identified causes underlying this encephalopathy (Table 6.5).

Progressive myoclonic epilepsies

This term is used to describe a specific phenotype which can be caused by a variety of genetically determined neurological disorders. The predominant clinical feature is the presence of severe myoclonic seizures which evolve progressively and which are associated with other features depending on the underlying cause. In most parts of the world there are six common underlying conditions: mitochondrial disorders, Unverricht–Lundborg disease,

Table 6.4 Causes of West syndrome

- Neurocutaneous syndromes (especially tuberous sclerosis, Sturge–Weber syndrome: 7–25% of all cases)
- Cortical dysplasia (many types: 10% of all cases)
- Congenital chromosomal disorders (many types)
- Inherited metabolic disorders (many types)
- Mitochondrial disease
- Neonatal and infantile infections (15% of all cases)
- Hypoxic–ischaemic encephalopathy
- Tumours and vascular disorders
- Trauma
- Degenerative disorders

Table 6.5 Causes of Lennox–Gastaut syndrome

- Cortical dysplasia (many types)
- Neurocutaneous syndromes (tuberous sclerosis, Sturge–Weber, other forms)
- Cerebral tumour (including hypothalamic hamartoma)
- Inherited metabolic disorders (various types)
- Ischaemic–hypoxic and perinatal injury
- Congenital chromosomal disorders (many types)
- Trauma
- Cerebral infection

dentato-rubro-pallido-luysian atrophy (DRPLA), Lafora body disease, neuronal ceroid lipofuscinosis, and sialidosis. These conditions are rare, and progressive myoclonic epilepsies account for less than 1% of all referrals to tertiary epilepsy services. The investigations to elucidate their underlying causes are outlined in Chapter 11 (Table 11.11).

Neurocutaneous disorders

Epilepsy is a prominent feature of most of the neurocutaneous conditions. Tuberous sclerosis complex, Sturge–Weber syndrome, and neurofibromatosis (type 1) are the most commonly encountered. Rarer conditions include hypo-melanosis of Ito, epidermal naevus syndrome, hereditary haemorrhagic telangiectasia, Parry–Romberg syndrome, midline linear naevus syndrome, incontinentia pigmenti, and Klippel–Trénaunay–Weber syndrome (11).

Tuberous sclerosis

Tuberous sclerosis or tuberous sclerosis complex (TSC) is a common and important cause of epilepsy (12). The incidence may be as high as 1 in 5800 live births and there is a high spontaneous mutation rate (1 in 25,000). It is inherited in an autosomal dominant fashion, and is usually caused by mutations of the *TSC1* or *TSC2* genes, both tumour suppressor genes. To date, about 300 unique *TSC1* or *TSC2* mutations have been identified in nearly 400 separate patients/families and there is also a significant degree of mosaicism which complicates genetic assessment. The manifestations of the condition are very variable, but epilepsy is present in 80%. It can take the form of neonatal seizures, West syndrome, Lennox–Gastaut syndrome, or as adult-onset partial or generalized seizures. About two-thirds of patients present with seizures before the age of 2 years. About 25% of all cases of West syndrome are due to TSC. The diagnostic criteria are shown in Table 6.6.

Neurofibromatosis

Neurofibromatosis type 1 (NF1) is a common, dominantly inherited genetic disorder, occurring in about 1 in 3000 live births (13). Almost half of all cases are new mutations and the new mutation rate for the *NF1* gene is about 1 in 10,000, amongst the highest known for any human gene. Many different mutations have been reported in this large gene, and although the penetrance is essentially complete, the clinical manifestations are extremely variable. The incidence of epilepsy is about 5–10%. The clinical features include: six or more café au lait macules over 5 mm in greatest diameter in prepubertal individuals and over 15 mm in greatest diameter in postpubertal individual, two or more neurofibromas of any type or one plexiform neurofibroma, freckling in the axillary or inguinal regions, optic glioma, Lisch nodules (iris hamartomas), and bone lesion such as sphenoid dysplasia or thinning of the long bone cortex, and pseudarthrosis. Epilepsy occurs but is less common in neurofibromatosis type 2.

Table 6.6 Diagnostic criteria of tuberous sclerosis complex

- Major features
- Facial angiofibromas or forehead plaque
- Non-traumatic ungual or periungual fibromas
- Hypomelanotic macules (3 or more)
- Shagreen patch (connective tissue naevus)
- Multiple retinal nodular hamartomas
- Cortical tuber
- Subependymal nodule
- Subependymal giant cell astrocytoma
- Cardiac rhabdomyoma, single or multiple
- Lymphangiomyomatosis
- Renal angiomyolipoma
- Minor features
- Multiple randomly distributed pits in dental enamel
- Hamartomatous rectal polyps
- Bone cysts
- Cerebral white matter radial migration lines
- Gingival fibromas
- Non-renal hamartoma
- Retinal achromic patch
- 'Confetti' skin lesions
- Multiple renal cysts
- Definite TSC: 2 major features or 1 major feature, plus 2 minor features
- Probable TSC: 1 major feature plus 1 minor feature
- Possible TSC: 1 major feature or 2 or more minor features

Sturge–Weber syndrome

This is the third neurocutaneous syndrome in which epilepsy is a prominent feature. The clinical features are a unilateral or bilateral port wine naevus, epilepsy, hemiparesis, mental impairment, and ocular signs (14). Seventy per cent of patients with Sturge–Weber syndrome develop seizures within the first year of life and almost all have developed epilepsy before the age of 4 years.

Other single-gene disorders

In addition to the conditions already mentioned, there are many other single-gene and chromosomal disorders in which epilepsy is part of the phenotype. Most are rare or very rare, manifest initially in childhood, and present for diagnosis to paediatric neurological services rather than to an epilepsy specialist, and in only a few of these conditions does the epilepsy have distinctive features or is a predominant or consistent feature. Almost all are associated with learning disabilities and other neurological features (the features of which vary with the specific condition) and epilepsy is only one symptom of a much broader clinical picture. Conditions in which epilepsy is a prominent feature include Angelman syndrome, Rett syndrome, lysosomal storage or transport disorders, peroxisomal, pyridoxine-dependent disorders, inherited disorders of cobalamin and folate metabolism, amino acid and organic acid disorders, neuroacanthocytosis, porphyrias, urea cycle disorders, and Wilson disease (see also Chapter 11).

Angelman syndrome

This condition, with a frequency of about 1 in every 10,000–20,000 births, accounts for about 6% of all those with mental retardation and epilepsy. There is a rather characteristic phenotype with dysmorphic features, learning disability, severe epilepsy, a characteristic motor disturbance with 'puppet-like' movements due to truncal ataxia and titubation, a happy demeanour, and speech disturbance. Epilepsy is present in 85–90% of cases. In about 80% of cases defects are present in the chromosome 15q11–q13 region, and involve a deletion, maternal disomy, imprinting defect, or, rarely, translocation. This region contains a cluster of GABA receptor subunit genes. Iatrogenic mutations in the *UBE3A* gene are found in about 10% of cases.

Rett syndrome

This is an X-linked dominant disorder, almost always presenting in females. The defect is in the *MECP2* gene, which controls RNA production. Birth and development in the first 6 months are normal. In the classic phenotype, the children then decline with severe mental regression with autistic features, motor disturbances with highly characteristic manual stereotypies, and eventually total quadraparesis, apnoeic attacks, and a complex disturbance of breathing and a tendency for gastric regurgitation. Short stature, wasting, and microcephaly are typical. Language is severely affected and speech may cease altogether. Epilepsy occurs in over 50% of identified cases, and tends to develop when the disease has stabilized. It has recently become clear that the phenotype is much wider than in the classic descriptions, and it is recognized that some adult women with only mild intellectual disability have the same genetic defect. Occasional male cases survive who have either a 47,XXY karyotype or somatic mosaicism (those with 47,XY and *MECP2* mutations die in the first years of life).

Disorders of chromosome structure

Epilepsy is also a feature of two common chromosomal abnormalities: Down syndrome and fragile X syndrome (15, 16). It also takes a highly characteristic form in the rare ring chromosome 20. Other uncommon chromosomal abnormalities in which epilepsy is found include trisomy 12p, 8, 13; ring chromosome 14; partial monosomy 4p (Wolf–Hirschhorn syndrome); inverted duplication of pericentromeric chromosome 15; and Klinefelter syndrome (where epilepsy occurs in about 10% of cases). In all these conditions, there are additional behavioural and intellectual disabilities and characteristic dysmorphic features. The seizures often take multiple forms, including myoclonus, and are of variable severity. Genetic testing is available for most conditions.

Down syndrome

The Down phenotype occurs in about 1 in every 650 live births. It is usually caused by trisomy of chromosome 21, and triplication of 21q22.3 results in the typical phenotype. In 95% of cases the cause is a non-disjunction, and in about 4% an unbalanced translocation. About 1% of cases are due to mosaicism. The risk of trisomy increases with maternal age. Epilepsy is present in up to 12% of cases and EEG abnormalities in more than 20%.

Fragile X syndrome

Fragile X syndrome is a condition due to an increased number of CGG repeats (typically more than 200) in the *FMR1* gene (at Xq27.3) accompanied by aberrant methylation of the gene (17). It is an X-linked condition in which males have more severe symptoms. It is diagnosed in about 1 in 4000 male births, and carrier rates in females (CAG repeats of approx 50–200) may be as high as 1 in 250. Seizures are present in one-quarter of cases and can take various forms. Repeat numbers vary, and mosaicism is common, and these may account for the variable clinical features.

Ring chromosome 20

This is a rare condition, but one in which epilepsy is the predominant feature and it has a highly characteristic phenotype. Seizures typically take the form of long episodes of non-convulsive status epilepticus characterized by confusion, staring, perioral and eyelid myoclonus, and with a highly characteristic EEG. The locus of fusion between the deleted short and long arms of the chromosome is at p13q13, p13q13.3.3, or p13q13.33. Mosaicism is common and the condition can develop at any age and varies considerable in severity.

Cortical dysplasia

Cortical dysplasia (synonyms: cortical dysgenesis, malformations of cortical development) is a term that is applied to developmental disorders of the cortex producing structural change (Table 6.7) (18, 19). A minority of these conditions are caused by identifiable genetic abnormalities, others by environmental influences such as infection, trauma, hypoxia, or exposure to drugs or toxins, but in most instances the cause is unclear. Cortical malformations can be due to abnormal neuronal and glial proliferation, abnormal neuronal migration, or abnormal synaptogenesis, cortical organization, or programmed cell death. Epilepsy is a predominant symptom, and occasionally the only symptoms (particularly in adult-onset epilepsy due to cortical dysplasia). Usually, though, there is also learning disability which can be severe and focal neurological signs.

Table 6.7 Types of cortical dysplasia

Abnormalities of gyration
◆ Agyria (lissencephaly), macrogyria, pachygyria spectrum (focal or diffuse) (*LIS1, RELN, ARX*, and *DCX* genes) ◆ Polymicrogyria ◆ Cobblestone complex (*FCMD* gene) ◆ Schizencephaly (*EMX2* gene) ◆ Minor gyral abnormalities
Heterotopias
◆ Periventricular nodular heterotopia (*FLNA* gene) ◆ Subcortical nodular heterotopia ◆ Subcortical band heterotopia (*DCX* and *LIS1* genes)
Other gross malformations
◆ Megalencephaly and hemimegalencephaly ◆ Agenesis of corpus callosum ◆ Anencephaly and holoprosencephaly ◆ Microcephaly
Cortical dysgenesis associated with neoplasia
◆ DNET ◆ Ganglioglioma ◆ Gangliocytoma
Other cortical dysplasias
◆ Hypothalamic hamartoma ◆ Focal cortical dysplasia ◆ Tuberous sclerosis (*TSC1* and *TSC2* genes)
Microdysgenesis

(From reference 38.)

Symptomatic epilepsy due to acquired causes

Almost any condition affecting the cerebral grey matter can result in epilepsy. The seizures in symptomatic and acquired epilepsy usually but not always take a partial or secondarily generalized form, and there are often no particularly distinctive features associated with any particular cause. The seizures also may have a strongly 'provoked' element, as may those in idiopathic epilepsy (20).

The epilepsies in acute cerebral conditions—for example, stroke, head injury, or infections—share a number of general features. The epilepsies are often divided into 'early' (i.e. seizures occurring within a week of the insult) and 'late' (i.e. chronic epilepsy developing later). There is often a 'silent period' between the injury and the onset of late epilepsy. Presumably, epileptogenic processes are developing during this period, and this raises the possibility of neuroprotective interventions to inhibit these processes and prevent later epilepsy. Antiepileptic drug therapy will prevent early epilepsy but does not reduce the frequency of late seizures. Early seizures are often not followed by late epilepsy—a fact that is important to emphasize to patients.

Hippocampal sclerosis

Hippocampal sclerosis is the most common cause of temporal lobe epilepsy, and has a rather typical clinical form (21–23). The principal pathological abnormality is atrophy and neuronal cell loss and gliosis in the CA1 and CA3 regions and in the hilar region of dentate gyrus, and relative sparing of the CA2 region. There is extensive synaptic rearrangement, including re-current innervation of dentate granule cells by their own neurons ('mossy fibre' innervation).

Hippocampal sclerosis can be caused in a variety of ways including cerebral trauma, infection (encephalitis or meningitis), vascular damage, or toxins (e.g. domoic acid). Familial genetic forms also exist. However, there is a clear association with a history of childhood febrile convulsions, and it is widely believed that the most common cause of hippocampal sclerosis is a prolonged or complex childhood febrile convulsion which causes excitotoxic damage acutely to the hippocampus and results in later hippocampal sclerosis and then temporal lobe epilepsy.

Prenatal or perinatal injury

In the past, epilepsy has often been attributed to perinatal injury, although it is now recognized that this is a misattribution, and many such cases have had in fact other genetic or developmental causes. In controlled studies, only severe perinatal insults have been found to increase the risk of subsequent epilepsy (e.g. perinatal haemorrhage, ischaemic–hypoxic encephalopathy). Less severe injuries such as toxaemia, eclampsia, forceps delivery, being born with the 'cord round the neck', low birth weight, or prematurity have only a very modest association, if any, with subsequent epilepsy.

Post-vaccination encephalitic encephalomyelitis

There has been controversy about a possible role of vaccination (particularly pertussis vaccination) in the causation of childhood encephalopathy and subsequent epilepsy (24). There is now a general consensus that the risk of vaccine-induced encephalopathy and/or epilepsy is extremely low. Risk estimates include: risk of a febrile seizure 1 per 19,496 pertussis vaccinations; risk of an afebrile seizure 1 per 76,133 vaccinations; risk of encephalopathy 0–3 cases per million vaccinations. Some cases of apparent vaccination injury in fact carry an inherited genetic defect of the *SCNIA* gene which is the root cause of the epilepsy.

Post-traumatic epilepsy

Head trauma is an important cause of epilepsy. Identified head injury accounts for about 6% of all cases of epilepsy. It is customary to draw distinctions between open head injury, where the dura is breached, and closed head injury, where there is no dural breach, and also between civilian and military head injury, the latter due to blast and high-velocity injuries.

Post-traumatic seizures are traditionally subdivided into immediate, early, and late categories. Immediate seizures are defined as those that occur within the first 24 hours after injury (these seizures are sometimes excluded from the early post-traumatic estimates), early seizures are those that occur within the first week, and late seizures those that occur after 1 week. About 5% of all those admitted to hospital with head injury experience early seizures, and they are more common in children than adults.

About 25% of those with early seizures develop late seizures. Commonly, late seizures develop in the months after a head injury and 57% of late seizures occur within a year, but the risk of developing seizures remains elevated for the first 5–10 years after the injury.

Closed head injuries are usually caused by road traffic accidents, falls, assault, or sporting injuries. In mild head injury, defined as head injury without skull fracture and with less than 30 minutes of post-traumatic amnesia, the risk of epilepsy is very small. Moderate head injury, defined as a head injury complicated by skull fracture and/or post-traumatic amnesia for more than 30 minutes, is followed by epilepsy in about 1–4% of cases. Severe closed head injury, defined as a head injury with post-traumatic amnesia of more than 24 hours, intracranial haematoma, and/or depressed skull fracture has been found in most studies to be followed by epilepsy in about 10–15% of patients. In a recent, very large population-based study of children and young adults, the relative risk for epilepsy was 2.22 (95% confidence interval (CI) 2.07–2.38) in the presence of mild brain injury and 7.40 (95% CI 6.16–8.89) in the presence of severe brain injury (25). Open head injury is a more potent cause of epilepsy. Between 30–50% of patients in penetrating wartime injuries suffer subsequent epilepsy. In Jennet's study from Glasgow of patients admitted to hospital, after head injury, the risk of late epilepsy was: 25% if early epilepsy was present and 3% if not; 35% if there is an intracranial haematoma and about 5% if not; 17% if there is a depressed skull facture and 4% if not. If there is neither haematoma nor depressed skull fracture, the risk of epilepsy is 1% if there were no early seizures and 26% if there were early seizures (26).

Epilepsy due to brain tumours

Brain tumours are responsible for about 5–10% of all newly diagnosed cases of epilepsy (27). The rate is greatest in adults, and about one-quarter of adults presenting with newly developing focal epilepsy have an underlying tumour, compared to less than 5% in children. The frequency of seizures is high in tumours in the frontal, central, and temporal regions, lower in posterior cortically placed tumours and very low in subcortical tumours. Epilepsy occurs in

92% of those with oligodendrogliomas, 70% of those with astrocytomas, and 37% of those with glioblastomas. Epilepsy is the first symptom of meningioma in 20–50% of cases. In slow-growing tumours, the history of epilepsy will often have extended for decades, sometimes even into infancy.

In hospital-based studies of chronic epilepsy due to cerebral tumours, oligodendrogliomas account for between 10–40% of cases, dysembryoplastic neuroepithelial tumours (DNETs) for 10–30%, astrocytomas for 10–30%, and gangliogliomas or hamartomas each for between 10–20%. Hypothalamic hamartomas are a rare tumour, but one with a characteristic phenotype. They usually present in young children with gelastic seizures, learning disability, behavioural disturbance, and later with precocious puberty.

Epilepsy following cerebral infection

Encephalitis is a potent cause of epilepsy (28). The risk of developing chronic epilepsy following encephalitis is estimated to be 16-fold greater than that in the general population and 4.2 times greater after bacterial meningitis, and 2.3 times greater after aseptic meningitis. The increased risk is highest during the first 5 years after infection, but remains elevated for up to 15 years. The commonest serious viral encephalitis is due to herpes simplex virus type-1 (HSV-1) and this frequently results in severe and intractable epilepsy. The incidence of severe HSV-1 encephalitis is about 1 per million persons per year. Pyogenic brain abscess is a now uncommon but serious cause of infective epilepsy. Commonly isolated organisms are streptococci, including aerobic, anaerobic, and microaerophilic types. *Streptococcus pneumoniae* is a rarer cause of brain abscesses, which are often the sequel to occult cerebrospinal fluid rhinorrhoea and also to pneumococcal pneumonia in elderly patients. Enteric bacteria and *Bacteroides* are isolated in 20–40% of cases and often in mixed culture. Staphylococcal abscesses account for 10–15% of cases and are usually caused by penetrating head injury or bacteraemia secondary to endocarditis. Clostridial infections are most often post-traumatic. Very rarely, brain abscess can be caused by fungi such as *Actinomyces* or *Nocardia*.

The frequency of post-infective epilepsy also varies according to geographic region. In Africa, for instance, malaria is a particularly common cause with seizures and typically status epilepticus in the acute phase of cerebral malaria, and there is a 9–11-fold (CI 2–18) increase in risk of chronic epilepsy in children with a history of malaria. Neurocysticercosis is the most common parasitic disease of the central nervous system (CNS) and a major cause of epilepsy in endemic areas such as Mexico, India, and China. The brain cysts can be single or multiple. Epilepsy is the commonest clinical manifestation and usual presenting feature. Diagnosis is made by imaging and by serological tests. Epilepsy is also frequently the presenting symptom of tuberculoma. Tuberculoma account for about 3% of all cerebral mass lesions in India, for instance, and 13% of all cerebral lesions in HIV-infected patients. Diagnosis depends on the clinical context, imaging, serology, and histological examination of biopsy material.

Epilepsy due to cerebrovascular disease

Stroke is the most commonly identified cause of epilepsy in the elderly, and occult stroke also explains the occurrence of many cases of apparently cryptogenic epilepsies in aged individuals (29). A history of stroke has been found to be associated with an increased lifetime occurrence of epilepsy (odds ration (OR) 3.3; 95% CI 1.3–8.5). Status epilepticus occurs in the acute phase of about 1% of all strokes, and 20% of status epilepticus is due to stroke. In cerebral haemorrhage, epilepsy is more common after large haemorrhages and haemorrhages which involve the cerebral cortex, and less common in deep haematomas and rare after subtentorial haemorrhage (30). The epilepsy almost always develops within 2 years of the haemorrhage and the risk of epilepsy is about 1%. Twenty to 34% of patients develop seizures after subarachnoid haemorrhage. Epilepsy occurs in about 6% of patients within 12 months and 11% within 5 years of a stroke due to cerebral infarction. The risk of epilepsy is about 17–20 times greater than in non-stroke controls. Factors associated with a greater risk of epilepsy have been the subject of several studies, and are: severity, size of infarct, haemorrhagic transformation, a cortical (as opposed to subcortical) site of the stroke, and, in some studies, embolism as a cause of the stroke.

Late-onset epilepsy can be the first manifestation of occult cerebrovascular disease. Between 5–10% of patients presenting with stroke have a history of prior epileptic seizures in the recent past, and in the absence of other causes, new-onset seizures should prompt an emergency screen for vascular risk factors with the aim of preventing a stroke.

Between 17–36% of supratentorial arteriovenous malformations (AVMs) present with seizures, with or without associated neurological deficits, and 40–50% with haemorrhage. Smaller arterial AVMs (<3 cm diameter) are more likely to present with haemorrhage than large ones. Conversely, large and/or superficial malformations are more epileptogenic, as are AVMs in the temporal lobe. About 40% of patients with large anterior venous malformations have epilepsy, and epilepsy is the presenting symptom in about 20%. Small venous malformations do not usually result in any symptoms. The risk of haemorrhage from a venous angioma is lower than from an arterial angioma.

Cavernous haemangioma (cavernoma) account for 5–13% of vascular malformations of the CNS and are present in 0.02–0.13% of autopsy series. Patients present with seizures (40–70%), focal neurological deficits (35–50%), non-specific headaches (10–30%), and cerebral haemorrhage. Familial clustering can be found in 10–30% of cavernous haemangiomas, and familial cases have been found to be linked to genes at three different loci, the *CCM1*, *CCM2*, and *CCM3* genes. Forty per cent of familial cases are due to *CCM1*, with higher rates amongst Hispanic cases. Genetic testing is available. Appearances on magnetic resonance imaging are characteristic.

Epilepsy can also be a symptom of cortical venous infarcts, rheumatic heart disease, endocarditis, mitral valve prolapse, cardiac tumours and cardiac arrhythmia, or after carotid endarterectomy. Infarction is also an important cause for seizures in neonatal epilepsy. Epilepsy is also common in eclampsia, hypertensive encephalopathy, malignant hypertension, and in the anoxic encephalopathy which follows cardiac arrest or cardiopulmonary surgery. Unruptured aneurysms occasionally present as epilepsy, especially if large and if embedded in the temporal lobe—for instance, a giant middle cerebral or anterior communicating aneurysm. Epilepsy, with a vascular basis, also occurs in antiphospholipid syndrome, CADASIL (cerebral autosomal dominant arteriopathy with subcortical infarcts and leucoencephalopathy), Moya Moya disease, collagen disease (e.g. Ehlers–Danlos syndrome, Marfan syndrome), vasculitis, Behçet's disease, and amyloid angiography. Other rare causes of epilepsy include: temporal arteritis, polyarteritis nodosum, Takayasu disease, Fabry disease, and the hyperviscosity syndrome.

Epilepsy in inflammatory and immunological diseases of the nervous system

Epilepsy is common in inflammatory disease (31). The frequency of epilepsy in patients with multiple sclerosis is about three times that in the general population. In one study, the cumulative risk of epilepsy in patients with multiple sclerosis was found to be 1.1% at 5 years, 1.8% by 10 years, and 3.1% by 15 years. ADEM (acute disseminated encephalomyelitis) is an acute inflammatory demyelinating disorder which can follow systemic infections, and which is immunologically-mediated. Epilepsy is a feature of the acute attack, and occurs much more commonly than in an acute attack of multiple sclerosis.

Epilepsy can occur in all other forms of large-, medium-, or small-vessel vasculitis, sometimes on the basis of infarction. Seizures occur in about 25% of cases of systemic lupus erythematosus (SLE). Seizures can be the presenting symptom, and are particularly common in severe or chronic cases and in lupus-induced encephalopathy. Epilepsy occurs less often in other vasculitides such as Behçet's disease and in other 'connective tissue disorders' such as Sjögren syndrome and mixed connective tissue disease and Henoch–Schönlein purpura. Seizures are the commonest neurological complication of the inflammatory bowel diseases (ulcerative colitis and Crohn's disease) occurring in one series in 6% of cases. Epilepsy is also a prominent feature of Hashimoto's thyroiditis, a relapsing encephalopathy associated with high titres of thyroid antibody. There has been recent interest in the occurrence of epilepsy in the syndrome of limbic encephalitis, associated with high titres of antibodies against voltage-gated potassium channels and the acute encephalopathy associated with anti-NMDA receptor antibodies. In these immunologically mediated disease, epilepsy usually presents as a subacute illness, associated also with psychosis, neurological signs (e.g. ataxia), memory loss, and behavioural change. Other cases of limbic encephalitis have no detectable antibody present although in such cases the cause is likely to be an as yet unidentified antibody, and some are para-neoplastic (32).

Provoked epilepsy

In the 19th century, all epilepsies were considered to be in part caused by provoking (exciting factors) (33) and it has been only recently that the importance of provoking factors has been again recognized (34).

The term reflex epilepsy is used to describe cases in which seizures are evoked consistently by a specific environmental trigger. Simple reflex seizures are defined as those precipitated by elementary sensory stimuli (e.g. flashes of light, startle), and complex reflex seizures are those precipitated by more elaborate stimuli (e.g. specific pieces of music). The complex forms are much more heterogeneous and less well defined than the simple reflex epilepsies. The stimuli most reported to cause seizures include flashing lights and other visual stimuli, startle, eating, hot water, music, reading, and movement. The commonest reflex epilepsies are those induced by visual stimuli, such as flashing lights, bright lights, moving visual patterns (e.g. escalators), eye closure, moving from dark into bright light, and viewing specific objects or colours. The term photosensitive epilepsy should be confined to those individuals who show unequivocal EEG evidence of photosensitivity, and differentiated from other, usually more complex, cases in which seizures can be apparently precipitated by visual stimuli but in whom EEG evidence of photosensitivity can not be demonstrated. Photosensitivity (strictly defined) is present in a population with a frequency of about 1.1 per 100,000 persons, and 5.7 per 100,000 in the 7–19 years age range, and is strongly associated with epilepsy. About 3% of persons with epilepsy are photosensitive and have seizures induced by photic stimuli. Most patients with photosensitivity have the syndrome of IGE, although photosensitivity is also occurs in patients with focal epilepsy arising in the occipital region and occasionally in other conditions.

Many types of metabolic disturbances can cause epilepsy (35). The degree and rate of fall are important variables in determining whether seizures will occur. The more abnormal the level and the faster the rate of change of metabolic parameters, the higher the chance of a seizure. Seizures occur most commonly in hypoglycaemia, hyponatraemia, hypocalcaemia, hypercalcaemia, hypomagnesaemia, hypokalaemia, and hyperkalaemia. Ten per cent of patients with severe renal failure have seizures, caused either by the metabolic disturbance, renal encephalopathy, dialysis encephalopathy, or dialysis disequilibrium syndrome. Seizures are also a common occurrence in hepatic failure. Hepatic encephalopathy may be overlooked and routine liver function tests can be relatively normal. Hyperammonaemia is sometimes diagnostically helpful in detecting liver disease and can be a cause of seizures. Reye syndrome should be considered in children with liver failure where it is associated with aspirin intake. Hypoglycaemia is a potent cause of seizures—which can occur if the blood sugar levels fall below 2.2 mmol/L. This is commonly due to insulin or other hypoglycaemics but can also be due to insulinoma. Non-ketotic hyperglycaemia frequently causes seizures. Levels of blood sugar as low as 15–20 mmol/L can cause seizures if there is associated hyperosmolarity.

Alcohol abuse is a potent cause of epilepsy (36). Binge drinking can result in acute cerebral toxicity and seizures. Alcohol withdrawal in an alcohol-dependent person carries an even greater risk of seizures. Seizures can also be caused by the metabolic disturbances associated with binge drinking, the cerebral damage due to trauma, cerebral infection, subdural haematoma, the chronic neurotoxic effects of chronic alcohol exposure, or to acute Wernicke's encephalopathy due to thiamine deficiency.

Seizures can also be provoked by exposure to many different toxins, notably heavy metal or carbon monoxide poisoning. A wide range of drugs, toxins, and illicit compounds can cause acute symptomatic seizures and epilepsy although seizures accounted for less than 1% of 32,812 consecutive patients prospectively monitored for drug toxicity (37).

Acknowledgements

The text of this chapter is based partly on the following: Shorvon SD. *Epilepsy* (Oxford Neurology Library Series). Oxford: Oxford University Press, 2009; Shorvon SD. *Handbook of the Treatment of Epilepsy*. Oxford: Wiley-Blackwell, 2010; Shorvon SD, Andermann F, Guerrini R (eds). *The Causes of Epilepsy: Common and Uncommon Causes in Adults and Children*. Cambridge: Cambridge University Press, 2011. This work was undertaken at UCLH/UCL who received a proportion of funding from the Department of Health's NIHR Biomedical Research Centres funding scheme.

References

1. Shorvon SD, Andermann F, Guerrini R (eds) *The Causes of Epilepsy. Common and Uncommon Causes in Adults and Children*. Cambridge: Cambridge University Press, 2011. [The most comprehensive reference work on the topic of causation of epilepsy. Therein are detailed references to most causes of epilepsy. Details in this chapter are taken from various contributions and from the historical introduction of this reference work.
2. Shorvon SD. The etiologic classification of epilepsy. *Epilepsia* 2011; 52:1052–7.
3. Guerrini R, Shorvon SD, Andermann F. Introduction to the concept of genetic epilepsy. In: Shorvon SD, Andermann F, Guerrini R (eds) *The Causes of Epilepsy. Common and Uncommon Causes in Adults and Children*, pp. 43–62. Cambridge: Cambridge University Press, 2011.
4. Greenberg DA, Subaran R. Blinders, phenotype, and fashionable genetic analysis: a critical examination of the current state of epilepsy genetic studies. *Epilepsia* 2011; 52(1):1–9.
5. Lu Y, Wang X. Genes associated with idiopathic epilepsies: a current overview. *Neurol Res* 2009; 31(2):135–43.
6. Johnson MR, Shorvon SD. Heredity in epilepsy: Neurodevelopment, comorbidity, and the neurological trait. *Epilepsy Behav* 2011; 22:421–7.
7. Panayiotopoulos CP. *A Clinical Guide to Epileptic Syndromes and Their Treatment* (2nd edn). New York: Springer, 2007.
8. Stephani U. Typical semiology of benign childhood epilepsy with centrotemporal spikes (BCECTS). *Epileptic Disord* 2000; 2:S3–S4.
9. Fejerman N, Caraballo R, Tenembaum SN. Atypical evolutions of benign localization-related epilepsies in children: are they predictable? *Epilepsia* 2000; 41:380–90.
10. Pellock JM, Hrachovy R, Shinnar S, Baram TZ, Bettis D, Dlugos DJ, *et al.* Infantile spasms: a U.S. consensus report. *Epilepsia* 2010; 51:2175–89.
11. Arzimanoglou A, French J, Blume WT, Cross JH, Ernst JP, Feucht M, *et al.* Lennox-Gastaut syndrome: a consensus approach on diagnosis, assessment, management, and trial methodology. *Lancet Neurol* 2009; 8:82–93.
12. Jóźwiak S, Kotulska KS. Gene table: monogenic determined neurocutaneous disorders. *Eur J Paediatr Neurol* 2010; 14:449–51.
13. Orlova KA, Crino PB. The tuberous sclerosis complex. *Ann N Y Acad Sci* 2010; 1184:87–105.
14. Ferner RE. Neurofibromatosis 1 and neurofibromatosis 2: a twenty first century perspective. *Lancet Neurol* 2007; 6:340–51.
15. Comi AM. Presentation, diagnosis, pathophysiology, and treatment of the neurological features of Sturge–Weber syndrome. *Neurologist* 2011; 17:179–84.
16. Singh R, Gardner RJ, Crossland KM, Scheffer IE, Berkovic SF. Chromosomal abnormalities and epilepsy: a review for clinicians and gene hunters. *Epilepsia* 2002; 43:127–40.
17. Battaglia A, Guerrini R. Chromosomal disorders associated with epilepsy. *Epileptic Disord* 2005; 7:181–92.
18. Qiu LF, Hao YH, Li QZ, Xiong ZQ. Fragile X syndrome and epilepsy. *Neurosci Bull* 2008; 24:338–44.
19. Guerrini R, Marini C. Genetic malformations of cortical development. *Exp Brain Res* 2006; 173:322–33.
20. Mitchell KJ. The genetics of neurodevelopmental disease. *Curr Opin Neurobiol* 2011; 21:197–203.
21. Shorvon SD. Introduction to the concept of symptomatic epilepsy. In: Shorvon SD, Andermann F, Guerrini R (eds) *The Causes of Epilepsy. Common and Uncommon Causes in Adults and Children*, pp. 113–30. Cambridge: Cambridge University Press, 2011.
22. Sloviter RS. Hippocampal epileptogenesis in animal models of mesial temporal lobe epilepsy with hippocampal sclerosis: the importance of the 'latent period' and other concepts. *Epilepsia* 2008; 49 (Suppl 9):85–92.
23. Baulac S, Gourfinkel-An I, Nabbout R, Huberfeld G, Serratosa J, Leguern E, *et al.* Fever, genes, and epilepsy. *Lancet Neurol* 2004; 3:421–30.
24. Cendes F. Febrile seizures and mesial temporal sclerosis. *Curr Opin Neurol* 2004; 17:161–4.
25. Shorvon S, Berg A. Pertussis vaccination and epilepsy—an erratic history, new research and the mismatch between science and social policy. *Epilepsia* 2008; 49:219–25.
26. Christensen J, Pedersen MG, Pedersen CB, Sidenius P, Olsen J, Vestergaard M. Long-term risk of epilepsy after traumatic brain injury in children and young adults: a population-based cohort study. *Lancet* 2009; 373(9669):1105–10.
27. Jennett B. *Epilepsy After Non-Missile Head Injuries* (2nd edn). Chicago, IL: Year Book Medical, 1975.
28. Thomas DG, Graham DI. *Brain Tumours*. London: Butterworth-Heinemann, 1980.
29. Singhi P. Infectious causes of seizures and epilepsy in the developing world. *Dev Med Child Neurol* 2011; 53:600–9.
30. Menon B, Shorvon SD. Ischaemic stroke in adults and epilepsy. *Epilepsy Res* 2009; 87:1–11.
31. Gilmore E, Choi HA, Hirsch LJ, Claassen J. Seizures and CNS hemorrhage: spontaneous intracerebral and aneurysmal subarachnoid hemorrhage. *Neurologist* 2010; 16:165–75.
32. Lunn M. Inflammatory and immunological diseases of the central nervous system. In: Shorvon SD, Andermann F, Guerrini R (eds) *The Causes of Epilepsy. Common and Uncommon Causes in Adults and Children*, pp. 585–92. Cambridge: Cambridge University Press, 2011.
33. Dalmau J. Status epilepticus due to paraneoplastic and nonparaneoplastic encephalitides. *Epilepsia* 2009; 50(Suppl 12):58–60.
34. Shorvon SD. Historical introduction: The causes of epilepsy in the pre-molecular era (1860–1960). In: Shorvon SD, Andermann F, Guerrini R (eds) *The Causes of Epilepsy. Common and Uncommon Causes in Adults and Children*, pp. 1–20. Cambridge: Cambridge University Press, 2011.
35. Shorvon SD, Guerrini R, Andermann D. Introduction to the concept of provoked epilepsy. In: Shorvon SD, Andermann F, Guerrini R (eds) *The Causes of Epilepsy. Common and Uncommon Causes in Adults and Children*, pp. 625–30. Cambridge: Cambridge University Press, 2011.
36. Menon B, Shorvon SD. Electrolytes or sugar disturbance. In: Shorvon SD, Andermann F, Guerrini R (eds) *The Causes of Epilepsy. Common and Uncommon Causes in Adults and Children*, pp. 655–63. Cambridge: Cambridge University Press, 2011.
37. Shapiro M, Cole A. Alcohol and toxin-induced seizures. In: Shorvon SD, Andermann F, Guerrini R (eds) *The Causes of Epilepsy. Common and Uncommon Causes in Adults and Children*, pp. 674–82. Cambridge: Cambridge University Press, 2011.
38. Shorvon S. *Handbook of epilepsy treatment*. Oxford: Wiley Blackwell, 2010.

CHAPTER 7

Classification, Clinical Symptoms, and Syndromes

Renzo Guerrini and Carmen Barba

The classification of the epilepsies and of epilepsy syndromes has been a topic of much concern, and controversy for decades. In 1981 the International League Against Epilepsy (ILAE) Commission on Classification and Terminology proposed an International Classification of Epileptic Seizures (1). Seizures were classified as partial and generalized (Table 7.1). Seizures were defined as partial if the first clinical and electroencephalographic (EEG) signs indicated that initial activation was limited to part of one cerebral hemisphere. Partial seizures were classified in simple or complex on the basis of whether or not awareness was impaired during the attack. Seizures were considered as generalized if the first clinical and EEG changes indicated the initial involvement of both hemispheres.

To complement the Classification of Epileptic Seizures, in 1989 the ILAE Commission on Classification and Terminology proposed a Classification of Epilepsies and Epileptic Syndromes (2), conceived as a tool for characterizing epilepsies as different conditions and diseases responsible for seizure recurrence. However, since current knowledge of the mechanisms of epileptogenesis was considered too limited to draw a classification based upon pathogenesis, the Commission adopted a syndromic classification. A syndrome was considered as a group of signs and symptoms customarily occurring in association, including seizure types, clinical background, neurophysiological and neuroimaging findings and, often, outcome (Table 7.2). According to symptoms, epilepsies were classified as generalized and partial (or focal). Generalized epilepsies were defined as characterized by generalized seizures, bilateral motor manifestations, and generalized interictal and ictal EEG discharges. Partial epilepsies were those characterized by seizures originating from a circumscribed brain region, and by clinical manifestations consistent with a focal onset of the epileptic discharge, with or without subsequent spread, and by focal ictal or interictal EEG abnormalities. The 1989 Classification also divided the epilepsies by aetiology, into two broad categories: idiopathic and symptomatic epilepsies. Idiopathic epilepsies were defined by absence of any brain lesions, normal background EEG activity and interictal generalized spike and wave discharges. They were considered to be due to a genetic predisposition or to a specific mode of inheritance. Symptomatic epilepsies were considered the expression of a focal or diffuse brain lesion as demonstrated by clinical history, structural neuroimaging, EEG findings, or biological tests.

Since 1989, various attempts of revision of the 1989 classification system have been made. In 1998 Lüders and colleagues called for a seizure classification based exclusively on ictal clinical semiology, either as reported by the patients or observers or as documented directly during video monitoring (3). The classification proposal was based on the assumption that ictal symptoms were produced

Table 7.1 International classification of epileptic seizures

Partial (focal, local) seizures
I) Simple partial seizures (without impairment of consciousness):
With motor signs
With sensory symptoms
With autonomic symptoms or signs
With psychic symptoms
II) Complex partial seizures (with impairment of consciousness)
III) Simple partial onset followed by impairment of consciousness:
With simple partial features followed by impaired consciousness
With automatisms
With impairment of consciousness at onset
With impairment of consciousness only
With automatisms
IV) Partial seizures evolving to secondarily generalized seizures:
Simple partial seizures evolving to generalized seizures
Complex partial seizures evolving to generalized seizures
Simple partial seizures evolving to complex partial seizures evolving to generalized seizures
Generalized seizures
I) Absence seizures:
Absences
Atypical absences
II) Myoclonic seizures
III) Tonic seizures
IV) Atonic seizures
V) Clonic seizures
VI) Tonic–clonic seizures
Unclassified epileptic seizures (lack of information)

Reproduced from Commission on Classification and Terminology of the International League Against Epilepsy. Proposal for a revised clinical and electroencephalographic classification of epileptic seizures. *Epilepsia* 1981; 22:489–501. With permission from Wiley.

Table 7.2 International classification of epilepsies and epileptic syndromes

Localization-related (focal, local) epilepsies and epileptic syndromes
I) Idiopathic:
Benign childhood epilepsy with centrotemporal spikes
Childhood epilepsy with occipital paroxysms
Primary reading epilepsy
II) Symptomatic:
Chronic progressive epilepsia partialis continua of childhood
Epilepsy characterized by seizures with specific modes of precipitation
Syndromes of great individual variability which are based mainly on seizure types and other clinical features as well as anatomic localization and aetiology
III) Cryptogenic:
Cryptogenic epilepsies are presumed to be symptomatic and the aetiology is unknown
Generalized epilepsies/epileptic syndromes
I) Idiopathic:
Benign neonatal familial convulsions
Benign neonatal convulsions
Benign myoclonic epilepsies of infancy
Childhood absence epilepsy (pyknolepsy)
Juvenile absence epilepsy
Juvenile myoclonic epilepsy
Epilepsy with grand mal (GTC) seizures on awakening
Other idiopathic generalized epilepsies not defined above
Epilepsy with seizures precipitated by specific modes of activation
II) Cryptogenic[a] or symptomatic:
West syndrome
Lennox–Gastaut syndrome
Epilepsy with myoclonic-astatic seizures
Epilepsy with myoclonic absences
III) Symptomatic:
Non-specific aetiology
Early myoclonic encephalopathy
Early infantile encephalopathy with suppression-bursts
Other symptomatic generalized epilepsies not defined above
Specific syndromes
Epilepsies/epileptic syndromes undetermined as to whether focal or generalized
With both partial and generalized seizures:
Neonatal seizures
Severe myoclonic epilepsy in infancy
Epilepsy with continuous spike-waves during sleep
Acquired epileptic aphasia (Landau–Kleffner syndrome)
Other undetermined epilepsies not defined above
Without unequivocal generalized or focal features
Special syndromes
Situation-related seizures:
Febrile convulsions
Isolated seizure/status epilepticus
Seizures due to acute metabolic or toxic factors

[a] Use of the term 'Cryptogenic' is now discouraged, and should be substituted by 'presumed symptomatic'.

Reproduced from Commission on Classification and Terminology of the International League Against Epilepsy. Proposal for revised classification of epilepsies and epileptic syndromes. *Epilepsia* 1989; 30:389–99. With permission from Wiley.

by epileptic interference of one of four 'spheres': sensorial, consciousness, autonomic and motor. Accordingly, seizures were classified in four main categories: auras, dialeptic, autonomic, and motor seizures. EEG findings were taken into account to differentiate between epileptic and non-epileptic events (3). This approach, however, was criticized because, it was suggested, different epileptic syndromes, having different outcomes, can be associated with the same types of seizures and appropriate management of a given patient requires that the physician defines the epileptic syndrome.

In 2001 the ILAE Task Force on Classification and Terminology proposed a 'new diagnostic scheme for people with epileptic seizures and with epilepsy' (4), organized in five axes (Table 7.3). That report recommended the terms of 'simple' and 'complex' be avoided in classifying specific seizure types, while ictal impairment of consciousness be mentioned when occurring in individual seizures. The terms 'partial' and 'cryptogenic' were discouraged as they conveyed ambiguous implications and replaced with 'focal' and 'probably symptomatic', respectively. The 2001 Task Force warned against the previous dichotomy between the concepts of 'partial' versus 'generalized' abnormalities, which might lead to neglect a variety of conditions between focal and generalized epileptogenic dysfunctions such as diffuse hemispheric or multifocal abnormalities (4). Finally, the concept of epileptic encephalopathy was introduced, to designate a group of conditions in which the epileptiform activity may contribute to progressive cerebral dysfunction.

In 2006, the ILAE Task Force on Classification and Terminology (5) proposed new criteria for the identification of specific seizure types and epilepsy syndromes (see Tables 7.4 and 7.5), with epileptic seizures being classified according to pathophysiologic mechanisms, neuronal substrates, response to AEDs, and ictal EEG patterns. Epileptic syndromes were classified according to seizure type, age of onset, interictal EEG pattern, progressive nature, pathophysiological mechanisms, anatomical substrates, aetiological categories, genetic basis, and associated interictal signs and symptoms. In 2006, the ILAE Task Force concluded that because

Table 7.3 Proposed diagnostic scheme for people with epileptic seizures and with epilepsy

Axis 1: Ictal phenomenology, from the Glossary of Descriptive Ictal Terminology, can be used to describe ictal events with any degree of detail needed
Axis 2: Seizure type, from the List of Epileptic Seizures. Localization within the brain and precipitating stimuli for reflex seizures should be specified when appropriate
Axis 3: Syndrome, from the List of Epilepsy Syndromes, with the understanding that a syndromic diagnosis may not always be possible
Axis 4: Aetiology, from a Classification of Diseases Frequently Associated with Epileptic Seizures or Epilepsy Syndromes when possible, genetic defects, or specific pathologic substrates for symptomatic focal epilepsies
Axis 5: Impairment, this optional, but often useful, additional diagnostic parameter can be derived from an impairment classification adapted from the WHO ICIDH-2

Reproduced from Engel J Jr. A Proposed Diagnostic Scheme for People with Epileptic Seizures and with Epilepsy: Report of the ILAE Task Force on Classification and Terminology. *Epilepsia* 2001; 42:796–803. With permission from Wiley.

Table 7.4 Epilepsy syndromes by age of onset

Neonatal period
Benign familial neonatal seizures
Early myoclonic encephalopathy
Ohtahara syndrome
Infancy
Migrating partial seizures of infancy
West syndrome and infantile spasms
Myoclonic epilepsy in infancy
Benign infantile seizures
Dravet syndrome
Myoclonic encephalopathy in non-progressive disorders
Childhood
Early onset benign childhood occipital epilepsy (Panayiotopoulos type)
Epilepsy with myoclonic astatic seizures
Benign childhood epilepsy with centrotemporal spikes
Late onset childhood occipital epilepsy (Gastaut type)
Epilepsy with myoclonic absences
Lennox–Gastaut syndrome
Epileptic encephalopathy with continuous spike-and-wave during sleep, including Landau–Kleffner syndrome
Childhood absence epilepsy
Adolescence
Juvenile absence epilepsy
Juvenile myoclonic epilepsy
Progressive myoclonus epilepsies
Less specific age relationship
Autosomal-dominant nocturnal frontal lobe epilepsy
Familial temporal lobe epilepsies
Mesial temporal lobe epilepsy with hippocampal sclerosis
Rasmussen syndrome
Gelastic seizures with hypothalamic hamartoma
Special epilepsy conditions
Symptomatic focal epilepsies not otherwise specified
Epilepsy with generalized tonic–clonic seizures only
Reflex epilepsies
Febrile seizures plus
Familial focal epilepsy with variable foci
Conditions with epileptic seizures that do not require a diagnosis of epilepsy
Benign neonatal seizures
Febrile seizures

Reproduced from Engel J Jr. Report of the ILAE Classification Core Group. *Epilepsia* 2006; 47:1558–68. With permission from Wiley.

Table 7.5 Seizure types

Self-limited epileptic seizures
I. Generalized onset
A. Seizures with tonic and/or clonic manifestations
B. Absences
C. Myoclonic seizure types
D. Epileptic spasms
E. Atonic seizures
II. Focal onset (partial)
A. Local
1. Neocortical
2. Hippocampal and parahippocampal
B. With ipsilateral propagation to:
1. Neocortical areas (includes hemiclonic seizures)
2. Limbic areas (includes gelastic seizures)
C. With contralateral spread to:
1. Neocortical areas (hyperkinetic seizures)
2. Limbic areas (dyscognitive seizures with or without automatisms [psychomotor])
D. Secondarily generalized
1. Tonic–clonic seizures
2. Absence seizures
3. Epileptic spasms (unverified)
III. Neonatal seizures
Status epilepticus
I. Epilepsia partialis continua (EPC)
II. Supplementary motor area (SMA) status epilepticus
III. Aura continua
IV. Dyscognitive focal (psychomotor, complex partial) status epilepticus
V. Tonic–clonic status epilepticus
VI. Absence status epilepticus
VII. Myoclonic status epilepticus
VIII. Tonic status epilepticus

Reproduced from Engel J Jr. Report of the ILAE Classification Core Group. *Epilepsia* 2006; 47:1558–68. With permission from Wiley.

the 1989 Classification of epilepsy syndromes and epilepsies was generally accepted and workable, it would not be discarded unless, and until, clearly better classifications had been devised. The Task Force suggested retaining the terms of 'focal' and 'generalized,' due to the prevalent usage and therapeutic implications. Conversely, the term cryptogenic was again discouraged as it was unclear whether it should be limited to conditions that are probably symptomatic, as originally intended, or to all conditions with unknown aetiology, as habitually meant by epidemiologists.

Various suggestions for revising terms and concepts of the 1989 Classification were proposed in 2010 (6). Although no adequate knowledge was considered to be available to propose a new classification of the epilepsies new terms and concepts appeared to better reflect current knowledge. For instance, it was recommended that the terms of generalized and focal be abandoned, as this dichotomy was considered no longer meaningful except for some forms of epilepsy such as, for example, many of the encephalopathic conditions observed in infants and young children and some of the neurodegenerative disorders of later life. Considering aetiology, the terms idiopathic, symptomatic, and cryptogenic were considered unworkable and from the perspective of recent knowledge prompted by molecular genetics and neuroimaging, the Commission proposed the terms of genetic (epilepsy is a direct result of a genetic cause) and structural and metabolic (epilepsy is the secondary result of a separate structural or metabolic condition). These Commission proposals have prompted abundant controversies and criticisms. The suggestions for updating terminology and concepts or amending the list of syndromes were, in fact, rather limited. A number of concept categories had already been recognized and updated in the 2001 and 2006 Task force reports (4, 5) and had been reinforced over time (7). For example, the term 'cryptogenic' had been discouraged since 2001 (4). On the other hand, the main syndrome categories introduced in 1989 still appear reliable for clinical and epidemiological purposes. Adding a class of genetic epilepsies to the aetiological classification may be appropriate to those epilepsies that are a direct result of a known genetic defect, in which seizures are the core symptom of the disorder.

However, for the great majority of patients, the categories of idiopathic and symptomatic still have solid implications for diagnosis, management, and prognosis, and allow a large number of patients to be categorized in easily recognizable syndromes (7).

In view of the uncertainty related to the most recent proposed amendments to the classification system, we will describe here the main symptom categories and epileptic syndromes as listed in the 1989 classification and revised in the 2001 and 2006 Task force reports (8) (Table 7.6), however introducing the most relevant amongst the most recently formulated concepts.

Table 7.6 Epileptic syndromes and epilepsies

Idiopathic focal epilepsies
A) Benign infantile seizures (non-familial)
B) Benign childhood epilepsy with centrotemporal spikes
C) Early and late onset idiopathic occipital epilepsy
Symptomatic (or probably symptomatic) focal epilepsies
A) Lobar epilepsies
B) Migrating partial seizures of early infancy
Idiopathic generalized epilepsies
A) Benign myoclonic epilepsy in infancy
B) Childhood absence epilepsy
C) Juvenile absence epilepsy
D) Juvenile myoclonic epilepsy
E) Epilepsy with generalized tonic–clonic seizures only
F) Epilepsy with myoclonic astatic seizures
G) Epilepsy with myoclonic absences
Familial (autosomal dominant) epilepsies
A) Benign familial neonatal convulsions and benign familial infantile convulsions
B) Autosomal dominant nocturnal frontal lobe epilepsy
C) Familial lateral temporal lobe epilepsy
D) Generalized epilepsies with febrile seizures plus
Reflex epilepsies
A) Idiopathic photosensitive occipital lobe and other visual sensitive epilepsies
B) Startle epilepsy
Epileptic encephalopathies
A) Early myoclonic encephalopathy and Ohtahara syndrome
B) West syndrome
C) Dravet syndrome
D) Lennox–Gastaut syndrome
E) Landau–Kleffner syndrome
F) Epilepsy with continuous spike waves during slow-wave sleep
Progressive myoclonus epilepsies
A) Lafora disease
B) Unverricht–Lundborg disease
C) Mitochondrial encephalopathy
D) Late infantile, juvenile, and adult ceroid-lipofuscinosis
E) Sialidosis
Seizures not necessarily needing a diagnosis of epilepsy
A) Febrile seizures
B) Benign neonatal seizures
C) Isolated seizures/isolated status epilepticus
D) Drug or other chemically-induced seizures

Reprinted from Guerrini R. Epilepsy in children. *The Lancet* 2006; 367:499–524. Copyright (2006), with permission from Elsevier.

Epileptic seizures

Generalized onset

A) Seizures with tonic and/or clonic manifestations

I) Clonic seizures: clonic seizures are fast rhythmic events (1–2 Hz), often associated with impaired consciousness.

II) Tonic seizures: the mechanism of tonic seizures is probably not the same as that of the tonic phase of generalized tonic–clonic seizures. Generalized tonic seizures typically occur in Lennox–Gastaut syndrome and occasionally in epilepsy with myoclonic astatic (or myoclonic-atonic) seizures.

III) Generalized tonic–clonic seizures (GTCSs) have sudden onset with immediate loss of consciousness. There is a brief tonic phase (10–30 seconds) with whole body tonic contraction, associated with a loud scream and vegetative symptoms such as tachycardia, midriasis, increased blood pressure, and apnoea. Tongue biting if present, is produced at this stage. The clonic phase lasts around 30 seconds—1 minute and is characterized by bilateral clonic jerks that gradually decrease in intensity and frequency. The postictal phase, which can last for several minutes up to hours, is characterized by initial mydriasis, body relaxation, hypotonia, and sleep. Urination if present, takes place at this stage. Finally the patient gradually recovers and appears confused, presenting sometimes with automatisms, headache, and muscle aches.

B) Myoclonic seizures

Myoclonic seizures are manifested as brief symmetrical muscular jerks of variable intensity. Proximal muscles such as girdle muscles are mostly involved. During stronger attacks, there is possibility of the patient falling over, but quickly recovering. The patient is usually conscious during the jerks. Myoclonic seizures may often be triggered by photic stimulation.

C) Absences

Typical absence seizures are brief (5–12 seconds). They appear mostly in children and are clinically characterized by sudden interruption of ongoing activity and staring straight ahead or drifting upwards. There is complete loss of awareness during the seizure. The onset and offset is sharp. Possible associated manifestations include slight rhythmic (3 Hz) eyelid myoclonus, slight decrement or increment of muscle tone, simple gestural automatisms (if the absence is of long duration), and, rarely, vegetative symptoms (urinary incontinence, pupil dilatation, pallor, flushing, tachycardia, change in blood pressure). Absence seizures can be easily produced if the child is asked to hyperventilate. Concomitant EEG abnormalities are typical generalized spike-and wave discharge at 3 Hz.

D) Epileptic spasms

These consist of a brief (0.5–2 second) tonic contraction of the neck and trunk in flexion, extension or in a mixed flexed-extended posture. They occur most commonly in clusters upon awakening. Each cluster consists of several spasms the intensity and frequency of which follow an increasing-plateau-decreasing pattern. Therefore the first spasms in a cluster can be barely visible, presenting a forced opening of the eyes or slight nodding of the head. Ictal EEG is characterized by pseudo-periodic slow polyphasic EEG discharges that are concomitant to spasms. EEG activity related to spasms can also be a bilateral electrodecremental pattern. Electromyographic activity from deltoid and neck muscles shows a characteristic rhomboid pattern during the spasm, usually lasting 0.5–2 seconds.

E) Atonic seizures

Atonic seizures are characterized by decrease or complete inhibition of postural tone. They manifest as head nodding, dropping of the jaw or of a limb, or falls. The patient can then lie motionless on the ground or promptly resume the posture. Pure atonic seizures are rare. Ictal EEG is usually characterized by a generalized slow spike-and-wave discharge.

Focal onset

(For a detailed description see 'A) Lobar epilepsies' section.)

A) Focal sensory seizures.

I) With elementary sensory (visual, somatosensory, vestibular, olfactory, gustatory, or auditory) symptoms as produced by activation of primary sensory cortices (e.g. occipital and parietal lobe seizures).

II) With experiential symptoms. These are complex, formed, distorted and/or multimodal sensory symptoms, usually implying seizure initiation in association cortices, such as the temporo-parieto-occipital junction.

B) Focal motor seizures.

I) With elementary clonic motor signs.

II) With asymmetric tonic motor seizures (e.g. supplementary motor seizures).

III) With typical (temporal lobe) automatisms (e.g. mesial temporal lobe seizures).

IV) With hyperkinetic automatisms.

V) With focal negative myoclonus.

VI) With inhibitory motor seizures.

Epilepsies and epileptic syndromes (Table 7.6)

Idiopathic focal epilepsies and syndromes

A) Benign infantile seizures (non-familial)

Watanabe described infants with complex partial seizures or partial seizures with secondary generalization, with normal development before seizure onset and a benign outcome (9, 10). Clinical and EEG features are similar to those of benign familial infantile seizures and of sporadic benign infantile seizures (11).

B) Benign epilepsy of childhood with centrotemporal spikes (BECTS)

BECTS is the most frequent epilepsy syndrome in childhood. Age at seizure onset ranges between 3–13 years. Prognosis is excellent with remission by adolescence (12). Seizures are typically hemifacial, involving mainly the lips, tongue, and pharyngeal-laryngeal muscles. Sensory symptoms can involve the same body parts as motor phenomena. Sometimes the homolateral upper limb is involved. Attacks are typically sleep-related, appearing within the first 30 minutes after falling asleep in most cases. They often determine arousal with ictal anarthria, while the child is fully aware. Secondary generalization can supervene but is rare. Typically parents are awakened by a grunting sound. They find the child dribbling profusely and unable to speak. Interictal EEG shows typical high amplitude, slow biphasic centrotemporal spikes, with a characteristic tangential dipolar distribution. Spikes greatly increase in frequency and often become bilateral during sleep.

AED treatment can be avoided if seizures are brief and limited to sleep. If treatment is necessary carbamazepine or valproate are preferred (8).

C) Idiopathic childhood occipital epilepsy (ICOE)

ICOE was originally described by Gastaut in 1982 as an idiopathic partial epilepsy with visual seizures (illusions, elementary hallucinations, ictal blindness) evolving either to hemiclonic or complex partial seizures, with or without secondary generalization, with age of onset between 15 months and 17 years. In around 25% of Gastaut's patients, a migraine-type postictal headache was reported (13). Interictal EEG showed normal background activity, with high amplitude, unilateral or bilateral, synchronous or asynchronous, occipital spike-and-wave discharges, facilitated by eye closure. Outcome was generally favourable with remission before adulthood.

A subset of children with ICOE present brief or prolonged sleep-related seizures characterized by tonic eye and head deviation, vomiting, and eventually hemiclonic or secondary generalization (14) The age at seizure onset is between 2–8 years. Prognosis is excellent with remission by the age of 12 and with most children having suffered only one seizure. This form of early onset idiopathic occipital epilepsy is also referred to as 'Panayiotopoulos syndrome' (15) or benign childhood seizure susceptibility syndrome.

The EEG abnormalities in this syndrome are not as specific as those of BECTS; in fact similar abnormalities can be observed in cryptogenic or symptomatic focal epilepsies with less favourable prognosis (16).

Symptomatic (or probably symptomatic) focal epilepsies

A) Lobar epilepsies

They represent the majority of focal epilepsies and are defined according to seizure semiology pointing to an anatomic location. Since epileptic discharges can spread, it is important to relay on the very first manifestations of a seizure to correctly localize its onset. However, defining the area of onset of focal seizures based on clinical and surface EEG findings alone may be very difficult when neuroimaging is normal. In addition, defining lobar origin may be a misleading process, as the epileptogenic area may not respect the anatomic limits of the cerebral lobes, seizure spread from clinically silent areas may be rapid, producing unresponsiveness before subjective symptoms are reported or memorized.

Temporal lobe epilepsies are the most frequent type of focal epilepsies (17). Onset is most often during childhood or early adulthood. Seizures are simple or complex partial and are of relatively long duration (1–2 min). Their onset is characterized by visceral symptoms (rising epigastric sensation, thoracic constriction, hot or cold sensation, olfactory hallucinations) or by psychic or affective symptoms (dreamy state, déjà-vu, déjà-vecu), usually accompanied or followed by vegetative manifestations (pallor, flushing, tachycardia, poly- or bradypnea, piloerection, mydriasis, or sweating).

Disruption of consciousness or 'unresponsiveness' appears later and can fluctuate. Sometimes it is not present at all even during automatisms that consist of oro-alimentary behaviour (lip-smacking, swallowing) or gestural automatisms (18). Late somatomotor manifestations such as dystonic posturing of the upper limb contralateral to the epileptic discharge may reflect the ictal spread to extratemporal cortical regions or activation of subcortical efferent systems. The postictal phase is characterized by prolonged confusion, occasionally accompanied by walking. Aphasia is observed when the dominant hemisphere is involved.

Lateral or neocortical temporal lobe epilepsy is characterized by auditory hallucinations or pseudovertigo and by aphasic speech arrest.

Mesial temporal lobe epilepsy is manifested by a highly characteristic ictal pattern, including epigastic sensation, psycho-motor arrest and staring, associated with mastication, lip smacking, and later gestural automatisms in the upper limb homolateral to the epileptic discharges. Hippocampal sclerosis or other mesial temporal lesions are frequently found on magnetic resonance imaging (MRI). Interictal EEGs can be normal or show unilateral or bilateral temporal abnormalities.

Frontal lobe epilepsies are also frequent (19). Seizures are usually brief (seconds to tens of seconds) and sleep-related. They are often manifested in clusters and are highly stereotyped in the same patient. Tonic or postural manifestations can cause disabling drop attacks. Consciousness disruption is highly variable but post-ictal recovery is usually fast. Some patients describe psychic symptoms such as forced thought. Secondary generalization is common. Subjective symptoms are usually ill defined but cephalic, thoracic or abdominal sensations are reported by some patients.

Posterior frontal lobe seizures—seizures originating from the supplementary motor area are characterized by speech arrest or palilalia (involuntary repetition of the same words or sentences, when the dominant hemisphere is involved), followed by abduction and elevation of the upper limb contralateral to epileptic discharge and version of head and eyes to same side (fencing posture). When the dorsolateral convexity is involved, a contralateral tonic posturing is observed. Frequently the discharge becomes bilateral with secondary generalization. The involvement of Brodmann's area 4 produces contralateral focal clonic movements. Speech arrest without loss of consciousness is observed when epileptic activity spreads to the foot of the third frontal gyrus.

Intermediate frontal lobe seizures are associated with a very fast spread of the epileptic discharge to other frontal lobe areas. Bilateral tonic manifestations appear suddenly, and can cause drop attacks. Axial tonic seizures with flexion of head and trunk associated with facial grimacing are typical. The patient can continuously moan and present apnoea, due to tonic diaphragm contraction.

Anterior frontal lobe seizures have a longer duration than other frontal seizures. Secondary generalization is rare. An automatic motor activity appears at seizure onset and involves either the upper limbs (fingers snapping, arms windmilling), or lower limbs (cycling, rhythmic flexion–extension) or girdles (rocking of pelvis, sexual automatisms). Verbal stereotypies are sometimes observed.

Involvement of specific frontal areas can be suspected when clustering of characteristic symptoms occurs. Forced thought or isolated alteration of awareness (frontal pseudo-absences) point to the fronto-polar area. Olfactory hallucinations with intense fear, bradycardia and micturition suggest the involvement of fronto-orbital regions. Complex and frantic motor behaviour with screaming and facial expression suggesting terror or rage are typical of anterior gyrus cinguli involvement.

Interictal EEG can be normal, but it is sometimes characterized by widespread abnormalities that enable neither lateralization nor localization.

Central region epilepsies are emanating from the perirolandic cortex (20). Typical signs include clonic motor or elementary sensory phenomena involving the contralateral hemibody with or without march. Secondary generalization is rare. Some of the seizures originating from this region can be precipitated by sensory or proprioceptive stimulations.

Seizures originating from the opercular-insular region are characterized by oro-alimentary manifestations such as mastication, swallowing, and salivation. Gustative hallucinations or illusions can be associated. Interictal or ictal abnormalities can be very mild. Seizures arising from the insula may also mimic temporomesial (21) and frontal nocturnal hypermotor seizures (22).

Parietal lobe epilepsies are rare (23). Fast spreading of epileptic discharges to contiguous lobes (frontal, temporal or occipital) can mask the initial signs or symptoms. Alteration of high cortical functions such as limb movement sensation, and autoscopia (seeing of one's own body image) can be the manifestation of non-dominant hemisphere involvement. In some patients unilateral spatial agnosia can only be recognized because they tend to look preferentially to one side that is homolateral to the epileptic discharge. Visual illusions (macropsia, micropsia, metamorphospia) are present when posterior parietal cortex or the parietal-occipital junction is involved. Clear rotatory vertigo is associated to an epileptic discharge in the inferior parietal region or the temporoparietal junction. Slow rotation of the body towards the same side of the epileptic discharge and dystonic posturing of the contralateral upper limb, is usually due to involvement of inferior parietal cortex. Interictal and ictal EEG abnormalities may be widespread involving central, parietal, temporal, and occipital regions.

Occipital lobe epilepsies are uncommon and difficult to correctly identify since rapid spreading of the epileptic discharge to contiguous lobes may mask initial symptoms (16). Elementary visual hallucinations (coloured blobs, flashes of light) associated to peri-ictal peripheral visual field deficit (hemianopia) are typical and testify the involvement of the contralateral pericalcarin region. Ictal or postictal headache are often observed. Eye movements are frequent in the course of the seizure. They can be phasic (oculo-clonic movement or 'epileptic nystagmus') or tonic (slow version of the eyes contralateral to the epileptic discharge). Occipital lobe seizures can rapidly propagate to the frontal region, causing the patient to fall, or to the mesial temporal lobe. Interictal EEG abnormalities involve the posterior regions and are usually enhanced during eye-closure.

B) Migrating partial seizures of early infancy

It has been proposed that occurrence of almost continuous migrating focal seizures, combined with multifocal ictal EEG discharges, and progressive deterioration of acquired skills, with onset in the first 6 months of life, represent an epilepsy syndrome (24). Seizures are markedly drug resistant and outcome is severe. The aetiology is so far unknown, but it is likely that multiple aetiologies can cause a similar picture.

Idiopathic generalized epilepsies

Idiopathic generalized epilepsies (IGEs) are frequent and usually, but not necessarily, have a favourable outcome. Common characteristics to all IGEs syndromes include generalized tonic–clonic, absence, and myoclonic seizures. Their onset is from infancy to adolescence. A family history of epilepsy is frequent. IGEs have complex inheritance and are likely to be caused by the combined interaction of two or more genes (25). Sporadic cases are common and affected families are usually small (26). Interictal EEG shows generalized spike-and-wave discharges at a frequency higher than 3 Hz. Drug treatment, especially valproic acid, is effective in most patients.

A) Benign myoclonic epilepsy in infants (BMEI)

This is a rare syndrome characterized by brief generalized myoclonic seizures with onset during the first or second year of life in otherwise normal children (27). Valproic acid is effective in controlling jerks. The appropriateness of the term 'benign' for this syndrome is questioned as a number of children exhibiting the clinical presentation of the BMEI will subsequently develop behavioural or cognitive problems and, sometimes, GTCSs in adolescence. Ictal EEG shows generalized polyspike-and-wave discharges, which are time-locked with the myoclonic jerks. Interictal abnormalities are rare.

B) Childhood absence epilepsy (CAE)

This is a frequent form of IGE with onset in otherwise healthy school-aged children. Clinical presentation is with frequent typical absence seizures. Interictal EEG shows normal background activity and generalized 3 Hz, spike-and-wave discharges, which translate into a clinical seizure when their duration outlasts 4–5 seconds.

Evolution is usually though not uniformly benign. Treatment with AEDs (valproic acid, ethosuximide, or lamotrigine) usually controls absence seizures, which tend to disappear in adolescence. Phenobarbitone and carbamazepine are not effective and can even increase seizure frequency (28). GTCSs can appear from adolescence in some patients. Late onset (above age 8), initial drug resistance, and photosensitivity are more likely to be associated with a less benign prognosis (see 'C) Juvenile absence epilepsy (JAE)' section). Absence seizures are also observed in other rare syndromes, which are not included in the classification such as eye-lid myoclonus with absences and perioral myoclonus with absences.

C) Juvenile absence epilepsy (JAE)

This syndrome has its onset around puberty and is characterized by rare typical absence seizures that cluster upon awakening (29). In 80% of patients, GTCSs are also present. They are usually rare and tend to appear after sleep deprivation, valproic acid is often effective. Ictal EEG can show either a typical 3 Hz or a faster (4–5 Hz) spike-and-wave discharge.

D) Juvenile myoclonic epilepsy (JME)

This syndrome represents about 3% of all patients with epilepsy referred to different epilepsy centres in Europe (30). Its onset is between age 6–25 years with a peak incidence between 12–17 years. Myoclonic jerks are always present. They usually involve the face and the upper limbs. Consciousness is retained but the patient can fall to the ground if the lower limbs are involved. They are typically experienced as tiny jerks that interfere with fine motor tasks in the minutes that follow awakening.

GTCSs are observed in 90% of patients and are sometimes preceded by a crescendo of bilateral jerks. Patients are most often brought to medical attention after a GTCS, while myoclonic seizures can go unnoticed for months or even years. Ten to 15% of patients also exhibit brief absence seizures. Visual sensitivity is present in 30–40% of patients. Sleep deprivation and alcohol intake are precipitating factors, especially for GTCSs. Interictal EEG shows generalized or asymmetric polyspike-and-wave discharges at 3 Hz or faster. Myoclonic jerks are time-locked to polyspike-and-wave complexes. A characteristic increase in polyspike-and-wave discharges is observed upon awakening (31). JME is genetically determined. Three to 9% of patients with JME carry dominant mutations of the *EFHC1* gene, which causes reversal of *EFHC1*-induced neuronal cell death and *EFHC1*-dependent increase of R-type Ca^+ current (32). One family with dominant JME harboured a mutation in the α1 subunit of the $GABA_A$ receptor gene (*GABRA1*) (33).

Response to treatment (valproic acid, primidone, benzodiazepines) is usually good but JME is a pharmaco-dependent type of epilepsy. Withdrawal of AEDs is associated to relapse in 90% of patients, even late in life (34). Carbamazepine use in patients with JME is sometimes associated to seizure-worsening, rarely escalating to status epilepticus (35).

E) Epilepsy with generalized tonic–clonic seizures only

GTC seizures take mostly or exclusively place within 2 hours from awakening or during evening time relaxation. Sleep deprivation, high alcohol intake, and induced arousals from sleep are all triggering factors. Interictal EEG can be normal or show generalized spike/polyspike-and-wave discharges that are increased upon awakening (31). As JAE, JME, and GMA represent a syndrome spectrum partially overlapping in age of onset, seizure types, and response to medication, the term IGEs with variable phenotypes has been suggested as all inclusive (4).

F) Epilepsy with myoclonic-astatic seizures (MAE)

This syndrome has its onset between 6 months and 6 years of age with a prominence in boys (36). A genetic predisposition is present, whose nosological boundaries are not well defined. Overlapping of some of the typical clinical manifestations with those of other severe childhood epilepsies (Lennox–Gastaut syndrome (LGS) and Dravet syndrome) is possible. Affected children exhibit atonic or myoclonic-atonic seizures and absence seizures with a clonic or tonic component. GTCSs are also present in most patients. Tonic seizures can appear late in the course, particularly in drug-resistant children. Non-convulsive myoclonic status with prolonged unresponsiveness can be observed in around 30–35% of children. Interictal EEG, normal at onset, shows generalized spike/polyspike-and-wave discharges later during the course. Outcome is unpredictable. Remission within a few months or years with normal cognition is possible even after a severe course (37). About 30% of children experience an epileptic encephalopathy with long lasting intractability and cognitive impairment.

G) Epilepsy with myoclonic absences (EMA)

This is a rare disorder (around 0.5–1% of all patients with epilepsy) with onset around age 7 (38). Children present with myoclonic absences that appear several times per day, as episodes of interruption of ongoing activity associated to rhythmic jerks in axial muscles causing a movement of shoulders, head and arms. Ictal EEG shows generalized 3 Hz spike-and-wave discharges resembling those of CAE, synchronous with myoclonic jerks. Prognosis is variable ranging from poor with evolution to different seizure types and mental retardation to very good with remission. A combination of different AEDs (valproic acid + ethosuximide or lamotrigine) is the most effective treatment (39).

Familial (autosomal dominant) epilepsies

A) Benign familial neonatal convulsions

Benign familial convulsions of the neonatal and infantile period encompass distinct age-related disorders. Benign familial neonatal convulsions are highly penetrant, with short lasting seizures beginning between a few days of life and 3 months. A few patients will manifest isolated seizures later in life. This disorder is associated with mutations of K^+ channel genes *KCNQ3* and *KCNQ2* (40, 41). Benign infantile convulsions are characterized by seizures between 4 and 8 months of age, often occurring in families. There is no known gene defect. Benign familial neonatal-infantile seizures begin between day 2 and 7 months of age, and are associated with *SCN2A* gene mutations (42).

B) Autosomal dominant nocturnal frontal lobe epilepsy (ADNFLE)

This syndrome is characterized by clusters of nocturnal motor seizures, which are often stereotyped and brief (5 seconds to a few minutes). They vary from simple arousals from sleep to dramatic, often bizarre, hyperkinetic events with tonic or dystonic posturing. ADNFLE is inherited as an autosomal dominant trait; penetrance is estimated at 70%. The genes known to be associated with ADNFLE are CHRNA4, encoding the α4 subunit of the neuronal nicotinic acetylcholine receptor (nAChR); CHRNB2, encoding the β2 subunit and CHRNA2, encoding for the α2 subunit (43).

C) Familial lateral temporal lobe epilepsy

This epilepsy syndrome is characterized by clinical manifestations usually beginning in childhood or adolescence as auditory hallucinations, often with associated olfactory, vertiginous, or visual symptoms (41). Mutations of *LGI1/epitempin*, the leucine-rich glioma-inactivated 1 gene have been identified in many families (44).

D) Generalized epilepsy with febrile seizures plus

This term designates a spectrum of epilepsy phenotypes including febrile seizures (FSs) and mild to severe generalized epilepsies (45). FSs are present in most of patients. FS+ are fever-related seizures continuing over the age of 6 or in association to afebrile GTCSs. FS+ may be associated with absence, myoclonic, or atonic seizures. Inheritance is autosomal dominant with 60% penetrance, including FSs and FS+. Mutations of β1 and α1 voltage-gated sodium channel subunit genes (*SCN1B*, *SCN1A*) account for 17% of generalized epilepsy with FS+ (46). Genetic heterogeneity is confirmed by the finding of mutations in the γ2 subunit $GABA_A$ receptor gene (*GABRG2*) in rare families (47).

Reflex epilepsies

A) Visual sensitive epilepsy

Visual sensitive epilepsy is a common manifestation of IGEs, but it can also be found in other generalized as well as focal epilepsies. In pure photosensitive IGEs, seizures are exclusively triggered by photic stimuli such as sunlight through tree foliage, sunlight reflected from water surfaces, stroboscopic light in discos, and television (TV) or computer screens. Seizure types are GTC (84% of patients), absence (6%), focal (2.5%), and myoclonic (1.5%) (48). EEG shows characteristics overlapping IGEs. The photosensitivity range (the lowest and highest IPS frequency capable of generating a photoparoxysmal response) should be carefully defined as it correlates with the likelihood experiencing seizures. Antiepileptic drug (AED) treatment can indeed be ineffective if patients are very sensitive to light or indulge in self-inducing seizures. It is essential to teach patients to avoid causative stimuli and/or to occlude one eye in front of them. Dark lenses can sometimes be beneficial. Some patients are exclusively sensitive to high-contrast patterns (blinds, wallpaper). In photosensitive occipital lobe epilepsy focal seizures can be induced by photic stimulation (video-games, TV) (49). They are characterized by visual symptoms lasting up to several minutes (colourful blobs, flashing lights, followed by amaurosis), followed by vegetative symptoms and headache.

B) Startle-induced epilepsy

This affects infants, children, or young adults with static or progressive encephalopathy. It is rarely observed in individuals without a brain lesion. An unexpected noise or a sudden movement can induce a focal or generalized, usually tonic seizure (50). Spontaneous seizures also occur in 40–95% of patients. An epileptogenic network involving the central cortex or the supplementary motor area is often demonstrated.

Progressive myoclonus epilepsies

Progressive myoclonus epilepsies (PMEs) are a group of aetiologically heterogeneous conditions characterized by multifocal and generalized myoclonic jerks, GTCSs, or clonic-tonic–clonic seizures, photosensitivity, progressive cognitive deterioration, and cerebellar and extrapyramidal signs. The different syndromes are identified by age at onset and rate of progression of symptoms. They include Lafora disease, Unverricht–Lundborg disease, myoclonus epilepsy with red ragged fibres (MERRF), early infantile, late infantile, juvenile, and adult ceroid-lipofuscinosis, and sialidosis (51). Many patients with PMEs do not receive an aetiological diagnosis (see Chapter 6).

Epileptic encephalopathies

Epileptic encephalopathies (EEs) are conditions in which seizures, the epileptiform abnormalities, or both, contribute to the progressive disturbance in cerebral function. About 40% of all epilepsies occurring in the first 3 years of life fit this definition (52). Epileptic encephalopathies may appear in children with normal early development and no brain lesions, in which case cognitive impairment is usually attributed to epilepsy. When a clinically manifest epileptogenic brain lesion is present, spread of epileptic activity to intact, remote areas is believed to amplify its clinical consequences.

Vigorous early treatment is often advocated. However, for most EEs there are no established endpoints for medical treatment and drug adjustments are empirically established. When an epileptogenic lesion is present and drugs fail, surgical approach can be successful. They are described in Chapter 15 and include:

- Early myoclonic encephalopathy and Ohtahara syndrome.
- West syndrome.
- Dravet syndrome.

- Lennox–Gastaut syndrome.
- Landau–Kleffner syndrome.
- Epilepsy with continuous spike waves during slow-wave sleep.
- Early onset epileptic encephalopathies caused by single gene mutations (*ARX, CDKL5, MECP2, FOXG1, STBPX, GLUT1*).

Conditions with epileptic seizures that do not require a diagnosis of epilepsy

Transient and reversible epileptogenic conditions are also known as situation-related seizures. They are not epilepsies stricto sensu, but seizures can relapse once the patient is re-exposed to the provoking factor.

A) Febrile seizures (FSs)

FSs are epileptic seizures that appear during a febrile illness, not associated to intracranial infection or other defined causes of seizures, in a normal child aged between age 3 months and 5 years. FSs are common and affect between 2–5% of children below age 5. Genetic factors are involved with both autosomal dominant and polygenic inheritance. During FSs most children have respiratory tract infections. There is a significant risk of occurrence in the 24 hours that follow the DPT (diphtheria, tetanus, and pertussis) vaccine and in the 8–14 days following the MMR (measles, mumps and rubella) vaccine (53).

Epilepsy will develop in only 5% of children who have had FSs (54).

Neuroimaging should be reserved to children with prolonged postictal unresponsiveness or focal deficits (55).

Simple FSs appear after the first year of life and bear an excellent prognosis. They are characterized by bilateral clonic or tonic–clonic movements, lasting less than 15 minutes, not relapsing during the same febrile illness, and not followed by postictal deficit. Seizures take place within 24 hours from fever onset at peak temperature or during defervescence. EEG is not useful in evaluating children with simple FSs. Temperature control is the best prophylaxis. Subsequent epilepsy is observed in less than 2.4% of cases.

Complicated FSs appear within the first year of life in children who frequently have a family history of epilepsy. They represent a febrile status epilepticus characterized by lateralized, prolonged (>15 minute), clonic seizures, often relapsing during the same febrile illness and followed by postictal paresis. Acute treatment with intrarectal diazepam should be used to stop the seizures. A complete neurological work-up, including EEG lumbar puncture and neuroimaging, should be considered if an intracerebral infection is suspected. Epilepsy can develop in up to 50% of children, particularly if prolonged relapsing seizures followed by postictal paresis are observed.

B) Benign neonatal seizures (BNSs)

These are self-limited events without sequelae.

C) Isolated seizures/isolated status epilepticus

These can appear in a patient without a family history of epilepsy and can remain an isolated event, not developing into an epilepsy syndrome. Isolated simple partial seizures can frequently be observed in adolescents.

D) Seizures due to acute metabolic or toxic factors

They are very frequent and usually do not need a chronic AED treatment.

References

1. Commission on Classification and Terminology of the International League Against Epilepsy. Proposal for a revised clinical and electroencephalographic classification of epileptic seizures. *Epilepsia* 1981; 22:489–501.
2. Commission on Classification and Terminology of the International League Against Epilepsy. Proposal for revised classification of epilepsies and epileptic syndromes. *Epilepsia* 1989; 30:389–99.
3. Lüders H, Acharya J, Baumgartner C, Benbadis S, Bleasel A, Burgess R, *et al.* Semiological seizure classification. *Epilepsia* 1998; 39:1006–13.
4. Engel J Jr. A proposed diagnostic scheme for people with epileptic seizures and with epilepsy: Report of the ILAE Task Force on Classification and Terminology. *Epilepsia* 2001; 42:796–803.
5. Engel J Jr. Report of the ILAE Classification Core Group. *Epilepsia* 2006; 47:1558–68.
6. Berg AT, Berkovic SF, Brodie MJ. Revised terminology and concepts for organization of seizures and epilepsies: Report of the ILAE Commission on Classification and Terminology, 2005–2009. *Epilepsia* 2010; 51:676–85.
7. Guerrini R. Classification concepts and terminology: Is clinical description assertive and laboratory testing objective? *Epilepsia* 2010; 51:718–20.
8. Guerrini R. Epilepsy in children. *Lancet* 2006; 367:499–524.
9. Watanabe K, Yamamoto N, Negoro T, Takahashi I, Aso K, Maehara M. Benign infantile epilepsy with complex partial seizures. *J Clin Neurophysiol* 1990; 7:409–16.
10. Watanabe K, Negoro T, Aso K. Benign partial epilepsy with secondarily generalised seizures in infancy. *Epilepsia* 1993; 34:635–8.
11. Saadeldin IY, Housawi Y, Al Nemri A, Al Hifzi I. Benign familial and non-familial infantile seizures (Fukuyama-Watanabe-Vigevano syndrome): a study of 14 cases from Saudi Arabia. *Brain Dev* 2010; 32:378–84.
12. Lerman P. Benign partial epilepsy with centro-temporal spikes. In: Roger J, Bureau M, Dravet C, Dreifuss FE, Perret A, Wolf P (eds) *Epileptic Syndromes in Infancy, Childhood and Adolescence*, pp. 189–200. London: John Libbey, 1992.
13. Gastaut H. Benign epilepsy of childhood with occipital paroxysms. In: Roger J, Bureau M, Dravet C, Dreifuss FE, Perret A, Wolf P (eds) *Epileptic Syndromes in Infancy, Childhood and Adolescence*, pp. 201–17. London: John Libbey, 1992.
14. Ferrie CD, Beaumanoir A, Guerrini R, Kivity S, Vigevano F, Takaishi Y, *et al.* Early-onset benign occipital seizure susceptibility syndrome. *Epilepsia* 1997; 38:285–93.
15. Panayiotopoulos CP, Michael M, Sanders S, Valeta T, Koutroumanidis M. Benign childhood focal epilepsies: assessment of established and newly recognized syndromes. *Brain* 2008; 131:2264–86.
16. Guerrini R, Parmeggiani L, Berta E, Munari C. Occipital lobe seizures. In: Oxbury JM, Polkey CE, Duchowny MS (eds) *Intractable Focal Epilepsy: Medical and Surgical Treatment*, pp. 77–89. London: Saunders, 2000.
17. Bancaud J. Sémiologie clinique des crises épileptiques d'origine temporale. *Revue Neurologique* 1987; 143:392–400.
18. Munari C, Bancaud J, Bonis A, Buser P, Talairach J, Szikla G, *et al.* Impairment of consciousness in temporal lobe seizures: a stereoelectroencephalographic study. In: Canger R, Angeleri F, Penry JK (eds) *Advances in Epileptology: XI Epilepsy International Symposium*, pp. 111–14. New York: Raven Press, 1980.
19. Bancaud J, Talairach J. Clinical semiology of frontal lobe seizures. *Adv Neurology* 1992; 57:3–58.
20. Chauvel P, Trottier S, Vignal JP, Bancaud J. Somatomotor seizures of frontal lobe origin. *Adv Neurology* 1992; 57:185–232.
21. Isnard J, Guénot M, Ostrowsky K, Sindou M, Mauguière F. The role of the insular cortex in temporal lobe epilepsy. *Ann Neurol* 2000; 48:614–23.

22. Ryvlin P, Minotti L, Demarquay G, Hirsch E, Arzimanoglou A, Hoffman D, *et al.* Nocturnal hypermotor seizures, suggesting frontal lobe epilepsy, can originate in the insula. *Epilepsia* 2006; 47:755–65.
23. Salanova V, Andermann F, Rasmussen T, Olivier A, Quesney LF. Parietal lobe epilepsy. Clinical manifestations and outcome in 82 patients treated surgically between 1929 and 1988. *Brain* 1995; 118:607–27.
24. Coppola G. Malignant migrating partial seizures in infancy: an epilepsy syndrome of unknown etiology. *Epilepsia* 2009; 50:49–51.
25. Berkovic SF, Scheffer IE. Genetics of the epilepsies. *Epilepsia* 2001; 42:16–23.
26. Italian League Against Epilepsy Genetic Collaborative Group. Concordance of clinical forms of epilepsy in families with several affected members. *Epilepsia* 1993; 34:819–26.
27. Dravet C, Bureau M, Roger J. Benign myoclonic epilepsy in infants. In: Roger J, Bureau M, Dravet C, Dreifuss FE, Perret A, Wolf P (eds) *Epileptic Syndromes in Infancy, Childhood and Adolescence,* pp. 67–74. London: John Libbey, 1992.
28. Guerrini R, Belmonte A, Genton P. Antiepileptic drug-induced worsening of seizures in children. *Epilepsia* 1998; 39:S2–10.
29. Wolf P. Juvenile absence epilepsy. In: Roger J, Bureau M, Dravet C, Dreifuss FE, Perret A, Wolf P (eds) *Epileptic Syndromes in Infancy, Childhood and Adolescence,* pp. 307–12. London: John Libbey, 1992.
30. Wolf P. Juvenile myoclonic epilepsy. In: Roger J, Bureau M, Dravet C, Dreifuss FE, Perret A, Wolf P (eds) *Epileptic Syndromes in Infancy, Childhood and Adolescence,* pp. 313–27. London: John Libbey, 1992.
31. Fittipaldi F, Currà A, Fusco L, Ruggeri S, Manfredi M. EEG discharges on awakening: a marker of idiopathic generalised epilepsy. *Neurology* 2001; 56:123–6.
32. Medina MT, Suzuki T, Alonso ME, *et al.* Impairment of consciousness in temporal lobe seizures: a stereoelectroencephalographic study. In: Canger R, Angeleri F, Penry JK (eds) *Advances in Epileptology: XI Epilepsy International Symposium,* pp. 111–14. New York: Raven Press, 1980.
33. Cossette P, Liu L, Brisebois K, Dong H, Dong H, Lortie A, Vanasse M, *et al.* Mutation of GABRA1 in an autosomal dominant form of juvenile myoclonic epilepsy. *Nat Genet* 2002; 31:184–9.
34. Nicolson A, Appleton RE, Chadwick DW, Smith DF. The relationship between treatment with valproate, lamotrigine, and topiramate and the prognosis of the idiopathic generalised epilepsies. *J Neurol Neurosurg Psychiatry* 2004; 75:75–9.
35. Genton P, Gelisse P, Thomas P, Dravet C. Do carbamazepine and phenytoin aggravate juvenile myoclonic epilepsy? *Neurology* 2000; 55:1106–9.
36. Doose H. Myoclonic astatic epilepsy. In: Roger J, Bureau M, Dravet C, Dreifuss FE, Perret A, Wolf P (eds) *Epileptic Syndromes in Infancy, Childhood and Adolescence,* pp. 103–14. London: John Libbey, 1992.
37. Oguni H, Tanaka T, Hayashi K, Funatsuka M, Sakauchi M, Shirakawa S, *et al.* Treatment and long-term prognosis of myoclonic-astatic epilepsy of early childhood. *Neuropediatrics* 2002; 33:122–32.
38. Tassinari CA, Bureau M, and Thomas P. Epilepsy with myoclonic absences. In: Roger J, Bureau M, Dravet C, Dreifuss FE, Perret A, Wolf P (eds) *Epileptic Syndromes in Infancy, Childhood and Adolescence,* pp. 151–60. London: John Libbey, 1992.
39. Bureau M, Tassinari CA. Epilepsy with myoclonic absences. In: Roger J, Bureau M, Dravet Ch, Genton P., Tassinari CA, Wolf P (eds) *Epileptic Syndromes in Infancy, Childhood and Adolescence* (3rd edn), pp. 305–12. London: John Libbey, 2002.
40. Dedek K, Kunath B, Kananura C, Reuner U, Jentsch TJ, Steinlein OK. Myokymia and neonatal epilepsy caused by a mutation in the voltage sensor of the KCNQ2 K+ channel. *Proc Natl Acad Sci U S A* 2001; 98:12272–7.
41. Singh NA, Charlier C, Stauffer D, DuPont BR, Leach RJ, Melis R, *et al.* A novel potassium channel gene, KCNQ2, is mutated in an inherited epilepsy of newborns. *Nat Genet* 1998; 18:25–9.
42. Berkovic SF, Heron SE, Giordano L, Marini C, Guerrini R, Kaplan RE, *et al.* Benign familial neonatal-infantile seizures: characterization of a new sodium channelopathy. *Ann Neurol* 2004; 55:550–7.
43. Marini C, Guerrini R. The role of the nicotinic acetylcholine receptors in sleep-related epilepsy. *Biochem Pharmacol* 2007; 74:1308–14.
44. Kalachikov S, Evgrafov O, Ross B, Winawer M, Barker-Cummings C, Martinelli Boneschi F, *et al.* Mutations in LGI1 cause autosomal-dominant partial epilepsy with auditory features. *Nat Genet* 2002; 30:335–41.
45. Scheffer IE, Berkovic SF. Generalised epilepsy with febrile seizures plus. A genetic disorder with heterogeneous clinical phenotypes. *Brain* 1997; 120:479–90.
46. Bonanni P, Malcarne M, Moro F, Veggiotti P, Buti D, Ferrari AR, *et al.* Generalised epilepsy with febrile seizures plus (GEFS+): clinical spectrum in seven Italian families unrelated to SCN1A, SCN1B, and GABRG2 gene mutations. *Epilepsia* 2004; 45:149–58.
47. Baulac S, Huberfeld G, Gourfinkel-An I, Mitropoulou G, Beranger A, Prud'homme JF, *et al.* First genetic evidence of GABA(A) receptor dysfunction in epilepsy: a mutation in the gamma2-subunit gene. *Nat Genet* 2001; 28:46–8.
48. Binnie CD, Jeavons PM. Photosensitive epilepsy. In: Roger J, Bureau M, Dravet C, Dreifuss FE, Perret A, Wolf P (eds) *Epileptic Syndromes in Infancy, Childhood and Adolescence*, pp. 299–305. London: John Libbey, 1992.
49. Guerrini R, Dravet C, Genton P *et al.* Idiopathic photosensitive occipital lobe epilepsy. *Epilepsia* 1995; 36:883–91.
50. Rosenow F, Lüders HO. Startle-induced seizures. In: Lüders HO, Noachtar S (eds) *Epileptic Seizures. Pathophysiology and Clinical Semiology*, pp. 585–92. New York: Churchill Livingstone, 2000.
51. Roger J, Genton P, Bureau M, Dravet C. Progressive myoclonus epilepsies in childhood and adolescence. In: Roger J, Bureau M, Dravet C, Dreifuss FE, Perret A, Wolf P (eds) *Epileptic Syndromes in Infancy, Childhood and Adolescence*, pp. 381–400. London: John Libbey, 1992.
52. Dalla Bernardina B, Colamaria V, Capovilla G, Bondavalli S. Nosological classification of epilepsies in the first three years of life. In: Nistico G, Di Perri R, Meinardi H (eds) *Epilepsy: An Update on Research and Therapy*, pp.165–183. New York: Alan Liss, 1983.
53. Barlow WE, Davis RL, Glasser JW, Rhodes PH, Thompson RS, Mullooly JP, *et al.* The risk of seizures after receipt of whole-cell pertussis or measles, mumps and rubella vaccine. *New Eng J Med* 2001; 345:656–1.
54. O'Donohoe N. Febrile convulsions. In: Roger J, Bureau M, Dravet C, Dreifuss FE, Perret A, Wolf P (eds) *Epileptic Syndromes in Infancy, Childhood and Adolescence*, pp. 45–52. London: John Libbey, 1992.
55. Wallace S. Febrile seizures: In: Wallace SJ, Farrell K (eds) *Epilepsy in Children* (2nd edn), pp. 123–30. London: Arnold, 2004.

CHAPTER 8

Differential Diagnosis of Epilepsy

Kristina Malmgren, Markus Reuber, and Richard Appleton

Introduction

A comprehensive discussion of the differential diagnosis of epilepsy cannot be limited to the description of the range of superficially similar disorders but must include an account of the diagnostic process for paroxysmal events in general, the criteria for the diagnosis of epileptic seizures, and the problem of misdiagnosis. In this chapter we will focus on the differential diagnosis of paroxysmal manifestations as they present in outpatient clinics or emergency rooms. We will not cover special situations such as status epilepticus or the epileptic encephalopathies, nor will we discuss underlying pathologies or acute symptomatic seizures. Whilst the most important differential diagnoses listed in Table 8.1 will be discussed in greater depth, less important diagnoses will be covered more briefly; and the least common or important will not be addressed at all.

The choice of treatment for paroxysmal neurological symptoms crucially depends on an accurate diagnosis. Often treatment will have to be administered in the absence of complete diagnostic certainty. It is best to think of the diagnosis of seizure disorders as a process rather than a single event. This process begins with the first meeting between the patient and the diagnostician, continues as more information becomes available from tests and further seizure accounts, and does not stop once an initial treatment decision has been made. The diagnosis may even remain uncertain in a specialist clinic. Limited evidence suggests that acknowledging diagnostic uncertainty in epilepsy can reduce misdiagnosis rates (1). Understandably, patients and their families (and frequently their doctors), want to have a definitive diagnosis. The doctor, wanting to comply with this request, may 'rush into' a diagnosis. However, clinicians should resist this temptation and admit to uncertainty.

The rates of misdiagnosis of seizures and epilepsy vary widely in different studies and depend on the clinical setting. In a primary care-based study in adults from the UK, 23% of 214 patients were found to have been misdiagnosed (2). Another UK study in which patients registered as having epilepsy in their primary care records were reviewed in a specialist clinic reported that 16.3% of 275 patients were misdiagnosed (3). The diagnostic error rate in patients originally thought to have epilepsy by neurologists was lower (5.6%) than that initially 'diagnosed' by non-specialists (19.3%), confirming the importance of the level of experience of the treating physician. There have also been several hospital-based studies on misdiagnosis of epilepsy in children. A prospective Dutch study in which experienced neuropaediatricians used defined criteria and consensus discussions to make diagnoses reported a rate of false-positive errors in 4.6% of cases (4), while a Danish study found that 30% of 184 children referred from their local paediatricians to a tertiary referral centre because of 'drug-resistant epilepsy' did not have epilepsy at all (5).

'Gold standard' diagnoses of epilepsy can be achieved by simultaneous video-electroencephalogram (EEG) recording, although even this test will only capture a limited number of seizures, and inter-rater agreement on video-EEG data is only moderate if experienced clinicians are asked to rate seizure recordings without knowing anything about the patient's history or subjective seizure experience (6). In clinical practice, video-EEG can only prove the diagnosis in a small minority of cases. Most patients do not have sufficiently regular seizures to allow ictal recordings (7), and some have seizures not reliably associated with scalp EEG changes (such as frontal lobe seizures or seizures without impairment of consciousness).

Surprisingly, there are no generally accepted and validated diagnostic criteria for the diagnosis of epilepsy at present. A study in adult patients has shown that the use of diagnostic criteria formulated in simple descriptive terms and a consensus discussion between neurologists improved the diagnostic agreement (8). In children the inter-rater agreement on the diagnosis of a first seizure has been shown to be no more than moderate, but the use of a panel of paediatric neurologists increased inter-rater agreement considerably (4).

The consequences of misdiagnosis may be far-reaching: an erroneous diagnosis of epilepsy may cause psychosocial and socioeconomic problems (e g loss of employment and driving restrictions for adults, unnecessary limitations of activities both in and out of school for children) and results in patients being treated with inappropriate or ineffective drugs, potentially resulting in side effects or teratogenicity. If a diagnosis of epilepsy is incorrectly made in a patient where the reason for paroxysmal attacks is a cardiac disorder, the consequences may be fatal (9). Death can also result from the inappropriate use of emergency interventions for people with psychogenic non-epileptic seizures (PNESs) (10).

Table 8.1 Differential diagnosis of paroxysmal neurological disorders

In adults and adolescents
◆ Syncope:
▪ Neurovasogenic ▪ Cardiac causes
◆ Psychogenic attack:
▪ Psychogenic non-epileptic seizure ▪ Depersonalization/derealization ▪ Panic attack ▪ Hyperventilation attack
◆ Sleep disorders:
▪ Parasomnias ▪ Narcolepsy with cataplexy
◆ Movement disorders:
▪ Paroxysmal dyskinesias ▪ Myoclonus ▪ Hyperekplexia
◆ Transient ischaemic attack
◆ Migraine
◆ Transient global amnesia
◆ Metabolic disorders:
▪ Hypo/hyperglycaemia ▪ Electrolyte disturbances
Additional differential diagnoses in children
◆ Physiological startle response
◆ Benign neonatal sleep myoclonus
◆ Shuddering or shivering attacks
◆ Extreme gastro-oesphageal reflux (Sandifer syndrome)
◆ Decerebrate (extensor) posturing (caused by cerebellar tonsillar herniation in acute hydrocephalus or raised intracranial pressure caused by meningitis/ encephalitis)
◆ Dystonic spasms in severe, four-limb spastic/dyskinetic cerebral palsy
◆ Opsoclonus-myoclonus syndrome
◆ Paroxysmal extreme pain syndrome
◆ Münchhausen by proxy
◆ 'Thought arrest' or day-dreaming

Diagnostic process

Diagnosticians have to consider a wide range of causes for paroxysmal neurological symptoms (see Table 8.1), however, the diagnostic process for patients presenting with transient loss of consciousness (TLOC) can follow a simple pragmatic decision tree in most cases (see Fig. 8.1).

The relative frequency of diagnoses made in medical settings does not reflect population incidence rates: One neurologist with a special interest in seizure disorders was able to reach a diagnosis in 87% of 158 consecutive cases. The most common diagnoses were epilepsy (43%), syncope (25%), and PNES (12%); 7% of patients received other diagnoses (11). A study which captured 350 consecutive TLOC presentations to doctors (in primary care, emergency care, and specialist clinics) in a geographically limited area of the Netherlands yielded similar numbers (12). If presentations to doctors mirrored population incidence rates, patients with syncope would be seen more commonly and patients with PNES less commonly.

The differential diagnosis of epilepsy in children is as large as that in adults, and establishing the correct diagnosis is particularly difficult in children under the age of 5 years. In the under-5s, the most important differential diagnoses include reflex anoxic seizures, tic or behavioural mannerism, day-dreaming, self-gratification, or fabricated illness. In older children, additional diagnoses include vaso-vagal syncope, cardiac arrhythmias, PNES, or paroxysmal dyskinesia.

The first step in the diagnostic process is the conversation between a healthcare professional and the patient. If the patient is a child, this conversation must always, wherever possible, involve the child, as well as parents or carers. Diagnostically relevant information is not limited to the description of the onset, course and offset of the patient's paroxysmal symptoms. The precise circumstances in which the symptoms occurred also have to be considered, the past medical history, family history, and current medication may give important diagnostic clues. A witness account should be sought if at all possible—even if the patient does not think that consciousness was impaired. The failure to seek and take account of a witness's description of the attacks has been identified as one of the commonest reasons for misdiagnoses (13).

Taking the history

The process of recording the patient's history should begin with a period of attentive listening. Giving the patient time and space to produce an account of their complaint without early interruption allows the healthcare professional not only to pay attention to factual features described by patients and witnesses but also to observe diagnostically relevant interactional behaviours of the patient and accompanying others (14). Documentation of the detailed description of the attack, using the patient's own words if possible, is of critical importance. Epileptic seizures and syncopal TLOC tend to be more stereotyped, whereas PNES are more likely to change with time.

What differentiates the three most common causes of TLOC: seizures, syncope, or PNES?

Factual distinguishing features

Table 8.2 provides an overview of semiological features, which may be helpful in distinguishing between the three most common causes of TLOC.

There is some evidence that factual information clusters can help clinicians to distinguish reliably between epilepsy and syncope (15-17) and between cardiac and reflex syncope (18). Clinical experience suggests that clusters of clinical details in the seizure description may also allow healthcare professionals to differentiate between PNES and epilepsy, although taken on their own, questions about seizures from sleep, ictal injuries or tongue biting have little differentiating value (19).

Situation in which the attack occurred

Most patients with epilepsy recognize triggers for their seizures or situations in which seizures are more likely to occur but the accuracy of these subjective observations is difficult to assess (20). In several idiopathic generalized epilepsy syndromes seizures typically occur within an hour or so of waking (21). Seizures are very closely

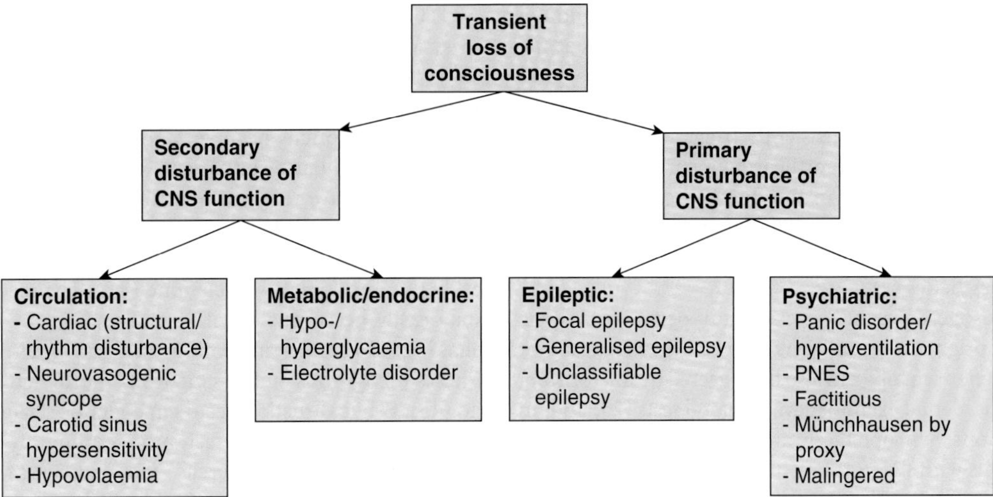

Fig. 8.1 A simple approach to the commonest causes of transient loss of consciousness.

Table 8.2 Semiological features which may help to distinguish between the three most common causes of transient loss of consciousness

Observation	Generalized tonic–clonic seizures	Syncope	Psychogenic non-epileptic seizures
Gradual onset	Focal onset possible (aura, duration typically <30 seconds)	Common (presyncopal symptoms, duration often minutes)	Not infrequent (often lasting several minutes)
Motor activity	Typical seizure patterns (tonic, clonic, tonic–clonic)	Myoclonic jerks common (short duration, rapid recovery) after loss of postural tone	Commonly undulating motor activity with sudden pauses but stable frequency
Asynchronous arm and leg movements	Unusual	Not rare (multifocal myoclonus)	Common
Purposeful movements	Very rare	Rare	Occasional
Rhythmic pelvic movements	Rare	Never	Occasional
Opisthotonus, 'arc de cercle'	Very rare	Occasional ('decerebrate' posturing)	Occasional
Prolonged ictal atonia	Very rare	Not >60 seconds	Occasional
Skin	Cyanosis common	Pallor, sweating	No cyanosis despite long seizure duration
Ictal crying	Very rare	Very rare	Occasional
Closed eyes	Rare	Rare	Very common
Resistance to eye opening	Very rare	Very rare	Common
Maintained pupillary light reflex	Often abolished	Common	Very common
Ictal reactivity	Rarely preserved	Rarely preserved	Occasionally partially preserved
Ictal incontinence	Not rare	Rare	Not rare
Seizure duration >2 minutes	Uncommon	Very uncommon (only if patient supported in upright posture)	Common
Postictal reorientation	Mostly over minutes	<1 minute (exception: head injury caused by collapse/patient maintained in upright position)	Often unexpectedly quick or slow
Tongue biting	Not infrequent (lateral)	Occasional (tip)	Occasional (tip)
Injury	Common (burns)	Rare	Common
Seizures at night (from 'sleep')	Common	Rare	Not rare

associated with menstruation in catamenial epilepsy (although patients with PNES may also report an increase of seizures at the time of their periods). In addition to photically-induced seizures (which are not uncommon), there are other, rare, reflex epilepsies in which epileptic seizures are consistently triggered by particular activities (such as reading, eating, or hearing a particular piece of music) (22). Seizures occurring in the doctor's office are more commonly reported by patients with PNES than patients with epilepsy (23). PNES are also particularly likely to occur after medical procedures or anaesthetics (24).

Reflex (neurovasogenic) syncope classically occurs when the patient has been upright and is more likely when they are also hot and dehydrated. Reflex syncope can also be triggered by micturition, coughing, emotions, dental examination, or blood tests (25) and, in children, vaccinations. Syncope rarely arises from sleep (26). One-half of adult patients with PNES (as many as patients with epilepsy) describe attacks from sleep, although video-EEG observation reveals that patients are usually awake at the start of the attacks. However, PNES are unlikely if attacks exclusively occur from sleep (27, 28). PNES from apparent sleep are also uncommon in children.

Attack onset

The onset of an epileptic seizure may be sudden or gradual (over seconds or even minutes). Symptoms such as déjà or jamais vu, olfactory and gustatory hallucinations, or rising epigastric sensations commonly feature in patients' accounts of partial epileptic seizures (especially seizures of temporal lobe origin) but are not specific for this disorder—they are also frequently reported by patients with PNES (29). These symptoms are more likely to point to a diagnosis of epilepsy if patients highlight that the precise nature of what they experience is difficult to explain (30). Idiopathic generalized tonic–clonic seizures (GTCSs) may be preceded by series of myoclonic seizures.

The combination of a sensation of feeling hot, sweaty, lightheaded, visual (seeing stars, vision going white, black, grey, becoming blurred or closing in) and auditory symptoms (sounds seeming distant, muffled or distorted) is so characteristic that these symptoms are often summarized as 'pre-syncopal', i.e. warning symptoms of syncope (25).

The onset of a PNES is more commonly gradual than that of epileptic seizures (31, 32). Although about half of patients with PNES will claim that their seizures tend to come out of the blue (29), PNES can be preceded by a prodrome of symptoms of physiological arousal (heart racing, dry mouth, tremor, sweaty hands) and typically with little cognitive awareness of anxiety (33).

During the attack

Whereas there is a gradual decline in the frequency and increase in amplitude of muscle contractions during the clonic phase of GTCS, jerking in PNES with significant motor activity is tremor-like and tends only to involve changes in amplitude. The onset and offset of the jerks in a PNES is usually sudden, unlike the more characteristic crescendo and decrescendo seen in a GTCS. Frequency remains unchanged throughout the attacks (34). Myoclonus or repeated jerks (clonic movements) during syncope are common, as is vocalization, brief limb posturing, upward and/or lateral deviation of the eyes, and eyelid flickering (35). Cyanosis is more common in epilepsy than syncope or PNES (36).

GTCSs typically last 50–90 seconds (37). Loss of consciousness in syncopal attacks typically lasts less than 1 minute, unless the subject is maintained in an upright posture. PNES typically last longer than epileptic seizures (31, 37, 38). Prolonged PNES treated as status epilepticus occur in about one-third of PNES-patients, and over one-quarter of patients diagnosed with PNES at an epilepsy centre have received intensive care treatment for presumed status epilepticus at least once (39, 40). Several types of PNES can be differentiated, the commonest resembling GTCS or manifesting as TLOC and loss of muscle tone (41). The second type of PNES may easily be confused with syncope (42). In convulsive PNES, shaking is often asynchronous and asymmetrical (37, 43, 44). Phases of vigorous and less vigorous motor activity can come and go (45). Pelvic thrusting occurs in epileptic seizures, particularly of frontal lobe origin, but is seen more commonly in PNES (37, 46). Ophisthotonus ('arc de cercle') may be seen (43). The head may shake from side to side (37, 47). Eyes and mouth are more likely to be closed than in epileptic seizures (48–50). Ictal crying or verbal communication may be observed (37, 51, 52).

The end of the attack

Whilst epileptic seizures tend to cause positive neurological symptoms during the ictus these are often followed by negative symptoms in the postictal phase. Postictal disorientation and anterograde amnesia (typically lasting for minutes) are most common, but focal weakness (Todd's paresis) is also well recognized.

Postictal symptoms tend to be shorter and less marked in patients with PNES (53), although prolonged dissociative states are not uncommon. The absence of postictal disorientation or amnesia after an episode of loss of consciousness associated with collapse is suggestive of syncope (16, 17), but prolonged syncopal episodes can result in a more extensive period of confusion. Recurrence of TLOC on rapid resumption of an upright posture is typical of syncope.

Minor injury, including carpet burns, bruising, and lacerations, are common in PNES, and neither a history of such injuries nor of urinary incontinence distinguishes securely between PNES and epileptic seizures (54). However, in children, these physical symptoms (and particularly carpet friction burns and urinary incontinence) are very rare and typically limited to patients with more chronic and refractory PNES. Severe lateral tongues bites are more likely in epileptic seizures although tongue biting is also reported frequently by patients with PNES and can occur in syncope (23, 29).

Past medical history

Patients' previous interactions with health services can give important diagnostic clues.

Table 8.3 lists features from the medical history that can help to determine the likelihood of the three most common causes of TLOC. Epileptic seizures may develop after stroke, brain injuries, or infections, and, in children, prolonged (complex) febrile seizures and may complicate systemic disorders. Patients with cardiac syncope often have a history of other cardiac symptoms (18). Patients with PNES often have a history of other unexplained physical symptoms including pain and fibromyalgia (23), and may have much more voluminous health records than other people of the same age and gender (55).

Table 8.3 Features in the medical history that help to determine the likelihood of epilepsy, syncope, and psychogenic non-epileptic seizure (PNES)

Feature in history	Epileptic seizures	Syncope	PNES
Manifestation <10 years of age	Common	Occasional	Unusual
Change of seizures semiology	Rare	Rare	Occasional (more dramatic with time)
High seizure frequency	Occasional	Rare	Common
Recurrent seizure status	Rare	Never	Common
Worsening with antiepileptic drugs	Rare	Rare	Occasional
Seizure provocation	Rare (e.g. photosensitive epilepsy)	Common (e.g. pain, fear)	Not rare (arguments, stress, doctor's office)
Seizures in front of a doctor	Unusual	Common (blood tests)	Common
Multiple unexplained physical symptoms	Rare	Rare	Common
Multiple surgical procedures and investigations	Rare	Rare	Common
Psychiatric treatment	Rare	Rare	Common
Vascular risk factors, history of heart disease	Rare (except in elderly patients)	Not rare (common in patients with cardiogenic syncope)	Rare
Sexual and physical abuse	Rare	Rare	Common
History of suicide attempts	Rare	Rare	Common
History of alcohol excess	Not uncommon	Infrequent	Not uncommon
History of learning disability/other CNS disorder	Not uncommon	Rare	Not uncommon

Interactional distinguishing features

The differences in TLOC presentations are not limited to *what* patients say but also *how* they interact with their doctor (30). A number of interactive and linguistic features have been described which may be used to differentiate between patients with epilepsy and PNES (Table 8.4) (56).

Patients with epilepsy tend to give (unprompted) detailed accounts of the symptoms of their seizures, which are characterized by significant formulation effort (hesitations, re-starts, reformulations, etc.) and may include meta-analytic comments such as 'this is really difficult to explain', clear contours of the period of impaired consciousness ('the last thing I remember...', 'the next thing I remember...'), or volunteered descriptions of seizure-suppression attempts. In contrast, patients with PNES resist the doctor's focus on specific attacks (57). Instead they tend to highlight the adverse consequences of their seizures and the dangerous or embarrassing situations in which seizures occurred (58). Rather than making recurrent and complex attempts to communicate an experience to the interviewer which is clearly difficult to share interindividually, their accounts of attacks often remain limited to 'holistic' statements such as 'I was out' or 'I don't remember anything'.

Taking the history in children

Much of the history-taking approach in adults also applies to children and the history must include the periods before, during, and

Table 8.4 Interactional and linguistic features which can help in the differentiation of epileptic seizures and psychogenic non-epileptic seizure (PNES)

Feature	Epilepsy	PNES
Subjective seizure symptoms	Volunteered, detailed	Avoided, no detail
Formulation work	Extensive	Practically absent
Seizure suppression attempts	Volunteered	Not mentioned
Gaps in consciousness	Exact description	Little description
Metaphors	Seizure as independently acting agent, patient often depicted as 'victim' of the seizure	Seizures as a place or space, which patients travel through
Seizure labels	No resistance to use of 'medical' labels (e.g. 'seizures', 'grand mal' for episodes)	Resistance to the use of 'medical' labels (e.g. seizure). Preference of lay terms ('fit', 'blackout')

after the episodes. In particular, specific questions should be asked about whether there was a likely or even possible trigger for the episodes. In the active, high-achieving teenager (most often female) with PNES, a relatively common trigger is a new activity or pursuit that proves to be the 'final straw'; rather than appearing to fail at this activity, the child becomes sick and is therefore unable to participate—and not just in this new activity but everything else. PNES is a common manifestation of this behaviour. Clearly, most of the history will be obtained from the child's parents or carers but it is crucial to always ask the child themselves about any aspects of the episodes. Even young children may be able to provide valuable information that may actually confirm the nature of the paroxysmal episodes. If the parent or carer has not actually witnessed the child's episodes then it is important to obtain information from those who have observed them. This may include contacting or talking with another family member, friend, schoolteacher, or other individuals, such as a swimming pool attendant or lifeguard. The sort of information—and how it is given to the doctor—that may suggest an adult is experiencing PNES, may similarly be heard from a mother who is fabricating her child's 'seizures' with the child being a victim of Münchhausen syndrome by proxy.

Examination

Ictal examination

The observation and examination of a patient during a seizure is rarely possible, especially in patients first presenting with seizures. However, the observation of closed eyes during the seizure, resisted eye opening, gaze avoidance, retained pupillary light reflex, semi-purposeful movements, responsiveness to tickle or corneal reflex, and normal plantar responses would be very helpful and support a diagnosis of PNES rather than epilepsy (59, 60). Examination findings during a faint may include abnormalities of heart rhythm and hypotension. The examination soon after a GTCS may show evidence of a severe (typically lateral) tongue bite, bruising or skeletal injury, and petechial haemorrhages around the eyes or in the conjunctiva.

Interictal examination

Interictal examination findings in patients with epilepsy may provide a clue to the underlying pathology (e.g. focal central nervous system dysfunction, neurocutaneous syndromes, intracranial space occupation). Patients with syncope may have a postural blood pressure drop, a cardiac murmur or arrhythmia. However, in one consecutive case series of 158 adult patients attending a TLOC clinic, physical examination findings did not contribute to the diagnosis in a single case (11). A brief screen for adverse life events and psychiatric morbidity may yield potential aetiological factors in patients with PNES (61), although rates of adverse life events and mental illness are also higher in patients with epilepsy and patients with refractory syncope than in the general population (62, 63).

Examination in children

The examination findings in children, both interictally and ictally, will generally be similar to those described in adults. Young children will often be distressed following a GTCS and will usually sleep; this is unlikely if the child has experienced a syncopal attack or a PNES. Increasingly, parents will attend the first new patient appointment with a video of their child's episodes which may prove diagnostic, particularly if the history is vague or the episodes are difficult to describe. This is particularly useful for episodes that occur from sleep, the rarer paroxysmal dyskinesias, and also PNES.

Investigations

Interictal tests

Interictal tests are greatly overrated in the differential diagnosis of TLOC. 'Brain tests' are often normal in patients with epilepsy, 'cardiac tests' are often normal in patients with syncope. In the series of 158 consecutive outpatients cited previously, interictal EEG only changed the diagnosis in one patient. Neuroimaging revealed a relevant abnormality in 12/43 scanned (27.9%) (11).

Electroencephalography

The EEG is a very useful test in the classification of the epilepsy syndrome, but the role of the EEG in the initial diagnosis of patients who have experienced a TLOC is controversial. There is a risk of non-experts overinterpreting the diagnostic significance of non-specific EEG changes (13): in one study such changes were seen in 55% of adults with a clinical diagnosis of epilepsy but also in 45% of people who had experienced syncope (15). Another study found non-specific EEG changes in 18% of adults with PNES (64).

As in adults, the EEG is an often over-used investigation in children. In view of the normal maturation of the EEG, which ranges from preterm through infancy and early childhood to the adult pattern by 12–14 years, there is an even greater danger of misinterpreting children's EEGs. It is of concern that in the UK, approximately half of the clinicians who routinely report paediatric EEGs have not received formal training in paediatric electroencephalography (65, 66). In addition, many paediatricians continue to believe that the EEG is a 'diagnostic test' for epilepsy and hold on to the erroneous belief that the child's paroxysmal episodes cannot be epileptic if the EEG is normal and conversely that the episodes must be epileptic if the EEG is abnormal.

Neuroimaging

Neuroimaging is never a diagnostic test for epilepsy, and even if abnormal does not necessarily mean that the patient's paroxysmal episodes are epileptic. However, neuroimaging should be carried out in all patients with suspected epilepsy to exclude underlying pathology (with the exception of those with a clear history and typical EEG changes of idiopathic generalized epilepsy). In one study, nearly 30% of MRI scans in adults with a clinical diagnosis of epilepsy showed abnormalities, but abnormalities were also seen in 4% of MRI scans in patients with syncope (12). One study described abnormalities in 27% of adults with PNES (67). As the quality of MRI scans improves, the risk of identifying non-specific changes and misinterpreting these as potential causes of epileptic seizures is likely to increase.

In children with early-onset seizures (specifically myoclonic, tonic, or focal seizures and infantile spasms), or in adolescents aged older than 14 years with a new focal epilepsy, neuroimaging is also mandatory and may identify an underlying structural lesion, including cortical dysplasia, a neuronal migration abnormality, neurocutaneous disorders, and, rarely (in contrast to adults), a tumour.

Cardiac investigations

Electrocardiography (ECG) is recommended in all adults presenting with TLOC because it is risk free and will identify patients with abnormal cardiac conduction syndromes which can imitate epileptic seizures or PNES (such as the long QT-syndrome) (68). It also helps to stratify patients into those with possible cardiac syncope who should be investigated further and those with neurovasogenic/unexplained syncope in whom further cardiological tests are unlikely to yield an explanation for the TLOC (69).

Cardiac arrhythmias are an uncommon cause of TLOC or 'drop attacks' (tonic or atonic seizures) in children under 10 years of age. However, an ECG should always be undertaken wherever there is a history of events that seem to be closely related to vigorous exercise or a sudden shock or startle. If the ECG is normal but the level of suspicion of a cardiac cause remains high, children should be referred for a formal cardiac opinion.

Ictal tests

Tests which observe attacks themselves (such as video-telemetry, ambulatory EEG, prolonged ECG, tilt-table tests or even home video recordings) are much more specific in the differential diagnosis of TLOC than interictal tests (70–72). However, these tests are also much less sensitive and rarely help in patients first presenting with seizures. Tests which use different forms of symptom provocation may increase the yield of time-limited brief outpatient procedures. Photic stimulation and hyperventilation lead to a small increase in the yield of routine EEG examination for epileptiform EEG changes, but (in combination with suggestion) provoke a typical PNES in around 50% of adult patients (73). Like syncope, PNES may also be provoked by tilt-table examinations (74).

Suggestion during a routine EEG rarely induces or provokes a PNES in children. Video-EEG may prove diagnostic in differentiating epileptic seizures from PNES or parasomnias but clearly only if the child experiences their habitual episodes during the recording. Ambulatory EEG is less useful than video-EEG, first because of considerable movement artefact or 'equipment failure' (both of which are common in this age group) and second because there is no video-footage of the clinical events. Where there is a high index of suspicion of fabricated seizures (Münchhausen by proxy), inpatient video-EEG telemetry is the investigation of choice.

Differential diagnoses of epilepsy

Syncope

Syncope is a sudden, transient, self-limited loss of consciousness, usually leading to falling. The onset of syncope is relatively rapid, and the subsequent recovery is spontaneous, complete, and relatively prompt. The underlying mechanism is transient global cerebral hypoperfusion (75). Syncope can be related to a range of triggers and mechanisms (Table 8.2) (76). A diagnosis of 'syncope' is therefore incomplete and must be combined with a determination of the likely underlying mechanism. The most important distinction is that between reflex or neurovasogenic (60–70%) and cardiac causes (10–20%) (69, 77, 78). Carotid sinus hypersensitivity (CSH) causes a particular form of neurovasogenic syncope in which hypotension and/or cardiac inhibition are triggered by stimulation of the carotid baroreceptors in the neck. CSH is particularly common in older patients (79). Cardiac syncope is more likely if there is a history of heart disease, if syncope was exercise-related or occurred from the supine position, if there is a shorter history of attacks, and an absence of pre-syncopal symptoms (18). The diagnostic evaluation of neurovasogenic syncope can be limited to the exclusion of risk factors for cardiac syncope by means of the patient's history and a routine ECG test. If in doubt, tilt-table testing can be helpful (80). A diagnosis of CSH can be established by performing carotid sinus massage under blood pressure and ECG monitoring. Patients with possible cardiac syncope need to be investigated further with echocardiography, and prolonged ECG recordings (possibly using implantable loop recorders which can continue to monitor the patient for intermittent arrhythmias for over 18 months) (71). One study showed that cardiac syncope may be under-recognized in seizure clinics and should always be considered as a possible diagnosis in patients whose apparently epileptic seizures fail to respond to antiepileptic drugs (9).

Psychogenic attacks

Psychogenic non-epileptic seizures

PNESs are episodes of altered movement, sensation, or experience resembling epileptic seizures but not associated with ictal electrical discharges in the brain (81). Attacks are interpreted as a dissociative or conversion response to distress in the current diagnostic manuals (82–84). In the ICD-10 (International Statistical Classification of Diseases and Related Health Problems, 10th revision), PNESs are described as involving 'partial or complete loss of the normal integration between memories of the part, awareness of identity and immediate sensations, and control of bodily movements' (84). Most PNESs are characterized by impairment of consciousness, collapse, and shaking of the limbs lasting for several minutes (81). A number of biographical, psychological, physiological, sociological, and financial factors including trauma and neglect in earlier life, adverse life events in adulthood, personality pathology, and inadequate coping skills can predispose to, precipitate and perpetuate PNESs (85). PNESs often occur in the context of comorbid psychopathology. Most PNESs are not considered to be under patients' volitional control although the distinction from attacks occurring in the context of factitious disorder or malingering is difficult (86).

Dissociative disorders

There are other, non-convulsive manifestations of dissociation (disruption in the usually integrated functions of consciousness, memory, identity, or perception) which can be mistaken for epileptic seizures. Simple partial seizures may involve feelings of depersonalization or derealization which can also occur as isolated dissociative symptoms in the absence of epileptic discharges in the brain (87). A dissociative aetiology is more likely if these symptoms are related to stressful events, if there is a history of other dissociative phenomena and if there are no associated symptoms of epilepsy (such as olfactory hallucinations, déjà vu or jamais vu experience) or investigation findings making epilepsy more likely (88). Complex partial seizures or transient epileptic amnesia may be difficult to distinguish from dissociative amnesia. Both may be characterized by decreased recall of autobiographical knowledge although only the latter typically involves the lack of recollection of traumatic events. Complex partial (non-convulsive) status epilepticus may only be distinguishable from brief periods of dissociative fugue (unexpected travel away from home or place of daily activities with lack of recall of identity) because of other signs or symptoms suggestive of epilepsy (such as automatisms or incontinence), because there are more definite epileptic seizures at other times, or because patients carried out more complex social or other activities, which are unlikely to have been completed in complex partial status epilepticus.

Panic disorder

Panic disorder is characterized by unpredictable, recurrent attacks of severe anxiety not restricted to any particular situation or circumstance. Dominant symptoms vary but sudden onset palpitations, chest pain, choking, dizziness, feelings of unreality (depersonalization/derealization) are common. Almost invariably patients have a secondary fear of dying, losing control, or going mad. Attacks last for minutes or longer. Many patients develop an urge to leave the situation in which the attack has occurred. Similar circumstances may be avoided in the future. In between attacks most patients are relatively asymptomatic although a degree of anticipatory anxiety (fear of further attacks) is common. Impairment of consciousness is not a feature of panic attacks (84), although it may be difficult to draw a line between feelings of unreality and more profound symptoms of dissociation (and PNES). Panic symptoms can also occur as a result of epileptic discharges, for instance in the amygdala and other parts of the limbic system. Table 8.5 lists a number of features, which can help in the differentiation of panic disorders and focal epilepsy.

Hyperventilation

Hyperventilation is defined as breathing in excess of the metabolic needs of the body, eliminating more carbon dioxide (CO_2) than is produced, and resulting in respiratory alkalosis. The reduction in blood CO_2 levels produces vasoconstriction and secondary hypoxia in the brain. Clinically, hyperventilation is associated with perioral and acral paraesthesiae, stiffness, clumsiness, dysarthria and carpopedal spasms. Symptoms are usually bilateral but can only manifest on one side. If maintained for long enough, hyperventilation can cause syncope or provoked epileptic seizures (89). It can link anxiety with physical and cognitive symptoms, which can easily be mistaken for epileptic seizures. Diagnostic confusion with epilepsy is particularly likely when sensory and motor symptoms are unilateral. Several studies suggest that cerebral anxiety networks are particularly sensitive to carbon dioxide fluctuations in patients with panic disorder. The diagnosis of hyperventilation related attacks is made more likely by elevated scores on the Nijmegen Hyperventilation Questionnaire (90), or the provocation of typical symptoms during a hyperventilation tests (maintaining a respiratory rate of 30/minute for 4 minutes).

Sleep disorders

Parasomnias

The diagnosis of paroxysmal nocturnal events often represents a clinical challenge, with the distinction between nocturnal epilepsy and non-epileptic sleep-related disorders causing the greatest

Table 8.5 Differential diagnosis of panic attacks and ictal anxiety caused by focal epileptic seizures (from Schoendienst and Reuber, 2007)

	Primary panic attack	**Focal epileptic seizure with ictal anxiety**
Clinical features		
Consciousness	Alert	May progress to impairment
Duration	5–10 minutes	0.5–2 minutes
Automatisms	Very rare	Common with progression to CPS
Nocturnal attacks	Occur from state of wakefulness	May wake patient up
Subjective symptoms		
Déjà vu, hallucinations	Very rare	>5%
Depressive symptoms	Common, severity associated	Not uncommon, severity not associated
Anticipatory anxiety	Very common	Can occur but not common
Relation to 'normal' anxiety	No clear subjective difference between 'normal' fear and panic states	Clear difference between 'normal' and ictal fear
Investigations		
Interictal EEG	Usually normal	Often abnormal
Ictal EEG	Usually normal	Usually abnormal (may be normal in SPS)
MRI of temporal structures	Usually normal	Often abnormal
Linguistic and interactional features in the history		
Anxiety symptoms as a topic	Usually volunteered	Not volunteered without prompting
Anxiety symptoms	Discussed extensively Volunteered quickly Self-initiated as a topic Frequent use of formulaic expressions Are described as focused on particular objects	Discussed sparingly Hesitant disclosure Often not discussed without prompting Apparently difficult to describe, descriptions characterized by high formulation effort. Ictal fear is described as non-specific untargeted anxiety.

difficulties. Epileptic seizures of frontal lobe origin often occur during sleep (non-rapid eye movement (NREM) light sleep). Some patients only have sleep-related epileptic seizures and fulfil the criteria for nocturnal frontal lobe epilepsy (NFLE). NFLE is most likely to be confused with NREM arousal parasomnias. NREM arousal parasomnias are paroxysmal behaviours without conscious awareness, usually arising from NREM deep sleep. They have a broad spectrum of clinical manifestations (91–93). In clinical practice the NREM arousal disorders are subdivided into three main forms: confusional arousals, sleep walking (somnambulism), and sleep terrors (pavor nocturnus). Common underlying mechanisms are believed to be responsible and patients may display features of several subtypes (sometimes also associated with obstructive sleep apnoea). The motor patterns observed during these events such as wandering, semipurposeful automatisms, and motor agitation may be seen also in epileptic seizures, and furthermore most descriptions of arousal disorders in the literature are not based on video-EEG or polysomnography recordings (93). A simple questionnaire has been developed to help with this particular differential diagnosis (the Frontal Lobe Epilepsy and Parasomnias (FLEP) scale) (94). A subsequent study based on the systematic semiological evaluation of video-EEG recorded parasomnias and NFLE seizures in 44 patients (120 events) has provided further evidence (95). Sixty-nine elemental semiological features were identified and cluster analysis was applied to the data set. Elemental clinical features strongly favouring a diagnosis of parasomnias included crying or sobbing, waxing and waning pattern, interactive behaviour, failure to wake after the event, prolonged duration (>2 minutes), and indistinct offset. In contrast, bicycling movements, thrashing, grunting, grimacing, and dystonic posturing clearly favoured NFLE. On the basis of this data set the authors developed a diagnostic classification tree based on video features only, which correctly classified 94% of the events (Fig. 8.2). This may be useful not only in the assessment of video-EEG monitoring data, but also in assessing home video recordings.

The similarities between features seen in parasomnias and NFLE as well as the fact that the disorders not uncommonly may coexist underlie a hypothesis that the disorders may have a common pathogenic background (96, 97).

Narcolepsy

Narcolepsy is a disorder of the regulation of sleep and wakefulness (98), mostly starting in adolescence. Patients have excessive daytime sleepiness (EDS) with or without irresistible sleep attacks and fractionated nocturnal sleep. They may also have episodes with sleepiness or 'micro-sleeps' with automatic behaviour. These episodes may be mistaken for absences or complex partial seizures with ambulatory automatisms, but typically patients come round from 'micro-sleep' refreshed and not confused or tired.

Most narcolepsy patients also have cataplexy (70%) which is characterized by a sudden loss of postural muscle tone, and may result in sudden falls with retained consciousness. The episodes are provoked by intense emotions, specifically laughter or anger, and may last seconds to several minutes. Cataplectic attacks may be both partial and complete. The partial attacks are usually very short, most often affect the jaw and the face and the return of muscle function is abrupt (99). The episodes of cataplexy are sometimes misdiagnosed as either focal or 'drop' (atonic or astatic) epileptic seizures. Other symptoms of narcolepsy include hallucinations and/or paralysis when falling asleep or on waking. The diagnosis of narcolepsy rests on clinical ground supported by sleep investigations (polysomnography followed by a multiple sleep latency test). Auxiliary laboratory tests can help differentiating between patients with or without cataplexy (almost all patients of Western European ancestry with narcolepsy and cataplexy are HLA DQB1*0602 positive and have low cerebrospinal fluid hypocretin-1 values) (98). Taking a careful history revealing the disabling EDS as well as the other symptoms will clarify the diagnosis.

Movement disorders

Paroxysmal dyskinesias

Paroxysmal dyskinesias (PDs) are a group of rare hyperkinetic movement disorders characterized by brief intermittent dyskinetic movements. The clinical features of the involuntary abnormal

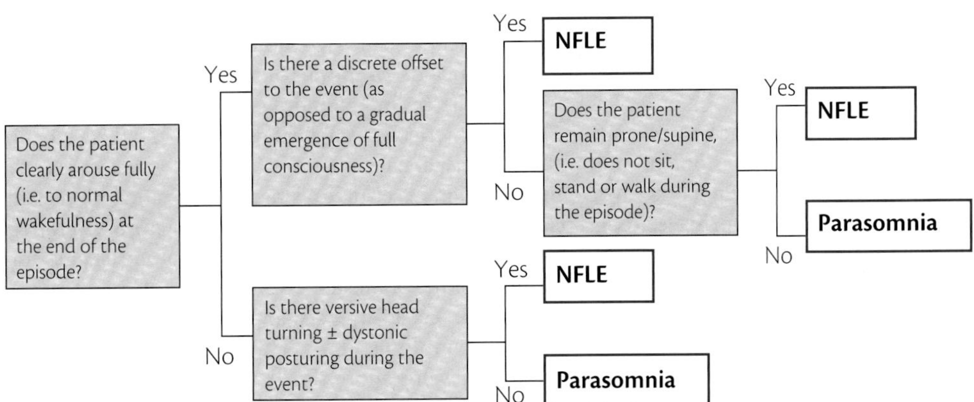

Fig. 8.2 Chi-squared automatic interaction detector tree analysis. Figure taken from Derry et al. (95) showing a diagnostic classification tree, based on video features only. This algorithm correctly identified 94% of the 120 nocturnal events in the study. NFLE, nocturnal frontal lobe epilepsy.

movements include dystonia, chorea, athetosis, ballism, or combinations of these symptoms (100). PD can occur in isolation or in association with epilepsy. Age of onset is usually below 20 years and there is often a family history although there are also sporadic cases. The attacks are brief, they may be uni-or bilateral, there is usually no loss of consciousness, and neurological status is typically normal between attacks. The most common type of PD is paroxysmal kinesigenic dyskinesia where the attacks are triggered by sudden voluntary movements. In a study of 121 affected individuals the mean delay from seeking medical advice to correct diagnosis was 4.8 years and alternative diagnoses given included epilepsy, psychogenic seizures, tics, anxiety, and malingering (101). As in epilepsy, diagnosis is based mainly on a carefully taken history. However, it may be difficult for both the person but also, where the patient is a child, for their carers to accurately describe the movements. In this situation video-footage of the episodes may prove diagnostic. The movement disorder in the genetic condition glucose transporter (GLUT1) deficiency may also be misdiagnosed as epilepsy; however, it is also important to appreciate that both epilepsy and a movement disorder may occur simultaneously in this condition.

Myoclonus

Myoclonus is a clinical sign that may be found in a number of different diseases, as an epileptic phenomenon or related to non-epileptic motor system disorders. Myoclonus is defined as sudden brief muscle jerks. The duration of movements is rarely longer than 100 msec and it is usually a positive phenomenon, resulting in synchronized muscle contractions. Negative myoclonus consists of a sudden brief loss of muscle tone which can be demonstrated by loss in electromyography activity. Myoclonic jerks can occur with dysfunction in cortical, brainstem, or spinal motor systems and may also be psychogenic (102, 103). Most causes of myoclonus are symptomatic, including posthypoxic or toxic-metabolic states, storage disease and neurodegenerative disorders. In an epidemiological study from Minnesota, US, the annual average incidence of myoclonus of any cause was 1.3 cases per 100,000 person-years (104). Symptomatic myoclonus was the most common aetiological category (72%), followed by epileptic myoclonus (17%) and essential myoclonus (11%).

Given the large number of possible causes of myoclonus, it is essential to take a good history including age of onset, family history, the character of myoclonus, precipitating factors, and presence of associated symptoms and signs. The physical examination can give important clues. Myoclonus at rest indicates a spinal or brainstem cause, whereas action-induced myoclonus points to a cortical origin. Electrophysiology is very helpful in detecting the level of origin of myoclonus (105).

In epilepsy, myoclonus may occur as one component of a seizure, as the only seizure manifestation, or as one of multiple seizure types within an epileptic syndrome. Epileptic myoclonus is accompanied by a generalized ictal epileptiform electroencephalographic discharge, but the myoclonus itself may be generalized, segmental, or focal (106). Myoclonus can appear in the generalized epilepsy syndromes (e g juvenile myoclonic epilepsy), symptomatic generalized epilepsies and the progressive myoclonic epilepsies (as in PME, e.g. Unverricht–Lundborg disease) but can also occur in focal epilepsy, often from a frontal focus.

The aetiology of myoclonus tends to be easier to determine if it occurs as one part of a syndrome than if myoclonus appears in isolation.

Transient ischaemic attacks

Whereas most epileptic seizures are characterized by predominantly 'positive' ictal features (e.g. excessive movement, sensory, visual, or auditory hallucinations), most transient ischaemic attacks (TIAs) involve 'negative' features (e.g. weakness, loss of sensation, loss of speech). TIAs are rarely associated with impairment of consciousness. However, especially in elderly patients with a history of cerebrovascular disease, it is not uncommon that focal seizures are mistaken for TIAs even though loss of consciousness is clearly described. In the case of brief attacks of sensory symptoms or aphasia without loss of consciousness it may be more difficult to differentiate between an epileptic or vascular origin, although epileptic seizures are usually of shorter duration. Limb-shaking TIAs pose a particular diagnostic challenge. Limb-shaking is a specific clinical feature of TIA that has been associated with a high-grade stenosis or occlusion of the internal carotid artery. Limb-shaking is characterized by brief, jerky, coarse involuntary movements involving an arm or a leg (107). In a study of the clinical characteristics of limb-shaking in 34 affected individuals the attacks were shown usually to last less than 5 minutes and were often accompanied by paresis of the involved limb. The symptoms were often precipitated by specific circumstances that may lower cerebral blood flow in patients with occlusion of the internal carotid artery (e.g. rising or exercise) (108). Other aspects that have been described as helpful in the differential diagnosis from focal seizures are lack of involvement of the face or trunk, absence of a march of symptoms, and of epileptiform activity on EEG (109).

Migraine

There are clinical similarities between migraine with visual aura and occipital epilepsy with simple partial seizures (especially when these seizures are followed by a postictal headache which may be indistinguishable from migraine). However, several studies have also identified diagnostically helpful differences (110): migrainous auras are more likely to start in the centre of the visual field, spread outwards over the course of minutes, and involve one hemifield. Epileptic auras tend to start in the periphery, move, split, or spread (possibly to the whole visual field) over the course of seconds. Although other visual phenomena are possible, migrainous auras are more likely to be black and white and produce linear patterns (111). Most elementary visual auras caused by epileptic seizures involve colourful rounded forms. Migraines also tend to be less frequent than epileptic seizures. Both can be associated with temporary blindness although this is more likely to affect the whole visual field in epilepsy than migraine. Other clinical pointers to epilepsy include symptoms of spread of the ictal discharges to other parts of the brain (including secondary GTCS), ictal gaze deviation or interictal visual field defects (112). It is recognized that elementary visual hallucinations (and ictal visual loss) can also be a manifestation of seizures primarily originating in the temporal lobes (113).

Basilar migraine may also be mistaken for epilepsy. In this form of migraine neurological symptoms suggest primary involvement of the brain stem. Basilar migraine can cause loss of consciousness preceded by vertigo, tinnitus, hypo-acusis, and bilateral visual symptoms (114). However, attacks of basilar migraine tend to develop more slowly than epileptic seizures and last longer. The symptoms listed here may also be associated with other brainstem signs unlikely in epileptic seizures (such as ataxia or diplopia). Clinical cases in which epileptic seizures seem to develop out of typical migraines also exist ('migralepsy').

Transient global amnesia

The syndrome of transient global amnesia (TGA) is defined by a sudden onset of an anterograde and retrograde amnesia lasting up to 24 hours. The memory impairment consists of a profound reduction of anterograde and a milder reduction of retrograde episodic memory, including executive functions and recognition (for references see (115). Typically patients recover (although they do not tend to retrieve memories of the period of amnesia) and a recent meta-analysis including 25 studies could not find long-term differences in cognitive performance between patients and healthy controls (116). Most attacks occur in people aged 50–70 years and occurrence below the age of 40 is rare, as is recurrence. There is, however, some evidence of association between younger patients and history of migraine and a case series of five patients with TGA who had previously successfully undergone temporal lobe resection for epilepsy suggests that epilepsy surgery in the temporal lobes may increase the vulnerability for TGA (117).

Precipitating factors described for TGA include physical exertion, emotional or psychological stress, pain, medical procedures, and sexual intercourse. The diagnosis is primarily clinical, using the following criteria (118): 1) anterograde amnesia witnessed by an observer; 2) no clouding of consciousness or loss of personal identity; 3) cognitive impairment limited to amnesia; 4) no focal neurological or epileptic signs; 5) no recent history of head trauma or seizures; and 5) resolution of symptoms within 24 hours. The exact pathophysiology of TGA is not clear although a number of neuroimaging studies have shown mesiotemporal abnormalities (for references see (119)).

The main differential diagnostic problem in relation to epilepsy concerns transient epileptic amnesia—TEA. This is a recently delineated neurological condition occurring in middle age and presenting with amnesic attacks (120). Butler described a series of 50 patients with TEA with detailed clinical and EEG data (121). They found that their patients with TEA had a mean onset of 62 years, similar to TGA. The amnesic episodes were rather more frequent (median 12/year) and shorter than TGA, although in general longer than epileptic seizures (median duration 30–60 minutes), and transient amnesia was the most prominent feature of the episodes. The amnesic attacks were characterized by mixed anterograde and retrograde amnesia, sometimes with repetitive questioning. Epileptiform activity on EEG was present in 37% of the patients and some patients had features indicative of focal epilepsy, e.g. olfactory hallucinations, oral automatisms, or brief periods of unresponsiveness. However, epilepsy was the initial specialist diagnosis in only 12 of 50 cases. Forty of the 50 patients described persistent memory difficulties. Importantly, attacks ceased on anticonvulsant medication in 44 of 47 treated patients. Attacks commonly occurred on waking, a helpful diagnostic clue.

Metabolic and endocrine disorders

The metabolic or endocrine problem most likely to cause confusion with epilepsy is hypoglycaemia. Episodic hypoglycaemia sufficient to cause neurological symptoms is most likely to occur in patients with diabetes mellitus (due to overmedication), alcoholism, or sepsis (122). However, it is particularly likely to cause diagnostic confusion in patients with insulinomas who develop hypoglycaemic attacks without identifiable precipitants (123). Autonomic symptoms of hypoglycaemia such as hunger, palpitations, tremor, or sweating can help with the diagnosis but may be less prominent than neurological symptoms confusion, impairment of consciousness (including symptomatic GTCS), odd behaviour, speech difficulties, and incoordination.

There are several other endocrine disorders, which can cause episodic symptoms such as flushing, tachycardia, tremor, and anxiety and which may be mistaken for simple partial seizures especially of temporal lobe origin (83). These include carcinoid syndrome, systemic mast cell disease, phaeochromocytoma, medullary carcinoma of the thyroid, pancreatic islet-cell tumours, renal cell carcinoma—or even menopausal hypo-oestrogenaemia. In children and adolescents, hypocalcaemia may also induce symptoms that mimic seizures, typically tonic or focal seizures; unfortunately, hypocalcaemia may also cause genuine epileptic seizures, although this is typically in young infants.

Common differential diagnoses in children

Many of the conditions seen in adults and described in this chapter also occur in children and particularly children over 10 years of age. Cardiac arrhythmias resulting in drop attacks tend to occur in older children (>12 years of age) and TIAs are extremely uncommon. PNES is less commonly seen in children and is rare under 9 years of age. The most common 'seizure' type in PNES is tonic–clonic-like followed by atonic-like seizures (drop or 'swoon'-type seizures). Paroxysmal movement disorders, including simple or complex motor tics and stereotypies are relatively common and are often misdiagnosed as focal or myoclonic seizures. Parasomnias are a common phenomenon in children, and particularly arising from NREM-sleep resulting in night terrors or rhythmic body-rocking or head-banging behaviours. Self-gratification is a common and normal behaviour in infants and young children and may persist well into late childhood, although by this stage children are much more self-conscious and it is unlikely to be witnessed. However, the behaviour may continue to be manifest in public places in children with learning difficulties or autism. Self-gratification is more likely to be seen when the child is bored or relaxed; specific situations include in a busy classroom or when watching television. Children can either assume dystonic or tonic postures with crossing of their legs or, less frequently, clonic movements of their legs usually in association with rhythmic rocking of the body and facial flushing. They may also appear to be 'absent' and unresponsive although they can usually be distracted out of them, but usually only temporarily. Predictably, these characteristic features may lead to a diagnosis of absence, complex partial seizure, or, rarely, tonic seizures.

Less common differential diagnoses in children

There is a wide range of other maturational (and therefore normal) phenomena but also a number of uncommon or rare non-physiological conditions that may be misdiagnosed as epilepsy, and usually as myoclonic, tonic, or complex partial seizures (see Fig. 8.1).

Fabricated or fictitious illness (also known as Münchhausen syndrome by proxy (124, 125)) is a relatively uncommon but almost certainly under-recognized phenomenon and represents a form of child abuse or 'non-accidental injury'. Syncope and seizures are the most common presentation of this condition. The parent, most often (but not invariably) the mother, fabricates a history that her child is experiencing seizures. Less commonly, this fabrication is more sinister in that the parent is actively doing something to the child which induces a 'seizure'. This may be by suffocation (causing an anoxic seizure), giving the child salt (causing a hypernatraemic seizure), or by overdosing the child with antiepileptic medication that has been erroneously prescribed for the child's 'epilepsy'. In addition, antiepileptic medication may cause side effects including ataxia or dyskinesia which may in turn be misdiagnosed as another type of seizure or an underlying neurodegenerative disorder leading to spiralling inappropriate investigation and overtreatment. A number of features should raise concern that the child's paroxysmal episodes are likely to be fabricated:

- The history of the events is—and remains persistently—vague.
- The person who has witnessed the events seems to be only the mother (or involved parent), despite the fact that the episodes are reported to occur every week or every day.
- The history is convincing of epilepsy but repeated EEGs are normal.
- The episodes continue on appropriate antiepileptic medication despite the fact that the child is considered to have a benign epilepsy syndrome.
- The parent provides a number of excuses for not being able to video a typical episode despite their very frequent occurrence (excuses include: 'I didn't have time to video them'; 'I was too upset'; 'She [the daughter] didn't want me to video her'; 'She [the daughter] was too embarrassed').
- The parent often has a history of either mental health or chronic, non-specific illnesses.

References

1. Beach R, Reading R. The importance of acknowledging clinical uncertainty in the diagnosis of epilepsy and non-epileptic events. *Arch Dis Child* 2005; 90(12):1219–22.
2. Scheepers B, Clough P, Pickles C. The misdiagnosis of epilepsy: findings of a population study. *Seizure* 1998; 7(5):403–6.
3. Leach JP, Lauder R, Nicolson A, Smith DF. Epilepsy in the UK: misdiagnosis, mistreatment and undertreatment. *Seizure* 2005; 14(7):514–20.
4. Stroink H, van Donselaar CA, Geerts AT, Peters AC, Brouwer OF, van Nieuwenhuizen O, *et al.* Interrater agreement of the diagnosis and classification of a first seizure in childhood. The Dutch Study of Epilepsy in Childhood. *J Neurol Neurosurg Psychiatry* 2004; 75(2):241–5.
5. Uldall P, Alving J, Hansen LK, Kibaek M, Buchholt J. The misdiagnosis of epilepsy in children admitted to a tertiary epilepsy centre with paroxysmal events. *Arch Dis Child* 2006; 91(3):219–21.
6. Benbadis SR, LaFrance WC Jr, Papandonatos GD, Korabathina K, Lin K, Kraemer HC, *et al.* Interrater reliability of EEG-video monitoring. *Neurology* 2009; 73(11):843–6.
7. Jacoby A, Baker GA, Steen N, Potts P, Chadwick DW. The clinical course of epilepsy and its psychosocial correlates: findings from a U.K. Community study. *Epilepsia* 1996; 37(2):148–61.
8. van Donselaar CA, Geerts AT, Meulstee J, Habbema JD, Staal A. Reliability of the diagnosis of a first seizure. *Neurology* 1989; 39(2 Pt 1):267–71.
9. Zaidi A, Clough P, Cooper P, Scheepers B, Fitzpatrick AP. Misdiagnosis of epilepsy: Many seizure-like attacks have a cardiovascular cause. *J Am Coll Cardiol* 2000; 36(1):181–4.
10. Reuber M, Baker GA, Gill R, Smith DF, Chadwick D. Failure to recognize psychogenic nonepileptic seizures may cause death. *Neurology* 2004; 62(5):834–5.
11. Angus-Leppan H. Diagnosing epilepsy in neurology clinics: A prospective study. *Seizure* 2008; 17(5):431–6.
12. Kotsopoulos IA, de Krom MC, Kessels FG, Lodder J, Troost J, Twellaar M, *et al.* The diagnosis of epileptic and non-epileptic seizures. *Epilepsy Res* 2003; 57(1):59–67.
13. Smith D, Defalla BA, Chadwick DW. The misdiagnosis of epilepsy and the management of refractory epilepsy in a specialist clinic. *Q J Med* 1999; 92(1):15–23.
14. Plug L, Reuber M. Making the diagnosis in patients with blackouts: it's all in the history. *Pract Neurol* 2009; 9(1):4–15.
15. Hoefnagels WAJ, Padberg GW, Overweg J, Roos RAC, van Dijk JG. Syncope or seizure? the diagnostic value of the EEG and hyperventilation test in transient loss of consciousness. *J Neurol, Neurosurg, Psychiatry* 1991; 54(11):953–6.
16. Hoefnagels WAJ, Padberg GW, Overweg J, von der Velde EA, Roos RAC. Transient loss of consciousness: the value of the history for distinguishing seizure from syncope. *J Neurol* 1991; 238:39–43.
17. Sheldon R, Rose S, Ritchie D, Conolly SJ, Koshman ML, Lee MA, *et al.* Historical criteria that distinguish syncope from seizures. *J Am Coll Cardiol* 2002; 40(1):142–8.
18. Alboni P, Brignole M, Menozzi C, Raviele A, Del Rosso A, Dinelli M, *et al.* Diagnostic value of history in patients with syncope with or without heart disease. *J Am Coll Cardiol* 2001; 37(7):1921–8.
19. Syed TU, LaFrance WC Jr, Kahriman ES, Hasan SN, Rajasekaran V, Gulati D, *et al.* Can semiology predict psychogenic nonepileptic seizures. *Ann Neurol* 2011; 69(6):997–1004.
20. Frucht MM, Quigg M, Schwaner C, Fountain NB. Distribution of seizure precipitants among epilepsy syndromes. *Epilepsia* 2000; 41(12):1534–9.
21. Pavlova MK, Shea SA, Scheer FA, Bromfield EB. Is there a circadian variation of epileptiform abnormalities in idiopathic generalized epilepsy? *Epilepsy Behav* 2009; 16(3):461–7.
22. Xue LY, Ritaccio AL. Reflex seizures and reflex epilepsy. *Am J Electroneurodiagnostic Technol* 2006; 46(1):39–48.
23. Benbadis SR. A spell in the epilepsy clinic and a history of 'chronic pain' or 'fibromyalgia' independently predict a diagnosis of psychogenic seizures. *Epilepsy Behav* 2005; 6(2):264–5.
24. Reuber M, Enright SM, Goulding PJ. Postoperative pseudostatus: not everything that shakes is epilepsy. *Anaesthesia* 2000; 55(1):74–8.
25. Colman N, Nahm K, van Dijk JG, Reitsma JB, Wieling W, Kaufmann H. Diagnostic value of history taking in reflex syncope. *Clin Autonomic Res* 2004; 14(Suppl 1):1/37–1/44.
26. Krediet CTP, Jardine DL, Cortelli P, Visman AGR, Wieling W. Vasovagal syncope interrupting sleep? *Heart* 2004; 90:e25.
27. Benbadis SR, Lancman ME, King LM, Swanson SJ. Preictal pseudosleep: a new finding in psychogenic seizures. *Neurology* 1996; 47(1):63–7.
28. Duncan R, Oto M, Russel AJ, Conway P. Pseudosleep events in patients with psychogenic non-epileptic seizures: prevalence and associations. *J Neurol Neurosurg Psychiatry* 2004; 75(7):1009–12.
29. Reuber M, Jamnadas-Khoda J, Broadhurst M, Grunewald R, Howell S, Koepp, M, *et al.* Psychogenic non-epileptic seizures: seizure manifestations reported by patients and witnesses. *Epilepsia* 2011; 52(11):2028–35.
30. Schwabe M, Reuber M, Schoendienst M, Guelich E. Listening to people with seizures: how can Conversation Analysis help in the differential diagnosis of seizure disorders. *Commun Med* 2008; 5(1): 59–72.
31. Luther JS, McNamara JO, Carwile S, Miller P, Hope V. Pseudoepileptic seizures: methods and video analysis to aid diagnosis. *AnnNeurol* 1982; 12(5):458–62.
32. Meierkord H, Will B, Fish D, Shorvon S. The clinical features and prognosis of pseudoseizures diagnosed using video-EEG telemetry. *Neurology* 1991; 41(10):1643–6.

33. Goldstein LH, Mellers JD. Ictal symptoms of anxiety, avoidance behaviour, and dissociation in patients with dissociative seizures. *J Neurol Neurosurg Psychiatry* 2006; 77(5):616–21.
34. Vinton A, Carino J, Vogrin S, Macgregor L, Kilpatrick C, Matkovic Z, *et al.* 'Convulsive' nonepileptic seizures have a characteristic pattern of rhythmic artifact distinguishing them from epileptic seizures. *Epilepsia* 2004; 45(11):1344–50.
35. Lempert T, Bauer M, Schmidt D. Syncope: a videometric analysis of 56 episodes of transient cerebral hypoxia. *Ann Neurol* 1994; 36:233–7.
36. James MR, Marshall H, Carew-McColl M. Pulse oximetry during apparent tonic-clonic seizures. *Lancet* 1991; 337(8738):394–5.
37. Gates JR, Ramani V, Whalen S, Loewenson R. Ictal characteristics of pseudoseizures. *Arch Neurol* 1985; 42(12):1183–7.
38. Selai CE, Elstner K, Trimble MR. Quality of life pre and post epilepsy surgery. *Epilepsy Res* 2000; 38(1):67–74.
39. Dworetzky BA, Bubrick EJ, Szaflarski JP. Nonepileptic psychogenic status: markedly prolonged psychogenic nonepileptic seizures. *Epilepsy Behav* 2010; 19(1):65–8.
40. Reuber M. Psychogenic nonepileptic seizures—a comprehensive review. *Adv Clin Neurosci* 2003; 13:175–204.
41. Groppel G, Kapitany T, Baumgartner C. Cluster analysis of clinical seizure semiology of psychogenic nonepileptic seizures. *Epilepsia* 2000; 41(5):610–4.
42. Benbadis SR, Chichkova R. Psychogenic pseudosyncope: an underestimated and provable diagnosis. *Epilepsy Behav* 2006; 9(1):106–10.
43. Gulick TA, Spinks IP, King DW. Pseudoseizures: ictal phenomena. *Neurology* 1982; 32(1):24–30.
44. Leis AA, Ross MA. Psychogenic seizures. *Neurology* 1992; 42(5):1128– 9.
45. Leis AA, Ross MA, Summers AK. Psychogenic seizures: ictal characteristics and diagnostic pitfalls. *Neurology* 1992; 42(1):95–9.
46. Geyer JD, Payne TA, Drury I. The value of pelvic thrusting in the diagnosis of seizures and pseudoseizures. *Neurology* 2000; 54(1):227–9.
47. Groppel G, Pataraia E, Olbrich A, Bacher J, Leutmezer F, Aull S, *et al.* Clinical symptoms in psychogenic seizures. *Wien Klin Wochenschr* 1999; 111(12):469–75.
48. Chung SG, P; Kirlin, KA. Ictal eye closure is a reliable indicator for psychogenic nonepileptic seizures. *Neurology* 2006; 66:1730–1.
49. DeToledo JC, Ramsay RE. Patterns of involvement of facial muscles during epileptic and nonepileptic events: review of 654 events. *Neurology* 1996; 47(3):621–5.
50. Fluegel D, Bauer J, Kaeseborn U, Burr W, Elger CE. Closed eyes during a seizure indicate psychogenic etiology: a study with suggestive seizure provocation. *J Epilepsy* 1996; 9:165–9.
51. Bergen D, Ristanovic R. Weeping as a common element of pseudoseizures. *Arch Neurol* 1993; 50(10):1059–60.
52. Walczak TS, Bogolioubov A. Weeping during psychogenic nonepileptic seizures. *Epilepsia* 1996; 37:208–10.
53. Ettinger AB, Weisbrot DM, Nolan E, Devinsky O. Postictal symptoms help distinguish patients with epileptic seizures from those with non-epileptic seizures. *Seizure* 1999; 8(3):149–51.
54. Peguero E, Abou-Khalil B, Fakhoury T, Mathews G. Self-injury and incontinence in psychogenic seizures. *Epilepsia* 1995; 36(6):586–91.
55. Williams C, House AO. Heavy hospital case notes: a simple case finding method for psychiatric problems. *Ir J Psychol Med* 1999; 16:123–6.
56. Schwabe M, Howell SJ, Reuber M. Differential diagnosis of seizure disorders: a conversation analytic approach. *Soc Sci Med* 2007; 65(4):712–24.
57. Plug L, Sharrack B, Reuber M. Conversation analysis can help in the distinction of epileptic and non-epileptic seizure disorders: a case comparison. *Seizure* 2009; 18:43–50.
58. Reuber M, Monzoni C, Sharrack B, Plug L. Using Conversation Analysis to distinguish between epilepsy and non-epileptic seizures: a prospective blinded multirater study. *Epilepsy Behav* 2009; 16(1):139–44.
59. Reuber M, Elger CE. Psychogenic nonepileptic seizures: review and update. *Epilepsy Behav* 2003; 4(3):205–16.
60. Syed TU, Arozullah AM, Suciu GP, Toub J, Kim H, Dougherty ML, *et al.* Do observer and self-reports of ictal eye closure predict psychogenic nonepileptic seizures? *Epilepsia* 2008; 49(5):898–904.
61. Bowman ES, Markand ON. Psychodynamics and psychiatric diagnoses of pseudoseizure subjects. *Am J Psychiatry* 1996; 153(1):57–63.
62. Gracie J, Newton JL, Norton M, Baker C, Freeston M. The role of psychological factors in response to treatment in neurocardiogenic (vasovagal) syncope. *Europace* 2006; 8(8):636–43.
63. Jones JE, Hermann BP, Barry JJ, Gilliam F, Kanner AM, Meador KJ. Clinical assessment of Axis I psychiatric morbidity in chronic epilepsy: a multicenter investigation. *J Neuropsychiatry Clin Neurosci* 2005; 17(2):172–9.
64. Reuber M, Fernandez G, Bauer J, Singh DD, Elger CE. Interictal EEG abnormalities in patients with psychogenic non-epileptic seizures. *Epilepsia* 2002; 43:1013–20.
65. Ganesan K, Appleton R, Tedman B. EEG departments in Great Britain: a survey of practice. *Seizure* 2006; 15(5):307–12.
66. Tan M, Appleton R, Tedman B. Paediatric EEGs: what NICE didn't say. *Arch Dis Child* 2008; 93(5):366–8.
67. Reuber M, Fernandez G, Helmstaedter C, Qurishi A, Elger CE. Evidence of brain abnormality in patients with psychogenic nonepileptic seizures. *Epilepsy Behav* 2002; 3:246–8.
68. Marsh E, O'Callaghan P, Smith P. The humble electrocardiogram. *Pract Neurol* 2008; 8(1):46–59.
69. Sarasin FP, Louis-Simonet M, Carballo D, Slama S, Rajeswaran A, Metzger JT, *et al.* Prospective evaluation of patients with syncope: a population-based study. *Am J Med* 2001; 111(3):177–84.
70. Benbadis SR, O'Neill E, Tatum WO, Heriaud L. Outcome of prolonged video-EEG monitoring at a typical referral epilepsy center. *Epilepsia* 2004; 45(9):1150–3.
71. Krahn AD, Klein GJ, Yee R, Skanes AC. The use of monitoring strategies in patients with unexplained syncope—role of the external and implantable loop recorder. *Clin Auton Res* 2004; 14(Suppl. 1):55–61.
72. Samuel M, Duncan JS. Use of the hand held video camcorder in the evaluation of seizures. *J Neurol Neurosurg Psychiatry* 1994; 57(11):1417–8.
73. McGonigal A, Oto M, Russel AJ, Greene J, Duncan R. Outpatient video EEG recording in the diagnosis of non-epileptic seizures: a randomized controlled trial of simple suggestion techniques. *J Neurol Neurosurg Psychiatry* 2002; 72(4):549–51.
74. Grubb BP, Gerard G, Wolfe DA, Samoil D, Davenport CW, Homan RW, *et al.* Syncope and seizures of psychogenic origin: identification with head- upright tilt table testing. *Clin Cardiol* 1992; 15(11):839–42.
75. Brignole M, Alboni P, Benditt DG, Bergfeldt L, Blanc JJ, Thomsen PE, *et al.* Guidelines on management (diagnosis and treatment) of syncope-update 2004. Executive Summary. *Eur Heart J* 2004; 25(22):2054–72.
76. Hainsworth R. Pathophysiology of syncope. *Clin Auton Res* 2004; 14(Suppl. 1):I/18–I/24.
77. Ammirati F, Colivicchi F, Santini M. Diagnosing syncope in clinical practice. Implementation of a simplified diagnostic algorithm in a multicentre prospective trial—the OESIL 2 study (Osservatorio Epidemiologico della Sincope nel Lazio). *Eur Heart J* 2000; 21(11): 935–40.
78. Blanc JJ, L'Her C, Touiza A, Garo B, L'Her E, Mansourati J. Prospective evaluation and outcome of patients admitted for syncope over a 1 year period. *Eur Heart J* 2002; 23(10):815–20.
79. Kenny RA, Richardson DA, Steen N, Bexton RS, Shaw FE, Bond J. Carotid sinus syndrome: a modifiable risk factor for nonaccidental falls in older adults (SAFE PACE). *J Am Coll Cardiol* 2001; 38(5):1491–6.

80. Mathias CJ. Role of autonomic evaluation in the diagnosis and management of syncope. *Clin Auton Res* 2004; 14(Suppl 1):45–54.
81. Reuber M. Psychogenic nonepileptic seizures: answers and questions. *Epilepsy Behav* 2008; 12:622–35.
82. American Psychiatric Association. *Diagnostic and Statistical Manual of Mental Disorders*. Washington, DC: APA, 1994.
83. Brick JF, Crosby TW. Hot flash epilepsy. *South Med J* 1988; 81(1):98.
84. World Health Organization. *The ICD-10 Classification of Mental and Behavioural Disorders: Clinical Descriptions and Diagnostic Guidelines*. Geneva: WHO, 1992.
85. Reuber M. The etiology of psychogenic non-epileptic seizures: toward a biopsychosocial model. *Neurol Clin* 2009; 27(4):909–24.
86. Reuber M, Zeidler M, Chataway J, Sadler M. Munchausen syndrome by phone. *Lancet* 2000; 365:1358.
87. Devinsky O, Putnam F, Grafman J, Bromfield E, Theodore WH. Dissociative states and epilepsy. *Neurology* 1989; 39(6):835–40.
88. Bowman ES, Coons PM. The differential diagnosis of epilepsy, pseudoseizures, dissociative identity disorder, and dissociative disorder not otherwise specified. *Bull Menninger Clin* 2000; 64(2):164–80.
89. Macefield G, Burke D. Paraesthesiae and tetany induced by voluntary hyperventilation. Increased excitability of human cutaneous and motor axons. *Brain* 1991; 114(Pt 1B):527–40.
90. van Dixhoorn JD, H.J. Efficacy of the Nijmegen Questionnaire in recognition of the hyperventilation syndrome. *J Psychosom Res* 1985; 29(2):199–206.
91. Provini F, Plazzi G, Tinuper P, Vandi S, Lugaresi E, Montagna P. Nocturnal frontal lobe epilepsy. A clinical and polygraphic overview of 100 consecutive cases. *Brain* 1999; 122(Pt 6):1017–31.
92. Zucconi M, Ferini-Strambi L. NREM parasomnias: arousal disorders and differentiation from nocturnal frontal lobe epilepsy. *Clin Neurophysiol* 2000; 111(Suppl 2):S129–35.
93. Derry CP, Duncan JS, Berkovic SF. Paroxysmal motor disorders of sleep: the clinical spectrum and differentiation from epilepsy. *Epilepsia* 2006; 47(11):1775–91.
94. Derry CP, Davey M, Johns M, Kron K, Glencross D, Marini C, *et al.* Distinguishing sleep disorders from seizures: diagnosing bumps in the night. *Arch Neurol* 2006; 63(5):705–9.
95. Derry CP, Harvey AS, Walker MC, Duncan JS, Berkovic SF. NREM arousal parasomnias and their distinction from nocturnal frontal lobe epilepsy: a video EEG analysis. *Sleep* 2009; 32(12):1637–44.
96. Tassinari CA, Cantalupo G, Hogl B, Cortelli P, Tassi L, Francione S, *et al.* Neuroethological approach to frontolimbic epileptic seizures and parasomnias: The same central pattern generators for the same behaviours. *Rev Neurol (Paris)* 2009; 165(10):762–8.
97. Bisulli F, Vignatelli L, Naldi I, Licchetta L, Provini F, Plazzi G, *et al.* Increased frequency of arousal parasomnias in families with nocturnal frontal lobe epilepsy: a common mechanism? *Epilepsia* 2010; 51(9):1852–60.
98. Billiard M. Diagnosis of narcolepsy and idiopathic hypersomnia. An update based on the International classification of sleep disorders, 2nd edition. *Sleep Med Rev* 2007; 11(5):377–88.
99. Overeem S, van Nues SJ, van der Zande WL, Donjacour CE, van Mierlo P, Lammers GJ. The clinical features of cataplexy: a questionnaire study in narcolepsy patients with and without hypocretin-1 deficiency. *Sleep Med* 2011; 12(1):12–8.
100. Unterberger I, Trinka E. Diagnosis and treatment of paroxysmal dyskinesias revisited. *Ther Adv Neurol Disord* 2008; 1(2):4–11.
101. Bruno MK, Hallett M, Gwinn-Hardy K, Sorensen B, Considine E, Tucker S, *et al.* Clinical evaluation of idiopathic paroxysmal kinesigenic dyskinesia: new diagnostic criteria. *Neurology* 2004; 63(12):2280–7.
102. Fahn S. Overview, history, and classification of myoclonus. *Adv Neurol* 2002; 89:13–7.
103. Kojovic M, Cordivari C, Bhatia K. Myoclonic disorders: a practical approach for diagnosis and treatment. *Ther Adv Neurol Disord* 2011; 4(1):47–62.
104. Caviness JN, Alving LI, Maraganore DM, Black RA, McDonnell SK, Rocca WA. The incidence and prevalence of myoclonus in Olmsted County, Minnesota. *Mayo Clin Proc* 1999; 74(6):565–9.
105. Shibasaki H. Electrophysiological studies of myoclonus. *Muscle Nerve* 2000; 23(3):321–35.
106. Caviness JN, Brown P. Myoclonus: current concepts and recent advances. *Lancet Neurol* 2004; 3(10):598–607.
107. Fisher CM. Concerning recurrent transient cerebral ischemic attacks. *Can Med Assoc J* 1962; 86:1091–9.
108. Persoon S, Kappelle LJ, Klijn CJ. Limb-shaking transient ischaemic attacks in patients with internal carotid artery occlusion: a case-control study. *Brain* 2010; 133(Pt 3):915–22.
109. Schulz UG, Rothwell PM. Transient ischaemic attacks mimicking focal motor seizures. *Postgrad Med J* 2002; 78(918):246–7.
110. Panayiotopoulos CP. Elementary visual hallucinations, blindness, and headache in idiopathic occipital epilepsy: differentiation from migraine. *J Neurol Neurosurg Psychiatry* 1999; 66(4):536–40.
111. Panayiotopoulos CP. Elementary visual hallucinations in migraine and epilepsy. *J Neurol Neurosurg Psychiatry* 1994; 57(11):1371–4.
112. Blume WT, Wiebe S, Tapsell LM. Occipital epilepsy: lateral versus mesial. *Brain* 2005; 128(Pt 5):1209–25.
113. Bien CG, Benninger FO, Urbach H, Schramm J, Kurthen M, Elger CE. Localizing value of epileptic visual auras. *Brain* 2000; 123 (Pt 2):244–53.
114. Kirchmann M, Thomsen LL, Olesen J. Basilar-type migraine: clinical, epidemiologic, and genetic features. *Neurology* 2006; 66(6):880–6.
115. Bartsch T, Deuschl G. Transient global amnesia: functional anatomy and clinical implications. *Lancet Neurol* 2010; 9(2):205–14.
116. Jager T, Bazner H, Kliegel M, Szabo K, Hennerici MG. The transience and nature of cognitive impairments in transient global amnesia: a meta-analysis. *J Clin Exp Neuropsychol* 2009; 31(1):8–19.
117. Dupont S, Samson S, Baulac M. Is anterior temporal lobectomy a precipitating factor for transient global amnesia? *J Neurol Neurosurg Psychiatry* 2008; 79(3):309–11.
118. Hodges JR, Warlow CP. Syndromes of transient amnesia: towards a classification. A study of 153 cases. *J Neurol Neurosurg Psychiatry* 1990; 53(10):834–43.
119. Shekhar R. Transient global amnesia—a review. *Int J Clin Pract* 2008; 62(6):939–42.
120. Kapur N. Transient epileptic amnesia—a clinical update and a reformulation. *J Neurol Neurosurg Psychiatry* 1993; 56(11): 1184–90.
121. Butler CR, Graham KS, Hodges JR, Kapur N, Wardlaw JM, Zeman AZ. The syndrome of transient epileptic amnesia. *Ann Neurol* 2007; 61(6):587–98.
122. Malouf R, Brust JC. Hypoglycemia: causes, neurological manifestations, and outcome. *Ann Neurol* 1985; 17(5):421–30.
123. Dizon AM, Kowalyk S, Hoogwerf BJ. Neuroglycopenic and other symptoms in patients with insulinomas. *Am J Med* 1999; 106(3): 307–10.
124. Martinovic Z. Fictitious epilepsy in Munchausen syndrome by proxy: family psychodynamics. *Seizure* 1995; 4(2):129–34.
125. Meadow R. Fictitious epilepsy. *Lancet* 1984; 1:25–8.

CHAPTER 9

The Electroencephalogram in the Investigation of Epilepsy

Stephan U. Schuele, Adriana C. Bermeo, and Samden D. Lhatoo

History of the electroencephalogram

Typical for revolutionary innovations, the electroencephalogram (EEG) conquered the medical world within a decade. In 1929, Hans Berger reported on the first recordings of the human EEG (1). His discovery became widely accepted through the corroborating studies of Adrian and Matthews published 5 years later (2). In 1935, Foerster and Altenburger performed the first intraoperative electrocortigogram (ECoG) from the human brain and by 1939, Penfield reported the first case of invasive monitoring for epilepsy surgery (3).

The early years of clinical EEG were dominated by two schools, one led by Frederick A. Gibbs and his wife Erna L. Gibbs in Boston, US, the other by Herbert H. Jasper in Montreal, Canada. Gibbs and Gibbs had the concept of epilepsy as a 'dysrhythmia' of the brain. They postulated that epilepsies could be classified based on pathognomonic interictal EEG findings. They deserve credit for describing the classical 3Hz spike and wave pattern seen with absence epilepsy but also erroneously assumed that rhythmic midtemporal theta known as 'psychomotor variant' is predictive of psychomotor epilepsy (4). Gibbs and Gibbs emphasized the use of the ear reference which is well suited to visualize the typical aspects of generalized 3 Hz spike and wave discharges but also led them to mislocalize patients with temporal lobe epilepsy due to the proximity of the abnormal activity to the ear reference. Jasper and colleagues preferred the use of a bipolar montage which is more sensitive for focal epileptiform discharges. The Montreal school pioneered the localization of interictal and ictal activity for surgical evaluation in collaboration with Wilder Penfield (5, 6).

In the pre-magnetic resonance imaging (MRI) era, epilepsy surgery almost always required an invasive evaluation which was initially limited to intraoperative recordings using subdural electrodes. In the late 1960s, the first implantable subdural strip electrodes were introduced in North America allowing seizure recording outside the operating room (7). At the same time in France, Tailarach and Bancaud introduced a stereotactic method to accurately place intracerebral depth electrodes, which could be left in place for several days and allowed a systematic exploration of seizure onset and propagation (8). Over the subsequent half a century, these techniques have further evolved and thinner electrode plates and depth diameters, MRI compatible platinum electrodes, amplifiers allowing 256 and more channel inputs, and sampling rates of 1 kHz and more are now widely available for the invasive recording of epilepsy patients.

In the pre-digital era, simultaneous recording and correlation of EEG and video was a major challenge. The first closed-circuit television (CCTV) for simultaneous recording of EEG and video was reported in 1966 and similar analogue recording systems were used for the next three decades (9). Since the 1990s, digital recording equipment has almost completely replaced analogue systems. Long-term monitoring is becoming increasingly available not only as a tool for presurgical evaluation, but also as the diagnostic method of choice for patients with treatment resistant seizures (10). In the last few years, central servers and remote access within and from outside the hospital has permitted an increasing number of intensive care units to offer continuous EEG monitoring for (subclinical) seizure detection and management, further expanding the role of EEG in neurological practice.

Physiological basis of the EEG

The main generators of the scalp EEG are excitatory and inhibitory postsynaptic potentials. EEG surface activity depends on the summation of the local field potentials which is enhanced in perpendicular oriented apical dendrites of pyramidal neurons close to the surface. In addition to orientation and location, the size of the neuronal population necessary to show synchronized activity is estimated at 6 cm^2 or more to become visible on the surface EEG (11, 12) (Fig. 9.1).

The cellular correlate of interictal epileptiform activity is a paroxysmal depolarization shift (PDS) which results in the initiation of a high-frequency burst of action potentials followed by a prolonged hyperpolarization. The cardinal features of interictal epileptiform abnormalities visible on surface EEG mimic the cellular processes and consist of a paroxysmal interruption of the existing background activity, an initial sharp wave (80–200 ms duration) or spike (40–80 ms) deflection corresponding to a summation of postsynaptic potentials. This is followed by a prominent slow wave, which reflects the cellular hyperpolarization. The transition from single PDS generating interictal spikes to a full electrographic

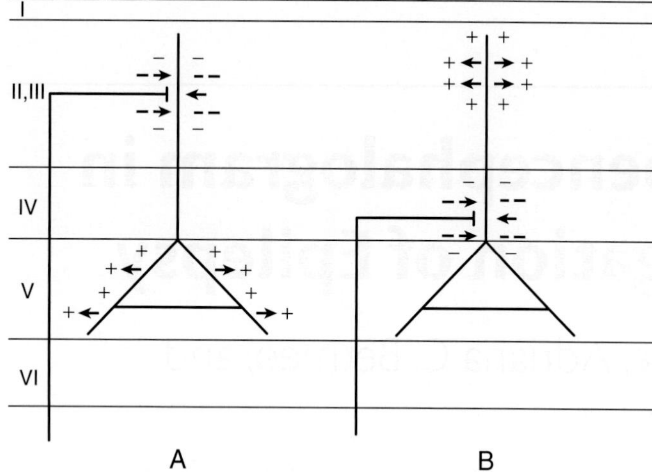

Fig. 9.1 Generation of extracellular voltage fields from graded synaptic activity. A) Excitatory postsynaptic potential (EPSP) at the apical dendrite is associated with a flow of positive ions into the cell (an active current sink) and an extracellular negative field. A passive current source at the level of the cell body and basal dendrites is associated with an extracellular positive field. B) EPSP on the proximal apical dendrite at the level of cortical layer IV is associated with an active current sink and an extracellular negative field. A passive current source at the distal apical dendrite in layers II and III is associated with an extracellular positive field. With permission from Ebersole, 2003 (13).

seizure is associated with the gradual loss of the afterhyperpolarization and the progressive appearance of an increasingly prolonged depolarization shift which leads to synchronized recruitment of additional neuronal population (14).

Indication for EEG studies

The indications for an EEG depend on the study type and clinical context:

Routine outpatient EEG:

- To determine the type of epilepsy (focal vs. generalized onset seizures, specific epilepsy syndrome).
- To prognosticate risk of seizure recurrence (after a first unprovoked seizure or prior to weaning medications).
- For the differential diagnosis of paroxysmal events which could be epileptic or non-epileptic (e.g. syncope, movement disorders, migraine, non-physiological events).

Ambulatory EEG:

- To increase the yield to detect interictal epileptiform abnormalities in patients with normal routine EEG.
- For the diagnostic evaluation of patients with events which are frequent enough and do not require medication tapering.
- To determine seizure frequency in patients who are unable to report their events (subclinical events, patients unaware of unwitnessed clinical events) to guide treatment and lifestyle restrictions.

Inpatient EEG:

- For evaluation of patients with unexplained altered mental status.
- For prognostication for patients in coma.
- As confirmatory testing for patients with a clinical exam ± apnea test consistent with 'brain death'.

Inpatient continuous (video) EEG monitoring:

- Epilepsy monitoring unit (usually associated with medication tapering)
  - Diagnostic evaluation of patients with intractable seizures for more than 1 year.
  - Rapid treatment changes in patients with poorly controlled seizures.
  - Presurgical evaluation of potential surgical candidates (non-invasive and invasive).

Intensive care unit:

- Detection of subclinical seizures in patient with altered mental status:
  - after convulsive status epilepticus.
  - after an acute brain insult (trauma, haemorrhage, anoxic injury).
- Monitoring of patients in burst suppression.
- Procedures:
  - Carotid endarterectomy, aneurysm surgery, balloon occlusion.
  - Wada test.

Scalp EEG

Recording techniques

Placement: EEG electrodes are placed according to the 10–20 system. This allows proportional coverage of individual head sizes using the 10th and 20th percentile of a particular distance defined by anatomical landmarks (nasion to inion and pre-auricular to pre-auricular point) (15).

Many centres use the new nomenclature: T7 (instead of T3) and P7 (instead of T5) for the left temporoparietal electrodes and T8 (instead of T4) and P8 (instead of T6) for the right temporoparietal electrodes (16). Paste is mostly used for 20–30 minute EEG recordings. Collodium is paramount to assure persistent quality for multihour or -day recordings.

Standard setting: the standard low frequency filter for routine EEG is 1 Hz and the high-frequency filter 70 Hz. A notch filter (60 Hz in the US and 50 Hz in Europe) can be used to reduce electrical interference. Sensitivity is initially set at 7 μV/mm. Electrode impedance should be at least 100 ohms and no more than 5 kohms.

Montages: digital recording offers the ability to change the montage setting during review. Most laboratories have a set of standard montages which should at minimum include a longitudinal bipolar (double banana), referential, and transverse bipolar montage.

Localization

EEG channels have two inputs, the second one being either a reference (referential montage) or the next electrode in line (bipolar montage).

Rules of localization: Fig. 9.2 (two channel bipolar montage) depicts that a deflection can be the result of a single generator over

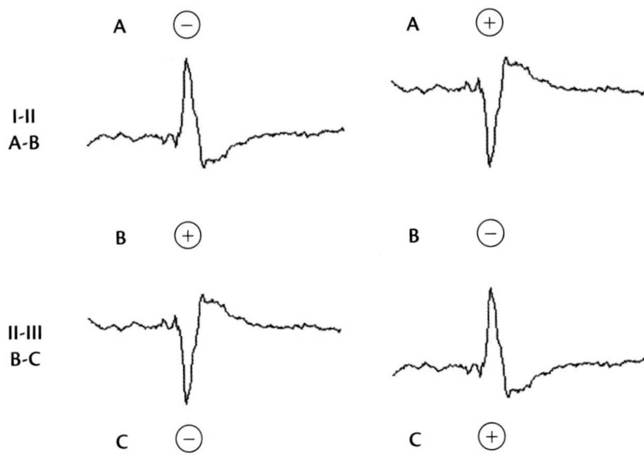

Fig. 9.2 Polarity convention: left column—the negative (upward) deflection in channel 1 (input A minus input B) is caused either by a relative negativity over input A or a relative positivity over input B. Right column—the positive (downward) deflection in channel 1 is caused either by a relative positivity over input A or a relative negativity over input B. Phase reversal channel 1 and 2: left column—the positive phase reversal over B is either due to a positive generator over B or two negative generators over A and C. Right column—the negative phase reversal over B is either due to a negative generator over B or two positive generators over A and C. In clinical practice, we are usually dealing with a single and mostly negative generator, i.e. the scenario indicated by column 2 with a negative generator over B.

the phase reversal or two generators of opposite polarity at the end of the 3-electrode chain. Biologically most plausible is a single, usually negative generator (Fig. 9.2 example on the right).

The presence or absence of a phase reversal determines the maximum of the electrical activity not only in bipolar but also referential montage configurations (Table 9.1).

Choice of reference: ideally, the chosen reference is not involved in the activity to be mapped. In that case, all channels will point in one direction (upward deflection when recording a negative generator). If the reference is involved and close to the maximum (e.g. temporal sharp wave in an ipsilateral ear reference), some deflections will go up and other down in relation to the reference and it can be difficult to visualize the maximum and the associated voltage field.

Phase reversal: it is important to note that phase reversals are not equivalent with abnormalities. They are simply indicators of the field maximum seen with normal and abnormal electrical activity.

Limitations of scalp EEG

Resolution: scalp recordings cannot detect electrical synchronization of less than 6 cm^2 of cortex, and have often poor resolution of cortex which is not covered by an electrode (e.g. mesial and basal cortex). Given the minimum amount of cortex required to be detectable on surface EEG, one can argue that the description 'focal' is not appropriate and 'regional' is a better term for surface abnormalities. Even the absence of EEG changes during a seizure does not exclude the diagnosis of epilepsy: only 20–30% of focal seizures without loss of consciousness have an EEG correlate on scalp EEG (17). On the other hand, in seizures with altered responsiveness ictal EEG changes are seen in 85–95% of cases and the lack thereof is highly suspicious of a non-epileptic phenomenon (18).

Sampling: a routine EEG captures only 20–30 minutes and sporadic or state dependent interictal epileptiform abnormalities may easily be missed. In serial EEG recordings, 50% of patients with epilepsy were found to have epileptiform abnormalities on the first EEG, 84% by the third EEG, and in 92% by the fourth EEG (19). A similar sampling phenomenon can be seen during continuous EEG monitoring in the intensive care unit during which seizures in patients with non-convulsive status are mostly captured within the first 1–2 hours of recording. However, 12% of patients with non-convulsive seizures will not be detected until the second monitoring day (20).

Methods to increase the yield of a routine EEG

- *Sleep deprivation:* the major benefit of sleep deprivation is probably that it ensures that the patient falls asleep during the recording the next morning although the sleep deprivation by itself may have some additional effect. Recording of sleep enhances the yield of the EEG to capture epileptiform abnormalities particularly in young patients and patients with generalized epilepsy syndromes (21).
- *Hyperventilation:* the physiological response to hyperventilation is a rhythmic polymorphic delta slowing (not to be overinterpreted as evidence of a generalized abnormality!). Hyperventilation can bring out epileptiform activity in 10% of generalized epilepsies and rarely in focal epilepsies. It may induce absence seizures in 50% of childhood absence epilepsies.
- *Photic stimulation:*
  - Photic driving is composed of rhythmic activity elicited over the posterior regions often at a stimulation frequency close to normal posterior background. Photic driving is a non-specific finding without clinical relevance.
  - Photoparoxysmal response: spike-and-waves or polyspike-and-waves triggered by photic stimulation. A type I response—non-sustained and limited to posterior head region—is in more than half of patients not associated with epilepsy. A type II—outlasting the stimulus and generalized in distribution—is

Table 9.1 Rules of localization

Montage type	Phase reversal	Conclusion	Common clinical situation, assuming a single generator
Bipolar	**No**	Maximum activity is located at the end of the chain	Generalized slowing, maximum (negativity) frontal
	Yes	Maximum activity is located over the phase reversal	Posterior alpha activity, maximum P7/P8 (Fig. 9.3A) Spike/sharp wave, maximum over the phase reversal
Referential	**No**	Reference electrode is either maximum or minimum	Maximum is indicated by the largest upward deflection
	Yes	Reference electrode is neither maximum nor minimum	Maximum is indicated by the largest upward deflection

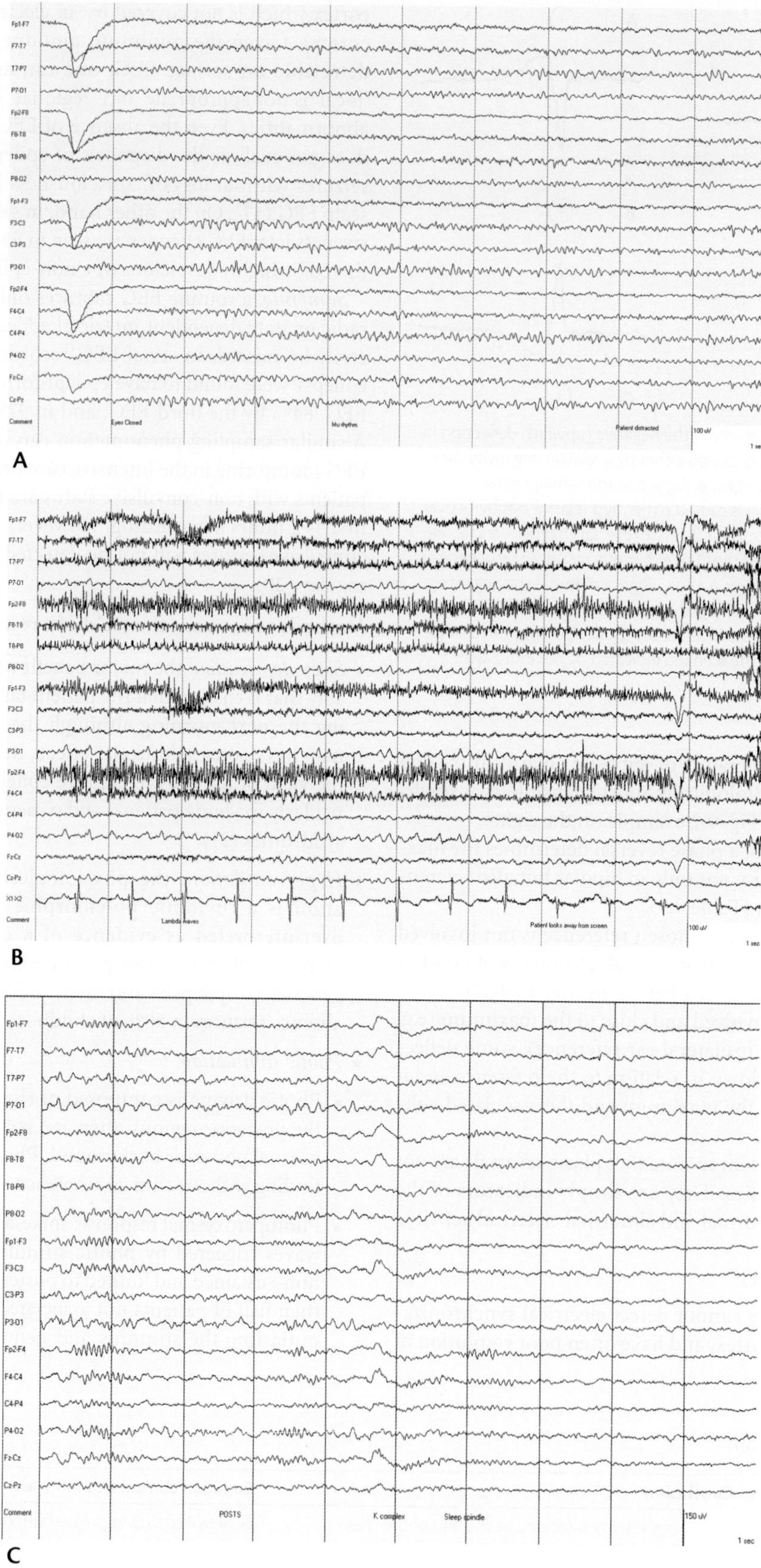

Fig. 9.3 Normal EEG activity. A) Mu rhythm: 7–12 Hz, comb-like activity, attenuated by thought or movements. Seen in 20% of normal individuals. B) Lambda waves: bi-or triphasic (check mark appearance) elicited by looking at a patterned design in a well-illuminated room in this case a computer screen. C) Sleep stage II: sleep spindles, K complex and posterior sharp transients of sleep (POSTS) are seen.

abnormal and a typical finding for genetic epilepsies in particular juvenile myoclonic epilepsy (JME).

- Photomyoclonic response: brief repetitive spikes generated by contraction of muscles of the face or scalp that are driven by the photic stimulation; seen in normal and epileptic patients.

Normal EEG

Normal activity and a number of physiological variants can be confused with abnormal activity and may lead to overinterpretation of the EEG (22; Table 9.2).

Table 9.2 Normal EEG activity and benign variants

Normal activity	
Awake	
Alpha rhythm	8–13 Hz, typically 15–45 μV in adults
Beta rhythm	> 13 Hz and < 40 Hz, typically < 20 μV
Mu rhythm (Fig. 9.3A)	20% of normal individuals. 7–12 Hz, comb-like, attenuated by thought or movements
Theta	> 4 Hz and < 8 Hz. More pronounced in drowsiness Normal intermittent temporal slowing (2–6 waves, theta range) over age 40 years
Posterior slow waves of youth	Most common in children and adolescents. Seen in 15% of young adults
Lambda waves (Fig. 9.3B)	Bi-or triphasic (check mark appearance) elicited by looking at a patterned design in a well-illuminated room
Sleep (Fig. 9.3AC)	
Vertex waves (stage I)	Diphasic, sharp transients with negative polarity
Positive occipital sharp transient of sleep (POSTS)	
Sleep spindles (stage II)	Sigmoid activity, 0.5–2 s in adults, 10–14 Hz, 20–40 μV
K complex	Diphasic
Benign variants (22)	
Subclinical rhythmic electrographic discharge in adults (SREDA)	Rare. Rhythmic sharply contoured 5–7 Hz theta waves, widespread, bilaterally synchronous, posterior head regions
Midline theta	Rhythmic sinusoidal, archiform theta over FZ/CZ
Frontal arousal rhythm	Trains of monophasic 7–10 Hz activity bifrontal
14 and 6 positive bursts	'Ctenoids'—comb (Greek). 0.5–1 s duration of 14 and 6 Hz positive spikes
Small sharp spikes (SSS, Fig. 9.4A)	Low amplitude (50 μV) and duration (<50 ms), anterior to midtemporal
6 Hz spike and wave	'Phantom spike and wave'-spike <25 μV compared to slow wave
Wicket spikes (Fig. 9.4B)	Monophasic, arciform 6–11 Hz, isolated or in trains, anterior to mid temporal. 1–3% of normal individuals
Rhythmic midtemporal discharges (RMTD)	'Psychomotor variant'. Drowsiness. Midtemporal train of rhythmic theta activity, lasting up to 10 s, variable morphology, often with a notched appearance. 0.5%

Physiological artefacts: ocular, cardiac, myogenic, glossokinetic, and others.

Interictal abnormalities

Non-epileptiform abnormalities

Slowing

- Generalized slowing indicates a diffuse dysfunction (Fig. 9.5A) which correlates clinically with an encephalopathy.
  - Intermittent generalized slowing is typical for a mild encephalopathy, continuous slowing (usually with loss of posterior background activity) indicates a moderate or severe encephalopathy.
  - Other patterns seen in comatose patients include *background suppression* (amplitude <10 μV), *burst suppression* and *alpha, theta or delta coma* consistent of diffuse, uniform, unreactive activity in that particular frequency range.
- Focal slowing indicates focal dysfunction.
  - Intermittent focal slowing, particularly over the temporal region can be normal in drowsiness, young individuals or patients over 40 years.
  - Continuous focal slowing is a reliable indicator for a focal structural abnormality (Fig. 9.5B).
  - Intermittent rhythmic focal slowing may represent an electrographic seizure equivalent particularly if associated with a clinical correlate.

Asymmetries

Alpha rhythm asymmetries up to 50% occur normally with the right side often higher than the left.

- Increase: increased amplitude is seen after burr holes or craniotomies known as breach rhythm (Fig. 9.5B).
- Decrease: reduction in amplitude may occur because of cortex injury or fluid collection between the cortex surface and the electrodes (e.g. subdural haemorrhage).
- Frequency asymmetry: hemispheric background frequencies should be within 1 Hz; frequency asymmetry is a non specific finding.

Generalized periodic discharges

This includes a heterogeneous group of abnormalities:

- Generalized (epileptiform) discharges after an anoxic injury often associated with myoclonic seizures.
- Triphasic waves typical for a metabolic encephalopathy (Fig. 9.5A).
- Periodic discharges recurring every 1–2 seconds typical for patients with Creutzfeldt–Jakob disease.

Epileptiform abnormalities

- Focal spikes and sharp waves are the hallmark of epilepsies with focal seizures (Fig. 9.6A).
  - Epileptiform abnormalities are seen in 80–90% of epileptic patients with focal seizures and are detected in less than 1–2% of the normal population.
  - Generalized or multifocal spikes or sharp waves, generalized spike and wave complexes and polyspikes are reliable indicators of epilepsies with generalized seizures (Fig. 9.6B).

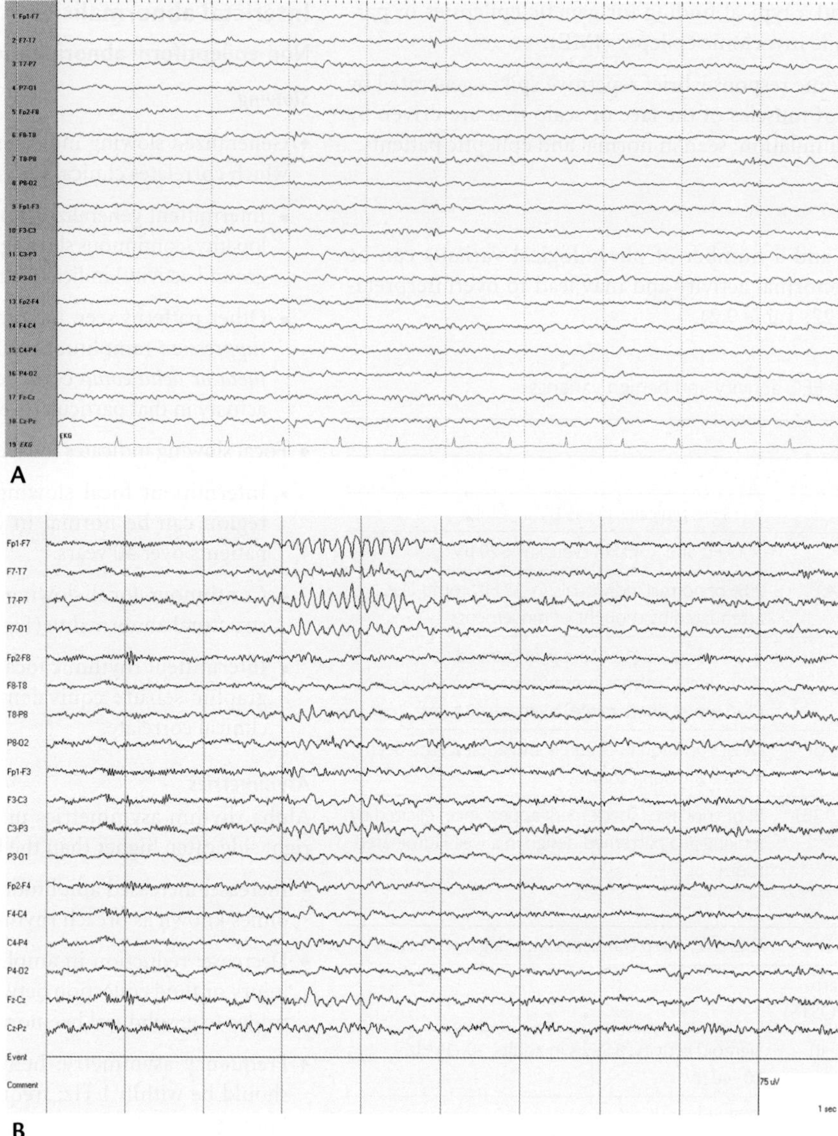

Fig. 9.4 Benign variants. A) Small sharp spikes: low amplitude (<50 μV) and duration (<50 ms), anterior to midtemporal. B) Wicket spikes: monophasic, arciform 6–11 Hz, isolated or in trains, anterior to mid temporal. Seen in 1–3% of normal individuals.

- In combination with a normal awake and sleep background, generalized 3–4 Hz spike and wave complexes and polyspikes are typical for a group of genetic epilepsy syndromes: childhood absence epilepsy (CAE), juvenile absence epilepsy (JAE), juvenile myoclonic epilepsy (JME).
- Generalized epileptiform discharges are less specific than focal epileptiform discharges and 10–20% of patients with generalized epileptiform discharges, recorded either spontaneously or triggered with photic stimulation or hyperventilation, have no history of seizures.

◆ Periodic lateralized epileptiform discharges (Fig. 9.6C): lateralized (and sometimes focal) epileptiform discharges that occur repetitively and semiperiodic every 1–5 seconds; they are usually seen in the context of acute or subacute focal cortical injury.

Ictal patterns

EEG seizures can be classified based on onset and early evolution into focal (or regional), lateralized, generalized, or non-localizable seizure patterns.

Focal seizures

Focal seizure patterns are characterized by rhythmic, often sinusoidal activity in the beta, alpha, or theta range or by repetitive discharges with evolve in frequency, amplitude, or distribution (Fig. 9.7A). They often start with a generalized desynchronization of the background and end with irregular slow activity, in secondarily generalized seizure often more pronounced over the site of onset. The ictal pattern is commonly not detectable during the aura but emerges with alteration of consciousness indicating a necessary spread outside the onset zone for the ictal discharge to become visible on scalp recordings. Hence, interictal epileptiform

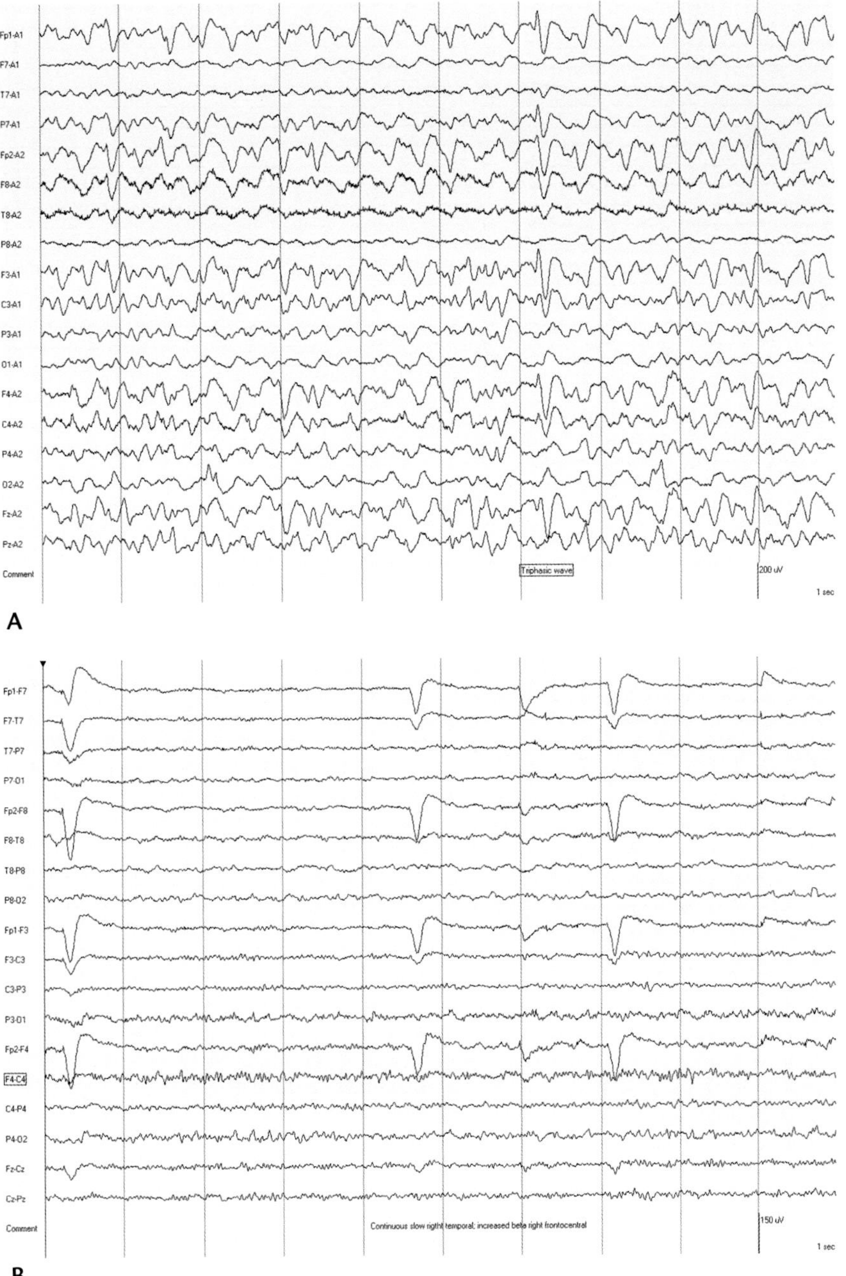

Fig. 9.5 Slowing. A) Generalized slowing and triphasic waves. Referential montage. Generalized 2–3 Hz slowing, maximum frontal. In second 7, a triphasic wave is seen. B) Focal slowing and asymmetry. Continuous irregular slowing is seen over the right temporoparietal region. Increased beta activity is noted over the right frontocentral area. Patient status post right-sided craniotomy for a right anterior temporal resection.

activity often provides a more accurate localization of the epileptogenic zone.

The localizing value of the ictal EEG depends on the region of onset. Most temporal lobe epilepsies have localized EEG findings, seen in 90% of mesial temporal lobe epilepsies and 75% of neocortical temporal lobe seizures which may present with a lateralized rather than focal/regional onset (23). A rhythmic theta pattern at onset is highly specific for temporal and exceedingly rare in extratemporal lobe epilepsies.

Frontal lobe epilepsies, particularly from the mesial structures tend to present with a diffuse suppression or generalized EEG onset and only around a third of cases have a localized EEG seizure pattern. This is further complicated by the fact that interictal epileptiform discharges in frontal lobe epilepsies can present in a generalized distribution, a phenomenon called secondary bilateral hypersynchrony.

Parietal and occipital lobe epilepsies show a localized onset pattern in up to half of the cases. However, similar to mesial frontal lobe epilepsies, occipital lobe seizures can be falsely localized to the contralateral site due to the orientation of the ictal vector. In addition, parieto-occipital lobe epilepsies have a tendency to spread rapidly into either the ipsilateral or contralateral frontal or temporal lobe or may even present with a generalized seizure pattern.

Generalized seizures

The EEG in generalized seizures often correlates with the seizure type. In the subgroup of genetic epilepsies, i.e. CAE, JAE, JME, the interictal EEG findings usually mimic the ictal EEG pattern.

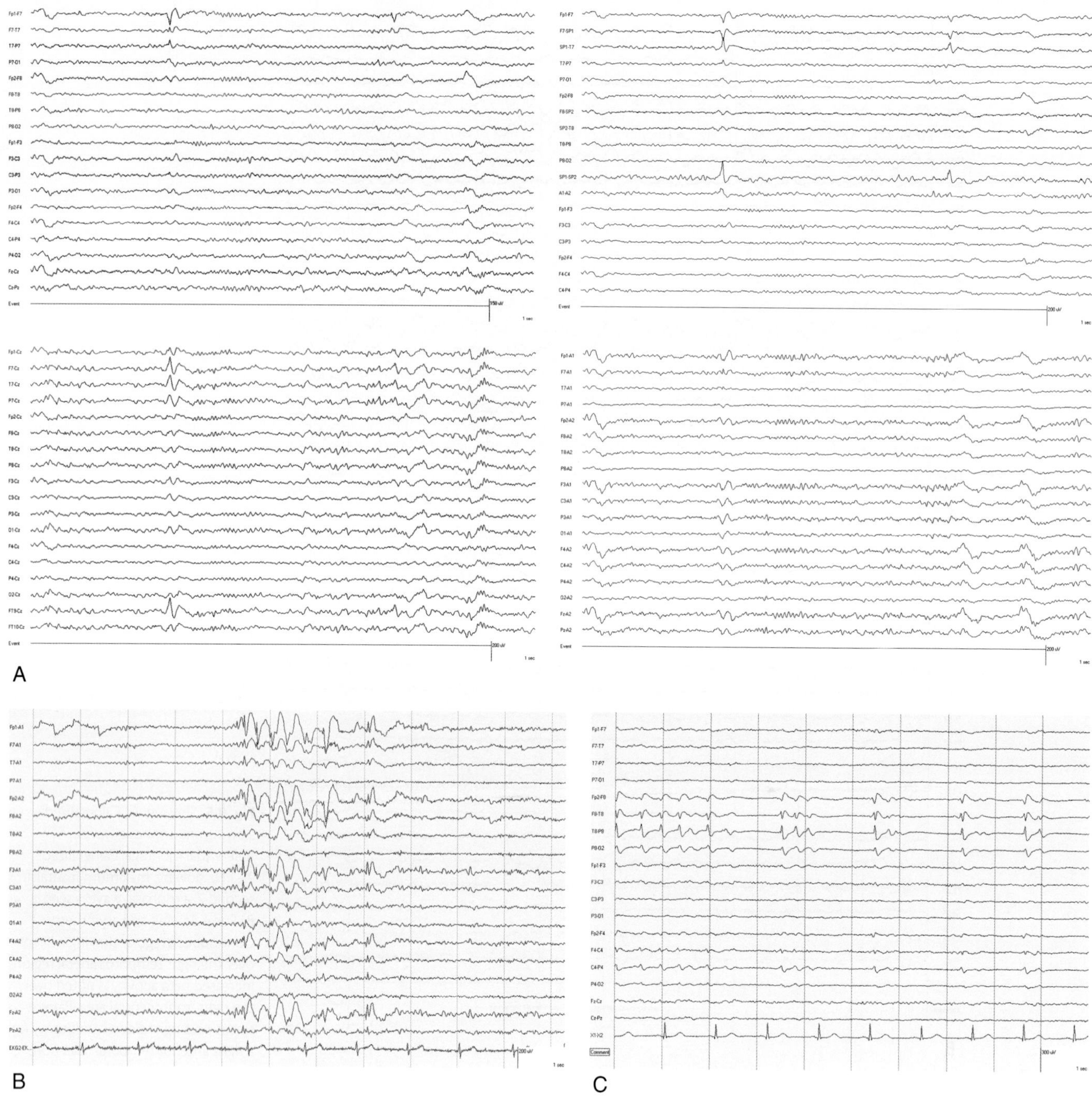

Fig. 9.6 Interictal epileptiform abnormalities. A) Left anterior temporal sharp wave (bipolar montage without and with sphenoidal—upper panel; referential montage to Vertex and Ear reference—lower panel). B) Generalized 2–3 Hz (poly)spike and wave complex in a patient with genetic generalized epilepsy. Referential montage. C) Periodic lateralized epileptiform discharges (PLEDS). Trains of 2 Hz lateralized semiperiodic epileptiform discharges over the right hemisphere, maximum T8 (phase reversal).

- The EEG during typical *absence seizures* in CAE and JAE shows the same 2.5–3.5 Hz spike and wave pattern which is seen interictally. Ictal burst are usually longer than asymptomatic interictal activity. However, even short bursts of 1–2 seconds duration can lead to symptoms and vice versa, patients with prolonged runs of 3 Hz spike and wave activity lasting 30 seconds and more can remain symptom free despite careful testing.
- The EEG during *myoclonic seizures* in JME typically shows a burst of polyspike and wave discharge in the 3–4 Hz range. The burst can outlast the initial myoclonic activity and be associated with staring and unresponsiveness. Seizures are triggered by sleep deprivation and often occur after awakening.
- *Generalized tonic–clonic seizures* associated with CAE and JME are often preceded by an absence or myoclonic seizure with corresponding EEG changes as previously outlined (Fig. 9.7B). The tonic phase is mostly obscured by a dense electromyography (EMG) artefact but if not, may show a brief attenuation and low voltage fast followed typically by a sharply contoured, rhythmic

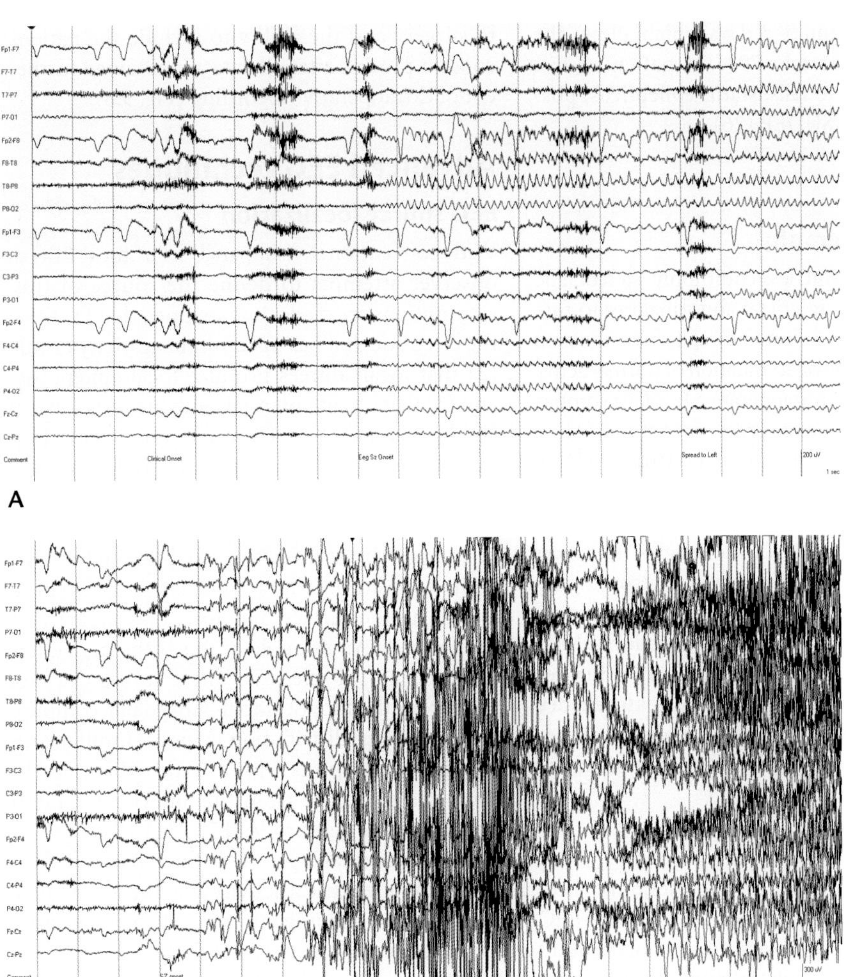

Fig. 9.7 Ictal pattern. A) Focal seizure. 20 s page. Five seconds after clinical onset, abrupt appearance of sharply contoured, rhythmic theta activity over the right temporal region spreading 8 s later into the left temporal area. B) Generalized seizure. At second 4, sudden appearance of diffuse polyspikes and low voltage fast activity, progressively obscured by irregular 2–3 Hz EMG correlated with myoclonic jerks followed by dense EMG artefact indicating tonic muscle activity.

activity in the alpha range coinciding with the tonic phase of the seizure. The rhythmic activity progressively slows down and at 4–5 Hz, a polyspike and wave pattern emerges accompanied by clonic jerking which becomes progressively more irregular. In about one-half of the patients the seizures end with a diffuse suppression, followed by a period of irregular generalized slowing.

- *Atonic* and *tonic seizures* are typical for Lennox–Gastaut syndrome and a variety of EEG seizure pattern have been described. Most typically, the seizures are associated with a voltage attenuation or electrodecremental response with or without visible superimposed low voltage fast. A generalized (poly)spike and wave complex can precede the event and a brief period of generalized slowing is usually seen after the event.

Video EEG monitoring

In the past, patients were usually referred to an epilepsy centre with a video EEG monitoring unit for a presurgical evaluation assuming that they are potential surgical candidates. However, selection criteria who constitutes a good surgical candidate (e.g. suspected epileptogenic zone based on semiology and interictal EEG, lesion on epilepsy protocol MRI), depend on a high level of expertise and technical infrastructure. It has become evident that 25% of patients treated for intractable seizures for many years by their neurologists or primary care physician have non-epileptic events. A referral for patients who continue to have seizures after 1 year of medical treatment to an epilepsy centre is therefore recommended to avoid long-term morbidity and mismanagement (24).

For most patients admitted to an epilepsy monitoring unit, tapering of medications is necessary to record seizures in a reasonable amount of time. This requires continuous nursing supervision and technical support to assure patient safety and optimized data utilization. Placement of additional electrodes over the area of interest (anterior temporal electrodes, sphenoidal electrodes) can be helpful to increase the yield of interictal abnormalities and to facilitate source localization. The goal is usually to record 2–3 typical events. Standardized testing during the event is mandatory to demonstrate the subjective symptoms, ictal and postictal lateralizing signs (ictal speech and postictal aphasia, Todd paralysis), to examine the level of consciousness, and to correlate clinical findings with the EEG. It is important to determine if the patient is aware of the events to assess the reliability of the patient's seizure account. For many patients, seeing their own seizure can be helpful to understand the impact of a seizure on their functioning and to facilitate their decision-making for surgery and adherence to medical management.

The typical length of stay is around 3–5 days which allows the recording of seizures in approximately 70% of patients (25). Complications are rare and related to falls, status epilepticus, postictal psychosis, and, in rare events, SUDEP (26).

Invasive EEG

Intraoperative electrocorticography

Intraoperative ECoG with subdural and, less commonly, stereotactic depth electrodes attempts to capture interictal abnormalities to further delineate the irritative cortex (as indicated by spikes) or the area of dysfunction (represented by slowing or attenuation of normal activity). The additional procedural risk of intraoperative ECoG is comparably small and usually extends the time of surgery by not more than 30–60 minutes. In many lesional (mesial temporal sclerosis (MTS), cavernous malformations, low grade tumours) and non-lesional (non-dominant) temporal lobe cases, intraoperative ECoG can be a useful adjustment to delineate the extent of the surgical resection without the risks associated with extraoperative invasive recordings.

For these patients, functional mapping can be often accomplished preoperatively through Wada testing or functional MRI (fMRI). If necessary, the relation to eloquent cortex can be further defined through central sulcus mapping with somatosensory evoked potentials or electrical cortical stimulation under anaesthesia (recording motor response from EMG electrodes) or in the awake patient (for language mapping).

Extraoperative invasive recording

Extraoperative invasive monitoring either through subdural electrode placement or a depth electrode exploration with 'stereo'-EEG is the preferred approach to invasive epilepsy surgery in many adult centres (7, 8). Particularly non-lesional extratemporal, dominant temporal, or bitemporal lobe cases and the group of patients with suspected dual pathology, post-traumatic epilepsy, or focal cortical dysplasia benefit from the invasive definition of the ictal onset area. Sampling of interictal epileptiform activity to delineate the irritative cortex is often more reliable outside the operation room with all its pitfalls in terms of time constraint and the effect of anaesthesia. A more systematic and reproducible functional mapping prior to surgery and the ability to include the patient in the informed consent process after all data are obtained further adds to the benefit of extraoperative recording (Fig. 9.8).

Advanced EEG techniques

EEG source localization

With conventional visual analysis of focal EEG activity, where the observer attempts to define the source of this activity, certain assumptions are made. It is assumed that (1) the source lies close to the electrode that has maximum negativity or minimum positivity; (2) that focal sources produce focal epileptiform abnormalities; and (3) that broad potential fields are indicative of diffuse or multifocal generators (27) However, this is not always true and clear exceptions to these assumptions are frequently found in clinical practice when depth electrodes are used to localize EEG activity because generators of EEG activity are dipolar with a field potential of one polarity at the active synaptic site (current sink) and a field of the opposite polarity at a distant site (current source) (28). What is seen on the surface therefore, may arise from a distant and/or deep source. An example of this is the mesial temporal EEG spike of hippocampal sclerosis. These spikes can be demonstrated to arise from the hippocampal–amygdalar complex with depth electrodes. Voltage distribution maps of simultaneous scalp recordings of these same spikes with a standard surface EEG montage will show these to arise from the anterior temporal or antero-basal temporal lobe (electrodes F7, T3, FT9). EEG source localization (EEG source imaging, ESI) is therefore aimed at locating the true generator of electrical activity as a direct or indirect indicator of the individual's epileptogenic zone. This is important in the characterization of a focal epilepsy although ESI techniques are also capable of source localizing eloquent cortex through analysis of evoked potentials. See Figs 9.9 and 9.10.

Sophisticated mathematical modelling techniques and algorithms are used to determine ESI and several commercially available software programs incorporate these for clinical and research usage. With both ESI and source imaging with magnetoencephalography, two important concepts require consideration—the forward and inverse problems; the 'solutions' to which add complexity

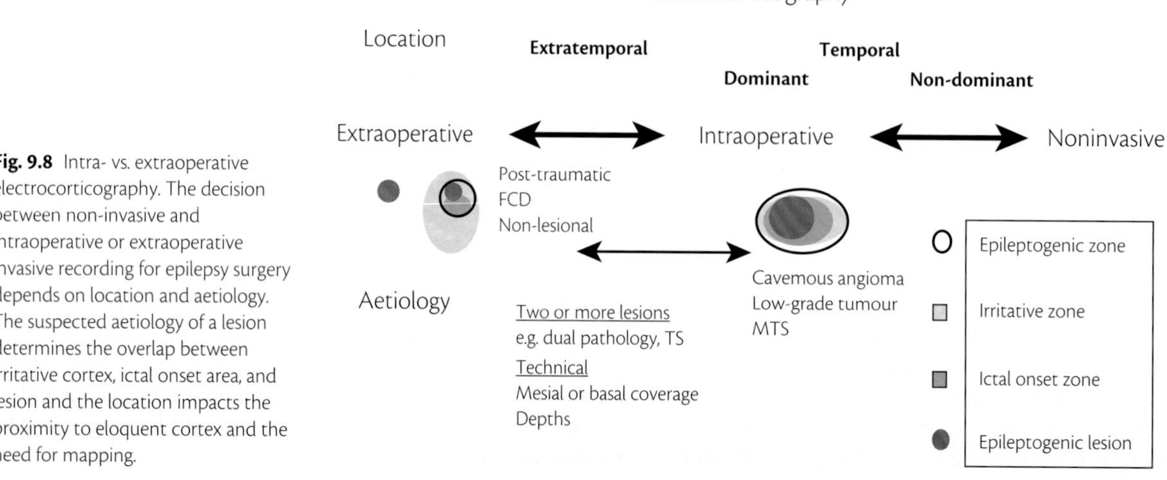

Fig. 9.8 Intra- vs. extraoperative electrocorticography. The decision between non-invasive and intraoperative or extraoperative invasive recording for epilepsy surgery depends on location and aetiology. The suspected aetiology of a lesion determines the overlap between irritative cortex, ictal onset area, and lesion and the location impacts the proximity to eloquent cortex and the need for mapping.

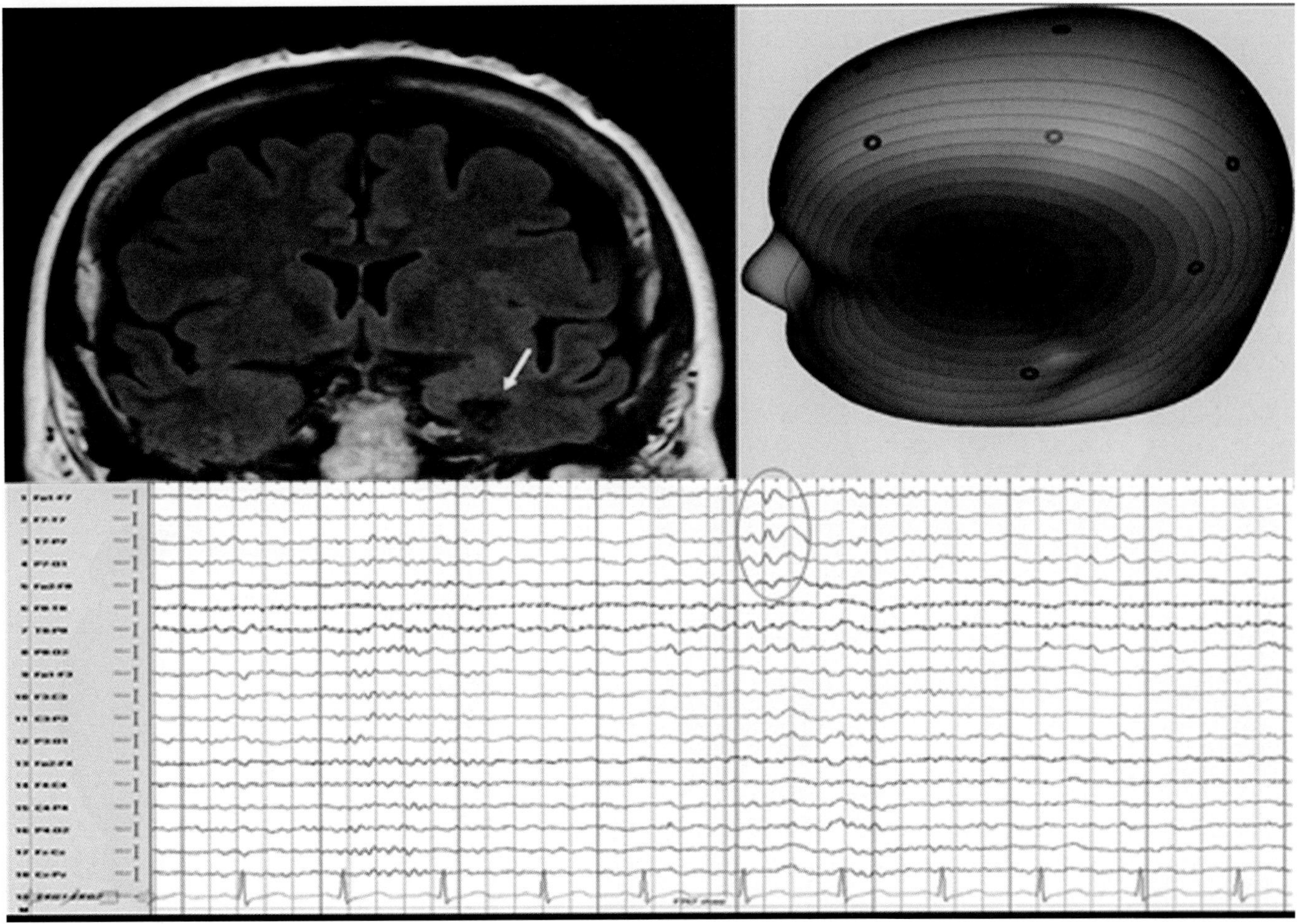

Fig. 9.9 A patient with a left temporal lobe epilepsy due to a mesial temporal cavernoma (top right—white arrow). The EEG shows a left temporal spike with a surface voltage distribution as seen in the top left figure.

to the modelling techniques and algorithms used. The forward problem refers to the problem of accurate localization of a field potential at the recording scalp electrodes for a given dipole source. This is made difficult by the fact that there are intervening physiological planes with varying tissue anisotropy (brain, cerebrospinal fluid, meninges, skull) and additionally, head shapes and sizes vary from individual to individual. Conversely, the inverse problem refers to the problem of working backwards from the field potential recorded at the scalp electrodes to identifying its source. The source can be a fixed, moving, or rotating dipole source, multiple dipoles or a distributed source and different algorithms are used for different situations. Clinical validation for these techniques is slowly building evidence for the utility of ESI (29), particularly in source localizing the interictal spike. Source localization of the ictal discharge is less convincingly studied.

Typically, EEG data is acquired using scalp electrodes in standard 10–20, 10–10 or 'high-density' electrode arrays. Although there is evidence that the accuracy of ESI yield is directly proportional to the number of electrodes used, the optimum is uncertain and beyond a certain number, a law of diminishing returns is likely. The epileptiform spike is then analysed singly or in averaged form by ESI software using one or more modelling techniques and algorithms. This is then pictorially represented on an MRI image, demonstrating localization in relation to surrounding brain structures. To lend confidence to ESI accuracy, it is essential that two important criteria are fulfilled. Firstly that the electrode positions incorporated into analysis are the subject's rather than the software's default positions. Secondly, the MRI images should be the patient's own images rather than the default software images. Non-fulfilment of either of these caveats can result in inaccurate results.

High-frequency recording

High-frequency oscillations (HFOs) within the spectral frequencies of 80–600 Hz can be recorded during invasive EEG in humans (Fig. 9.11). These high-frequency signals are thought to represent short-term neuronal synchronization of action potentials. In the last decade increased attention has been given to these EEG elements as they are thought to be potential markers of epileptogenic brain tissue or epileptogenic networks. HFOs can be recorded from normal and pathologic brain tissue with a tendency for the faster HFOs (fast ripples 200–600 Hz) to be more likely present on pathologic epileptogenic areas whereas ripples in the 80–200 Hz range may be more likely found in specific structures of normal cerebral cortex (30–32).

Although HFOs are generated in very small and limited regions of the cortex, both ictal and interictal HFOs can be recorded with

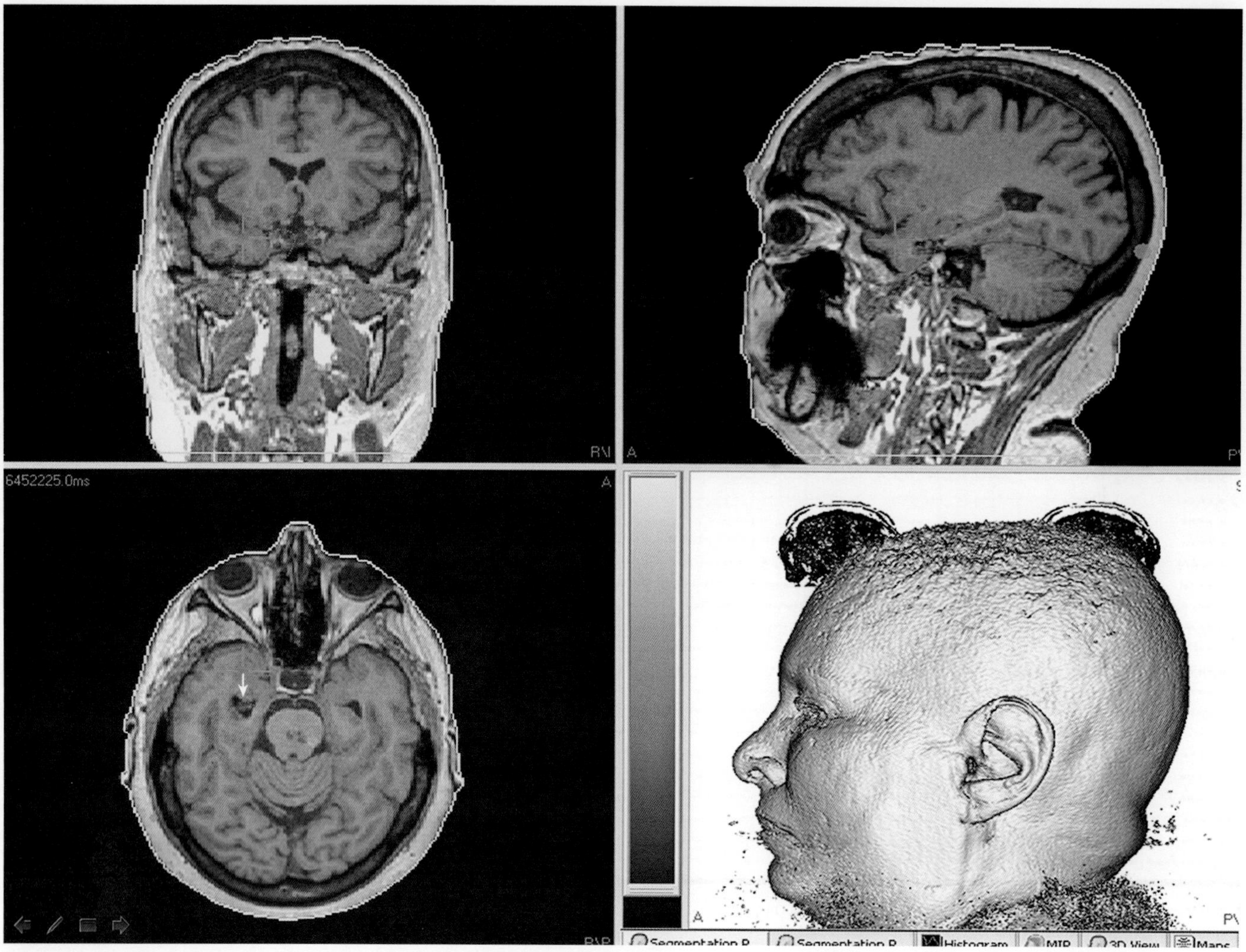

Fig. 9.10 (See also Colour plate 5.) EEG source localization in the same patient shows source localization of the spike to a dipole cluster (in red) in the close vicinity of the cavernoma (white arrow).

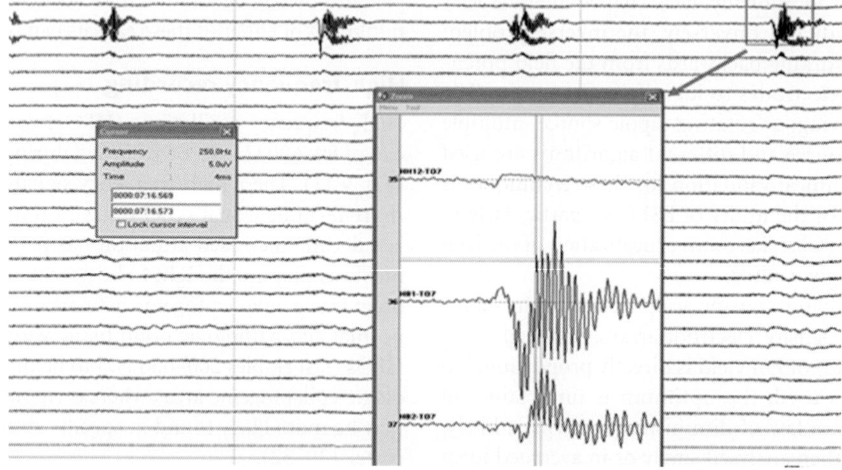

Fig. 9.11 Abnormal high-frequency oscillations of 250 Hz superimposed on interictal spikes seen in the hippocampal body depth electrodes of a patient with left mesial temporal lobe epilepsy.

standard depth and subdural macroelectrodes during invasive video EEG recordings of patients with focal epilepsy (32, 33). Elevated sampling frequencies (>1000 Hz), opening of high-frequency filters, and time stretching displays are necessary for recording and visual analysis.

Interictal HFOs are seen on top of spikes or independent from traditional EEG spikes and are considered an independently generated interictal epileptiform abnormality in invasive EEG recordings. It has been postulated that the association of spikes with HFOs may result helpful in differentiating interictal spikes arising from epileptogenic tissue from interictal spikes of unclear significance. HFOs can also be seen as an ictal phenomenon at the EEG onset of seizures where they usually have a restricted field and are found more likely in electrodes involved in the seizure onset zone than in electrodes where seizures propagate.

Several clinical studies support the role of interictal as well as ictal HFOs as biological markers of epileptogenic cortex. Interictal HFOs tend to be more geographically restricted to the seizure onset zone than interictal spikes are and more limited to the seizure onset zone independently of the type and extension of the brain lesion (34, 35). Interictal HFOs are a more specific marker of ictal onset than spikes and HFOs become more abundant in the period of time preceding a seizure and as antiepileptic medications are tapered down in the context of presurgical VEEG evaluation (33).

The clinical utility of identifying the unique characteristics of pathologic HFOs resides in the fact that these may help identify the epileptogenic zone which is the main objective of most invasive video EEG evaluation in patients with localization related epilepsy. Jacobs et al. was able to demonstrate that patients who have a larger proportion of HFO generating cortical areas surgically removed went on to have better postoperative outcome (36).

References

1. Berger H. Über das elektrenkephalogramm des menschen. *Arch Psychiat Nervenkr* 1929; 87:527–70.
2. Adrian ED, Matthews BHC. The berger rhythm. Potential changes from the occipital lobe in man. *Brain*. 1934; 57:355–85.
3. Foerster O, Altenburger H. Elektrobiologische vorgaenge an der menschlichen hirnrinde. *Dtsch Z Nervenheilk* 1935; 135:277–88.
4. Gibbs FA, Davis H. Changes in the human electroencephalogram associated with loss of consciousness. *Am J Physiol* 1935; 113:49–50.
5. Jasper HH, Carmichal L. Electrical potentials from the intact human brain. *Science* 1935; 81:51–3.
6. Feindel W, Leblanc R, de Almeida AN. Epilepsy surgery: Historical highlights 1909–2009. *Epilepsia* 2009; 50(Suppl 3):131–51.
7. Nair DR, Burgess R, McIntyre CC, Luders H. Chronic subdural electrodes in the management of epilepsy. *Clin Neurophysiol* 2008; 119(1):11–28.
8. Talairach J, Bancaud J. Stereotactic approach to epilepsy: Methodology of anatomo-functiona-stereotactic investigations. *Prog Neurol Surg* 1973; 5:297–354.
9. Goldensohn ES. Simultaneous recording of EEG and clinical seizures using kinescope. *Electroencephalogr Clin Neurophysiol* 1966; 21:623.
10. Velis D, Plouin P, Gotman J, da Silva FL, ILAE DMC Subcommittee on Neurophysiology. Recommendations regarding the requirements and applications for long-term recordings in epilepsy. *Epilepsia* 2007; 48(2):379–84.
11. Cooper R, Winter AL, Crow HJ, Walter WG. Comparison of subcortical, cortical and scalp activity using chronically indwelling electrodes in man. *Electroencephalogr Clin* Neurophysiol 1965; 18:217–28.
12. Tao JX, Ray A, Hawes-Ebersole S, Ebersole JS. Intracranial EEG substrates of scalp EEG interictal spikes. *Epilepsia* 2005; 46(5):669–76.
13. Ebersole JS. Cortical generators and EEG voltage fields. In: Ebersole JS, Pedley TA (eds) *Current practice of clincial electroencephalography* (3rd edn), pp. 12–31. Philadelphia, PA: Lippincott Williams & Wilkins, 2003.
14. McCormick DA, Contreras D. On the cellular and network bases of epileptic seizures. *Annu Rev Physiol* 2001; 63:815–46.
15. Malmivuo J, Plonsey R. Electroencephalography. In: *Bioelectromagnet ism – principles and applications of bioloelectric and biomagnetic fields*, pp. 257–64. New York: Oxford University Press, 1995.
16. American Clinical Neurophysiology Society. Guideline 5: Guidelines for standard electrode position nomenclature. *J Clin Neurophysiol* 2006; 23(2):107–10.
17. Devinsky O, Kelley K, Porter RJ, Theodore WH. Clinical and electroencephalographic features of simple partial seizures. *Neurology* 1988; 38(9):1347–52.
18. Verma A, Radtke R. EEG of partial seizures. *J Clin Neurophysiol* 2006; 23(4):333–9.
19. Salinsky M, Kanter R, Dasheiff RM. Effectiveness of multiple EEGs in supporting the diagnosis of epilepsy: An operational curve. *Epilepsia* 1987; 28(4):331–4.
20. Claassen J, Mayer SA, Kowalski RG, Emerson RG, Hirsch LJ. Detection of electrographic seizures with continuous EEG monitoring in critically ill patients. *Neurology* 2004; 62(10):1743–8.
21. Mendez OE, Brenner RP. Increasing the yield of EEG. *J Clin Neurophysiol* 2006; 23(4):282–93.
22. Klass DW, Westmoreland BF. Nonepileptogenic epileptiform electroencephalographic activity. *Ann Neurol* 1985; 18(6):627–35.
23. Foldvary N, Klem G, Hammel J, Bingaman W, Najm I, Luders H. The localizing value of ictal EEG in focal epilepsy. *Neurology* 2001; 57(11):2022–8.
24. Labiner DM, Bagic AI, Herman ST, Fountain NB, Walczak TS, Gumnit RJ, *et al.* Essential services, personnel, and facilities in specialized epilepsy centers—revised 2010 guidelines. *Epilepsia* 2010; 51(11):2322–33.
25. Friedman DE, Hirsch LJ. How long does it take to make an accurate diagnosis in an epilepsy monitoring unit? *J Clin Neurophysiol* 2009; 26(4):213–17.
26. Noe KH, Drazkowski JF. Safety of long-term video-electroencephalo graphic monitoring for evaluation of epilepsy. *Mayo Clin Proc* 2009; 84(6):495–500.
27. Rose S, Ebersole JS. Advances in spike localization with EEG dipole modeling. *Clin EEG Neurosci* 2009; 40(4):281–7.
28. Brazier MA. The electrical fields at the surface of the head during sleep. *Electroencephalogr Clin Neurophysiol* 1949; 1(2):195–204.
29. Plummer C, Harvey AS, Cook M. EEG source localization in focal epilepsy: Where are we now? *Epilepsia* 2008; 49(2):201–18.
30. Engel J, Jr, Bragin A, Staba R, Mody I. High-frequency oscillations: What is normal and what is not? *Epilepsia* 2009; 50(4):598–604.
31. Gotman J. High frequency oscillations: The new EEG frontier? *Epilepsia* 2010; 51(Suppl 1):63–5.
32. Urrestarazu E, Chander R, Dubeau F, Gotman J. Interictal high-frequency oscillations (100–500 hz) in the intracerebral EEG of epileptic patients. *Brain* 2007; 130(Pt 9):2354–66.
33. Khosravani H, Mehrotra N, Rigby M, Hader WJ, Pinnegar CR, Pillay N, *et al.* Spatial localization and time-dependant changes of electrographic high frequency oscillations in human temporal lobe epilepsy. *Epilepsia* 2009; 50(4):605–16.
34. Jacobs J, LeVan P, Chander R, Hall J, Dubeau F, Gotman J. Interictal high-frequency oscillations (80–500 hz) are an indicator of seizure onset areas independent of spikes in the human epileptic brain. *Epilepsia* 2008; 49(11):1893–907.
35. Jacobs J, Levan P, Chatillon CE, Olivier A, Dubeau F, Gotman J. High frequency oscillations in intracranial EEGs mark epileptogenicity rather than lesion type. *Brain* 2009; 132(Pt 4):1022–37.
36. Jacobs J, Zijlmans M, Zelmann R, Chatillon CE, Hall J, Olivier A, et al. High-frequency electroencephalographic oscillations correlate with outcome of epilepsy surgery. *Ann Neurol* 2010; 67(2):209–20.

CHAPTER 10

Neuroimaging in the Investigation of Epilepsy

Trevor T.-J. Chong and Mark Cook

Introduction

Modern clinical neurology has at its disposal a myriad of neuroimaging techniques to study the brains of patients *in vivo*. The *raison d'etre* for neuroimaging in clinical epilepsy is to localize an epileptogenic focus (Table 10.1) with the ultimate goal of resecting it, while minimizing the extent to which normal brain tissue is excised. Typically, the work-up of a patient with epilepsy will initially include long-term video electroencephalography (EEG), as well as structural and functional neuroimaging. If the sum of these data converges upon a single ictal focus, then surgical treatment might be undertaken with the aid of electrocorticography (ECoG).

In this review, we provide a brief overview of the current imaging modalities available to the modern epileptologist. Due to space constraints, this review does not aim to be comprehensive; rather, our overarching goal is to summarize the current status of the available neuroimaging techniques, with an emphasis on their clinical application and limitations in evaluating patients with epilepsy. We conclude with a general discussion on the relative utility of each modality individually and when applied together.

Structural imaging

Magnetic resonance imaging

In patients who present acutely with a first-episode seizure, computed tomography (CT) is an efficient first-line investigation which can exclude many acute neurological problems requiring urgent intervention, such as an intracerebral haemorrhage or abscess. CT has a number of advantages, including low cost, accessibility, efficiency and ease of use, but its sensitivity in unselected patients with epilepsy is less than 30% (3). Today, due to its greater spatial resolution, magnetic resonance imaging (MRI) has overtaken CT as the mainstay of imaging in patients who are not acutely unwell. In fact, the International League Against Epilepsy (ILAE) has long stated that 'Everybody with epilepsy should have, in the ideal situation, a high-quality MRI' (4).

The diagnostic yield of MRI depends on several factors; for example, the patient population, the pathological substrate, the quality of the scanner, the imaging protocols, and the experience of the interpreting physician. With regards to the patient population, the yield for identifying putative lesions is around 12.7–14% in patients with newly diagnosed epilepsy (5) or a first seizure (6), but rises to 65–83% in patient groups with intractable temporal lobe epilepsy (TLE) who are being considered for surgery (7–9). It is worth noting that, despite its superior spatial resolution, MRI can still miss more subtle structural lesions, such as small areas of cortical dysplasia (10).

Standard scanning protocols can be insufficient to detect the majority of lesions in patients with refractory epilepsy (11), so imaging protocols should be tailored to the clinical scenario (12). A screening protocol for epilepsy should include at least axial T1- and T2-weighted images, proton density sequences, and fluid attenuated inversion recovery (FLAIR) sequences (Fig. 10.1). T1-weighted images provide good definition of the normal anatomy and grey–white matter differentiation; T2-weighted images allow better visualization of focal pathology; and FLAIR sequences provide high lesion contrast in areas close to cerebrospinal

Table 10.1 Description of zones and lesions of the cortex of patients with epilepsy

Zone	Definition
Irritative zone	Region of cortex that generates interictal epileptiform discharge on EEG or MEG
Seizure onset/ pacemaker zone	Region of cortex from which the clinical seizures originate
Ictal symptomatic zone	Region of cortex that generates the initial seizure symptomatology
Functional deficit zone	Region of cortex that, in the interictal period, is functioning abnormally, as indicated by neuropsychological examination, neuropsychological testing and functional imaging or non-epileptiform EEG or MEG abnormalities.
Epileptogenic lesion	Structural lesion causally related to the epilepsy
Epileptogenic zone	Region of cortex that is indispensable for seizure generation. By definition, complete removal is both necessary and sufficient for seizure freedom
Eloquent cortex	Region of cortex that is indispensable for defined cortical functions

Adapted from Lüders and Awad (1, 2).

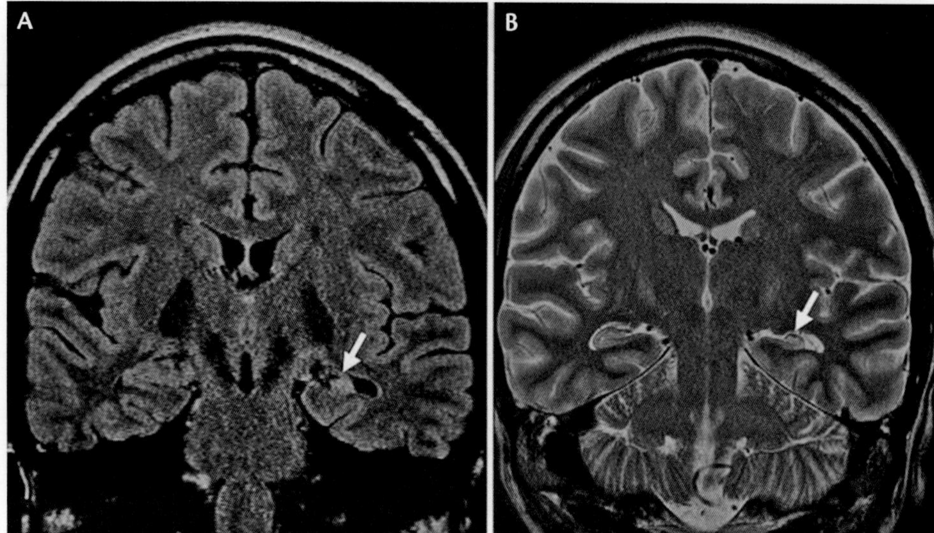

Fig. 10.1 Structural MRI of a patient with left temporal lobe epilepsy secondary to hippocampal sclerosis. A) Coronal FLAIR and (B) T2-weighted images showing increased signal and loss of internal structure of the left hippocampus (arrows). From Deblaere K, Achten E. Structural magnetic resonance imaging in epilepsy. *European Radiology* 2008; 18:119–29.

fluid (CSF). These sequences should be acquired in at least two orthogonal planes covering the whole brain, with the minimum achievable slice thickness. In particular, the acquisition of T2-weighted or FLAIR images in the coronal plane perpendicular to the long axis of the hippocampus is critical to adequately visualize mesial temporal structures. Usually the administration of gadolinium is unnecessary in an initial scan, unless indicated in the clinical history (e.g. a suspicion of a mass lesion or vascular lesion) (13).

In addition to the aforementioned sequences, an optimized epilepsy protocol should also comprise a high-resolution (ideally slice thickness <1.5 mm), three-dimensional, T1-weighted, gradient echo volume acquisition (14, 15). This can be accomplished with a magnetization-prepared rapid acquisition with gradient echo (MPRAGE) sequence, or spoiled gradient recalled (SpGR). This acquisition allows viewing of multiplanar images; avoids partial volume effects in detecting malformations of cortical development; and can correct for coronal head rotation. In addition, a further gradient echo T2 image (T2*) or susceptibility weighted image (SWI) can be acquired to detect haemosiderin deposits, small cavernomas, or vascular anomalies. More recently, a new technique in MRI acquisition has been described (the PROPELLER sequence), which images hippocampal structures with greater spatial resolution (16). New morphometric methods are also being developed to automatically measure brain structures (17).

The precise definition of 'a high-quality MRI,' as suggested by the ILAE (4), obviously changes with time. In fact, further technical and methodological advances in MRI have meant that some patients with previously unremarkable imaging have been shown to have identifiable lesions in newer scanners with more advanced protocols. From a technical perspective, the use of higher field strength magnets (e.g. 3 Tesla) and/or phased array surface coils (18, 19) has been shown to increase the yield of structural MRI. Together, these advances have led some authors to advocate that patients with previously unremarkable MRI scans be rescanned as more advanced equipment and methods become available (20). One of the problems that this field will face in the future will be how to differentiate the epileptogenic potential of more subtle lesions detected with more advanced imaging techniques. This will necessitate garnering converging evidence using other forms of imaging, as will be discussed in later sections.

Voxel-based morphometry

The principal shortcoming of attempting to quantify more subtle structural abnormalities on individual MRIs is that a volume of interest must first be defined (e.g. the hippocampus), and manual volumetry typically requires approximately 30 minutes of interactive time. In the research domain, voxel-based morphometry (VBM) is an MRI analysis technique which attempts to objectively and automatically identify morphological abnormalities across a group of patients with epilepsy. Typically in VBM, T1-weighted volumetric MRI scans are acquired for individual patients, and these images subsequently undergo spatial normalization, tissue segmentation, and spatial smoothing in order to warp patients' brains to a standard space (Fig. 10.2). Statistical tests are then performed across all voxels in the image to identify volume differences between the patient group and a reference population. The advantage of this approach is that it can detect regional changes in tissue volume or density objectively and automatically, without needing to specify a priori which brain areas to examine (22, 23).

Several attempts have been made to improve on the standard approach, including tensor-based morphometry, which employs more detailed warping procedures (24); cortical thickness mapping, in which grey matter thickness is compared across the brain surface; and voxel-based relaxometry to compare T2 signal between subjects (25). In general, VBM and its derivatives have provided interesting data showing the widespread structural changes that occur in epilepsy. For example, one study showed that patients with mesial TLE had widespread grey matter changes which extended to the thalamus, limbic system, and cerebellum, while patients with cryptogenic TLE had grey matter loss in the temporal, frontal and orbitofrontal cortices (26).

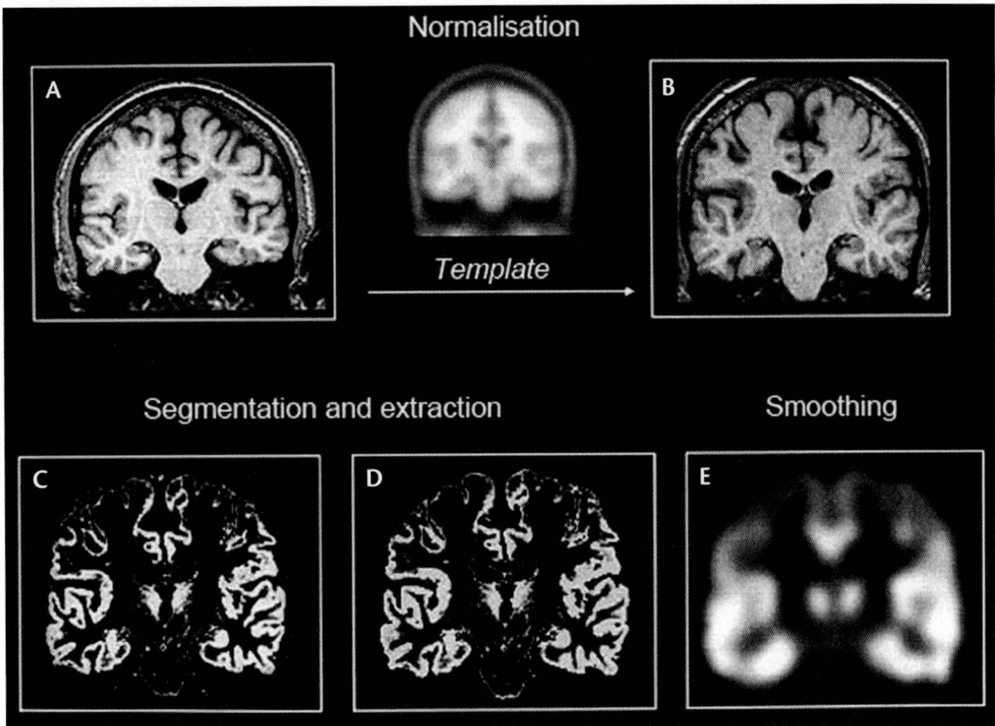

Fig.10.2 The process of spatial pre-processing for voxel-based morphometry. A) Raw images are normalized to stereotaxic space (B) using the 305 normal data set of Montreal Neurological Institute (Template). C) Grey matter is automatically segmented from normalized images using a combined voxel intensity and a priori knowledge approach. D) An extraction technique removes non-grey-matter voxels. E) Normalized grey matter images are smoothed with an isotropic Gaussian kernel with full-width half-maximum of 10 mm. There is bilateral hippocampal pathology and diminished left parahippocampal-fusiform grey/white matter differentiation is visible in all stages. Adapted from Keller S, et al. Voxel based morphometry of grey matter abnormalities in patients with medically intractable temporal lobe epilepsy: effects of side of seizure onset and epilepsy duration *Journal of Neurology, Neurosurgery and Psychiatry* 2002; 73(6):648–55.

However, it is crucial to note the mathematical assumptions and caveats underlying the VBM approach. Broadly speaking, the notion of intersubject spatial normalization is inherently problematic (27), given the morphometric (especially gyral) variations between individuals. At best, one may assume that there are minimal differences in the brains of mesial TLE patients, but those of other groups of patients with focal epilepsy may be even more heterogeneous. Even within individuals, normalization accuracy is likely to vary between brain regions, being poorer in more highly convoluted areas of cortex. Furthermore, although the preprocessing of images is largely automated, there is latitude for the experimenter to vary the method of brain segmentation; the kernel size during spatial smoothing; intersubject spatial normalization; and the final methods of statistical analysis. These factors likely result in varying statistical sensitivity across the brain (23, 28), and underlie the inconsistencies across studies. Consequently, although VBM remains popular in basic and clinical neuroscience, it has had very limited application in clinical decision-making. In the future, it may be possible to improve specificity of VBM by using large control groups, and by looking for overlapping or coincident abnormalities in the same brain region with more than one imaging modality (29).

Diffusion tensor imaging and tractography

In a routine MRI, the contribution of diffusion or Brownian motion on the overall signal intensity is relatively small (causing a signal attenuation of <2%). However, by incorporating pulsed magnetic field gradients into a standard spin echo sequence, one can acquire images that are sensitive to the diffusion properties of water. By using this phenomenon, diffusion tensor imaging (DTI) aims to measure the movement of water molecules (i.e. the overall magnitude of diffusion), expressed as mean diffusivity (MD) or an apparent diffusion coefficient (ADC) (31). The tendency of water molecules to diffuse in one direction over another is expressed as fractional anisotropy (FA). ADC and FA represent the two key parameters in DTI. Increases in ADC and reductions in FA are thought to relate to neuronal loss, gliosis, axonal or myelin abnormalities, abnormal connections between brain regions, and/or structural disorganization, which may not be visible on conventional MRI (32).

Identification of local abnormalities

The main applications of DTI in epilepsy are twofold: first, to identify local abnormalities in the epileptogenic zone; and, second, to identify white matter tracts. With regards to the first aim, the assumption is that diffusion abnormalities will reflect a deranged microstructural arrangement of cerebral tissue and thus help localize epileptic foci in patients with unremarkable structural scans. DTI studies have been conducted in patients following status epilepticus or single seizures (33–36), as well as in the interictal period—overall, these studies have shown that DTI may indeed confer additional sensitivity over conventional MRI in the identification of occult structural abnormalities (37–39).

However, the correlation between diffusion abnormalities and seizure localization with EEG has yielded discrepant findings (40, 41). Broadly speaking, the issue with many of these studies is that they contain only a small number of patients and utilize various methods of analysis, which make it difficult to compare their results. Furthermore, those studies that have examined patients in the immediate postictal period have included patients who had had varying seizure durations and intervals from seizure to scan; factors which would have clearly affected the nature and degree of diffusivity changes.

Tractography

A second application of DTI is tractography, which ultimately aims to infer the structural connectivity between different regions of the brain (Fig. 10.3). Tractography is based on the principle that water molecules diffuse along a path parallel, rather than perpendicular, to those of the myelinated nerve fibre tracts which contain them. Specifically, directional information obtained in each voxel is used to generate virtual, three-dimensional white matter maps. Each of the surrounding voxels is then considered in turn for connection to the central voxel by assessing their diffusion properties, specifically with regards to their shape (quantitative diffusion anisotropy measures) and orientation (principal eigenvector map) (42).

In epilepsy, tractography has been used: (1) to assess the pathophysiology of chronic epilepsy on white matter tracts; (2) to investigate the effect of TLE on the reorganization of language function; (3) to evaluate the structural changes caused by surgery; and (4) to predict the effects of surgery (43). Clinically, tractographic data, in combination with functional activation studies, could potentially guide surgical procedures by delineating areas of eloquent cortex and principal white matter connections (44–47). As an example, one study measured the volume of tracts connected with a frontal lobe speech region identified using fMRI, which allowed the authors to predict the severity of naming deficits after temporal lobe surgery (48). Similarly, another study showed that damage to the DTI-identified tract corresponding to the loop of Meyer correlated with postoperative field defects in mesial TLE (MTLE) patients (49). The promise of tractography in the future would be to identify the white matter connections that need to be transected to functionally isolate the seizure focus, which may reduce the risks of surgical complications.

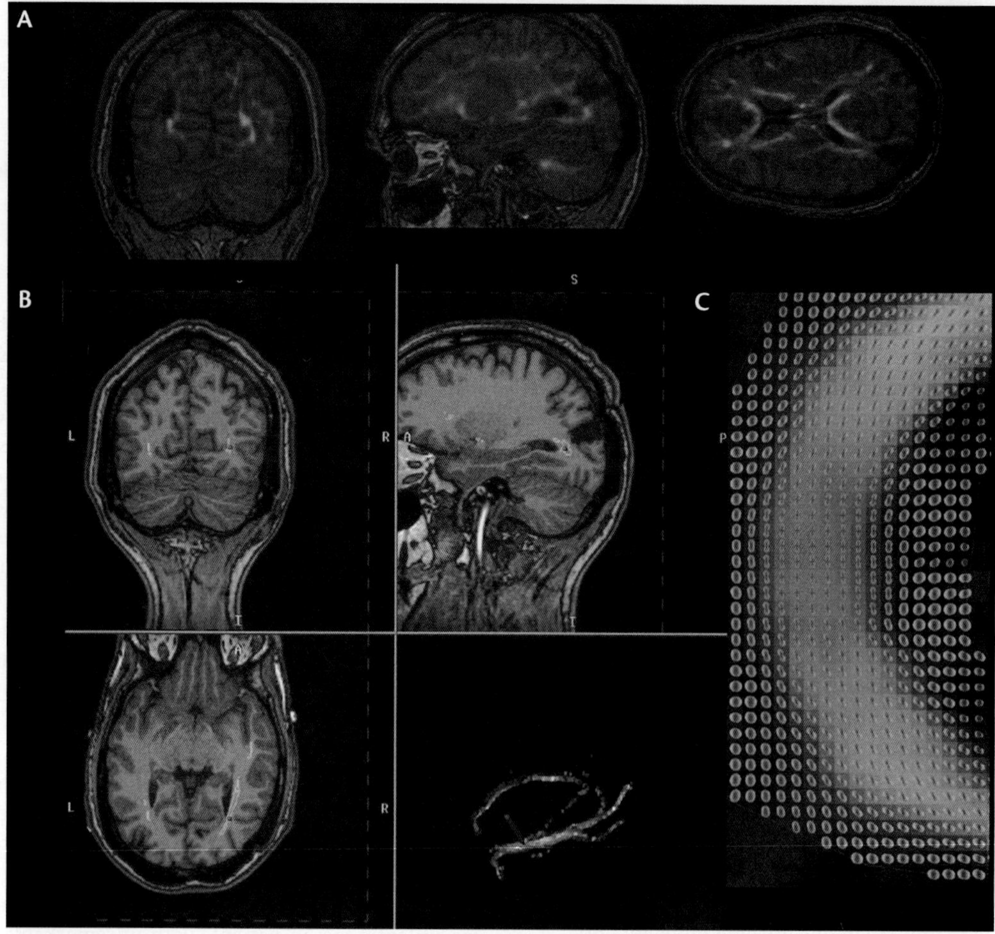

Fig. 10.3 (Also see Colour plate 6.) Tractography of the optic radiations in a patient who underwent resection of a cavernoma located in the right parieto-occipital cortex. A) Diffusion-weighted images with 30 directions were acquired and co-registered to the patient's MPRAGE, with colour fractional anisotropy (FA) corresponding to tensor orientations. B) Tractography was incorporated into a Stealth neuronavigation system for the operative procedure. The optic radiations are indicated in yellow. C) A zoomed region of interest from the splenium of the corpus callosum is displayed, with the individual superquadratic glyphs from each voxel indicating principal orientation. Each glyph incorporates directional information (blue = inferior/superior; green = anterior–posterior; red = left–right). These orientations are useful in reviewing the quality of tractography results. Reproduced with permission of Simon Vogrin.

However, several issues currently limit the more widespread application of tractography. From a practical point of view, DTI and tractography are currently very time-consuming processes but, with increases in computing power, this should become less of an issue. Another problem is methodological: typically, the size of a single voxel is 2–3 mm^3, a volume which contains thousands of axons. Most methods assume that fibres at each voxel are adequately described by a single orientation estimate, but the complexity of subcortical white matter tracts, particularly at points of fibre kissing or crossing, may vary between individuals. In recent times, newer algorithms (50) and diffusion models (51–54) have been developed in an attempt to overcome these problems, and improvements in orientation (55) and spatial resolution (56) should see advances in this area in the near future. Nevertheless, it is in principle challenging to validate tractographic methods, as prior anatomical knowledge is required to confirm trajectories (57–59). It should also be remembered that tractography cannot at present distinguish between afferent and efferent pathways.

A challenge surrounds the difficulty in quantifying tractographic data. Until recently, tractographic analysis has relied on visual assessment of fibre trajectories and comparison with control subjects or atlases (i.e. it is necessary to have prior anatomical knowledge (59)). Several recent studies have made important advances in this regard (60, 61). Nevertheless, an ongoing methodological constraint is the lack of an absolute metric to evaluate connectivity, given the wide intersubject variation and intrasubject uncertainty with respect to the course and trajectory of the major white matter tracts (61).

Functional modalities

Single-photon emission computed tomography

Functional imaging has the advantage of localizing epileptogenic foci even in areas that are morphologically inconspicuous. In a single-photon emission computed tomography (SPECT) study, patients are injected with a photon-emitting radioisotope attached to molecules designed to label the brain areas of interest (62). The distribution of radioisotope is then detected by a gamma camera, which allows a quantitative assessment of regional cerebral blood flow. All of the radiolabelled compounds that are in use today share the common properties of having a small molecular size and being lipophilic. These properties allow them to readily cross the blood–brain barrier and subsequently accumulate in the brain parenchyma for long enough to permit image acquisition (63). In practice, the vast majority of studies use radiolabelled technetium (Tc), in the form of ^{99m}Tc-hexamethylpropyleneamineoxime (^{99m}Tc-HMPAO) or ^{99m}Tc-ethyl cysteinate diethylester (^{99m}Tc-ECD). The peak uptake of these compounds occurs at approximately 2 minutes after injection. Importantly, they are not redistributed to other brain areas, and therefore the administration of these tracers provides us with a snapshot of the cerebral circulation at the time of injection. These tracers remain stable for up to at least two hours, thus permitting delayed acquisition of the SPECT images.

Ictal versus interictal SPECT

The radiolabelled tracer can be delivered either during a seizure (ictal SPECT) or in the absence of seizure activity (interictal SPECT) (Fig. 10.4). A priori, one might expect ictal SPECTs to result in greater yields of seizure localization than interictal SPECTs, and current data indeed reflect this prediction. Specifically, studies on patients with TLE have shown sensitivities of between 73–97% for ictal SPECTs, compared to around 50% for interictal SPECTs (64–67). In some cases, the re-evaluation of MRI prompted by an abnormal SPECT result has revealed a subtle structural lesion. Despite the promising data for ictal SPECTs in TLE, it is worth noting that the sensitivity of ictal SPECTs appears to be lower with in patients with extratemporal seizure foci (66%), but fewer data are available (66, 68).

Subtraction SPECT

In order to maximize the yield of a SPECT study, the pattern of interictal activity can be subtracted from that of ictal activity ('subtraction SPECT') to reveal foci of hyperperfusion during the time of the seizure (Fig. 10.4). An alternative approach is to compare the activity on an ictal SPECT image to that of a control database. These subtraction images can then be co-registered with high-resolution structural images on MRI ('subtraction ictal SPECT coregistered to MRI', SISCOM), which further improves our ability to localize the epileptogenic focus (69–74). In fact, current data show that the SISCOM technique has an impressive positive predictive value for surgical outcome if the hyperperfused area is fully resected (73–75). In one study, 75% of patients whose SISCOM findings fell within the margins of the resected tissue or in the disconnected hemisphere were seizure-free following surgery. All (100%) of those whose SISCOM findings fell outside the margins of surgery continued to have seizures (76). It is worth noting, however, that, although SISCOM is a strong predictor of surgical outcome, its relative advantage to other methods (such as MRI or intracranial EEG) is still debatable (the role of SISCOM in large case series are described in (70, 77)).

Limitations

The main practical difficulty of acquiring an accurate ictal SPECT relates to its poor temporal resolution. The value of an ictal SPECT is heavily contingent on the timing of radiocontrast administration due to the rapid propagation of seizure activity from the original focus to adjacent areas, and the accompanying rapidly evolving haemodynamic changes (78).Specifically, in temporal lobe epilepsy, the initial ictal hyperperfusion of the mesial and anterotemporal temporal lobes occurs immediately after seizure onset (79). However, within 1–2 minutes following the termination of the seizure, the lateral temporal neocortex becomes intensely hypoperfused, and this hypoperfusion then spreads over the next few minutes to the mesial temporal areas (the 'postictal switch' (80)). Over the next 15 minutes, perfusion in these areas is then restored until it reaches the interictal state of mild hypoperfusion.

This implies a very narrow window within which the radioisotope needs to be administered. In practice, there is usually a delay before the delivery of the tracer, which takes a further 30 seconds to cross the blood–brain barrier if it is administered peripherally. Furthermore only 70% of the radioisotope will be taken up at first pass. One study suggested that an injection time of less than 20 seconds after seizure onset is an important predictor of accurate localization, which is obviously difficult to achieve in practice (77).

In summary, therefore, in those cases in which the administration of radiotracer is less than optimal, the interpretation of the subsequent SPECT images becomes complicated by two issues. First, the ictal SPECT hyperperfusion patterns often contain both

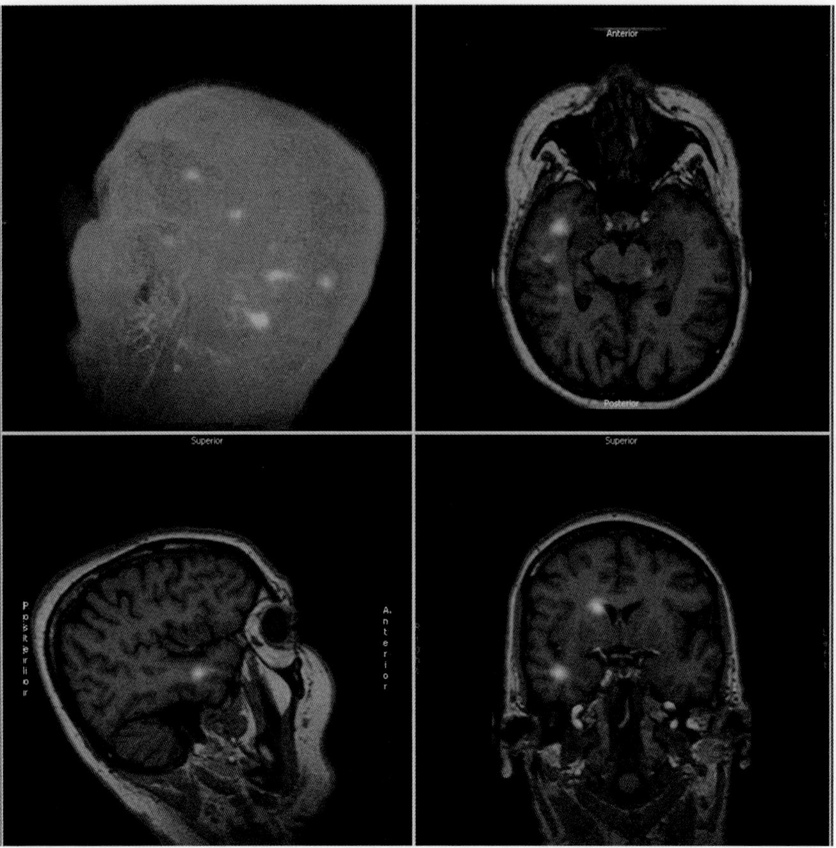

Fig. 10.4 (Also see Colour plate 7.) SISCOM data from a patient with focal epilepsy of the right temporal lobe. Interictal ^{99m}Tc-ECD SPECT activity was subtracted from ictal activity, and then co-registered to the patient's MRI. Reproduced with permission of Simon Vogrin.

the ictal onset zone and the seizure propagation pathways (81). In practice, the ictal onset zone is often considered the region with the largest and most intense hyperperfusion, but the false positive results that subsequently occur therefore make SPECT less reliable than other imaging modalities in predicting surgical outcome. Second, postictal switching can result in false localization or lateralization of the ictal focus when the delay between seizure onset and tracer application is too long. For example, a recent study showed that patients with supplementary motor area seizures had ictal SPECTs which falsely localized to bilateral anterior cingulate cortex (82). Together, this implies that patients may need their epileptogenic focus to be more precisely delineated with other methods, such as intracranial EEG.

Positron emission tomography

As with SPECT, positron emission tomography (PET) potentially provides information about seizure localization that may not be gleaned from conventional MRI sequences alone. The goal of a PET study is to detect areas of relative hypometabolism, which are presumed to reflect focal functional disturbances of cerebral activity associated with the ictal onset zone. The underlying pathophysiology leading to this hypometabolism is incompletely understood, and has been related to neuronal loss, diaschisis, inhibitory processes, or a reduction in synaptic density.

In a PET study, patients are injected with a radioactive ligand, the nature of which is determined by the target areas to be imaged. The most common radioisotope in clinical use today is 2-(^{18}F) fluoro-2-deoxy-D-glucose ((^{18}F) FDG). FDG follows the topographic distribution of glucose uptake in the brain, and therefore provides an estimate of the rate of regional glucose metabolism. It is therefore considered an indirect marker of neuronal activity. In contrast to SPECT, PET isotopes emit positrons, which travel a short distance before colliding with an electron. These particles are then mutually annihilated, resulting in the emission of a pair of photons which travel in diametrically opposite directions, and which are detected by the PET scanners.

Focal areas of reduced FDG uptake tend to correlate with the focus of seizure activity, even in the presence of grossly normal structural imaging with MRI (83, 84) (Fig. 10.5). In TLE, comparison with the contralateral side has been useful in localizing the epileptogenic focus. The sensitivity of PET in patients with TLE is in the order of 70–90% (85–90). Much of this variability is related to the heterogeneity of the epilepsy, rather than technical factors such as differences in quality or specifications of the PET camera (91). Some reports suggest that the sensitivity of PET is increased when seizures are more frequent or when performed soon after a seizure has occurred.

In contrast to patients with TLE, the sensitivity for seizure localization in extra-TLE is significantly lower, in the order of 30–60% (86, 92–96). An exception may be patients with cortical dysplasia, in whom the reported sensitivity of PET varies between 60–92%. In general, however, the sample sizes tend to be smaller in this population of extra-TLE patients, and less data are available.

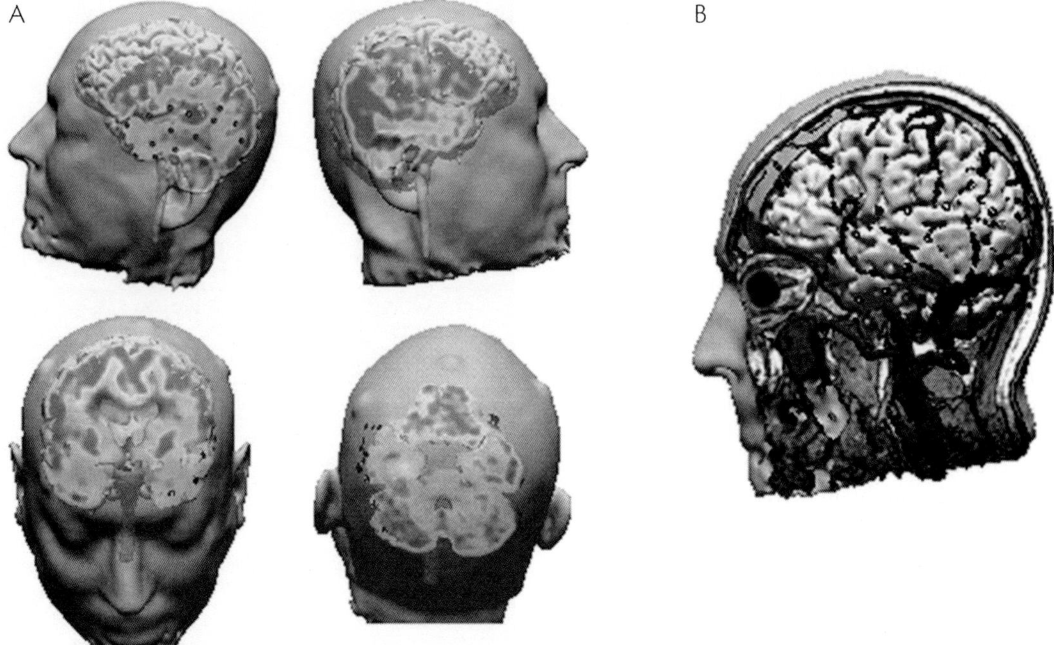

Fig. 10.5 (Also see Colour plate 8.) Multimodal imaging used in the presurgical planning of a patient with temporal lobe epilepsy. A) Coronal, sagittal, and axial slices from the patient's (^{18}F) FDG PET study, co-registered with the patient's MRI to plan for the placement of intracranial electrodes (blue dots). These images demonstrate reduced FDG tracer uptake in the left temporal lobe. B) Cortical reconstruction demonstrating the venous distribution (purple) from a magnetic resonance venogram co-registered to the same patient's 3D MPRAGE volume. Reproduced with permission of Simon Vogrin.

PET ligands other than (^{18}F) FDG

In addition to (^{18}F) FDG, several other radioisotopes are used to better understand the neurobiology and functional changes associated with different subtypes of epilepsy, although most of these are not used in routine clinical practice. These radiotracers differ according to the target receptor to which the tracer is sensitive. For example, alpha-methyl-L-tryptophan (AMT) is a tracer for tryptophan metabolism (83); and other ligands have been used which bind to opioid receptors (97), histamine H1 receptors (98), N-methyl-D-aspartate (NMDA) receptors (99), and peripheral benzodiazepine receptors (100).

^{11}C-flumazenil is notable for its capacity to bind to the $GABA_A$ receptor complex, the concentration of which appears to be lower in epileptogenic foci relative to the homologous region on the contralateral hemisphere and the remaining neocortex (101). Some data show that the distribution of ^{11}C-flumazenil PET was more accurate than (^{18}F) FDG-PET for the localization of seizure onset in patients with extra-TLE (102), and suggests ^{11}C-flumazenil to be a viable alternative or adjunct marker in identifying epileptogenic regions (103). Furthermore, the degree of gamma-aminobutyric acid (GABA) receptor reduction showed a positive correlation with seizure frequency. This implies that inhibitory mechanisms are disturbed in the epileptogenic focus (104), and that ^{11}C-flumazenil could act as a biochemical marker of epileptogenicity.

However, ^{11}C-flumazenil abnormalities tend to be functional, transient, and seizure-related. In particular, one study showed that the most accurate seizure localization with ^{11}C-flumazenil occurred with scans that occurred at the shortest interictal period (105). This is related to the short half-life of ^{11}C (20 minutes), which necessitates rapid acquisition of the PET scan after seizure onset. Consequently, ^{11}C-flumazenil-PET is not routine, and its clinical utility remains controversial (106, 107). Nevertheless, regardless of whether ^{11}C-flumazenil is superior to (^{18}F) FDG-PET, it may provide useful data complementary to those of (^{18}F) FDG-PET and MRI (86).

Limitations

As in SPECT, the extent of (^{18}F) FDG uptake usually extends beyond the seizure focus, and it is limited by weak temporal and spatial resolution. For example, it is not unusual for patients with TLE to also demonstrate hypometabolism of their frontal lobes, which may represent inhibitory phenomena induced by the epileptogenic focus (108). The authors of one study compared pre- and postoperative (^{18}F) FDG-PET scans in patients with MTLE-hippocampal sclerosis who were rendered seizure-free after surgery (109). In this study, there were postoperative increases in (^{18}F) FDG metabolism in the propagation pathways of ictal and interictal epileptic discharges (e.g. temporal white matter, inferior precentral gyrus, anterior cingulate gyrus), suggesting that hypometabolism in these regions was functional, seizure-related, and reversible. Thus, a 'PETectomy' (i.e. resecting the area of temporal lobe hypometabolism visible on a PET (110)) would result in resection of larger areas of tissue than is necessary. In general, these data suggest that PET alone is less useful for precise neuroanatomical localization.

Furthermore, it is worth noting the temporal limitations of PET imaging. First, the temporal dynamics of PET are slower than the blood flow changes detected with SPECT. In addition, the half-life of the ^{18}F label (110 minutes) is relatively short and, in contrast to the radiolabelled technetium used in SPECT, there is prolonged cerebral uptake of (^{18}F) FDG, which leads to significant contamination caused by seizure propagation. Together, these imply that PETs can only reliably image the interictal state, unlike SPECT. Some authors have, however, attempted to obtain ictal PETs in rare cases of epilepsia partialis continua.

Functional magnetic resonance imaging

There are many cases in which the epileptogenic zone is near the eloquent cortex, in which case it is likely that the resection margin will encroach upon functional brain tissue, and there is a risk of postoperative neurological deficit. Although the gold standard for functional mapping remains intraoperative cortical stimulation, this is often impractical. Functional magnetic resonance imaging (fMRI) has become a widely acceptable technique to non-invasively map brain function in normal and diseased brains. It involves detecting dynamic changes in the relative concentrations of oxy- and deoxyhaemoglobin during brain activity, and to use these microvascular blood-oxygen level dependent (BOLD) changes as a surrogate measure for neuronal function. In the epilepsy population, it has been used to non-invasively map sensory, motor, language, and memory functions for presurgical planning.

One of the key uses of fMRI in epilepsy is to lateralize language function, a goal which has been traditionally accomplished with the intracortical amobarbital (Wada) test. The reported concordance between fMRI and the Wada test is variable, but is generally 90% or higher, and fMRI is currently thought of as a valid alternative to the latter test (111–115). Various paradigms are in use, including verbal fluency and language comprehension. The most reliable fMRI data are in sensory and motor tasks (116–118), which result in excellent agreement with intraoperative cortical mapping (119, 120) (Fig. 10.6). In addition, fMRI may be able to visualize the functional anatomy of memory tasks (121), the assessment of which is critical prior to planning anterior temporal lobe resection.

When compared with the 'gold standard' of electrocortical stimulation, the specificity of fMRI in one study was 67% and sensitivity greater than 90% (122). Differences may have been due to the inability of electrocortical stimulation to map deep sulcal areas, coregistration errors in fMRI, BOLD identification of draining veins rather than capillaries, or the threshold used for processing the fMR images.

Although the use of fMRI has become widespread, it is worth noting several caveats in the interpretation of its data. First, there are the limitations imposed by the neurophysiological underpinnings of the fMRI technique. The BOLD signal depends on a complex cascade of phenomena which couple a change in neuronal activity to a change in cerebral haemodynamics. Thus, the BOLD response is merely a surrogate measure of synaptic activity and, in the pathological brain, it is unclear whether the normal mechanisms of neurovascular coupling still hold. In addition, an altered BOLD response can be the result of alterations in the blood flow to an area (such as occurs with vascular malformations (123), a large tumour with mass effect and oedema (112), or in the postictal state (124)). Such alterations in cerebral haemodynamics could therefore be misinterpreted as functional activation of a particular area (125).

A second group of factors are technical. Some of the brain regions of most interest in epilepsy, such as the inferior frontal lobes and mesial temporal lobes (including the hippocampus), are susceptible to geometric distortions and signal loss during typical fMRI acquisition sequences, especially at higher field strength (126–128).

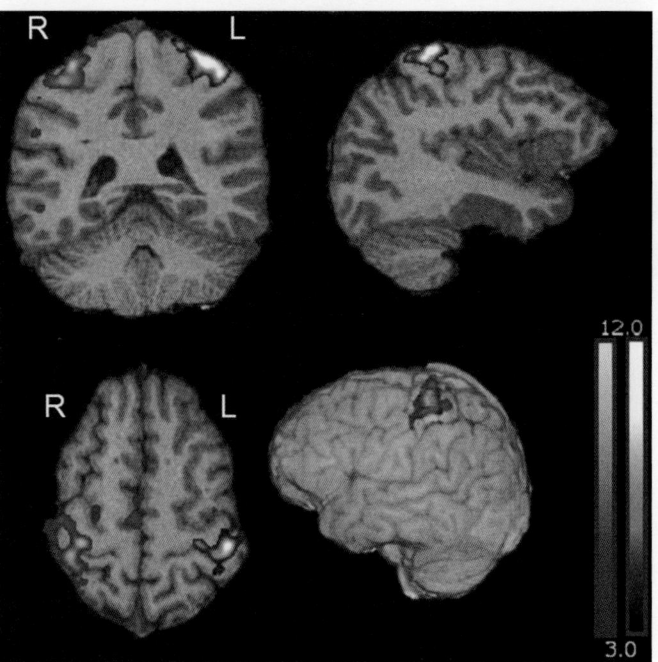

Fig. 10.6 (Also see Colour plate 9.) FMRI scans acquired from an individual subject during a finger-tapping task. Coronal, sagittal, and axial sections, as well as a rendered whole brain, show motor regions which are active during tapping with fingers of the left (blue) and right (red) hands. Images were acquired with a 1.5 T MRI scanner, and activations are shown at a statistical cluster threshold of $z = 3.0$. Subject's right is figure left. Reproduced with permission of Simon Vogrin.

Third, the nature of the task, and the selection of an appropriate baseline condition, is critical in deriving accurate activations, especially when it comes to more complex cognitive functions, such as language or memory. FMRI has been used extensively in the cognitive neuroscience literature, and there are a multitude of tasks that have been devised to probe the various cognitive domains. A priori, one may expect different paradigms to activate different brain region, and indeed the lack of protocol standardization for the various cognitive functions has led to greater variability in functional localization. For example, no standardized fMRI paradigm has been validated which can identify the ability of the unresected side to sustain memory postoperatively and predict postoperative memory performance. More broadly, a shortcoming of fMRI is that the activations that are identified in any given task imply that those areas are implicated in that task, but a causal relationship cannot be drawn.

Finally, the analysis of the tasks themselves is far from standardized, and the activations will vary depending on such factors as the haemodynamic response function model that is chosen (129), and the statistical threshold that is arbitrarily set by the particular laboratory. More broadly on this point, one should not neglect the philosophical differences in analysing fMRI data between the clinical and research domains—the emphasis in research is to avoid false positive (Type I) errors, which leads to more conservative statistical thresholds being favoured. Conversely, in clinical neurology, the priority is to identify all brain regions involved in a particular task, and as a result more liberal statistical thresholds may be set to avoid false negatives.

EEG-fMRI

Simultaneous EEG and fMRI is a rapidly evolving technique which offers the hope of combining two modalities with complementary strengths. EEG, of course, has excellent temporal resolution, in the order of milliseconds, but has poor spatial resolution, as the exact location of neuronal currents varies with individual geometry and conductivity, and the limited number of EEG channels. In comparison, fMRI has good spatial resolution, but its temporal resolution is limited by the haemodynamic (BOLD) response, which typically follows a neural stimulus by 2–6 seconds. Each of these modalities is based on fundamentally different neurophysiological principles (with EEG measuring electrical activity and fMRI measuring BOLD responses); thus, applied together, they may be able to offer converging evidence in seizure localization.

The general approach to EEG-fMRI is to map regional changes in BOLD signal that are time-locked to interictal epileptiform discharges (IEDs) identified on the simultaneously recorded EEG (129, 130) (Fig. 10.7). Of course, there are inherent technical

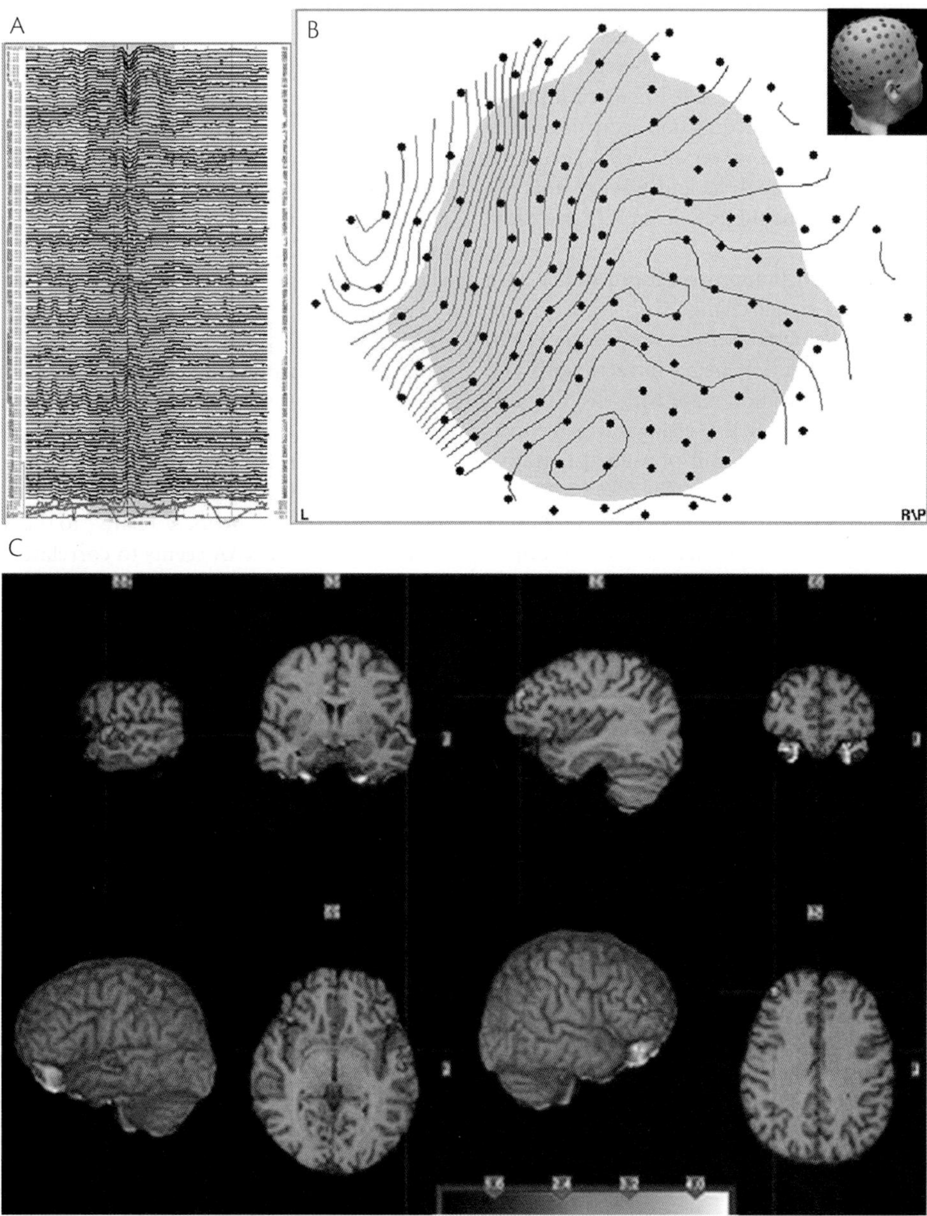

Fig. 10.7 (Also see Colour plate 10.) Upper panel) EEG-fMRI findings from a patient with left temporal lobe epilepsy. 128-channel EEG recorded in the MRI scanner showing left temporal spikes (A). The large gradient artefact was filtered, leaving, nevertheless, some transient waveforms. The epileptic discharges of this patient could be identified unambiguously from their morphology and spatial distribution (B). Lower panel) During a 35 minute simultaneous EEG-fMRI session, there were 11 interictal discharges which were localized to the left superior temporal gyrus (C). These activations were modelled using a multi-haemodynamic response function approach, including regressors for head movement. Three principal clusters were found—in the left superior temporal gyrus, the left precentral gyrus, and right frontal lobe, with the former two activations correlating with the patient's seizure semiology. With permission from Vogrin, S. et al. ESI and fMRI of interictal and ictal epileptic discharges. *International Journal of Bioelectromagnetism* 2011; 13(4):S261–7.

difficulties related to minimizing the electromagnetic noise during simultaneous acquisition of EEG and fMRI data. Traditionally, conventional 'spike-triggered' studies involve an expert observer visually identifying interictal epileptiform activity on scalp EEG, and manually triggering image acquisition (131–133). Those EEG events are then convolved with a model of the haemodynamic response function, which provides a regressor for a general linear model analysis of the fMRI data. Images associated with interictal discharges are then compared to those without visible interictal discharges. The next advance in data acquisition was periodic imaging, in which fMRI image acquisition was alternated with EEG epochs in order to minimize image artefact (134). Such protocols have allowed high-frequency EEG (in the gamma range or higher) to be recorded and mapped to thalamocortical circuits in normals (135), and these high-frequency oscillations may potentially be of relevance in epilepsy as well. Today we are able to record simultaneous EEG-fMRI without gaps in the acquisition sequence. With these new techniques have also come newer analysis algorithms, such as independent components analysis and wavelet analysis (136), which are able to minimize the subjectivity in IED classification by automating that process.

In order to validate the EEG-fMRI approach, most studies have studied IED-correlated BOLD signal change with invasive and non-invasive methods of localizing the seizure onset zone (137), with the 'gold standard' for validation being intracranial EEG. Comparison of the IED-BOLD activation maps with electro-clinical data on seizure onset has revealed BOLD changes which correspond to the source of spiking activity and presumed irritative zone, with a concordance rate of approximately 70% (130, 131, 138–141). This implies, however, that distant positive BOLD responses have also been found in areas unrelated or not implicated in the individual patient's pathology—for example, one study showed occipital coactivation with frontal IEDs (142). The assumption in most studies is that positive BOLD changes generally reflect increases in neuronal activity, and in fact previous reports suggest seizures and IEDs are indeed associated with a positive BOLD response (143). This has led some authors to focus their attention on regions with the most significant BOLD response to assess concordance (138), while others considered all areas with a positive BOLD response (130, 131, 140). However, the relationship between BOLD and IED is not clear-cut, and lack of activation does not allow any firm inferences to be drawn. It is worth noting also that the significance and neurophysiological mechanism of negative BOLD responses, especially with respect to IEDs, remains unclear, and its localizing value is contentious (144–149).

Just as simultaneous EEG-fMRI has the potential to combine the strengths of each modality, so are its limitations amplified. The analysis of combined EEG-fMRI data relies on the assumption that there is normal haemodynamic response function (HRF)-coupling in generalized spike-wave discharges (for which there actually appears to be some preliminary evidence (150)). In addition, as in standalone fMRI, the final outcome depends on the specific HRF that is chosen to model the data (129). Furthermore, while EEG may complement the poor temporal resolution of fMRI, ultimately, the delay of the HRF still limits interpretation of the data. Simultaneous EEG-fMRI relies on recordings of IEDs which occur during the scanning period (a problem shared with MEG and standard EEG), and therefore requires patients to have a reasonably active resting EEG. In most studies reported, this is often the case (131, 138), but this could very well represent a selection bias. In a recent paper, events were captured in only 40% of patients (137).

In sum, the precise clinical role of EEG-fMRI remains to be defined. While the aforementioned imaging modalities are informative in the majority of patients, at present the greatest utility of EEG-fMRI is in patients for whom other source localization techniques have failed to identify a single circumscribed focus.

Magnetic resonance spectroscopy

As has been clear from the experience with PET and SPECT, biochemical and metabolic abnormalities can occur in the absence of visible structural abnormalities on MRI. Magnetic resonance spectroscopy (MRS) is a tool that aims to detect changes in cerebral energy metabolism, which may occur in the absence of any obvious structural changes. It is based on the hypothesis that the epileptogenic focus is associated with long-term changes of metabolite concentrations (152). By detecting the magnetic resonance signals from phosphorus (^{31}P) or single proton (^{1}H) entities (153), MRS aims to infer the presence of various neural metabolites, such as N-acetylaspartate (NAA), creatine (Cr), choline compounds (signal intensities of $-CH_3$ groups), glutamate (Glu), glutamine (Gln), lactate (-CH doublet), and GABA (Fig. 10.8).

Proton MRS can lateralize an epileptic lesion in more than 85% of MTL epilepsies, but its ability to lateralize extra-TLE is somewhat less (e.g. around 50% in one study of patients with frontal lobe epilepsy (154)). NAA is generally considered a marker for neuronal disease and is usually reduced in pathological conditions that lead to neuronal damage. In the initial studies on epilepsy, the critical finding was reduced signal intensities of NAA on the side ipsilateral to the seizure focus relative to the contralateral side. This focal reduction of NAA seems to correlate well with EEG abnormalities and the severity of cell loss, as verified by histological samples obtained from the resected hippocampi of patients with MTS. Although the proportion of neurons in MTS that are lost is between 30–50%, there may, in addition, be underlying neuronal and glial dysfunction that contribute to the NAA changes on MRS. Glutamate and glutamine have also been found to be elevated in the temporal lobe ipsilateral to the seizure focus, including in patients with normal structural scans. It is important to note, however, that the spatial resolution of MRS is low.

MRS has also been used to measure the changes in neural metabolites as a result of anticonvulsant medications or surgical resection. For example, GABA is the major inhibitory neurotransmitter in humans, and is the target of several anticonvulsant drugs (e.g. vigabatrin, gabapentin, topiramate, zonisamide). In contrast, glutamate is a key excitatory neurotransmitter, and intracellular glutamate concentrations are elevated in the epileptogenic human hippocampus and neocortex (153). Although the precise fluctuations in neurotransmitter concentrations with long-term anticonvulsant therapy are still unclear, in the future GABA and glutamate imaging may allow us to individualize anticonvulsant therapy. For example, a patient with low GABA levels may benefit from an anticonvulsant that increases cellular GABA or decreases cellular glutamate.

Currently, the clinical application of MRS is limited by several technical factors, not least of which is lack of availability and expertise. Despite the relative success of MRS in the research domain, it continues to have problems with sensitivity when applied to clinical populations. Examples of factors which limit its widespread application as a diagnostic tool include long acquisition times

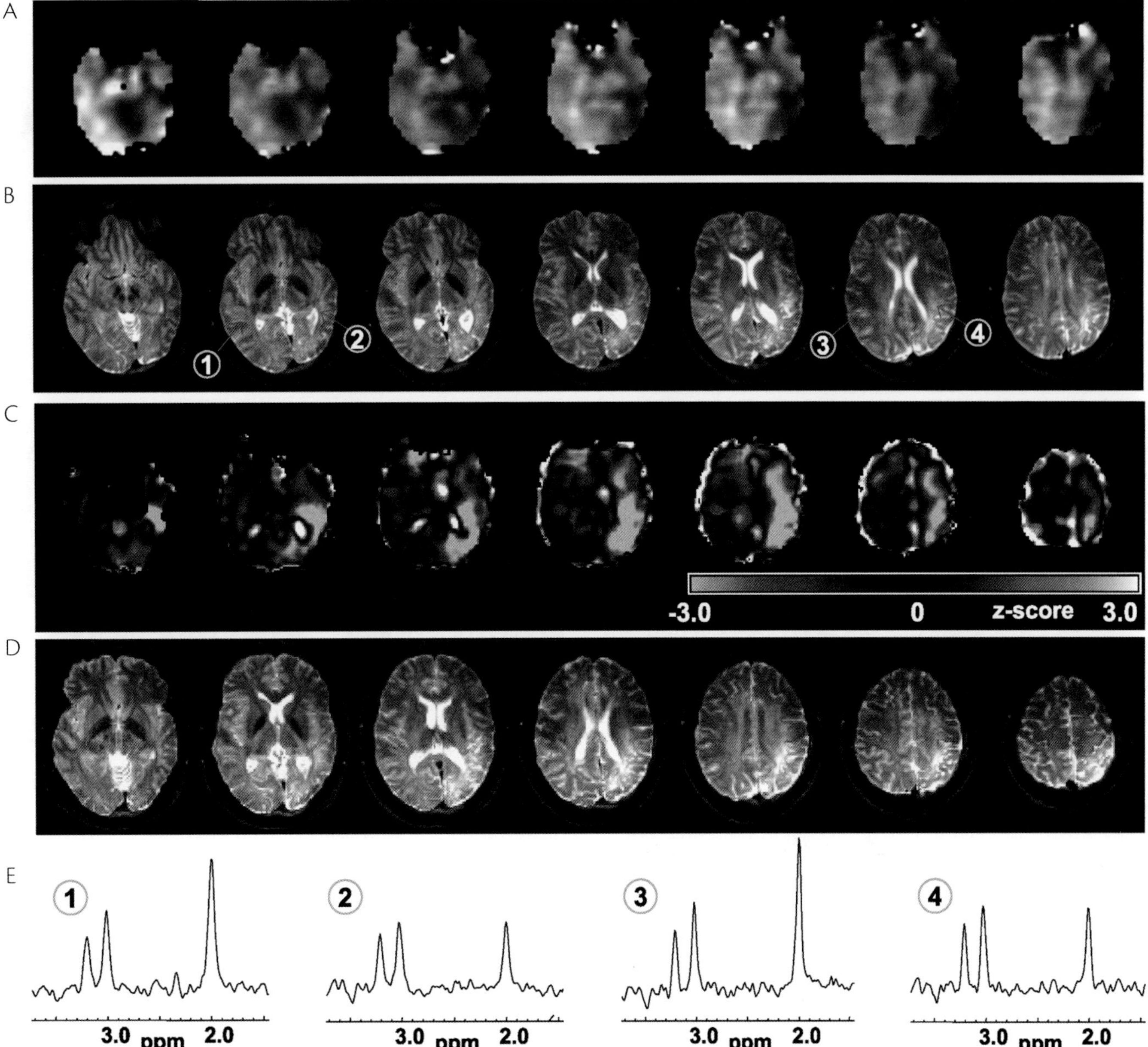

Fig. 10.8 (Also see Colour plate 11.) Magnetic resonance spectroscopy data from a single subject. A) NAA/Cr images at 7 axial slices. B) T2-weighted images corresponding to the centre of the metabolite image slice. C) *z*-score images for NAA/Cr in the standard spatial reference frame. D) T2-MRI following affine registration to the standard spatial reference frame. E) Spectra from the locations indicated in (B). From Maudsley A, et al. Application of volumetric MR spectroscopic imaging for localization of neocortical epilepsy. *Epilepsy Res* 2010; 88(2–3):127–38.

when using conventional phase-encoding; loss of spectral information from magnetic-susceptibility-induced spectral line broadening; image distortions extending from the large subcutaneous lipid signals or unsuppressed water; and limitations on signal quality and spatial resolution due to poor detection sensitivity.

Magnetoencephalography

In conjunction with the aforementioned techniques, magnetoencephalography (MEG) is emerging as an important tool in identifying the source of interictal discharges (156). EEG and MEG are complementary techniques—whereas scalp EEG detects extracellular volume currents produced by post-synaptic potentials, MEG uses a superconducting quantum interference device (SQUID) to amplify the small magnetic fields generated by small intraneuronal electric currents. In contrast to EEG, which is sensitive to both radial and tangential activity, MEG is maximally sensitive to dipoles oriented tangentially to the brain surface, which therefore correspond to sulcal activity. Being complementary techniques, EEG and MEG may also be simultaneously performed to provide converging evidence in localizing a seizure focus (Fig. 10.9).

Relative to EEG alone, however, MEG offers several potential advantages. For example, in contrast to the electrical fields measured by EEG, the magnetic currents that are recorded by MEG are less distorted by the tissue layers separating the brain and

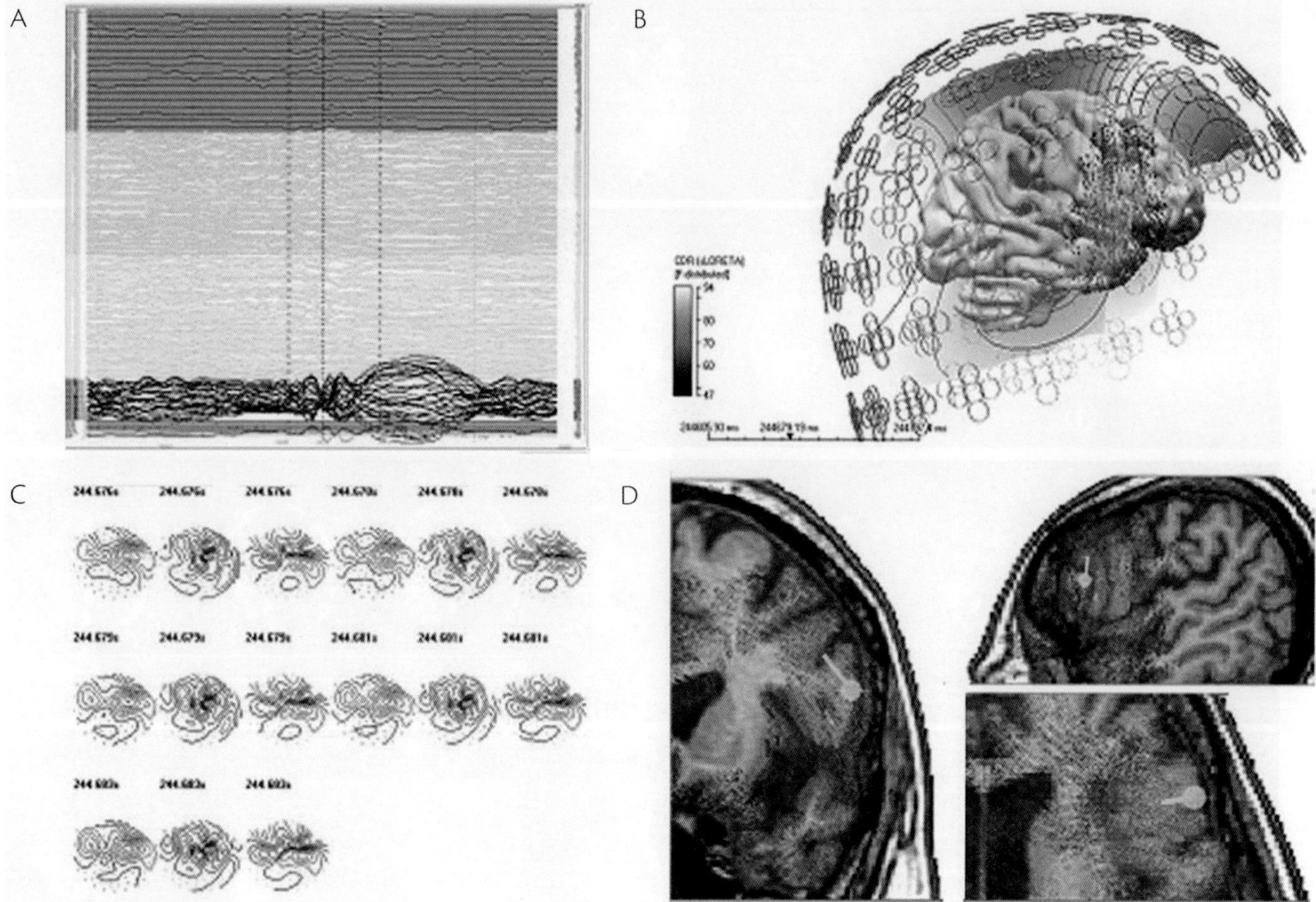

Fig. 10.9 (Also see Colour plate 12.) A polyphasic spike-and-slow wave interictal discharge recorded by simultaneous EEG-MEG. A) The 306 magnetometers and gradiometers (green traces) and 34 EEG electrodes (dark blue traces) demonstrate high spatial coverage in (B) the reconstructed model. C) Comparison of individual magnetometer and orthogonal gradiometer field maps correspond to (D) a standardized low-resolution brain electromagnetic tomography (sLORETA) analysis of the distributed dipolar source orientation strength and equivalent current dipole (green dipole). Reproduced with permission of Simon Vogrin.

scalp surface (157). Consequently, there is less spatial blurring of these signals, and MEG may therefore more reliably localize brain activity, at a spatial resolution of 2–3 mm (cf. 7–10 mm with EEG) (158, 159). Furthermore, MEG is less susceptible to variation in head geometry compared to EEG, and can be better estimated using the simple spherical model. MEG requires 3–4 cm^2 of synchronized cortical activity to detect an epileptic spike (160, 161), whereas 6–20 cm^2 is required for scalp EEGs (162, 163).

In comparison to other functional neuroimaging techniques, MEG has excellent temporal resolution. When MEG source localization is coregistered on patients' structural MRIs (a process known as magnetic source imaging, MSI), the magnetic dipole representing an epileptiform discharge can be visualized on the patient's MRI scan, thus affording good spatial resolution as well (164, 165).

MEG plays two roles in presurgical evaluation. First, it is useful in identifying the epileptogenic focus itself. In the case of MRI-negative cases, MEG can assist in detecting the ictal source, and MEG-guided reviews of MRI have revealed subtle abnormalities not initially seen in around 17.5% of cases (166, 167). On the other extreme, MEG can be used to identify the epileptogenic focus in patients with multiple intracerebral lesions (e.g. tuberous sclerosis or multiple cavernomas) or lesions of undetermined significance (165). In addition, MEG can be used as a non-invasive alternative to ECoG in the 20–60% of patients who have had previously unsuccessful epilepsy surgery (168–171). In such patients, scalp EEG is often distorted by scalp scarring, skull defects, and CSF collections. MEG may therefore offer more accurate localization than scalp EEG. In addition, it is a good alternative to those patients who have postoperative dural adhesions which hinder the insertion of invasive intracranial electrodes. Due to the need to minimize head movements during recordings, most MEG studies have predominantly aimed to localize interictal events. Some authors have documented ictal events as well, but obviously this is not possible in the majority of cases, due to the associated head movements.

In terms of the sensitivity of MEG, one large series of 455 epilepsy patients who were evaluated preoperatively demonstrated an average sensitivity of 70% (165). Among patients who underwent surgical therapy, MSI successfully localized a lesion in 89%, supplied additional information in 35%, and provided information that was crucial to medical decision-making in 10% (165). Some studies suggest that MEG has specific advantages for spike detection in extratemporal epilepsies, particularly those that lie superficially on the brain's surface (e.g. one study showed a sensitivity in MTLE of 50% compared to 92% for extra-TLE) (85). This is related to the fact that only 3.5–4 cm^2 of synchronized activity from the lateral neocortex is required to produce a detectable MEG signal, compared to 6–8 cm^2 in MTLE (160, 172).

The second role of MEG is to investigate the function of cortical areas near the epileptogenic focus (similar to evoked potentials and fMRI). In order to avoid postoperative neurological deficits, MEG can be used to delineate adjacent areas of eloquent cortex in sensorimotor, language, and visual areas. In localizing the primary sensorimotor cortex, MEG is able to delineate the central sulcus by identifying the somatosensory-evoked magnetic field, which is accurate in approximately 90% of patients when referenced against direct cortical stimulation through electrocorticography. Language mapping can be determined by MEG with various language paradigms (e.g. word recognition, silent reading, picture naming, verb generation), with similarly high concordant rates of 75–95% when referenced against Wada testing (173).

The application of MEG is limited by its availability—there are only approximately 100 MEG installations available for medical use worldwide. Its set-up is limited by the costs associated in constructing a shielded room with high-permeability metals to reduce competing ambient magnetic noise, as the epileptiform spikes detected by MEG are 10^{-9} smaller than environmentally generated magnetic noise.

Discussion

Approximately 15% of epileptic surgical candidates are rejected on the basis that an epileptogenic focus cannot be delineated (174). With the constant advances in neuroimaging, it is foreseeable that this proportion will drop, and that those who do undergo surgery will do so with less risk to their areas of eloquent cortex. With the gamut of technologies that are available to the modern epileptologist, the question of how to approach a patient with epilepsy becomes a difficult one, and one that varies between institutions based on the available expertise and equipment. Each of the techniques discussed has its limitations. EEG and MEG are insensitive to deeper sources. PET and SPECT reveal regional, rather than local, abnormalities, and lack the spatial resolution of MRI. MRI has the best spatial resolution in detecting structural lesions, but may still miss more subtle lesions (10). Furthermore, a lesion that is detected does not necessarily indicate an epileptic focus and, conversely, patients without an identifiable structural lesion on MRI can nevertheless be successful surgical candidates (175).

The issue that will become even more relevant in the future will be how to establish which lesions identified with more advanced MRI technology are epileptogenic. Combining the strengths and weaknesses of each modality could potentially result in more robust data compared to each modality on their own, and in fact current attempts at seizure localization usually involve multiple technologies, either separately (e.g. SISCOM, MSI) or concurrently (e.g. EEG-fMRI, EEG-MEG), with the aim of finding converging evidence for a single, resectable seizure focus.

High-resolution structural MRI forms the basis on which the findings of other functional imaging modalities can be coregistered. SISCOM, of course, is a long-established technique, but there have also been attempts to coregister FDG-PET and MRI prior to surgical resection (176) (Fig. 10.5), which has shown potential for improved sensitivity and specificity compared to either technology alone. From a research perspective, combining the principles of PET and MRI could also prove a powerful approach. By labelling ligands and tracers with magnetic nanoparticles, it may be possible to combine the ability of PET to identify specific receptors with the high spatial resolution of MRI. A proof of principle was recently reported with magnetic nanoparticles labelled with AMT in an animal model (177).

With regards to DTI, there have been recent attempts to correlate diffusion abnormalities with intracranial EEG recordings (40, 178), and DTI has also been used to add details to head models in EEG source localization (179–181). The combination of tractography, EEG and fMRI has been shown to delineate the pathways through which epileptic activity propagates (182). Taking parsimony to its logical extreme, some authors have even speculated on the potential for coregistering structural MRI, DTI, SPECT, PET, fMRI, EEG, and MEG across a single platform.

The major difficulty in evaluating neuroimaging modalities in the work-up of a patient with epilepsy is the lack of clinical data from large, randomized controlled trials to guide imaging decisions. In fact, very few rigorous studies have examined the cost–benefit or predictive value of neuroimaging in clinical practice. In 2004, the UK's National Institute for Health and Clinical Excellence failed to identify any study of neuroimaging in epilepsy that achieved more than Grade III clinical evidence (183). Since then, a meta-analysis of localization accuracy, cost-effectiveness, and predictive value of neuroimaging in presurgical evaluation was highly critical, commenting on the poor quality of all existing studies, which the authors concluded were unable to usefully inform clinical practice (184). To this end, an important recent study recruited a large cohort of presurgical patients, who were initially subjected to non-invasive evaluation, followed by intracranial EEG, and finally surgery. This study assessed the additional predictive value of FDG-PET, ictal SPECT, and MSI against intracranial EEG (185) and the outcome of epilepsy surgery (186). The data showed that all three modalities were of benefit in predicting seizure-freedom following surgery, but that MSI had the greatest sensitivity for detecting the seizure onset zone as confirmed by intracranial EEG. FDG-PET and ictal SPECT nevertheless had independent predictive value for seizure-free postsurgical outcome.

Future studies along similar lines will be important in filling the existing evidence gap, especially given resource limitations which behove us to establish which investigations are cost-effective, and which are optional or even redundant. However, in practice, measuring non-invasive techniques against the yardstick of intracranial EEG is not possible, as many patients do not undergo invasive studies, and in any case intracranial EEGs sample only a limited part of the brain. Furthermore, there is the difficulty of designing large-scale randomized controlled trials to recruit a sufficient number of patients and achieve adequate follow-up when the background is that of an ever-changing neuroimaging landscape. Thus, the rapid advances in neuroimaging imply that a long-term study examining surgical outcome may only inform the use of outdated technology by the time it is completed. This fact notwithstanding, such studies could nevertheless prove useful, as is evidenced by our current ongoing use of older imaging modalities such as PET and SPECT.

The advances in neuroimaging techniques have also made the standardization of studies difficult. The wide variations in data analysis for many of the more modern modalities have led to many methodological inconsistencies between studies. Future studies need to clarify not only the sensitivity and specificity of individual techniques and analysis algorithms, but also the reproducibility of findings both within and between centres, the positive predictive value for important clinical outcomes, the economic value of each modality, and, more broadly, the independent value of neuroimaging over other modalities (such as EEG and neuropsychometry). Although many clinicians would feel disinclined to merely replicate previous findings, it can only be with such replication that one can establish a genuine trend, especially given the small numbers of subjects that are usually involved. Thus, future studies will probably see multicentre collaborations in order to recruit sufficient numbers of patients and to pool collective resources.

It is certainly an exciting time for neuroimaging in epilepsy. However, the translation of the many small studies in the literature into clinical practice should proceed cautiously, due to the limitations of each modality, and the lack of a strong (Class I) evidence base for any given approach. For now, the newer neuroimaging modalities remain auxiliary techniques as part of a multimodality and multidisciplinary assessment, which should include a thorough clinical evaluation, neuropsychological testing, neuropsychiatric evaluation, interictal and ictal EEG recordings, optimal conventional imaging with MRI, and possibly MEG, PET, or SPECT scanning.

Acknowledgements

The authors wish to thank Simon Vogrin for contributing Figs 10.3–10. 7 and 10.9 to this chapter.

References

1. Lüders H, Awad I. *Conceptual considerations*. In: Lüders H (ed) *Epilepsy Surgery*, p. 51–62. New York: Raven Press, 1992.
2. Rosenow F, Lüders H. Presurgical evaluation of epilepsy. *Brain* 2001; 124:1683–700.
3. Gastaut H, Gastaut J. Computerized transverse axial tomography in epilepsy. *Epilepsia* 1976; 17:325–64.
4. International League Against Epilepsy. Recommendations for neuroimaging of patients with epilepsy. Commission on neuroimaging of the International League Against Epilepsy. *Epilepsia* 1997; 38:1255–6.
5. Berg AT, Testa FM, Levy SR, Shinnar S. Neuroimaging in children with newly diagnosed epilepsy: A community-based study. *Pediatrics* 2000; 106:527–32.
6. King MA, Newton MR, Jackson GD, Fitt GJ, Mitchell LA, Silvapulle MJ, *et al.* Epileptology of the first-seizure presentation: a clinical, electroencephalogrpahic, and magnetic resonance imaging study of 300 consecutive patients. *Lancet* 1998; 352(9133):1007–11.
7. Cakirer S, Ba ak M, Mutlu A, Galip GM. MR imaging in the presurgical workup of patients with drug-resistant epilepsy. *Am J Neuroradiol* 2004; 25:919–26.
8. Cakirer S, Ba ak M, Mutlu A, Galip GM. MR imaging in epilepsy that is refractory to medical therapy. *European Radiol* 2002; 12:549–58.
9. Matsuda K, Mihara T, Tottori T, Otubo T, Usui N, Baba K, *et al.* Magnetic resonance imaging in 120 patients with intractable partial seizures: a preoperative assessment. *Neuroradiology* 2005; 47:352–61.
10. Matsuda K, Mihara T, Tottori T, Otubo T, Usui N, Baba K, *et al.* Neuroradiologic findings in focal cortical dysplasia: histologic correlation with surgically resected specimens. *Epilepsia* 2001; 42(s6):29–36.
11. von Oertzen J, Urbach H, Blümcke I, Reuber M, Träber F, Peveling T, *et al.* Time-efficient relaxometry of the entire hippocampus is feasible in temporal lobe epilepsy. *Neurology* 2002; 58:257–64.
12. Urbach H. Imaging of the epilepsies. *European Radiol* 2005; 15:494–500.
13. Elster A, Mirza W. MR imaging in chronic partial epilepsy: role of contrast enhancement. *Am J Neuroradiol* 1991; 12(1):165–70.
14. Widjaja E, Raybaud C. Advances in neuroimaging in patients with epilepsy. *Neurosurg Focus* 2008; 25(3: E3):1–11.
15. Salmenpera T, Duncan J. Imaging in epilepsy. *J Neurol Neurosurg Psychiatry* 2005; 76(Suppl III):2–10.
16. Eriksson SH, Thom M, Bartlett PA, Symms MR, McEvoy AW, Sisodiya SM, *et al.* PROPELLER MRI visualizes detailed pathology of hippocampal sclerosis. *Epilepsia* 2008; 49(1):33–9.
17. Bonilha L, Halford JJ, Rorden C, Roberts DR, Rumboldt Z, Eckert MA. Automated MRI analysis for identification of hippocampal atrophy in temporal lobe epilepsy. *Epilepsia* 2008; 50(2):228–33.
18. Knake S, Triantafyllou C, Wald LL, Wiggins G, Kirk GP, Larsson PG, *et al.* 3T phased array MRI improves the presurgical evaluation in focal epilepsies: a prospective study. *Neurology* 2005; 65:1026–31.
19. Strandberg M, Larsson EM, Backman S, Källén K. Pre-surgical epilepsy evaluation using 3T MRI. Do surface coils provide additional information? *Epileptic Disord* 2008; 10(2):83–92.
20. Duncan J. The current status of neuroimaging for epilepsy. *Curr Opin Neurol* 2009; 22:179–84.
21. Deblaere K, Achten E. Structural magnetic resonance imaging in epilepsy. *European Radiol* 2008; 18:119–29.
22. Wright IC, McGuire PK, Poline JB, Travere JM, Murray RM, Frith CD, *et al.* A voxel-based method for the statistical analysis of gray and white matter density applied to schizophrenia. *Neuroimage* 1995; 2:244–52.
23. Ashburner J, Friston K. Voxel-based morphometry—the methods. *Neuroimage* 2000; 11:805–21.
24. Chung MK, Worsley KJ, Paus T, Cherif C, Collins DL, Giedd JN, *et al.* A unified statistical approach to deformation-based morphometry. *Neuroimage* 2001; 14(3):595–606.
25. Abbott DF, Pell GS, Pardoe H, Jackson GD. Voxel-based iterative sensitiviy (VBIS) analysis: methods and a validation of intensity scaling for T2-weighted imaging of hippocampal sclerosis. *Neuroimage* 2009; 44:812–19.
26. Riederer F, Lanzenberger R, Kaya M, Prayer D, Serles W, Baumgartner C. Network atrophy in temporal lobe epilepsy. *Neurology* 2008; 71(6):419–25.
27. Bookstein F. 'Voxel-based morphometry' should not be used with imperfectly registered images. *Neuroimage* 2001; 14:1454–62.
28. Crum WR, Griffin LD, Hill DL, Hawkes DJ. Zen and the art of medical image registration: correspondence, homology, and quality. *Neuroimage* 2003; 20(3):1425–37.
29. Richardson M. Current themes in neuroimaging of epilepsy: Brain networks, dynamic phenomena, and clinical evidence. *Clin Neurophysiol* 2010; 121:1153–75.
30. Keller SS, Wieshmann UC, Mackay CE, Denby CE, Webb J, Roberts N. Voxel based morphometry of grey matter abnormalities in patients with medically intractable temporal lobe epilepsy: effects of side of seizure onset and epilepsy duration. *J Neurol Neurosurg Psychiatry* 2002; 73(6):648–55.
31. Hajnal J, Doran M, Hall AS, Collins AG, Oatridge A, Pennock JM, *et al.* MR imaging of anisotropically restricted diffusion of water in the nervous system: technical, anatomic, and pathologic considerations. *J Comput Assist Tomogr* 1991; 15(1):1–18.
32. Rugg-Gunn F. Diffusion imaging in epilepsy. *Expert Rev Neurother* 2007; 7(8):1043–54.
33. Chu K, Kang DW, Kim JY, Chang KH, Lee SK. Diffusion-weighted magnetic resonance imaging in nonconvulsive status epilepticus. *Arch Neurol* 2001; 58(6):993–8.
34. Kim JA, Chung JI, Yoon PH, Kim DI, Chung TS, Kim EJ, *et al.* Transient MR signal changes in patients with generalized tonicoclonic seizure or status epilepticus: periictal diffusion-weighted imaging. *Am J Neuroradiol* 2001; 22(6):1149–60.

35. Parmar H, Lim SH, Tan NC, Lim CC. Acute symptomatic seizures and hippocampus damage: DWI and MRS findings. *Neurology* 2006; 66(11):1732–35.
36. Diehl B, Symms MR, Boulby PA, Salmenpera T, Wheeler-Kingshott CA, Barker GJ, *et al.* Postictal diffusion tensor imaging. *Epilepsy Res* 2005; 65(3):137–46.
37. Salmenpera TM, Simister RJ, Bartlett P, Symms MR, Boulby PA, *et al.* High-resolution diffusion tensor imaging of the hippocampus in temporal lobe epilepsy. *Epilepsy* Res 2006; 71:102–6.
38. Goncalves Pereira P, Oliveira E, Rosado P. Apparent diffusion coefficient mapping of the hippocampus and the amygdala in the pharmaco-resistant temporal lobe epilepsy. *Am J Neuroradiol* 2006; 27:671–83.
39. Kimiwada T, Juhász C, Makki M, Muzik O, Chugani DC, Asano E, *et al.* Hippocampal and thalamic diffusion abnormalities in children with temporal lobe epilepsy. *Epilepsia* 2006; 47:167–75.
40. Guye M, Ranjeva JP, Bartolomei F, Confort-Gouny S, McGonigal A, Régis J, *et al.* What is the significance of interictal water diffusion changes in frontal lobe epilepsies? *Neuroimage* 2007; 35:28–37.
41. Thivard L, Hombrouck J, du Montcel ST, Delmaire C, Cohen L, Samson S, *et al.* Productive and perceptive language reorganization in temporal lobe epilepsy. *Neuroimage* 2005; 24:841–51.
42. Mori S, van Zijl P. Fiber tracking: principles and strategies—a technical review. *NMR in Biomedicine* 2002; 15:468–80.
43. Yogarajah M, Duncan J. Diffusion-based magnetic resonance imaging and tractography in epilepsy. *Epilepsia* 2008; 49(2):189–200.
44. Stefan H, Nimsky C, Scheler G, Rampp S, Hopfengärtner R, Hammen T, *et al.* Periventricular nodular heterotopia: a challenge for epilepsy surgery. *Seizure* 2007; 16(1):81–6.
45. Nimsky C, Ganslandt O, Merhof D, Sorensen AG, Fahlbusch R. Intraoperative visualization of the pyramidal tract by diffusion-tensor-imaging-based fiber tracking. *Neuroimage* 2006; 30(4):1219–29.
46. Catani M, Howard RJ, Pajevic S, Jones DK. Virtual in vivo interactive dissection of white matter fasciculi in the human brain. *Neuroimage* 2002; 17(1):77–94.
47. Guye M, Parker GJ, Symms M, Boulby P, Wheeler-Kingshott CA, Salek-Haddadi A, *et al.* Combined functional MRI and tractography to demonstrate the connectivity of the human primary motor cortex in vivo. *Neuroimage* 2003; 19(4):1349–60.
48. Powell HW, Parker GJ, Alexander DC, Symms MR, Boulby PA, Barker GJ, *et al.* Imaging language pathways predicts postoperative naming defects. *J Neurol Neurosurg Psychiatry* 2008; 79:327–30.
49. Powell HW, Parker GJ, Alexander DC, Symms MR, Boulby PA, Wheeler-Kingshott CA, *et al.* MR tractography predicts visual field defects following temporal lobe resection. *Neurology* 2005; 65:596–9.
50. Parker G, Alexander D. Probabilistic anatomical connectivity derived from the microscopic persistent angular structure of cerebral tissue. *Philos Trans R Soc Lond B Biol Sci* 2005; 460:893–902.
51. Tournier JD, Calamante F, Gadian DG, Connelly A. Direct estimation of the fiber orientation density function from diffusion-weighted MRI data using spherical deconvolution. *Neuroimage* 2004; 23:1176–85.
52. Tuch D. Q-ball imaging. *Magn Res Med* 2004; 52:1358–72.
53. Alexander D. Multiple-fiber reconstruction algorithms for diffusion MRI. *Ann N Y Acad Sci* 2005; 1064:113–33.
54. Perrin M, Poupon C, Rieul B, Leroux P, Constantinesco A, Mangin JF, *et al.* Validation of q-ball imaging with a diffusion fibre-crossing phantom on a clinical scanner. *Philos Trans R Soc Lond B Biol Sci* 2005; 360:881–91.
55. Tuch DS, Reese TG, Wiegell MR, Makris N, Belliveau JW, Wedeen VJ. High angular resolution diffusion imaging reveals intravoxel white matter fiber heterogeneity. *Magn Res Med* 2002; 48:577–82.
56. Nunes RG, Jezzard P, Behrens TE, Clare S. Self-navigates multishot echo-planar pulse sequence for high-resolution diffusion-weighted imaging. *Magn Res Med* 2005; 53:1474–8.
57. Hagmann P, Thiran JP, Jonasson L, Vandergheynst P, Clarke S, Maeder P, *et al.* DTI mapping of human brain connectivity: statistical fibre tracking and virtual dissection. *Neuroimage* 2003; 19(3):545–54.
58. Parker GJ, Stephan KE, Barker GJ, Rowe JB, MacManus DG, Wheeler-Kingshott CA, *et al.* Initial demonstration of in vivo tracing of axonal projections in the macaque brain and comparison with the human brain using diffusion tensor imaging and fast marching tractography. *Neuroimage* 2002; 15(4):797–809.
59. Hagler DJ Jr, Ahmadi ME, Kuperman J, Holland D, McDonald CR, Halgren E, *et al.* Automated white-matter tractography using a probabilistic diffusion tensor atlas: Application to temporal lobe epilepsy. *Hum Brain Mapp* 2009; 30(5):1535–47.
60. Ciccarelli O, Parker GJ, Toosy AT, Wheeler-Kingshott CA, Barker GJ, Boulby PA, *et al.* From diffusion tractography to quantitative white matter tract measures: a reproducibility study. *Neuroimage* 2003; 18:348–59.
61. Jones D. Determining and visualizing uncertainty in estimates of fiber orientation from diffusion tensor MRI. *Magn Res Med* 2003; 49:7–12.
62. la Fougère C, Rominger A, Förster S, Geisler J, Bartenstein P. PET and SPECT in epilepsy: A critical review. *Epilepsy Behav* 2009; 15:50–5.
63. Neirinckx RD, Canning LR, Piper IM, Nowotnik DP, Pickett RD, Holmes RA, *et al.* Technetium-99m d,l-HM-PAO: A new radiopharmaceutical for SPECT imaging of regional cerebral blood perfusion. *J Nucl Med* 1987; 28(2):191–202.
64. Spanaki MV, Spencer SS, Corsi M, MacMullan J, Seibyl J, Zubal IG. Sensitivity and specificity of quantitate difference SPECT analysis in seizure localization. *J Nucl Med* 1999; 40:730–6.
65. Devous MD Sr, Thisted RA, Morgan GF, Leroy RF, Rowe CC. SPECT brain imaging in epilepsy: a meta-analysis. *J Nucl Med* 1998; 39:285–93.
66. Weil S, Noachtar S, Arnold S, Yousry TA, Winkler PA, Tatsch K. Ictal ECD-SPECT differentiates between temporal and extratemporal epilepsy: confirmation by excellent postoperative seizure control. *Nucl Med Commun* 2001; 22:233–7.
67. Zaknun JJ, Bal C, Maes A, Tepmongkol S, Vazquez S, Dupont P, *et al.* Comparative analysis of MR imaging, ictal SPECT and EEG in temporal lobe epilepsy: a prospective IAEA multi-center study. *Eur J Nucl Med Mol Imaging* 2008; 35:107–15.
68. Lee JJ, Lee SK, Lee SY, Park KI, Kim DW, Lee DS, *et al.* Seizure, Frontal lobe epilepsy: clinical characteristics, surgical outcomes and diagnostic modalities. *Seizure* 2008; 17:514–23.
69. Ahnlide JA, Rosén I, Lindén-Mickelsson Tech P, Källén K. Does SISCOM contribute to favorable seizure outcome after epilepsy surgery? *Epilepsia* 2007; 48:579–88.
70. Matsuda H, Matsuda K, Nakamura F, Kameyama S, Masuda H, Otsuki T, *et al.* Contribution of subtraction ictal SPECT coregistered to MRI to epilepsy surgery: a multicenter study. *Ann Nucl Med* 2009; 23:283–91.
71. Kaiboriboon K, Lowe VJ, Chantarujikapong SI, Hogan RE. The usefulness of subtraction ictal SPECT coregistered to MRI in single- and dual-headed SPECT cameras in partial epilepsy. *Epilepsia* 2002; 43:408–14.
72. O'Brien T. SPECT: methodology. *Adv Neurol* 2002; 83:11–32.
73. O'Brien TJ, So EL, Cascino GD, Hauser MF, Marsh WR, Meyer FB, *et al.* Subtraction SPECT coregistered to MRI in focal malformations of cortical development: localization of the epileptogenic zone in epilepsy surgery candidates. *Epilepsia* 2004; 45:367–76.
74. O'Brien TJ, So EL, Mullan BP, Cascino GD, Hauser MF, Brinkmann BH, *et al.* Subtraction peri-ictal SPECT is predictive of extratemporal epilepsy surgery outcome. *Neurology* 2000; 55:1668–77.
75. O'Brien TJ, So EL, Mullan BP, Hauser MF, Brinkmann BH, Bohnen NI, *et al.* Subtraction ictal SPECT co-registered to MRI improves clinical usefulness of SPECT in localizing the surgical seizure focus. *Neurology* 1998; 50:445–54.
76. Wichert-Ana L, de Azevedo-Marques PM, Oliveira LF, Terra-Bustamante VC, Fernandes RM, Santos AC, *et al.* Interictal hyperemia

correlates with epileptogenicity in polymicrogyric cortex. *Epilepsy Res* 2008; 79:39–48.

77. Lee SK, Lee SY, Yun CH, Lee HY, Lee JS, Lee DS. Ictal SPECT in neocortical epilepsies: clinical usefulness and factors affecting the pattern of hyperperfusion. *Neuroradiology* 2006; 48:678–84.
78. Van Paesschen W. Ictal SPECT. *Epilepsia* 2004; 45(Suppl. 4):35–40.
79. Kazemi N, O'Brien TJ, Cascino GD, So LS. Single photon emission computed tomography. In: Engel J Jr, Pedley T (eds) *Epilepsy: A Comprehensive Textbook*, pp. 965–74. Philadelphia, PA: Lippincott Williams & Wilkins, 2008.
80. Newton MR, Berkovic SF, Austin MC, Reutens DC, McKay WJ, Bladin PF. Dystonia, clinical lateralization, and regional blood flow changes in temporal lobe seizures. *Neurology* 1992; 42:371–7.
81. Dupont P, Van Paesschen W, Palmini A, Ambayi R, Van Loon J, Goffin J, *et al.* Ictal perfusion patterns associated with single MRI-visible focal dysplastic lesions: Implications for the noninvasive delineation of the epileptogenic zone. *Epilepsia* 2006; 47(9):1550–7.
82. Fukuda M, Masuda H, Honma J, Kameyama S, Tanaka R. Ictal SPECT analyzed by three-dimensional stereotactic surface projection in frontal lobe epilepsy patients. *Epilepsy Res* 2006; 68:95–102.
83. Chugani DC, Chugani HT, Muzik O, Shah JR, Shah AK, Canady A, *et al.* Imaging epileptogenic tubers in children with tuberous sclerosis complex using alpha-(11C)methyl-L-tryptophan positron emission tomography. *Ann Neurol* 1998; 44:858–66.
84. da Silva EA, Chugani DC, Muzik O, Chugani HT. Identification of frontal lobe epileptic foci in children using positron emission tomography. *Epilepsia* 1997; 38:1198–1208.
85. Knowlton RC, Laxer KD, Aminoff MJ, Roberts TP, Wong ST, Rowley HA. Magnetoencephalography in partial epilepsy: clinical yield and localization accuracy. *Ann Neurol* 1997; 42:622–31.
86. Ryvlin P, Bouvard S, Le Bars D, De Lamérie G, Grégoire MC, Kahane P, *et al.* Clinical utility of flumazenil-PET versus (18F) fluorodeoxyglucose-PET and MRI in refractory partial epilepsy: a prospective study in 100 patients. *Brain* 1998; 121(11):2067–81.
87. Valk PE, Laxer KD, Barbaro NM, Knezevic S, Dillon WP, Budinger TF. High-resolution (2.6 mm) PET in partial complex epilepsy associated with mesial temporal sclerosis. *Radiology* 1993; 186:55–8.
88. Gaillard WD, Bhatia S, Bookheimer SY, Fazilat S, Sato S, Theodore WH. FDG-PET and volumetric MRI in the evaluation of patients with partial epilepsy. *Neurology* 1995; 45:123–6.
89. Ryvlin P, Philippon B, Cinotti L, Froment JC, Le Bars D, Mauguière F. Functional neuroimaging strategy in temporal lobe epilepsy: a comparative study of 18 FDG-PET and 99m Tc-HMPAO-SPECT. *Ann Neurol* 1992; 31:650–6.
90. Swartz B, Tomiyasu U, Delgado E. Neuroimaging in temporal lobe epilepsy: test sensitivity and relationships to pathology and postoperative outcome. *Epilepsia* 1992; 33:624–34.
91. Henry T, Engel J, Mazziotta J. Clinical evaluation of interictal fluorine-18-fluorodeoxyglucose PET in partial epilepsy. *J Nucl Med* 1993; 34:1892–8.
92. Drzezga A, Arnold S, Minoshima S, Noachtar S, Szecsi J, Winkler P, *et al.* 18F-FDG PET studies in patients with extratemporal and temporal epilepsy: evaluation of an observer-independent analysis. *J Nucl Med* 1999; 40:737–46.
93. Arnold S, Schlaug G, Niemann H, Ebner A, Lüders H, Witte OW, *et al.* Topography of interictal glucose hypometabolism in unilateral mesiotemporal epilepsy. *Neurology* 1996; 46:1422–30.
94. Gambhir S, Singh Sethi R, Deswal S. Incidental detection of a single brain metastasis from breast carcinoma during Tc-99m MIBI scintimammography. *Clin Nucl Med* 2001; 26:883–4.
95. Juhász C, Chugani DC, Muzik O, Shah A, Shah J, Watson C, *et al.* Relationship of flumazenil and glucose PET abnormalities to neocortical epilepsy surgery outcome. *Neurology* 2001; 56:1650–8.
96. Won HJ, Chang KH, Cheon JE, Kim HD, Lee DS, Han MH, *et al.* Comparison of MR imaging with PET and ictal SPECT in 118 patients with intractable epilepsy. *Am J Neuroradiol* 1999; 20:593–9.
97. Frost JJ, Mayberg HS, Fisher RS, Douglass KH, Dannals RF, Links JM, *et al.* Mu-opiate receptors measured by positron emission tomography are increased in temporal lobe epilepsy. *Ann Neurol* 1988; 23:231–7.
98. Iinuma K, Yokoyama H, Otsuki T, Yanai K, Watanabe T, Ido T, *et al.* Histamine H1-receptors are increased in parietal epilepsy: A PET Study. *Lancet* 1993; 341:238.
99. Kumlien E, Hartvig P, Valind S, Oye I, Tedroff J, Långström B. NMDA-receptor activity visualized with (S)-(N-methyl-11C) ketamine and positron emission tomography in patients with medial temporal lobe epilepsy. *Epilepsia* 1999; 40(1):30–7.
100. Sauvageau A, Desjardins P, Lozeva V, Rose C, Hazell AS, Bouthillier A, *et al.* Increased expression of 'peripheral-type' benzodiazepine receptors in human temporal lobe epilepsy: Implications for PET imaging of hippocampal sclerosis. *Metab Brain* Dis 2002; 17(1):3–11.
101. Savic I, Persson A, Roland P, Pauli S, Sedvall G, Widén L. In-vivo demonstration of reduced benzodiazepine receptor binding in human epileptic foci. *Lancet* 1988; 2:863–6.
102. Muzik O, da Silva EA, Juhasz C, Chugani DC, Shah J, Nagy F, *et al.* Intracranial EEG versus flumazenil and glucose PET in children with extratemporal lobe epilepsy. *Neurology* 2000; 54:171–9.
103. Savic I, Thorell J, Roland P. (11C)Flumazenil positron emission tomography visualizes frontal epileptogenic regions. *Epilepsia* 1995; 36:1225–32.
104. Savic I, Svanborg E, Thorell J. Cortical benzodiazepine receptor changes are related to frequency of partial seizures: a positron emission tomography study. *Epilepsia* 1996; 37:236–44.
105. Bouvard S, Costes N, Bonnefoi F, Lavenne F, Mauguière F, Delforge J, *et al.* Seizure-related short-term plasticity of benzodiazepine receptors in partial epilepsy: a (11C)flumazenil-PET study. *Brain* 2005; 128:1330–43.
106. Koepp MJ, Hammers A, Labbé C, Woermann FG, Brooks DJ, Duncan JS. 11C-flumazenil PET in patients with refractory temporal lobe epilepsy and normal MRI. *Neurology* 2000; 54:332–9.
107. Kaneko K, Sasaki M, Morioka T, Koga H, Abe K, Sawamoto H, *et al.* Pre-surgical identification of epileptogenic areas in temporal lobe epilepsy by 123I-iomazenil SPECT: a comparison with IMP SPECT and FDG PET. *Nucl Med Comm* 2006; 2006(27):893–9.
108. Nelissen N, Van Paesschen W, Baete K, Van Laere K, Palmini A, *et al.* Correlations of interictal FDG-PET metabolism and ictal SPECT perfusion changes in human temporal lobe epilepsy with hippocampal sclerosis. *Neuroimage* 2006; 32(2):684–95.
109. Joo EY, Hong SB, Han HJ, Tae WS, Kim JH, Han SJ, *et al.* Postoperative alteration of cerebral glucose metabolism in mesial temporal lobe epilepsy. *Brain* 2005; 128(8):1802–10.
110. Vinton AB, Carne R, Hicks RJ, Desmond PM, Kilpatrick C, Kaye AH, *et al.* The extent of resection of FDG-PET hypometabolism relates to outcome of temporal lobectomy. *Brain* 2006; 130(2):548–60.
111. Benson RR, FitzGerald DB, LeSueur LL, Kennedy DN, Kwong KK, Buchbinder BR, *et al.* Language dominance determined by whole brain functional MRI in patients with brain lesions. *Neurology* 1999; 52:798–809.
112. Gaillard WD, Balsamo L, Xu B, Grandin CB, Braniecki SH, Papero PH, *et al.* Language dominance in partial epilepsy patients identified with an fMRI reading task. *Neurology* 2002; 59:256–65.
113. Lehéricy S, Cohen L, Bazin B, Samson S, Giacomini E, Rougetet R, *et al.* Functional MR evaluation of temporal and frontal language dominance compared with the Wada test. *Neurology* 2000; 54:1625–33.
114. Woermann FG, Jokeit H, Luerding R, Freitag H, Schulz R, Guertler S, *et al.* Language lateralization by Wada test and fMRI in 100 patients with epilepsy. *Neurology* 2003; 61:699–701.
115. Yetkin FZ, Swanson S, Fischer M, Akansel G, Morris G, Mueller W, *et al.* Functional MR of frontal lobe activation: comparison with Wada language results. *Am J Neuroradiol* 1998; 19(6):1095–8.

116. Hammeke TA, Yetkin FZ, Mueller WM, Morris GL, Haughton VM, Rao SM, *et al.* Functional magnetic resonance imaging of somatosensory stimulation. *Neurosurgery*, 1994; 35:677–81.
117. Kim SG, Ashe J, Georgopoulos AP, Merkle H, Ellermann JM, Menon RS, *et al.* Functional imaging of human motor cortex at high magnetic field. *J Neurophysiol* 1993; 69(1):297–302.
118. Rao SM, Binder JR, Bandettini PA, Hammeke TA, Yetkin FZ, Jesmanowicz A, *et al.* Functional magnetic resonance imaging of complex human movements. *Neurology* 1993; 42:2311–18.
119. Yetkin FZ, Mueller WM, Morris GL, McAuliffe TL, Ulmer JL, Cox RW, *et al.* Functional MR activation correlated with intraoperative cortical mapping. *Am J Neuroradiol* 1997; 18:1311–15.
120. Yousry TA, Schmid UD, Jassoy AG, Schmidt D, Eisner WE, Reulen HJ, *et al.* Topography of the cortical motor hand area: prospective study with functional MR imaging and direct motor mapping at surgery. *Radiology* 1995; 195:23–9.
121. Binder JR, Swanson SJ, Sabsevitz DS, Hammeke TA, Raghavan M, Mueller WM. A comparison of two fMRI methods for predicting verbal memory decline after left temporal lobectomy: language lateralization versus hippocampal activation asymmetry. *Epilepsia* 2010; 51(4):618–26.
122. Bookheimer SY, Zeffiro TA, Blaxton T, Malow BA, Gaillard WD, Sato S, *et al.* A direct comparison of PET activation and electrocortical stimulation mapping for language localization. *Neurology* 1997; 48:1056–65.
123. Lehéricy S, Biondi A, Sourour N, Vlaicu M, du Montcel ST, Cohen L, *et al.* Arteriovenous brain malformations: is functional MR imaging reliable for studying language reorganization in patients? Initial observations. *Radiology* 2002; 223:672–82.
124. Jayakar P, Bernal B, Santiago Medina L, Altman N. False lateralization of language cortex on functional MRI after a cluster of focal seizures. *Neurology* 2002; 58:490–2.
125. Wellmer J, Weber B, Urbach H, Reul J, Fernandez G, Elger CE. Cerebral lesions can impair fMRI-based language lateralization. *Epilepsia* 2009; 50(10):2213–23.
126. Jezzard P, Clare S. Sources of distortion in functional MRI data. *Hum Brain Mapp* 1999; 8:80–5.
127. Ances BM, Leontiev O, Perthen JE, Liang C, Lansing AE, Buxton RB. Regional differences in the coupling of cerebral blood flow and oxygen metabolism changes in response to activation: implications for BOLD-fMRI. *Neuroimage* 2008; 39:1510–21.
128. Restom K, Perthen JE, Liu TT. Calibrated fMRI in the medial temporal lobe during a memory-encoding task. *Neuroimage* 2008; 40:1495–502.
129. Bénar CG, Gross DW, Wang Y, Petre V, Pike B, Dubeau F, *et al.* The BOLD response to interictal epileptiform discharges. *Neuroimage* 2002; 3:1182–92.
130. Krakow K, Woermann FG, Symms MR, Allen PJ, Lemieux L, Barker GJ, *et al.* EEG-triggered functional MRI of interictal epileptiform activity in patients with partial seizures. *Brain* 1999; 122(9):1679–88.
131. Al-Asmi A, Bénar CG, Gross DW, Khani YA, Andermann F, Pike B, *et al.* fMRI activation in continuous and spike-triggered EEG-fMRI studies of epileptic spikes. *Epilepsia* 2003; 44(10):1328–39.
132. Warach S, Ives JR, Schlaug G, Patel MR, Darby DG, Thangaraj V, *et al.* EEG-triggered echo-planar functional MRI in epilepsy. *Neurology* 1996; 47(1):89–93.
133. Seeck M, Lazeyras F, Michel CM, Blanke O, Gericke CA, Ives J, *et al.* Noninvasive epileptic focus localization using EEG-triggered functional MRI and electromagnetic tomography. *Electroencephalogr Clinl Neurophysiol* 1998; 106(6): 508–12.
134. Lemieux L, Salek-Haddadi A, Josephs O, Allen P, Toms N, Scott C, *et al.* Event-related fMRI with simultaneous and continuous EEG: description of the method and initial case report. *Neuroimage* 2001; 14(3):780–7.
135. Ritter P, Freyer F, Curio G, Villringer A. High-frequency (600 Hz) population spikes in human EEG delineate thalamic and cortical fMRI activation sites. *Neuroimage* 2008; 42:483–90.
136. Formaggio E, Storti SF, Bertoldo A, Manganotti P, Fiaschi A, Toffolo GM. Integrating EEG and fMRI in epilepsy. *Neuroimage* 2011; 54:2719–31.
137. Thornton R, Laufs H, Rodionov R, Cannadathu S, Carmichael DW, Vulliemoz S, *et al.* EEG correlated functional MRI and postoperative outcome in focal epilepsy. *J Neurol Neurosurg Psychiatry* 2010; 81: 922–7.
138. Salek-Haddadi A, Diehl B, Hamandi K, Merschhemke M, Liston A, Friston K, *et al.* Hemodynamic correlates of epileptiform discharges: an EEG-fMRI study of 63 patients with focal epilepsy. *Brain Res* 2006; 1088:148–66.
139. Bénar CG, Grova C, Kobayashi E, Bagshaw AP, Aghakhani Y, Dubeau F, *et al.* EEG-fMRI of epileptic spikes: Concordance with EEG source localization and intracranial EEG. *Neuroimage* 2006; 30:1161–70.
140. Lazeyras F, Blanke O, Perrig S, Zimine I, Golay X, Delavelle J, *et al.* EEG-triggered functional MRI in patients with pharmacoresistant epilepsy. *J Magn Res Imaging* 2000; 12:177–85.
141. Zimine I, Seghier ML, Seeck M, Lazeyras F. Brain activation using triggered event-related fMRI. *Neuroimage* 2003; 18:410–15.
142. Kobayashi E, Bagshaw AP, Bénar CG, Aghakhani Y, Andermann F, Dubeau F, *et al.* Temporal and extratemporal BOLD responses to temporal lobe interictal spikes. *Epilepsia* 2006; 2:343–54.
143. Salek-Haddadi A, Friston KJ, Lemieux L, Fish DR. Studying spontaneous EEG activity with fMRI. *Brain Res Rev* 2003; 43:110–33.
144. Carmichael DW, Hamandi K, Laufs H, Duncan JS, Thomas DL, Lemieux L. An investigation of the relationship between BOLD and perfusion signal changes during epileptic generalised spike wave activity. *Magn Res Imaging* 2008; 26:870–3.
145. Kobayashi E, Bagshaw AP, Grova C, Gotman J, Dubeau F. Grey matter heterotopia: what EEG-fMRI can tell us about epileptogenicity of neuronal migration disorders. *Brain* 2006; 129(2):366–74.
146. Stefanovic B, Warnking JM, Kobayashi E, Bagshaw AP, Hawco C, Dubeau F, *et al.* Hemodynamic and metabolic responses to activation, deactivation and epileptic discharges. *Neuroimage* 2005; 28:205–15.
147. Shmuel A, Yacoub E, Pfeuffer J, Van de Moortele PF, Adriany G, Hu X, *et al.* Sustained negative BOLD, blood flow and oxygen consumption response and its coupling to the positive response in the human brain. *Neuron* 2002; 36:1195–210.
148. Parkes LM, Fries P, Kerskens CM, Norris DG. Reduced BOLD response to periodic visual stimulation. *Neuroimage* 2004; 21(1):236–43.
149. Kobayashi E, Bagshaw AP, Grova C, Dubeau F, Gotman J. Negative BOLD responses to epileptic spikes. *Hum Brain Mapp* 2006; 27:488–97.
150. Hamandi K, Laufs H, Nöth U, Carmichael DW, Duncan JS, Lemieux L. BOLD and perfusion changes during epileptic generalised spike wave activity. *Neuroimage* 2008; 39:608–18.
151. Vogrin S, Lau S, Haueisen J, Cook M. ESI and fMRI of interictal and ictal epileptic discharges. *Int J Bioelectromagn* 2001; 13(4):S261–7.
152. Pan J, Williamson A, Cavus I. Neurometabolism in human epilepsy. *Epilepsia* 2008; 49(S3):S31–41.
153. Laxer K. Clinical applications of magnetic resonance spectroscopy. *Epilepsia* 1997; 38(S4):S13–17.
154. Garcia PA, Laxer KD, van der Grond J, Hugg JW, Matson GB, Weiner MW. Proton magnetic resonance spectroscopic imaging in patients with frontal lobe epilepsy. *Ann Neurol* 1995. 37(2):279–81.
155. Maudsley A, Domenig C, Ramsay RE, Bowen BC. Application of volumetric MR spectroscopic imaging for localization of neocortical epilepsy. *Epilepsy Res* 2010; 88(2–3):127–38.
156. Ikeda A, Nagamine T, Kunieda T, Ohara S, Shibasaki H. Magnetoencephalography (MEG): its clinical usefulness in epilepsy surgery. In: Lüders H (ed) *Epilepsy surgery*, pp. 441–50. Philadelphia, PA: Lippincott Williams & Wilkins, 2001.

157. Ricci GB, Romani GL, Salustri C, Pizzella V, Torrioli G, Buonomo S, *et al.* Study of focal epilepsy by multichannel neuromagnetic measurements. *Electroencephalogr Clin Neurophysiol* 1987; 66(4): 358–68.

158. Leahy RM, Mosher JC, Spencer ME, Huang MX, Lewine JD. A study of dipole localization accuracy for MEG and EEG using a human skull phantom. *Electroencephalogr Clin Neurophysiol* 1998; 107:159–73.

159. Otsubo H, Oishi M, Snead O. *Magnetoencephalography*. In: Miller J, Silbergeld D (eds) *Epilepsy Surgery: Principles and Controversies*, p. 752–67. New York: Taylor and Francis Group, 2006.

160. Mikuni N, Nagamine T, Ikeda A, Terada K, Taki W, Kimura J, *et al.* Simultaneous recording of epileptiform discharges by MEG and subdural electrodes in temporal lobe epilepsy. *Neuroimage* 1997; 5:298–306.

161. Oishi M, Otsubo H, Kameyama S, Wachi M, Tanaka K, Masuda H, *et al.* Ictal magnetoencephalographic discharges from elementary visual hallucinations of status epilepticus. *J Neurol Neurosurg Psychiatry* 2003; 74:525–7.

162. Tao JX, Ray A, Hawes-Ebersole S, Ebersole JS. Intracranial EEG substrates of scalp EEG interictal spikes. *Epilepsia* 2005; 46:669–76.

163. Cooper R, Winter AL, Crow HJ, Walter WG. Comparison of subcortical, cortical and scalp activity using chronically indwelling electrodes in man. *Electroencephalogr Clin Neurophysiol* 1965; 22:153–8.

164. Lee D. High-resolution magnetic resonance imaging (MRI), surface coil MRI, and magnetoencephalography. *Adv Neurol* 2006; 97:279–83.

165. Stefan H, Hummel C, Scheler G, Genow A, Druschky K, Tilz C, *et al.* Magnetic brain source imaging of focal epileptic activity: a synopsis of 455 cases. *Brain* 2003; 126:2396–405.

166. Funke M, Lewine J, Orrison W. MEG-guided identification of structural brain lesions in patients with neocortical epilepsy. In: Nowak H, Haueisen J, Giessler F, Huonker R (eds) *BIOMAG 2002: Proceedings of the 13th International Conference on Biomagnetism*, pp. 212–15. Berlin: VDE Verlag GmBH, 2005.

167. Moore KR, Funke ME, Constantino T, Katzman GL, Lewine JD. Magnetoencephalographically directed review of high spatial-resolution surface-coil MR images improves lesion detection in patients with extratemporal epilepsy. *Radiology* 2002; 225:880–7.

168. Engel J Jr, Van Ness PC, Rasmussen TB, Ojemann LM. Outcome with respect to epileptic seizures. In: Engel J (ed) *Surgical Treatment of the Epilepsies*, pp. 609–21. New York: Raven Press, 1993.

169. Munari, C, Broggi G, Scerrati M. Epilepsy surgery: guidelines for minimum standard equipment and organization. *J Neurosurg Sci* 2000; 44:173–6.

170. Mohamed IS, Otsubo H, Ochi A, Elliott I, Donner E, Chuang S, *et al.* Utility of magnetoencephalography in the evaluation of recurrent seizures after epilepsy surgery. *Epilepsia* 2007; 48:2150–9.

171. Salanova, V, Markand O, Worth R. Longitudinal follow-up in 145 patients with medically refractory temporal lobe epilepsy treated surgically between 1984 and 1995. *Epilepsia* 1999; 40:1417–23.

172. Baumgartner C, Barth DS, Levesque MF, Sutherling WW. Detection of epileptiform discharges on magnetoencephalography in comparison to invasive measurements. In: Hoke M, Erne S, Okada Y, Romani G (eds) *Biomagnetism: Clinical Aspects*, pp.67–71. Amsterdam: Elsevier, 1992.

173. Papanicolaou AC, Simos PG, Breier JI, Zouridakis G, Willmore LJ, Wheless JW, *et al.* Magnetoencephalographic mapping of the language-specific cortex. *J Neurosurg* 1999; 90:85–93.

174. Berg AT, Vickrey BG, Langfitt JT, Sperling MR, Walczak TS, Shinnar S, *et al.* The multicenter study of epilepsy surgery: recruitment and selection for surgery. *Epilepsia* 2003; 11:1425–33.

175. Alarcón G, Valentín A, Watt C, Selway RP, Lacruz ME, Elwes RD, *et al.* Is it worth pursuing epilepsy surgery for epilepsy in patients with normal neuroimaging? *J Neurol Neurosurg Psychiatry* 2006; 4:474–80.

176. Murphy MA, O'Brien TJ, Morris K, Cook MJ. Multi-modality image-guided surgery for the treatment of medically refractory epilepsy. *J Neurosurg* 2004; 100:452–62.

177. Akhtari M, Bragin A, Cohen M, Moats R, Brenker F, Lynch MD, *et al.* Functionalised magnetonanoparticles for MRI diagnosis and localization in epilepsy. *Epilepsia* 2008; 49(8):1419–30.

178. Thivard L, Adam C, Hasboun D, Clémenceau S, Dezamis E, Lehéricy S, *et al.* Interictal diffusion MRI in partial epilepsies explored with intracerebral electrodes. *Brain* 2006; 129(2):375–85.

179. Wolters CH, Anwander A, Tricoche X, Weinstein D, Koch MA, MacLeod RS. Influence of tissue conductivity anisotropy on EEG/MEG field and return current computation in a realistic head model: za simulation and visualization study using high-resolution finite element modeling. *Neuroimage* 2006; 30:813–26.

180. Rullmann M, Anwander A, Dannhauer M, Warfield SK, Duffy FH, Wolters CH. EEG source analysis of epileptiform activity using a 1 mm anisotropic hexahedra finite element head model. *Neuroimage* 2009; 44:399–410.

181. Hallez H, Vanrumste B, Van Hese P, D'Asseler Y, Lemahieu I, Van de Walle R. A finite difference method with reciprocity used to incorporate anisotropy in electroencephalogram dipole source localization. *Phys Med Biol* 2005; 50:3787–806.

182. Hamandi K, Powell HW, Laufs H, Symms MR, Barker GJ, Parker GJ, *et al.* Combined EEG-fMRI and tractography to visualise propagation of epileptic activity. *J Neurol Neurosurg Psychiatry* 2007; 79(5):594–7.

183. Stokes T, Shaw EJ, Juarez-Garcia A, Camosso-Stefinovic J, Baker R. *Clinical guidelines and evidence review for the epilepsies: diagnosis and management in adults and children in primary and secondary care.* London: Royal College of General Practitioners, 2004.

184. Whiting P, Gupta R, Burch J, Mota RE, Wright K, Marson A, *et al.* A systematic review of the effectiveness and cost-effectiveness of neuroimaging assessments used to visualise the seizure focus in people with refractory epilepsy being considered for surgery. *Health Technol Assess* 2006; 10(4):1–250, iii–iv.

185. Knowlton RC, Elgavish RA, Limdi N, Bartolucci A, Ojha B, Blount J, *et al.* Functional imaging: I. Relative predictive value of intracraninal electroencephalography. *Ann Neurol* 2008; 64:25–34.

186. Knowlton RC, Elgavish RA, Bartolucci A, Ojha B, Limdi N, Blount J, *et al.* Functional imaging: II. Prediction of epilepsy surgery outcome. *Ann Neurol* 2008; 64:35–41.

CHAPTER 11

The Biochemical, Haematological, Histological, Immunological, and Genetic Investigation of Epilepsy

Simon Shorvon

In most patients with newly diagnosed epilepsy, a number of simple tests are routinely carried out. These are listed in Table 11.1, and the neurophysiological and imaging tests are described in more detail in Chapters 1 and 10. Depending on the clinical context, however, other tests are sometimes needed to establish the cause of epilepsy. In this chapter a range of laboratory investigations which are used in the investigation of the cause of epilepsy in selected patients, are outlined. Tests for cerebral infection depend on locality and clinical context, and are not included here.

It must be also strongly emphasized that a detailed clinical history, including the family history, and examination, including a search for associated neurological or systemic disturbances, are as important in assessing cause as any test. The value of many of the tests listed here is dependent on clinical context. Failure to account for the clinical context may lead to misinterpretation and erroneous conclusions.

A detailed discussion of the indications, interpretation, and place of these tests in clinical practice is beyond the scope of this short chapter. It is intended here simply to provide brief lists of available tests. The lists are not exhaustive, but cover many tests used in specialist clinical practice to identify epilepsy aetiology. Some of the conditions being investigated are extremely rare, and others more common.

Biochemical tests in urine and blood

Urinary biochemical tests

Table 11.2 lists a variety of urine investigations for biochemical defects which might present with epilepsy or include epilepsy in the presentation. Most of these conditions are relevant mainly in paediatric epileptology and will be seldom helpful in adults. Exceptions to this rule are the tests for Wilson disease, ornithine transcarbamylase deficiency, porphyria (and rarely others) which can present at any age. Many of these tests are prone to false positives, and are affected by renal dysfunction, or in some cases exogenous substances. Thus, abnormalities should be interpreted with care and assessment should be carried out in consultation with a clinical chemical biochemist. In all the conditions listed, there are other clinical signs or associated clinical symptoms.

Blood biochemistry

In Table 11.3 are listed some of the biochemical tests in blood which can be helpful in diagnosing patients with epilepsy. As with the urinary tests, many of the conditions being sought are rare and relevant mainly to paediatric epileptology. Some of the abnormalities can be detected by urinary analysis also, although blood biochemistry in most cases is more reliable and more sensitive.

Porphyria is a not uncommon cause of epilepsy in some parts of the world and the biochemical investigation is crucial in its diagnosis and characterization. In Table 11.4 are listed urinary, faecal, and serum tests which can be helpful in differentiating the types of porphyria in which epilepsy is a common presentation.

Haematological tests

A variety of disorders can be detected by haematological examination of a blood sample (Table 11.5).

Table 11.1 Minimum dataset of screening investigations to be carried out in most cases of newly diagnosed epilepsy where the cause is not immediately apparent

Electroencephalogram (EEG)
Magnetic resonance imaging (MRI) scan (and in some cases, computed tomographic (CT) scanning)
Electrocardiogram (routine ECG in all cases, and in selected cases more extensive cardiological investigation)
Full blood count and differential
Biochemical tests including urea, electrolytes, sugar, liver function tests, thyroid function, and autoimmune screen

Table 11.2 Urinary biochemical tests that can be helpful in determining the cause of epilepsy

Investigation	Condition being tested for	Clinical epilepsy presentation
Alpha-aminoadipic semialdehyde (α-AASA)	Pyridoxine-dependent epilepsy	Neonatal seizures and later refractory epilepsy in childhood
Acylcarnitines	Disorders of fatty acid oxidation or organic acidurias	Acute metabolic encephalopathy and epilepsy with learning disability and often other signs
Amino acids[a]	Various metabolic deficiency states-aminoacidopathies (phenylketonuria, homocysteinuria, pyridoxal phosphate-responsive epilepsy)	Epilepsy with learning disability and often other signs
Copper	Wilson disease	Epilepsy can be a feature but usually subordinated to movement disorder or hepatic dysfunction
Creatine	Creatine synthesis disorders	Early epilepsy, movement disorders, and developmental delay
Glycosaminoglycans	Mucopolysaccharidoses (e.g. MPS II, Hunter, MPS III, Sanfilippo)	Developmental delay and regression, epilepsy, dysostosis
Guanidinoacetate	Creatine synthesis disorders	Early epilepsy, movement disorders and developmental delay
Oligosaccharides	Oligosaccharidoses (e.g. mannosidosis, sialidosis, fucosidosis)	Learning disability, skeletal deformities and myoclonic epilepsy
Organic acids (carboxylic acids)	Organic acidurias (e.g. glutaric aciduria type 1, propionic acidaemia, methylmalonic acidaemia). Fatty acid oxidation disorders	Encephalopathy, movement disorders and epilepsy
Orotic acid	Some urea cycle defects (e.g. ornithine transcarbamylase deficiency)	Encephalopathy (precipitated by intercurrent illness, fasting, protein load, valproate)
Porphyrins	Porphyria (see Table 11.4)	Seizures, often precipitated by exogenous cause
Pterins	Disorders of biogenic amine metabolism (e.g. tetrahydrobiopterin deficiency disorders)	Developmental delay and seizures
Purine and pyrimidine metabolites	Disorders of purine or pyrimidine metabolism	Psychomotor retardation and epilepsy
Uracil	Ornithine transcarbamylase deficiency or disorders of pyrimidine metabolism	Encephalopathy (precipitated by intercurrent illness, fasting, protein load, valproate)
Uric acid	Disorders of purine metabolism (e.g. Lesch–Nyhan syndrome)	Psychomotor retardation and epilepsy

[a] The presence of amino acids in the urine depends on the renal threshold, and so decreases or mild elevations will only be seen in blood (plasma). For that reason diagnosis of phenylketonuria (and most other aminoacidopathies) is nowadays always made in blood/plasma. Similarly, if homocysteinuria is suspected, measurement of plasma homocysteine is preferable, though some labs still use the urine nitroprusside test as a non-quantitative screen for homocysteinuria. The main use of urine amino acids is to look for renal transport defects associated with aminoaciduria, e.g. cystinuria.

Cerebrospinal fluid examination

Cerebrospinal fluid (CSF) examination has a limited role in the diagnosis of biochemical disorders and should be ordered usually after consultation with a chemical biochemist. Most of the conditions being sought are rare and CSF examination complements other investigations. The range of tests is listed in Table 11.6.

CSF examination has a more important role in the investigation of infectious and immunological disease (see also Table 11.8).

Histological investigations and biopsy

In Table 11.7, some of the more common biopsies carried out in patients presenting with epilepsy (almost always associated with other features) are listed. These tend to be confirmatory tests undertaken fairly late in the course of investigation, and should be arranged after full consultation with the neuropathological department. A detailed discussion of the histological findings in cerebral tumours, cerebral malformations, or other structural lesions is beyond the scope of this chapter.

Immunological investigations

The range of identifiable immunological causes of epilepsy has increased in recent years. These now form an important group of conditions, presenting in childhood or adult life, and seizures can be a prominent or presenting feature. The range of tests is outlined in Table 11.8.

Genetic investigations

Many epilepsies have a genetic basis, although often this is complex. For a number of well-defined conditions, genetic testing is widely available, but for most of genes, genetic testing is only available in a limited fashion, and is furthermore expensive. For many of these, cheaper diagnostic alternatives exist. Some of the commoner available genetic tests are given in the tables, according to phenotype. It should be recognized, however, that as testing becomes more widely used, the recognized phenotype associated with genetic defects invariably broadens, and no simple correspondence between genotype and phenotype is found. The same

Table 11.3 Blood biochemical tests that can be helpful in determining the cause of epilepsy

Investigation	Condition being tested for	Clinical epilepsy presentation
Alpha-aminoadipic semialdehyde (α-AASA)	Pyridoxine-dependent epilepsy	Neonatal seizures and later refractory epilepsy in childhood
Acylcarnitines and carnitine levels	Disorders of fatty acid oxidation or organic acidurias	Acute metabolic encephalopathy
Amino acids	Various aminoacidopathies (e.g. phenylketonuria, homocysteinaemia [classical homocysteinuria, cobalamin metabolism defects])	Epilepsy with learning disability and often other signs
Ammonia	Urea cycle defects (e.g. ornithine transcarbamylase deficiency). Some organic acidurias or fatty acid oxidation defects	Encephalopathy (precipitated by intercurrent illness, fasting, protein load, valproate)
Ceruloplasmin	Menkes disease, Wilson disease	Epilepsy, mental regression, neurological signs, hair changes
Calcium	Hypocalcaemia, hypoparathyroidism, pseudo-hypoparathyroidism, DiGeorge syndrome	Neonatal seizures, other epilepsy, learning disability, other neurological signs
Copper	Menkes disease, Wilson disease	Epilepsy, mental regression, neurological signs, hair changes
Creatinine	Creatine deficiency syndromes (GAMT, AGAT, and transporter deficiency)	Epilepsy, learning disability
Folate (serum folate and red cell folate)	Folate deficiency including the rare inherited metabolic diseases of folate malabsorption and metabolism	Megaloblastic anaemia or macrocytosis will be present in most cases. Seizures can be present, usually associated with other features depending on cause.
Glucose	Hypoglycaemia (various causes)	Epilepsy, acute encephalopathy
Homocysteine	Classical homocysteinuria, cobalamin absorption/metabolism defects, defects of folate metabolism, sulphite oxidase and molybdenum cofactor deficiencies	Seizures and other signs depending on condition
Lactate	Mitochondrial disorders (various types)	Acute encephalopathy with seizures, myoclonic seizures, other neurological signs
Magnesium	Low magnesium	Neonatal seizures
Vitamin B_{12} (cobalamin) and where appropriate methylmalonic acid and homocysteine	Vitamin B_{12} deficiency (various causes, including the rare inherited disorders of cobalamin absorption, transport, uptake and metabolism)	Seizures are occasionally present as part of the phenotype
Vitamin B_1 (thiamine)	Vitamin B_1 deficiency (various causes)	Seizures are occasionally present as part of the phenotype
Liver function tests	POLG related disorders	Regression with seizures and myoclonus
	Hepatic failure of various causes (including alcoholic liver disease)	Variable phenotype frequently with epilepsy and/or myoclonus
Renal function tests	Renal failure of various causes	Seizures are occasionally present as part of the phenotype
Thyroid function levels	Hypothyroidism	Presentation with other features and on occasion seizures
Uric acid	Disorders of purine metabolism (e.g. Lesch–Nyhan syndrome)	Psychomotor retardation and epilepsy
Enzyme activities: for instance, hexosaminidase A and B	Hexosaminidase deficiencies	Wide neurological phenotype with occasional epilepsy

genotype can result in different phenotypes (phenotypic heterogeneity) and identical phenotypes may be due to different genotypes (genetic heterogeneity).

Pure epilepsies

There are a number of so-called 'pure epilepsies' in which epilepsy is the only or the predominant feature of the genetic defect (15 genes have been identified). Some of these syndromes are shown in Table 11.9. Genetic testing of the *SCN1A* gene is fairly widely available, but not of the other genes. These are all familial epilepsies, and are rare (sometimes only reported in a single family), and these genes are not routinely tested.

Cortical dysplasias

In some patients with epilepsy, a cortical dysplasia can be identified. Some have intellectual impairment or other neurological signs, but in others epilepsy can be the only or the most prominent findings. Some of the genes associated with cortical dysplasia are shown

Table 11.4 The diagnostic tests in the acute porphyrias associated with epilepsy

	Urine ALA and PBG levels	Urine porphyrin levels	Faecal porphyrin levels	Red cell porphyrin levels
Acute intermittent porphyria	Normal	Increased URO (may be normal if not in an acute attack)	Normal	Normal
Variegate porphyria	Increased (may be normal if not in an acute attack)	Increased COPRO	Increased CPPRO and PROTO	Normal
Hereditary coproporphyria	Increased (may be normal if not in an acute attack)	Increased COPRO	Increased CPPRO	Normal

ALA, amino levulinic acid; COPRO, coproporphyrins; PBG, porphobilinogen; PROTO, protoporphyrins; URO, uroporphyrins.

From Dean G, Shorvon S. Porphyria. In: Shorvon SD, Guerrini R, Andermann F. *The Causes of Epilepsy: common and uncommon causes in adults and children*, pp. 231–6. Cambridge: Cambridge University Press, 2011.

Table 11.5 Haematological tests that can be helpful in determining the cause of epilepsy

Investigation	Condition being tested for	Clinical epilepsy presentation
Full blood count, differential	Various disorders	Abnormalities are associated with a variety of conditions which can result in epilepsy, and should prompt an extensive search, both for primary conditions and also for conditions in which abnormalities are secondary consequences of other disorders
Acanthocytes	Neuroacanthocytosis	Progressive myoclonic epilepsy, other neurological signs
Macrocytosis	B_{12} and folate deficiency and alcoholism	Seizures are an occasional feature of B_{12} or folate deficiency, and are common in alcoholism
Sickle-cell	Sickle-cell disease and sickle cell trait	Seizures can result from cerebrovascular consequences
White cell count and differential	Various haematological, immunological, infective disorders	Seizures can be a symptom in a variety of disorders of white-cell production and also lymphomas
Vacuolated lymphocytes	Lysosomal storage disorders including the neuronal ceroid lipofuscinoses and the sphingolipidoses	The neuronal lipofuscinoses can present as progressive myoclonic epilepsy, seizures are less common features of lysosomal disorders
Platelet abnormalities and other abnormalities of the clotting cascade	Various disorders	Seizures can be a symptom in a variety of haematological and clotting disorders, leading to haemorrhagic stroke or sinus thrombosis. Autoimmune thrombocytopenia. Vitamin K deficiency in neonates

Table 11.6 Tests of the cerebrospinal fluid that can be helpful in determining the cause of epilepsy

Investigation	Conditions being tested for	Clinical epilepsy presentation
Alpha-aminoadipic semialdehyde (α-AASA)	Pyridoxine deficient seizures	Neonatal seizures and refractory seizures in childhood
Serine and glycine	Disorders of serine biosynthesis	Neonatal seizures and encephalopathies
Glucose	GLUT-1 deficiency	Epilepsy, myoclonus, regression, behavioural and movement disorders
Lactate	Mitochondrial disorders (various types)	Acute encephalopathy with seizures, myoclonic seizures, other neurological signs
5-methyl-tetrahydrofolate (5-MTHF)	Cerebral folate deficiency states (e.g. 5-MTHF reductase deficiency)	Epilepsy, regression, and other neurological signs
Pyridoxal 5′-phosphate (PLP)	Pyridox(am)ine phosphate oxidase (PNPO) deficiency	Neonatal seizures

CSF creatine can be used diagnostically, but now is replaced by largely MRS and the estimation of GAA and creatine in urine.

Table 11.7 Histological tests which can be helpful in identifying the cause of epilepsy

Tissue	Conditions being tested for	Comments
Brain	Otherwise undiagnosed structural or degenerative disorders of brain: examples include cerebral tumours, infective lesions, inflammatory lesions, cerebral malformations, mitochondrial and other genetic disorders, SSPE where CSF is negative, Rasmussen's encephalitis, Creutzfeldt–Jakob disease, primary cerebral or granulomatous disorders	Neurological features in which epilepsy is often a prominent feature.
Bone marrow	Niemann–Pick type C, malignancies, and marrow aplasia	In Niemann-Pick type C, the marrow characteristically shows sea-blue histiocytes and foamy cells
Conjunctiva	Mucoliposis IV	Multilaminate bodies—but this test is now rarely used
Hair	Menkes disease	Epilepsy is a feature associated with other neurological features
Liver (including copper assay)	Wilson disease	Epilepsy is an occasional symptom associated with other features
Liver (including respiratory chain analysis and electron microscopy)	Mitochondrial disease	Hepatic failure can be a presenting feature, and epilepsy can be present
Muscle (including respiratory chain enzyme analysis)	Mitochondrial disease	Epilepsy amongst other neurological features. Also, progressive myoclonic epilepsy
Liver biopsy	Glycogen storage diseases, SLE, and other systemic diseases	Neurological features can include epilepsy
Skin	Lafora body disease, SLE, neurofibromatosis, and other systemic diseases	A cause of progressive myoclonic epilepsy
Fibroblasts—for assay of enzymes	Many enzymes (including: methylmalonic CoA mutase and methionine synthetase, methylcobalamin and adenosylcobamain synthesis)	

Table 11.8 Immunological tests which can be helpful in identifying the cause of epilepsy

Test	Conditions being tested for	Comments
Antiadenylate kinase 5 antibodies	Limbic encephalitis	Reported very rarely
Antiglycine receptor antibodies	Limbic encephalitis	Reported very rarely
Antinuclear antibodies (ANA), aniphospholipid antibodies (aPL), LA (lupus anticoagulant), antiglutamate receptor antibodies, anti-NR2 antibodies, anti-N-methyl-D-aspartate (NMDA) antibodies	Systemic lupus erythematosus and antiphospholipid syndrome (and other collagen vascular diseases)	Lupus not infrequently presents as epilepsy
Anti- NMDA antibodies	Acute encephalopathy and limbic encephalitis (often associated with ovarian teratoma)	Presents with characteristic form of status epilepticus
Anti-*Saccharomyces cerevisiae antibodies*	Crohn's disease	Seizures rare in Crohn's disease
IgA antibodies to endomysium, gliadin and reticulin	Coeliac disease	Highly sensitive and specific (but can be negative in cases on dietary treatment)
Oligoclonal bands in CSF (unmatched in serum)	Various auto-immune and infective and para-infective disorders, multiple sclerosis	Oligoclonal bands (unmatched in serum) imply immunological cause but not specific
Oligoclonal bands in CSF	Rasmussen's encephalitis	Positive in only some cases
Protoplasmic staining antineutrophil cytoplasmic antibodies (p-ANCA)	Ulcerative colitis	Epilepsy rare in ulcerative colitis
Thyroid peroxidase antibodies (TPO)	Hashimoto encephalitis (steroid responsive encephalopathy associated with auto-immune thyroiditis; STREAT)	Seizures and status are common presentations of Hashimoto's encephalitis
Voltage-gated potassium channel antibodies (VGKC)	Limbic encephalitis	
Intracellular antibodies (e.g. anti-Hu, anti-Ma-2, etc)	Limbic encephalitis, especially paraneoplastic	
Antibodies against glutamic acid decarboxylase (anti-GAD antibodies)	Stiff person syndrome, and other neurological syndromes	
Other antineuronal antibodies		

Table 11.9 Pure epilepsies—genetic abnormalities

Syndrome	Commonly involved genes
Generalized epilepsy with febrile seizures plus (GEFS+)	*SCN1A, SCN1B, GABRG2*
Severe myoclonic epilepsy of infancy (SMEI; Dravet syndrome)	*SCN1A, GABRG2*
Benign familial neonatal seizures (BFNS)	*KCNQ2, KNCQ3*
Benign familial neonatal-infantile seizures (BFNIS)	*SCN2A*
Autosomal dominant nocturnal frontal lobe epilepsy (ADNFLE)	*CHRNA4, CHRNB2, CHRNA2*
Autosomal dominant temporal lobe epilepsy	*LGI1*

Note: other pure epilepsy genes include: *KCNA1, GABRA1, EFCH1, PCDH19, ATP1A2.*

Table 11.10 Cortical dysplasia—gene mutations

Type of cortical dysplasia	Genes carrying mutations
Agyria–pachygyria, band spectrum and lissencephaly (various types)	*LIS1, DCX, ARX, RELN, TUBA1A, POMT1, POMT2, FKRP, FKTN*
Periventricular nodular heterotopia	*FLNA*
Periventricular nodular heterotopia with other associations	*FMR1, ARFGEF2, LRP2, KIAA1803, ASXL2*
Polymicrogyria (various types)	*SRPX2, TBR2, PAX6, TUBB2B, GPRS6, RAB3GAP1, KIAA1279, COL19A1*
Schizencephaly	*EMX2*
Tuberous sclerosis	
Agenesis of the corpus callosum	*ARX, ZEB2, 1q44 deletions,*

in Table 11.10, but a few of these are relatively routinely tested as the diagnosis is usually made by neuroimaging or neuropathology.

Progressive myoclonic epilepsies

This is a syndrome which is often susceptible to genetic testing. The common causes and the genetic and laboratory tests are summarized in Table 11.11.

Syndromes with chromosomal disorders

Epilepsy is sometimes a feature of chromosomal disorders which can be detected by karyotyping. All are invariably associated with learning disability (usually severe) and other clinical features. The most commonly identifiable are shown in Table 11.12. Genetic and prenatal testing are widely available. Where mosaicism is common,

Table 11.11 The progressive myoclonic epilepsies (PMEs)

Disease		Age at onset	Suggestive clinical features	Suggestive laboratory features	Genetics	Gene
Unverricht–Lundborg disease		8–13 years	Myoclonus, mild dementia and ataxia	None identified	AR	*EPM1*
Lafora body disease		10–18 years	Severe myoclonus, occipital seizures, inexorable dementia, Lafora bodies	Lafora bodies in axillary skin biopsies	AR	*EPM2A EPM2B*
Myoclonus epilepsy and ragged red fibres (MERRF)		Variable	Deafness, optic atrophy, myopathy, myoclonus	Muscle biopsy showing ragged red fibres and histochemical changes. Also, increased level of pyruvate and lactate (blood and CSF)	Mitochondrial	*tRNAlys*
Sialidoses	Type I	8–20 years	Severe myoclonus, tonic–clonic seizures, ataxia, cherry-red spot, visual failure	Elevated urinary sialyloligosaccharides, deficiency of neuroaminidase in leucocytes and cultured skin fibroblasts	AR	*NEU*
	Type II	10–30 years	Severe myoclonus, ataxia, cherry-red spot, visual failure, dysmorphic features, hearing loss	Elevated urinary sialyloligosaccharides, deficiency of neuroaminidase and b-galactosidase in leucocytes and cultured skin fibroblasts	AR	*PPGB*
Neuronal ceroid lipofuscinoses	CLN2	2.4–4 years	Myoclonic, tonic–clonic, atonic or atypical absence seizures, psychomotor delay and ataxia, visual failure	Curvilinear, rectilinear or fingerprint lipidic inclusions in skin biopsy at electron microscopy	AR	*TPP1*
	CNL3	5–10 years	Myoclonus and tonic–clonic seizures, macular degeneration, optic atrophy, dementia		AR	*CLN3*
	CNL4	15–50 years	Generalized seizures, myoclonic jerks, extrapyramidal symptoms		AR/AD	–
Dentato-rubro-pallido-luysian atrophy (DRPLA)		Variable	Seizures, myoclonus, ataxia, chorea, dementia	None identified	AD	*ATN1 (CAG repeat disorder)*

NB These are the more common causes of this rare syndrome. A similar clinical picture of can also be due to other conditions, although often with other features present. Conditions which have been reported include: biotin-responsive progressive myoclonus; infantile and other variants of neuronal ceroid lipofuscinosis; coeliac disease; Gaucher disease; GM2 gangliosidosis (juvenile type); hexosaminidase deficiency; Huntington disease; Hallervorden–Spatz disease; neuroserpin inclusion body disease; juvenile neuroaxonal dystrophy; Menkes disease.

Adapted from: Shorvon S. *Handbook of Epilepsy Treatment*. Oxford: Wiley-Blackwell Publishing, 2010

Table 11.12 Some chromosomal disorders causing epilepsy

Down syndrome (trisomy 21)
Fragile X syndrome (loss of function mutation of *FMR1* gene)
Wolf–Hirschhorn syndrome (deletion of 4p)
Inc dup(15) syndrome (inverted duplicated chromosome 15)
Ring chromosome 20

for instance in Ring chromosome 20 Syndrome, at least 100 mitoses may need to be examined before excluding the condition.

Neurocutaneous syndromes

There are two common neurocutaneous syndromes, causing epilepsy, with a known genetic basis—tuberous sclerosis and neurofibromatosis type 1. Approximately 85% of patients with tuberose sclerosis can be found to have a mutation in either the *TSC1* or *TSC2* genes. Molecular genetic testing for diagnostic confirmation and prenatal testing of the *TSC1* and *TSC2* genes is available but complicated by the large size of the two genes, the large number of disease-causing mutations, and the high rate of somatic mosaicism (10–25%). Other screening tests include: clinical examination, dermatological examination and examination with Wood's light, biopsy, ophthalmological examination, renal ultrasound, and other imaging. Mutations in the *NF1* gene is the cause of neurofibromatosis type 1. Genetic linkage has been found in other much rarer neurocutaneous syndromes including: hypomelanosis of Ito, incontinentia pigment, nevus sebaceous syndrome, and Parry–Romberg syndrome.

Other single-gene disorders resulting in epilepsy

There are over 120 single gene disorders which result in epilepsy, and in which the gene has been identified. Some of the more common disorders, for which genetic testing is available, are listed in Table 11.13. Almost all are associated with intellectual impairment and often with other neurological features. DNA analysis can be carried out for all these conditions, although alternative methods of diagnosis (clinical and biochemical) are more commonly employed in many cases.

Some illustrative examples of single-gene disorders of metabolism

These examples are given here to illustrate the complexity of single-gene disorders which can cause epilepsy. These conditions are all rare, often have a family history, present usually in infancy or childhood and are associated with a constellation of neurological and non-neurological features. There diagnostic evaluation should be conducted in specialized paediatric units with expertise in clinical biochemistry, neuropathology, and neurogenetics.

Urea cycle disorders

There are six inherited urea cycle defects, in which deficiency can produce seizures: N-acetyl glutamate synthetase (NAGS; a cofactor), carbamoylphosphate synthetase I deficiency (CPS1 deficiency), ornithine transcarbamylase deficiency (OTC deficiency), citrulinemia type 1 (ASS1 deficiency), argininosuccinic aciduria (ASL deficiency), arginase deficiency (hyperargininaemia; ARG deficiency). Defects

Table 11.13 Other single-gene disorders causing epilepsy

Condition	Gene
Angelman syndrome[a]	*UBE3A* (due to deletions in 15q11–q13 region)
Lysosomal storage or transport disorders	Various
Neuroacanthocytosis	*VPS13A*
Organic acid, amino acid and peroxisomal disorders	Various
Porphyria	*ALAD, ALAS2, CPOX, FECH, HMBS, PPOX, UROD, or UROS.*
Pyridoxine-dependent epilepsy	*ALDH7A1, PNPO*
Rett syndrome	*MECP2. CDKL5*
Urea cycle disorders	*CPS1, OTC. ASS1, ASL, ARG1, NAGS*
Wilson disease	*ATP7B*
Inherited disorders of cobalamin and folate metabolism[b]	*MMACHC, MMADHC, MTRR, LMBRD1, MTR, SLC46A1, FTCD, MTHFR, GRT*

[a] In about 80% of cases defects are present in the chromosome 15q11–q13 region, and involve a deletion, maternal disomy, imprinting defect or rarely translocation. This region contains a cluster of GABA receptor subunit genes. Iatrogenic mutations in the *UBE3A* gene are found in about 10% of cases. Diagnostic genetic testing is available. About 80% of cases can be identified via the methylation test, and mutation testing of the *UBE3A* gene can be used in cases where the methylation test is negative.

[b] Two inherited disorders of folate and seven inherited disorders of cobalamin deficiency are recognized. Seizures can occur in any of these, although are generally more prominent in the folate deficiency states.

result in the failure to metabolize nitrogen from the breakdown of protein. Severe deficiency results in infantile death, but milder or partial deficiency can present at any age. Typical symptoms include a loss of appetite, vomiting, lethargy, seizures, disorders of sleep, behavioural change, delusions, hallucinations and psychosis. The EEG shows an encephalopathic pattern. Diagnosis is made by the finding of a high plasma ammonia (>150 μmol/L), with normal plasma sugar and anion gap, in the presence of a chronic or subacute encephalopathy. Measurements of plasma amino acids analysis (citrulline, arginine, alanine, asparagine, glutamine) and urinary orotic acid can distinguish between the specific disorders, The definitive diagnosis is by molecular genetic analysis

Peroxisomal disorders

The peroxisome is an organelle present in almost all nucleated cells. It is responsible for the metabolism of fatty acids and phospholipids amongst other metabolic processes. Seizures are common in some of these conditions, but are invariably associated with other prominent and severe neurological features (the range of symptoms depend on the specific defect). There are 17 peroxisomal disorders, which have been categorized into four diagnostic groups. Those in which epilepsy is a particularly prominent symptom are Zellweger syndrome, the adrenoleucodystrophies, and glutaric aciduria type III.

1. Peroxisome biogenesis disorders (PBDs)—these include: cerebro-hepatic-renal (Zellweger) syndrome (ZS, ZWS1), neonatal adrenoleucodystrophy (NALD), and infantile Refsum disease (IRD). In these disorders the process of peroxisomal assembly is

disrupted and all peroxisomal function is absent or deficient. In all these, plasma concentrations of VLCFAs (very long chain fatty acids) are elevated. Other biochemical abnormalities (including erythrocyte plasmalogen, plasma bile-acid intermediates, pristanic acid, and phytanic acid) can be detected in blood and or urine and confirmed in cultured fibroblasts.

2. Rhizomelic chondrodysplasia punctata (RCDP; three types). In these cases, plasmalogen level in erythrocytes is the diagnostic test, confirmed by enzyme analysis and DNA analysis.
3. All types of X-linked adrenoleucodystrophy (X-ALD). These are most common peroxisomal disorder and the diagnostic screening test is elevated VLCFAs followed by molecular analysis.
4. Refsum, AMACR (alpha-methylacyl-CoA racemase), hyperoxaluria type I, glutaric aciduria type III, mevalonate kinase deficiency, acatalasaemia. These conditions are heterogenous. In Refsum disease, an elevated serum level of phytanic acid is reliable in diagnosis. Liver biopsy is needed in hyperoxaluria type I for enzymatic assay. In glutaric aciduria type III, there is persistent elevation of glutaric acid excretion. In mevalonate kinase deficiency there is increased urinary excretion of mevalonic acid. In AMACR increased levels of pristanic acid can be detected and confirmed by enzymatic and molecular assays.

Lysosomal storage disorders

More than 50 lysosomal storage disorders exist. These include: the glycogen storage diseases, the mucopolysaccharidoses, the mucolipidoses, the oligosaccharidoses (including sialidosis), lipidoses (including Niemann–Pick disease types C and D, and NCL), sphingolipidoses (including: Niemann–Pick disease types A and B, Gaucher, Krabbe, Fabry, GM1 and GM2 gangliosidosis, metachromatic leucodystrophy galactosialidosis) and lysosomal transport diseases. The conditions are characterized by progressive neurological disorders with symptoms which include epilepsy, developmental delay, hypotonia, epilepsy (complex partial or myoclonic), peripheral neuropathy, intellectual disability, ataxia, and/or spasticity. There are also dysmorphic features, bony abnormalities, organomegaly, cardiac and ophthalmic signs. Screening can be performed via skeletal radiography to look for evidence of dysostosis multiplex, abdominal ultrasonography to identify hepatosplenomegaly, and echocardiography to evaluate for cardiac involvement. Ophthalmologic examination may reveal corneal clouding or cherry-red spot. A peripheral blood smear may reveal white blood cell vacuoles (granular, fingerprint lipid whorls, zebra bodies, or autophagic vacuoles). Urine can be screened for elevated excretion of oligosaccharides (oligosaccharidoses) and glycosaminoglycans (mucopolysaccharidoses). Blood chitotriosidase (an enzymatic marker of macrophage activation) may be elevated. Assay of enzymatic activity in peripheral white blood cells provides a definitive diagnosis. Confirmatory DNA mutation analysis can helpful.

Probably the most common of these diseases causing epilepsy is Neimann–Pick Type C, and the diagnosis is confirmed by bone marrow biopsy which shows lipid-laden histiocytes, the biochemical demonstration of impaired cholesterol esterification and positive filipin staining in cultured fibroblasts.

Acknowledgements

This work was undertaken at UCLH/UCL who received a proportion of funding from the Department of Health's NIHR Biomedical Research Centres funding scheme.

Further reading

The following are general sources for, and provide further details of, the investigations listed in this chapter:

Human Metabolome Database: http://www.hmdb.ca

King MD, Stephenson JBP. *A handbook of neurological investigation in children.* Oxford: Wiley-Blackwell, 2009.

Metabolic and genetic disease information centre: http://www.metagene.de/program/s.prg?id=1943

OMIM, Online Mendelian Inheritance in Man: http://www.ncbi.nlm.nih.gov/omim

Shorvon SD. *Handbook of the treatment of epilepsy* (3rd edn). Oxford: Wiley-Blackwell Publishing, 2010.

Shorvon SD, Guerrini R, Andermann F. *The Causes of Epilepsy: Common and uncommon causes in adults and children.* Cambridge:Cambridge University Press, 2011.

CHAPTER 12

Non-Pharmacological Therapy of Epilepsy

Peter Wolf, Katia Lin, and Marina Nikanorova

Epilepsy may be defined conceptually as 'an enduring predisposition to generate seizures' requiring 'the occurrence of at least one epileptic seizure' (1) or operationally as 'a condition characterized by recurrent unprovoked seizures' (2). Both definitions imply an indication for treatment but not for a specific type of treatment. Pharmacotherapy, if possible with one antiepileptic drug (AED) in monotherapy, is considered the standard treatment for the majority of the affected persons. The method of continuous administration of AEDs is closely related to the view that epileptic seizures are spontaneous and unpredictable. This may be correct in most cases but other possibilities exist and allow different approaches addressing the prevention or arrest of individual seizure events by various means.

In some patients, pharmacotherapy fails (3) and treatment alternatives become desirable. Surgical treatment and stimulation methods have their own chapters in this book, but specific diets are another possibility and are in some cases more effective than drugs.

The widely varied approaches which are the subject of this chapter, have in common that they give the patients a much more active role in the treatment of their condition than both drug treatment and surgery.

Individual seizures as targets of intervention

Theoretical background

A diagnosis of epilepsy does not indicate that the seizure susceptibility of the affected individual is always more or less identical. Some people have seizures only in sleep, others only soon after waking up. Cyclic recurrence of seizures is a well-known pattern where a few days of high seizure susceptibility alternate with intervals of up to some weeks without seizures. In women, seizure susceptibility may be related to the menstrual cycle, which is called catamenial epilepsy (4).

In addition, exogenous modulators of seizure activity exist, such as disturbances of sleep–waking cycle, increased alcohol intake, or extraordinary stress (5, 6). Lifestyle issues such as social habits like party-going, or long-distance air travel may be relevant (7). Therapeutic interventions can focus on endogenous and exogenous facilitating factors of seizures.

Generalized tonic–clonic seizures (GTCSs) may start with prodromes (8), a series of minor seizure-like absences or myoclonic seizures, or auras of variable length. Intervention may be possible during the prodromal phase to prevent the convulsive seizures.

In an important group of patients, seizures are habitually and reproducibly precipitated by specific sensory or cognitive stimuli, which is termed reflex epilepsy (9). The most common and best-known variety is photosensitivity (10). It is less well known that the same triggers can also inhibit seizures (11). Prevention and inhibition of reflex seizures is another possible non-pharmacological approach to the treatment of epilepsy.

Behaviour modification

The comprehensive care of people with epilepsy (PWE) should start with careful history taking and the thorough identification of seizure-inducing factors, which may alert the patient to the importance of such factors and how to avoid them, or to take specific countermeasures that may prevent a seizure. Habitual triggering factors of seizures include irregular sleep habits, inconsiderate consumption of alcoholic beverages and recreational drugs, excessive psychophysical stress, and others. According to Aird (5) addressing these factors contributed to 'appreciable benefit' in 43%, and seizure control in 17% of 500 patients with refractory seizures. Instructions on these aspects are a central part of a patient education programme that in a controlled investigation has been shown to significantly improve treatment success (12). This approach depends, as much as pharmacotherapy, on patients' adherence to the regimen. But many patients appreciate being given some responsibility for their treatment and cooperate very well.

Typically, this approach is part of a comprehensive therapy programme. Here it can make the difference between becoming seizure free or not, and can sometimes ensure success with a lower dose of AEDs. In selected patient groups, behaviour modification may be the only treatment.

Of 25 prospective patients who, for various reasons (AED failure in 11), did not accept pharmacotherapy (6), 16 were advised and instructed about systematic avoidance of seizure-provoking factors. After follow-up for 2 years or more, seven of them had remained seizure free. Most responders had mild idiopathic generalized epilepsies.

Table 12.1 Possible applications of acute drug administration

- *Status epilepticus*, any type
- Febrile (and non-febrile) convulsions in children
- Seizure clusters (habitual or at AED withdrawal)
- Catamenial epilepsy
- Prophylaxis of seizures at perceived risk:
  - AED withdrawal
  - Lifestyle situations
  - Unavoidable disturbance of sleep
  - Long-distance travel
  - Reflex seizures
- Individual triggers
- Response to 'warnings'
- Getting prepared for a situation where a seizure must by no means occur (job interview, social occasions)

Acute drug administration

Strictly speaking, acute drug administration (ADA) is not a non-pharmacological therapy, but it is fundamentally different from usual antiepileptic pharmacotherapy, and primarily a variety of behavioural intervention because it is based on the patients' (and their carers') identification of an imminent risk, and their response to it.

The topic was recently reviewed by Wolf (13). Apart from *status epilepticus*, the indications are listed in Table 12.1. ADA is most often used in combination with continuous AED treatment where it can make the difference between becoming seizure free or not; allow for a lower dose of continuous AEDs; or prevent clusters of seizures and prolonged seizures (e.g. prolonged febrile seizures). ADA can be used as monotherapy in the occasional instances that all seizures occur in situations of identified risk where they can be prevented (14).

The drugs used for ADA in the vast majority are benzodiazepines (BZDs), i.e. drugs with a strong antiepileptic action that are not commonly used for continuous AED treatment because of frequent development of secondary tolerance. The choice of BZDs will depend upon their routes of administration, speed and duration of their action, and their availability (not all BZDs are available in all countries). Intravenous administration is not considered here. Some basic pharmacokinetic facts for the choice of drug are presented in Table 12.2.

- Oral clobazam or diazepam is indicated when no immediate effect is required but medium duration action is desired: seizure prevention at perceived risks (sleep deprivation, jet lag, party, etc.) or preparing for socially sensitive situations; prevention of clusters of seizures after a first seizure.
- Rectal diazepam or clonazepam is used when rapid effect is required: prolonged febrile (and non-febrile) seizures; incipient *status epilepticus*; prevention of impending convulsive seizure at identified prodromes of any kind.
- Buccal or nasal midazolam or lorazepam: same indications as rectal diazepam but with circumstances where this route of administration is more rapid, easier to apply, or better acceptable. Midazolam when very short action is desired.

Arrest of incipient seizure activity

The seizure events of some patients don't have a rapid or immediate onset but evolve over periods of seconds to some minutes, sometimes more. This applies both to generalized and focal epilepsies.

The GTCSs of some patients with idiopathic generalized epilepsy are habitually preceded by repetitive absences or myoclonic seizures. If patients or their carers are aware of this relationship, they can use the minor seizures as an indicator of an impending convulsive seizure and possibly prevent it. Which acute drug is used will depend on what, in the patient's experience, is the shortest interval between the onset of minor seizures and the GTCS. If it is less than 20–30 minutes, rectal, buccal or nasal BZD administration would apply. If it is longer, an oral BZD will be used.

Focal seizures typically originate in a restricted local neuronal network from where they spread to other parts in the same hemisphere, sometimes to both. This evolution takes an amount of time which interindividually is variable but intraindividually rather constant and can sometimes be used to intervene, typically with a rapidly acting BZD. However, even the very rapid routes of BZD administration take some 3–5 min to act effectively, which is too slow for many of these situations, and interventions with more immediate impact would be welcome.

It is known that about two-thirds of patients with focal epilepsies develop spontaneous manoeuvres to arrest or counteract incipient seizures (15, 16), in up to 80% with success (17). This was a well-established therapeutic approach before the advent of modern pharmacotherapy (18) and is still a treatment option for the rare patients who decline AED therapy (6). Successful cure of epilepsy with systematic seizure arrest by an olfactory stimulus was described in detail by Efron (19, 20).

Table 12.2 Pharmacokinetic key data

Drug	Route	Onset action	Peak level	Half-life
Diazepam	Oral	15–20 min	30–60 min	20–50 hrs
	Rectal	<5 min	10–20 min	20–50 hrs
Clonazepam	Rectal	6–10 min	10–40 min	20–50 hrs
Clobazam[a]	Oral	15–20 min	1–2.5 hrs	20–40 hrs
Midazolam	Buccal	<5 min	20–30 min	1–3 hrs
Lorazepam	Nasal	<5 min	15–60 min	12–16 hrs

[a] Slow active metabolite.

Seizure prodromes

The term prodrome is used for 'warnings' that in some patients habitually precede a seizure for more than 1 hour. In the majority, they express minimal or 'subclinical' status-like seizure activity such as absence status or aura status (8). Prodromes offer excellent conditions for ADA with an oral BZD. In practice, it is often necessary to get relatives or carers involved because reduced awareness and reactivity may be part of the prodromal symptoms.

Reflex seizures and reflex epilepsies

The reproducibility of some patients' seizures by well-defined triggers can sometimes provide possibilities of targeted prevention.

Definition, precipitating stimuli, clinical manifestations, and diagnosis

Reflex seizures

Reflex, stimulus-sensitive, triggered, or sensory-evoked epileptic seizures are synonyms (21) and they represent seizures that are 'objectively and consistently evoked by a specific afferent stimulus or by activity of the patient' (22). The afferent stimuli may be elementary/unstructured (e.g. light flashes) or elaborated/structured (e.g. a particular musical work). Activities may be elementary (e.g. a particular movement) or elaborate (e.g. involving visuomotor coordination) (22). Reflex seizures may occur in patients with focal and generalized epilepsy syndromes who also get spontaneous seizures. Isolated reflex seizures can also occur in situations that do not necessarily require a diagnosis of epilepsy (21).

Visual stimuli are the most common external factors triggering seizures in humans. They may include: flickering lights/intermittent photic stimulation, flickering sunlight, artificial light, television, Pokémon cartoon, videogames; and also, specific visual patterns (geometric), striped patterns as from Venetian blind, clothes (23–25). In addition, many other precipitating stimuli were also described: higher mental activities such as calculation, reading, speaking, writing, and other language functions, praxis, thinking, decision-making, and neuropsychological electroencephalogram (EEG) activation (26–30); unexpected touch or noise and startle (31); somatosensory or proprioceptive stimuli; micturition (32, 33); music (34); eating (35); tooth-brushing (36); and hot water. Reflex epileptic mechanisms were recently extensively reviewed by Wolf and Koepp (9).

The epileptic response may consist of clinical seizures—generalized (absences, myoclonia, GTCSs) or focal (e.g. visual, motor, or somatosensory)—or of epileptiform EEG patterns (subclinical or ictal), alone or in combination. The role of the EEG is fundamental in establishing the relationship between the precipitating stimulus and the reflex seizures (21).

Reflex triggers of seizures need to be distinguished from factors that temporarily increase seizure propensity such as intense emotional stress, sleep deprivation and tiredness, fever, menstruation, alcohol consumption, and many others.

Reflex epilepsies

Reflex epilepsies constitute epileptic syndromes in which all epileptic seizures are precipitated by sensory stimuli, and the 2006 International League Against Epilepsy Commission on Classification and Terminology Report (37) listed idiopathic photosensitive occipital lobe epilepsy (IPOLE), primary reading epilepsy (PRE), and hot-water epilepsy (HWE) as reflex epilepsies. These are summarized in Table 12.3, but there may be others. A variety of HWE in infants was described by Plouin and Vigevano (48), and the large population of photosensitive subjects includes a small group with triggered GTCS only and no spontaneous seizures. These are generally not considered as representing a separate syndrome but may be therapeutically addressed differently from patients with both spontaneous and reflex seizures.

Pathophysiology of reflex epileptic ictogenesis

With elementary stimuli the latency from the stimulus onset to the clinical or EEG response is typically short (1–3 seconds) and with complex stimuli, longer (usually some up to many minutes).

A complex interaction between factors and stimuli from the endogenous (e.g. hormones, electrolytes, state of consciousness, and body temperature) and exogenous environment (e.g. sensory, electrical, and biochemical) may lower the seizure threshold, selectively activate ictogenesis in specific hyperexcitable cortical systems or functional networks, and provoke the initiation of a seizure (21, 49, 50).

Whereas the anatomical substrate of ictogenesis in many reflex epilepsies remains poorly understood, in others recent EEG and sophisticated neuroimaging studies (positron emission tomography, single-photon emission computed tomography, EEG/electromyography-functional magnetic resonance imaging) have highlighted the important role of corticoreticular and corticocortical circuitry, including the occipitotemporal regions in the generation of seizures in PRE (41, 51), photoparoxysmal response generated in an hyperexcitable occipital cortex and participation of frontorolandic regions in IPOLE (10, 24), ictal hypermetabolic uptake in the medial temporal structures and hypothalamus in HWE (52), these areas correspond only to a part of the neural network that underlies the function of reading, vision, or thermoregulation, which are complex processes that comprise different functions of the brain and are integrated into a network that expands over different brain areas. According to Moeller et al. (53), the generation of spikes and waves in the photoparoxysmal response is an intracortical event different from the corticothalamic circuit producing spontaneous spikes and waves in absence epilepsies. Considering these aspects, reflex epilepsies could be considered excellent models of 'system epilepsies', in which seizures are the result of hyperexcitability of a network of either genetic or acquired origin, with possible age-related clinical expression, and give rise to an epileptic process after the stimulus specific for that area is applied (30, 49, 54, 55).

The importance of reflex mechanisms recognition in the comprehensive treatment of patients with epilepsy

The arrest of seizure activity at the stage of the aura (i.e. at the stage of locally restricted neuronal discharge) can be achieved both by non-specific (i.e. relaxation, concentration techniques or both, biofeedback, vagal nerve stimulation) and by specific focus-targeted sensory or cognitive inputs. Specific focus-targeted inputs activate circumscribed cortical areas that are not yet involved in the epileptic discharge but are likely to become it during its spread from the primary epileptic focus to other areas and, eventually, both cerebral hemispheres (30, 49).

Table 12.3 Reflex epilepsy syndromes recognized by the ILAE Commission on Classification and Terminology Report (25)

	IPOLE (10, 21, 24, 37, 38)	PRE (27, 39, 40)	HWE (41–46)
Synonyms	–	–	Water-immersion epilepsy, bathing epilepsy
First reported	Guerrini et al. (1995)	Bickford et al. (1956)	Allen (1945)
Definition	All seizures induced by photic stimuli, particularly videogames and TV	Seizures occurring in relation to reading (especially aloud), progressing to a GTCS if stimulus continued	CFS precipitated by bathing with hot water (40–50°C) poured over the head
Prevalence	0.4% of all epilepsies	Very low	6.9% of all epilepsies in the Bangalore community (60/100,000)
Age of onset	Late childhood or puberty	Late puberty	13.4 ± 11.1 (SD) years (44)
M:F	1:2	1.8:1	2–2.5:1
Seizures	Auras of colourful elementary circular, bright or flashing, visual hallucinations often associated with conscious tonic head and eye version. Blurring of vision or blindness has also been reported. Visual symptoms may be isolated, usually lasting for seconds, frequently 1–3 min and rarely longer (5–15 min) in which case other symptoms also occur (autonomic, mainly retching and ictal vomiting, and, rarely, secondary GTCS)	SFS characterized by myoclonia in the jaw or orofacial muscles, sometimes with involvement of arms, progressing to a GTCS if reading continues. Occasionally, transient cognitive impairment with the jerks. Rarely partial seizures with ictal dyslexia or alexia, speech arrest. Bilateral brachial myoclonia may also occur. Absences uncommon	CFS with or without secondary GTCS, initiating with fixed look, fear, dysphasia, visual and auditory hallucinations associated with complex automatisms, lasting 30 s to 3 min. Primary GTCS have also been reported in 1/3 of cases
Neurological examination	Normal	Normal	Normal
EEG	Interictal: uni- or bilateral spontaneous synchronous or asynchronous occipital spikes or spike-waves and/or generalized spike and wave discharges Ictal: IPS (5–40 Hz) elicits abnormal EEG paroxysms of spikes or polyspikes confined to the occipital regions or generalized photoparoxysmal responses of spikes or polyspikes and slow waves that predominate in the posterior regions	Interictal: normal Ictal: very brief 3–6 Hz bilateral and synchronous spikes or spike-waves maximal in the dominant occipital and parietal areas, evoked paroxysmal rhythmic theta activity or spikes over one or both frontocentral, centroparietal, or temporoparietal regions in association with jaw jerks. The left > right hemisphere is involved when activity is unilateral, but bilateral jaw jerks may be associated with unilateral discharges. Also, uni-, bilateral or asymmetric myoclonia and bilaterally synchronous spike and wave activity may be associated	Interictal: usually normal, but 15–20% might show diffuse abnormalities, and lateralized or localized spike discharges Ictal: left or right temporal rhythmic delta activity, sharp and slow waves in the left hemisphere or bilateral spikes
Neuroimaging	No structural lesions on MRI	No structural lesions on MRI	No structural lesions on MRI
Genetics	Unclear—probably genetically determined	Unclear—probably genetically determined	Two gene loci described in families with autosomal dominant occurrence (45, 46)
Management	Avoidance of precipitating factors is essential, particularly to videogames and TV. Avoid stroboscope lights, looking away, covering one eye, wearing polarized or coloured glasses, watching TV from a distance of at least 2 m, viewing a 100 Hz television set are often effective. Sodium valproate, clonazepam, clobazam No deterioration in neurological status and good prognosis	Avoidance of precipitating factors. Valproate or small doses (0.5–1 mg) of clonazepam No deterioration in neurological status and good prognosis	Avoid precipitant stimuli (prefer warm water for a head bath or sponging with hot towels). Phenytoin or carbamazepine. Prophylaxis with benzodiazepines (clobazam 5–10 mg 1.5–2 h before a head bath) No deterioration in neurological status and good prognosis

CF, complex focal seizures; EEG, electroencephalogram; F, female; GTCS, generalized tonic–clonic seizures; HWE, hot-water epilepsy; ILAE, International League Against Epilepsy; IPOLE, idiopathic photosensitive occipital lobe epilepsy; IPS, intermittent photic stimulation; M, male; MRI, magnetic resonance imaging; PRE, primary reading epilepsy; SD, standard deviation; SFS, simple focal seizures

In some patients, the same stimulus can both precipitate and abort a seizure. The type of response to the stimulus largely depends on the state of cortical activation at the moment the input is given: while an input meeting a pool of potentially ictogenic neurons in the resting condition or at the intermediate state of activation of the neuronal membrane may precipitate a seizure; seizure interruption may occur when epileptic discharge has already begun or a critical mass of neurons responding to a stimulus strong enough may block the spread of seizure activity (49).

Because of their variability from patient to patient, as well as their variability with time in the same patient, combined with the emphasis on AED therapy in modern epilepsy care, the utility of these factors that may modify ictal susceptibility of patients has been neglected in the current management of PWE (5).

Specific non-pharmacological measures for prevention and inhibition of reflex seizures and epilepsies

Visually-induced seizures are by far the most common reflex seizures. Changes in luminance, contrast, pattern, and colour can provoke seizures in photosensitive individuals. Although no randomized controlled trials, or controlled comparative clinical trials to evaluate pharmacological and non-pharmacological treatments have been performed, data on efficacy depending on series of patients have allowed the implementation of diverse preventive measures for photosensitive epilepsies. The modern environment is a rich source of potentially seizure-triggering visual stimuli, to which people are increasingly exposed at all ages worldwide, such as televisions (TVs), computers, video games, discotheque lights, Venetian blinds, striped walls, rolling stairs, striped clothing, and sunlight reflected from snow or the sea or interrupted by trees during a ride in a car or train, dysfunctioning fluorescent lighting, etc. (10, 23, 25).

In these cases, avoidance of potentially provocative visual stimuli is the mainstay of treatment. Protection against the stimulus by its modification or attenuation has especially been used for photosensitivity. It was reviewed by Covanis et al. (56) and is summarized in Table 12.4. Successful use of dark and coloured glasses or filters has been described by several authors (57–60). For TV-sensitive patients, a 100 Hz screen is less provocative than a 50 Hz screen. (61).The effectiveness of stimulus avoidance and modification will depend on the individual's degree of photosensitivity (Table 12.4). Patients with seizures exclusively triggered by visual stimuli, such as TV or flickering sunlight (also called 'pure photosensitive epilepsy'), may be treated without AEDs. For most patients, however, non-pharmacological approaches are combined with AEDs, since avoidance of provocative visual stimuli in modern daily life is becoming increasingly difficult (56).

Deconditioning: rather systematic attempts at treating reflex epilepsies, such as photosensitive seizures, by deconditioning methods were undertaken with some success by Forster (62), who applied standardized methods of deconditioning, e.g. by starting intermittent photic stimulation with reduced light intensity or with subthreshold flickering frequencies and then gradually increasing the intensity. However, his findings were not replicated and are today largely forgotten. Wolf and Dockweiler (63) reported successful deconditioning in a patient with tonic versive seizures precipitated by touch. Deconditioning seems to be a useful approach in selected cases only and requires a tailored intervention taking care of the individual circumstances.

Table 12.4 Non-pharmacological preventive measures for visually induced seizures

- Looking away or avoiding the source of stimuli, such as discotheque lighting, striped clothing, and other striped patterns; sunlight on water; flickering sunlight; sudden changes in light and contrast; and flashing TV programmes and videogames (49)
- Closing or monocular occlusion with the palm of a hand so as to prevent light reaching the retina of one eye. Other alternative methods are the use of dark or coloured glasses (dark blue/green or precision tints), or the use of polarized glasses which are effective in reducing the diffusion of light (49, 50)
- Use small TV, 12-inch set and viewing from a distance of at least three times the width of the TV screen in a well-lit room (6, 49)
- Use preferably liquid crystal display computers or TV; 100 Hz TV set (120 Hz in North America) will increase the frequency of the flickering screen from 50 Hz (60 Hz in North America) to 100 Hz (120 Hz in North America) and make sensitivity to whole-screen flicker or the pattern of vibrating lines less likely and the image more stable (51)
- Use of temporal optical filters or video-hazard blocker to avoid TV flicker- and pattern-induced seizures (52, 53)
- Avoid adjusting the controls or fast-forwarding the video and keep at a distance from the screen by using remote control (49)

Behavioural therapy: antistress, cognitive behavioural therapy, and relaxation programmes were applied for preventing seizures precipitated by higher mental activities (64, 65).

Stimulus avoidance: most patients with PRE get a series of orofacial myocloni before developing a GTCS. They can learn to stop reading at the first myoclonus and thus avoid major seizures. This can be used as a monotherapeutic approach (27), but for patients who have experienced rapid development of GTCSs or who need to read a lot this is not sufficient and they will need pharmacotherapy.

Briefer and less vigorous tooth-brushing has been recommended for PWE with a slow precipitation of seizures only by vigorous tooth-brushing (36), and the introduction of an urinary catheter to suppress micturition-induced reflex seizures (32).

Stimulus attenuation and sensory protection: its role in photosensitivity is described in an earlier section. Patients with the infantile type of HWE (48) are susceptible to water with a temperature above 37.5°C. As these infants don't have spontaneous seizures and the condition is age-limited, treatment consisting in bathing them in water below this temperature is sufficient.

In the variety of HWE in older children, adolescents, and adults (42, 43), the patients get seizures when hot water is poured over their head ('head bath'). The non-pharmacological treatment consists of using lukewarm water for head bath or sponging the head with hot towels, avoiding pouring water over the head (66).

Acute drug prevention: Dhanaraj and Jayavelu (47) reported 10 patients with the last-mentioned type of HWE who were successfully treated only by intake of 10 mg clobazam 1½ hour before a head bath. However, with daily or *quasi*-daily application of clobazam, tolerance is likely to develop because of the accumulation of the active metabolite desmethylclobazam with a half-life of about 50 hours. Midazolam seems to be a better choice for this condition where it could be applied orally since no immediate action is required.

Diets

The history of the treatment of epilepsy starts many centuries before the advent of modern pharmacotherapy. Diets were an important part of therapy, and still after the introduction of the first effective AED, bromide, diets were discussed in textbooks in relation to theories about metabolic and nutritional causes of seizures (67). In a chronic condition with a substantial rate of pharmacoresistance, there will always be an interest in alternative treatments. On the Internet, always a mine of alternative approaches, recommendations can be found, e.g. of glutamate aspartate restricted diet, and a detailed discussion of nutritional factors supposed to have an influence on epilepsy and their possible control (68). One diet (with two variants) stands out because it is today scientifically well established.

The ketogenic diet

The ketogenic diet is a high-fat, low-to-adequate protein, low-carbohydrate diet which is used as a therapeutic alternative to AEDs in epilepsy treatment. Historically, fasting can be considered its precursor. The first modern use of starvation as a treatment for epilepsy was recorded in 1911 by two Parisian physicians, Guelpa and Marie, who treated 20 patients with epilepsy and reported the decrease of seizure severity during treatment. Later on, several similar attempts have been made in the US by Dr Hugh W. Conklin and Bernard Macfadden (69)

The beginning of ketogenic diet use in epilepsy treatment was in 1921, when Dr Wilder in the Mayo Clinic proposed producing ketonaemia by other means than fasting. He suggested that the diet should be as effective as fasting and could be maintained for a much longer period of time (69).

However, further development of the new AEDs, such as phenytoin and later valproate, was associated with a decline of interest in the ketogenic diet. Nevertheless, the ketogenic diet has experienced a re-emergence in recent years, and now it is available in more than 45 countries (69, 70).

Types of ketogenic diet

Three types of ketogenic diet are currently used for epilepsy treatment (71): the classical ketogenic diet, modified Atkins diet, and ketogenic diet with medium-chain triglycerides.

The classical ketogenic diet is constituted from normal foods and involves utilization of the long-chain triglycerides. It has a ratio of fat to protein plus carbohydrate of 4:1. The two other diets are less restrictive than the traditional ketogenic diet. The modified Atkins diet has a ketogenic ratio of 0.9:1, and the ketogenic diet with medium-chain triglycerides is a variant with the ketogenic ratio 1.2:1. It is an option for patients who can tolerate more calories, have a large appetite, or who cannot accept the restrictions of the classical ketogenic diet. All three types of the ketogenic diet showed comparable efficacy in the treatment of childhood epilepsy (72–74).

Indications for use

Although a ketogenic diet might be effective in a broad range of medically refractory epilepsies, it is most often used for the treatment of generalized epilepsies. The particular benefit of the ketogenic diet has been identified in myoclonic-astatic epilepsy, Dravet syndrome, and infantile spasms (71).

A ketogenic diet is effective in up to 54–60% of patients with myoclonic-astatic epilepsy (75–78). In the series of Oguni et al. (75), a significant decrease in myoclonic and atonic seizures was observed in 15 out of 26 patients. In the study by Caraballo et al. (77), after 18 months after the diet initiation two of six children became seizure-free, two demonstrated seizure reduction of 75% or more, and two patients of 50–74% reduction.

In Dravet syndrome, as shown in one case series, the ketogenic diet resulted in greater than 75% improvement in 50% of patients, while another case series showed greater than 50% improvement in seizure frequency in over 60% of children (79–81). However, all the studies were retrospective and in none of them was a direct comparison of the diet efficacy and AEDs performed.

A ketogenic diet might be also beneficial in infantile spasms refractory to vigabatrin and corticosteroids (81–83). A comparative assessment of the ketogenic diet versus adrenocorticotropic hormone (ACTH) demonstrated that complete seizure control after 1 month of therapy was achieved in 62% and 90% of children respectively. The ketogenic diet had fewer side effects than ACTH but ACTH normalized EEG more rapidly (83). In their prospective study, Hong et al. (82) reported that greater than 50% spasm improvement occurred in 64% of patients at 6 months and 77% after 1–2 years. Thirty-eight (37%) became spasm-free for at least a 6-month period within a median 2.4 months of starting the ketogenic diet.

Ketogenic diet is elective therapy for several metabolic conditions (71): glucose transporter type I (GLUT-I) deficiency, pyruvate dehydrogenase deficiency, phosphofruktokinase deficiency and glycogenosis type V (MacArdle disease). In these disorders the ketogenic diet provides an alternative source of energy for the brain, in GLUT-I deficiency syndrome in the form of ketone bodies and beta-hydroxybutirate, in pyruvate dehydrogenase deficiency an alternative source of acetyl-CoA, thus controlling seizures and improving the general condition of patients (71, 84).

Contraindications

Ketogenic diet is contraindicated in the following conditions (71):

- Primary carnitine deficiency
- Carnitine palmitoyltransferase deficiency type I or II
- Carnitine translocase deficiency
- Defects of beta-oxidation
- Pyruvate carboxylase deficiency
- Porphyria.

Initiating the ketogenic diet in patients with these conditions might cause a severe deterioration or devastating catabolic crisis. Therefore, before diet administration, all patients should be screened for disorders of fatty acid transport and disturbances of beta-oxidation.

Mechanisms of action

The mechanisms underlying the efficacy of the ketogenic diet are still not completely understood. Many hypotheses have been developed and tested, however, none of them gives complete explanation. One of the theories suggested is that ketone bodies could have a direct anticonvulsant effect but most studies have failed to observe it (85). The modulation of the neurotransmitter system by the ketogenic diet has also been discussed. Nevertheless, data confirming this hypothesis is lacking. There is evidence indicating that the ketogenic diet enhances energy production in the brain, and as a consequence the brain tissue becomes more resistant to metabolic stress (86). The author proposed that enhancements in metabolism, induced by the ketogenic diet, compensate for metabolic deficits exhibited within epileptic foci and transient failures of gamma-aminobutyric acidergic inhibition. Weinshenker (85) reported the involvement of noradrenaline to the anticonvulsant effect of the ketogenic diet, although noting that its presence is rather 'permissive' than an integral part of the direct anticonvulsant mechanism.

Implementation and management of the ketogenic diet

The International Ketogenic Diet Study Group has recently elaborated recommendations for the optimal clinical management of children receiving the ketogenic diet (71). Before starting the ketogenic diet a clinical consultation is needed. The purpose of it is to give the family or carers complete information about the ketogenic diet, to review the current antiepileptic treatment, and determine carbohydrate content, to make the decision regarding which type of diet should be chosen.

The following laboratory tests are recommended to be performed before diet initiation:

- Complete blood count with platelets
- Electrolytes (serum bicarbonate, total protein, calcium, zinc, selenium, magnesium, phosphate)
- Liver and kidney tests (albumin, aspartate transaminase, alanine transaminase, blood urea nitrogen, creatinine)
- Fasting lipid profile
- Serum acylcarnitine level
- Urinalysis
- Urine calcium and creatinine
- Urine organic acids
- Serum amino acids.

The procedure usually begins with an initial fasting period. In many countries this takes place at the hospital since the child can experience side effects, such as hypoglycaemia, acidosis, vomiting. The fasting period varies from 12–48 hours. While staying at the hospital the parents/carers are taught to calculate, weigh, and prepare meals. However, some studies demonstrated that fasting is not necessary to achieve ketosis, and the gradual initiation of the ketogenic diet without fasting is associated with less side effects but the same seizure control within the first 3 months (87, 88).

The concomitant AEDs are not changed in the first months after diet initiation, whereas they can be reduced or sometimes withdrawn after several months of seizure control by the ketogenic diet. Ketogenic diets contain limited quantities of fruits, vegetables, and insufficient amounts of calcium and vitamins D and B. Therefore, dietary supplementation is needed. A child on the ketogenic diet should be seen by a neurologist and a dietician at least every 3 months during the first year on the diet. At each visit a laboratory assessment should be performed (complete blood count with platelets, electrolytes, serum liver and kidney parameters, fasting lipid profile, serum acylcarnitine, urinalysis, and urine calcium and creatinine). Between the visits, parents evaluate urine ketosis several times per week.

Adverse effects

The most frequently observed side effects of the ketogenic diet are: gastrointestinal disturbances (constipation, vomiting, diarrhoea, abdominal pain), hypercholesterolaemia, kidney stones, and growth failure. Gastrointestinal symptoms have been reported in 12–50% of children, and hypercholesterolemia in 14–59% of patients (80, 89). Kidney stones occur in 5–7% of children. Risk factors include young age, family history of kidney stones, and urine calcium/creatinine ratio of more than 0.2 (90). Oral potassium citrate significantly decreases the risk of kidney stone formation. A number of studies have demonstrated the slowed growth of patients on the ketogenic diet. The majority of children were below the 10th percentile for height at diet follow-up (80, 91, 92). Growth problems were independent from the type of diet, mean age, diet duration, protein, and energy intake per body weight (73, 92). However, one recent study, evaluating the long-term outcomes of the ketogenic diet, reported the improvement of growth after diet discontinuation (93).

Ketogenic diet discontinuation

The ketogenic diet should not be discontinued before at least a mean of 3.5 months of use (71). In patients with more than 50% seizure reduction the ketogenic diet can be discontinued after 2 years, whereas in patients with almost complete seizure control it can be used for a longer period, up to 6–12 years (89). Typically the ketogenic diet is tapered off slowly, over 2–3 months. The ketogenic ratio gradually decreases from 4:1 to 3:1 to 2:1. Ketogenic food is then continued with free fluid intake and amount of calories. Usual food can be reintroduced after the ketosis is lost.

References

1. Fisher RS, van Emde Boas W, Blume W, Elger C, Genton P, Lee P, *et al.* Epileptic seizures and epilepsy: Definitions proposed by the ILAE and IBE. *Epilepsia* 2005; 46:470–2.
2. Hauser WA, Annegers JF, Kurland LT. Prevalence of epilepsy in Rochester, Minnesota: 1940-1980. *Epilepsia* 1991; 32:429–45.
3. Ad hoc Task Force of the ILAE Commission on Therapeutic Strategies. Definition of drug resistant epilepsy: consensus proposal. *Epilepsia* 2010;51:1069–77.
4. Foldvary-Schaefer N, Falcone T. Catamenial epilepsy. Pathophysiology, diagnosis, and management. *Neurology* 2003; 61(Suppl 2):S2–S15.
5. Aird RB. The importance of seizure-inducing factors in the control of refractory forms of epilepsy. *Epilepsia* 1983; 24:567–83.
6. Wolf P, Okujava N. Possibilities of non-pharmacological conservative treatment of epilepsy. *Seizure* 1999; 8:45–52.
7. Trevorrow T. Air travel and seizure frequency for individuals with epilepsy. *Seizure* 2006; 15:320–7.
8. Scaramelli A, Braga P, Avellanal A, Bogacz A, Camejo C, Rega I, *et al.* Prodromal symptoms in epileptic patients: clinical characterization of the pre-ictal phase. *Seizure* 2009; 18:246–50.
9. Wolf P, Koepp M (2012). Reflex epilepsies. In: Handbook of Clinical Neurology, Vol.107, *Epilepsy*, Part I (H Stefan & WH Theodore, eds). Edinburgh: Elsevier (in press).
10. Kasteleijn-Nolst Trenité DGA. Photosensitivity, visually sensitive seizures and epilepsies. *Epilepsy Res* 2006; 70(Suppl 1): 269–79.
11. Beniczky S, Guaranha MSB, Conradsen I, Singh MB, Rutar V, Lorber B, Braga P, Bogacz Fressola A, Inoue Y, Yacubian EMT, Wolf P.

Modulation of epileptiform discharges in juvenile myoclonic epilepsy: An investigation of reflex epileptic traits. *Epilepsia* 2012; 53: 832–9.
12. May TW, Pfäfflin M. The efficacy of an educational treatment program for patients with epilepsy (MOSES): results of a controlled, randomized study. *Epilepsia* 2002; 43:539–49.
13. Wolf P. Acute drug administration in epilepsy. A review. *CNS Neurosci Ther* 2011; 17:442–8.
14. Wolf P. Acute administration of benzodiazepines as part of treatment strategies for epilepsy. *CNS Neurosci Ther* 2011; 17:214–20.
15. Paulson GW. Inhibition of seizures. *Dis Nerv Syst* 1963; 24:657–64.
16. Cull CA, Fowler M, Brown SW. Perceived self-control of seizures in young people with epilepsy. *Seizure* 1996; 5:131–8.
17. Lee SA, No YJ. Perceived self-control of seizures in patients with uncontrolled partial epilepsy. *Seizure* 2005; 14:100–5.
18. Gowers WR. *Epilepsy and other convulsive diseases*. London: Churchill, 1881.
19. Efron R. The effect of olfactory stimuli in arresting uncinate fits. *Brain* 1956; 79:267–81.
20. Efron R. The conditioned inhibition of uncinate fits. *Brain* 1957; 80:251–62.
21. Panayiotopoulos CP. *A clinical guide to epileptic syndromes and their treatment: based on the new ILAE diagnostic scheme*. Oxford: Bladon Medical Publishing, 2002.
22. Blume WT, Lüders HO, Mizrahi E, Tassinari C, van Emde Boas W, Engel J Jr. Glossary of descriptive terminology for ictal semiology: report of the ILAE task force on classification and terminology. *Epilepsia* 2001; 42:1212–8.
23. Wilkins AJ, Andermann F, Ives J. Stripes, complex cells and seizures: an attempt to determine the locus and nature of the trigger mechanism in pattern-sensitive epilepsy. *Brain* 1975; 98:365–80.
24. Parra J, Kalitzin SN, Silva FHL. Photosensitivity and visually induced seizures. *Curr Opin Neurol* 2005; 18:155–9.
25. Kasteleijn-Nolst Trenité DGA, Van der Beld G, Heyndrickx I, Groen P. Visual stimuli in daily life. *Epilepsia* 2004; 45(Suppl 1):2–6.
26. Wilkins AJ, Zifkin B, Andermann F, McGovern E. Seizures induced by thinking. *Ann Neurol* 1982; 11:608–12.
27. Wolf P. Reading epilepsy. In: Roger J, Bureau M, Dravet CH, Dreifuss FE, Perret A, Wolf P (eds) *Epileptic syndromes in infancy, childhood and adolescence* (2nd edn), pp. 281–98. London: J. Libbey, 1992.
28. Inoue Y, Seino M, Tanaka M, Kubota H, Yamakaku K, Yagi K. *Epilepsy with praxis-induced epilepsy*. In: Wolf P (ed) *Epileptic seizures and syndromes*, pp. 81–91. London: John Libbey, 1994.
29. Matsuoka H, Takahashi T, Sasaki M, Matsumoto K, Yoshida S, Numachi Y, *et al.* Neuropsychological EEG activation in patients with epilepsy. *Brain* 2000, 123(2):318–30.
30. Ferlazzo E, Zifkin BG, Andermann E, Andermann F. Cortical triggers in generalized reflex seizures and epilepsies. *Brain* 2005; 128(4):700–10.
31. Alajouanine T, Gastaut H. La syncinésie-sursaut et l'épilepsie sursaut à déclenchement sensoriel ou sensitif inopiné. Les faits anatomo-cliniques (15 observations). *Rev Neurol* 1955; 93:29–41.
32. Glass HC, Prieur B, Molnar C, Hamiwka L, Wirrell E. Micturition and emotion-induced reflex epilepsy: case report and review of the literature. *Epilepsia* 2006; 47(12):2180–2.
33. Okumura A, Kondo Y, Tsuji T, Ikuta T, Negoro T, Kato K, *et al.* Micturition induced seizures: ictal EEG and subtraction ictal SPECT findings. *Epilepsy Res* 2007; 73(1): 119–21.
34. Wieser HG, Hungerbuhler H, Siegel AM, Buck A. Musicogenic epilepsy: review of the literature and case report with ictal single photon emission computed tomography. *Epilepsia* 1997; 38:200–7.
35. Scollo-Lavizzari G, Hess R. Sensory precipitation of epileptic seizures. Report on two unusual cases. *Epilepsia* 1967; 8:157–61.
36. Koutroumanidis M, Pearce R, Sadoh DR, Panayiotopoulos CP. Tooth brushing-induced seizures: a case report. *Epilepsia* 2001; 42(5):686–8.
37. Engel J Jr. Report of the ILAE Classification Core Group. *Epilepsia* 2006; 47(9):1558–68.
38. Guerrini R, Dravet C, Genton P, Bureau M, Bonanni P, Ferrari AR, *et al.* Idiopathic photosensitive occipital lobe epilepsy. *Epilepsia* 1995; 36(9):883–91.
39. Taylor I, Marini C, Johnson MR, Turner S, Berkovic SF, Scheffer IE. Juvenile myoclonic epilepsy and idiopathic photosensitive occipital lobe epilepsy: is there overlap? *Brain* 2004; 127(8):1878–86.
40. Bickford RG, Whelan JL, Klass DW, Corbin KB. Reading epilepsy: clinical and electrographic studies of a new syndrome. *Trans Am Neurol Assoc* 1956; 81(1):100–2.
41. Koutroumanidis M, Koepp MJ, Richardson MP, Camfield C, Agathonikou A, Ried S, *et al.* The variants of reading epilepsy: a clinical and video-EEG study of 17 patients with reading-induced seizures. *Brain* 1998; 121(8):1409–27.
42. Allen IM. Observation on cases of reflex epilepsy. *N Z Med J* 1945; 44:135–42.
43. Mani KS, Gopalakrishnan PN, Vyas JN, Pillai MS. Hot-water epilepsy: a peculiar type of reflex epilepsy, a preliminary report. *Neurology (India)* 1968; 16(3):107–10.
44. Satishchandra P, Shivaramakrishnana A, Kaliaperumal VG, Schoemberg BS. Hot-water epilepsy: A variant of reflex epilepsy in Southern India. *Epilepsia* 1988; 29:52–6.
45. Ratnapriya R, Satishchandra P, Dilip S, Gadre G, Anand A. Familial autosomal dominant reflex epilepsy triggered by hot water maps to 4q24–q28. *Hum Genet* 2009; 126:677–83.
46. Ratnapriya R, Satishchandra P, Kumar SD, Gadre G, Reddy R, Anand A. A locus for autosomal dominant reflex epilepsy precipitated by hot water maps at chromosome 10q21.3–q22.3. *Hum Genet* 2009; 125:541–9.
47. Dhanaraj M, Jayavelu A. Prophylactic use of clobazam in hot water epilepsy. *J Assoc Physicians India* 2003; 51:43–4.
48. Plouin P, Vigevano F. Reflex seizures in infancy. In: Wolf P, Inoue Y, Zifkin B (eds) *Reflex epilepsies: progress in understanding*, pp. 115–22. Montrouge: John Libbey Eurotext, 2004.
49. Wolf P. From precipitation to inhibition of seizures: rationale of a therapeutic paradigm. *Epilepsia* 2005; 46(Suppl 1):15–6.
50. Zifkin BG. Some lessons from reflex seizures. *Epilepsia* 2010; 51(Suppl 1):43–4.
51. Salek-Haddadi A, Mayer T, Hamandi K, Symms M, Josephs O, Fluegel D, *et al.* Imaging seizure activity: a combined EEG/EMG-fMRI study in reading epilepsy. *Epilepsia* 2009; 50(2):256–64.
52. Satishchandra P, Kallur KG, Jayakumar PN. Inter-ictal and ictal 99m TC ECD SPECT scan in hot-water epilepsy. *Epilepsia* 2001; 42(Suppl 7), 158.
53. Moeller F, Siebner HR, Ahlgrimm N, Wolff S, Muhle H, Granert O, *et al.* fMRI activation during spike and wave discharges evoked by photic stimulation. *NeuroImage* 2009; 48:682–95.
54. Avanzini G, Manganotti P, Meletti S, Moshé SL, Panzica F, Wolf P, Capovilla G. The system epilepsies: A pathophysiological hypothesis. *Epilepsia* 2012; 53: 771–8.
55. Striano P, Striano S. Reading epilepsy and its variants: a model for system epilepsy. *Epilepsy Behav* 2011; 20(3):591.
56. Covanis A, Stodieck SRG, Wilkins AJ. Treatment of photosensitivity. *Epilepsia* 2004; 45(Suppl. 1):40–5.
57. Wilkins AJ, Baker A, Amin D, Smith S, Bradford J, Zaiwalla Z, *et al.* Treatment of photosensitive epilepsy using coloured glasses. *Seizure* 1999; 8(8):444–9.
58. Takahashi Y, Sato T, Goto K, Fujino M, Fujiwara T, Yamaga M, *et al.* Optical filters inhibiting television-induced photosensitive seizures. *Neurology* 2001; 57(10):1767–73.
59. Takahashi T, Kamijo K, Takaki Y, Yamazaki T. Suppressive efficacies by adaptive temporal filtering system on photoparoxysmal response elicited by flickering pattern stimulation. *Epilepsia* 2002; 43(5): 530–4.

60. Capovilla G, Gambardella A, Rubboli G, Beccaria F, Montagnini A, Aguglia U, *et al.* Suppressive efficacy by a commercially available blue lens on PPR in 610 photosensitive epilepsy patients. *Epilepsia* 2006; 47:529–33.
61. Ricci S, Vigevano F, Manfredi M, Kasteleijn-Nolst Trenité DG. Epilepsy provoked by television and video games: safety of 100-Hz screens. *Neurology* 1998; 50(3):790–3.
62. Forster FM. Reflex epilepsy. *Behavioral Therapy and Conditional Reflexes.* Springfield, IL: Thomas, 1977.
63. Wolf P, Dockweiler U. Deconditioning therapy in a patient with versive seizures precipitated by touch. In: Beaumanoir A, Gastaut H, Naquet R (eds) *Reflex seizures and reflex epilepsies*, pp. 447–51. Genève: Médecine & Hygiène, 1989.
64. Dahl JA, Brorson LO, Melin L. Effects of a broad-spectrum behavioural medicine treatment program on children with refractory epileptic seizures.: an 8-year follow-up. *Epilepsia* 1992; 33:98–102.
65. Martinovic Z. Adjunctive behavioural treatment in adolescents and young adults with juvenile myoclonic epilepsy. *Seizure* 2001; 10:42–47.
66. Satishchandra P. Hot-water epilepsy. *Epilepsia* 2003; 44(Suppl 1): 29–32.
67. Turner WA. *Epilepsy—A study of the idiopathic disease.* London: Macmillan, 1907
68. Wilson L. *Epilepsy and seizures.* The Center for Development, 2011. http://www.drlwilson.com/articles/epilepsy.htm
69. Wheless JW. History of the ketogenic diet. *Epilepsia* 2008; 49 (Suppl. 8):3–5.
70. Kossoff EH, McGrogan JR. Worldwide use of the ketogenic diet. *Epilepsia* 2005;46(2):280–9.
71. Kossoff EH, Zupec-Kania BA, Amark PE, Ballaban-Gil KR, Christina Bergqvist AG, Blackford R, *et al.* Optimal management of children receiving the ketogenic diet: Recommendations of the International Ketogenic Diet Study Group. *Epilepsia* 2009; 50(2):304–17.
72. Liu YC. Medium-chain triglyceride (MCT) ketogenic therapy. *Epilepsia* 2008;49 (Suppl. 8):33–6.
73. Neal EG, Chaffe H, Schwartz RH, Lawson MS, Edwards N, Fitzsimmons G, *et al.* A randomized trial of classical and medium-chain triglyceride ketogenic diets in the treatment of childhood epilepsy. *Epilepsia* 2009; 50(5):1109–17.
74. Miranda MJ, Mortensen M, Povlsen JH, Nielsen H, Beniczky S. Danish study of a Modified Atkins diet for medically intractable epilepsy in children: Can we achieve the same results as with the classical ketogenic diet? *Seizure* 2011; 20(2):151–5.
75. Oguni H, Tanaka T, Hayashi K, Funatsuka M, Sakauchi M, Shirakawa S, *et al.* Treatment and long-term prognosis of myoclonic-astatic epilepsy of early childhood. *Neuropediatrics* 2002; 33(3):122–32.
76. Laux LC, Devonshire KA, Kelley KR, Goldstein J, Nordli DR Jr. Efficacy of the ketogenic diet in myoclonic epilepsy of Doose. *Epilepsia* 2004; 45(Suppl. 7):251.
77. Caraballo RH, Cersosimo RO, Sakr D, Cresta A, Escobal N, Fejerman N. Ketogenic diet in patients with myoclonic-astatic epilepsy. *Epileptic Disord* 2006; 8(2):151–5.
78. Kilaru S, Bergqvist AG. Current treatment of myoclonic astatic epilepsy: clinical experience at the Children's Hospital of Philadelphia. *Epilepsia* 2007; 48(9):1703–7.
79. Caraballo RH, Cersosimo RO, Sakr D, Cresta A, Escobal N, Fejerman N. Ketogenic diet in patients with Dravet syndrome. *Epilepsia* 2005; 46(9):1539–44.
80. Kang HC, Kim YJ, Kim DW, Kim HD. Efficacy and safety of the ketogenic diet for intractable childhood epilepsy: Korean multicenter experience. *Epilepsia* 2005; 46(2):272–9.
81. Dressler A, Stöcklin B, Reithofer E, Benninger F, Freilinger M, Hauser E, *et al.* Long-term outcome and tolerability of the ketogenic diet in drug-resistant childhood epilepsy: the Austrian experience. *Seizure* 2010; 19(7):404–8.
82. Hong AM, Turner Z, Hamdy RF, Kossoff EH. Infantile spasms treated with the ketogenic diet: prospective single-center experience in 104 consecutive infants. *Epilepsia* 2010; 51(8):1403–7.
83. Kossoff EH, Hedderick EF, Turner Z, Freeman JM. A case-control evaluation of the ketogenic diet versus ACTH for new-onset infantile spasms. *Epilepsia* 2008; 49(9):1504–9.
84. Klepper J. Glucose transporter deficiency syndrome (GLUTIDS) and the ketogenic diet. *Epilepsia* 2008; 49(Suppl. 8):46–9.
85. Weinshenker D. The contribution of norepinephrine and orexigenic neuropeptides to the anticonvulsant effect of the ketogenic diet. *Epilepsia* 2008; 49(Suppl. 8):104–7.
86. Bough K. Energy metabolism as part of the anticonvulsant mechanism of the ketogenic diet. *Epilepsia* 2008; 49 (Suppl.8):91–3.
87. Kim DW, Kang HC, Park JC, Kim HD. Benefits of the non-fasting ketogenic diet compared with the initial fasting ketogenic diet. *Pediatrics* 2004; 114(6):1627–30.
88. Bergqvist AG, Shall JI, Gallagher PR, Cnaan A, Stallings VA. Fasting versus gradual initiation of the ketogenic diet: a prospective, randomized clinical trial of efficacy. *Epilepsia* 2005; 46(11):1810–19.
89. Groesbeck DK, Bluml RM, Kossoff EH. Long-term use of the ketogenic diet in the treatment of epilepsy. *Dev Med Child Neurol* 2006; 48(12): 978–81.
90. Furth SL, Casey JC, Pyzik PL, Neu AM, Docimo SG, Vining EP, *et al.* Risk factors for urolithiasis in children on the ketogenic diet. *Pediatr Nephrol* 2000; 15(1–2):125–8.
91. Vining EP, Pyzik PL, McGrogan J, Hladky H, Anand A, Kriegler S, *et al.* Growth of children on the ketogenic diet. *Dev Med Child Neurol*, 44(12):796–802.
92. Williams S, Basualdo-Hammond C, Curtis R, Schuller R. Growth retardation in children with epilepsy on the ketogenic diet: a retrospective chart review. *J Am Diet Assoc* 2002; 102(3):405–7.
93. Patel A, Pyzik PL, Turner Z, Rubenstein JE, Kossoff EH. Long-term outcomes of children treated with the ketogenic diet in the past. *Epilepsia* 2010; 51(7):1277–82.

CHAPTER 13

Reproductive Aspects of Epilepsy

Michael R. Johnson and John J. Craig

Introduction

Although reproductive aspects should be important for both men and women with epilepsy almost all attention has concentrated on women, in particular those of childbearing age. In this chapter we will cover the important reproductive issues that apply to both men and women with epilepsy. However, since it is the management of women with epilepsy of childbearing age, especially those who contemplate pregnancy, or who become pregnant, that causes most concern, the topics covered in this chapter will tend to focus on the issues relating to the management of women with epilepsy.

There are many important topics when considering the reproductive aspects of epilepsy (Table 13.1). In this chapter we will discuss the interactions between reproductive hormones and epilepsy, including the effects of epilepsy and antiepileptic drugs (AEDs) on reproductive hormones, the effects of reproductive hormones on epilepsy (catamenial epilepsy), and the interactions between AEDs and hormonal contraception. We will also consider teratogenicity and perinatal outcomes, concentrating on the risks for major congenital malformations (MCMs) and the effects of AEDs on cognitive function and behaviour. Lastly, we will consider the relevant management issues in pregnancy and lactation, not forgetting the importance of optimal preconceptual counselling.

Epilepsy and antiepileptic drugs and their relationship to reproductive hormones

Epilepsy and AEDs are associated with changes in hormones that may contribute to reproductive and sexual dysfunction in both men and women, as well as abnormalities of bone health. Female sexual hormones may also affect the seizure threshold in women resulting in a greater likelihood of seizures at certain times of the menstrual cycle (catamenial epilepsy).

Hormonal alterations that occur following seizures include changes in prolactin, luteinizing hormone, and follicle stimulating hormone (1). These changes may occur as a consequence of both generalized and focal seizures and are thought to arise as a result of connections between the hypothalamic–pituitary axis and areas of the brain involved in seizures. The precise hormonal mechanisms remain somewhat unclear and are reviewed in detail elsewhere (1–3). These hormonal changes may result in reproductive dysfunction in women with epilepsy, with the most common disorders being polycystic ovarian syndrome (PCOS) and hypothalamic amenorrhea (1, 4).

PCOS is defined as the presence of: (1) multiple follicular cysts, (2) ovulatory dysfunction (oligo-ovulation and anovulation), and (3) clinical or serological evidence of hyperandrogenism (3). PCOS is associated with secondary health consequences including insulin resistance and obesity. It is estimated that PCOS occurs in about 5% of women without epilepsy but in up to 20% of women with epilepsy. The relationship between PCOS and epilepsy is complicated by the potentially confounding effects of antiepileptic medication on female sexual hormones. Since the original observation by Isojarvi and colleagues (5) that sodium valproate may be associated with an increased incidence of PCOS, cross sectional studies have produced conflicting results, demonstrating both a significant association between valproate and PCOS or reporting no significant association (3). In contrast to valproate, data relating to carbamazepine and lamotrigine have failed to show an increased prevalence of PCOS in women taking these AEDs (3). To date, there is little evidence relating to the risks of PCOS with long-term treatment with levetiracetam (6). To address the conflicting results of cross sectional studies of valproate, Morrell and colleagues (7) conducted an important prospective, randomized, longitudinal evaluation of the impact of valproate on the development of PCOS. In this study, women with epilepsy and regular menstrual cycles were randomized to treatment with valproate or lamotrigine and followed for 12 months. Women initiating valproate were significantly more likely to develop PCOS than those taking lamotrigine (9% vs. 2% respectively, $p = 0.007$). These observations together

Table 13.1 Reproductive topics in epilepsy to be considered

The effects of AEDs on appearance
The effect of hormones on seizure control
The effects of epilepsy and AEDs on fertility
The effects of AEDs on contraception and vice versa
The effects of pregnancy on AEDs and seizure control
The effects of epilepsy and AEDs on pregnancy including fetal development

with other data showing that valproate-associated changes are reversible when valproate is discontinued (8, 9) suggest that a reasonable treatment option in women who develop PCOS and/or ovulatory dysfunction whilst taking valproate is to consider alternative AED therapy, bearing in mind the importance of seizure control in epilepsy and the suitability of a particular AED to an individual's epilepsy.

As well as seizures having effects on neuroendocrine function, exacerbation of epilepsy itself may occur as a result of menstrual cycle-related changes in reproductive hormones (catamenial epilepsy). There is no agreement on the degree of seizure exacerbation required to meet a definition of catamenial epilepsy and therefore reliable epidemiological estimates on prevalence are lacking. Using a definition for catamenial epilepsy that 75% or more of seizures had to occur within 4 days before and within 6 days of the onset of menstruation, it was shown that only five of 40 (12.5%) women met this criterion (10). In contrast, 31 of 40 (78%) claimed that most of their seizures occurred around the time of menstruation. Physiological changes to gamma-aminobutyric acid A ($GABA_A$) receptor function as a result of withdrawal of progesterone and its active metabolite allopregnanolone at the time of menstruation provide one possible mechanism for menstrual exacerbation of seizures (11), although other mechanisms are postulated (4). Regardless of the cause of catamenial epilepsy, the primary therapeutic aim where catamenial exacerbation of seizures is present remains control of epilepsy with standard chronic AED therapy. Clobazam or acetazolamide given intermittently around the time of menstruation have been tried, but good evidence for the benefit of this approach is lacking. Seven out of 11 women with uncontrolled seizures given intramuscular medroxyprogesterone reported fewer seizures (12), but larger well-controlled studies on the benefits of hormonal manipulation in catamenial epilepsy are lacking (and would be well worth doing).

In addition to the effects of epilepsy on reproductive hormones, AED exposure may affect reproductive hormones in both men and women. In a study of 85 men with focal epilepsy, the enzyme-inducing AEDs carbamazepine and phenytoin were associated with reduced bioavailable testosterone and reduced levels of sexual function (13). Similarly, enzyme-inducing AEDs are associated with reduced levels of oestrogens and androgens and an increased incidence of sexual dysfunction in women (14, 15). In contrast, valproate is associated with increased androgen concentrations (16). Other factors contributing to an increased incidence of sexual dysfunction in men and women with epilepsy include the stress of living with a chronic illness and the persisting social stigma associated with epilepsy. Despite awareness of hormonal issues occurring as a result of treatment with AEDs (17), there is no consensus regarding their management. Although several studies suggest the adverse effects of AEDs on reproductive hormones may be reversible on AED withdrawal, any potential benefits in reproductive and sexual health from AED withdrawal (or switch to alternative AED) must be very carefully weighed against the increased risk of harm from uncontrolled seizures.

It is increasingly recognized that alterations of reproductive hormones by AEDs may have adverse consequences for bone health (2, 18). Whilst the negative impact on bone health may be a consequence of increased clearance of vitamin D by cytochrome P450 enzyme-inducing AEDs, it is clear that non-enzyme-inducing AEDs including valproate (19, 20), clonazepam, and gabapentin (21) may also be associated with an increased fracture risk. There is limited data on other commonly used AEDs, although drugs such as topiramate, zonisamide, and acetazolamide that inhibit carbonic anhydrase may theoretically affect bone health by inducing a metabolic acidosis (18). There are no clinical studies on levetiracetam although animal data suggest levetiracetam may reduce bone strength without altering bone mass density (22). Unfortunately, as with concerns regarding AEDs and reproductive health, in respect of bone health, there are insufficient data to make firm recommendations for the screening, prevention, or treatment of patients taking AEDs. One might reasonably conclude, however, that all people taking enzyme-inducing AEDs should be counselled about the risks for bone disease and encouraged to adopt a lifestyle that maximizes bone health (regular exercise, avoidance of smoking, adequate dietary calcium and vitamin D intake, etc.). Screening for osteoporosis or vitamin D deficiency can be justified if patients taking enzyme-inducing AEDs have additional risk factors for osteoporosis (e.g. older age, postmenopausal, previous fracture, smoking history, low body mass index, or sedentary lifestyle) (18), and the UK Medicines and Healthcare products Regulatory Agency advises that vitamin D supplementation should be considered for such at-risk patients on long-term enzyme-inducing AEDs or sodium valproate (http://www.mhra.gov.uk/Publications/Safetyguidance/index.htm).

Hormonal contraception in epilepsy

Contraception in women with epilepsy is a topic of great practical importance. Plenty of guidelines exist to assist the clinician including those of the UK National Institute for Health and Clinical Excellence (NICE) epilepsy guidelines (http://guidance.nice.org.uk), the Scottish Intercollegiate Guidelines Network (SIGN) guidelines on the diagnosis and management of adults with epilepsy (http://www.sign.ac.uk/guidelines/fulltext/70/index.html), primary care guidelines on the management of epilepsy in women from the Royal Society of Medicine (http:// http://www.rsm.ac.uk/media/pr160.php), Guidelines from the Royal College of Obstetricians and Gynaecologists Faculty of Sexual and Reproductive Healthcare Clinical Effectiveness Unit, as well as several excellent journal articles to which the reader is referred (e.g. 23, 24). Therefore, within this section we seek only to highlight the key points that guide choice of hormonal contraception in women of childbearing potential with epilepsy, and to discuss some of the more recent or contentious issues of practical importance.

Of prime importance are considerations relating to the prescription of oral contraceptives in women taking hepatic enzyme (particularly the cytochrome P450 CYP3A4 isoenzyme) inducing AEDs (phenytoin, carbamazepine, eslicarbazepine, oxcarbazepine, barbiturates). Topiramate is a CYP3A4 inducer but warrants special mention and is discussed separately later in the chapter. Women using hepatic enzyme-inducing AEDs who wish to use hormonal contraception should be advised against the use of lower-dose progestogen-only methods (i.e. the progestogen-only pill (POP) and the progestogen-only implant). Oral contraceptives that combine an oestrogen and progestogen (combined oral contraceptive pills or COCPs) may be used, but since the clearance of oestradiol is increased by enzyme-inducing AEDs, a COCP containing a minimum 50 micrograms of oestradiol is recommended. The presence of breakthrough bleeding should be taken as an indication of inadequate contraception even in the setting of an increased dose of oestradiol. In the presence of breakthrough bleeding, higher doses of oestradiol can be used to achieve adequate contraceptive effect, but even in the absence of breakthrough bleeding women on enzyme-inducing AEDs still need to be informed that there is a higher risk of contraceptive failure compared to the general population taking the COCP. Because of the potentially serious consequences of unwanted pregnancy the additional consistent use of condoms is recommended in women on enzyme-inducing AEDs choosing combined hormonal oral contraception.

Non-enzyme-inducing AEDs (clobazam, levetiracetam, gabapentin, valproate, lacosamide, pregabalin, vigabatrin, zonisamide) have no effect on contraceptive efficacy and so the standard COCP with 30 micrograms of oestradiol can be used, as well as standard low-dose progestogen methods such as the POP or progestogen-only implant.

Topiramate and lamotrigine require special discussion. Topiramate is a CYP3A4 inducer, but the contraceptive efficacy of the COCP is thought not to be affected at monotherapy doses less than 200 mg/day (25). Even so, it is the practice of the authors of this chapter to recommend consistent additional use of condoms even at doses of topiramate less than 200 mg/day. Low-dose progestogen methods (such as the progesterone-only oral contraceptive) are not recommended when topiramate is being taken. The situation for lamotrigine is more complex. Lamotrigine is metabolized by the UDP-glucuronyl transferases and there is no evidence that lamotrigine induces cytochrome P450 enzymes. In a study of 16 female volunteers, co-administration of lamotrigine (up to 300 mg/day) had no effect on the pharmacokinetics of the ethinyloestradiol component of a COCP but a modest increase in the clearance of the levonorgestral component was observed (and some volunteers reported vaginal bleeding), but with no corresponding hormonal evidence that suppression of ovulation had not been maintained (26). However, as a consequence of this data, the manufacturer of lamotrigine released new guidance and the Summary of Product Characteristics (SPC) now comments that the 'possibility of reduced contraceptive effectiveness cannot be excluded'. It would seem sensible therefore for prescribers of the COCP with lamotrigine to warn their patients that reduced contraceptive effectiveness cannot be excluded and recommend the consistent use of condoms in addition to the COCP. A second issue relating to co-administration of the COCP with lamotrigine and which also warrants specialist discussion is the important effect the COCP has on systemic lamotrigine levels. Thus, plasma lamotrigine levels are approximately halved by co-administration of the COCP (27). This may result in reduced seizure control after the addition of the COCP or conversely may result in lamotrigine toxicity following removal of the COCP. Therefore, substantial care should be taken when introducing the COCP in someone who is seizure free on a stable dose of lamotrigine or withdrawal of the COCP in patients on lamotrigine.

Taking all this into account the Faculty of Sexual and Reproductive Healthcare (FSRH) Clinical Effectiveness Unit of the Royal College of Obstetricians and Gynaecologists recently updated their guidance on AEDs and contraception to include lamotrigine as a 'condition' where the 'theoretical or proven risks of the COCP generally outweigh the advantages' stating (in the context of lamotrigine therapy) that the 'provision of the COCP requires expert clinical judgement and/or referral to a specialist provider, since the use of the method is not usually recommended unless other methods are not available or not acceptable' (http://www.ffprhc.org.uk). In contrast to the advice relating to the COCP, the United Kingdom Medical Eligibility Criteria for Contraceptive Use (UKMEC) categories for anticonvulsant therapy and contraception list lamotrigine therapy as a condition for which there is *no* restriction on the use of either the POP or progestogen-only implant (http://www.ffprhc.org.uk). Based on the results of the Siddhu study, however (26), there must be some doubt over the effectiveness of progestogen-only methods of contraception in women taking lamotrigine.

For enzyme-inducing AEDs, the efficacy of the progestogen-only injectable depot medroxyprogesterone acetate (DMPA) is not reduced. The rate limiting step for the clearance of medroxyprogesterone (Depo-Provera®) is hepatic blood flow, and so enzyme-inducing AEDs should have no effect. Reflecting this, the SPC for Depo-Provera® recommends no dosing adjustment for Depo-Provera® in patients receiving enzyme-inducing AEDs, yet the SIGN and NICE guidelines recommend a reduced dosing interval of 10 weeks instead of 12.

In conclusion, for women on long-term enzyme-inducing AEDs, methods such as DMPA or intrauterine methods such as levonorgestrel-releasing intrauterine or copper-bearing intrauterine systems (which are not discussed in detail here but where, like DMPA, there are no restrictions on use in conjunction with enzyme-inducing AEDs) may represent the most reliable contraceptive options.

Teratogenicity and perinatal outcomes

Role of the epilepsy pregnancy registry

Bearing in mind the risks to the fetus from *in utero* exposure to AEDs it is important to have as much information as possible on the safety, or otherwise, of these drugs. Since it would generally be considered unethical to carry out randomized controlled drug trials on women who could become pregnant (indeed women with epilepsy of childbearing years are often actively excluded from many of the pharmaceutical drug trials), and current post-marketing surveillance programmes are not organized in such a fashion as to be able to provide information of fetal risks, it seems logical, given that women are already becoming pregnant on AEDs, either singly or in combination, to gather data by whatever means possible.

In recent years this has been attempted with the establishment of prospective epilepsy and pregnancy registries. A number of registries exist, all of which have the principal aim of collecting as much information as possible on the outcomes of pregnancies exposed to AEDs. Some caveats about the information generated must be appreciated. Principally, the information does not apply to randomly assigned treatments. Instead treatment will have been at the discretion of the treating physician who will have chosen particular regimens for specific reasons. At its simplest level, like may not be being compared with like, with it being difficult if not impossible to account for the effects of confounding variables. Reporting is often selective, depending on the type of registry and its catchment area, and therefore the results may not be representative of the broader population with epilepsy. Most also do not include a control population, although some gather information on women with epilepsy who are not taking AEDs during pregnancy.

Nevertheless, despite these provisos, prospective pregnancy registries probably offer the only hope of providing any useful information, in an acceptable time frame, to guide women with epilepsy and those looking after them of the risks of MCMs for particular AEDs or combinations (Table 13.2).

Existing pregnancy registries are either sponsored by individual pharmaceutical companies and therefore focus on a single AED or represent the efforts of independent researchers based in one or multiple countries who collect outcome data on all available AEDs. Their methodologies (28), while varying somewhat, are broadly similar in that they aim to collect information on pregnancies that have been exposed to AEDs, or not, in any combination and which have been identified before the outcome of the pregnancy is known. In addition to collecting demographic details, information is collected on drug exposure, including folate, history of exposure to other teratogens, epilepsy history and seizure control during pregnancy, past pregnancy details, and family history of adverse pregnancy outcomes. At a predefined time period, or time periods, information is then collected on pregnancy outcome.

The effects of antiepilepsy drugs on the developing fetus/embryo

When considering the risks to the fetus these are usually taken to be the risk of:

1. MCMs, in other words malformations of such significance that they require medical or surgical intervention.
2. Minor abnormalities, which while occasionally disfiguring, do not require intervention.
3. Cognitive and behavioural delay/upset.
4. Intra-uterine growth retardation.

Most research has concentrated on the risk of MCM, although increasing data are emerging on the cognitive and behavioural impact of *in utero* AED exposure. While it is clearly difficult to compare the impact of adverse pregnancy outcomes, as serious as MCMs can be, they can often be detected *in utero* presenting pregnant women with choices. Occasionally they can also be rectified at birth or thereafter. Neither can yet be claimed for any effects on cognitive development or behaviour.

In contrast to many other potential teratogens, which may be given for short periods or can be stopped when the woman becomes pregnant, AEDs usually have to be taken throughout the pregnancy and so the embryo/fetus is chronically exposed. The timing of exposure is also important with MCMs resulting from exposure in the first trimester. In contrast any effect on cognitive functioning and growth extends throughout the pregnancy and possibly even beyond birth.

The effects of seizures

The fetus seems relatively resistant to the effects of seizures although anecdotal evidence suggests that tonic–clonic seizures may cause fetal bradycardia or miscarriage. There is no evidence that simple partial, complex partial, absence, or myoclonic seizures are harmful to the fetus. Prospective studies have not found an association between tonic–clonic seizures and malformations, (29, 30), although one study reported a reduced verbal intelligent quotient in infants exposed to more than five tonic–clonic seizures in pregnancy (31). Nevertheless the risk of seizure recurrence, injury, status epilepticus, or even death needs to be considered. Status epilepticus in pregnancy has been felt to be particularly dangerous to both mother and baby. Among 29 cases of status epilepticus occurring during pregnancy nine of the mothers and 14 of the fetuses died (32). In contrast, in a prospective study where there were 36 cases (1.8%) of status epilepticus, (one-third were convulsive in type) occurring in 1956 pregnancies, there was one still-birth which occurred around the time of status epilepticus, one spontaneous abortion occurring long after the period of status epilepticus, and no cases of maternal mortality (33).

Antiepilepsy drugs and major congenital malformations

There is good evidence from human pregnancies that AEDs have an effect on fetal and embryonic development. It is a consistent finding that women with epilepsy who are not taking AEDs have a lower risk of having children with MCMs than those who are (34). It has consistently been reported that women who take polytherapy are more at risk than those who take monotherapy (35–37). Animal studies have also demonstrated teratogenicity with all of the older AEDs and some of the more recently introduced ones (38).

Overall, women with epilepsy who are taking an AED in monotherapy have at least a 2–3 times increased risk over the background population of having an infant with a MCM. This is equivalent to a 4–9% chance of a major congenital malformation for each pregnancy (34, 35, 39, 40, 41). The risk of MCMs is higher for pregnancies exposed to polytherapy and increases the more AEDs are taken (34, 37, 39, 40–44) (Table 13.3).

With regard the safety of individual AEDs taken in monotherapy, there is evidence from multiple sources of differences between AEDs, with the greatest risks being found for valproate. Data are now also available for the newer AEDs, with most outcomes being reported for lamotrigine (45).

When considering the risk for MCM with AED exposure it is important not only to consider the total risk but also the types of MCM that occur.

The *North American AED Pregnancy Registry* published data on 146 women who had used phenobarbital as monotherapy during the first trimester of pregnancy. The MCM rate among 77 exposed pregnancies was 6.5% (95% confidence interval (CI) 2.1%–14.5%), significantly more than the background risk of 1.62% (relative risk 4.2, 95% CI 1.5–9.4%, 1-sided P = 0.001) (46).

The risk of MCM for phenytoin has been reported to be 3.4% and 3.7% in 87 (37) and 82 (41) pregnancies respectively. In a systematic

Table 13.2 Epilepsy and pregnancy registers—advantages and disadvantages

- Pharmaceutical company (e.g. GSK, UCB-Pharma)
- National (USA, UK & Ireland, Australia, India)
- Multinational (EURAP)

Potential disadvantages	Potential advantages
◆ Not randomized	◆ Prospective/observational
◆ No control population	◆ Reflect current practice
◆ Selective reporting	◆ Broad based
◆ Heterogeneous populations	◆ Adequate numbers recruited
◆ Incomplete confounding variables studied	◆ Homogeneous population

review of 1198 pregnancies exposed to phenytoin a higher MCM rate of 7.4% (95% CI 3.6–11.1) was reported (47). Phenobarbital, primidone, and phenytoin have been associated with congenital heart defects and facial clefts (48). A few studies have found a positive dose-response with barbiturates. Phenytoin has also been implicated as causing urogenital defects, and dysmorphic facial and other features such as distal phalangeal hypoplasia (49).

The risks for MCMs with carbamazepine are less clear. In one case–control study the MCM rate for infants exposed to carbamazepine was found to be approximately twice that of control group (relative risk 2.24; 95% CI 1.1–4.56) (50). In contrast, an increased risk was not found by the *UK Epilepsy and Pregnancy Register*, where the MCM rate for 927 prospectively collected carbamazepine monotherapy exposures pregnancies was 2.2% (41). Carbamazepine has been reported to be associated neural tube defects, at a rate of anything from 0.2–1% of exposed pregnancies as well as heart defects, inguinal hernia, hypospadias, and hip dislocations (51). There have also been reports of reduced head circumference, weight, and length at birth. In a recent systematic review and case–control study the EUROCAT Antiepileptic Study Working Group reported that for carbamazepine, teratogenicity appeared to be relatively specific to spina bifida (52).

Valproate has consistently been shown to be associated with the greatest risk for MCM. The *North American Pregnancy Registry* described 16 major malformations among 149 valproate-exposed women (10.7%; 95% CI 6.3–16.9%). Compared with a background prevalence of 1.62% for major malformations, they calculated a relative risk for major malformations in valproate exposed pregnancies of 7.3 (95% CI 4.4–12.2%) (53). The *Australian Pregnancy Registry for Women on Anti-epileptic Medication* revealed an even higher malformation rate of 15.2%% for pregnancies exposed to valproate in monotherapy (n = 224) (54). That valproate was associated with the highest MCM rate compared with other commonly used AEDs alone was shown by the *UK Epilepsy and Pregnancy* Register: of 762 pregnancies exposed to valproate alone, 6.2% had a major malformation (41). The risk of MCM is dose dependent with valproate with total daily doses over 1000 mg being associated with a higher risk of MCMs (41, 54). There is some evidence of a pharmacogenetic susceptibility to the teratogenic effects of valproate both, from human reports (55, 56) and preclinical studies (57). Preclinical studies have also suggested that for valproate high peak plasma concentrations are associated with an increased risk of malformations (58). Thus, it has been suggested that a sustained-release preparation may be preferable, with the total daily dose being divided into two or three administrations per day.

Exposure to valproate in early pregnancy is associated with significantly increased risks for spina bifida, atrial septal defects, cleft palate, hypospadias, and craniosynostosis (59). The risk of spina bifida (1–2%) (41, 60, 61) is dose dependent, with the greatest risk for those exposed to doses of greater than 1000 mg per day. Skeletal defects, including radial ray aplasia, rib and vertebral anomalies (62), and polydactyly have also been reported.

Considering the newer AEDs, most human data are available for lamotrigine. The *International Lamotrigine Pregnancy Registry* recently reported a MCM rate of 2.2% (95% CI 1.6–3.1%) among 1558 first trimester lamotrigine-exposed pregnancies (45). For polytherapy outcomes containing lamotrigine, the occurrence of birth defects varied according to whether sodium valproate was included in the polytherapy regimen. For combinations containing sodium valproate in addition to lamotrigine (n = 150) the rate of major birth defects was 10.7% (95% CI 6.4–17.0%). This compared with a rate of 2.8% (95% CI 1.5–5.0%) for polytherapy combinations which included lamotrigine but not sodium valproate (n = 430). No distinctive pattern of malformations was reported in this study. Data from the *UK Epilepsy and Pregnancy Register* revealed a similar malformation rate for pregnancies exposed to lamotrigine alone, with 21 of 647 (3.2%) infants having a MCM. A positive dose-response was seen, with 5.4% of pregnancies exposed to more than 200 mg a day of lamotrigine having a major congenital malformation (41). This rate was not that different for that observed by the same investigators for pregnancies exposed to less than 1000 mg a day of valproate (41). A positive dose response for lamotrigine has not however been reported by the International Lamotrigine Registry (45, 63) or the North American Pregnancy Register, who found a MCM rate of 2.3% among 684 infants exposed to lamotrigine in monotherapy (64). A 10.4-fold (95% CI 4.3–24.9) increase in the rate of clefting abnormalities was noted in the North American Pregnancy Registry (64). In contrast the UK Epilepsy and Pregnancy Register (65) and the European Surveillance of Congenital Anomalies found no evidence of increased isolated orofacial clefts relative to other MCMs for lamotrigine (66).

Reported data on the other new AEDs are sparse. A report of 55 exposures to oxcarbazepine (35 monotherapy and 20 polytherapy) noted only one major malformation (67). Six malformations from the outcomes of the 248 monotherapy exposures to oxcarbazepine (2.4%), either reported in the literature or held by the Novartis Germany database have been reported (68). In a post-marketing surveillance study of gabapentin as add-on therapy for 3100 patients in England no congenital abnormalities were seen in the 11 infants born to women who used gabapentin in the first-trimester of pregnancy (69). In the tiagabine clinical trials 22 patients who received the drug became pregnant, of whom nine carried to term. In one of these a hip displacement was noted, though this was a breech delivery (70). The UK Epilepsy and Pregnancy Register reported on 203 pregnancies exposed to topiramate. Of the 70 cases that had just received topiramate, three (4.8%) had a MCM, of which two were clefting abnormalities and one a case of hypospadias (71). In contrast, in another study of 52 pregnancies exposed to topiramate, no concerns were raised (72). With regards to levetiracetam, published cases are limited. Three small reports of pregnancies exposed to levetiracetam have not raised any obvious concerns (73–75). The UK Epilepsy and Pregnancy Register have reported on 362 pregnancies exposed to levetiracetam. There were no MCMs among the 133 monotherapy exposures and nine among the 229 exposed to levetiracetam as part of a polytherapy regimen (76).

The North American AED Pregnancy Registry has published data in abstract form for 197 monotherapy exposures to both topiramate and levetiracetam in which eight and four MCMs were noted respectively equating to rates of 4.1% and 2.0%. In keeping with results from the UK two of the eight MCMs with topiramate were cleft lip deformities (77).

For zonisamide, data for exposed pregnancies are even more limited. The only published report includes 25 pregnancies (78). Considering some concerns were expressed in this small study, not to have further information from many more pregnancies is clearly of concern in itself.

For all the newer AEDs, preclinical models are therefore of interest. In these studies topiramate was teratogenic in mice, rats, and rabbits at high doses, with limb and digital malformations, including right-sided ectrodactyly being observed in rats and rib and vertebral malformations in rabbits. Vigabatrin was also shown to be teratogenic in rabbits, inducing cleft defects. Gabapentin was associated with skeletal malformations, including delayed ossification of the calcaneus and hindlimb digits in mice, and incomplete fusion of skull bones and sternebrae in rats. However, the type and incidence of these abnormalities were not felt to be indicative of developmental toxicity. Tiagabine, oxcarbazepine, and levetiracetam have not been shown to be teratogenic.

Interpreting MCM rates in pregnancies exposed to combination therapy is difficult. Critically, emerging data from the pregnancy registries mostly show that combinations containing valproate carry the highest risk (41, 45, 79).

Antiepileptic drugs and minor abnormalities

Children of women with epilepsy, whether or not they are taking AEDs, are at increased risk of minor anomalies (80). Specific AED-related fetal syndromes have been suggested for most of the older AEDs (49, 81, 82). The types of abnormalities have included minor craniofacial and digital anomalies and growth retardation. Except for valproate (81, 83, and Table 13.4), there is no convincing evidence that a specific syndrome is associated with a specific AED, hence the term 'fetal-AED' syndrome may be more appropriate for other AEDs. It is unclear what the influence is of other variables, such as maternal epilepsy and hereditary factors. In any case minor abnormalities have mostly been felt in themselves to cause little disability. This opinion is however changing so that facial dysmorphism is increasingly felt to predict cognitive and behavioural upset (31, 84).

Effects of antiepileptic drugs on cognitive functioning

The effects of *in utero* exposure to AEDs on cognitive functioning and behaviour have not been studied as comprehensively as studies on MCMs. An early Cochrane review concluded that the majority of studies in this area were of limited quality with little evidence implicating one drug over another with respect to a detrimental effect on development (85). However, more recent studies have begun to clarify the impact of AEDs on neurodevelopment.

Studies have shown mean intelligent quotient (IQ) to be significantly lower in the children of women with epilepsy compared with controls (86–89). In one study, 24% of AED exposed infants had a developmental disorder compared with 10.5% of non-exposed siblings (88). In another study from India, children of mothers with epilepsy had significantly lower full-scale IQs and language development compared with children that had not been exposed to AEDs (89). While it has been suggested that these findings are independent of AED exposure, a growing body of evidence suggests AEDs do carry risks. Although valproate has been reported as having the most detrimental effect, other AEDs including carbamazepine and phenytoin may also have an adverse effect (88).

In a retrospective observational study, 16% of 224 children who had been exposed to AEDs prenatally had additional educational needs compared with 11% of 176 exposed to no drugs (odds ratio 1.49, 95% CI 0.83–2.67%) (90). A total of 30% of those exposed to valproate, and 20% exposed to polytherapy containing valproate, had additional educational needs. This compared with 3.2% and 6.5% exposed to carbamazepine and other monotherapy regimens, respectively. These results compare with rates for developmental delay for infants exposed prenatally to carbamazepine of between 8% and 20% (86, 91, 92).

In a more thorough investigation of partly the same cohort of children Adab et al. found that verbal IQ was significantly lower in children exposed to valproate monotherapy (mean 83.6, 95% CI 78.2–89.0%; n = 41) than in unexposed children (90.9, CI 87.2–94.6%; n = 80) or in children exposed to carbamazepine (94.1, CI 89.6–98.5; n = 52) or phenytoin (98.5, CI 90.6–106.4; n = 21) (31). Doses of valproate above 800 mg/day were associated with lower verbal IQ than lower doses. Using multiple regression analysis it was found that in addition to valproate exposure, five or more tonic–clonic seizures in pregnancy and low maternal IQ were also associated with lower verbal IQ in the offspring.

In a study from Finland among a small number of exposed infants, full scale IQ was low (<80) in four of 21 infants that had been exposed to valproate (19%) and exceptionally low (<70) in two infants (10%). Of note, the mothers of the valproate exposed group performed significantly worse on IQ tests and also had significantly lower educational levels (93).

Using an Indian adaptation of the Bayley Scale of Infant Development, motor and mental development were measured in 395 infants born to women with epilepsy (94). In addition to paediatricians being blinded to AED exposure, multiple confounders were taken into account. Unfortunately these did not include maternal IQ. Valproate was associated with significantly lower mental and motor developmental scores compared with carbamazepine, but not with other AEDs used in monotherapy. While maternal educational status was significantly correlated with motor development in infants, mental development was not. The importance of including parental variables was shown in a prior study from the same group where low maternal IQ and maternal education as well as AED exposure were found to be associated with significant impairment of intellectual and language functions in children of mothers with epilepsy (89). In a study that recruited cases that had been identified prospectively through the UK Epilepsy and Pregnancy Register exposure to valproate and to a lesser extent carbamazepine, but not lamotrigine, had a significant detrimental effect on neurodevelopment, when compared with a control population (95).

The prospective Neurodevelopmental Effects of Antiepileptic drugs (NEAD) study applied the Bayley Mental Developmental Scale at 3 years in 309 children born to mothers taking AEDs (96). In the NEAD study, the valproate group global IQ was reduced by 9 points compared with the lamotrigine group, 7 points compared with the phenytoin group and 6 points compared with the carbamazepine group. The association between valproate use and global IQ was dose dependent: children born to mothers taking a valproate dose of less than 1000 mg per day had a global IQ that was not significantly different to that in children born to mothers taking carbamazepine, lamotrigine, or phenytoin. In a further study in the same cohort (97), dose-related effects of AED exposure on both verbal and non-verbal cognitive ability was assessed using a variety of measures. At the time of assessment (mean age 3 years), infants exposed to valproate scored worse on tests of verbal and non-verbal functioning (scores adjusted for maternal IQ, maternal age, dose, race, alcohol, and folic acid use during pregnancy). In contrast, carbamazepine was negatively associated with verbal performance (language abilities) only, and no significant effects were observed for lamotrigine or phenytoin. A dose dependent relationship was present for lower verbal and non-verbal abilities with valproate and for lower verbal abilities in children born to mothers taking carbamazepine. Other groups have also reported that valproate is associated with worse cognitive outcomes, especially in regards to language skills and also that the effect is dose related (98–100).

Further research is required on this important topic. As has been stated, and excepting the improvement in methodologies of recent studies, most studies have involved the analysis of relatively small, non-population based samples, have lacked randomization, have often lost enrolled subjects over time, have assessed children at a very young age and have not taken account of important confounding variables (101). However, at this stage it might be reasonable to conclude that valproate is associated with greater risks to cognitive ability (particularly verbal abilities) than either carbamazepine, lamotrigine, or phenytoin. What it is unclear, though, is whether there is a 'safe' dose for valproate, below which the risk of cognitive impairment (as well MCMs) is equivalent to other AEDs. In terms of clinical management therefore, it seems that valproate is a poor first choice for most women of childbearing potential (97), and for those women where the benefits of valproate in terms of seizure control are judged to outweigh the risks the correct dose should be the lowest dose that adequately controls the seizures.

Data for the other newer AEDs are restricted to Levetiracetam. In a study from the Liverpool and Manchester Neurodevelopmental Group and the UK and Epilepsy Pregnancy Register which compared cognitive development in children exposed to levetiracetam and valproate, children exposed to levetiracetam *in utero* were not at an increased risk of delayed early development compared with control children. In contrast those exposed to valproate scored significantly worse (102).

Management of women with epilepsy before, during, and after pregnancy

Preconception counselling should be available to all women with epilepsy contemplating pregnancy. This should start at the time of diagnosis and at subsequent reviews. While it may not always be appropriate to discuss the many relevant issues (for example, in paediatric practice) it should certainly be considered in female adolescents with epilepsy, including those whose care is being transferred from a paediatrician to an adult physician. The fact that the relevant issues have been discussed should always be clearly recorded in the notes.

Where resources permit, an organized joint obstetric/neurology preconceptual service should be available to allow rapid assessment of women actively contemplating pregnancy and to coordinate care during pregnancy. This may not always be possible. Nevertheless, a reconfiguration of clinics and additional resources to allow for this service should be actively considered.

During counselling a re-evaluation of the diagnosis and the need for continued antiepilepsy medication should take place. Consideration should be given to the AED and indeed the dosage of any AED that is prescribed. The risks and benefits of reducing or changing medication should be fully discussed with each individual patient. Other areas that need to be covered are contraception, fertility, and the use of folic acid.

Folic acid

The prescription of folic acid before conception and at least until the end of the first trimester is recommended in patients taking antiepileptic medication, as it is for all women. This followed the recognition that there is an increased risk of neural tube defects in children born to mothers taking AEDs, in particular sodium valproate and carbamazepine (60, 61, 103). Large community-based studies have demonstrated a reduction in the rate of neural tube defects in women taking folic acid preconceptually (104, 105). It has been inferred from this that folic acid will protect women with epilepsy who are also at increased risk of this complication. The optimum dosage of folic acid remains undetermined. Community-based studies have used dosages ranging from 0.5–4.0 mg daily, the higher dosage being suggested for women considered at higher risk. It is the higher dosage that is generally recommended in the UK for women with epilepsy (5 mg daily).

Some concerns have been raised that folic acid may exacerbate seizures but these fears have been generally felt to be unfounded. There is no evidence that folic acid confers additional protection against neural tube defects or other malformations seen in association with AEDs. There is some evidence that the neural tube defects which occur in association with sodium valproate are different from those seen in the general population. They tend to be low lumbar or sacral in site (106). Other abnormalities are less common and the defect may be the result of altered canalization rather than folding of the developing neural crest. It remains uncertain as to whether folic acid will protect against this form of neural tube defect (107) or other defects associated with AEDs (108). The potential effect of folate supplementation was reported for 4680 cases from the UK Epilepsy and Pregnancy Register (109). While those women who received preconceptual folic acid, approximately three-quarters of whom received 5 mg each day, appeared more likely to have a child with a MCM than those who did not (3.9% vs. 2.2%; odds ratio 1.8 (95% CI 1.2–2.5)), the rate of neural tube defects for valproate-exposed pregnancies, while raised, was about half that in folate-exposed compared with those not exposed to folate (0.8% vs. 1.6%). Since this is the very reason that high-dose folate is advocated in AED-exposed pregnancies, despite the lack of evidence for folate having additional protective effects, current guidelines should continue to be observed, at least for those pregnancies exposed to valproate. Furthermore, preconceptual folate use has been reported to be associated with higher verbal outcomes (97).

Monitoring pregnancy in women with epilepsy

Ideally, pregnancies in women with epilepsy should be supervised in an obstetric unit, with access to high-resolution ultrasound scanning and the full range of prenatal tests, which has access to a physician with specialist expertise in epilepsy. Where the latter is not available an obstetrician who specializes in medically complicated pregnancies should be identified.

Effects of pregnancy on epilepsy

It is generally held that women with well-controlled epilepsy are unlikely to experience a significant change in their seizure frequency during pregnancy. This was confirmed by the EURAP study group, who reported the outcomes of 1956 prospectively studied pregnancies. Using first trimester as reference, seizure control remained unchanged throughout pregnancy in 63.6%, of whom 92.7% were seizure free during the entire pregnancy (33). Loss of seizure control was associated with a history of localization-related epilepsy, being on more than one AED, and taking oxcarbazepine in pregnancy.

Reasons for loss of seizure control are varied. Poor compliance with AED treatment because of nausea or the fear of harm from AEDs to the fetus can result in loss of control. Measuring compliance is problematic and monitoring serum levels or self-reporting may not be reliable. The ability to study longer-term compliance is therefore of interest. In one study that measured AED levels in hair samples it was shown that 15% of pregnant women had little or no AED in their proximal compared with distal hair measurements of AEDs (110).

During pregnancy total serum AED levels may fall with less marked reductions in non-protein bound (free) drug concentrations (111, 112) (Table 13.5). Many factors may contribute to this fall including increased metabolism/excretion, increased plasma volume, and reduced protein binding. Total AED concentrations do not predict response during pregnancy and therefore if serum assessments are to be made, measurement of the unbound fraction is the method of choice (113). This is especially relevant for those AEDs, such as valproate and phenytoin, that are moderately or highly protein bound.

Several studies have demonstrated pronounced alterations in the pharmacokinetics of lamotrigine during pregnancy (114–118). Apparent clearance increases steadily throughout pregnancy, peaking at about the 32nd week of gestation, when a 330% increase from baseline has been observed. The observed fall in lamotrigine levels during pregnancy has been reported as being associated with a decline in seizure control.

There is currently no consensus on how best to monitor AED levels during pregnancy. It has previously been advocated that a baseline, preconception, unbound (free) AED level, repeated at the beginning of each trimester and in the last 4 weeks of pregnancy should be the minimum level of monitoring (119). More frequent measurements will be necessary if seizure control deteriorates, side effects ensue, or compliance is an issue. For most AEDs routine monitoring of serum levels is probably not necessary.

Table 13.3 MCM rates for AEDs—comparing monotherapy and polytherapy exposures

Reference	% MCM	
	Monotherapy	Polytherapy
Samren et al. 1997	8.0	9.8
Olafsson et al. 1998	3.4	8.7
Canger et al. 1999	5.7	5.3
Kaneko et al. 1999	7.8	9.6 (2 AEDs), 11.5 (3 AEDs), 13.5 (4 AEDs), 15.4 (5 AEDs)
Samren et al. 1999	3.3	4.7 (2 AEDs), 4.4 (3 AEDs), 8 (4+ AEDs)
Holmes et al. 2001	4.5	8.6
Kaaja et al. 2003	3.2	5.8 (2 AEDs), 8.3 (3 + AEDs)
Morrow et al. 2006	3.7	6.0

For lamotrigine, however, some are of the opinion that close monitoring is mandatory and that drug levels should be increased if serum levels fall, to prevent deterioration in seizure control (120). That close monitoring may be effective at minimizing seizure deterioration was shown in 42 women receiving lamotrigine where monthly monitoring and dose adjustment was associated with only 19% having an increased seizure frequency (121). Whether such practices expose the fetus to additional risks has not been established.

Most women with epilepsy will have a normal uncomplicated vaginal delivery. However, in approximately 2–4% the stress of labour may result in an increased risk of seizures during labour or in the following 24 hours (33). Tonic–clonic seizures may result in fetal hypoxia and it is therefore generally recommended that delivery takes place in a unit equipped with facilities for maternal and neonatal resuscitation. Factors that increase the risk of seizures such as sleep deprivation, pain, overbreathing, and emotional distress should be reduced as much as possible and early consideration given for epidural anaesthesia. The analgesic pethidine may have a proconvulsant effect and is best avoided if possible.

AEDs should be continued throughout labour. If necessary, all AEDs can be given by nasogastric tube; phenytoin, sodium valproate, phenobarbitone, levetiracetam, diazepam, and clonazepam can be given parenterally and carbamazepine rectally.

Seizures in labour should be terminated as soon as possible using intravenous lorazepam or diazepam. For persisting seizures treatment should be for status epilepticus and delivery expedited. Where there is doubt about whether seizures are due to eclampsia or epilepsy a slow bolus of 4 mg of magnesium sulphate over 3–5 minutes, followed by 1 mg/hour for 24 hours is recommended in addition to intravenous lorazepam or diazepam (http://www.sign.ac.uk/guidelines/fulltext/70/index.html).

AED levels revert to prepregnancy levels after birth at a variable rate (115). Hence, if the dose of an AED has been increased during pregnancy because of falling AED levels it may be useful to measure serum levels repeatedly during the first 6–8 weeks after delivery to anticipate and manage the potential development of drug toxicity. However, the decision to reduce the AED dosage following delivery back to the preconception dosage, and the rate of dose reduction, should be made on an individual basis and with great care. In particular, if the increase in dose has resulted in a sustained improvement in seizure control with no evidence of toxicity the dose should not be changed. If the dose of AED has been increased during pregnancy and a decision is subsequently taken to reduce the dose back to preconceptual levels postpartum, then substantial care should be taken as too rapid a dose reduction may result in uncontrolled seizures and maternal harm.

The effects of epilepsy and antiepileptic drugs on pregnancy

The over-representation of epilepsy as one of the leading indirect causes of maternal mortality in pregnancy raises significant concerns. The confidential enquiries into maternal deaths in the UK, covering the period from 1985–1999 identified that maternal mortality was over-represented among women with epilepsy, with over a 10-fold increased risk compared with what might be expected considering the prevalence of epilepsy. While the reasons for the increased risk are not fully understood follow up reports have consistently reported that SUDEP accounts for most of the excess deaths.

For the period 2000–2002, of the 10 out of the 13 epilepsy-related deaths (of 256 deaths) that had a postmortem examination, nine cases were felt either to have died, or probably to have died from SUDEP. In two out of the seven cases where blood levels of AEDs were measured there was no measurable trace of AEDs. In the most recent report spanning 2006–2008, 14 of the 261 maternal deaths were recorded as being due to epilepsy (122). Of the 14, nine were taking lamotrigine, none of whom had their AED level measured in pregnancy and 11 were felt to have died as a result of SUDEP. Of the five that had AED levels measured at autopsy, three had a subtherapeutic level and two a low level. Of note, the proportion of deaths felt to be due to epilepsy has not increased over the years studied.

Data on whether women with epilepsy are at increased risk of obstetric complications are conflicting. Complications reported include an increased rate of vaginal bleeding, spontaneous abortion, pre-eclampsia, and premature or prolonged labour. Higher frequencies of labour induction and artificial labour have also been reported, but whether this is due to a greater frequency of medical indications or is due to increased concern on the part of obstetricians or mothers-to-be is uncertain. The adverse outcomes most consistently reported are increased stillbirths and neonatal deaths, although there is some evidence that the latter has been improving. That women with epilepsy who have seizures during pregnancy may also be more likely to have preterm, small or low birth weight babies compared with women without epilepsy has been shown in a study from Taiwan (123).

Vitamin K

Since 1958 over 40 cases of neonatal bleeding associated with maternal AED treatment have been reported (124). It is felt that this is due to reduced clotting factors, consequent to increased vitamin K clearance by hepatic enzyme-inducing AEDs such as phenytoin, phenobarbital, and carbamazepine. Newborn infants that have been exposed to enzyme-inducing AEDs *in utero* may show increased levels of PIVKA II (protein induced by vitamin K absence of factor II), an indirect marker of vitamin K deficiency (125, 126). While there is no evidence directly linking this biochemical marker to a clinically increased risk of bleeding in the neonate, its suppression with vitamin K_1 supplementation given as 10 mg orally each day from the 36th week of gestation (127) has resulted in early guidelines for best practice advocating maternal supplementation with vitamin K_1, with all infants also being given 1 mg vitamin K_1 intramuscularly at birth (119, 128). However, the results of the only case–control study performed did not show that there was an increased risk for bleeding in infants exposed *in utero* to enzyme-inducing AEDs (mainly carbamazepine and phenytoin) (129) although it was felt that supplementation might be necessary in selected cases, such as when prematurity was anticipated or there was a history of maternal alcohol abuse. Based on this report and a further review of all available literature the American Academy of Neurology updated its recommendations in 2009, stating that there was currently inadequate evidence to determine if newborns of women with epilepsy taking AEDs had a substantially increased risk of haemorrhagic complications (130). At present giving oral supplementation with vitamin K is not possible in the UK as there is currently no orally available preparation that can be prescribed for this indication. At birth it is recommended that infants receive vitamin K, with 1 mg of vitamin K given intramuscularly (as is the case for all newborns).

Table 13.4 Features of fetal valproate syndrome

- Tall forehead
- Medial eyebrow deficiency
- Flat nasal bridge
- Broad nasal root
- Shallow philtrum
- Long upper lip
- Thin vermillion border

Management of the postpartum period

Breastfeeding should be encouraged and may even have the additional advantage that it ensures the baby is withdrawn gradually from being exposed to AED therapy. AEDs are excreted in breast milk at a level inversely proportional to the degree of maternal serum protein binding (131–137). Hence the amount transferred to the infant in breast milk varies substantially between AEDs (Table 13.6). Concentrations of AEDs can differ substantially between the start and end of a meal, and between the right and left breast depending on the fat and protein contents of the milk. For some AEDs, such as phenobarbital and primidone, reduced neonatal serum protein binding and immature elimination mechanisms can result in drug accumulation. This can result in sedation of the infant and necessitate the discontinuation of breastfeeding. For most AEDs including phenytoin, carbamazepine, and valproate, breastfeeding is usually without problems as these drugs are highly protein bound and therefore are poorly excreted into breast milk. Information on the concentration in breast milk of the newer AEDs is rather limited, however preliminary data indicate that lamotrigine passes into breast milk in significant levels. When combined with the effects of immature hepatic uridine diphosphate glucuronyltransferase enzyme systems neonatal exposure to lamotrigine might result in high blood concentrations in some infants, a problem that could be compounded if valproate is also taken (138). For levetiracetam, plasma concentrations in breastfed infants are low despite extensive transfer of levetiracetam into breast milk (139).

There have been some concerns that breastfeeding during AED therapy might have a detrimental effect on cognitive development. Data from the Neurodevelopmental Effects of Antiepileptic Drugs Study is reassuring, albeit the numbers studied were small. Intelligent quotients for breastfed children did not differ from

Table 13.5 Pharmacokinetics of antiepileptic drugs in pregnancy

Antiepileptic drug	Decrease in total plasma concentration (%)	Decrease in free concentration (%)
Phenobarbital	55	50
Phenytoin	61	18
Carbamazepine	10–40	4
Valproate	39	25
Lamotrigine	40–60	
Oxcarbazepine MHD	36–50	
Levetiracetam	50–60	

MHD = monohydroxy metabolite.

Table 13.6 Antiepileptic drugs studied in breast milk as a proportion of blood levels

Antiepileptic drug (reference)	Proportion appearing in breast milk (%)
Valproate (131)	3
Phenytoin (132)	18–45
Carbamazepine (133)	36
Phenobarbitone (134)	36
Lamotrigine (115)	61
Gabapentin (137)	70–130
Primidone (134)	72
Ethosuximide (135)	86
Topiramate (136)	86
Levetiracetam (139)	105

those that were not breastfed either for all AEDs combined or for those exposed to the individual AEDs studied (phenytoin, carbamazepine, lamotrigine, or valproate) (140).

Risk of injury to the infant largely depends on seizure type and frequency. Any such risk can be minimized if time is allocated to training mothers with epilepsy on safe handling, bathing techniques, feeding, and safe practice around the home.

The postnatal check in addition to providing a chance to examine the infant for any abnormalities also offers an opportunity to discuss contraception, the need for planning future pregnancies, folate requirements and risks associated with AEDs in pregnancy.

References

1. Luef G. Hormonal alterations following seizures. *Epilepsy Behav* 2010; 19:131–3.
2. Pack AM, Reddy DS, Duncan S, Herzog A. Neuroendocrinological aspects of epilepsy: Important issues and trends for future research. *Epilepsy Behav* 2011; 94:102–22.
3. Verrotti A, D'Egidio C, Mohn A, Coppola G, Parisi P, Chiarelli F. Antiepileptic drugs, sex hormones, and PCOS. *Epilepsia* 2011; 52(2):199–211.
4. Pack AM. Implications of hormonal and neuro-endocrine changes associated with seizures and antiepilepsy drugs: a clinical perspective. *Epilepsia* 2010; 51(Suppl. 3):150–3.
5. Isojärvi JI, Laatikainen TJ, Pakarinen AJ, Juntunen KT, Myllyla VV. Polycystic ovaries and hyperandrogenism in women taking valproate for epilepsy. *N Engl J Med* 1993; 329:1383–8.
6. Tauboll E, Gregoraszczuk EL, Tworzydø A, Wójtowicz AK, Ropstad E. Comparison of reproductive effects of levetiracetam and valproate studied in prepubertal porcine ovarian follicular cells. *Epilepsia* 2006; 47:1580–3.
7. Morrell MJ, Hayes FJ, Sluss PM, Adams JM, Bhatt M, Ozkara C, *et al.* Hyperandrogenism, ovulatory dysfunction, and polycystic ovary syndrome with valproate versus lamotrigine. *Ann Neurol* 2008; 64:200–11.
8. Isojärvi JI, Rättyä J, Myllylä VV, Knip M, Koivunen R, Pakarinen AJ, *et al.* Valproate, lamotrigine, and insulin-mediated risks in women with epilepsy. *Ann Neurol* 1998; 43:446–51.
9. Mikkonen K, Vainionpää LK, Pakarinen AJ, Knip M, Järvelä IY, Tapanainen JS, *et al.* Long-term reproductive endocrine health in young women with epilepsy during puberty. *Neurology* 2004; 62(3):445–50.
10. Duncan S, Read CL, Brodie MJ. How common is catamenial epilepsy? *Epilepsia* 1993; 34:827–31.
11. Reddy DS, Rogawski MA. Neurosteriod replacement therapy for catamenial epilepsy. *Neurotherapeutics* 2009; 6:392–401.
12. Mattson RH, Cramer JA, Caldwell BV, Siconolfi BC. Treatment of seizures with medroxyprogesterone acetate: preliminary report. *Neurology* 1984; 34:1255–8.
13. Herzog AG, Drislane FW, Schomer DL, Pennell PB, Bromfield EB, Dworetzky BA, *et al.* Differential effects of antiepileptic drugs on neuroactive steroids in men with epilepsy. *Epilepsia* 2006; 47:1945–8.
14. Herzog AG, Coleman AE, Jacobs AR, Klein P, Friedman MN, Drislane FW, Schomer DL. Relationship of sexual dysfunction to epilepsy laterality and reproductive hormone levels in women. *Epilepsy Behav* 2003; 4:407–13.
15. Morrell MJ, Flynn KL, Done S, Flaster E, Kalayjian L, Pack AM. Sexual dysfunction, sex steroid hormone abnormalities, and depression in women with epilepsy treated with antiepilepsy drugs. *Epilepsy Behav* 2005; 6:360–5.
16. Isojärvi J. Disorders of reproduction in patients with epilepsy: antiepileptic drug related mechanisms. *Seizure* 2008; 17:141–4.
17. Luef G. Female issues in epilepsy: a critical review. *Epilepsy Behav* 2009; 15:78–82.
18. Nakken KO, Tauboll E. Bone loss associated with use of antiepileptic drugs. *Expert Opin Drug Saf* 2010; 9(4):561–71.
19. Sato Y, Kondo I, Ishida S, Motooka H, Takayama K, Tomita Y, Maeda H, *et al.* Decreased bone mass and increased bone turnover with valproate therapy in adults with epilepsy. *Neurology* 2001; 57:445–9.
20. Boluk A, Guzelipek M, Savli H, Temel I, Ozi ik HI, Kaygusuz A. The effect of valproate on bone mineral density in adult epileptic patients. *Pharmacol Res* 2004; 50(1):93–7.
21. Jette N, Lix LM, Metge CJ, Prior HJ, McChesney J, Leslie WD. Association of antiepileptic drugs with non-traumatic fractures: a population based analysis. *Arch Neurol* 2011; 68:107–12.
22. Nissen-Meyer LS, Svalheim S, Tauboll E, Reppe S, Lekva T, Solberg LB, *et al.* Levetiracetam, phenytoin, and valproate act differently on rat bone mass, structure, and metabolism. *Epilepsia* 2007; 48(10):1850–60.
23. O'Brien MD and Gilmour-White SK. Management of epilepsy in women. *Postgrad Med J* 2005; 81:278–85.
24. O'Brien MD, Guillebaud J. Contraception for women with epilepsy. *Epilepsia* 2006; 47(9):1419–22.
25. Doose DR, Wang SS, Padmanabhan M, Schwabe S, Jacobs D, Bialer M. Effect of topiramate or carbamazepine on the pharmacokinetics of an oral contraceptive containing norethindrone and ethinyl estradiol in healthy obese and nonobese female subjects. *Epilepsia* 2003; 44:540–9.
26. Sidhu J, Job S, Singh S, Phillipson R. The pharmacokinetic and pharmacodynamic consequences of the co-administration of lamotrigine and a combined oral contraceptive in healthy female subjects. *Br J Clin Pharmacol* 2006; 61:191–9.
27. Sabers A, Bucholt JM, Uldall P, Hansen EL. Lamotrigine plasma levels reduced by oral contraceptives. *Epilepsy Res* 2001; 47:151–4.
28. Tomson T, Battino D, Craig J, Hernandez-Diaz S, Holmes LB, Lindhout D, *et al.* Pregnancy registries : differences, similarities, and possible harmonization. *Epilepsia* 2010; 51(5):909–15.
29. Gaily E, Granstrom ML, Hiilesmaa V, Bardy A. Minor abnormalities in children of mothers with epilepsy. *Journal of Paediatrics* 1988; 112:520–9.
30. Steegers-Theunissen RP, Renier WO, Borm GF, Thomas CM, Merkus HM, Op de Coul DA, *et al.* Factors influencing the risk of abnormal pregnancy outcome in epileptic women: a multi centre prospective study. *Epilepsy Res* 1994; 18:261–9.
31. Adab N, Kini U, Vinten J, Ayres J, Baker G, Clayton-Smith J, *et al.* The longer term outcome of children born to mothers with epilepsy. *J Neurol Neurosurg Psychiatry* 2004; 75:1575–83.
32. Teramo K, Hiilesmaa V. Pregnancy and fetal complications in epileptic pregnancies. In: Janz D, Dam M, Richens A, Bossi L, Helge H, Schmidt D (eds) *Epilepsy, Pregnancy and the Child*, pp. 53–9. New York: Raven Press, 1982.

33. The EURAP Study Group. Seizure control and treatment in pregnancy. Observations from the EURAP Epilepsy Pregnancy Registry. *Neurology* 2006; 66:354–60.
34. Samren EB, Van Duijn CM, Christiaens L, Hofman A, Lindhout D. Antiepileptic drug regimes and major congenital abnormalities in the offspring. *Ann Neurol* 1999; 46:739–46.
35. Delgado-Escuta AV, Janz D. Consensus guidelines: preconception counselling, management, and care of the pregnant woman with epilepsy. *Neurology* 1992; 42 (Suppl 5):149–60.
36. Janz D. Are antiepileptic drugs harmful when taken during pregnancy? *J Perinat Med* 1994; 22:367–77.
37. Holmes LB, Harvey EA, Coull BA, Huntington KB, Khoshbin S, Hayes AM, *et al.* The teratogenicity of anticonvulsant drugs. *N Engl J Med* 2001; 344:1132–38.
38. Finnell RH, Dansky LV. Parental epilepsy, anticonvulsant drugs, and reproductive outcome: epidemiologic and experimental findings spanning three decades; 1: animal studies. *Reprod Toxicol* 1991; 5:281–99.
39. Samren EB, Van Duijin C, Koch S, Hiilesmaa VK, Klepel H, Bardy AH, *et al.* Maternal use of antiepileptic drugs and the risk of major congenital malformations: a joint European prospective study of human teratogenesis associated with maternal epilepsy. *Epilepsia* 1997; 38:981–90.
40. Olafsson E, Hallgrimsson JT, Hauser WA, Ludvigsson P, Gudmundsson G. Pregnancies of women with epilepsy: a population-based study in Iceland. *Epilepsia* 1998; 39:887–92.
41. Morrow J, Russell A, Guthrie E, Parsons L, Robertson I, Waddell R, *et al.* Malformation risks of antiepileptic drugs in pregnancy: a prospective study from the UK Epilepsy and Pregnancy Register. *J Neurol Neurosurg Psychiatry* 2006; 77:193–8.
42. Canger R, Battino D, Canevini MP, Fumarola C, Guidolin L, Vignoli A, *et al.* Malformations in offspring of women with epilepsy: a prospective study. *Epilepsia* 1999; 40:1231–6.
43. Kaneko S, Battino D, Andermann E, Wada K, Kan R, Takeda A, *et al.* Congenital malformations due to antiepileptic drugs. *Epilepsy Res* 1999; 33:145–8.
44. Kaaja E, Kaaja R, Hiilessmaa V. Major malformations in offspring of women with epilepsy. *Neurology* 2003; 60:575–9.
45. Cunnington MC, Weil JG, Messenheimer JA, Ferber S, Yerby M, Tennis P. Final results from 18 years of the International Lamotrigine Pregnancy Registry. *Neurology* 2011; 76:1817–23.
46. Holmes LB, Wysznski DF, Lieberman E, for the AED Pregnancy Registry. The AED (Antiepileptic Drug) Pregnancy Registry: a 6-year experience. *Arch Neurol* 2004; 61:673–8.
47. Meador K, Reynolds MW, Crean S, Fahrbach K, Probst C. Pregnancy outcomes in women with epilepsy: a systematic review and meta-analysis of published pregnancy registries and cohorts. *Epilepsy Res* 2008; 81(1):1–13.
48. Arpino C, Brescianini S, Robert E, Castilla EE, Cocchi G, Cornel MC, *et al.* Teratogenic effects of antiepileptic drugs: use of an international database on malformations and drug exposure (MADRE). *Epilepsia* 2000; 41:1436–43.
49. Hanson JW, Smith DW. The fetal hydantoin syndrome. *J Pediatr* 1975; 87:285–90.
50. Diav-Citron O, Shechtman S, Arnon J, Ornoy A. Is carbamazepine teratogenic? A prospective controlled study of 210 pregnancies. *Neurology* 2001; 57:321–24.
51. Granstrom ML, Hiilesmaan VK. Malformations and minor anomalies in children of epileptic mothers: preliminary results of the prospective Helsinki study. In: Janz D, Dam M, Richens A, Bossi L, Helge H and Schmidt D (eds) *Epilepsy, Pregnancy and the Child*, pp. 251–258. New York: Raven Press, 1992.
52. Jentinik J, Dolk H, Loane MA, Morris JK, Wellesley D, Garne E, De Jong-Van Den Berg L for the EUROCAT antiepileptic study working group. Intrauterine exposure to carbamazepine and specific congenital malformations: systematic review and case-control study. *BMJ* 2010; 341:c6581.
53. Wysznski D, Nambisan M, Surve T, Alsdorf R, Smith C, Holmes L for the Antiepileptic Drug Pregnancy Registry. Increased risk of major malformations in offspring exposed to valproate during pregnancy. *Neurology* 2005; 64:961–5.
54. Vajda FJ, Graham JE, Hitchcock AA, O'Brien TJ, Lander CM, Eadie MJ. Is lamotrigine a significant human teratogen? Observations from the Australian Pregnancy Register. *Seizure* 2010; 19:558–61.
55. Duncan S, Mercho S, Lopes-Cendes I, Seni MH, Benjamin A, Dubeau F, *et al.* Repeated neural tube defects and valproate monotherapy suggest a pharmacogenetic abnormality. *Epilepsia* 2001; 42:750–53.
56. Malm H, Kajantie E, Kivirikko S. Valproate embryopathy in three sets of siblings: Further proof of hereditary susceptibility. *Neurology* 2002; 59:630–3.
57. Faiella A, Wernig M, Consalez GC. A mouse model for valproate teratogenicity: parental effects, homeotic transformations, and altered HOX expression. *Hum Molecular Genet* 2000; 9:227–36.
58. Nau H. Teratogenic valproic acid concentrations: infusion by implanted minipumps vs conventional injection regimen in the mouse. *Toxicol Appl Pharmacol* 1985; 80:243–50.
59. Jentinik J, Loane MA, Dolk H, Barisic I, Garne E, Morris JK, *et al.* for the EUROCAT Antiepileptic Study Working Group. Valproic acid monotherapy in pregnancy and major congenital malformations. *N Engl J Med* 2010; 362:2185–93.
60. Omtzigt JG, Los FJ, Grobbee DE, Pijpers L, Jahoda MG, Brandenburg H, *et al.* The risk of spina bifida aperta after first-trimester exposure to valproate in a prenatal cohort. *Neurology* 1992; 42(suppl 5):119–25.
61. Lindhout D, Omtzigt JGC, Cornel MC. Spectrum of neural-tube defects in 34 infants prenatally exposed to antiepileptic drugs. *Neurology* 1992; 42(suppl 5):111–18.
62. Koch S, Losche G, Jager-Roman E, Jakob S, Rating D, Deichl A, *et al.* Major birth malformations and antiepileptic drugs. *Neurology* 1992; 42(suppl 5):83–8.
63. Cunnington M, Ferber S, Quartey G. Effect of dose on the frequency of major birth defects following fetal exposure to lamotrigine monotherapy in an international observational study. *Epilepsia* 2007; 48:1207–10.
64. Holmes LB, Baldwin EJ, Smith CR, Habecker E, Glassman L, Wong SL, *et al.* Increased frequency of isolated cleft palate in infants exposed to lamotrigine during pregnancy. *Neurology* 2008; 70:2152–8.
65. Hunt SJ, Craig JJ, Morrow JI. Increased frequency of isolated cleft palate in infants exposed to lamotrigine during pregnancy. *Neurology* 2009; 72(12):1108.
66. Dolk H, Jentinik J, Loane M, Morris J, Jong-Van Den Berg LT. On behalf of the EUROCAT Antiepileptic Drug Working Group. Does lamotrigine use in pregnancy increase orofacial cleft risk relative to other malformations? *Neurology* 2008; 71:706–7.
67. Meischenguiser R, D'Giano CH, Ferraro SM. Oxcarbazepine in pregnancy: clinical experience in Argentina. *Epilepsy Behav* 2004; 5:163–7.
68. Montouris G. Safety of the newer antiepileptic drug oxcarbazepine during pregnancy. Curr *Med Res Opin* 2005; 21:693–702.
69. Wilton LV, Shakir S. A post-marketing surveillance study of gabapentin as add-on therapy for 3,100 patients in England. *Epilepsia* 2002; 43:951–5.
70. Leppik I, Gram L, Deaton R, Sommerville K. Safety of tiagabine: summary of 53 trials. *Epilepsy Res* 1999; 33:235–46.
71. Hunt S, Russell A, Smithson WH, Parsons L, Robertson I, Waddell R, *et al.* Topiramate in pregnancy: preliminary experience from the UK Epilepsy and Pregnancy Register. *Neurology* 2008; 22:272–6.
72. Ornoy A, Zvi N, Arnon J, Wajnberg R, Schechtman S, Diav-Citron O. The outcome of pregnancy following topiramate treatment: A study on 52 pregnancies. *Reprod Toxicol* 2008; 25:388–9.
73. Long L. Levetiracetam monotherapy during pregnancy: a case series. *Epilepsy Behav* 2003; 4:447–8.

74. Ten Berg K, Samren EB, VanAN Oppen AC, Engelsman M, Lindhout D. Levetiracetam use and pregnancy outcome. *Reprod Toxicol* 2005; 20:175–8.
75. Hunt S, Craig J, Russell A, Guthrie E, Parsons L, Robertson I, *et al.* Levetiracetam in pregnancy: preliminary experience from the UK Epilepsy and Pregnancy Register. *Neurology* 2006; 67:1876–9.
76. Kennedy F, Morrow J, Hunt S, Russell A, Smithson WH, Parsons P, *et al.* Malformation risks of anti-epileptic drugs in pregnancy: an update from the UK Epilepsy and Pregnancy Register. *J Neurol Neurosurg Psychiatry* 2010; 81:e18.
77. Holmes LB, Smith CR, Hernandez-Diaz S. Pregnancy Registries: Larger sample sizes essential. *Birth Defects Res A* 2008; 82:307.
78. Kondo T, Kaneko T, Amano Y, Egawa I. Preliminary report on teratogenic effects of zonisamide in the offspring of treated women with epilepsy. *Epilepsia* 1996; 37:1242–4.
79. Vajda FJE, Hitchcock AA, Graham J, O'Brien TJ, Lander CM, Eadie MJ. The teratogenic risk of antiepileptic drug polytherapy. *Epilepsia* 2010; 51:805–10.
80. Nulman I, Scolnik D, Chitayat D, Farkas L, Koren G. Findings in children exposed in utero to phenytoin and carbamazepine monotherapy: independent effects of epilepsy and medications. *Am J Med Genet* 1997; 68:18–24.
81. Diliberti JH, Farndon PA, Dennis NR, Curry CJR. The fetal valproate syndrome. *Am J Med Genet* 1984; 19:473 –81.
82. Rudd NL, Freedom RM. A possible primidone embryopathy. *J Pediatr* 1979; 94:835–7.
83. Jager-Roman E, Deichl A, Hartmann AM, Koch S, Rating D, *et al.* Fetal growth, major malformations, and minor anomalies in infants born to women receiving valproic acid. *J Pedriatr* 1986; 108:997–1004.
84. Kini U, Adab N, Vinten J, Fryer J. Clayton-Smith J and on behalf of the Liverpool and Manchester Neurodevelopment Study Group Dysmorphic features: an important clue to the diagnosis and severity of fetal anticonvulsant syndrome. *Arch Dis Fetal Neonatal Ed* 2006; 91:90–5.
85. Adab N, Tudur SC, Vinten J, Williamson P, Winterbottom J. Common antiepileptic drugs in pregnancy in women with epilepsy (Cochrane review). In: *The Cochrane Library*. Chichester: John Wiley & Sons, Ltd; Issue 3, 2003.
86. Gaily E, Kantola-Scorsa E, Granstrom ML. Intelligence of children of epileptic mothers. *J Pediatr* 1998; 113:677–84.
87. Scolnik D, Nulman I, Rovet J, Gladstone D, Czuchta D, Gardner HA, *et al.* Neurodevelopment of children exposed in utero to phenytoin and carbamazepine monotherapy. *JAMA* 1994; 271:767–70.
88. Dean JCS, Hailey H, Moore SJ, Lloyd DJ, Turnpenny PD, Little J. Long term health and neurodevelopment in children exposed to antiepileptic drugs before birth. *J Med Genet* 2002; 39:251–9.
89. Thomas SV, Sukumaran S, Lukose N, George A, Sarma PS. Intellectual and language functions in children in mothers with epilepsy. *Epilepsia* 2007; 48:2234–40.
90. Adab N, Jacoby A, Smith D, Chadwick D. Additional educational needs in children born to mothers with epilepsy. *J Neurol Neurosurg Psychiatry* 2001; 70:15–21.
91. Jones KLJ, Lacro RV, Johnson KA, Adams J. Pattern of malformations in the children of women treated with carbamazepine during pregnancy. *N Eng J Med* 1989; 320:1661–6.
92. Ornoy A, Cohen E. Outcome of children born to epileptic mothers treated with carbamazepine during pregnancy. *Arch Dis Child* 1996; 75:517–20.
93. Eriksson K, Viinikainen K, Monkkonen A, Aikiä M, Nieminen P, Heinonen S, *et al.* Children exposed to valproate in utero-population based evaluation of risks and confounding factors for long-term neurocognitive development. *Epilepsy Res* 2005; 65:189–200.
94. Thomas SV, Ajaykumar B, Sindhu L, Nair MK, George B, Sarma PS. Motor and mental development of infants exposed to antiepileptic drugs in utero. *Epilepsy Behav* 2008; 13:229–36.
95. Cummings C, Stewart M, Stevenson M, Morrow J, Nelson J. Neurodevelopment of children exposed in utero to lamotrigine, sodium valproate and carbamazepine. *Arch Dis Child* 2011; 96:643–7.
96. Meador KJ, Baker GA, Browning N, Clayton-Smith J, Combs-Cantrell DT, Cohen M, *et al.* Cognitive function at 3 years of age after fetal exposure to antiepileptic drugs. *N Engl J Med* 2009; 360:1597–605.
97. Meador KJ, Baker GA, Browning N, Cohen MJ, Clayton-Smith J, Kalayjian LA, *et al.* for the NEAD Study Group. Foetal antiepileptic drug exposure and verbal versus non-verbal abilities at three years of age. *Brain* 2011; 134:396–404.
98. McVearry KM, Gaillard WD, Van Meter J, Meador KJ. A prospective study of cognitive fluency and originality in children exposed in utero to carbamazepine, lamotrigine, or valproate monotherapy. *Epilepsy Behav* 2009; 16:609–16.
99. Bromley RL, Mawer G, Love J, Kelly J, Purdy L, McEwan L, *et al.* Early cognitive development in children born to women with epilepsy: a prospective report. *Epilepsia* 2010; 51:2058–65.
100. Nadebaum C, Anderson VA, Vajda F, Reutens DC, Barton S, Wood AG. Language skills of school-aged children prenatally exposed to antiepileptic drugs. *Neurology* 2011; 76:719–26.
101. Nicolai J, Vles JS, Aldenkamp AP. Neurodevelopmental delay in children exposed to anti-epileptic drugs in utero: a critical review directed at structural study-bias. *J Neurol Sci* 2008; 271:1–14.
102. Shallcross R, Bromley RL, Irwin B, Bonnett LJ, Morrow J, Baker GA on behalf of the Liverpool Manchester Neurodevelopment Group and the UK Epilepsy and Pregnancy Register. Child development following in utero exposure. Levetiracetam vs sodium valproate. *Neurology* 2011; 76:383–9.
103. Rosa FW. Spina bifida in infants of women treated with carbamazepine during pregnancy. *N Eng J Med* 1991; 324:674–7.
104. Medical research council research group(MRC) vitamin study research group. Prevention of neural-tube defects: results of the Medical research council vitamin study. *Lancet* 1991; 338:131–7.
105. Czeizel AE, Dudas I. Prevention of the first occurrence of neural-tube defects by periconceptual vitamin supplementation. *N Eng J Med* 1992; 327:1832–5.
106. Van Allen MI, Kalousek DK, Chernoff GF, Juriloff D, Harris M, McGillivray BC, *et al.* Evidence for multi-site closure of the neural tube in humans. *Am J Med Genet* 1993; 47:723–43.
107. Craig J, Morrison P, Morrow J, Patterson V. Failure of periconceptual folic acid to prevent a neural tube defect in the offspring of a mother taking sodium valproate. *Seizure* 1999; 8:253–4.
108. Hernandez-Diaz S, Werler MM, Walker AM, Mitchell AA. Folic acid antagonists during pregnancy and the risk of birth defects. *N Engl J Med* 2000; 343:1608–14.
109. Morrow JI, Hunt SJ, Russell AJ, Smithson WH, Parsons L, Robertson I, *et al.* Folic acid use and congenital malformations in offspring of women with epilepsy. A prospective study from the UK Epilepsy and Pregnancy Register. *J Neurol Neurosurg Psychiatry* 2008; 80:506–11.
110. Williams J, Myson V, Sterard S, Jones G, Wilson JF, Kerr MP, *et al.* Self-discontinuation of antiepileptic medication in pregnancy: detection by hair analysis. *Epilepsia* 2002; 43:824–31.
111. Perucca E, Crema A. Plasma protein binding of drugs in pregnancy. *Clin Pharmacokinet* 1982; 7:336–52.
112. Lander CM, Eadie MJ. Plasma antiepileptic drug concentrations during pregnancy. *Epilepsia* 1991; 32:257–66.
113. Yerby MS, Friel PN, McCCormack K. Antiepileptic drug disposition during pregnancy. *Neurology* 1992; 42(Suppl 5):12–16.
114. Tomson T, Ohman I, Vitols S. Lamotrigine in pregnancy and lactation: a case report. *Epilepsia* 1997; 38:1039–41.
115. Ohman I, Vitols S, Tomson T. Lamotrigine in pregnancy: pharmacokinetics during delivery, in the neonate, and during lactation. *Epilepsia* 2000; 41:709–13.
116. Tran TA, Leppik IE, Blesi K, Sathanandan ST, Remmel R. Lamotrigine clearance during pregnancy. *Neurology* 2002; 59:251–5.

117. Pennell PB, Newport DJ, Stowe ZN, Helmers SL, Montgomery JQ, Henry TR. The impact of pregnancy and childbirth on the metabolism of lamotrigine. *Neurology* 2004; 62:292–5.
118. De Haan GJ, Edelbroek P, Segers J, Engelsman M, Lindhout D, Dévilé-Notschaele M, *et al.* Gestation-induced changes in lamotrigine pharmacokinetics: a monotherapy study. *Neurology* 2004; 63:571–3.
119. Quality standards subcommittee of the American Academy of Neurology. Practice parameter: Management issues for women with epilepsy (summary statement). *Neurology* 1998; 51:944–48.
120. Pennell PB, Peng L, Newport DJ, Ritchie JC, Koganti A, Holley DK, *et al.* Lamotrigine in pregnancy. Clearance, therapeutic drug monitoring and seizure frequency. *Neurology* 2008; 70:2130–6.
121. Sabers A, Petrenaite V. Seizure frequency in pregnant women treated with lamotrigine monotherapy. *Epilepsia* 2009; 50:2163–6.
122. Cantwell R, Clutton-Brock T, Cooper G, Dawson A, Drife J, Garrod D, *et al.* Saving Mothers' Lives: Reviewing maternal deaths to make motherhood safer: 2006–2008. The Eighth Report of the Confidential Enquiries into Maternal Deaths in the United Kingdom. *BJOG* 2011; 118(suppl 1):1–203.
123. Chen Y-H, Chiou H-Y, Lin H-C, Lin H-L. Affect of seizures during gestation on pregnancy outcomes in women with epilepsy. *Arch Neurol* 2009; 66:979–84.
124. Laosombat V. Hemorrhagic disease of the newborn after maternal anticonvulsant therapy: a case report and literature review. *J Med Assoc Thai* 1988; 71:643–8.
125. Cornelissen M, Steegers-Theunissen R, Kollee L, Eskes T, Vogels-Mentink G, Motohara K, *et al.* Increased incidence of neonatal vitamin K deficiency resulting from maternal anticonvulsant therapy. *Am J Obstet Gynecol* 1993; 168:923–8.
126. Howe AM, Oakes DJ, Woodman PDC, Webster WS. Prothrombin and PIVKA-II levels in cord blood from newborns exposed to anticonvulsants during pregnancy. *Epilepsia* 1999; 40:980–4.
127. Cornelissen M, Steegers-Theunissen R, Kollee L, Eskes T, Motohara K, Monnens L. Supplementation of vitamin K in pregnant women receiving anticonvulsant therapy prevents neonatal vitamin K deficiency. *Am J Obstet Gynecol* 1993; 168:884–8.
128. Crawford P, Appleton R, Betts T, Duncan J, Guthrie E, Morrow J. Best practice guidelines for the management of women with epilepsy. *Seizure* 1999; 8:201–17.
129. Kaaja E, Kaaja R, Matila R, Hiilesmaa V. Enzyme-inducing antiepileptic drugs in pregnancy and the risk of bleeding in the neonate. *Neurology* 2002; 58:549–53.
130. Harden CL, Pennell PB, Koppel BS, Hovinga CA, Gidal B, Meador KJ, *et al.* Practice parameter update : management issues for women with epilepsy – focus on pregnancy (an evidence-based review): vitamin K, folic acid, blood levels, and breastfeeding: report of the Quality Standards Subcommittee and Therapeutics and Technology Assessment Subcommittee of the American Academy of Neurology and American Epilepsy Society. *Neurology* 2009; 73(2):142–9.
131. Nau H, Rating D, Koch S, Hauser I, Helge H. Valproic acid and its metabolites: placental transfer, neonatal pharmacokinetics, transfer via mother's milk and clinical status in neonates of epileptic mothers. *J Pharmacol Exp Ther* 1981; 219:768 –77.
132. Mirkin BL. Diphenylhydantoin: placental transfer, fetal localization, neonatal metabolism and possible teratogenic effects. *J Pediatr* 1971; 78:329–37.
133. Froescher W, Eichelbaum N, Niesen M, Dietrich K, Rausch. Carbamazepine levels in breast milk. *Ther Drug Monit* 1984; 6:266–71.
134. Kuhnz W, Koch S, Helge H, Nau H. Primidone and phenobarbital during lactation period in epileptic women: total and free drug levels in the nursed infants and their effects on neonatal behavior. *Dev Pharmacol Ther* 1988; 11:147–54.
135. Kuhnz W, Koch S, Jakob S, Hartmann A, Helge H, Nau H. Ethosuximide in epileptic women during pregnancy and lactation period: placental transfer, serum concentrations in nursed infants and clinical status. *Br J Clin Pharmacol* 1984; 18:671–7.
136. Ohman I, Vitols S, Luef G, Soderfeldt B, Tomson T, Söderfeldt B, Tomson T. Topiramate kinetics during delivery, lactation and in the neonate: preliminary observations. *Epilepsia* 2002; 43:1157–60.
137. Ohman I, Vitols S, Tomson T. Pharmacokinetics of gabapentin during delivery, in the neonatal period and lactation: does fetal accumulation occur during pregnancy? *Epilepsia*2005; 46:1621–4.
138. Berry DJ. The distribution of lamotrigine throughout pregnancy. *Ther Drug Monit* 1999; 21:450.
139. Tomson T, Palm R, Kallen K, Ben-Menachem E, Söderfeldt B, Danielsson B, *et al.* Pharmacokinetics of Levetiracetam during pregnancy, delivery, in the neonatal period, and lactation. *Epilepsia* 2007; 48:1111–16.
140. Meador KJ, Baker GA, BrowningR N, *et al* on behalf of NEAD Study Group. Effects of breastfeeding in children of women taking antiepileptic drugs. *Neurology* 2010; 75:1954–60.

CHAPTER 14

Neonatal Seizures and Infantile-Onset Epilepsies

Elia Pestana Knight and Ingrid E.B. Tuxhorn

Introduction

Seizures in the newborn and infant are generally of ominous significance and highly associated with acute neurological injury, morbidity, and mortality. They manifest with unique clinical and electrical features quite different from seizures in older children and adults. The neurologist as well as neonatalogist who is well versed with the clinical and electrographic characteristics of neonatal seizures and epilepsies has an important role to play in the early diagnosis and management that may impact the short- and long-term prognosis. In this chapter we will review the clinical significance of neonatal and infantile seizures and epilepsies, the pathophysiology of the clinical and electrographic phenotypes relevant for accurate diagnosis, current evidence-based treatments, aetiologies, and management options on the horizon to potentially improve neurological outcomes.

Incidence

Neonatal seizures are common neurocritical events affecting approximately 1–4/1000 live term births requiring expert neurological care by experienced and trained paediatric neurologists (1–3). In the US, of the approximately 4 million live births annually, there are 3700–15,000 term infants with neonatal seizures each year.

The neonatal period is one of the highest risk periods for seizures and the incidence of seizures in the first 28 days of life is reported to range between 1–5% (1.5–5.5 per 1000 neonates) from different countries (4–10). Most occur within the first week of life. Conceptual age and birth weight has been determined a specific risk factor for incidence with up to 57 per 1000 in very-low-birth-weight (<1500 g), dropping to 5 per 1000 in low-birth-weight (1500–2499 g) to 3 per 1000 in normal-weight-newborns (2500–3999 g) (11). Under conceptual age of 30 weeks seizures were seen in 4% and over 30 weeks in 1.5% in another study.

Definitions and concepts

As neonatal seizures are frequently encountered in the newborn in the neonatal intensive care unit particularly in the setting of hypoxic-ischaemic encephalopathy (HIE) and can be extremely subtle to the extent of not being clinically observable in nearly half of affected neonates, there needs to be a high index of suspicion for clinical or subclinical seizures to make the diagnosis (3).

Concepts underlying the definition of neonatal seizures may have several important practical consequences (7):

- A definition of neonatal seizures that is limited to purely clinical criteria will:
  - Result in the exclusion of pure electroencephalographic seizures not associated with a clinic seizure event which may apply to the majority of neonatal seizures.
  - Result in missing subtle behavioural and autonomic clinical seizure events that may or may not be associated with electrographic seizure discharges.
  - Result in the erroneous diagnosis of other neonatal paroxysmal disorders as neonatal seizure events such as normal awake/sleep paroxysmal behaviours, e.g. sleep myoclonus and abnormal movements such as dystonia or choreoathetosis, jitteriness, and tremors.
- A definition of neonatal seizures that is limited to purely electrographic criteria will:
  - Exclude subtle clinical seizures that do not have an electroencephalographic correlate which may be seen in the setting of electroclinical dissociation after initiation of treatment with antiepileptic drugs (AEDs) or when seizures originate and remain localized in deeper brain structures rather than spreading to involve the more superficial cortical neuronal networks (8, 9).

The realization that neonatal seizures have distinct clinical and electrographic phenotypes that may occur independently has led to a broader more inclusive definition of any paroxysmal alteration of neurological behaviour or function and electroencephalographic function seen in newborns and infants from the time of birth until 44 weeks of conceptional age, which is defined as the gestational age plus the chronological age (10, 11). Besides the clinical implications described earlier, the broader definition is also important for meaningful epidemiological and clinical research of neonatal seizures to improve management and outcome (12).

Classification of neonatal seizures in the International League Against Epilepsy schemas

The unique aspects of definition of neonatal seizures are also reflected in the attempts to include them in the seizure and epileptic syndrome classifications of the International League Against Epilepsy (ILAE) over the past 30 years. Generally applying the various syndromic classifications of the ILAE to neonatal seizures has its limitations, as most neonatal seizures are acute reactions and symptomatic, and are usually a direct consequence of a specific aetiology. On the syndromic level there are currently five well-defined neonatal epilepsy syndromes: benign neonatal convulsions, benign familial neonatal convulsions (BFNCs), early myoclonic epilepsy (EME), early infantile epileptic encephalopathy (EIEE), and migrating partial seizures of infancy which we will discuss later in this chapter.

Table 14.1 Various published classification schemas for neonatal seizures

Year	Source (reference)	Classification
1981	Commission on Classification and Terminology of the International League Against Epilepsy (13)	Focal seizures Generalized seizures Unclassified seizures Neonatal seizures
1987	Mizrahi and Kellaway (20)	I. Seizures with a close association to EEG seizure discharges A. Focal clonic 1. Unifocal 2. Multifocal a. Alternating b. Migrating 3. Hemiconvulsive 4. Axial B. Myoclonic 1. Generalized 2. Focal C. Focal tonic 1. Asymmetric truncal 2. Eye deviation D. Apnoea II. Seizures with an inconsistent or no relationship to EEG seizures discharges A. Motor automatisms: 1. Oral-buccal-lingual movements 2. Ocular signs 3. Progression movements: a. Pedalling b. Stepping c. Rotary arm movements 4. Complex purposeless movements B. Generalized tonic: 1. Extensor 2. Flexor 3. Mixed extensor/flexor C. Myoclonic: 1. Generalized 2. Focal 3. Fragmentary III. Infantile spasms IV. EEG seizures without clinical seizures
2008	Volpe (29)	Subtle Clonic: Focal Multifocal Tonic: Focal Multifocal Myoclonic
2010	Berg et al. (18)	Generalized seizures: Tonic–clonic (in any combination) Absence: Typical Atypical Absence with special features Myoclonic absence Eyelid myoclonia Myoclonic: Myoclonic Myoclonic atonic Myoclonic tonic Clonic Tonic Atonic Focal seizures Unknown: Epileptic spasms *Eliminates neonatal seizures as a separate category. Recommends that neonatal seizure be classified within the available categories of the classification of seizures*

Tables 14.1 and 14.2 show the placement of neonatal seizures in the different classification schemes that have been proposed by the classification commissions of the ILAE.

The 1981 seizure classification from the Commission on Classification and Terminology of the ILAE (13) included neonatal seizures in the group of unclassified epileptic seizures. In 1989, the Commission on Classification and Terminology of the ILAE proposed a new classification for epilepsies and epileptic syndromes. In this classification, neonatal seizures were included under the undetermined category of epilepsies with both generalized and focal seizures (14). Revisions of the prior classifications placed neonatal seizures into an independent category as the defining features were considered to be sufficiently unique (15–17). The latest proposal for seizure and epilepsy syndrome classification of the ILAE eliminates neonatal seizures as a separate category and recommends that neonatal seizure be classified within the available categories of the classification of seizures (18). In this scheme many types of neonatal seizures, e.g. subtle seizures will have to be classified as unknown or undetermined. Nevertheless, specific neonatal electroclinical syndromes that are usually rare (e.g. benign familial neonatal epilepsy, early myoclonic encephalopathy and Ohtahara syndrome) are placed in the electroclinical syndrome classification based on age of onset in the neonatal period. Benign neonatal seizures, together with febrile seizures, were included within the conditions of epileptic seizures that traditionally are not diagnosed as

Table 14.2 Neonatal seizures: placement in different epilepsy syndrome classification schemes

Year	Source (reference)	Classification
1989	Commission on Classification and Terminology of the International League Against Epilepsy (14)	1.0 Localization-related epilepsies and syndromes 2.0 Generalized epilepsies and syndromes 3.0 Epilepsies and syndromes undetermined whether focal or generalized 3.1. With both generalized and focal seizures—neonatal seizures 3.2. Without equivocal generalized or focal features 4.0 Special syndromes
2001 2006	Engel (15) Engel (16)	*Proposes a five-axis classification: Axis 1—ictal phenomenology; Axis 2—seizure type; Axis 3—syndrome; Axis 4—aetiology; Axis 5—impairment* *Epilepsy syndromes and related conditions:* Benign familial neonatal seizures Early myoclonic encephalopathy Ohtahara syndrome Conditions with epileptic seizures that do not require a diagnosis of epilepsy: Benign neonatal seizures Single seizures or isolated cluster of seizures Rarely repeated seizures (oligoepilepsy)
2006	Engel (17)	*Epileptic syndromes by age of onset and related conditions* Neonatal period: Benign familial neonatal seizures (BFNS) Early myoclonic encephalopathy (EME) Ohtahara syndrome Infancy Childhood Adolescence Less specific age relationship Special epilepsy conditions Conditions with epileptic seizures that do not require a diagnosis of epilepsy: Benign neonatal seizures (BNS) Febrile seizures (FS)
2010	Berg et al. (18)	*Epileptic syndromes by age of onset and related conditions* Neonatal period: Benign familial neonatal seizures (BFNS) Early myoclonic encephalopathy (EME) Ohtahara syndrome Infancy Childhood Adolescence Less specific age relationship Distinctive constellations Epilepsies attributed to and organized by structural-metabolic causes Angioma Epilepsies of unknown cause Conditions with epileptic seizures that are traditionally not diagnosed as a form of epilepsy per se Benign neonatal seizures (BNS) Febrile seizures (FS)

forms of epilepsy. It is in this category where many of the patients with neonatal seizures could be placed (19).

The validity and limitations in applying the current 1981 and 1989 classification to neonates have been documented in a number of neonatal seizures studies (19–21).

Watanabe et al. (21) followed a group of mainly term neonates who presented with neonatal seizures and developed epilepsy within the first month of life. The study found that 84% of the patients who had seizure onset within the neonatal period had partial seizures and 12% had generalized seizures regardless of the type of epilepsy syndrome whether idiopathic, symptomatic, or cryptogenic). Only 4% of the infants had mixed seizures. When the 1989 classification was applied to the different epilepsy syndrome with onset during the neonatal period, it became very clear that most of the syndromes were incorrectly placed under generalized epilepsies even when their predominant seizure type was partial (84%). Only patients with early infantile epileptic encephalopathy had generalized seizures as the main seizure type (5/8 patients). Another important finding of the study is the dynamic evolution over time of symptomatic neonatal seizures when the 1989 Classification was applied at different times of follow-up. This topic will be further covered under the prognosis section.

The study of Mastangelo et al. (19) also documented the limitations of the 1989 Classification for classifying epilepsies with onset in the neonatal period. Only six out of the 94 infants with neonatal seizures were correctly classified at the end of the neonatal period. Application of the 2001 multidimensional classification improved the yield of classification of 74 out of the 94 neonates.

A number of authors have suggested also including the aetiology in addition to the electroclinical and age-dependent features in the classification of neonatal seizures as this strongly drives prognosis. Simon Shorvon proposed an aetiological classification of epilepsy in which neonatal seizures are included in predominately acquired perinatal and infantile causes (22). A multidimensional classification for neonatal seizures proposed by Scher (9) combines the electroclinical (Axis 1—accuracy of diagnosis), neuroimaging (Axis 2—brain region-specific), maturational stage (Axis 3—maturational context) and the aetiology (Axis 4—aetiology specific). This multidimensional classification for neonatal seizures adds the neuroimaging data that is now routinely available and prenatal and postnatal maturational changes in the classification of neonatal seizures. However, there is a need for follow-up studies to validate the utility of this classification from a clinical outcome and research perspective.

Classifying the clinical semiology of neonatal seizures

There are a number of published clinical classifications of neonatal seizures (10, 12, 23–28). While earlier classifications emphasized the clinical differences between seizures in the neonate and those seen in older children—typically clonic or tonic in neonates not tonic–clonic as in the older child, uni- or multifocal, and myoclonic—the minimal or subtle (also termed anarchic) features frequently seen in neonatal behaviour were later recognized and include oral-buccal-lingual movements, movements of progression, and random eye movements. These were first considered to be purely epileptic in origin but have subsequently been attributed to brainstem release phenomena (20). Clinically, the most widely used classifications of neonatal seizures have been proposed by Volpe (29) and Mizrahi and Kellaway in 1987 (20). Table 14.1 includes these classifications within the different existing and proposed seizure classification. Volpe's classification is based mainly on clinical semiological features observed in the ill neonates during the seizures while Mizrahi and Kellaway's classification of neonatal seizures also includes the EEG findings in addition to the observed semiological features. The results of the Mizrahi and Kellaway study highlighted key characteristics that are very important for diagnosis and management. Seventy-five per cent of the neonates (265) enrolled in the study (349 infants) had clinical features suspicious for seizures that turned out not to be seizures. Fifteen per cent (11 infants) of the 71 neonates with seizures had only electroencephalographic (EEG) seizures while twenty-two per cent (30 infants) of the 71 neonates had more than one type of clinical seizure and some of the different types of seizures overlapped or occurred at the same time. Myoclonic seizures had a poor prognosis, regardless of correlation with EEG seizures and were associated with significant neurological morbidity and high mortality when compared to clonic seizures. Tremors were seen in 13 out of 349 neonates and correlated with altered neurological function but were not generally a seizure symptom. Some abnormal movements were considered 'clinical seizures' that had a poor temporal correlation with EEG seizures (see Table 14.1). The newborns with these findings had significant neurological morbidity (50%) and mortality (20%) noted prior or at the time of hospital discharge. These abnormal movements may represent abnormal extrapyramidal movements rather than seizures given the vulnerability of the basal ganglia to anoxic injury during the newborn period and imply more diffuse and severe brain injury. This is a hypothesis that needs to be explored using modern neuroimaging modalities in larger patient series.

Clinical description of neonatal seizures (20, 29):

1. Subtle seizures: subtle seizures include sudden or paroxysmal changes in behaviour, motor, or autonomic function. Some of the manifestations seen during these seizures can be ocular, oral-buccal-lingual, unusual limbs movements, and autonomic changes. The ocular movements may include horizontal eye deviations, jerking of the eyes, roving eye movements, sustained eye opening, staring, ocular fixation, or nystagmus. The oral-buccal-lingual movements include chewing, sucking, tongue protrusion, crying, and grimacing. Limb movements may include pedalling, bicycling, stepping, rowing, swimming, boxing, hooking, and other more non-specific movements. Autonomic changes may include apnoeas, tachypnoea, hiccups, or haemodynamic changes such as tachycardia, bradycardia, and hypertension. In general, subtle seizures have a poor correlation with electrographic seizure discharges in neonates.
2. Clonic seizures: clonic seizures in the neonate are slow rhythmic jerking movements that can be localized to a limb or side of the body or multifocal. When clonic seizures are focal, there is typically a repetitive jerking of one arm or leg, one side of the face, neck, or trunk or entire one side of the body. Typically, the clonic limb movements cannot be suppressed by restraint. This helps to differential focal clonic seizures from tremors or jitteriness. When the seizures are multifocal clonic, they involve more than one limb on both sides of the body in a simultaneous and progressive fashion. Typically these clonic movements do not exhibit a 'Jacksonian march'. For example, clonic movements can be seen initially in the left arms, then in the right leg, and then in the left leg, etc. Clonic seizures, particularly focal clonic seizures, have a high correlation with contralateral electrographic seizure patterns and underlying structural abnormalities as the aetiology.
3. Tonic seizures: focal tonic seizures are characterized by a persistent posturing of a limb, trunk, or neck. Focal tonic seizures tend to be correlated with electrographic seizure patterns. Generalized tonic seizures are described as tonic contraction of both upper and lower extremities. The tonic contraction can include extension of the upper and lower extremities or a combination of upper extremities flexion with lower extremities extension. Generalized tonic seizures are poorly correlated with electrographic seizure patterns and respond poorly to antiepileptic medications. The differential diagnosis of generalized tonic seizures includes decerebrate and decorticate posturing, opisthotonos, and hyperekplexia.
4. Myoclonic seizures: may be focal, multifocal, and generalized. Focal myoclonic seizures are limited to a segment of the body or limb while multifocal myoclonic seizures characteristically involve irregular and asynchronous jerking of different parts of the body. Generalized myoclonic seizures are described as brief or sudden jerking movements of both upper and lower extremities. In general, myoclonic seizures are poorly correlation with electrographic seizure patterns in the EEG. However, generalized myoclonic seizures are more closely correlated with EEG seizures than focal or multifocal myoclonic seizures.

Neonatal status epilepticus

Neonatal status epilepticus has been defined as a single seizure lasting more than 30 minutes or multiple seizures that account for 30 minutes over 1-hour period or recurrent seizures seen in more than 50% of a 1–3-hour record (30–33). Neonatal status epilepticus was thought to be a rare event in neonates and in 1987 Clancy and Legido reported seizures lasting more than 30 minutes in only 0.4% of the neonatal EEGs they reviewed (30). More recent studies report neonatal status epilepticus in up to 12–24% of the neonates with seizures (3, 31, 34, 35).

The prognosis of neonatal status epilepticus is generally grave. Pisani et al. reported near 20% mortality and near 50% of adverse neurological outcome at age 2 years in infants who suffered neonatal status epilepticus (31). It appears to also signal a poorer prognosis in full-term babies for an adverse neurological outcome, while in the preterm baby under 29 weeks it is a risk factor for subsequent epilepsy (31, 32). Similarly, more severe neonatal seizures were associated with a poor long-term prognosis at age 4 years in a group of neonates with HIE (36).

EEG biomarkers and characteristics

In theory, neonatal seizures are clinical paroxysmal events temporally associated with electrical seizure patterns. This overlap of clinical and electrical activity is present in electroclinical seizures, but there is ample evidence that clinical seizures may occur without electrical seizures and electrical seizures may occur without clinical seizures in the neonate (Fig. 14.1). Electrographic seizures without corresponding clinical manifestations have been recorded in 44–66% of neonates with seizures (3, 30, 34, 37). This number was lower but still 15% in the study of Mizrahi and Kellaway when the inclusion criterion was clinical suspicion of neonatal seizures by the referring physician (20). The number of subclinical neonatal seizures can be higher when studying special population of neonates (37). For instance, 100% of seizures were subclinical in neonates who had heart surgery (38). On the other hand, when neonatal seizures are suspected in infants who are exhibiting abnormal or unusual movements, as determined by the observation of medical personnel, there may be an overdiagnosis of seizures. Around 70% of the movements identified as seizures by medical personnel had no EEG correlate in the study of Murray et al. (37). In the study of Mizrahi and Kellaway, over 70% of the neonates with clinical suspicion of seizures, did not have seizures recorded during continuous video-EEG (20).

This data confirms that a high degree of suspicion is important for early identification of clinical and subclinical neonatal seizures on the one hand but that the accuracy of identifying a clinical event as a seizure may be low. Neonates at higher risk for seizures are those with: severe asphyxia and/or on cooling protocol, neonates with rhythmic body movements or unexplained apneas, encephalopathic neonates, critically ill neonates on ventilator or with neuromuscular blockade and neonates with moderate to severe abnormalities on routine EEG.

Vulnerable neonates may have a high seizure burden as documented in several studies of special patient populations. In the study of Murray et al., 526 neonatal seizures were recorded in 12 infants (37). Clancy et al. recorded 1429 electrographic seizures in 21 infants who had heart surgery (38) while Shellhaas et al. recorded 851 neonatal seizures in 125 continuous EEGs. This study estimated a neonatal seizure burden of seven seizures per hour (35).

Conventional EEG is the gold standard for confirming the diagnosis of neonatal seizures. In many centres, continuous EEG with video is used in the diagnosis and management of neonatal seizures. Amplitude-integrated EEG offers a less expensive screening tool for neonatal seizures and background abnormalities (39).

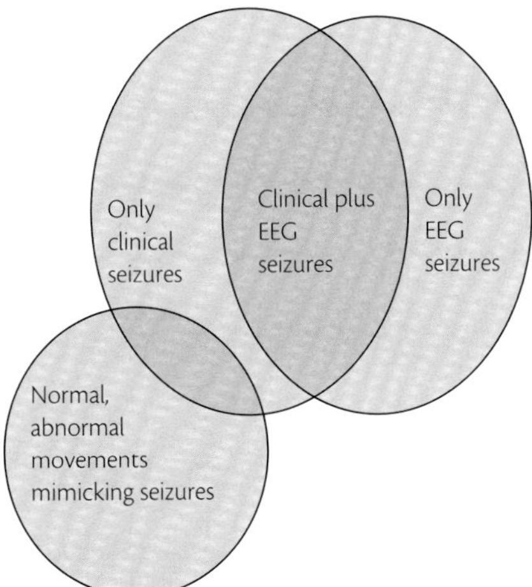

Fig. 14.1 Schematic diagram showing the interrelationship between clinical seizures, electrographic seizures, and neonatal movements.

Interictal EEG

Infants with normal background activity are much less likely to develop seizures compared to those with significant abnormalities. A severe background abnormality such as burst suppression or isoelectric background are indicators of a severe electrophysiological dysfunction signifying brain injury and encephalopathy and may point to a high risk for adverse neurological outcome or even death. In contrast, a near normal background activity despite the presence of seizures implies preserved brain neurophysiology and good chances for neurological functional recovery. Analysis of the EEG background in neonates with seizures adds important prognostic information for the treating physician. Elements that need to be considered in the EEG background analysis in the context of the infant's conceptual and corrected age include amplitude, continuity, frequency, symmetry, synchrony, interburst interval duration, reactivity, differentiation between awake and sleep cycles, and the presence of abnormal graphoelements. The background pattern can be present during the seizure and often is abnormal (35). In the study of Shellhaas et al., 15% of the neonatal with seizures had a normal EEG background. The EEG background was mildly abnormal in 23%, moderately abnormal in 32%, and severely abnormal in 30% (35). Neonatal EEG background has a good correlation with the neurodevelopmental outcome later in life.

Focal sharp waves may point to focal injury such as stroke, subarachnoid haemorrhage, malformations, or tumours. Multifocal sharp waves usually signify diffuse injury and epileptogenesis. Bicentral sharp waves have been described in hypocalcaemic seizures and vertex spikes have been described in maple syrup urine disease, periodic lateralized epileptiform discharges have been described in acute brain destruction due to herpes simplex virus encephalitis, stroke, and haemorrhage. Vertex spikes have been described in maple syrup urine disease and sinus venous thrombosis. Nevertheless, sharp waves in general have poor specificity regarding aetiology of neonatal seizures. Frontal sharp waves and sporadic centrotemporal sharp waves can be part of the normal background in the preterm, near-term, and term neonate.

The presence of a burst-suppression pattern is common in hypoxic neonatal ischaemic encephalopathy when it is usually transient and short lived. If it persists longer than 2 weeks it may signal the diagnosis of an early myoclonic encephalopathy or Ohtahara syndrome.

Ictal EEG

Neonatal seizures tend to have distinctive EEG characteristics of morphology, spatial distribution, and temporal evolution when compared to EEG seizures in older children and adults (39):

Neonatal EEG seizures have a sudden and clear onset, a clear middle with an evolution, and usually an abrupt cessation. The ictal pattern can be stereotypic but multiple different ictal patterns can be seen as well. The typical neonatal seizure begins as a low amplitude, sinusoidal rhythmic wave discharge (delta, theta, alpha, or beta frequencies) sometimes with spikes and sharp waves and as it evolves the amplitude increases and frequency decreases.

The ictal activity in the neonate is invariably focal, as the neonatal brain lacks the maturational organization for synchronization. Typically we will see the ictal discharge arising focally, e.g. in the temporal region, then migrating to adjacent electrodes (central, occipital, frontal) and then involving the whole hemisphere (hemiconvulsion) before also migrating from one hemisphere to another giving the EEG a more generalized appearance. Often the neonatal seizures are independent multifocal or simultaneous multifocal, but they also can be focal involving a single electrode (Figs 14.1 and 14.2). Around 80% of the electrographic seizures originate from the centrotemporal or midline vertex regions in neonates (35). Seizure discharges may be surface positive (Fig. 14.3). The minimal amplitude of the ictal pattern is generally at least 2 μV. The minimal duration of seizures is approximately 10 seconds (30, 40, 41). Rhythmic discharges lasting less than 10 seconds are known as brief ictal rhythmic electrographic discharges or BIRDs and were found in almost 20% of the neonatal polysomnograms recorded by Oliveira et al. (42). Even when brief, 15.9% of BIRDs have associated clinical manifestations (42). In this study, the presence of BIRDs was associated with leucomalacia and hypoglycaemia and with an abnormal developmental outcome. Nevertheless, the risk for postnatal seizures was not high for neonates with BIRDs (43).

The mean duration of seizures is around 90 seconds, although some studies report longer mean durations (30, 37). Minimal duration between two seizure patterns has to be 10 seconds or more to be considered as two independent seizures (Fig. 14.4). This definition was developed arbitrarily and is used as a measure of seizure burden in newer research studies.

In very sick neonates with severe encephalopathy marked by a depressed background activity, the ictal patterns may be of low voltage, quite focal, and of long duration with little or no spatial and morphological evolution of the pattern. These patterns are usually not associated with clinical seizures and are suggestive of a poor prognosis. Similarly, alpha seizures are characterized by sudden, rhythmic activity in the alpha frequency range of 8–12 Hz usually arising in the temporal regions and are frequently not associated with clinical signs signifying a poor prognosis in the face a diffuse encephalopathy (44, 45, 46).

A note on using amplitude integrated EEG

The amplitude integrated EEG (aEEG) is being applied increasingly in neonatal units to monitor sick neonates at the bedside. Usually two electrodes are used and the data acquired is compressed to provide information on the EEG background and to detect seizures (47, 48). However, current studies suggest that the seizure detection rate is low compared to conventional EEG. At this juncture, an EEG cannot replace conventional EEG but may provide useful complementary real-time information to guide management of the patient at the bedside.

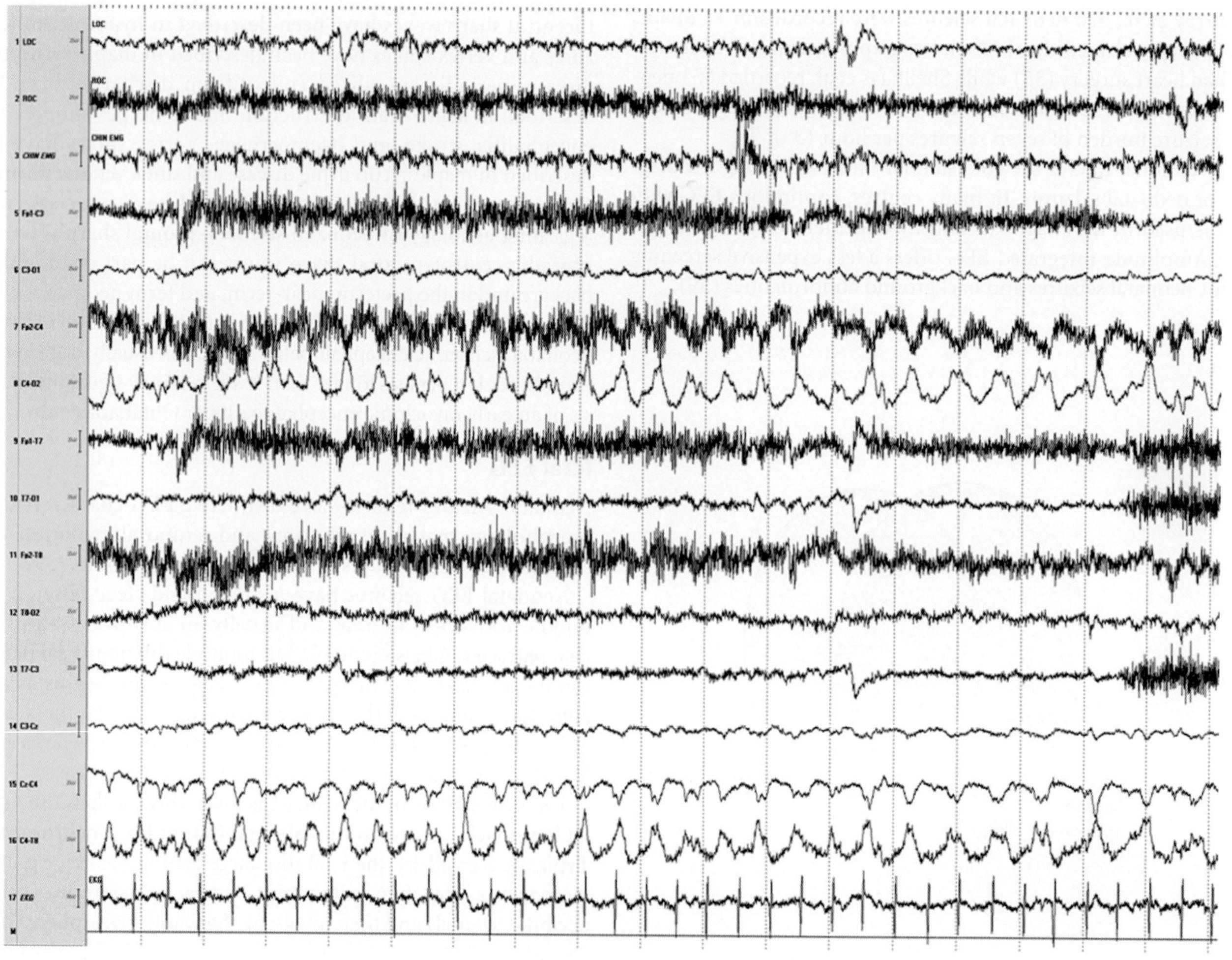

Fig. 14.2 This ictal EEG record shows a right frontal seizure discharge in a full term neonate with severe hypoxic ischemic encephalopathy.

Risk factors and aetiologies

Multiple antenatal and intrapartum risk factors have been associated with the risk of neonatal seizures in preterm and term newborns. Table 14.3 summarizes the results of the studies about risk for neonatal seizures published during and after year 2000 (49–53).

Consistently, older and newer studies have emphasized the association between low birth weight/prematurity and neonatal seizures (5, 6, 52).

The associations between race, gender, hospital where the birth took place, mode of delivery, and fetal distress with neonatal seizures have been more variable and probably dependent on the specific populations that were studied.

Maternal diabetes is a risk factor that can lead to neonatal seizures and epilepsy in neonates via different mechanisms. Chronic hyperglycaemia has a teratogenic effect in the developing brain. Neonates born to diabetic mothers have a higher incidence of systemic malformations than the general population, including central nervous system malformations (54). The variety of brain malformations includes holoprosencephaly, anencephaly, and malformations of cortical development (55). All these brain malformations can present with seizures in the neonatal period (56). Chronic hyperglycaemia can also lead to fetal hyperinsulinaemia and macrosomia. Macrosomic neonates are at high risk of acute metabolic problems frequently associated to neonatal seizures including hypoglycaemia, hypocalcaemia, hypomagnesaemia, respiratory distress, and asphyxia (57). Severe hypoglycaemia in the neonate can lead to metabolic stroke-like lesions, particularly in the parieto-occipital regions (29, 58, 59), and invariably results in epilepsy (60). Nevertheless, a similar pattern of posterior cerebral injury has also been reported in a neonate with ischaemia and severe hyperglycaemia, suggesting a vulnerability of this region of the brain to both extremes of abnormalities in the serum glucose (61).

Fever and maternal infections are also important risk factors associated with neonatal seizures (51, 62). Herpes simplex virus infection is a cause of neonatal seizures and chronic brain lesions secondary to this virus contribute to the development of epilepsy (63). Congenital infections, particularly the TORCH group, can lead to neonatal seizures and epilepsy (64) via disruption of organogenesis (65). In the particular case of congenital cytomegalovirus infection, the most common cause of congenital infection, there are no randomized controlled trials that evaluate the effect of antenatal interventions in the prevention of transmission of the cytomegalovirus from the mother to the fetus (66).

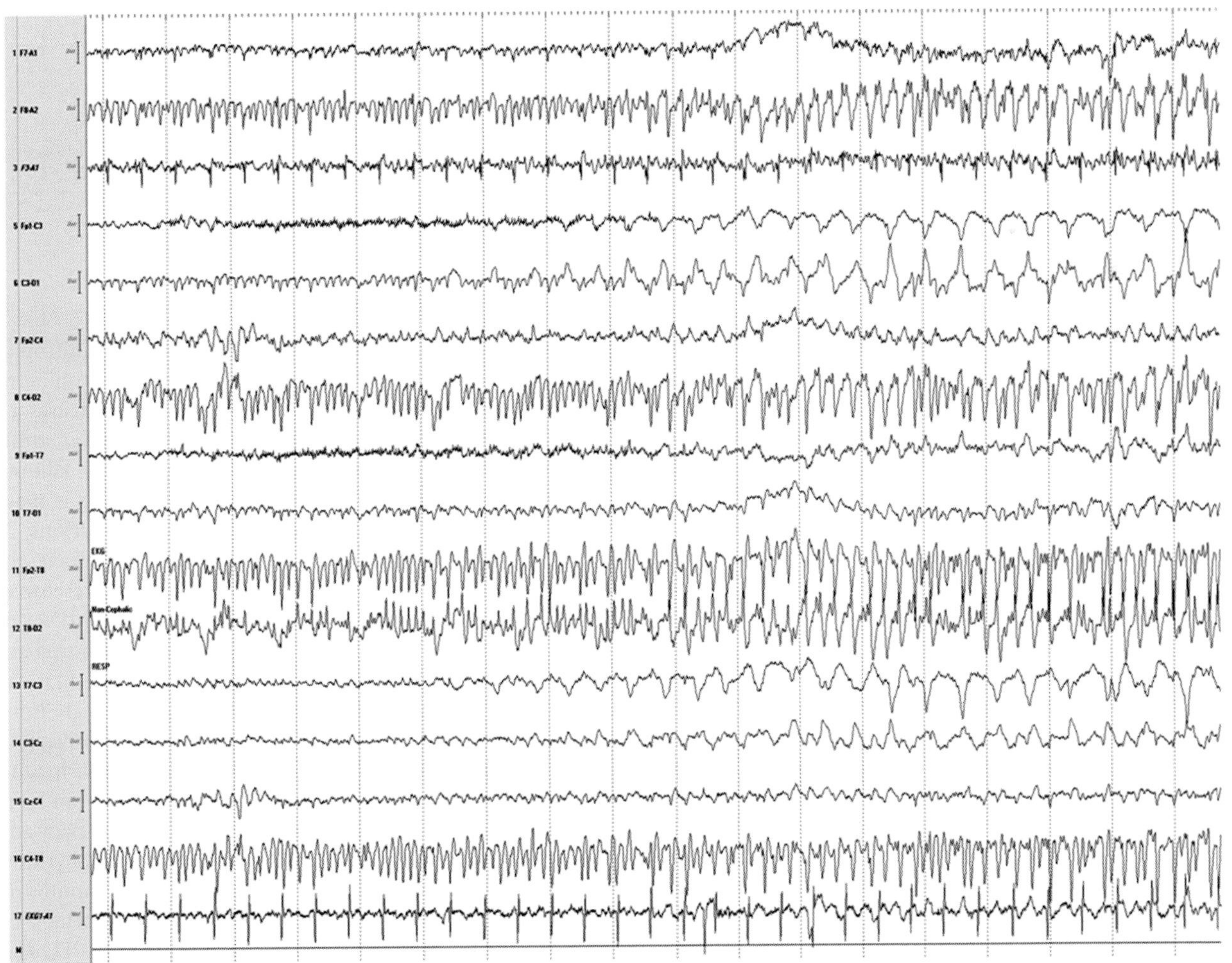

Fig. 14.3 This EEG record of the same patient shows ongoing right frontal seizure discharges with rhythmic spikes and simultaneous onset of a new left central seizure pattern.

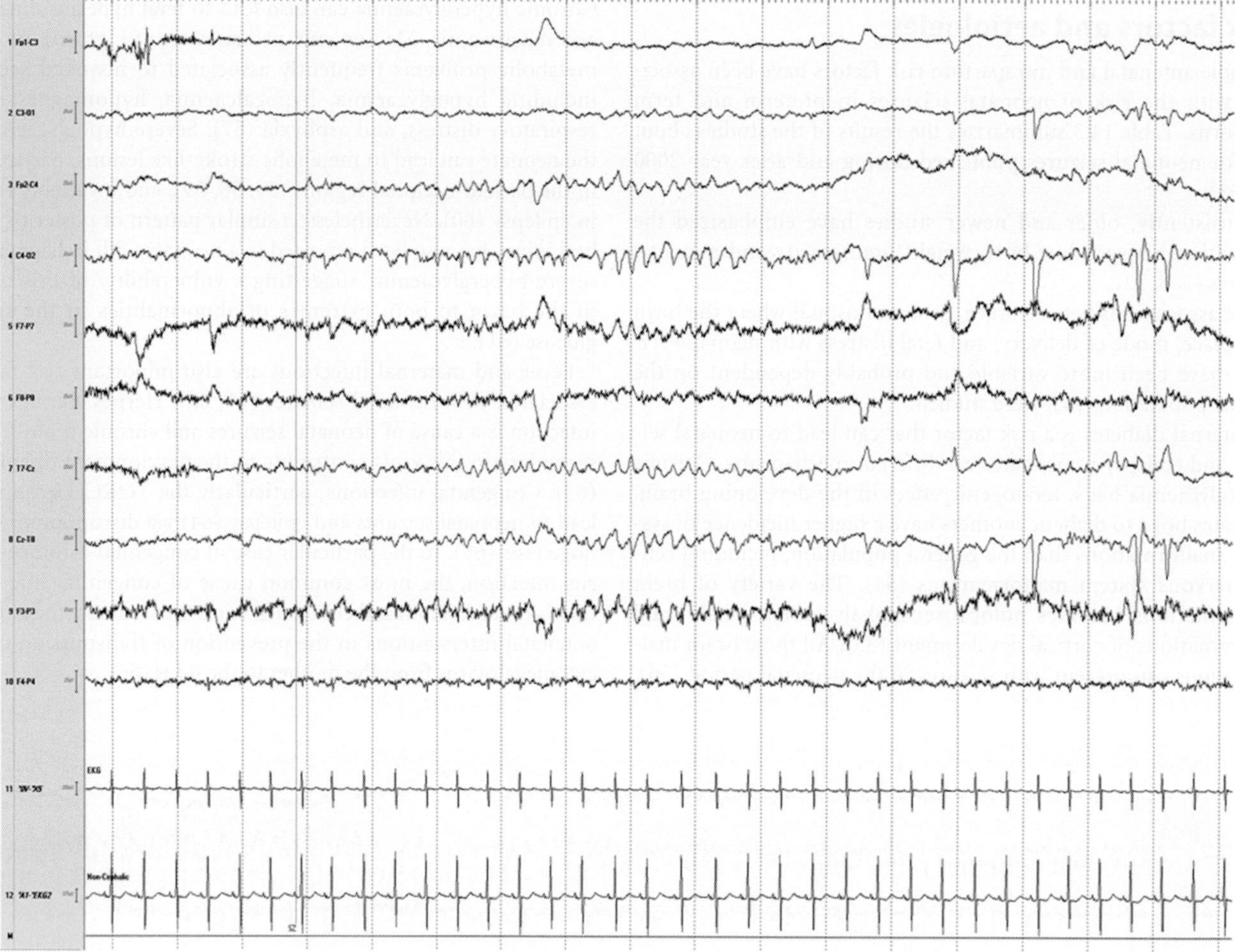

Fig. 14.4 This EEG record shows BIRDs with a positive polarity in the right central region followed by right occipital spikes.

Fig. 14.6 lists the aetiologies of neonatal seizures. Global hypoxic-ischaemia accounts for almost 40% of all neonatal seizures affecting term and preterm infants. Ischaemic infarcts, whether arterial or venous, account for near 20% of all cases of neonatal seizures each. Cerebral malformations, metabolic disturbances, infections, and inborn errors of the metabolism account for near 10% of the aetiologies. Although neonatal Group B streptococcal infections have been significantly reduced in the US, Canada, and other developed countries due to screening of pregnant women and strict surveillance (67, 68), this bacteria continues to be the leading cause of neonatal seizures in countries outside the US (69, 70).

Inborn errors of metabolism manifesting with an acute encephalopathy and neonatal seizures are rare but the more frequent ones include maple syrup urine disease, ketotic and non-ketotic hyperglycinaemia and urea cycle disorders, biotinidase deficiency, pyridoxine-dependent seizures, folinic acid responsive seizures, molybdenum cofactor, Menkes disease, phenylketonuria and tetrahydrobiopterin deficiency, and mitochondrial disorders. The acute encephalopathy is usually a prominent component in these disorders. Branched chain amino acids leucine, isoleucine, and valine are elevated in maple syrup urine disease due to a decarboxylation defect. After the first feeding and protein load the infant develops seizures, hypotonia, hypoglycaemia, and decreased responsiveness. The urine will test positive for 2,4-dinitrophenylhydrazine. The glycine encephalopathies are catastrophic metabolic encephalopathies presenting with intractable seizures, coma, apnoea, ophthalmoplegia which spares the pupils, stimulus-induced and spontaneous myoclonus, and multiorgan failure. The EEG shows severe burst suppression. The diagnosis is made by serum amino acid and specific enzyme determinations. Non-ketotic hyperglycinaemia is due to an inability to cleave glycine resulting in increased glycine levels in serum and cerebrospinal fluid. Treatment includes a N-methyl-D-aspartate (NMDA) antagonist, magnesium, sodium benzoate, and dextromethorphan. The urea cycle abnormalities present with seizures in the first days of life, coma, and prominent bulbar dysfunction and there is hyperammonaemia. In addition, biotinidase deficiency may begin in the first week of life with seizures and is associated with hypotonia, alopecia, and seborrhoeic dermatitis. The diagnosis can be made by measuring the biotinidase activity in the blood and daily administration of free biotin is the definitive treatment. Pyridoxine-dependent seizures usually appear within the first 3 months of life, the neonate is jittery, irritable, and presents with intractable clonic seizures. The diagnosis is likely when seizures and the EEG seizures remit within a few hours after 50–100 mg of pyridoxine has been administered intravenously. As lifelong treatment is necessary, this

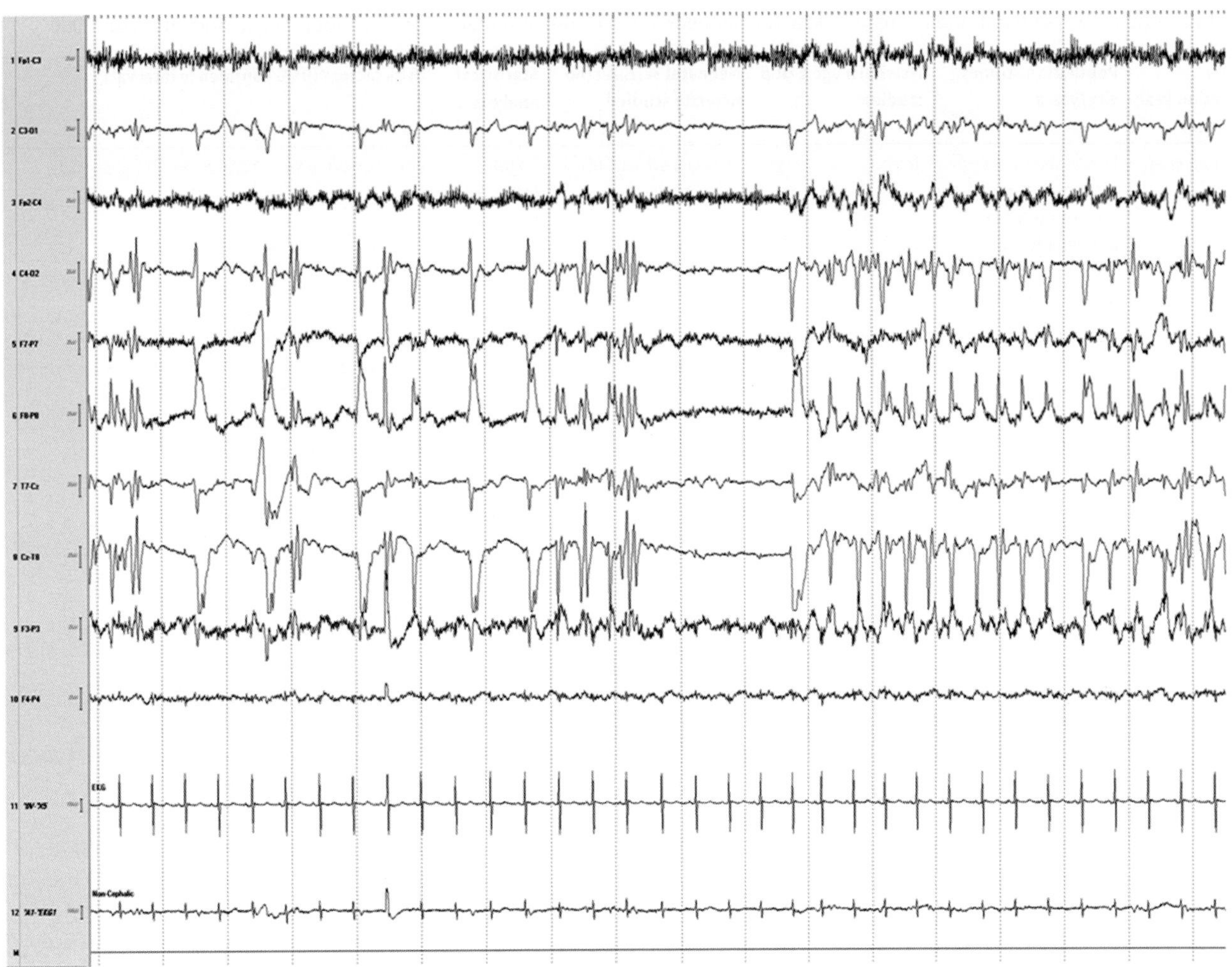

Fig. 14.5 This ictal EEG record of same patient shows brief cessation for 3 seconds followed by resumption of an EEG seizure. This is considered to be one seizure due to the short interval between the two EEG seizure patterns.

diagnosis should not be missed (71, 72). Folinic acid-responsive neonatal seizures appear unexpectedly during the first few hours of life in the term infant without the typical risk factors previously described. There is progressive brain atrophy and developmental delay and frequent episodes of status epilepticus. Cerebrospinal fluid analysis with high-performance liquid chromatography yields an unidentified compound which may be a marker for this condition. Treatment includes administration of 2.5 mg of folinic acid twice daily; some cases have been described to temporarily respond to pyridoxine. Gene mutations in antiquitin which leads to inactivation of pyridoxal phosphate (PLP) has been found in patients with pyridoxine-responsive seizures as well as folinic acid responsive seizures so that some authors recommend treating patients with antiquitin (alpha-aminoadipic semialdehyde dehydrogenase) deficiency with both pyridoxine and folinic acid (73, 74, 75). Poor feeding, jitteriness, a high-pitched cry, and intractable seizures are seen in molybdenum cofactor deficiency which can be detected by an abnormal sulphite test in a fresh urine sample and elevated xanthine, hypoxanthine, and diminished uric acid concentrations in the serum (76–78). The condition is due to mutations in genes producing substrates for molybdenum cofactor synthesis leading to cofactor deficiency, which interrupts proper function of the enzymes sulphite oxidase and xanthine dehydrogenase. This condition carries a poor prognosis without definitive treatments.

Considering that these disorders are relatively rare compared to structural abnormalities and acute/transient metabolic disorders such as glucose and electrolyte imbalances, a stepwise approach to the work-up as well as collaboration with the paediatric metabolic expert, geneticist, and paediatric neurologist is suggested to identify these inborn errors cost effectively. Newborn screen is also an important diagnostic tool when identifying the cause of neonatal seizures in some countries.

In approximately 10% of neonatal seizures, the aetiology remains unknown (79).

Pathophysiology

The neonatal brain compared to other periods in childhood may be selectively more vulnerable to generating seizures due to a relative imbalance between inhibition and excitation. This susceptibility

Table 14.3 Antenatal, perinatal, and neonatal risk factors for neonatal seizures. Summary of studies published in and after year 2000

Author/ publication year (reference)	Population studies/ city/years	Newborn age group studies	Neonatal seizures/no. neonate studied	Statistical analysis	Risk factors (95% confidence interval)
Lieberman et al., 2000 (51)	Hospital-based study/ term neonates with confirmed seizures at Brigham and Women's Hospital, Boston/1989–1996	Term	38 neonatal seizures 152 controls	Logistic regression	Intrapartum fever >100.4°F OR 3.4 (1.03–10.9)
Saliba et al., 2001 (52)	Population-based study/discharge diagnosis, birth and death certificates, Harris county, Texas/1992–1994	Preterm Term	48 neonatal seizures 9834 preterm 141 neonatal seizures 93,565 term	Multivariate analysis	Birth weight <1500 g RR 9.1 (4.7–17.5) Birth weight 1500–1999 g RR 3.4 (1.5–8.1) Male gender RR 1.8 (1.0–3.3) Small for gestational age OR 1.9 (1.2-2.9) Birth in level III: —Private/university RR 2.8 (1.5–5.0) —Public/university RR 1.5 (1.0–2.3) Maternal age 18–24 years RR 1.6 (1.1–2.3) Deliver via Caesarean section RR 2.2 (1.5–3.2)
Kohelet et al., 2006 (50)	Population-based study/Israel National Very Low Birthweight Infant Database, Israel/1995–2002	Very low birthweight infants with periventricular encephalomalacia, gestational age 24–36 weeks	102 with seizures 442 without seizures	Logistic regression	Necrotizing enterocolitis and surgery OR 2.84 (1.11–7.0) Intraventricular haemorrhage: —Grade 2–3 OR 2.18 (1.10–4.34) —Grade 4 OR 4.51 (2.13–9.7) Posthaemorrhagic hydrocephalus OR 2.22 (1.20–4.11) Sepsis OR 2.40 (1.39–4.20)
Hall et al., 2006 (49)	Population-based study/Colorado Birth Certificate Registry, Colorado/1989–2003	Term	567 with seizures 5667 controls	Logistic regression	Preexisting diabetes OR 4.32 (1.62–11.51) Herpes/vaginal delivery OR 2.92 (1.46–5.85) Cesarean section OR 1.69 (1.37–2.09) Fetal distress OR 5.08 (3.92–6.59)
Scher et al., 2008 (53)	Hospital-based study/Magee-Women's Hospital, Pittsburgh,/14-year period		193 EEG confirmed seizures: 78 preterm 115 full-term	Analysis of variance	No differences for intrapartum or neonatal factors (fetal distress, neonatal encephalopathy, gestational age, type of delivery, Caesarean section)

CI, confidence interval; OR, odd ratio; RR, relative risk.

may come as a consequence of delayed maturation of inhibitory circuits and precocious maturation of excitatory circuits (80). In addition, physiological brain plasticity during the neonatal period is characterized by florid growth of excitatory synapses and activity-dependent pruning, which may generate a 'pro-seizure' type of set up. This may be compounded by the paradoxical and transient excitatory effects of gamma-aminobutyric acid (GABA) (as opposed to inhibitory function in the older child's brain) in the developing brain (81). Further the chloride channel of the mature brain (KCC2) which pumps chloride out of the neuron resulting in hyperpolarization and inhibition is at low levels while the chloride transporter that moves chloride into the neurones (NKCC1 transporter) is at high levels. This results in neuronal depolarization and increased excitability when the ligand-dependent $GABA_A$ receptor

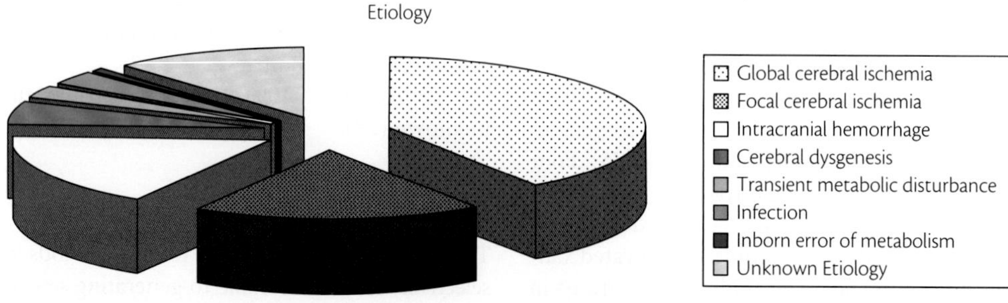

Fig. 14.6 Aetiologies of neonatal seizures.

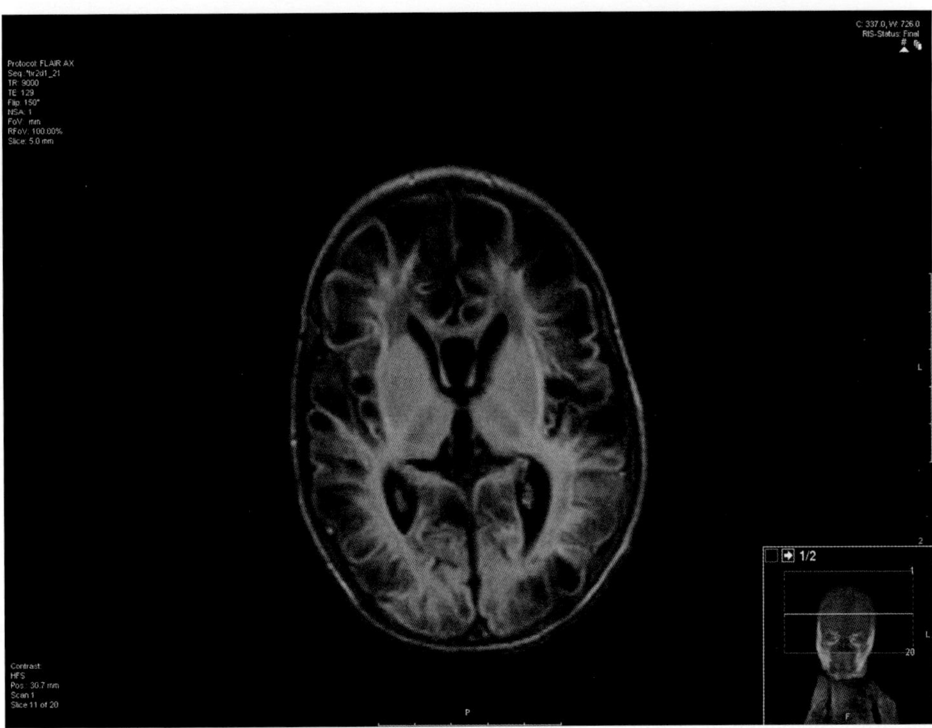

Fig. 14.7 MRI scan of the infant with severe HIE and neonatal seizures illustrated in Fig 2-5. There is severe diffuse multicystic encephalomalacia of both hemispheres and post ischemic changes of the basal ganglia and brain stem.

is activated in the immature brain. Based on animal studies, this excitation-to-inhibition switch is completed by postnatal day 14 which approximately reflects the maturational state of the human toddler (81, 82).

Finally, glutamatergic receptors that regulate neuronal excitability also undergo marked developmental changes in the immature neuron and may appear to further contribute to the increased seizure susceptibility of the human neonate. The NMDA receptor in the developing brain primarily expresses the NR2B subunit that prolongs the duration of the excitatory postsynaptic potentials. Increased excitability also results from a developmental over expression of the NR2C, NR2D, and NR3A subunits that demonstrate a reduced sensitivity to magnesium blockade (80).

Are neonatal seizures per se harmful to the developing brain?

The answer to this question remains controversial but there is some distinct evidence that seizures may not be as innocuous as once considered.

In experimental models the immature brain appears to be more resistant to some seizure-induced injury including acute cell loss than the mature brain (83). While the histological changes signifying damage from seizures in the immature brain appear minimal, seizures have been noted to induce abnormal neurogenesis, synaptogenesis, pruning, neuronal migration, alterations in receptor subunit composition, as well as gene expression for neurotransmitter receptors and transporters (84, 85). Holmes and colleagues have shown that recurrent seizures produce changes in the developing brain that result in increased risk for epilepsy and impaired learning and behaviour in animal models (86). This appears to be corroborated in a recent clinical study of metabolic magnetic resonance spectroscopy imaging of infants with HIE and seizures in which seizure severity was associated with an increased lactate/choline ratio which is an indicator of cerebral oxidative metabolism in the frontal lobe intervascular boundary zone, the lentiform nucleus, and the thalamus. In addition there was a reduced N-acetylaspartate/choline ratio as an indicator of neuronal damage in the frontal lobe (87). Currently no clinical outcome studies have measured the actual seizure burden to answer the question of impact of seizures per se on developmental outcome. A temperospatial analysis using conventional EEG to measure ictal time in various regions of interests rather than limiting the assessment to presence or absence and numeric counts of seizures has been suggested by Clancy (88).

Treatment

The management of neonatal seizures has changed very little in the last 10 years. Phenobarbital is still the first-line drug and the most commonly used drug (82%) for the treatment of neonatal seizures across the US despite its limited efficacy (89). Painter and collaborators documented that phenobarbital and phenytoin provided seizures control in little less than 50% of the treated neonates (89, 90). When used in combination, the efficacy increased to 60% (65). Lorazepam (9%) was used more frequently than phenytoin (2%) in five neonatal intensive care units included in one study that described the management approach of neonatal seizures in the US (90).

In addition to lorazepam, midazolam is another benzodiazepine used in the management of refractory neonatal seizures. Although some studies have a small sample size (91–93), all but one (69), reported full therapeutic response to bolus or continuous infusion of midazolam (66–70). Side effects included urinary retention and hypotension (94, 95). Hypotension was resolved when the dose of midazolam was adjusted (69) or treatment with ionotropic agents was added (95). One study reported mortality and poor neurological outcome in almost half of the neonates treated with midazolam (91). A less optimistic result with the use of midazolam (50% response) was reported in a study that compared this drug with lidocaine (77%) for the treatment of refractory neonatal seizures in the setting of HIE (96). The study suggested a better response to lidocaine for patients with more refractory seizures and more severe HIE. Another study also reported response of refractory neonatal seizures to lidocaine in three out of five treated patients (97). Lidocaine continuous infusion is the most common drug used for the treatment of refractory neonatal seizures in Europe (98). In Israel, lidocaine is more commonly recommended by neonatologists than neurologists for the treatment of refractory neonatal seizures (99). The efficacy and safety of lidocaine continuous infusion has been well studied in preterm and full term babies (100, 101). The main side effects of lidocaine continuous infusion is cardiac arrhythmia, therefore continuous cardiac monitoring as well as drug serum level monitoring is recommended (101, 102).

Newer AEDs are now being used for the management of refractory neonatal seizures. One survey of paediatric neurologists documented that over 70% recommended either topiramate (55%) or levetiracetam (47%) for the management of neonatal seizures (103). One small series reported seizure reduction or seizure control without side effects in four out of the six neonates who received topiramate for refractory seizures (104). Data on pharmacokinetics of topiramate, in neonates on whole-body hypothermia treatment for hypoxic-ischaemic encephalopathy, a common cause of neonatal seizures, documented slower absorption and elimination but good serum concentration at topiramate dose of 5 mg/kg/day (105). Some studies document good response of neonatal seizures to the administration of levetiracetam. In one retrospective study, levetiracetam provided seizure resolution in 64% of the neonates at 24 hours and 100% after 3 days of treatment (106). Another retrospective study documented seizure reduction of more than 50% in 35% of the neonates and seizure resolution in 30% of the neonates (107). The efficacy of levetiracetam in the control on neonatal seizures was persistent over time. Seventy-nine to 100% of neonates who received levetiracetam remained seizure free after 1 week of treatment (108, 109). Seizure remission remained 71% at 4 weeks in the study of Ramantani et al. (109) and 83% at 3 months in the study of Furwentsches et al. (108).

New therapeutic choices that take into account the physiopathology of neonatal seizures are on the horizon (110, 111). Bumetanide, a diuretic and NKCC1 inhibitor, provided significant seizures reduction in a neonate with refractory seizures (112) but data from larger studies is needed.

Treatment with AEDs may terminate clinical manifestations of a seizure while the electrographic seizure discharge continues leading to an uncoupling that has been found in up to 58% of patients in a study by Scher and colleagues (113). This phenomenon makes it important to document EEG remission of seizures in the course of medical therapy of the sick neonate who has been found to have seizures.

One reason for the electroclinical uncoupling may be the maturational switch from NKCC1 to KCC2 in a caudal–rostral fashion permitting antiseizure medication to be more effective at the brainstem and spinal cord level than the rostral level (114).

Prognosis and outcome

The outcome of children who suffered neonatal seizures has been of interest to the medical community for a long time. Older studies including data from 1956–1997 reported a normal outcome in 22–48% of the patients. Mortality was reported in 16–35% of the cases. Some degree of neurological impairment was seen in 30–49% (115). Postnatal epilepsy occurred in 20–56% of children who had neonatal seizures (115).

Table 14.4 summarizes the studies on neonatal outcome published from the year 2000 (31, 34, 36, 116–122). Recent studies report normal development in 14–68% of the patients with lower frequency in children who had neonatal seizures and were preterm or had extremely low birth weight. Mortality is relatively high (11–34%) for infants with neonatal seizures (20, 31), although, it has decreased in the last 20–30 years (29). Mortality seems to be higher in preterm babies with neonatal seizures. Morbidity is also high in children who had neonatal seizures (32–80%). Developmental delay (around 45%) and cerebral palsy (17–40%) dominate the spectrum of comorbidities. Other frequent consequences of neonatal seizure are mental retardation, learning disabilities, hearing and visual impairment, microcephaly, and failure to thrive.

Postnatal epilepsy can be found in 7–41% of children who had neonatal seizures. Watanabe et al. followed a group of children for 3 years who had neonatal seizures confirmed by EEG. Neonates who had infrequent and self-limited seizures and equivocal seizures were excluded from the study because not all neonatal seizures are related to epilepsy (21). Thirty-two per cent of the patients had idiopathic epilepsy, 58.6% had symptomatic epilepsy, and 9.4% had cryptogenic epilepsy. Follow-up of the neonates with symptomatic epilepsy documented that 41% of the patients developed West syndrome. In these patients, West syndrome evolved to symptomatic generalized or localization related epilepsy or Lennox–Gastaut syndrome (21).

There is controversy regarding whether neonatal seizures independently contribute to a poor neurodevelopmental outcome. Other factors that need to be considered are severity of EEG findings (both severity of seizures and severity of encephalopathy) and aetiology (29). The study of Glass et al. documented that severe seizures, in the setting of asphyxia, were an independent risk factor for poor cognitive and neurodevelopmental outcome at the end of a 4-year follow-up period (29, 36). The study of Kwon et al. (119) documented that when adjusted for hypothermia treatment and severity of encephalopathy, neonatal seizures were not independently associated with death, moderate to severe disability, and lower mental developmental score at age 18 months in children who had neonatal asphyxia. The main problem of both studies is that the diagnosis of seizures was clinical. Both studies did not use continuous EEG to assess for subclinical seizures. The main difference between the studies is not only in the follow-up time. The study of Glass et al. evaluated seizure severity and their contribution to neurodevelopment whereas the study of Kwon evaluated the presence of seizures regardless of the severity (104, 119). The question of whether neonatal seizures and their management contribute negatively to the neurodevelopmental outcome in addition

Table 14.4 Neonatal seizures outcome. Summary of studies published during and after the year 2000

Author/ publication year (reference)	Follow-up time	Population studied: main aetiologies	N	Normal	Death	Neurological impairment	Post-natal epilepsy
Iype et al., 2008 (118)	4 months	Term and preterm: 40.5% HIE 32.4% hypoglycaemia 10.8% benign neonatal seizure 8.1% unknown 47.2% multiple causes	135	68%	13.5%	32% neurological impairment 17% spasticity 7% abnormal vision 4% abnormal hearing	7%
McBride et al., 2000 (120)	12–18 months	Term and preterm: 23 asphyxia[a] 7 stroke 7 other 3 unknown	40	–	25%	47% CP[b] 30% no walking at 18 months 32% microcephaly 30% failure to thrive Bayley median score 89	–
Kwon et al., 2011 (119)	18 months	Term: HIE 44% had hypothermia therapy	127	–	–	62% death or moderate/severe disability[c] Bayley 75 ± 23 40% Bayley <70	–
Davis et al., 2010 (116)	18–22 months	Extremely low birth weight infants[d]	414	14%	22% (late death)	72% neurodevelopmental impairment 32% moderate–severe CP 55% Psychomotor Development Index <70 64% Mental Development Index <70 32% isolated developmental impairment 55% head circumference <10% 11% hearing impairment 43% vision impairment	16%
Pisani et al., 2007 (31)	24 months	Term and preterm: Neonatal status epilepticus vs. recurrent neonatal seizures 43.4% HIE 23% cerebral haemorrhage 33% others	106	34%	19%	47% adverse outcome (CP, DD, epilepsy, blindness, deafness, or death) 37% CP (19/39 CP + epilepsy) 34% DD (28/36 DD + CP)	18%
Pisani et al., 2008 (121)	30 months	Preterm: 50.9% HIE 29.4% cerebral haemorrhage 19.7% others	51	20%	34%	80% adverse outcome 40% CP (9/20 CP + epilepsy) 30% DD + CP 15% DD + CP + epilepsy	41.6% of neonatal status epilepticus
Nagarajan et al., 2011 (34)	2–6 years	≥32 weeks GA	43	26%	21%	76% neurodevelopmental impairment 32% CP	41%
Guillet and Kwon, 2007 (117)	Median age 32 months for phenobarbital at discharge group and 57 for no phenobarbital at discharge group	≥34 weeks GA: 30% HIE 16% stroke 6% bleed 48% other	132	–	3% (n=196)	19% CP 54% DD 24% seizure after discharge	16%
Glass et al., 2009 (36)	4 years	Term: HIE	143/50 lost to follow-up	–	11%	56% abnormal neurological exam FSIQ mean score 52	–
Ronen et al., 2007 (122)	10 years	Term and preterm: Variable	88	35%	24%	41% neurodevelopment impairment 25% CP 20% mental retardation 27% learning disorder	23%

CP, cerebral palsy; DD, developmental delay; FSIQ, Full Scale Intelligence Quotient; GA, gestational age; HIE, hypoxic-ischaemic encephalopathy

[a] Asphyxia and neonatal seizures were associated with microcephaly, severe cerebral palsy and failure to thrive

[b] Seizure severity was associated with severe cerebral palsy

[c] Seizures were not associated with death, or moderate or severe disability or lower Bayley when adjusted for treatment and severity of encephalopathy

[d] Seizures in extremely low birth weight infants are an independent risk factor for adverse neurodevelopmental outcome

to the hypoxic brain injury, still needs to be answered with a prospective multicenter study that includes continuous video-EEG so the real impact of subclinical seizures (the majority of the neonatal seizures) can be evaluated.

Neonatal and early infantile epilepsies

Two idiopathic epilepsy syndromes begin in the neonatal period: benign familial neonatal seizures and benign idiopathic neonatal seizures (120). In the study of Watanabe et al., 21% of the neonates had benign neonatal convulsions and 10% had benign familial neonatal convulsion (21).

Benign familial neonatal seizures

Benign familial neonatal seizures begin in the first week of life. The presentation of seizures peak around the 5th day of life (5th day fits). The clinical seizures are typically partial clonic with a migratory component. In the study of Watanabe et al., all the neonates with benign neonatal convulsions had partial seizures (21). Children with this epilepsy could also present with apnoeas and more rarely with tonic seizures or status epilepticus. Neurological exam is normal. EEG findings are variable from normal, to excessive discontinuity, focal or multifocal epileptiform discharges. There is no family history of epilepsy. Seizures have an excellent response to phenobarbital, phenytoin, and benzodiazepines. The prognosis is excellent with rare recurrence of seizures.

Benign neonatal familial convulsion

BNFC also presents within the first weeks of life. Associated seizure types include tonic, clonic, apnoeas with cyanosis, or other autonomic seizures. Seizures can be focal or multifocal. In the study of Watanabe et al., all but one neonate with BFNCs had partial seizures (21). Typically, the seizures are very brief. Frequency of seizures can be high at the time of presentation. The neurological exam and neurodevelopment is normal in these infants. EEG can be normal or show transient abnormalities including excessive epileptiform discharges. As familial epilepsy, there is a family history of seizures beginning in the neonatal period in other relatives. The inheritance is autosomal dominant with around 85% penetrance. Mutations in the voltage-gated potassium channels KCNQ2 in chromosome 20q13.3 and KCNQ3 on chromosome 8q24 are responsible for this epilepsy (121). Seizures resolve spontaneously by mid-infancy. When treatment is needed, phenobarbital has been the drug of choice. Ten to 16% of these patients can develop epilepsy later in life.

Two epileptic encephalopathies also present during the neonatal period: early infantile encephalopathy with burst suppression or Ohtahara syndrome, and early myoclonic encephalopathy (123–125).

Early infantile encephalopathy with burst suppression or Ohtahara syndrome

Early infantile encephalopathy with burst suppression or Ohtahara syndrome begins in the first few weeks of life with generalized or asymmetrical spasms and partial seizures. Neurodevelopment becomes abnormal with loss of milestones, hypotonia, spasticity, and abnormal movements. EEG is characterized by episodes of burst suppression that are persistent during awake and sleep stages. The aetiology is mainly related to cerebral malformations. Seizures are very refractory to treatment with adrenocorticotropic hormone (ACTH) or AEDs. Prognosis is poor. Clinically and electroencephalographically, most of the patients evolve into West syndrome with EEG hypsarrhythmia and later to Lennox–Gastaut syndrome (126–128).

Early myoclonic encephalopathy

Early myoclonic encephalopathy begins also in early infancy with myoclonic seizures and partial seizures. Spasms and tonic seizures can present later in the course of the disease. Neurodevelopment is also severely affects and neurological exam is abnormal. EEG shows burst suppression pattern is more predominant during sleep. This pattern persists during the patient's life. The aetiology of the syndrome is genetic or metabolic rather than structural. This syndrome typically does not evolve into West syndrome. Response to ACTH and AEDs is also very disappointing (127).

Migrating partial seizures

This entity was first described in 1995 and manifests with unprovoked, explosive electroclinical seizures and marked developmental dysfunction (129). This is seen in infants without prior neurological insults or evidence of cerebral dysgenesis who develop intractable near continual multifocal seizures that evolve across multiple regions of both hemispheres in an alternating and sequential fashion. The prognosis is poor with mortality in 1/3 of the patients and severe psychomotor retardation of the survivors.

Other infantile epilepsies that usually start beyond the neonatal period such as severe myoclonic epilepsy (Dravet syndrome), myoclonic epilepsy (Doose syndrome), and infantile spasms (West syndrome) are discussed in Chapter 15.

References

1. Allan WC, Sobel DB. Neonatal intensive care neurology. *Semin Pediatr Neurol* 2004; 11(2):119–28.
2. Glass HC, Bonifacio SL, Peloquin S, Shimotake T, Sehring S, Sun Y, *et al.* Neurocritical care for neonates. *Neurocrit Care* 2010; 12(3): 421–9.
3. Wusthoff CJ, Dlugos DJ, Gutierrez-Colina A, Wang A, Cook N, Donnelly M, *et al.* Electrographic seizures during therapeutic hypothermia for neonatal hypoxic-ischemic encephalopathy. *J Child Neurol* 2011; 26(6):724–8.
4. Eriksson M, Zetterstrom R. Neonatal convulsions. Incidence and causes in the Stockholm area. *Acta Paediatr Scand* 1979; 68(6):807–11.
5. Lanska MJ, Lanska DJ, Baumann RJ, Kryscio RJ. A population-based study of neonatal seizures in Fayette County, Kentucky. *Neurology* 1995; 45(4):724–32.
6. Ronen GM, Penney S, Andrews W. The epidemiology of clinical neonatal seizures in Newfoundland: a population-based study. *J Pediatr* 1999; 134(1):71–5.
7. Scher MS. Neonatal seizures. In: Taeusch HW, Ballard RA, Gleason CA (eds) *Avery's Diseases of the Newborn* (8th edn), pp. 1005–25. Philadelphia, PA: Elsevier Saunders, 2005.
8. Jensen FE. Neonatal seizures: an update on mechanisms and management. *Clin Perinatol* 2009; 36(4):881–900.
9. Weiner SP, Painter MJ, Geva D, Guthrie RD, Scher MS. Neonatal seizures: electroclinical dissociation. *Pediatr Neurol* 1991; 7(5):363–8.
10. Mizrahi EM. Neonatal seizures and neonatal epileptic syndromes. *Neurol Clinics* 2001; 19:427–63.
11. Sankar MJ, Agarwal R, Aggarwal R, Deorari AK, Paul VK. Seizures in the newborn. *Indian J Pediatr* 2008; 75(2):149–55.

12. Scher MS. Neonatal seizure classification: a fetal perspective concerning childhood epilepsy. *Epilepsy Res* 2006; 70(Suppl 1):S41–57.
13. Proposal for revised clinical and electroencephalographic classification of epileptic seizures. From the Commission on Classification and Terminology of the International League Against Epilepsy. *Epilepsia* 1981; 22(4):489–501.
14. Proposal for revised classification of epilepsies and epileptic syndromes. Commission on Classification and Terminology of the International League Against Epilepsy. *Epilepsia* 1989; 30(4):389–99.
15. Engel J Jr. A proposed diagnostic scheme for people with epileptic seizures and with epilepsy: report of the ILAE Task Force on Classification and Terminology. *Epilepsia* 2001; 42(6):796–803.
16. Engel J Jr. ILAE classification of epilepsy syndromes. *Epilepsy Res* 2006; 70(Suppl 1):S5–10.
17. Engel J Jr. Report of the ILAE classification core group. *Epilepsia* 2006; 47(9):1558–68.
18. Berg AT, Berkovic SF, Brodie MJ, Buchhalter J, Cross JH, van Emde BW, *et al.* Revised terminology and concepts for organization of seizures and epilepsies: report of the ILAE Commission on Classification and Terminology, 2005–2009. *Epilepsia* 2010; 51(4): 676–85.
19. Mastrangelo M, Van LA, Bray M, Pastorino G, Marini A, Mosca F. Epileptic seizures, epilepsy and epileptic syndromes in newborns: a nosological approach to 94 new cases by the 2001 proposed diagnostic scheme for people with epileptic seizures and with epilepsy. *Seizure* 2005; 14(5):304–11.
20. Mizrahi EM, Kellaway P. Characterization and classification of neonatal seizures. *Neurology* 1987; 37(12):1837–44.
21. Watanabe K, Miura K, Natsume J, Hayakawa F, Furune S, Okumura A. Epilepsies of neonatal onset: seizure type and evolution. *Dev Med Child Neurol* 1999; 41(5):318–22.
22. Shorvon SD. The etiologic classification of epilepsy. *Epilepsia* 2011; 52(6):1052–7.
23. Rose A. Lombroso C. A study of clinical, pathological and electroencephalographic features in 137 full-term babies with a long-term follow up. *Pediatrics* 1970; 45:404–25.
24. Dreyfus-Brisac C, Monod N. Electroclinical studies of status epilepticus and convulsions in the newborn. In: Kellaway P, Petersen I (eds) *Neurological and* Electroencephalographic Correlative Studies in Infancy, pp. 250–72. New York: Grune and Stratton, 1964.
25. Lombroso C. Seizures in the newborn. In: Vinken P, Bruyn G (eds) *The Epilepsies. Handbook of Clinical Neurophysiology*, Vol 15, pp. 189–218. Amsterdam: North Holland, 1974.
26. Volpe J. Neonatal seizures. *N Engl J Med* 1973; 289:413–16.
27. Watanabe K, Hara K, Miyazaki S. Electroclinical studies of seizures in the newborn. *Folia Psychiatr Neurol Jpn* 1977; 31:383–92.
28. Volpe J. Neonatal seizures: current concepts and revised classification. *Pediatrics* 1989; 84:422–8.
29. Volpe J. Neonatal seizures. In: Volpe JJ (ed) *Neurology of the Newborn* (5th edn), pp. 203–44. Philadelphia, PA: Saunders Elsevier, 2008.
30. Clancy RR, Legido A. The exact ictal and interictal duration of electroencephalographic neonatal seizures. *Epilepsia* 1987; 28(5): 537–41.
31. Pisani F, Cerminara C, Fusco C, Sisti L. Neonatal status epilepticus vs recurrent neonatal seizures: clinical findings and outcome. *Neurology* 2007; 69(23):2177–85.
32. Scher MS, Hamid MY, Steppe DA, Beggarly ME, Painter MJ. Ictal and interictal electrographic seizure durations in preterm and term neonates. *Epilepsia* 1993; 34(2):284–8.
33. Nash KB, Bonifacio SL, Glass HC, Sullivan JE, Barkovich AJ, Ferriero DM, *et al.* Video-EEG monitoring in newborns with hypoxic-ischemic encephalopathy treated with hypothermia. *Neurology* 2011; 76(6): 556–62.
34. Nagarajan L, Ghosh S, Palumbo L. Ictal electroencephalograms in neonatal seizures: characteristics and associations. *Pediatr Neurol* 2011; 45(1):11–16.
35. Shellhaas RA, Clancy RR. Characterization of neonatal seizures by conventional EEG and single-channel EEG. *Clin Neurophysiol* 2007; 118(10):2156–61.
36. Glass HC, Glidden D, Jeremy RJ, Barkovich AJ, Ferriero DM, Miller SP. Clinical neonatal seizures are independently associated with outcome in infants at risk for hypoxic-ischemic brain injury. *J Pediatr* 2009; 155(3):318–23.
37. Murray DM, Boylan GB, Ali I, Ryan CA, Murphy BP, Connolly S. Defining the gap between electrographic seizure burden, clinical expression and staff recognition of neonatal seizures. *Arch Dis Child Fetal Neonatal Ed* 2008; 93(3):F187–91.
38. Clancy RR, Sharif U, Ichord R, Spray TL, Nicolson S, Tabbutt S, *et al.* Electrographic neonatal seizures after infant heart surgery. *Epilepsia* 2005; 46(1):84.
39. Mizrahi EM, Hrachovy RA, Kellaway P. *Atlas of neonatal electroencephalography* (3rd edn). Philadelphia, PA: Lippincott Williams & Wilkins, 2004.
40. Scher MS, Beggarly M. Clinical significance of focal periodic discharges in neonates. *J Child Neurol* 1989; 4(3):175–85.
41. Shewmon DA. What is a neonatal seizure? Problems in definition and quantification for investigative and clinical purposes. *J Clin Neurophysiol* 1990; 7(3):315–68.
42. Oliveira AJ, Nunes ML, Haertel LM, Reis FM, da Costa JC. Duration of rhythmic EEG patterns in neonates: new evidence for clinical and prognostic significance of brief rhythmic discharges. *Clin Neurophysiol* 2000; 111(9):1646–53.
43. Nagarajan L, Palumbo L, Ghosh S. Brief electroencephalography rhythmic discharges (BERDs) in the neonate with seizures: their significance and prognostic implications. *J Child Neurol* 2011; 26(12):1529–33.
44. Knauss T, Carlson C. Neonatal paroxysmal monorhythmic alpha activity. *Arch Neurol* 1978; 35:104–7.
45. Willis J, Gould JB. Periodic alpha seizures with apnea in a newborn. *Dev Med Child Neurol* 1980; 22:214–22.
46. Watanabe K, Kuroyanagi M, Hara K, Miyazaki S. Neonatal seizures and subsequent epilepsy. *Brain Dev* 1982; 4:341–6.
47. Clancy RR, Dicker L, Cho S, Cook N, Nicolson SC, Wernovsky G, *et al.* Agreement between long-term neonatal background classification by conventional and amplitude-integrated EEG. *J Clin Neurophysiol* 2011; 28(1):1–9.
48. Shellhaas RA, Soaita AI, Clancy RR. Sensitivity of amplitude-integrated electroencephalography for neonatal seizure detection. *Pediatrics* 2007; 120(4):770–7.
49. Hall DA, Wadwa RP, Goldenberg NA, Norris JM. Maternal risk factors for term neonatal seizures: population-based study in Colorado, 1989–2003. *J Child Neurol* 2006; 21(9):795–8.
50. Kohelet D, Shochat R, Lusky A, Reichman B. Risk factors for seizures in very low birthweight infants with periventricular leukomalacia. *J Child Neurol* 2006; 21(11):965–70.
51. Lieberman E, Eichenwald E, Mathur G, Richardson D, Heffner L, Cohen A. Intrapartum fever and unexplained seizures in term infants. *Pediatrics* 2000; 106(5):983–8.
52. Saliba RM, Annegers FJ, Waller DK, Tyson JE, Mizrahi EM. Risk factors for neonatal seizures: a population-based study, Harris County, Texas, 1992–1994. *Am J Epidemiol* 2001; 154(1):14–20.
53. Scher MS, Steppe DA, Beggarly M. Timing of neonatal seizures and intrapartum obstetrical factors. *J Child Neurol* 2008; 23(6): 640–3.
54. Barnes-Powell LL. Infants of diabetic mothers: the effects of hyperglycemia on the fetus and neonate. *Neonatal Netw* 2007; 26(5):283–90.

55. Dheen ST, Tay SS, Boran J, Ting LW, Kumar SD, Fu J, *et al.* Recent studies on neural tube defects in embryos of diabetic pregnancy: an overview. *Curr Med Chem* 2009; 16(18):2345–54.
56. Kanekar S, Gent M. Malformations of cortical development. *Semin Ultrasound CT MR* 2011; 32(3):211–27.
57. Schwartz R, Teramo KA. Effects of diabetic pregnancy on the fetus and newborn. *Semin Perinatol* 2000; 24(2):120–35.
58. Vijay K, Agarwal A. Neonatal hypoglycemia resulting in occipital cerebral injury. *Pediatr Radiol* 2010; 40(Suppl 1):S178.
59. Karimzadeh P, Tabarestani S, Ghofrani M. Hypoglycemia-occipital syndrome: a specific neurologic syndrome following neonatal hypoglycemia? *J Child Neurol* 2011; 2:152–9.
60. Montassir H, Maegaki Y, Ohno K, Ogura K. Long term prognosis of symptomatic occipital lobe epilepsy secondary to neonatal hypoglycemia. *Epilepsy Res* 2010; 88(2–3):93–9.
61. Efron D, South M, Volpe JJ, Inder T. Cerebral injury in association with profound iatrogenic hyperglycemia in a neonate. *Eur J Paediatr Neurol* 2003; 7(4):167–71.
62. Lieberman E, Lang J, Richardson DK, Frigoletto FD, Heffner LJ, Cohen A. Intrapartum maternal fever and neonatal outcome. *Pediatrics* 2000; 105(1 Pt 1):8–13.
63. Caviness AC, Demmler GJ, Selwyn BJ. Clinical and laboratory features of neonatal herpes simplex virus infection: a case-control study. *Pediatr Infect Dis J* 2008; 27(5):425–30.
64. Lombardi G, Garofoli F, Stronati M. Congenital cytomegalovirus infection:treatment, sequelae and follow-up. *J Matern Fetal Neonatal Med* 2010; 23(Suppl 3):45.
65. Shet A. Congenital and perinatal infections: throwing new light with an old TORCH. *Indian J Pediatr* 2011; 78(1):88–95.
66. McCarthy FP, Giles ML, Rowlands S, Purcell KJ, Jones CA. Antenatal interventions for preventing the transmission of cytomegalovirus (CMV) from the mother to fetus during pregnancy and adverse outcomes in the congenitally infected infant. *Cochrane Database Syst Rev* 2011; 3:CD008371.
67. Bizzarro MJ, Raskind C, Baltimore RS, Gallagher PG. Seventy-five years of neonatal sepsis at Yale: 1928–2003. *Pediatrics* 2005; 116(3):595–602.
68. Sgro M, Shah PS, Campbell D, Tenuta A, Shivananda S, Lee SK. Early-onset neonatal sepsis: rate and organism pattern between 2003 and 2008. *J Perinatol* 2011 31(12):794–8.
69. Al-Taiar A, Hammoud MS, Thalib L, Isaacs D. Pattern and etiology of culture proven early-onset neonatal sepsis: a five-year prospective study. *Int J Infect Dis* 2011; 15(9):e631–4.
70. Barbadoro P, Marigliano A, Savini S, D'Errico MM, Prospero E. Group B Streptococcal sepsis: An old or ongoing threat? *Am J Infect Control* 2011; 39(8):e45–e48.
71. Clancy R, Chung HJ. EEG changes during recovery from acute severe neonatal citrullinemia. *Electroencephalogr Clin Neurophysiol* 1991; 78:222–7.
72. Pettit RE. Pyridoxine dependency seizures: report of a case with unusual features. *J Child Neurol* 1987; 2:38–41.
73. Chapman K, Mizrahi E, Clancy R, *et al.* Diagnosis and treatment of seizures in special clinical settings 'neonatal seizures'. In: *Wyllie's Treatment of Epilepsy*, pp. 419–20. Philadelphia, PA: Wolters, Kluwer, Lippincott Williams and Wilkins, 2006.
74. Nicolai J, van Kranen-Mastenbroek VH, Wevers RA, Hurkx WA, Vles JS. Folinic acid responsive seizures initially responsive to pyridoxine. *Pediatr Neurol* 2006; 34:164–7.
75. Gallagher RC, Van Hove JL, Scharer G, Hyland K, Plecko B, Waters PJ, *et al.* Folinic-acid responsive seizure are identical to pyridoxine-dependent epilepsy. *Ann Neurol* 2009; 65:550–6.
76. Slot HMJ, Overweg-Plandsoen WCG, Bakker HD, Abeling NG, Tamminga P, Barth PG, *et al.* Molybdenum cofactor deficiency; an easily missed caused of neonatal convulsions. *Neuropediatrics* 1993; 24:139–42.
77. Arnold GL, Greene CL, Stout JP, Goodman SI. Molybdenum cofactor deficiency. *Pediatr* 1993; 123:595–8.
78. Johnson JL. Prenatal diagnosis of molybdenum cofactor deficiency and isolated sulfite oxidase deficiency. *Proc Natl Acad Sci U S A* 2002; 23:6–8.
79. Tekgul H, Gauvreau K, Soul J, Murphy L, Robertson R, Stewart J, *et al.* The current etiologic profile and neurodevelopmental outcome of seizures in term newborn infants. *Pediatrics* 2006; 117(4):1270–80.
80. Johnston MV. Selective vulnerability in the neonatal brain. *Ann Neurol* 1998; 44:155–56.
81. Khazipov R, Khalilov I, Tyzio R, Morozova E, Ben-Ari Y, Holmes GL. Developmental changes in GABAergic actions and seizure susceptibility in the rat hippocampus. *Eur J Neurosci* 2004; 19: 590–600.
82. Tyzio R, Holmes GL, Ben-Ari Y, Khazipov R. Timing of the developmental switch in GABA, mediated signaling from excitation to inhibition in CA3 rat hippocampus using gramicidin perforated patch and extracellular recordings. *Epilepsia* 2007; 48 (suppl 5):96–105.
83. Haas KZ, Sperber EF, Opanashuk LA, Stanton PK, Moshé SL. Resistance of immature hippocampus to morphologic and physiologic alterations following status epilepticus or kindling. *Hippocampus* 2001; 11:615–25.
84. McCabe BK, Silveira DC, Cilio MR, Cha BH, Liu X, Sogawa Y, *et al.* Reduced neurogenesis after neonatal seizures. *J Neurosci* 2001; 21:2094–103.
85. Fando JL, Conn M, Wasterlain CG. Brain protein synthesis during neonatal seizures: an experimental study. *Exp Neurol* 1979; 63:220–8.
86. Holmes GL, Gairsa JL, Chevassus-Au-Louis N, Ben-Ari Y. Consequences of neonatal seizures in the rat: Morphological and behavioral effects. *Ann Neurol* 1998; 44:845–57.
87. Miller SP, Weiss J, Barnwell A, Ferriero DM, Latal-Hajnal B, Ferrer-Rogers A, *et al.* Seizure-associated brain injury in term newborns with perinatal asphyxia. *Neurology* 2002; 58(4):542–8.
88. Clancy RR. The contribution of EEG to the understanding of neonatal seizures. *Epilepsia* 1996; 37:S52–9.
89. Painter MJ, Scher MS, Stein AD, Armatti S, Wang Z, Gardiner JC, *et al.* Phenobarbital compared with phenytoin for the treatment of neonatal seizures. *N Engl J Med* 1999; 341(7):485–9.
90. Bartha AI, Shen J, Katz KH, Mischel RE, Yap KR, Ivacko JA, *et al.* Neonatal seizures: multicenter variability in current treatment practices. *Pediatr Neurol* 2007; 37(2):85–90.
91. Castro Conde JR, Hernandez Borges AA, Domenech ME, Gonzalez CC, Perera SR. Midazolam in neonatal seizures with no response to phenobarbital. *Neurology* 2005; 64(5):876–9.
92. Sheth RD, Buckley DJ, Gutierrez AR, Gingold M, Bodensteiner JB, Penney S. Midazolam in the treatment of refractory neonatal seizures. *Clin Neuropharmacol* 1996; 19(2):165–70.
93. Sirsi D, Nangia S, LaMothe J, Kosofsky BE, Solomon GE. Successful management of refractory neonatal seizures with midazolam. *J Child Neurol* 2008; 23(6):706–9.
94. Kawaguchi N, Imataka G, Suzumura H, Yamanouchi H. [Etiology and management of neonatal seizures—successful treatment by midazolam]. *No To Hattatsu* 2006; 38(1):5–9.
95. Hu KC, Chiu NC, Ho CS, Lee ST, Shen EY. Continuous midazolam infusion in the treatment of uncontrollable neonatal seizures. *Acta Paediatr Taiwan* 2003; 44(5):279–81.
96. Shany E, Benzaqen O, Watemberg N. Comparison of continuous drip of midazolam or lidocaine in the treatment of intractable neonatal seizures. *J Child Neurol* 2007; 22(3):255–9.
97. Boylan GB, Rennie JM, Chorley G, Pressler RM, Fox GF, Farrer K, *et al.* Second-line anticonvulsant treatment of neonatal seizures: a video-EEG monitoring study. *Neurology* 2004; 62(3):486–8.
98. Vento M, de Vries LS, Alberola A, Blennow M, Steggerda S, Greisen G, *et al.* Approach to seizures in the neonatal period: a European perspective. *Acta Paediatr* 2010; 99(4):497–501.

99. Bassan H, Bental Y, Shany E, Berger I, Froom P, Levi L, *et al.* Neonatal seizures: dilemmas in workup and management. *Pediatr Neurol* 2008; 38(6):415–21.
100. Malingre MM, Van Rooij LG, Rademaker CM, Toet MC, Ververs TF, van KC, *et al.* Development of an optimal lidocaine infusion strategy for neonatal seizures. *Eur J Pediatr* 2006; 165(9):598–604.
101. van den Broek MP, Huitema AD, van Hasselt JG, Groenendaal F, Toet MC, Egberts TC, *et al.* Lidocaine (lignocaine) dosing regimen based upon a population pharmacokinetic model for preterm and term neonates with seizures. *Clin Pharmacokinet* 2011; 50(7):461–9.
102. Van Rooij LG, Toet MC, Rademaker KM, Groenendaal F, de Vries LS. Cardiac arrhythmias in neonates receiving lidocaine as anticonvulsive treatment. *Eur J Pediatr* 2004; 163(11):637–41.
103. Silverstein FS, Ferriero DM. Off-label use of antiepileptic drugs for the treatment of neonatal seizures. *Pediatr Neurol* 2008 Aug; 39(2): 77–9.
104. Glass HC, Poulin C, Shevell MI. Topiramate for the treatment of neonatal seizures. *Pediatr Neurol* 2011; 44(6):439–42.
105. Filippi L, la MG, Fiorini P, Poggi C, Cavallaro G, Malvagia S, *et al.* Topiramate concentrations in neonates treated with prolonged whole body hypothermia for hypoxic ischemic encephalopathy. *Epilepsia* 2009; 50(11):2355–61.
106. Khan O, Chang E, Cipriani C, Wright C, Crisp E, Kirmani B. Use of intravenous levetiracetam for management of acute seizures in neonates. *Pediatr Neurol* 2011; 44(4):265–9.
107. Abend NS, Gutierrez-Colina AM, Monk HM, Dlugos DJ, Clancy RR. Levetiracetam for treatment of neonatal seizures. *J Child Neurol* 2011; 26(4):465–70.
108. Furwentsches A, Bussmann C, Ramantani G, Ebinger F, Philippi H, Poschl J, *et al.* Levetiracetam in the treatment of neonatal seizures: a pilot study. *Seizure* 2010; 19(3):185–9.
109. Ramantani G, Ikonomidou C, Walter B, Rating D, Dinger J. Levetiracetam: safety and efficacy in neonatal seizures. *Eur J Paediatr Neurol* 2011; 15(1):1–7.
110. Kahle KT, Staley KJ. The bumetanide-sensitive Na-K-2Cl cotransporter NKCC1 as a potential target of a novel mechanism-based treatment strategy for neonatal seizures. *Neurosurg Focus* 2008; 25(3):E22.
111. Silverstein FS, Jensen FE, Inder T, Hellstrom-Westas L, Hirtz D, Ferriero DM. Improving the treatment of neonatal seizures: National Institute of Neurological Disorders and Stroke workshop report. *J Pediatr* 2008; 153(1):12–15.
112. Kahle KT, Barnett SM, Sassower KC, Staley KJ. Decreased seizure activity in a human neonate treated with bumetanide, an inhibitor of the Na(+)-K(+)-2Cl(-) cotransporter NKCC1. *J Child Neurol* 2009; 24(5):572–6.
113. Scher MS, Alvin J, Gaus L, Minnigh B, Painter MJ, *et al.* Uncoupling of EEG-clinical neonatal seizures after antiepileptic drug use. *Pediatr Neurol* 2003; 28:277–80.
114. Dzhala VI, Talos DM, Sdrulla DA, Brumback AC, Mathews GC, Benke TA, *et al.* NKCC1 transporter facilitates seizures in the developing brain. *Nat Med* 2005; 11:1205–13.
115. Mizrahi EM. Acute and chronic effects of seizures in the developing brain: lessons from clinical experience. *Epilepsia* 1999; 40(Suppl 1): S42–50.
116. Davis AS, Hintz SR, Van Meurs KP, Li L, Das A, Stoll BJ, *et al.* Seizures in extremely low birth weight infants are associated with adverse outcome. *J Pediatr* 2010; 157(5):720–5.
117. Guillet R, Kwon J. Seizure recurrence and developmental disabilities after neonatal seizures: outcomes are unrelated to use of phenobarbital prophylaxis. *J Child Neurol* 2007; 22(4):389–95.
118. Iype M, Prasad M, Nair PM, Geetha S, Kailas L. The newborn with seizures—a follow-up study. *Indian Pediatr* 2008; 45(9):749–52.
119. Kwon JM, Guillet R, Shankaran S, Laptook AR, McDonald SA, Ehrenkranz RA, *et al.* Clinical seizures in neonatal hypoxic-ischemic encephalopathy have no independent impact on neurodevelopmental outcome: secondary analyses of data from the neonatal research network hypothermia trial. *J Child Neurol* 2011; 26(3):322–8.
120. McBride MC, Laroia N, Guillet R. Electrographic seizures in neonates correlate with poor neurodevelopmental outcome. *Neurology* 2000; 55(4):506–13.
121. Pisani F, Barilli AL, Sisti L, Bevilacqua G, Seri S. Preterm infants with video EEG confirmed seizures: outcome at 30 months of age. *Brain Dev* 2008; 30(1):20–30.
122. Ronen GM, Buckley D, Penney S, Streiner DL. Long-term prognosis in children with neonatal seizures: a population-based study. *Neurology* 2007; 69(19):1816–22.
123. Yamamoto H, Okumura A, Fukuda M. Epilepsies and epileptic syndromes starting in the neonatal period. *Brain Dev* 2011; 33(3): 213–20.
124. Burgess DL. Neonatal epilepsy syndromes and GEFS+: mechanistic considerations. *Epilepsia* 2005; 46(Suppl 10):51–8.
125. Ohtahara S, Yamatogi Y. Ohtahara syndrome: with special reference to its developmental aspects for differentiating from early myoclonic encephalopathy. *Epilepsy Res* 2006; 70(Suppl 1):S58–67.
126. Ohtahara S, Ishida T, Oka E, Yamatogi Y, Inoue H. On the specific age-dependent epileptic syndrome. The early-infantile epileptic encephalopathy with suppression burst. *No To Hattatsu* 1976; 8:270–80.
127. Djukic A, Lado FA, Shinnar S, Moshé SL. Are early myoclonic encephalopathy (EME) and the Ohtahara syndrome (EIEE) independent of each other? *Epilepsy Res* 2006; 70:68–76.
128. Kato M, Saitoh S, Kamei A, Shiraishi H, Ueda Y, Akasaka M, *et al.* A longer polyalanine expansion mutation in the ARC gene causes early infantile epileptic encephalopathy with suppression-burst pattern. (Ohtahara syndrome). *Am J Hum Genet* 2007; 81:361–6.
129. Coppola G, Plouin P, Chiron C, Robain O, Dulac O. Migrating partial seizures in infancy: a malignant disorder with developmental arrest. *Epilepsia* 1995; 36:1017–24.

CHAPTER 15

Epileptic Encephalopathies

Renzo Guerrini and Carla Marini

It has been recognized for many years that some patients with severe forms of epilepsy experience clinical deterioration even when an underlying progressive disease has been ruled out. There must therefore be an ongoing process, likely related to epilepsy, which causes a regress in neurological function. The term 'epileptic encephalopathy' has been initially used to designate Lennox–Gastaut syndrome (1) in which cognitive and behavioural deterioration are prominent manifestations and has over the years been better defined in its supposed pathophysiological bases as applicable to conditions in which seizures, the epileptiform abnormalities, or both, contribute to the progressive disturbance in cerebral function (2).

About 40% of all epilepsies occurring in the first 3 years of life fit this definition (3). However, the epileptic encephalopathies represent more a concept and an operational category than a syndrome spectrum. Some syndromes such as West syndrome, Dravet syndrome (severe myoclonic epilepsy), epilepsy with continuous spike and waves during sleep, Landau–Kleffner syndrome, and Lennox–Gastaut syndrome are always manifested as epileptic encephalopathies, irrespective from the underlying cause and severity of electroencephalogram (EEG) abnormalities. However, even syndromes with good outcome, such as benign rolandic epilepsy, may sometimes have a complicated evolution, with learning and language impairment, especially if severe spike and wave discharges appear on the EEG and persist for at least several months (4). Persistent spike-and-wave related anatomo-specific cortical dysfunction has been blamed for such an ominous evolution (5, 6). Other syndromes seem to have almost equal chances of either having a short course and a good outcome or precipitating within the spectrum of an epileptic encephalopathy. For example, myoclonic-astatic epilepsy might unpredictably evolve as an epileptic encephalopathy or rapidly remit without major consequences on cognitive outcome, irrespective from its initial clinical and EEG characteristics (7). In such cases it is often entirely unclear which factors, clinical or EEG, can be blamed for either outcome. Finally, a particular situation is represented by epileptic encephalopathies that appear in children with a highly epileptogenic, usually developmental, brain lesion, such as, for example, hemimegalencephaly, from which epileptic activity spreading to intact, remote areas interferes with their function and amplifies the clinical consequences of the malformation.

It is generally acknowledged that proper recognition and rationale treatment choices provide higher chances of reducing seizure severity and cognitive impairment in epileptic encephalopathies, although this is difficult to demonstrate unequivocally in relation to different aetiologies. Although vigorous early treatment is often advocated, for most conditions there are no established endpoints and drug choices are empirically made. Surgical treatment can be successful in selected cases. However, only in some surgically treatable syndromes early treatment has a definite effect on long-term prognosis (8). In many individuals the underlying cause, which often remains unrecognized, probably plays a greater part than is acknowledged in determining cognitive outcome.

Infantile spasms and West syndrome

Infantile spasms (IS) are typical of the first year of life, are usually resistant to conventional antiepileptic drugs and are associated with developmental delay, or deterioration. Interictal EEG is often 'hypsarrhythmic', with high voltage (up to 500 μV) slow waves, irregularly interspersed with spikes and sharp waves giving the EEG the appearance of a chaotic disorganization of electrogenesis. During slow sleep, bursts of more synchronous, polyspikes and waves often appear. In West syndrome spasms, hypsarrhythmia, and cognitive deterioration occur together. However, IS may also occur without the typical EEG features of West syndrome, especially in severe brain lesions, such as tuberous sclerosis or lissencephaly (9). Disappearance of social smile, loss of visual attention, or autistic withdrawal are often reported by the parents with the onset of spasms. However, developmental delay may predate the onset of spasms in up to 70% of children (10).

A cumulative incidence of 2.9 per 10,000 live births and an age-specific prevalence of 2.0 per 10,000 in 10-year-old children were observed in the US (11). Epileptic spasms can persist or, rarely, appear in older children.

IS are manifested as clusters of increasing-plateau -decreasing-intensity brisk (0.5–2.0 s) flexions or extensions of the neck, with abduction or adduction of the upper limbs and upward eye deviation that are repeated many times per day. After a series, the child is usually exhausted. Asymmetric spasms are often associated with a lateralized brain lesion (12), although unilateral lesions might cause symmetric spasms. Lateralized motor phenomena, including lateral or upward eye deviation and eyebrow contraction, and abduction of one shoulder, may sometimes constitute the entire series of spasms or initiate a series which will eventually develop into bilateral manifestations. Such lateralized manifestations are usually accompanied by asymmetric ictal EEG changes. Other seizure types can coexist.

Duration of spasms is variable, depending both on treatment and on their tendency to remit or evolve into other seizure types. Rapid spontaneous remission is rare. In about 50% of children, spasms disappear before the age of 3 years and in 90% before the age of 5 years (13). Misdiagnosis of colic, startles, Moro response, or shoulder shrugs is still frequent.

The initial diagnostic efforts directed at the causes of spasms may have immediate practical implications as symptomatic and cryptogenic spasms carry a different prognostic outlook and, in relation to specific aetiologies, may determine different therapeutic options. However, the terms symptomatic and cryptogenic have not been used uniformly. Most investigators define as symptomatic those cases in which an aetiological factor can be clearly identified. Others link symptomaticity to either or both abnormal development prior to the onset of spasms and clinical or imaging evidence of a brain lesion, with brain malformations and perinatal hypoxic-ischaemic encephalopathy being the most frequent causes. Cryptogenic spasms are those for which no cause can be identified, or development was normal before clinical onset. The term cryptogenic does not necessarily mean that no lesion is present; therefore, a difference of nature between cryptogenic and symptomatic cases is not clearly established. A few cases that are not included in the symptomatic group, despite increasingly accurate investigations, may belong to an 'idiopathic' group (14, 15).

A family history of IS is found in about 4% of the cases (16). Familial cases are probably the expression of several genetic disorders, some of which are well characterized, including leucodystrophy (17), tuberous sclerosis (18), X-linked lissencephaly and band heterotopia (19), X-linked mental retardation and IS due to mutations of the *ARX* gene (20, 21). Boys with X-linked IS due to *ARX* mutations usually have severe developmental delay and may have microcephaly. Onset of spasms is early and hypsarrhythmia is frequent (22, 23). A syndrome of early-onset IS, and severe quadriplegic dyskinesia, in which spasms tend to remit but episodes of status dystonicus complicate the course, has been associated with expansions in the first polyalanine tract of the *ARX* gene (21).

A syndrome with microcephaly and early-onset intractable seizures, including spasms with or without hypsarrhythmia, has been associated with mutations or deletions of the X-linked gene *CDKL5* (24–26). The syndrome is much more frequent in females. Infants with *CDKL5*-related early epileptic encephalopathy can present in the first year of life with an unusual electroclinical pattern of prolonged generalized tonic–clonic seizures (27). Patients harbouring deletions of chromosome 7q11.23 including the *MAGI2* gene, involved in regulation of trafficking, distribution, or function of the glutamate receptors, have infantile spasms (28). Mutations in *STXBP1* gene associated with Ohtahara syndrome can also cause infantile spasms (29).

A possibly recessive syndrome of early onset IS, often preceded and followed by other types of seizures, associated with hypsarrhythmia, facial dysmorphisms, optic atrophy, and peripheral oedema, has been reported from Finland as PEHO syndrome (progressive encephalopathy with oedema, hypsarrhythmia, and optic atrophy) (30). Cases exist outside Finland. Other genetic disorders are more rare and may be of recessive (31, 32) or of undetermined nature (33). IS and West syndrome have also been associated with various mitochondrial disorders, inherited disorders of metabolism, chromosomal abnormalities, and copy number variations (Table 15.1).

Prognosis of infantile spasms and West syndrome depends more on aetiology than on treatment. Unfavourable prognostic factors include symptomaticity, early onset (before 3 months), and pre-existing seizures other than spasms, an asymmetric EEG, and relapse after initial response to treatment (10). Adequate resolution requires the cessation of clinical spasms and normalization of EEG (34). Good prognostic indicators include no obvious aetiology, normal brain magnetic resonance imaging (MRI) (35) typical hypsarrhythmia, rapid response to treatment, and no regression after onset of spasms or its short duration (36). Overall, about 80% of patients have residual cognitive or behavioural impairment, but only one-third of cryptogenic cases do (36). About 50% of children will subsequently exhibit other epilepsy types.

Infantile spasms must be differentiated from rarer, earlier-onset conditions with ominous prognosis, such as the early infantile epileptic encephalopathy and the early myoclonic encephalopathy.

Vigabatrin (GVG) and adrenocorticotropic hormone (ACTH) have proven effective in a few controlled trials, but uncertainties remain regarding the best treatment. In three comparative studies, GVG was slightly less effective than, or as effective as ACTH (37–39), but possibly better tolerated (37). Two randomized trials reported a 78% responder rate (40), and a higher effectiveness of high doses (100–148 mg/kg per day) (41). Particular efficacy has been shown in children with tuberous sclerosis (42). Response to 100 mg/kg per day occurs within a few days. Some clinician considers GVG the first-line drug, despite the risk of visual field constriction (43). This side effect appears in 30–50% of patients having received a substantial drug load, but is not ascertainable in small children. According to the Vigabatrin Pediatric Advisory Group (2000) responders should receive GVG for no more than 6 months and non-responders should be switched to ACTH within 3 weeks. Transient MRI hyperintensities of globus pallidi, thalami, dentate nuclei, and cerebral peduncles have been described in infants treated with GVG for infantile spasms (44, 45). The meaning of these findings and how their report would affect treatment choices is still unclear. The United Kingdom IS Study (UKISS) comparing hormonal treatment against GVG showed that tetracosactide (synthetic ACTH) or prednisolone controlled spasms better than did vigabatrin initially, but not at 12–14 months of age (46). On 24-month follow-up cognitive outcome was better for the hormonal group. It is used in daily doses from 20 to 40 IU. An individualized regimen permits to keep dose-related side effects such as hypertension, brain shrinking, adrenal hypo-responsiveness, and cardiac hypertrophy to a minimum (47). Infections are an ominous complication of ACTH treatment and are responsible for most deaths (48). A 4–6-week duration of ACTH course is advisable. Spasms may respond within days but behavioural improvement needs several weeks. Relapse rate is 30%. A second cycle of ACTH is recommended in cases of relapse after an initial good response. High-dose oral prednisolone has been suggested as an alternative to ACTH, providing an equivalent efficacy, with reduced side effects and considerably lower cost (49). In a recent review of

Table 15.1 West syndrome and Lennox–Gastaut syndromes: aetiologies

Type of aetiology	Specific aetiology	Syndrome
Malformations of cortical development	◆ Focal cortical dysplasia	WS
	◆ Tuberous sclerosis *TSC1, TSC2* genes	WS-LGS
	◆ Lissencephaly *LIS1, DCX, ARX, TUBA1A*	WS-LGS
	◆ Subcortical band heterotopia *DCX, LIS1*	WS-LGS
	◆ Bilateral perisylvian polymicrogyria	WS
	◆ Bilateral frontoparietal polymicrogyria	WS
	GPR56	WS-LGS
	◆ Diffuse polymicrogyria *TUBB2B*	WS
	◆ Hemimegalencephaly	WS
	◆ Neurocutaneous disorders	IS
	◆ Aicardi syndrome	IS
	◆ Schizencephaly	IS
	◆ Periventricular heterotopia/ microcephaly *ARFGEF2*	WS
	◆ Holoprosencephaly *SIX3, SHH, TGIF, ZIC2, PTCH1, GLI2*	WS
Pre-, peri-, or postnatal damage	◆ Hypoxic ischaemic sequelae	WS
	◆ Haemorrhagic	WS
	◆ Fetal infections	WS-LGS
	◆ Postnatal infection (encephalitis and meningitis)	WS-LGS
	◆ Trauma	WS
	◆ Cardiac surgery with hypothermia	WS
Chromosomal abnormalities and copy number variations	◆ 15q11.2–q13.1 duplication	LGS
	◆ 4p- (Wolf–Hirshhorn syndrome)	LGS
	◆ invdup15	LGS
	◆ Angelman syndrome	WS
	◆ Down syndrome	WS-LGS
	◆ Miller–Dieker syndrome	WS-LGS
	◆ del1p36	WS
	◆ del 7q11.23–q21.1 (*MAGI2)*	WS
	◆ Pallister–Killian syndrome: mosaic 12p(i[12p])	IS
Inborn errors of metabolism	◆ Menkes disease	WS
	◆ Phenylketonuria	WS
	◆ Mitochondrial disease (NARP)	WS
	◆ Complex 1 deficiency	IS
	◆ Hypoglycaemia	WS
	◆ PEHO syndrome	WS
	◆ Non-ketotic hyperglycaemia	WS
	◆ Other organic acid disorders	WS
	◆ Pyridoxine dependency	IS
	◆ Biotinidase dependency	WS
	◆ Congenital disorders of glycosylation	WS
Vascular malformations	Sturge–Weber syndrome	WS-LGS
Brain tumours	All brain tumours	WS
Monogenic: non-malformative—non-metabolic	◆ ARX ◆ CDKL5 ◆ *STPBX1*	WS
No identifiable causes	About 40% positive family history of epilepsy	WS-LGS

Aetiologies are cumulatively intended for West syndrome, the infantile spasms an epileptic spasms and Lennox–Gastaut syndrome. The column legend indicates the prominent syndrome presentation. For example, girls with Aicardi syndrome exhibit infantile spasms, rather than West syndrome. However this distinction may not always be feasible.
IS, infantile spasms; LGS, Lennox–Gastaut syndrome; WS, West syndrome.

the literature the US Consensus report has suggested that a short course of high-dose ACTH (150 units/m^2/day in two divided doses for 2 weeks followed by a 2-week taper) and VGB 100 -150 mg/kg/ day demonstrated the best evidence for efficacy and a safe adverse event profile (50). Pyridoxine is a preferred agent in Japan but its use is not supported by controlled studies (51). Video-EEG monitoring is often necessary to show that the spasms have truly disappeared (50, 52).

Surgical treatment should be considered early when drug resistance is faced and focal epileptogenesis is shown. About 60% of operated children become seizure free; the best results are obtained when operating on small lesions (53). However, most children have large multilobar cortical dysplasia needing extensive resections, with limited cognitive improvement (8).

There is some evidence for use of the ketogenic diet in resistant spasms (49, 54).

Lennox–Gastaut syndrome

Lennox–Gastaut syndrome is characterized by intractable brief tonic and atonic seizures, atypical absences, and a generalized interictal EEG pattern of spike and slow wave discharges. It accounts for 2.9% of all childhood epilepsy (55). Incidence peaks between 3–5 years of age. Cognitive and psychiatric impairment is frequent. About 30% of cases occur *de novo* in previously healthy children. However, multiple aetiologies are observed in the remaining cases with neuronal migration disorders and hypoxic brain damage being the most frequent causes. About 40% of children have previous IS (10). Persistence of seizures in adulthood is frequent.

The term Lennox–Gastaut syndrome, which was adopted by the International League Against Epilepsy in 1989 (56), is still used loosely to designate children with multiple types of intractable seizures, which include drop attacks.

Cognitive impairment is often present before seizure onset but the proportion of mentally retarded patients increases, reaching up to 75–95% at 5 years from onset (57). Cognitive slowing is a constant element of the syndrome even in *de novo* cases.

About 80% of patients continue to have seizures later in life, with symptomatic origin and early onset having the poorest outcome (10). The core seizure types of the syndrome, including tonic, atonic seizures, atypical absences, and non-convulsive status are not always present at onset nor are interictal slow spike and wave discharges. Some authors consider fast (10 Hz) rhythms associated with tonic seizures or with minimal manifestations (such as a brief apnoea or upward eye deviation), especially during non-REM sleep, an essential diagnostic criterion (58).

Tonic seizures, with a 'sustained increase in muscle contraction lasting a few seconds to minutes' are the most characteristic type (59). Tonic seizures may be manifested as sudden drop attacks. During sleep, tonic seizures are usually manifested as full-blown stiffening of the whole body with abduction and elevation of the limbs. Atypical absences are difficult to identify due to their gradual onset and termination. Myoclonic seizures occur in a minority of patients. Between 50–75% of patients exhibit non-convulsive status, manifested as subcontinuous atypical absences with fluctuating responsiveness that may sometimes be interspersed with recurring brief tonic seizures (57). Non-convulsive status has been associated with worse cognitive outcome (60). Generalized tonic–clonic seizures or focal seizures may be present in a minority of patients.

The classic EEG feature of Lennox–Gastaut syndrome is the slow spike and wave pattern, often repeated in bilaterally synchronous complexes at 1–2 Hz. Generalized bursts of 'polyspikes' or fast rhythms (>10 Hz), also called generalized paroxysmal fast activity, are recorded during slow sleep. They occur as an interictal manifestation or are accompanied by a grading range of clinical manifestations. Sleep EEG recordings may be necessary to elicit their presence.

Drop-attacks are also observed in other epilepsy syndromes typical of childhood. In particular, children with myoclonic-astatic epilepsy, making differential diagnosis difficult (61). Difficult problems of differential diagnosis are sometimes posed by epilepsy with continuous spike and waves during sleep (62) and the atypical benign rolandic epilepsy (63). Children with this syndrome spectrum present with atypical and atonic absences that may cause repeated falls.

Lennox–Gastaut syndrome can appear in the absence of any obvious or suspected aetiology (cryptogenic), in otherwise healthy children or be symptomatic. Aetiology of Lennox–Gastaut syndrome is extremely heterogeneous (Table 15.1). Familial cases of Lennox–Gastaut syndrome have been associated with familial bilateral frontoparietal polymicrogyria due to *GPR56* gene mutations (64) and with familial pachygyria associated with *DCX* gene mutations (65). In many cases, brain imaging is normal and no aetiology is found. The multiple causes that can be related to the syndrome can influence prognosis or, sometimes, therapeutic strategies.

The optimum treatment for Lennox–Gastaut syndrome remains uncertain. Broad-spectrum drugs should be preferred (66). Only a few controlled studies are available, usually designed to evaluate efficacy of one drug on one or two types of seizures and no study is available investigating early overall effect of a given drug on the syndrome evolution. Randomized clinical trials in Lennox–Gastaut syndrome have been performed for lamotrigine (LTG), topiramate (TPM), felbamate, rufinamide, thyrotropin-releasing hormone (TRH) analogue, and cinromide (57). A Cochrane review (67) suggested that although no study to date has shown any one drug to be highly efficacious, rufinamide, LTG, TPM and felbamate might be helpful as add-on therapy. However, there is no guidance on how to combine these drugs and many researchers combine them with valproate (VPA), ethosuximide (ESM), or benzodiazepines, especially clobazam where available. However, treatment approaches are complicated by the potential of polytherapies for adverse events and seizure aggravation (10). It has been suggested that vagus nerve stimulation and the ketogenic diet can be useful in some cases (68). Corpus callosotomy might reduce seizures with drop attacks, with better results when performed at a younger age (69).

Landau–Kleffner syndrome and epilepsy with continuous spike and waves during slow wave sleep

In Landau–Kleffner and continuous spike and waves during slow wave sleep syndromes, frequent or persistent discharges, with or without accompanying seizures, cause impairment of cortical functions. These two syndromes, which may on occasion partially overlap, are non-convulsive age- related epileptic encephalopathies.

Landau–Kleffner syndrome is a rare, severely disabling disorder, with an insidious, or sudden, loss of language understanding (auditory agnosia), followed by progressive loss of verbal expression (70). Age at onset is between 3–7 years. Focal seizures represent the initial symptom in 60% of children, but are absent altogether in 25%. They have variable severity but remit before adulthood. EEG abnormalities predominate in the temporoparietal regions, bilaterally, or on either side (70). EEG discharges interfere with auditory-evoked responses (71), suggesting epilepsy-related dysfunction of auditory processing. Onset before age 5 years and persistent EEG anomalies over the language areas forecast a severe evolution. Although prognosis of aphasia is overall unpredictable, recovery without consequences is exceptional (72). No aetiology has been identified, although rare lesional cases have been reported.

Treatment efficacy has been empirically investigated. Large doses of ACTH or steroids for prolonged periods (>3 months) have a definite effect on EEG and language (73). Scattered reports indicate that benzodiazepines, VPA, ESM, and immunoglobulins may be useful. It has been suggested that surgical treatment with multiple subpial transections is followed by longlasting improvement in selected cases (74). However, the merit of this approach remains highly uncertain. Language therapy is indicated and alternatives to oral language should be offered to the most severely impaired children.

In epilepsy with continuous spike and wave discharges during slow sleep (or electrical status epilepticus during slow sleep), cognitive decline is associated with continuous sleep-related EEG discharges, persisting for months to years. The syndrome appears in previously healthy or in delayed children. Brain lesions, especially polymicrogyria (62) and porencephaly (75) are found in 30–50% of patients. Onset is insidious. Seizures start at 3–5 years as nocturnal and focal attacks and share similarities to those observed in rolandic epilepsy. After a few months, continuous spike and waves during slow sleep and atypical or atonic absences appear. There is marked decrease in intelligence quotient scores with attention deficit and hyperactivity, sometimes with language disturbances and autistic features. Long-term course of epilepsy is favourable, but cognitive impairment persists in most children. Earlier onset and long duration of typical sleep-related EEG abnormalities are major risk factors for a poor prognosis (76). The benign atypical partial epilepsy syndrome (63) bears a close relation to continuous spike and waves during slow wave sleep. Drug treatment is the same as in Landau–Kleffner syndrome as many aspects of these syndromes truly overlap (77).

Dravet syndrome (severe myoclonic epilepsy in infancy)

Dravet syndrome (DS), otherwise known as severe myoclonic epilepsy of infancy (SMEI) is an increasingly recognized epileptic encephalopathy where the clinical diagnosis can be genetically confirmed in around 80% of patients. The syndrome spectrum includes conditions with variable severity, all appearing in otherwise normal infants (81), spanning from the classical phenotype to 'borderline SMEI' (SMEB) in which patients share most but not all the characteristic clinical features (78).

Since its first descriptions DS has been increasingly recognized worldwide; yet it remains a rare disorder with an incidence probably less than 1 per 40,000 (79). The prevalence of Dravet syndrome in children with seizure onset in the first year of life varies between 3–8% (80, 81). The initial manifestations are generalized or unilateral clonic (hemiclonic with alternating side) seizures, typically triggered by fever. These seizures are often prolonged, tend to recur in clusters, and may evolve into status epilepticus. Vaccinations or hot water immersion can precipitate seizures through increase in body temperature.

Between ages 1–4 years other seizure types appear, including myoclonic, atypical absences, focal, and, exceptionally, tonic seizures. Myoclonic jerks can be massive and involve the whole body leading to falling or be barely visible, exhibiting a multifocal distribution. They are often precipitated by photic stimulation. Myoclonic jerks are inconstantly accompanied by time-locked paroxysmal EEG activity. Atypical absence seizures are present in 40–90% of patients (81) and can be associated with a prominent myoclonic component. Ictal EEG shows 2.5–3 Hz generalized spike and wave discharges. About 40% of patients experience non-convulsive status epilepticus or 'obtundation status' characterized by fluctuating unresponsiveness, with erratic myoclonic jerks. These episodes may last days and be particularly insidious. Ictal EEG shows diffuse slow waves intermingled with focal of diffuse spikes. More than 50% of patients have focal seizures. Convulsive seizures tend to be present throughout as generalized clonic or tonic clonic seizures, unilateral seizures with alternating side (81). Interictal EEG, normal at onset, subsequently shows generalized or multifocal paroxysmal activity. About 25% of children are photosensitive and may indulge in self-stimulation.

Early developmental skills and behaviour are usually normal. Around the second year of life, developmental slowing or stagnation becomes obvious in most patients (82, 83). Behavioural disturbances with hyperactivity and autistic traits are frequently reported. The frequency of convulsive seizures seems to correlate with the severity of developmental delay (82). An earlier onset of absence and myoclonic seizures carries a higher risk of severe cognitive impairment (83).

A family history of epilepsy is often found. Affected relatives most often exhibit epilepsy phenotypes consistent with the generalized epilepsy with febrile seizure plus (GEFS+) spectrum (84). Dravet syndrome has been associated with an overwhelmingly high number of *SCN1A* mutations (85, 86) (see Chapter 2). The frequency of detectable mutations is around 70–80% (87). Duplications and amplifications involving *SCN1A* are additional, rare, molecular mechanisms (88). Most mutations are *de novo*, but familial *SCN1A* mutations also occur (85, 89-91). Somatic mosaic mutations have been reported in some patients and should be considered when estimating the recurrence (92, 93).

Some general genotype–phenotype correlations have been suggested: truncating, nonsense, frame shift mutations, and partial or whole gene deletions are correlated with a classical Dravet syndrome phenotype and appear to have a significant correlation with an earlier age of seizures onset (94). The severity of the phenotypes is also correlated with *SCN1A* missense mutations falling into the pore forming region of the sodium channel while missense changes associated to the GEFS+ spectrum are nearly always localized outside the pore forming region (95).

Mutations of the *PCDH19* gene have been described in girls with early onset epileptic encephalopathy mimicking Dravet syndrome (96, 97). *PCDH19* encodes a protocadherin 19, a transmembrane protein of the cadherin family of calcium-dependent cell-cell adhesion molecules, which is strongly expressed in the central nervous system. *PCDH19* should be tested in patients with Dravet syndrome in whom no *SCN1A* abnormalities can be found. Despite intensive investigation, the aetiology of about 15% of patients sharing features with Dravet syndrome remains unknown.

Neuroradiological studies are unrevealing in most patients (98). In an extensive postmortem neuropathological study of three adult cases, no histological signature of the condition was identified (99).

At onset children are often regarded as having febrile seizures, only their frequent repetition, often with unilateral features, makes one suspect Dravet syndrome or GEFS+.

Seizures persist into adulthood but are less frequent, rarely prolonged and are usually confined to sleep (99, 100). Mortality rates are at around 16% (101), mainly as a result of sudden death or seizure-related accidents.

VPA, benzodiazepines, TPM, and levetiracetam have demonstrated some efficacy. Stiripentol, an inhibitor of the P450 cytochrome, was effective in combination with clobazam in two class I trials (102, 103). Stiripentol acts by increasing the concentration of norclobazam, an active metabolite of clobazam. Phenytoin (PHT), carbamazepine (CBZ), and LTG can worsen seizures and must be avoided (81, 104).

Myoclonic-astatic (or myoclonic-atonic) epilepsy

Myoclonic-astatic epilepsy is a generalized epilepsy syndrome with multiple seizure types, including myoclonic-astatic, absences, and tonic-clonic and eventually tonic seizures. Seizure onset is between 18–60 months and most children have normal developmental skills until then (7). The nosological limits of the disorders are difficult to determine and its course has variable severity, manifesting as an epileptic encephalopathy only in some cases. In a hospital population of children presenting their first seizure between age 1 and 10 years it was estimated that myoclonic-astatic epilepsy represented 2.2% (61). Sex ratio has been defined as 2.7–3:1 in favour of males (61, 105).

Genetic factors seem to play a major role. A family history of epilepsy was present in 32% of children described by Doose (1992) (105) and in 15% in the series from Kaminska et al. (1999) (61). Ten patients out of 88 belonging to families with the GEFS+ complex had myoclonic-astatic epilepsy (106-108). In two large series, 5% of children with myoclonic-astatic epilepsy had mutations of the *SLC2A1* gene (109), causing glucose transporter-1 (GLUT-1) deficiency. Diagnosing GLUT-1 deficiency, with chronic hypoglycorrhachia, has important therapeutic implications as this condition can be successfully treated with the ketogenic diet.

Myoclonic and myoclonic-astatic seizures are present in all children and are prominent in most. Clinically, myoclonic seizures are brief, generalized jerks, isolated or repeated in short series. A wide range of severity is observed, ranging from head nodding to falls with injury. The duration of these episodes is brief (0.3–1 seconds according to video-EEG analysis) (110). Falls can either be caused by massive myoclonic jerks or by from a post-myoclonic atonic component, or both. In some children, myoclonic seizures are also triggered by photic stimulation. Tonic–clonic seizures are the second most frequent seizure type, present in 75–95% of children (61, 105) and are usually the first manifestation to appear. Absence seizures are present in 62–89% of patients (61, 105). Most often, they present as atypical absences (105). Episodes of non-convulsive status, presenting as stupor and apathy, associated to multifocal, arrhythmic twitching might be present. CBZ and GVG treatment has been reported to precipitate non-convulsive status (111, 112). Tonic seizures have been described in 30–95% of patients (61, 105).

They can manifest as typical axial, tonic attacks during sleep or as tonic-vibratory seizures, especially at the end of night time sleep. Only about one-third of children with favourable course have tonic seizures (61). Febrile seizures, usually simple in type, are reported to precede non-febrile seizures in 11–28% of children (61, 105).

Background EEG activity is normal at seizure onset, although a characteristic 4–7 Hz, monomorphic theta activity with diffuse distribution, but prominent on centro-parietal areas, is often observed. Interictal abnormalities consist of bursts of 2–3 Hz generalized (poly) spike-and-wave discharges that increase during sleep (105). Myoclonic seizures are electrographically characterized by a generalized (poly) spike-and-wave complexes (110). A series of 2–3 jerks is most commonly observed. The atonic component of myoclonic-atonic seizures is accompanied by EMG inhibition, lasting 60–400 msec, time-locked to the onset of the slow wave (110, 113). Tonic seizures are accompanied by 10–15 Hz polyspike discharges lasting as long as the tonic contraction on EMG. Myoclonic status is associated to a chaotic EEG with independent spike-and-wave discharges, sometimes resembling hypsarrhythmia (105).

Evolution of myoclonic-astatic epilepsy can be either favourable with seizure remission within 3 years from onset and normal cognitive development or unfavourable with multiple drug-resistant seizure types and cognitive impairment (7, 61). There are no distinguishable cluster of clinical or EEG characteristics at epilepsy onset that can help predicting the outcome (61).

Myoclonic-astatic epilepsy must be differentiated from cryptogenic Lennox–Gastaut syndrome, and atypical benign rolandic epilepsy (63), and from epilepsy with continuous spike wave activity during slow sleep (114). Differential diagnosis is sometimes necessary with late infantile ceroid-lipofuscinosis at its clinical onset.

VPA is the first choice drug, because of its wide spectrum of action. No controlled trials are available, however. If VPA fails, a combination of VPA with LTG should be the next step. ESM can be effective, in particular when myoclonus and absence seizures are prominent in the clinical picture. Alternatively small doses of benzodiazepine associated to VPA can sometimes prove effective. LTG, which can aggravate some epilepsies with myoclonic seizures, such as Dravet syndrome and juvenile myoclonic epilepsy (104, 115) has however proven useful in myoclonic-astatic epilepsy (116). CBZ and GVG should be avoided due to their potential to precipitate non-convulsive status (61, 112, 117).

Encephalopathic childhood epilepsies associated with inherited metabolic disorders

Over 50 genetically determined metabolic diseases have been associated with seizures. Most present in infancy or childhood as intractable epilepsies and are, at their onset, difficult to distinguish from epileptic encephalopathies due to a non-progressive disorder, as those forms discussed earlier. However, they often present early in life with multiple seizure types and a few, if any, specific findings (118, 119). The degree of encephalopathy depends upon the severity of the metabolic defect. A metabolic disorder should be suspected when a specific aetiology or a well-recognized syndrome is not established or clinical worsening cannot be simply explained by the presence of severe epilepsy. Likewise, children having relatively few seizures who experience worsening of seizure and motor or cognitive impairment should be re-evaluated for possible metabolic defects.

Examples of metabolic disorders with specific treatments include pyridoxine-responsive epilepsies, central creatinine deficiency, phenylketonuria; glucose transporter deficiency syndrome (GLUT-1 DS), pyruvate dehydrogenase deficiency, disorders of lactic acidosis, biotinadase deficiency, Menkes disease.

Some peculiar EEG abnormalities may be helpful. A suppression burst pattern is noted in non-ketotic hyperglycinaemia, phenylketonuria, maple syrup urine disease, molybdenum cofactor deficiency, and disorders of biotin metabolism (120). A comb-like rhythm with 7–9 Hz central activity may be demonstrated in children with maple syrup urine disease, vertex positive spikes in sialidosis type 1, bi-occipital polymorphic delta activity in X-linked adrenal leucodystrophia, and 14–22 Hz persistent rhythm is frequently noted with infantile neuroaxonal dystrophy.

Numerous mitochondrial disorders are accompanied by encephalopathy and seizures. The best-known mitochondrial disorders transmitted with maternal inheritance are myoclonus epilepsy with ragged red fibres (MERRF) and mitochondrial encephalopathy, lactic acidosis and stroke-like episodes (MELAS). Other mitochondrial encephalopathies are associated with nuclear mutations rather than mitochondrial DNA mutation; they include Leigh syndrome, Alpers syndrome, and co-enzyme Q10 deficiency. These encephalopathic diseases have variable presentation with multisystemic involvement and epilepsy. Mitochondrial disorders are treated through metabolic therapy typically made up of cocktails containing co-enzyme Q10, L-carnitine, dichloroacetate, and multivitamins but the effects of such treatment approach to seizure severity has not been assessed (120).

Epileptic encephalopathies and multilobar brain malformations

A particular subgroup of epileptic encephalopathies are those that originate from the spreading to the whole brain of severe epileptic activity that originates from a large dysplastic cortical area. This is also the case of West syndrome in association with focal cortical dysplasia (FCD). However, there may be other forms of epileptic encephalopathies that are manifested with electroclinical characteristics which are more in relation to the specific aetiology than with a given epilepsy syndrome. The prototype of these conditions is hemimegalencephaly, a nosologically heterogeneous condition in which one cerebral hemisphere is enlarged and structurally abnormal. The abnormality is unilateral based on gross structure. The histopathological characteristics of hemimegalencephaly are similar to those of FCD, with which differences are more quantitative than qualitative. In the most severe cases one entire hemisphere is involved.

The clinical appearance of hemimegalencephaly ranges from cases with severe epileptic encephalopathy beginning in the neonatal period, to rare patients who may have normal cognitive level, with or without epilepsy. However, the most typical presentation is with hemiparesis and hemianopia, cognitive impairment, and early-onset seizures. The most severely affected children have almost continuous focal seizures, accompanied by infantile spasms

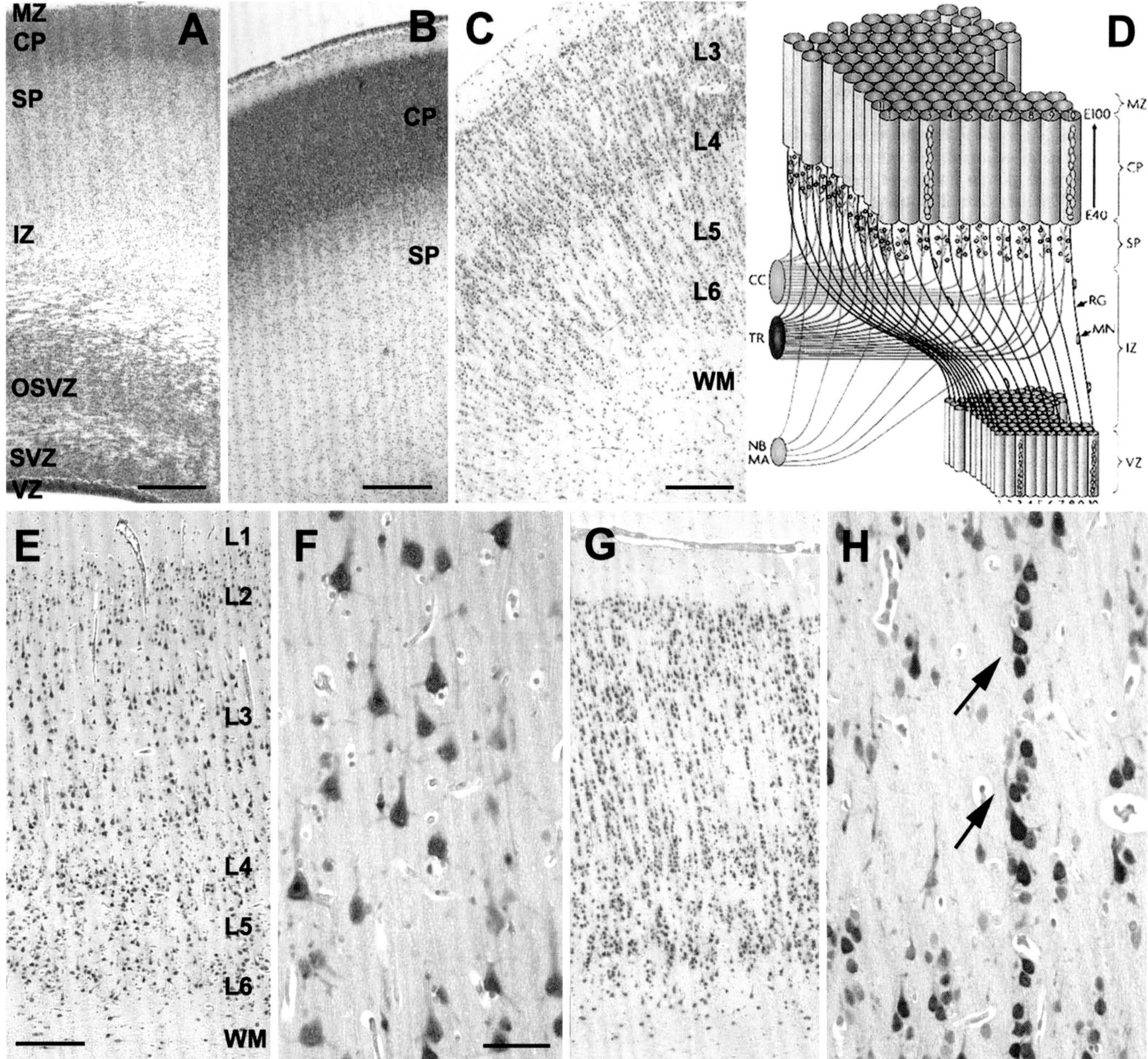

Colour plate 1 (See also Fig. 4.1.) FCD Type Ia compared to normal development and anatomy of the human neocortex. A) The developing human neocortex reviewed at 17th week of gestation (WoG). Cortical neurons (stained purple by thionine) arise from radial glial cells, the epithelial stem cells that line the ventricle. Radial glial cells in the ventricular zone (VZ) generate intermediate progenitor cells that migrate into the subventricular zone (SVZ). The outer subventricular zone (OSVZ) is massively expanding at this time period and most likely contribute to the evolutionary advance underlying cortical size and complexity in human brain (21). CP, cortical plate; IZ, intermediate zone; MZ, marginal zone; SP, subcortical plate (also see (D)). B) Expansion of the cortical plate at 19th WoG. Migrating neurons follow an inside-out pattern forming different pyramidal cell layers. C) The hexalaminar cortical architecture is fully developed in the premature brain (35th WoG), with prominent radial (vertical) columnar arrangements still being visible (4 μm thin paraffin sections were used for all preparations shown here). Note the similarity with a surgical specimens obtained from a 15-year-old child with epilepsy and FCD Type Ia (G–H). D) This well-recognized model of radial neuronal migration that underlies cortical organization is based on (20). The cohorts of neurons generated in the VZ traverse IZ and SP, containing 'waiting' afferents from several sources (cortico-cortical connections (CC), thalamic radiation (TR), nucleus basalis (NB), monoamine subcortical centers (MA)), and finally pass through the earlier generated deep layers before setting in at the interface between the cortical plate (CP) and marginal zone (MZ). MN, migrating neurons; RG, radial glial cell. E–F) Adult human temporal neocortex (NeuN immunohistochemistry). Scale bar in E = 200 μm (applies also to G); in F = 50 μm (applies also to (H)). G–H) Fifteen-year-old child with drug-resistant epilepsy and severe psycho-motor retardation. Seizure onset was recorded from only one hemisphere and histopathological analysis revealed persistent vertical microcolumns in the temporal and occipital lobe specimen. Note that neurons are also significantly smaller (arrow in (H)), compared to controls shown in (F). NeuN immunohistochemistry.

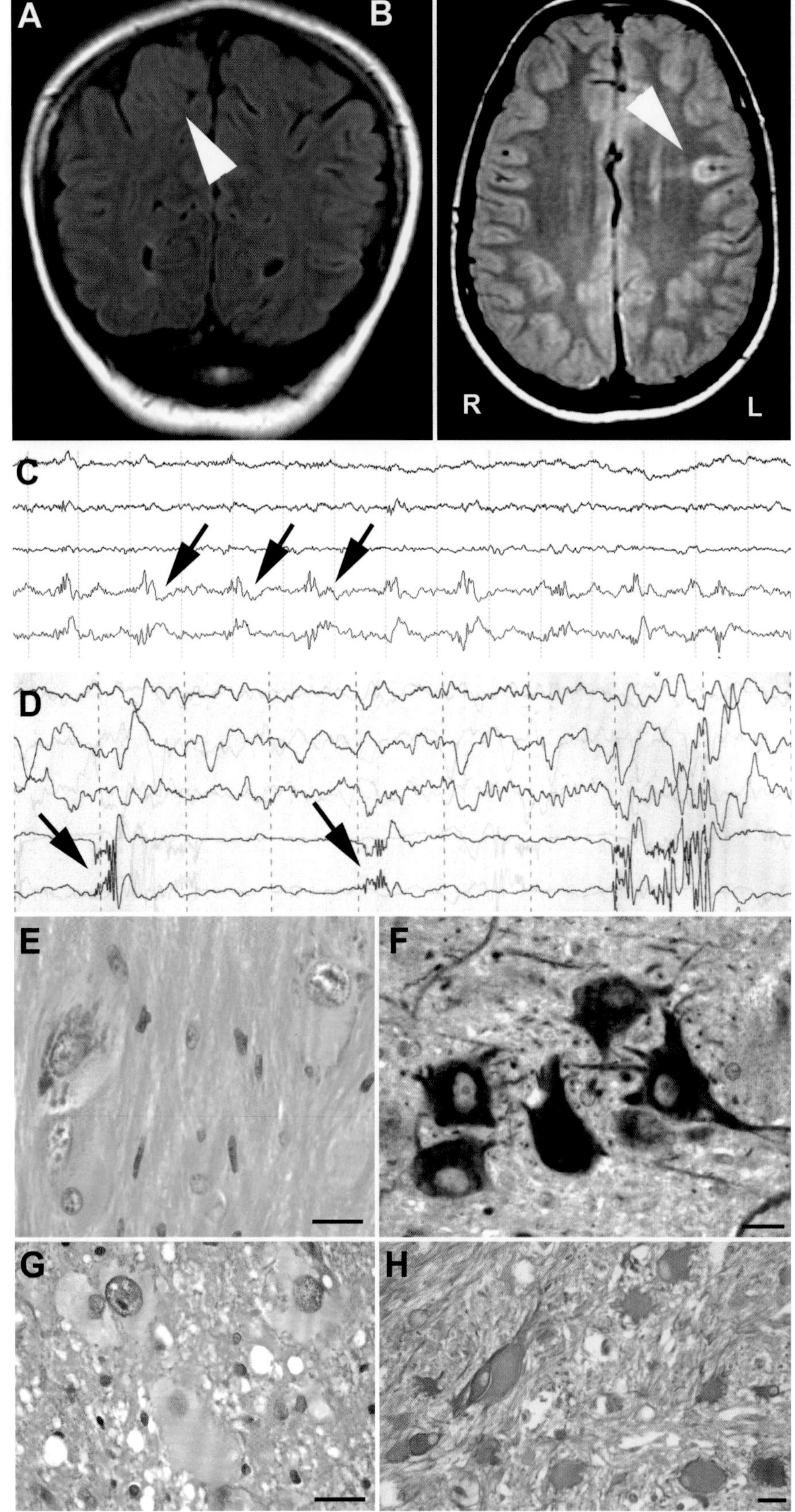

Colour plate 2 (See also Fig. 4.2.) Clinicopathological findings in FCD Type II. A) FCD Type IIa in an 18-year-old female patient with refractory seizures from age 5 years, that would start with sensory disturbance in the left foot. Coronal T2 FLAIR did not reveal definitely abnormal signal intensities, which is often reported for FCD Type IIa. Indeed, histopathological inspection showed characteristic hallmarks of FCD Type IIa (see (E) and (F)) in surgical specimen obtained from the indicated brain region (arrowhead). MRI figure kindly provided by Dr Duncan (London, UK). B) Proton density imaging reveals a hyperintense signal change in the left frontal lobe of the patient with drug-resistant seizures, tapering from the depth of the gyrus towards the ventricle ('transmantle sign', arrowhead). C) Interictal EEG recording from the scalp surface of the patient shown in (B). Arrows point to characteristic 'brushes', which can be often recognized in patients with FCD Type IIB. D) The peculiar electrographic pattern ('brushes') becomes more evident when recording is obtained from depth electrodes implanted into the lesion (patient with histopathologically confirmed FCD Type IIB). (C) and (D) were kindly provided by Dr Spreafico (Milan, Italy). E–F) Dysmorphic neurons revealed by HE (E), or neurofilament immunostaining (SMI311 (F)) are typical findings in FCD Type IIa and IIb. G–H) Balloon cells revealed by HE (H), or vimentin immunostaining (H) can be seen only in FCD Type IIb. Scale bars in (E)–(H) = 20 μm.

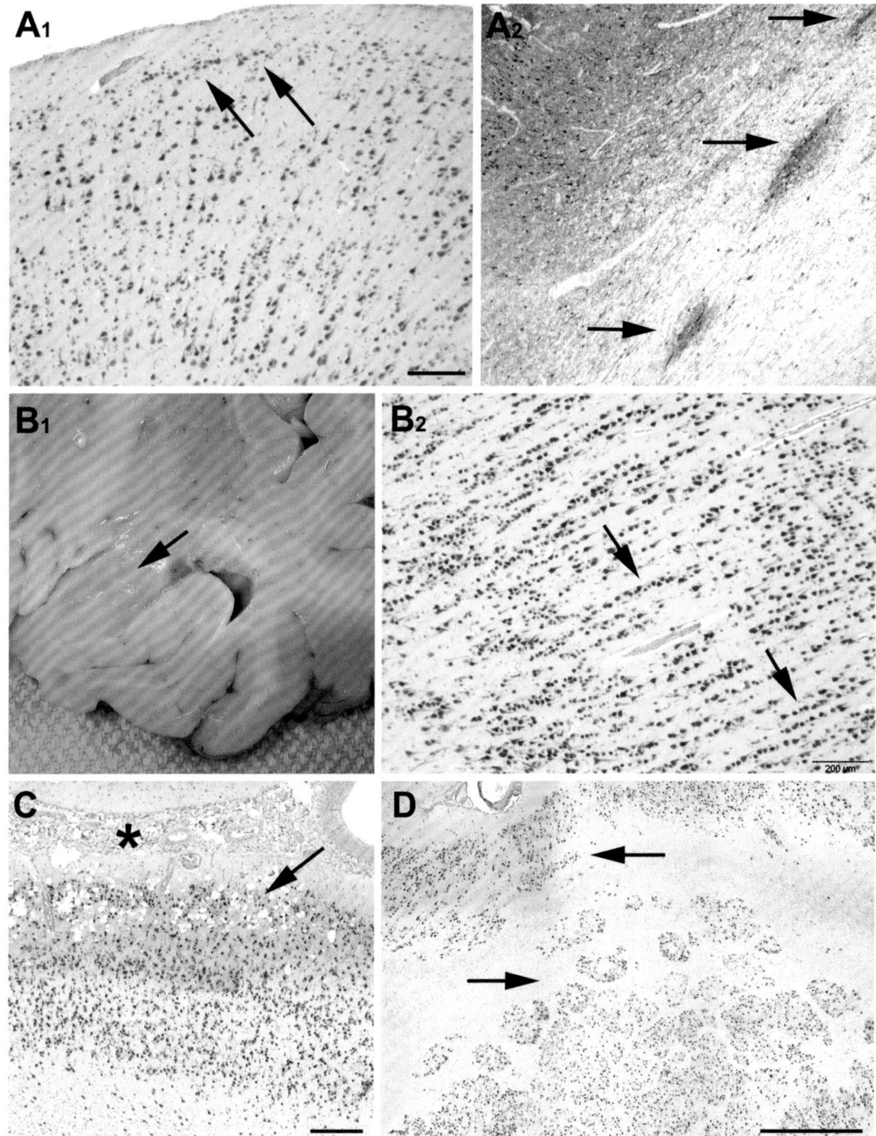

Colour plate 3 (See also Fig. 4.3.) Associated FCDs Type III. A1) This abnormal pattern of superficial cortical lamination (arrows) was associated with hippocampal sclerosis in an MTLE patient and should be diagnosed as FCD Type IIIa. It is similar to that described by Thom et al. as temporal lobe sclerosis (34). Scale bar = 200 µm (applies also to (A2) and (B2)). Another characteristic FCD Type IIIa pattern is that of heterotopic 'lentiform' neuronal islets in the white matter of the temporal lobe in MTLE-HS patients (A2). B1) Dysembryoplastic neuroepithelial tumour of the right mesial temporal lobe. Courtesy of Dr Macaulay (Halifax, Canada). B2) Persisting vertical microcolumns can be observed in the vicinity of long-term epilepsy associated tumours and should be diagnosed as FCD Type IIIb. C) Leptomeningeal vascular malformations (asterisk) usually associate with abnormal lamination in adjacent neocortex (FCD Type IIIc) marked by an arrow. D) These massive cortical lamination abnormalities were registered adjacent to a glial scar (acquired by perinatal head trauma) and classify as FCD Type IIId. Such lesions can be progressive in nature and were first described by Marin-Padilla et al. in 2002 (93).

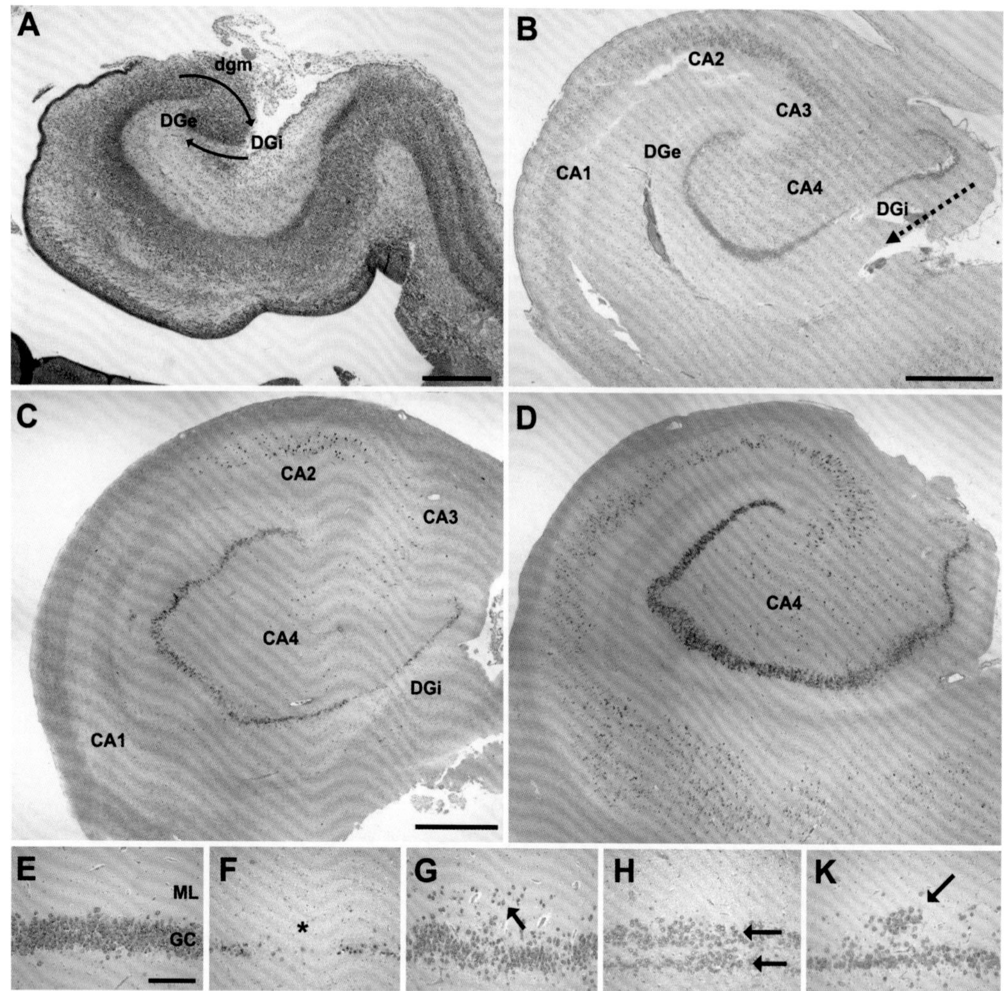

Colour plate 4 (See also Fig. 4.4.) Microscopic anatomy of the developing human hippocampus and in MTLE patients with hippocampal sclerosis. A) Human hippocampal development at 17th WoG. Scale bar = 500 µm. The figure should also illustrate the particular development of the dentate gyrus, which retains its neurogenic propensity throughout life. The dentate gyrus matrix is bending through the dentate notch and form the internal limb (DGi). From here, newly generated granule cells were continuously integrated and form the external limb (DGe) (64). B) Human hippocampus at birth (42nd WoG). Scale bar = 1 mm (applies also to (C) and (D)). All hippocampal sectors were clearly visible (CA1–4). The term 'hilus' should be restricted to the rodent hippocampus, and is not defined by Lorente de No (38). The same applies for the term 'endfolium', which is not a proper anatomical terminology for this region. The dashed line should indicate that the DGi is likely the portion of the DG maintaining its neurogenic capacity throughout life. C) Severe hippocampal sclerosis (HS Type 1b, Table 4.3) in an adult patient with febrile seizures at age 3 years and onset of spontaneous recurrent and drug-resistant seizures since his 14th year of life. NeuN immunohistochemistry with haematoxylin counterstaining (4 µm thin paraffin embedded section; applies to all images shown here). Note that restricted cell loss in DGi, compared to the mid portion or DG3 area. Experimental data has shown that this patterns correlates with the patient's ability to store and recall memory with this isolated hippocampus/hemisphere (Wada-testing; (58)). D) A patient with limbic encephalitis and late onset of her MTLE. The surgical specimen showed restricted cell loss within the CA4 region. This rare pattern is classified as atypical HS (Type 3, Table 4.3). E) Normal appearance of the human dentate gyrus with densely packed granule cells and sharp borders to subgranular and molecular layers (10× magnification, bar = 100µm, refers also to (F)–(K)). F) Granule cell pathology with significant granule cell loss indicated by thinning of dentate gyrus and cell free gaps (asterisk). G) Granule cell dispersion with spreading of granule cells into the molecular layer (arrow): H) Bilaminar architecture of the granule cell layer (arrows). K) granule cell dispersion with spreading of granule cell clusters into the molecular layer (arrow), as described by (62). GC, granule cell layer; ML, molecular layer.

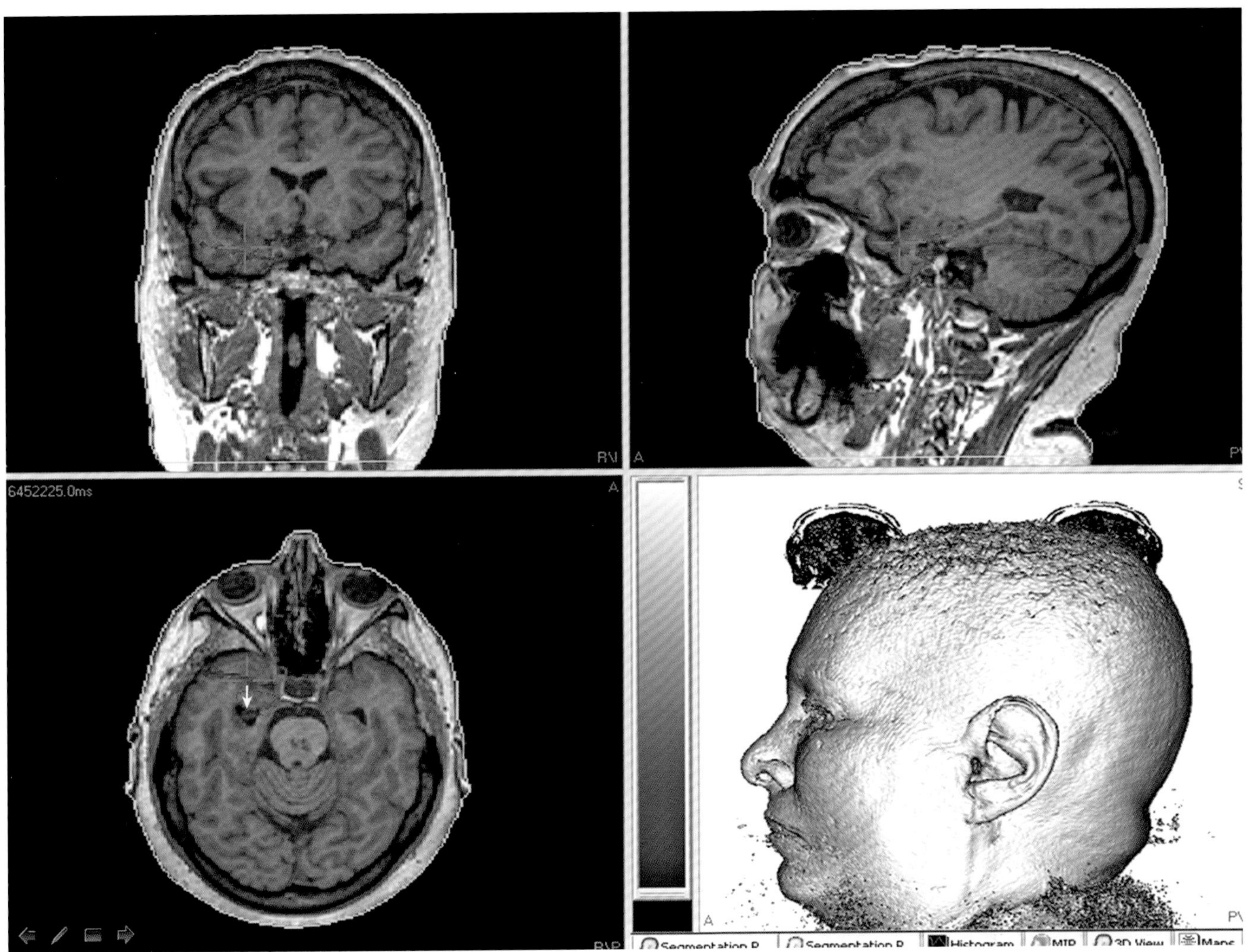

Colour plate 5 (See also Fig. 9.10.) EEG source localization in the same patient shows source localization of the spike to a dipole cluster (in red) in the close vicinity of the cavernoma (white arrow).

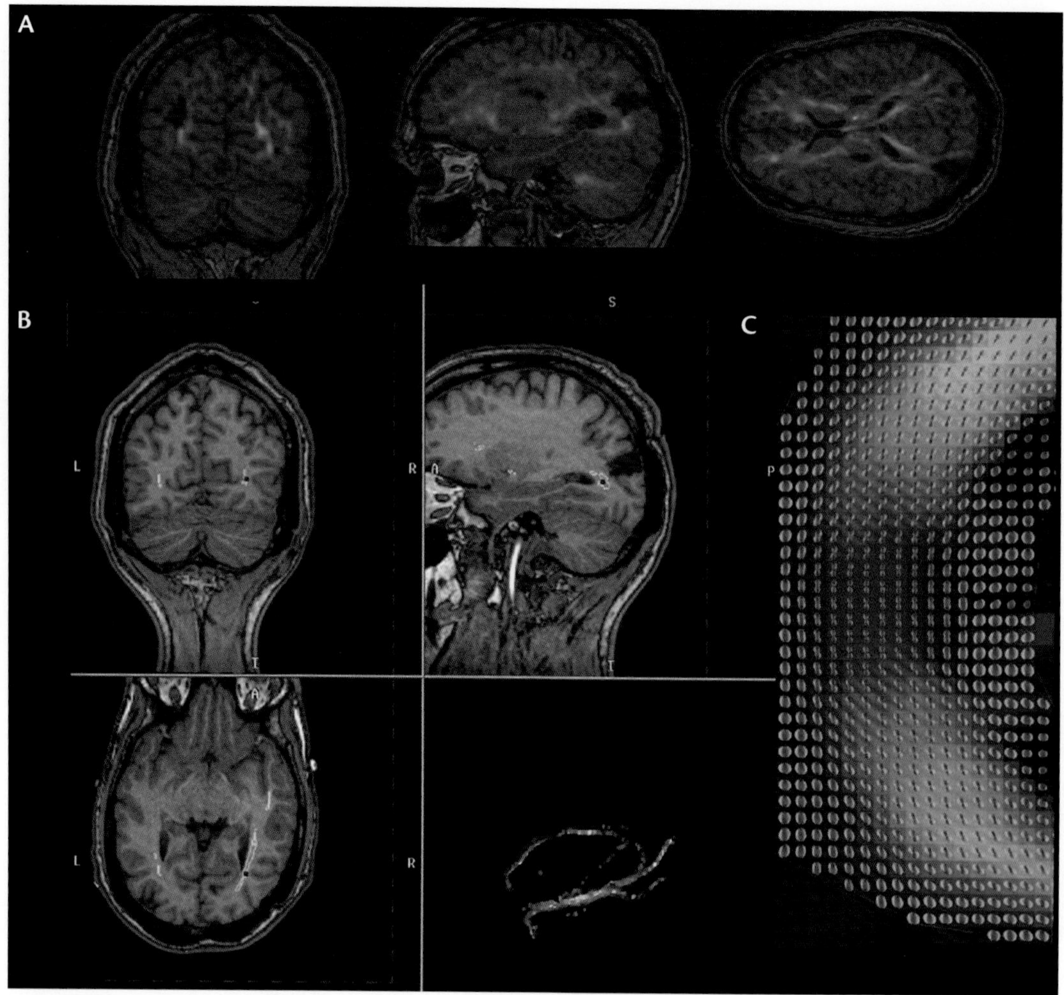

Colour plate 6 (Also see Fig. 10.3.) Tractography of the optic radiations in a patient who underwent resection of a cavernoma located in the right parieto-occipital cortex. A) Diffusion-weighted images with 30 directions were acquired and co-registered to the patient's MPRAGE, with colour fractional anisotropy (FA) corresponding to tensor orientations. B) Tractography was incorporated into a Stealth neuronavigation system for the operative procedure. The optic radiations are indicated in yellow. C) A zoomed region of interest from the splenium of the corpus callosum is displayed, with the individual superquadratic glyphs from each voxel indicating principal orientation. Each glyph incorporates directional information (blue = inferior/superior; green = anterior–posterior; red = left–right). These orientations are useful in reviewing the quality of tractography results. Reproduced with permission of Simon Vogrin.

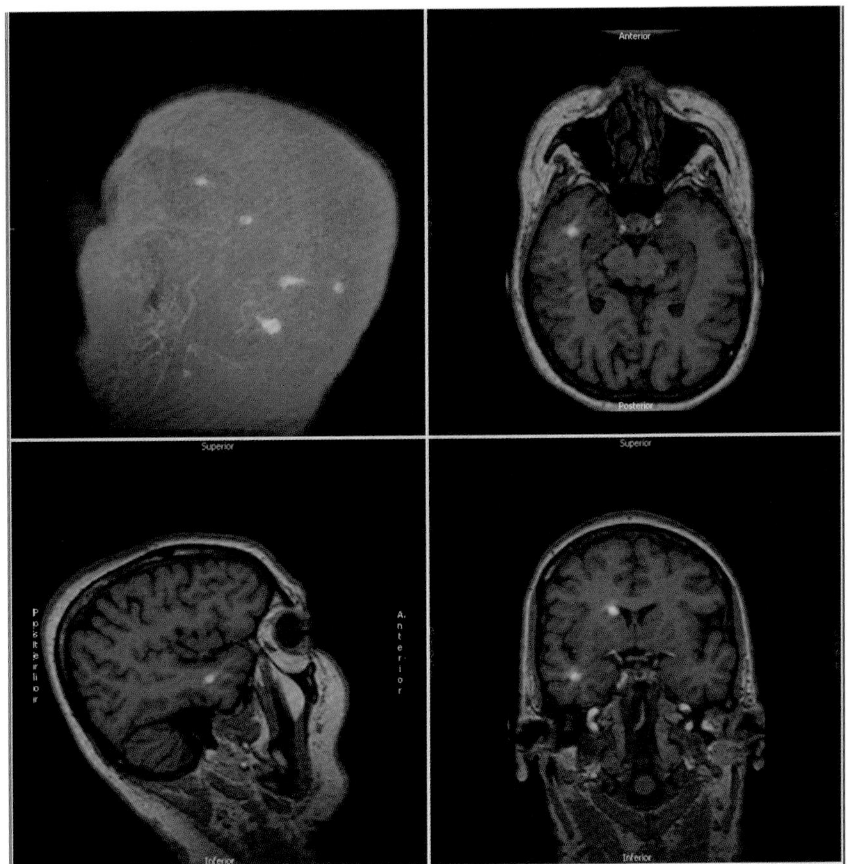

Colour plate 7 (Also see Fig. 10.4.) SISCOM data from a patient with focal epilepsy of the right temporal lobe. Interictal ^{99m}Tc-ECD SPECT activity was subtracted from ictal activity, and then co-registered to the patient's MRI. Reproduced with permission of Simon Vogrin.

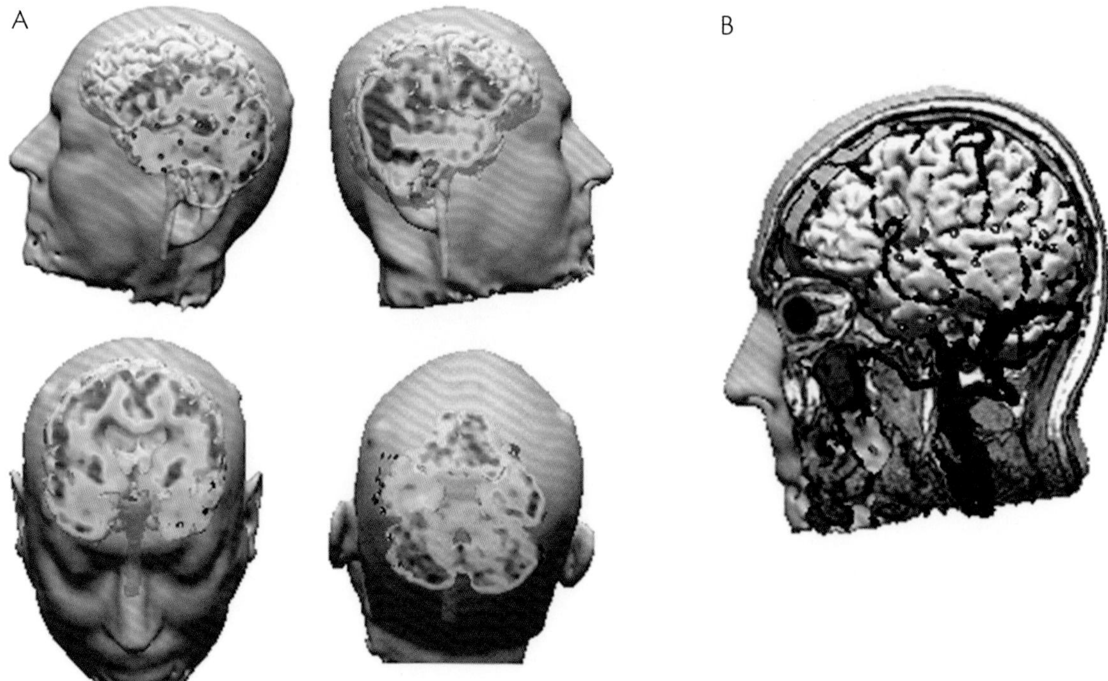

Colour plate 8 (Also see Fig. 10.5.) Multimodal imaging used in the presurgical planning of a patient with temporal lobe epilepsy. A) Coronal, sagittal, and axial slices from the patient's (^{18}F) FDG PET study, co-registered with the patient's MRI to plan for the placement of intracranial electrodes (blue dots). These images demonstrate reduced FDG tracer uptake in the left temporal lobe. B) Cortical reconstruction demonstrating the venous distribution (purple) from a magnetic resonance venogram co-registered to the same patient's 3D MPRAGE volume. Reproduced with permission of Simon Vogrin.

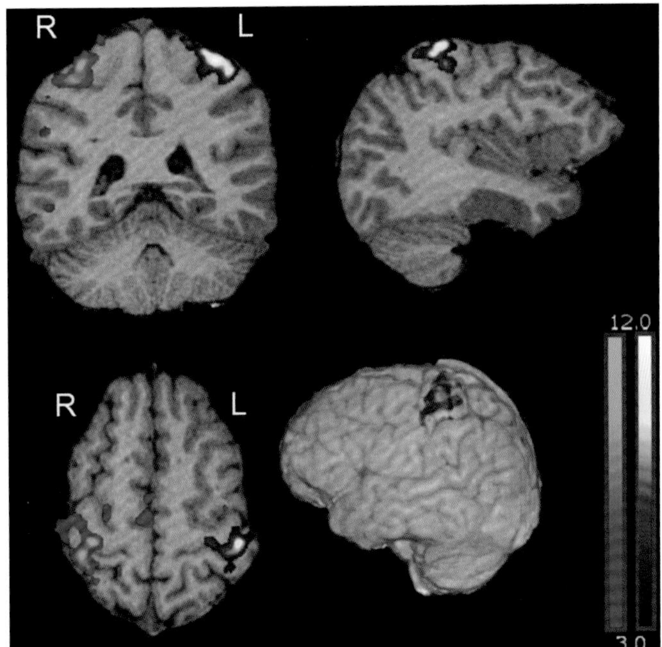

Colour plate 9 (Also see Fig. 10.6.) FMRI scans acquired from an individual subject during a finger-tapping task. Coronal, sagittal, and axial sections, as well as a rendered whole brain, show motor regions which are active during tapping with fingers of the left (blue) and right (red) hands. Images were acquired with a 1.5 T MRI scanner, and activations are shown at a statistical cluster threshold of z = 3.0. Subject's right is figure left. Reproduced with permission of Simon Vogrin.

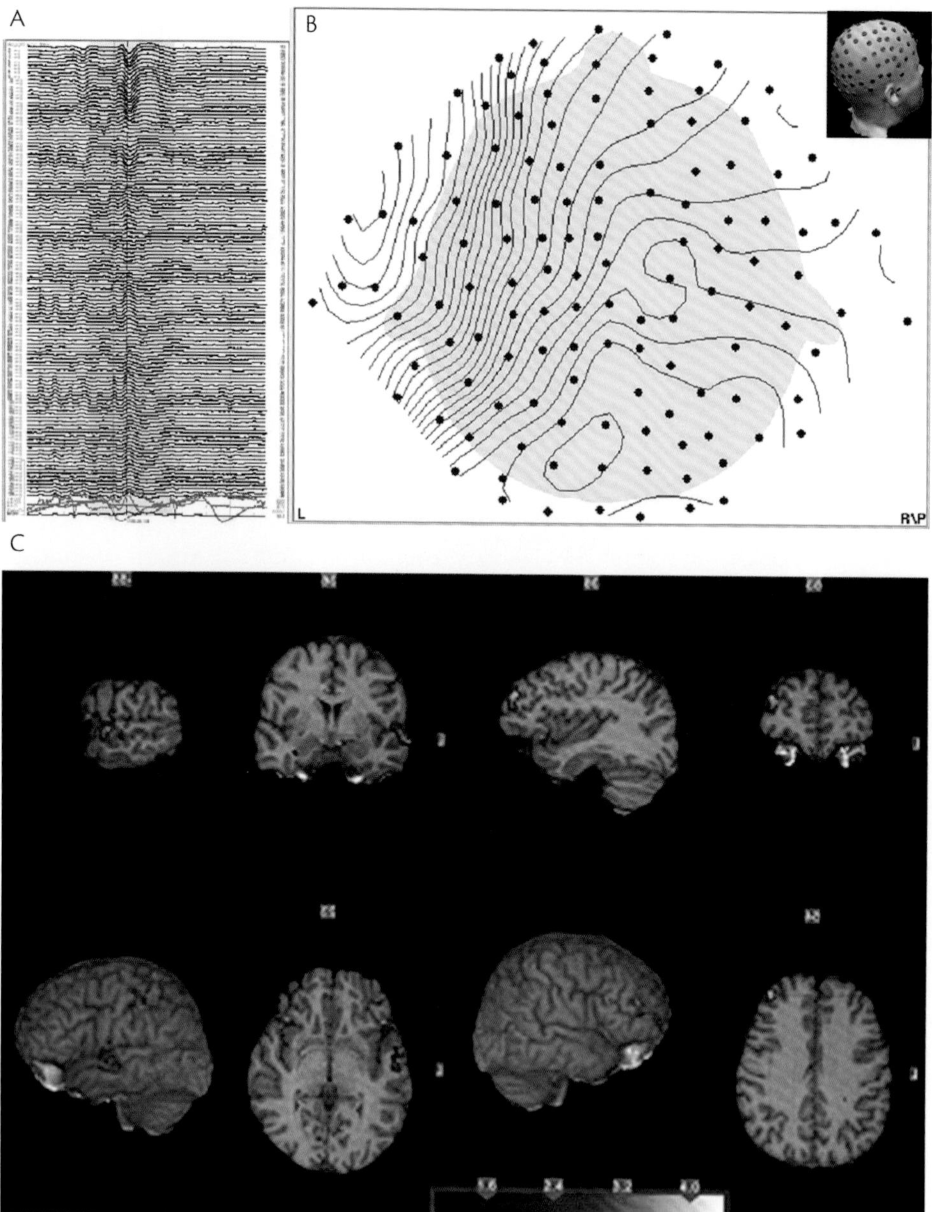

Colour plate 10 (Also see Fig. 10.7.) Upper panel) EEG-fMRI findings from a patient with left temporal lobe epilepsy. 128-channel EEG recorded in the MRI scanner showing left temporal spikes (A). The large gradient artefact was filtered, leaving, nevertheless, some transient waveforms. The epileptic discharges of this patient could be identified unambiguously from their morphology and spatial distribution (B). Lower panel) During a 35 minute simultaneous EEG-fMRI session, there were 11 interictal discharges which were localized to the left superior temporal gyrus (C). These activations were modelled using a multi-haemodynamic response function approach, including regressors for head movement. Three principal clusters were found—in the left superior temporal gyrus, the left precentral gyrus, and right frontal lobe, with the former two activations correlating with the patient's seizure semiology. With permission from Vogrin, S. et al. ESI and fMRI of interictal and ictal epileptic discharges. *International Journal of Bioelectromagnetism* 2011; 13(4):S261–7.

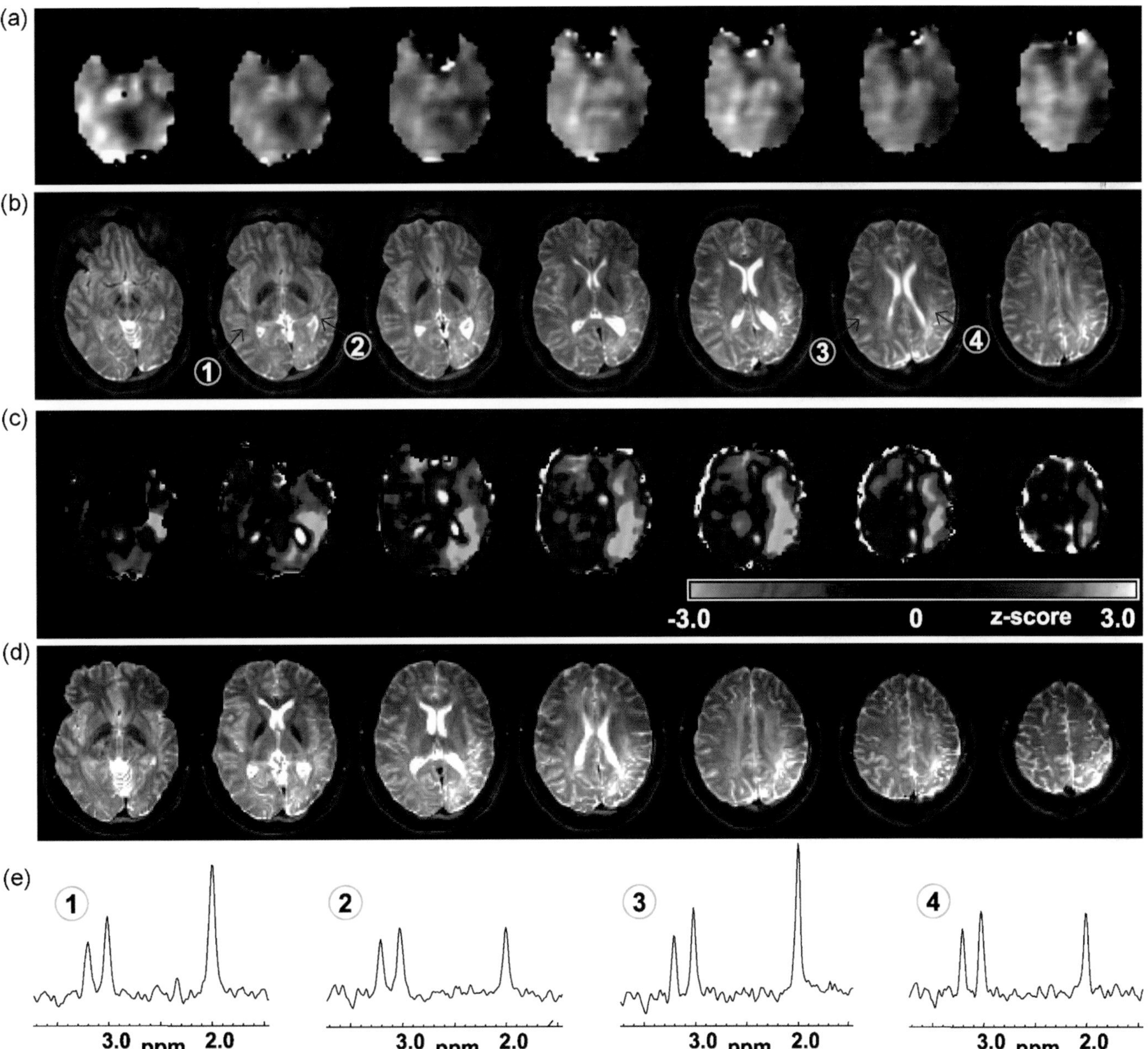

Colour plate 11 (Also see Fig. 10.8.) Magnetic resonance spectroscopy data from a single subject. A) NAA/Cr images at 7 axial slices. B) T2-weighted images corresponding to the centre of the metabolite image slice. C) z-score images for NAA/Cr in the standard spatial reference frame. D) T2-MRI following affine registration to the standard spatial reference frame. E) Spectra from the locations indicated in (B). From Maudsley A, et al. Application of volumetric MR spectroscopic imaging for localization of neocortical epilepsy. *Epilepsy Res* 2010; 88(2–3):127–38.

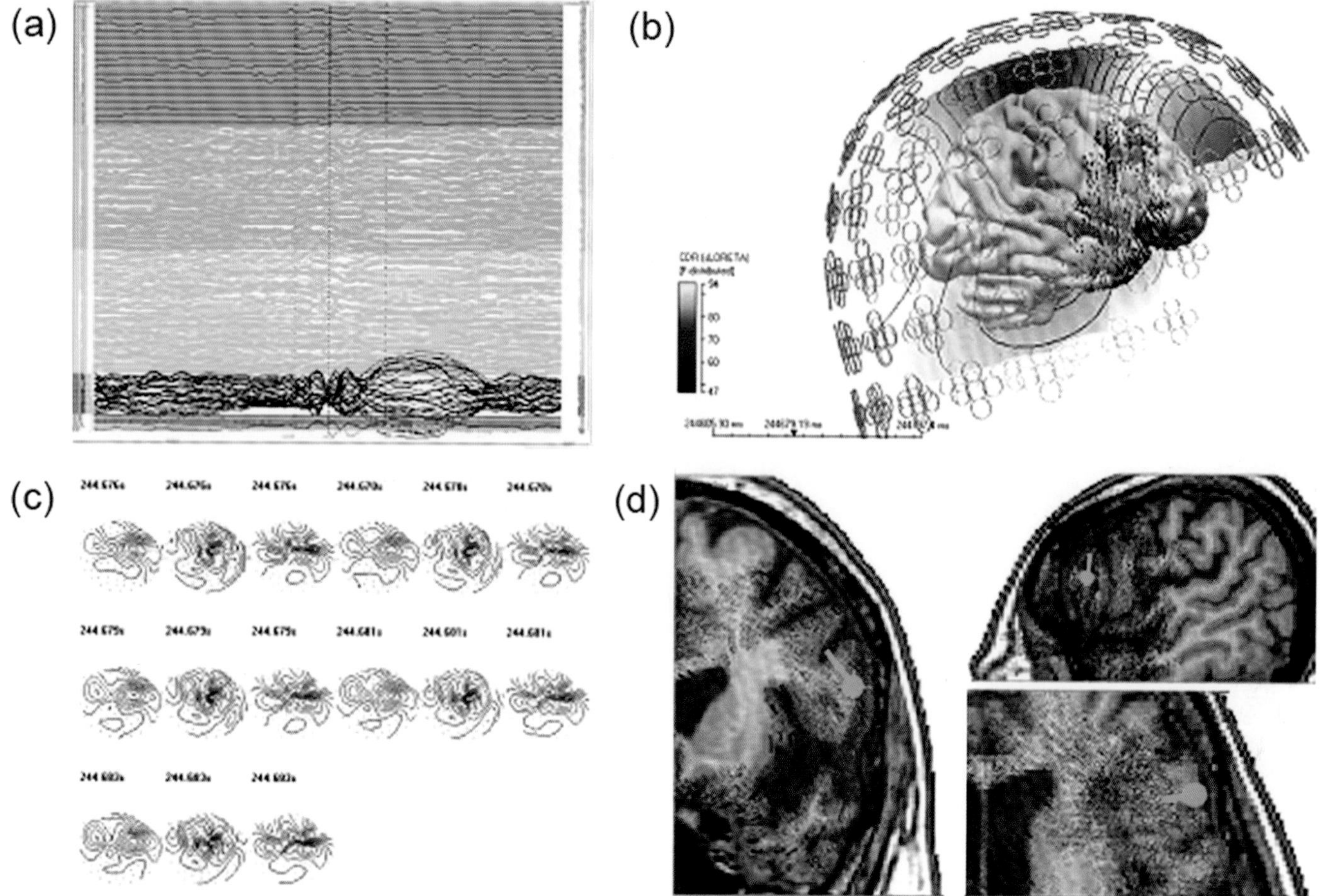

Colour plate 12 (Also see Fig. 10.9.) A polyphasic spike-and-slow wave interictal discharge recorded by simultaneous EEG-MEG. A) The 306 magnetometers and gradiometers (green traces) and 34 EEG electrodes (dark blue traces) demonstrate high spatial coverage in (B) the reconstructed model. C) Comparison of individual magnetometer and orthogonal gradiometer field maps correspond to (D) a standardized low-resolution brain electromagnetic tomography (sLORETA) analysis of the distributed dipolar source orientation strength and equivalent current dipole (green dipole). Reproduced with permission of Simon Vogrin.

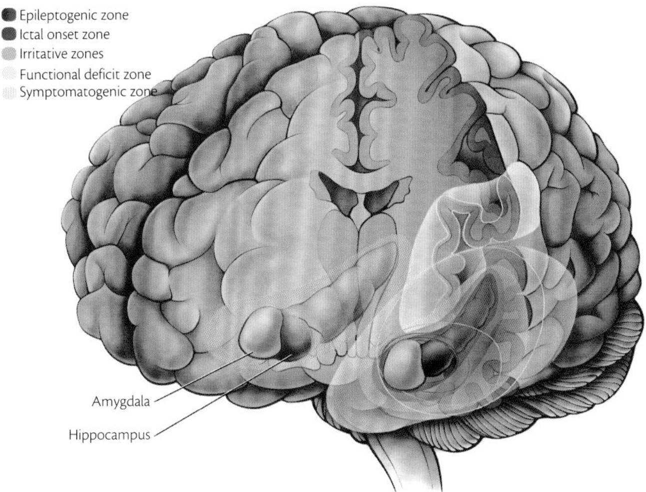

Colour plate 13 (Also see Fig. 27.2.) The epileptogenic zone and its relationship with related zones in a patient with left hippocampal sclerosis. These are: (1) Epileptogenic zone = left hippocampus and amygdala. (2) Epileptic lesion zone and ictal onset zone = left hippocampus. (3) Irritative zones = left and right hippocampus + adjacent temporal neocortex. (4) Functional deficit zone = left temporal lobe (reduced left temporal neuropsychological measures—e.g. verbal memory). (5) Symptomatogenic zone = left insula and lower motor strip (e.g. causing epigastric sensation followed by a right face clonic seizure). Copyright Samden D. Lhatoo.

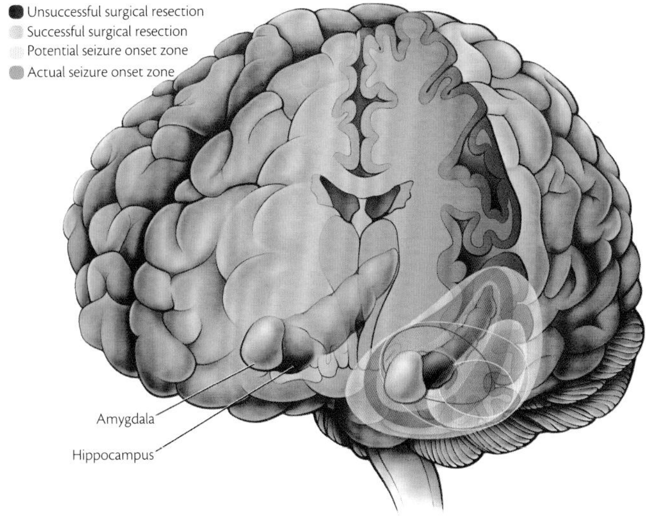

Colour plate 14 (Also see Fig. 27.3.) Surgical resection and the epileptogenic zone. Copyright Samden D. Lhatoo.

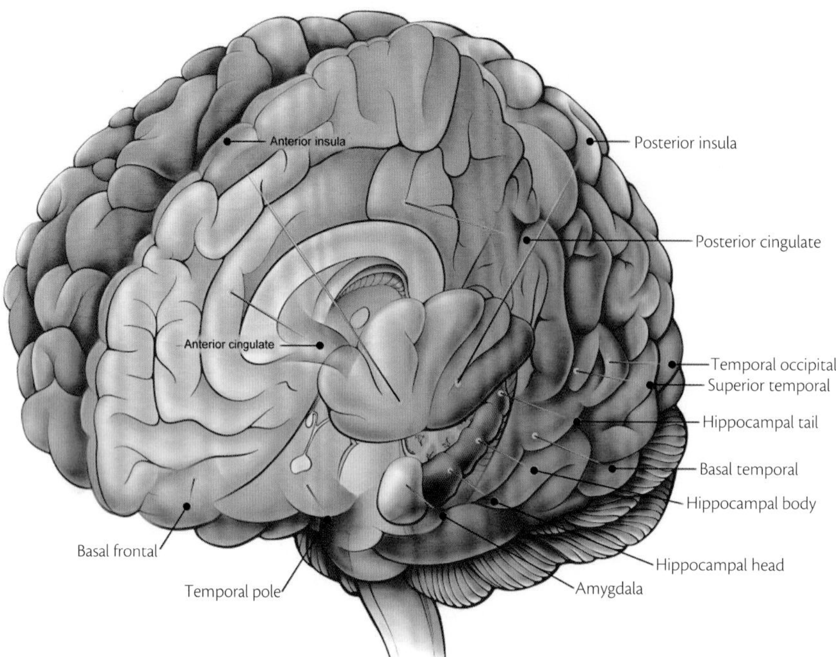

Colour plate 15 (Also see Fig. 27.5.) Diagrammatic representation of stereotactically implanted depth electrodes in a patient with lesion-negative temporal lobe epilepsy. Electrode labels denote the main anatomical structures targeted by the innermost electrode contacts. The outer contacts also sample cortex at or close to the point of electrode insertion. For example, the deep anterior insular contacts sample the anterior insular gyri whilst the superficial contacts of the same electrode sample the superior frontal gyrus where the electrode is inserted. Similarly, the deep contacts of the hippocampal body electrode sample the hippocampal body whilst the superficial contacts sample the lateral temporal neocortex in the middle temporal gyrus. Copyright Samden D. Lhatoo.

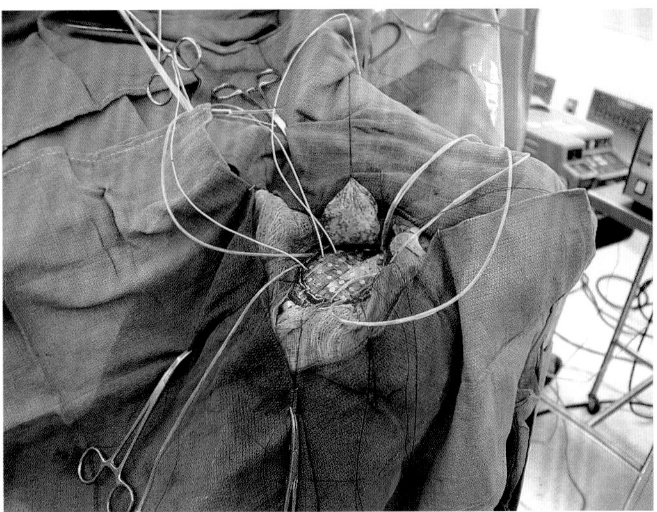

Colour plate 16 (Also see Fig. 27.6.) A right craniotomy with an 8 × 8 (64 electrode) grid covering the frontal and temporal areas of a patient with lesion negative right hemisphere epilepsy. Copyright Samden D. Lhatoo.

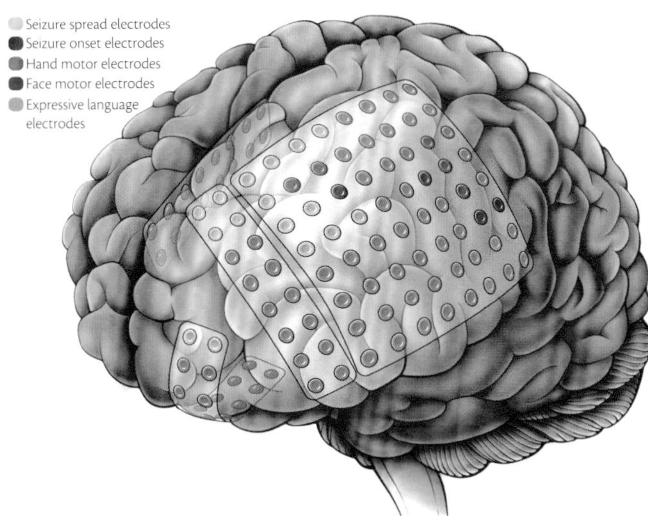

Colour plate 17 (Also see Fig. 27.8.) Brain map of a patient with left frontal lobe epilepsy showing the language, hand motor, and face motor areas with their relationship to the seizure onset (red) and seizure spread (yellow) electrodes. The ictal onset zone in this case therefore lies in the left superior frontal gyrus of the prefrontal cortex, is relatively distant from eloquent cortex and unlikely to cause deficits if resected. Copyright Samden D. Lhatoo.

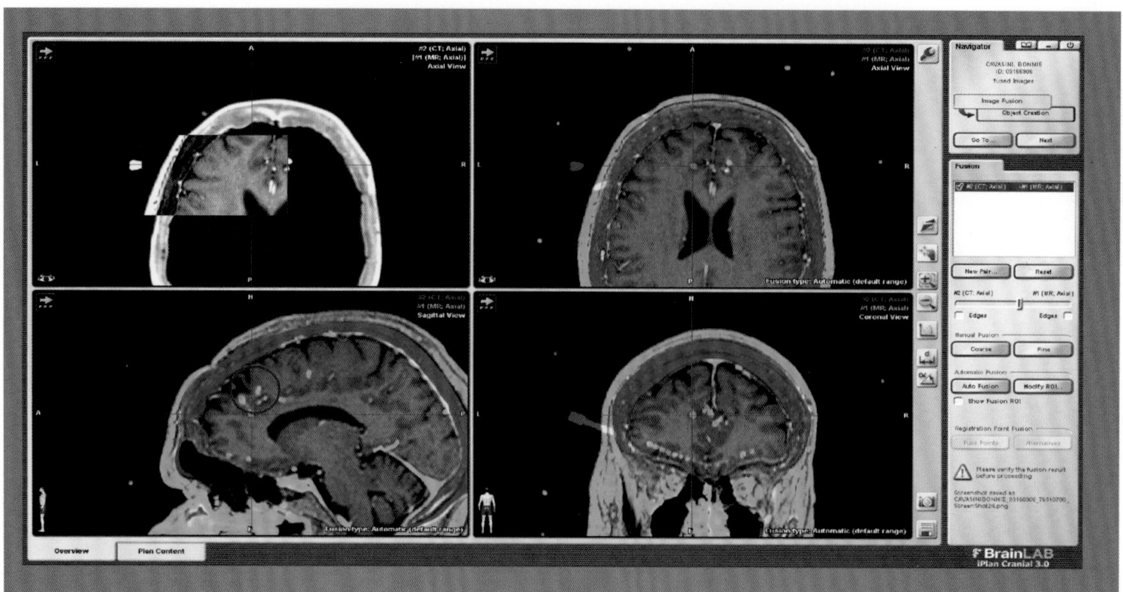

Colour plate 18 (See also Fig. 29.6.) Location of depth electrodes can be determined by the fusion of high-resolution CT images (taken after placing the electrodes) with preoperative MRI. The red circle shows the area of seizure onset around the right mesiofrontal lesion.

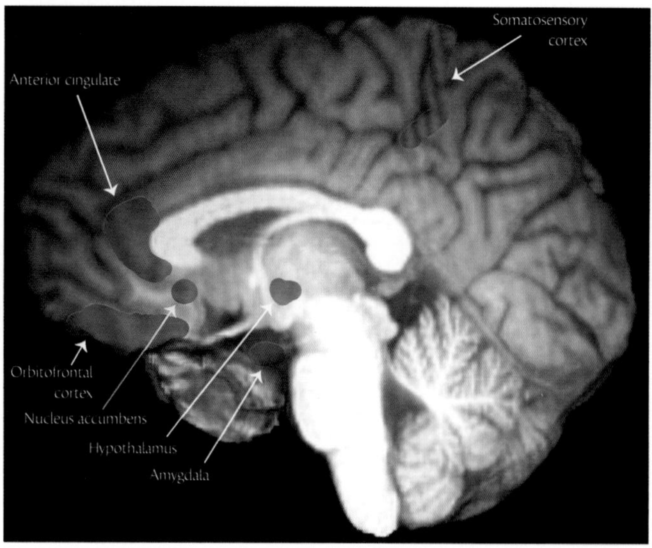

Colour plate 19 (See also Fig. 35.1.) Sagittal view of the right hemisphere of the brain showing overlapping regions of the sexual and affective networks (approximate locations shown with shading).

and a suppression-burst pattern on EEG (121). The healthy hemisphere is therefore connected with a structurally abnormal contralateral hemisphere that is highly epileptogenic. Early surgery with hemispherectomy often controls the seizures. Hemispherotomy (hemispheric disconnection) is preferred to functional or anatomical hemispherectomy in some centres. Behavioural and cognitive improvement has been reported but is usually moderate (8).

References

1. Gastaut H, Roger J, Soulayrol R, Tassinari CA, Regis H, Dravet C, *et al.* Childhood epileptic encephalopathy with diffuse slow spike-waves (otherwise known as 'petit mal variant') or Lennox Syndrome. *Epilepsia* 1966; 7:139–79.
2. Engel J Jr. A proposed diagnostic scheme for people with epileptic seizures and with epilepsy: report of the ILAE Task Force on Classification and Terminology. *Epilepsia* 2001; 42(6):796–803.
3. Dalla Bernardina B, Colamaria V, Capovilla G, Bondavalli S. Nosological classification of epilepsies in the first three years of life. In: Nistico G, Di Perri R, Meinardi H (eds) *Epilepsy: an update on research and therapy*, pp. 165–83. New York: Alan R. Liss, Inc., 1983.
4. Massa R, de Saint-Martin A, Carcangiu R, Rudolf G, Seegmuller C, Kleitz C, *et al.* EEG criteria predictive of complicated evolution in idiopathic rolandic epilepsy. *Neurology* 2001; 57(6):1071–9.
5. Piccirilli M, D'Alessandro P, Tiacci C, Ferroni A. Language lateralization in children with benign partial epilepsy. *Epilepsia* 1988; 29(1):19–25.
6. Shewmon DA, Erwin RJ. Focal spike-induced cerebral dysfunction is related to the after-coming slow wave. *Ann Neurol* 1988; 23(2):131–7.
7. Guerrini R, Aicardi J. Epileptic encephalopathies with myoclonic seizures in infants and children (severe myoclonic epilepsy and myoclonic-astatic epilepsy). *J Clin Neurophysiol* 2003; 20(6):449–61.
8. Pulsifer MB, Brandt J, Salorio CF, Vining EP, Carson BS, Freeman JM. The cognitive outcome of hemispherectomy in 71 children. *Epilepsia* 2004; 45(3):243–54.
9. Dulac O. Infantile spasms and West syndrome. In: Engel J Jr, Pedley TA (eds) *Epilepsy: a comprehensive textbook*, pp. 2277–83. Philadelphia, PA: Lippincott-Raven, 1997.
10. Guerrini R. Epilepsy in children. *Lancet* 2006; 367(9509):499–524.
11. Trevathan E, Murphy CC, Yeargin-Allsopp M. The descriptive epidemiology of infantile spasms among Atlanta children. *Epilepsia* 1999; 40(6):748–51.
12. Kramer U, Sue WC, Mikati MA. Focal features in West syndrome indicating candidacy for surgery. *Pediatr Neurol* 1997; 16(3):213–17.
13. Cowan LD, Hudson LS. The epidemiology and natural history of infantile spasms. *J Child Neurol* 1991; 6(4):355–64.
14. Dulac O, Plouin P, Jambaqué I, Motte J. Spasmes infantiles épileptiques bénins. *Rev EEG. Neurophysiol Clin* 1986; 16:371–82.
15. Vigevano F, Fusco L, Cusmai R, Claps D, Ricci S, Milani L. The idiopathic form of West syndrome. *Epilepsia* 1993; 34(4):743–6.
16. Sugai K, Fukuyama Y, Yasuda K, Fujimoto S, Ohtsu M, Ohta H, *et al.* Clinical and pedigree study on familial cases of West syndrome in Japan. *Brain Dev* 2001; 23(7):558–64.
17. Coleman M, Hart PN, Randall J, Lee J, Hijada D, Bratenahl CG. Serotonin levels in the blood and central nervous system of a patient with sudanophilic leukodystrophy. *Neuropadiatrie* 1977; 8(4):459–66.
18. Riikonen R. Infantile spasms: modern practical aspects. *Acta Paediatr Scand* 1984; 73(1):1–12.
19. Guerrini R, Carrozzo R. Epileptogenic brain malformations: clinical presentation, malformative patterns and indications for genetic testing. *Seizure* 2001; 10(7):532–43.
20. Stromme P, Mangelsdorf ME, Shaw MA, Lower KM, Lewis SM, Bruyere H, *et al.* Mutations in the human ortholog of Aristaless cause X-linked mental retardation and epilepsy. *Nat Genet* 2002; 30(4):441–5.
21. Guerrini R, Moro F, Kato M, Barkovich AJ, Shiihara T, McShane MA, *et al.* Expansion of the first PolyA tract of ARX causes infantile spasms and status dystonicus. *Neurology* 2007; 69(5):427–33.
22. Stromme P, Mangelsdorf ME, Scheffer IE, Gecz J. Infantile spasms, dystonia, and other X-linked phenotypes caused by mutations in Aristaless related homeobox gene, ARX. *Brain Dev* 2002; 24(5):266–8.
23. Kato M, Das S, Petras K, Sawaishi Y, Dobyns WB. Polyalanine expansion of ARX associated with cryptogenic West syndrome. *Neurology* 2003; 61(2):267–76.
24. Archer HL, Evans J, Edwards S, Colley J, Newbury-Ecob R, O'Callaghan F, *et al.* CDKL5 mutations cause infantile spasms, early onset seizures, and severe mental retardation in female patients. *J Med Genet* 2006; 43(9):729–34.
25. Mei D, Marini C, Novara F, Dalla Bernardina B, Granata T, Fontana E, Parrini E, Ferrari AR, Murgia A, Zuffardi O, Guerrini R. Xp22.3 genomic deletions involving the CDKL5 gene in girls with early onset epileptic encephalopathy. *Epilepsia* 2010;51:647–54.
26. Elia M, Falco M, Ferri R, Spalletta A, Bottitta M, Calabrese G, *et al.* CDKL5 mutations in boys with severe encephalopathy and early-onset intractable epilepsy. *Neurology* 2008; 71(13):997–9.
27. Melani F, Mei D, Pisano T, Savasta S, Franzoni E, Ferrari AR, *et al.* CDKL5 gene-related epileptic encephalopathy: electroclinical findings in the first year of life. *Dev Med Child Neurol*; 53(4):354–60.
28. Marshall CR, Young EJ, Pani AM, Freckmann ML, Lacassie Y, Howald C, *et al.* Infantile spasms is associated with deletion of the MAGI2 gene on chromosome 7q11.23-q21.11. *Am J Hum Genet* 2008; 83(1):106–11.
29. Otsuka M, Oguni H, Liang JS, Ikeda H, Imai K, Hirasawa K, *et al.* STXBP1 mutations cause not only Ohtahara syndrome but also West syndrome—result of Japanese cohort study. *Epilepsia* 2010; 51(12):2449–52.
30. Riikonen R. Epidemiological data of West syndrome in Finland. *Brain Dev* 2001; 23(7):539–41.
31. Ciardo F, Zamponi N, Specchio N, Parmeggiani L, Guerrini R. Autosomal recessive polymicrogyria with infantile spasms and limb deformities. *Neuropediatrics* 2001; 32(6):325–9.
32. Fleiszar KA, Daniel WL, Imrey PB. Genetic study of infantile spasm with hypsarrhythmia. *Epilepsia* 1977; 18(1):55–62.
33. Reiter E, Tiefenthaler M, Freillinger M, Bernert G, Seidl R, Hauser E. Familial idiopathic West syndrome. *J Child Neurol* 2000; 15(4):249–52.
34. Pellock JM, Hrachovy R, Shinnar S, Baram TZ, Bettis D, Dlugos DJ, *et al.* Infantile spasms: a U.S. consensus report. *Epilepsia*; 51(10):2175–89.
35. Saltik S, Kocer N, Dervent A. Informative value of magnetic resonance imaging and EEG in the prognosis of infantile spasms. *Epilepsia* 2002; 43(3):246–52.
36. Kivity S, Lerman P, Ariel R, Danziger Y, Mimouni M, Shinnar S. Long-term cognitive outcomes of a cohort of children with cryptogenic infantile spasms treated with high-dose adrenocorticotropic hormone. *Epilepsia* 2004; 45(3):255–62.
37. Vigevano F, Cilio MR. Vigabatrin versus ACTH as first-line treatment for infantile spasms: a randomized, prospective study. *Epilepsia* 1997; 38(12):1270–4.
38. Cossette P, Riviello JJ, Carmant L. ACTH versus vigabatrin therapy in infantile spasms: a retrospective study. *Neurology* 1999; 52(8):1691–4.
39. Lux AL, Edwards SW, Hancock E, Hancock E, Johnson AL, Kennedy CR, *et al.* The United Kingdom Infantile Spasms Study comparing vigabatrin with prednisolone or tetracosactide at 14 days: a multicentre, randomised controlled trial. *Lancet* 2004; 364(9447):1773–8.
40. Appleton RE, Peters AC, Mumford JP, Shaw DE. Randomised, placebo-controlled study of vigabatrin as first-line treatment of infantile spasms. *Epilepsia* 1999; 40(11):1627–33.
41. Elterman RD, Shields WD, Mansfield KA, Nakagawa J. Randomized trial of vigabatrin in patients with infantile spasms. *Neurology* 2001; 57(8):1416–21.

42. Jambaque I, Chiron C, Dumas C, Mumford J, Dulac O. Mental and behavioural outcome of infantile epilepsy treated by vigabatrin in tuberous sclerosis patients. *Epilepsy Res* 2000; 38(2–3):151–60.
43. Lewis H, Wallace SJ. Vigabatrin. *Dev Med Child Neurol* 2001; 43(12):833–5.
44. Milh M, Villeneuve N, Chapon F, Pineau S, Lamoureux S, Livet MO, *et al.* Transient brain magnetic resonance imaging hyperintensity in basal ganglia and brain stem of epileptic infants treated with vigabatrin. *J Child Neurol* 2009; 24(3):305–15.
45. Thelle T, Gammelgaard L, Hansen JK, Ostergaard JR. Reversible magnetic resonance imaging and spectroscopy abnormalities in the course of vigabatrin treatment for West syndrome. *Eur J Paediatr Neurol* 2011; 15(3):260–4.
46. Lux AL, Edwards SW, Hancock E, Johnson AL, Kennedy CR, Newton RW, *et al.* The United Kingdom Infantile Spasms Study (UKISS) comparing hormone treatment with vigabatrin on developmental and epilepsy outcomes to age 14 months: a multicentre randomised trial. *Lancet Neurol* 2005; 4(11):712–17.
47. Heiskala H, Riikonen R, Santavuori P, Simell O, Airaksinen E, Nuutila A, *et al.* West syndrome: individualized ACTH therapy. *Brain Dev* 1996; 18(6):456–60.
48. Wong M, Trevathan E. Infantile spasms. *Pediatr Neurol* 2001; 24(2):89–98.
49. Kossoff EH. Infantile spasms. *Neurologist* 2010; 16(2):69–75.
50. Pellock JM, Hrachovy R, Shinnar S, Baram TZ, Bettis D, Dlugos DJ, *et al.* Infantile spasms: a U.S. consensus report. *Epilepsia* 2010; 51(10):2175–89.
51. Mackay MT, Weiss SK, Adams-Webber T, Ashwal S, Stephens D, Ballaban-Gill K, *et al.* Practice parameter: medical treatment of infantile spasms: report of the American Academy of Neurology and the Child Neurology Society. *Neurology* 2004; 62(10):1668–81.
52. Gaily E, Liukkonen E, Paetau R, Rekola R, Granstrom ML. Infantile spasms: diagnosis and assessment of treatment response by video-EEG. *Dev Med Child Neurol* 2001; 43(10):658–67.
53. Asano E, Chugani DC, Juhasz C, Muzik O, Chugani HT. Surgical treatment of West syndrome. *Brain Dev* 2001; 23(7):668–76.
54. Kossoff EH, Pyzik PL, McGrogan JR, Vining EP, Freeman JM. Efficacy of the ketogenic diet for infantile spasms. *Pediatrics* 2002; 109(5):780–3.
55. Berg AT, Shinnar S, Levy SR, Testa FM, Smith-Rapaport, S, Beckerman, B. How well can epilepsy syndromes be identified at diagnosis? A reassessment two years after initial diagnosis. *Epilepsia* 2000; 41:1267–75.
56. ILAE. Commission on Classification and Terminology of the International League Against Epilepsy: Proposal for revised classification of epilepsies and epileptic syndromes. *Epilepsia* 1989; 30:389–99.
57. Arzimanoglou A, French J, Blume WT, Cross JH, Ernst JP, Feucht M, *et al.* Lennox–Gastaut syndrome: a consensus approach on diagnosis, assessment, management, and trial methodology. *Lancet Neurol* 2009; 8(1):82–93.
58. Genton P Guerrini R, Dravet C. The Lennox–Gastaut syndrome. In: Meinardi IH (ed) *The Epilepsies. Part II. Handbook of Clinical Neurology*, pp. 211–22. Amsterdam: Elsevier, 2000.
59. Blume WT. Lennox–Gastaut syndrome: potential mechanisms of cognitive regression. *Ment Retard Dev Disabil Res Rev* 2004; 10(2):150–3.
60. Hoffmann-Riem M, Diener W, Benninger C, Rating D, Unnebrink K, Stephani U, *et al.* Nonconvulsive status epilepticus—a possible cause of mental retardation in patients with Lennox–Gastaut syndrome. *Neuropediatrics* 2000; 31(4):169–74.
61. Kaminska A, Ickowicz A, Plouin P, Bru MF, Dellatolas G, Dulac O. Delineation of cryptogenic Lennox–Gastaut syndrome and myoclonic astatic epilepsy using multiple correspondence analysis. *Epilepsy Res* 1999; 36(1):15–29.
62. Guerrini R, Genton P, Bureau M, Parmeggiani A, Salas-Puig X, Santucci M, *et al.* Multilobar polymicrogyria, intractable drop attack seizures, and sleep-related electrical status epilepticus. *Neurology* 1998; 51(2):504–12.
63. Aicardi J, Chevrie JJ. Atypical benign partial epilepsy of childhood. *Dev Med Child Neurol* 1982; 24(3):281–92.
64. Parrini E, Ferrari AR, Dorn T, Walsh CA, Guerrini R. Bilateral frontoparietal polymicrogyria, Lennox–Gastaut syndrome, and GPR56 gene mutations. *Epilepsia* 2009; 50(6):1344–53.
65. Lawrence KM, Mei D, Newton MR, Leventer RJ, Guerrini R, Berkovic SF. Familial Lennox–Gastaut syndrome in male siblings with a novel DCX mutation and anterior pachygyria. *Epilepsia* 2010; 51(9):1902–5.
66. French JA, Kanner AM, Bautista J, Abou-Khalil B, Browne T, Harden CL, *et al.* Efficacy and tolerability of the new antiepileptic drugs II: treatment of refractory epilepsy: report of the Therapeutics and Technology Assessment Subcommittee and Quality Standards Subcommittee of the American Academy of Neurology and the American Epilepsy Society. *Neurology* 2004; 62(8):1261–73.
67. Hancock EC, Cross HH. Treatment of Lennox–Gastaut syndrome. *Cochrane Database Syst Rev* 2009; 3:CD003277.
68. Neal EG, Chaffe H, Schwartz RH, Lawson MS, Edwards N, Fitzsimmons G, *et al.* The ketogenic diet for the treatment of childhood epilepsy: a randomised controlled trial. *Lancet Neurol* 2008; 7(6):500–6.
69. Asadi-Pooya AA, Sharan A, Nei M, Sperling MR. Corpus callosotomy. *Epilepsy Behav* 2008; 13(2):271–8.
70. Deonna T. Cognitive and behavioral manifestations of epilepsy in children. In: Wallace SJ Farrell K (eds) *Epilepsy in children* (2nd edn), pp. 250–7. London: Arnold, 2004.
71. Seri S, Cerquiglini A, Pisani F. Spike-induced interference in auditory sensory processing in Landau–Kleffner syndrome. *Electroencephalogr Clin Neurophysiol* 1998; 108(5):506–10.
72. Duran MH, Guimaraes CA, Medeiros LL, Guerreiro MM. Landau–Kleffner syndrome: long-term follow-up. *Brain Dev* 2009; 31(1):58–63.
73. Buzatu M, Bulteau C, Altuzarra C, Dulac O, Van Bogaert P. Corticosteroids as treatment of epileptic syndromes with continuous spike-waves during slow-wave sleep. *Epilepsia* 2009; 50(Suppl 7): 68–72.
74. Grote CL, Van Slyke P, Hoeppner JA. Language outcome following multiple subpial transection for Landau–Kleffner syndrome. *Brain* 1999; 122(Pt 3):561–6.
75. Tassinari C, Rubboli G, Volpi L, Billard C. Electrical status epilepsticus during slow sleep (ESES or CSWS) including acquired epileptic aphasia (Landau–Kleffner syndrome). In: Roger J, Bureau M, Dravet C, Genton P, Tassinari CA, Wolf P (eds) *Epileptic syndromes in infancy, childhood and adolescence* (3rd edn), pp. 69–79. London: John Libbey, 2002.
76. Smith MC, Hoeppner TJ. Epileptic encephalopathy of late childhood: Landau–Kleffner syndrome and the syndrome of continuous spikes and waves during slow-wave sleep. *J Clin Neurophysiol* 2003; 20(6):462–72.
77. Hughes JR. A review of the relationships between Landau–Kleffner syndrome, electrical status epilepticus during sleep, and continuous spike-waves during sleep. *Epilepsy Behav* 2011; 20(2):247–53.
78. Guerrini R, Oguni H. Borderline Dravet syndrome: a useful diagnostic category? *Epilepsia* 2011; 52(Suppl 2):10–12.
79. Hurst DL. Epidemiology of severe myoclonic epilepsy of infancy. *Epilepsia* 1990; 31:397–400.
80. Yakoub M, Dulac O, Jambaque I, Chiron C, Plouin P. Early diagnosis of severe myoclonic epilepsy in infancy. *Brain and Development* 1992; 14:299–303.
81. Dravet C, Bureau, M, Oguni, H, Fukuyama, Y, Cokar, O. Severe myoclonic epilepsy in infancy (Dravet syndrome). In: Roger J, Bureau M, Dravet CH, Genton P, Tassinari CA, Wolf P (eds) *Epileptic*

syndromes in infancy, childhood and adolescence, pp. 89–113. London, Paris: John Libbey, 2005.

82. Wolff M, Casse-Perrot C, Dravet C. Severe myoclonic epilepsy of infants (Dravet syndrome): natural history and neuropsychological findings. *Epilepsia* 2006; 47(Suppl 2):45–8.
83. Ragona F, Granata T, Dalla Bernardina B, Offredi F, Darra F, Battaglia D, *et al.* Cognitive development in Dravet syndrome: a retrospective, multicenter study of 26 patients. *Epilepsia* 2011; 52(2):386–92.
84. Singh R, Scheffer IE, Whitehouse W, Harvey AS, Crossland KM, Berkovic SF. Severe myclonic epilepsy of infancy is part of the spectrum of generalized epilepsy with febile seizures plus (GEFS+). *Epilepsia* 1999; 40:175.
85. Claes L, Del-Favero J, Ceulemans B, Lagae L, Van Broeckhoven C, De Jonghe P. De novo mutations in the sodium-channel gene SCN1A cause severe myoclonic epilepsy of infancy. *Am J Hum Genet* 2001; 68(6):1327–32.
86. Mulley JC, Scheffer IE, Petrou S, Dibbens LM, Berkovic SF, Harkin LA. SCN1A mutations and epilepsy. *Hum Mutat* 2005; 25(6):535–42.
87. Marini C, Scheffer IE, Nabbout R, Suls A, De Jonghe P, Zara F, *et al.* The genetics of Dravet syndrome. *Epilepsia* 2011; 52(Suppl 2):24–9.
88. Marini C, Scheffer IE, Nabbout R, Mei D, Cox K, Dibbens LM, *et al.* SCN1A duplications and deletions detected in Dravet syndrome: implications for molecular diagnosis. *Epilepsia.* 2009; 50(7):1670–8.
89. Sugawara T, Mazaki-Miyazaki E, Fukushima K, Shimomura J, Fujiwara T, Hamano S, *et al.* Frequent mutations of SCN1A in severe myoclonic epilepsy in infancy. *Neurology* 2002; 58(7):1122–4.
90. Nabbout R, Gennaro E, Dalla Bernardina B, Dulac O, Madia F, Bertini E, *et al.* Spectrum of SCN1A mutations in severe myoclonic epilepsy of infancy. *Neurology* 2003; 60(12):1961–7.
91. Wallace RH, Hodgson BL, Grinton BE, Gardiner RM, Robinson R, Rodriguez-Casero V, *et al.* Sodium channel alpha1-subunit mutations in severe myoclonic epilepsy of infancy and infantile spasms. *Neurology* 2003; 61(6):765–9.
92. Depienne C, Arzimanoglou A, Trouillard O, Fedirko E, Baulac S, Saint-Martin C, *et al.* Parental mosaicism can cause recurrent transmission of SCN1A mutations associated with severe myoclonic epilepsy of infancy. *Hum Mutat* 2006; 27(4):389.
93. Marini C, Mei D, Helen Cross J, Guerrini R. Mosaic SCN1A mutation in familial severe myoclonic epilepsy of infancy. *Epilepsia* 2006; 47(10):1737–40.
94. Marini C, Mei D, Temudo T, Ferrari AR, Buti D, Dravet C, *et al.* Idiopathic epilepsies with seizures precipitated by fever and SCN1A abnormalities. *Epilepsia* 2007; 48(9):1678–85.
95. Meisler MH, Kearney JA. Sodium channel mutations in epilepsy and other neurological disorders. *J Clin Invest* 2005; 115(8):2010–17.
96. Depienne C, Bouteiller D, Keren B, Cheuret E, Poirier K, Trouillard O, *et al.* Sporadic infantile epileptic encephalopathy caused by mutations in PCDH19 resembles Dravet syndrome but mainly affects females. *PLoS Genet* 2009; 5(2):e1000381.
97. Marini C, Mei D, Parmeggiani L, Norci V, Calado E, Ferrari A, *et al.* Protocadherin 19 mutations in girls with infantile-onset epilepsy. *Neurology* 2010; 75(7):646–53.
98. Striano P, Mancardi MM, Biancheri R, Madia F, Gennaro E, Paravidino R, *et al.* Brain MRI findings in severe myoclonic epilepsy in infancy and genotype-phenotype correlations. *Epilepsia* 2007; 48(6):1092–96.
99. Catarino CB, Liu JY, Liagkouras I, Gibbons VS, Labrum RW, Ellis R, *et al.* Dravet syndrome as epileptic encephalopathy: evidence from long-term course and neuropathology. *Brain* 2011; 134(Pt 10): 2982–3010.
100. Jansen FE, Sadleir LG, Harkin LA, Vadlamudi L, McMahon JM, Mulley JC, *et al.* Severe myoclonic epilepsy of infancy (Dravet syndrome): recognition and diagnosis in adults. *Neurology* 2006; 67(12):2224–6.
101. Dravet C. Dravet syndrome history. *Dev Med Child Neurol* 2011; 53(Suppl 2):1–6.
102. Chiron C, Marchand MC, Tran A, Rey E, d'Athis P, Vincent J, *et al.* Stiripentol in severe myoclonic epilepsy in infancy: a randomised placebo-controlled syndrome-dedicated trial. STICLO study group. *Lancet* 2000; 356(9242):1638–42.
103. Kassai B, Chiron C, Augier S, Cucherat M, Rey E, Gueyffier F, *et al.* Severe myoclonic epilepsy in infancy: a systematic review and a meta-analysis of individual patient data. *Epilepsia* 2008; 49(2):343–8.
104. Guerrini R, Dravet C, Genton P, Belmonte A, Kaminska A, Dulac O. Lamotrigine and seizure aggravation in severe myoclonic epilepsy. *Epilepsia* 1998; 39s:508–12.
105. Doose H. Myoclonic-astatic epilepsy. *Epilepsy Res Suppl* 1992; 6:163–8.
106. Singh R, Scheffer IE, Crossland K, Berkovic SF. Generalized epilepsy with febrile seizures plus: a common childhood-onset genetic epilepsy syndrome. *Ann Neurol* 1999; 45(1):75–81.
107. Scheffer IE, Berkovic SF. Generalized epilepsy with febrile seizures plus. A genetic disorder with heterogeneous clinical phenotypes. *Brain* 1997; 120:479–90.
108. Singh R, Andermann E, Whitehouse WP, Harvey AS, Keene DL, Seni MH, *et al.* Severe myoclonic epilepsy of infancy: extended spectrum of GEFS+? *Epilepsia* 2001; 42(7):837–44.
109. Mullen SA, Marini C, Suls A, Mei D, Della Giustina E, Buti D, *et al.* Glucose transporter 1 deficiency as a treatable cause of myoclonic astatic epilepsy. *Arch Neurol* 2011; 68(9):1152–5.
110. Oguni H, Fukuyama Y, Imaizumi Y, Uehara T. Video-EEG analysis of drop seizures in myoclonic astatic epilepsy of early childhood (Doose syndrome). *Epilepsia* 1992; 33(5):805–13.
111. Guerrini R, Arzimanoglou A, Brouwer O. Rationale for treating epilepsy in children. *Epileptic Disord* 2002; 4(Suppl 2):S9–21.
112. Lortie A, Chiron C, Mumford J, Dulac O. The potential for increasing seizure frequency, relapse, and appearance of new seizure types with vigabatrin. *Neurology* 1993; 43(11 Suppl 5):S24–7.
113. Oguni H, Uehara T, Imai K, Osawa M. Atonic epileptic drop attacks associated with generalized spike-and-slow wave complexes: video-polygraphic study in two patients. *Epilepsia* 1997; 38(7):813–18.
114. Patry G, Lyagoubi S, Tassinari CA. Subclinical 'electrical status epilepticus' induced by sleep in children. *Arch Neurol* 1971; 24:242–52.
115. Biraben A, Allain H, Scarabin JM, Schuck S, Edan G. Exacerbation of juvenile myoclonic epilepsy with lamotrigine. *Neurology* 2000; 55(11):1758.
116. Dulac O, Kaminska A. Use of lamotrigine in Lennox–Gastaut and related epilepsy syndromes. *J Child Neurol* 1997; 12(Suppl 1): S23–8.
117. Guerrini R, Parmeggiani, L, Kaminska, A, Dulac, O. Myoclonic astatic epilepsy. In: Roger J, Bureau M, Dravet CH, Genton P, Tassinari CA, Wolf P (eds) *Epileptic syndromes in infancy, childhood and adolescence* (3rd edn), pp. 105–12. London and Paris: John Libbey, 2002.
118. Nordli D, DeVivo DC. Inherited metabolic disorders. In: Engel J, Pedley TA (eds) *Epilepsy: A Comprehensive Textbook* (2nd edn), pp. 2603–19. Philadelphia, PA: Wolters Klower, 2008:
119. Pellock J, Nordli DR, Dulac O. Drug treatment in children. In: Engel J, Pedley PT (eds) *Epilepsy: A Comprehensive Textbook* (2nd edn), pp, 1249–57. Philadelphia, PA: Wolters Klower, 2008.
120. Guerrini R, Pollock J. Epileptic encephalopathies. In: Stefan H, Theodore WH (eds) *Epilepsy. Handbook of Clinical Neurology.* London: Elsevier, in press.
121. Paladin F, Chiron C, Dulac O, Plouin P, Ponsot G. Electroencephalographic aspects of hemimegalencephaly. *Dev Med Child Neurol* 1989; 31(3):377–83.

CHAPTER 16

Principles of Treatment of Epilepsy in Children and Adolescents

Renzo Guerrini

General considerations

The bases for classifying epilepsy syndromes and treatment options of most syndromes of childhood and adolescence have been dealt with, in part, in Chapters 7 and 15. This chapter will be mainly devoted to principles of treatment in young patients with different types of epilepsy, excluding the epileptic encephalopathies and early childhood syndromes dealt with in these other chapters. Advances in clinical pharmacology, a better understanding of the molecular mechanisms involved in epileptogenesis, and a more precise diagnosis of the specific aetiologies and of epilepsy syndromes, have allowed more rational treatment choices. Childhood-onset epilepsies encompass all known seizure types: focal seizures, epileptic spasms, typical and atypical absences, myoclonic, tonic, atonic, clonic, and tonic–clonic seizures. Epilepsies starting in adolescence will manifest with focal, myoclonic, generalized tonic–clonic seizures (GTCSs) or, rarely, absence seizures. Atonic or tonic seizures very rarely start in adolescence. A syndrome-specific response to treatment has been demonstrated to occur in a few of these conditions, including responsiveness to drugs or drug-induced seizure aggravation (1). In a few instances specificity relates to the aetiology of epilepsy, not just its electroclinical pattern of presentation, but this is unusual. An example is infantile spasm secondary to tuberous sclerosis which shows the best response to vigabatrin treatment (2). Carbamazepine is highly effective in nocturnal frontal lobe epilepsy (3).

Knowledge of the main mechanisms of action and spectrum of efficacy of antiepileptic drugs (AEDs), and correct syndrome diagnosis are therefore essential for rationale treatment. However, efficacy and safety data emerging from AED trials in children is difficult to interpret. In most trials, different epilepsy syndromes and aetiologies are lumped together, and the studies were not designed in general to detect worsening of seizures or specific reactions in different syndromes. Furthermore, finding that two or more drugs are equivalent when compared to one another on 'newly diagnosed' cases, does not rule out the possibility that all drugs are relatively ineffective and that spontaneous remissions or improvements significantly influence the results. Information on drug safety in children is scanty as AEDs are marketed for children only if they appear promising in adults, with considerable delay.

When to start treatment

The decision to start treating a child with epilepsy should ideally be tailored to the individual patient. Some seizure types, such as absences, spasms, or tonic seizures, are always frequent and once their presence is ascertained, treatment should be started. Analogously, the aetiology of epilepsy should be taken into account, as some epileptogenic conditions, especially cortical dysplasia, are associated with a very high seizure recurrence risk and very low chances of prolonged remission. Some conditions appear to be scarcely influenced by AED treatment and this can be the case for both some 'benign' epilepsies and some 'severe encephalopathies'. Ambrosetto and Tassinari (4) showed no clear difference in the total number of seizures suffered by children with rolandic epilepsy, either treated or not. Treatment can be withheld without significant risk in many children with single unprovoked seizures, febrile convulsions, and in adolescents with isolated seizures (5).

However, there are paediatric epilepsy syndromes where delaying treatment may have devastating effects because ongoing clinical or subclinical epileptic activity exerts a disruptive interference on cognitive functioning. Although this is the case with most childhood epileptic encephalopathies, cognitive deterioration may be prominent even when seizures are rare (6).

The risk for accidental death related to severe seizures should also be considered, especially in the neurologically impaired (7).

Setting the targets of treatment: treating benign versus severe epilepsies

The initial approach and the targets of treatment differ considerably, in the most common forms of epilepsy (e.g. absence epilepsy or a mild form of focal epilepsy) and in the severe epileptic encephalopathies (often with multiple seizure types). In the first group, seizure control without adverse events, and in the most convenient and least expensive manner, are reasonable targets. Epileptic encephalopathies present completely different challenges to both the physician's preferences and the patient's efficacy and tolerability response. Vigorous early pharmacological or surgical treatment is often advocated on the assumption that epileptic activity would cause or worsen the encephalopathy per se. However, for many of these conditions there are no established endpoints of treatment and drug adjustments are very empirically established.

Cognitive and behavioural effects of antiepileptic drugs in children

Although a detrimental dose-dependent effect of some AEDs on cognitive functions is self-evident, only a few controlled studies have formally addressed this important point in children (8). Clear evidence has only been obtained about reduction of IQ scores and increased P300 wave latency, an electrophysiological measure of cognitive processing speed reduction, in children treated with phenobarbital (9, 10). Although such effects are believed to be reversible upon drug withdrawal, enduring consequences in academic achievement suggest that prolonged decreases in cognitive processing may not be compensated upon in prospect (10). Carbamazepine does not affect IQ (11), but may slightly impair children's memory, without affecting academic achievement (12, 13). Phenytoin might slightly affect IQ but its effects on academic achievement are unknown (8). The effects of valproate on memory are suggested to be less pronounced than those of phenytoin and carbamazepine (14) but might not have been adequately studied. The neuropsychological effects of new AEDs in children are largely unknown.

Lamotrigine, gabapentin, and levetiracetam, have been reported to increase the risk for aggressive behaviour, especially in cognitively impaired children (8).

Clinical characteristics and response to treatment of the epileptic syndromes of childhood and adolescence

The epileptic encephalopathies (infantile spasms, Lennox–Gastaut syndrome, Dravet syndrome, myoclonic-astatic epilepsy, and epilepsy with continuous spikes and waves during sleep) and their treatment are considered in Chapter 7.

Focal epilepsies and epileptic syndromes

Idiopathic focal epilepsies

Idiopathic focal epilepsies are the most frequently occurring epilepsy syndromes in children. They have an age-dependent course and may occur in more than one family member. Seizures are usually brief and can cluster at the onset. Response to AEDs is usually satisfactory but it is unclear whether treatment influences the long-term outcome. Therapy is not necessarily needed if seizures are infrequent, but is required if seizures are prolonged or if secondarily generalized. Parents usually accept withholding treatment if it is explained that the disorder is self-limiting and does not induce brain damage. Carbamazepine or valproate is usually the preferred option (15) but no controlled trials are available.

Benign epilepsy of childhood with centrotemporal spikes (BECTS) represents 8–23% of childhood epilepsies (16). Seizure onset is between 3–13 years. Prognosis is excellent with remission within adolescence in all patients (17). Typical seizures cause arousal soon after falling asleep, with lateralized facial contraction, anarthria, dribbling, and a grunting sound, without loss of consciousness. Sometimes the homolateral upper limb is involved. Secondary generalization can supervene. Interictal electroencephalogram (EEG) shows typical biphasic centrotemporal spikes, with a tangential dipolar distribution, which often become bilateral during sleep. The total number of seizures a child will suffer is variable but AED treatment can often be avoided (4). Atypical forms are not rare and can be associated with atonic seizures and unusual EEG characteristics (18). Some EEG features, particularly spike and wave discharges instead of the more typical rolandic sharp waves, may predict a complicated evolution, including a paradoxical aggravation under carbamazepine treatment (19).

Benign epilepsy of childhood with occipital paroxysms was originally described as a form of focal epilepsy with age at onset between 2–17 years, visual ictal symptoms, such as illusions, elementary hallucinations, and blindness, evolving either to hemiclonic or complex partial seizures with possible generalization and migraine-type postictal headache (20). Remission occurs by adulthood. Interictal EEG shows unilateral or bilateral occipital spike-and-waves, facilitated by eye closure. This forms accounts for no more than about 1% of epilepsies.

A different, more frequent form of childhood idiopathic occipital epilepsy, observed in about 3% of all children with epilepsy, appears between 2–8 years with prolonged seizures appearing during sleep, with tonic eye and head deviation, ictal vomiting, and hemiclonic jerks or generalization (21). Prominent autonomic manifestations and the inconstant presence of the typical occipital EEG abnormalities have cast some doubts on the occipital origin of seizures in all patients (22). Severe prolonged autonomic seizures may require differential diagnosis with acute symptomatic seizures or abdominal emergencies (23). Treatment is rarely necessary, with most children remitting by the age of 12, after presenting just a few seizures (21). EEG and clinical manifestations are not as specific and constantly present as those of BECTS (22, 24), which makes it mandatory to rule out a symptomatic origin.

Symptomatic focal epilepsies

Symptomatic focal epilepsies account for about 40% of all epilepsies in children (25) and are defined according to seizure semiology pointing to lobar location. However, the epileptogenic area itself can involve multilobar networks. Seizures can include a single symptom or have complex symptomatology. The sequence of events is related to the origin and propagation of the discharge but in young children ictal symptoms can be limited to reduced activity and interaction with motionless staring and unresponsiveness, which reflects extensive seizure spread but not the origin or distribution. Postictal sleepiness is frequent and has a major significance for differential diagnosis. The surface EEG may be misleading.

Attributing seizure origin to a specific area is difficult when neuroimaging is normal, unless a highly characteristic clustering of symptoms occurs. Focal symptomatic epilepsies are usually defined by seizure characteristics and only a few specific syndromes are identifiable.

Mesial temporal lobe epilepsy is the best defined focal symptomatic epilepsy syndrome. Most affected children have hippocampal sclerosis, which is visible on magnetic resonance imaging

(MRI) (26) and about 40% of these have a history of prolonged febrile convulsions (27). Seizures start in school age or earlier (28). Typical episodes include an initial rising epigastric sensation with fear, oro-alimentary automatisms (chewing, swallowing, lip smacking), alteration of consciousness with staring, and postictal confusion (29). Aphasia is often observed when the dominant hemisphere is involved. In infants and small children reduction of motor activity may be the prominent feature, without automatisms (so called 'hypomotor seizures') (30). Interictal EEGs can be normal or show unilateral or bilateral temporal abnormalities. Memory disturbances are common but are difficult to demonstrate before the child is of school age. Drug resistance is frequent. Anterior temporal lobectomy or more selective resections give excellent results in about 80% of children (29).

Frontal lobe epilepsy is relatively frequent in children. Seizures are usually sleep related and brief, lasting seconds to tens of seconds, with complex motor manifestations. They are highly stereotyped in the same patient. Arousal from sleep, with opening of the eyes and a frightened expression is often the first ictal manifestation (31). Consciousness disruption is variable but postictal recovery of awareness is usually fast. Subjective symptoms are ill defined. Onset of motor phenomena is with tonic asymmetric posturing or repetitive 'hyperkinetic' automatisms. Most children also exhibit organized movements of the proximal limbs (so-called '*hypermotor seizures*') (32). Epileptic nocturnal wanderings are longer attacks (2–3 minutes) with arousal from sleep and an ambulatory behaviour during which a frightened child may scream and attempt to escape (33). Ictal fear is often misdiagnosed as pavor nocturnus. Frontal lobe seizures in the awake child may cause violent drop attacks (34). Interictal and even ictal EEG is often normal, or shows abnormalities that enable neither lateralization nor localization (32).

Occipital lobe epilepsy of symptomatic origin may be difficult to diagnose in children because seizure spread masks initial symptoms (35). Ictal elementary visual hallucinations (coloured blobs, flashes of light) associated to peripheral visual field deficit (hemianopia) are typical (36). Lateral movements of the eyes, either oculoclonic or tonic, are frequent. Perinatal ischemic insults and cortical malformations are the most frequent causes (35). Sturge–Weber syndrome, coeliac disease, Lafora disease, and mitochondrial disorders also cause occipital seizures. Interictal EEG abnormalities are usually increased during eye-closure. Early differential diagnosis from idiopathic occipital epilepsy may be difficult and requires an MRI study.

Pharmacological treatment of focal epilepsies in children and adolescents

Monotherapy with valproate or carbamazepine have shown similar effectiveness and good tolerability in children with newly diagnosed focal epilepsy with or without secondary generalization (37). In one study, phenytoin, phenobarbital, carbamazepine, and valproate have comparable efficacy, with 20% of children being seizure free and 73% achieving a 1-year remission by 3 years of follow-up (38). However, the severe sedative side effects of phenobarbital and less good tolerability of phenytoin, make these two drugs unsuitable first choices. In two studies, vigabatrin had an efficacy comparable to carbamazepine, but was better tolerated (39, 40). However, the potential for irreversible visual field defects (41) now limits the use of vigabatrin to a few selected, very severe cases. Most of the newer drugs can also be used in monotherapy, but very few comparative controlled trials are available in children (42). Two class I studies used topiramate in children older than 3 years (43) or older than 6 years (44) with new or recently diagnosed focal epilepsy. In one study, higher doses of topiramate were more effective than lower doses (43). In the second study, topiramate at doses of 100 and 200 mg/day was equivalent in safety to 600 mg carbamazepine and 1250 mg valproate (44). Use of fixed doses, however, is flawed with respect to optimization dose studies. Oxcarbazepine and phenytoin had comparable efficacy, but the discontinuation rate was higher for phenytoin (45).

Studies on heterogeneous groups, such as it can be 'newly diagnosed focal epilepsy', may mask specific drug effects on aetiologically homogeneous syndromes. In spite of this limitation, from the range of available studies it is recommended that children with newly diagnosed focal epilepsy are initiated on either carbamazepine or valproate and that topiramate is considered as an alternative monotherapy (42). Lamotrigine and gabapentin are also potentially interesting initial monotherapies, although only two class I studies are available in adults, which did not include children. Evidence about the effectiveness of monotherapy with tiagabine, levetiracetam, and zonisamide is still insufficient.

Controlled trials in pharmacoresistant focal epilepsies have demonstrated the efficacy of add-on topiramate (46), lamotrigine (47), oxcarbazepine (48), gabapentin (49), and clobazam (50, 51). Development of tolerance after a few months seems to hamper the long-term use of clobazam. Evidence about add-on efficacy of levetiracetam, tiagabine, and zonisamide is insufficient.

While assessing the patient's response to the different drugs, it is wise to explore whether a surgical option is possible. However, as there are many drugs now available, a deadline of about 2 years (52) should be set within which surgery will be performed.

Idiopathic generalized epilepsies

Idiopathic generalized epilepsies (IGEs) are frequent and have an age at onset that spans from early childhood to adolescence. They are genetically determined (see Chapter 2). Due to the overlapping features between different IGEs, the term *IGEs with variable phenotypes* has been suggested as all inclusive (53, 54). Social adjustment is usually good but some patients experience learning difficulties. Seizures are primarily generalized absence, myoclonic and tonic–clonic. Interictal EEG abnormalities are generalized spike-and wave or polyspike-and wave discharges at 3 Hz.

Most patients respond to antiepileptic drugs, but response is drug specific. Valproate is effective in about 80% of patients (42) while other drugs for long term treatment, such as ethosuximide, lamotrigine, topiramate and levetiracetam have a more selective action. There is no evidence that any other drug is effective in the absence or myoclonic seizures (42) and some drugs precipitate or worsen these seizure types in specific syndromes (1).

Benign myoclonic epilepsy in infants (BMEI) represents less than 2% of the epilepsies beginning in the first 3 years of life (55). Generalized myoclonic seizures cause nodding or falls in otherwise normal infants. Generalized spike and wave discharges are rare interictally but are always present during jerks. Valproate is effective but treatment is not necessary in mild cases. Use of the term 'benign' is questionable (53) since at follow-up about half of the children have cognitive or behavioural disorders and some develop GTCSs. Distinction from mild forms of myoclonic astatic epilepsy is difficult and in some cases the two forms can merge (56).

Childhood absence epilepsy and juvenile absence epilepsy

Childhood absence epilepsy represents about 12% of childhood epilepsy (57). Onset is in school age. A genetic background is often observed (see Chapter 2). Very frequent, typical absence seizures (up to hundreds per day) are observed, lasting about 10 seconds, accompanied by rhythmic 3 Hz generalized spike and wave discharges. Absences disappear before adulthood in up to 90% of patients in which no other seizure types are associated (58). If absences persist, GTCSs usually appear. Early and late onset (below 4 years and above age 9), initial drug resistance, associated photosensitivity and subsequent appearance of other neurological symptoms are related to a less favourable prognosis (59, 60). Early-onset absence seizures may be an isolated expression of glucose transporter type1 (GLUT-1) deficiency syndrome, due to mutations of the *SLC2* gene (61). Recognition of this condition is particularly important as initiation of the ketogenic diet produces a dramatic clinical improvement (62).

Juvenile absence epilepsy starts around age 10–12. Its clinical manifestations and those of juvenile myoclonic epilepsy are partially overlapping. Absence seizures cluster upon awakening (63). GTCSs, often precipitated by sleep deprivation, occur in up to 80% of patients and photosensitivity in 20% (64). Absences tend to remit within a few years but GTCSs may recur, especially following sleep deprivation. The long-term prognosis is unclear.

In two early comparative trials, valproate and ethosuximide showed similar efficacy controlling absence seizures (65, 66). Lamotrigine was effective as monotherapy in a double blind trial of new-onset absence seizures (67) and was also effective as an add-on treatment of resistant absence seizures (68). However, such trials were not considered to provide sufficient evidence to inform clinical practice (69). A more recent trial confirmed previous results, showing that valproate and ethosuximide are more effective than lamotrigine but also suggested that ethosuximide has fewer adverse attentional effects than valproate (70). Some children may require combinations of drugs.

Epilepsy with myoclonic absences is a rare disorder (around 0.5–1% of epilepsy) with onset between age 1–12 years (71). About 50% of children have pre-existing cognitive impairment. Myoclonic absences appear several times per day, as rhythmic jerking of shoulders, head, and arms. Impairment of consciousness is variable. The EEG findings are identical to those in childhood absence epilepsy. Evolution to different seizure types with cognitive impairment occurs in about 60% of children. A combination of valproate and ethosuximide seems to be the most effective treatment (72). Myoclonic absences are also observed in symptomatic forms of epilepsies with variable aetiologies, where they represent just one seizure type, often amongst others.

Juvenile myoclonic epilepsy (JME) represents about 2% of epilepsies (57) and is a genetically determined syndrome (see Chapter 2). Peak incidence is between 12–18 years. The clinical presentation is often with myoclonic jerks which involve the proximal limbs and cause dropping of objects on awakening. GTCSs occur in 90% of patients, with an average frequency of two per year (73), often following sleep deprivation. It is not unusual that the myoclonic jerks are recognized for what they are only after a GTCS has occurred. About 35% of patients have absences and 5% photic-induced seizures. Interictal EEG abnormalities are characteristically activated upon awakening (74). AEDs control seizures in 85% of patients (73). Valproate is the drug of choice (75), but primidone, and benzodiazepines have proven useful alternatives (73). Add-on levetiracetam has been reported to reduce myoclonic jerks in one trial (76). Lamotrigine exacerbated GTCSs in some patients (77). Withdrawal of AEDs is associated to 90% relapse, even late in life (75). Seizure clusters or status epilepticus can be precipitated by withdrawal of effective drugs or by introducing carbamazepine (73), although carbamazepine can improve tonic–clonic seizures when these are refractory to other medication (78).

Epilepsy with seizures precipitated by light stimulation

Visual sensitive (or photosensitive) epilepsies are characterized by seizures precipitated by environmental photic stimuli (79). The age at onset peaks at 11 years. Sensitivity to visual stimuli is associated with the inability of the visual cortex to process afferent inputs of high luminance and contrast through the normal mechanisms of cortical gain control (80).

Photic-induced absences, myoclonic seizures, and GTCs are typically observed in the idiopathic generalized epilepsies and in Dravet syndrome (81) but can rarely be observed in patients with other types of epilepsy. Single or repeated seizures while playing video games or in front of the television (especially with a 50 Hz screen) can be observed in children without a history of spontaneous seizures. They manifest as either GTCSs or prolonged attacks with visual symptoms and vomiting (82). An outbreak was reported in Japan, where several hundred children and adolescents experienced a seizure while watching television broadcasting a popular cartoon (83). Self-induction is possible, especially in children with absences or myoclonic jerks who indulge in compulsively staring or blinking in front of light sources or contrasted patterns.

If attacks are infrequent, preventive measures can be sufficient. Video games should be avoided. The triggering power of 50 Hz television screens is lowered by increasing the ambient light and by watching at a distance greater than 2.5 metres; 100 Hz television screens are much less provocative (84). If treatment is necessary, sodium valproate is the drug of choice (85). Preliminary results have also been obtained with levetiracetam (86). Polarized glasses or optical filters for screens have proven helpful in severe cases (87, 88).

Ketogenic diet

The ketogenic diet is widely used to treat children with severe drug-resistant epilepsies, especially the epileptic encephalopathies (89) but no comparative trials are available. The diet has shown some efficacy in a randomized clinical trial and is worth trying in drug-resistant cases (90), although no specific syndrome has shown to respond better than others and assessment of risk and benefits requires further study. The mechanisms of action are not known but the predominantly fat nutrition maintains ketosis in the long term and high concentrations of ketone bodies have been correlated with better seizure control. The diet may result too restrictive, and cause diarrhoea, vitamin deficiency, renal stones, and cardiac complications (91).

Surgical treatment

Some of children who are refractory to AEDs may benefit from surgical treatment and the benefits of early intervention have been emphasized. However, the average delay from seizure onset to surgery is too long, ranging from 12–15 years (92).

The aim of surgery is to reach complete control or to significantly reduce seizure frequency, while minimizing the harmful effects of epileptic activity and of AEDs on cognitive functions. *Resective surgery,* implies removal of the neuronal aggregate that is responsible for seizure generation; *palliative* or *functional surgery* aims at preventing or limiting propagation of seizure activity, without targeting seizure control.

Identifying a child who can benefit from surgery involves several steps. Medical intractability should be ascertained, possibly limited to the more appropriate drugs. Idiopathic and non-lesional genetic epilepsies should be ruled out as surgery is contraindicated in these cases. The level of seizure-related disability should be established on the basis of each patient's clinical presentation.

Resective surgery

An intervention is only possible if no independent epileptogenicity is detected outside the planned resection area and if any resulting neurological deficit is no more invalidating than epilepsy itself. Clinical, video-EEG telemetry, neuropsychological assessment, and high-resolution MRI should provide a consistent localization of the epileptogenic zone, i.e. the network of abnormally behaving neurons, usually distributed within a relatively large brain volume (93). The epileptogenic zone includes the *ictal onset zone,* which is the neurophysiologically defined cortical area in which seizures are initiated, but does not necessarily correspond to the *epileptogenic lesion*, which is anatomically defined. Defining the *symptom-producing zone*, i.e. the area of the brain that produces initial clinical manifestations, the *zone of functional alteration,* which is outlined by functional techniques (e.g. by EEG, positron emission tomography (PET), or single-positron emission computed tomography (SPECT)), and the *irritative zone*, i.e. the area over which paroxysmal EEG activity is recorded, may help better delineate the epileptogenic zone. Removal of an epileptogenic lesion, without defining and removing the epileptogenic zone ('lesionectomy'), produces seizure control in a significant proportion of children (94) but delineation and removal of the entire epileptogenic zone, or at least the ictal onset zone, improves the outcome of lesionectomy. Surgery should be considered only very cautiously in the face of a normal high-resolution MRI scan (25).

In cooperative children, functional MRI is used to map the motor and sensory cortex and is now preferred to the Wada intracarotid amytal test for evaluating hemispheric language dominance (95). In selected cases, MRI spectroscopy, EEG triggered functional MRI, ictal and interictal SPECT, and PET can help improve the surgical planning. Intracranial EEG recordings are reserved to cases in which doubts persist on the localization and extension of the resection. Use of stereotactically implanted depth electrodes or subdural grids, depends on the preoperative hypothesis about seizure origin and propagation.

Anterior temporal lobectomy is the most common operation and provides the best results (29). Extratemporal cortical resections yield excellent results in well-selected lesional cases. Seizure freedom is higher after temporal resection (78%) than after extratemporal or multilobar resections (54%) and in children with tumours (82%) than in those with cortical malformations (52%) (96). Hemispherectomy (or hemispherotomy) controls seizures in about 82% of children with acquired lesions, in 50% of those with a progressive disorder, and in 31% of those with malformations (97). These results are obtained at the cost of worsening any pre-existing hemiplegia and visual field defect. Hemispherotomy (hemispheric disconnection) is now preferred to hemispherectomy in an increasing number of centres.

Palliative surgery

Corpus callosotomy is a midline disconnection procedure, aimed at inhibiting interhemispheric seizure spread in patients with disabling seizures with falls due to bilateral synchronization. In order to limit disconnection symptoms, the anterior two-thirds of the corpus are sectioned. Complete section can be carried out at a second operation if anterior resection is ineffective. Focal seizures may persist after the procedure but impairment related to falling to the ground can be reduced (98).

Vagus nerve stimulation is used as an adjunct to treat drug-resistant epilepsy. A stimulator is placed under the skin and emanates adjustable pulsed stimuli to an electrode that is wrapped around the left vagus nerve (99). Interesting results have been obtained in children with severe epilepsies that are not treatable by surgery but epilepsy syndromes that are likely to benefit electively are still undetermined. Adverse effects of hoarseness, cough, and pain are usually reasonably well tolerated.

References

1. Guerrini R, Belmonte A, Genton P. Antiepileptic drug-induced worsening of seizures in children. *Epilepsia* 1998; 39(suppl 3): 2–10.
2. Chiron C, Dumas C, Jambaque I, Mumford J, Dulac O. Randomised trial comparing vigabatrin and hydrocortisone in infantile spasms due to tuberous sclerosis. *Epilepsy Res* 1997; 26: 389–95.
3. Picard F, Bertrand S, Steinlein OK, Bertrand D. Mutated nicotinic receptors responsible for autosomal dominant nocturnal frontal lobe epilepsy are more sensitive to carbamazepine. *Epilepsia* 1999; 40:1198–209.
4. Ambrosetto G, Tassinari CA. Antiepileptic drug treatment of benign childhood epilepsy with rolandic spikes: Is it necessary? *Epilepsia* 1990; 31: 802–5.
5. Camfield PR, Camfield CS. Treatment of children with 'ordinary' epilepsy. *Epileptic Disord* 2000; 2:45–51.
6. Deonna T, Roulet-Perez E. Early-onset acquired epileptic aphasia (Landau-Kleffner syndrome, LKS) and regressive autistic disorders with epileptic EEG abnormalities: the continuing debate. *Brain Dev* 2010; 32(9):746–52.
7. Camfield CS, Camfield PR, Veugelers PJ. Death in children with epilepsy: a population-based study. *Lancet* 2002; 359:1891–5.
8. Loring DW, Meador KJ. Cognitive side effects of antiepileptic drugs in children. *Neurology* 2004; 62:872–7.
9. Farwell JR, Lee YJ, Hirtz DG, Sulzbacher SI, Ellenberg JH, Nelson KB. Phenobarbital for febrile seizures—effects on intelligence and on seizure recurrence. *N Engl J Med* 1990; 322:364–9.
10. Sulzbacher S, Farwell JR, Temkin N, Lu AS, Hirtz DG. Late cognitive effects of early treatment with phenobarbital. *Clin Pediatr* 1999; 38:387–94.
11. Riva D, Devoti M. Carbamazepine withdrawal in children with previous symptomatic partial epilepsy: effects on neuropsychologic function. *J Child Neurol* 1999; 14:357–62.
12. Seidel WT, Mitchell WG. Cognitive and behavioral effects of carbamazepine in children: data from benign rolandic epilepsy. *J Child Neurol* 1999; 14:716–23.
13. Bailet LL, Turk WR. The impact of childhood epilepsy on neurocognitive and behavioral performance: a prospective longitudinal study. *Epilepsia* 2000; 41:426–31.

14. Forsythe I, Butler R, Berg I, McGuire R. Cognitive impairment in new cases of epilepsy randomly assigned to carbamazepine, phenytoin and sodium valproate. *Dev Med Child Neurol* 1991; 33:524–34.
15. Lerman P. Benign partial epilepsy with centro-temporal spikes. In: Roger J, Bureau M, Dravet C, Dreifuss FE, Perret A, Wolf P (eds) *Epileptic Syndromes in Infancy, Childhood and Adolescence* (2nd edn), pp. 189–200. London: John Libbey, 1992.
16. Dalla Bernardina B, Sgro V, Fejerman N. Epilepsy with central temporal spikes and related syndromes. In: Roger J, Bureau M, Dravet C, Genton P, Tassinari CA, Wolf P (eds) *Epileptic Syndromes in Infancy, Childhood and Adolescence* (3rd edn), pp. 181–202. London: John Libbey, 2002.
17. Bouma PA, Bovenkerk AC, Westendorp RG, Brouwer OF. The course of benign partial epilepsy of childhood with centrotemporal spikes: a meta-analysis. *Neurology* 1997; 48:430–7.
18. Massa R, de Saint-Martin A, Carcangiu R, Rudolf G, Seegmuller C, Kleitz C, *et al.* EEG criteria predictive of cognitive complications in idiopathic focal epilepsy with rolandic spikes. *Neurology* 2001; 57: 1071–9.
19. Parmeggiani L, Seri S, Bonanni P, Guerrini R. Electrophysiological characterization of spontaneous and carbamazepine-induced epileptic negative myoclonus in benign childhood epilepsy with centro-temporal spikes. *Clin Neurophysiol* 2004; 115:50–8.
20. Gastaut H. Benign epilepsy of childhood with occipital paroxysms. In: Roger J, Dravet, C, Bureau M, Dreifuss FE, Perret A, Wolf P (eds) *Epileptic Syndromes in Infancy, Childhood and Adolescence* (2nd edn), pp. 201–17. London: John Libbey, 1992.
21. Ferrie CD, Beaumanoir A, Guerrini R, Kivity S, Vigevano F, Takaishi Y. Early-onset benign occipital seizure susceptibility syndrome. *Epilepsia* 1997; 38: 285–93.
22. Panayiotopoulos CP, Michael M, Sanders S, Valeta T, Koutroumanidis M. Benign childhood focal epilepsies: assessment of established and newly recognized syndromes. *Brain* 2008; 131:2264–86.
23. Arzimanoglou A, Guerrini R, Aicardi J. *Epilepsy in Children* (3rd edn). Philadelphia, PA: Lippincott-Williams & Wilkins, 2004.
24. Guerrini R, Belmonte A, Veggiotti P, Mattia D, Bonanni P. Delayed appearance of interictal EEG abnormalities in early onset childhood epilepsy with occipital paroxysms. *Brain Dev* 1997; 19:343–6.
25. Guerrini R. Epilepsy in children. *Lancet* 2006 11; 367:499–524.
26. Harvey AS, Berkovic SF, Wrennall JA, Hopkins IJ. Temporal lobe epilepsy in childhood: clinical, EEG, and neuroimaging findings and syndrome classification in a cohort with new-onset seizures. *Neurology* 1997; 49:960–8.
27. Kuks JBM, Cook MD, Fish DR, Stevens JM, Shorvon SD. Hippocampal sclerosis in epilepsy and childhood febrile seizures. *Lancet* 1993; 342: 1391–4.
28. Harvey AS, Grattan-Smith JD, Desmond PM, Chow CW, Berkovic SF. Febrile seizures and hippocampal sclerosis: frequent and related findings in intractable temporal lobe epilepsy of childhood. *Pediatr Neurol* 1995; 12: 201–6.
29. Mohamed A, Wyllie E, Ruggieri P, Kotagal P, Babb T, Hilbig A, *et al.* Temporal lobe epilepsy due to hippocampal sclerosis in pediatric candidates for epilepsy surgery. *Neurology* 2001; 56:1643–9.
30. Hamer HM, Wyllie E, Lüders HO, Kotagal P, Acharya J. Symptomatology of epileptic seizures in the first three years of life. *Epilepsia* 1999; 40: 837–44.
31. Vigevano F, Fusco L. Hypnic tonic postural seizures in healthy children provide evidence for a partial epileptic syndrome of frontal origin. *Epilepsia* 1993; 34: 110–19.
32. Holthausen H, Hoppe M. Hypermotor seizures. In: Lüders HO, Noachtar S (eds) *Epileptic Seizures: Pathophysiology and Clinical Semiology*, pp. 439–48. Philadelphia, PA: Churchill Livingstone, 2000.
33. Plazzi G, Tinuper P, Montagna P, Provini F, Lugaresi E. Epileptic nocturnal wandering. *Sleep* 1995; 18: 749–56.
34. Biraben A, Chauvel P. Falls in epileptic seizures with partial onset. In: Beaumanoir A, Andermann F, Avanzini G, Mira L (eds) *Falls in epileptic and non-epileptic seizures during childhood*, pp. 125–35. London: John Libbey & Company Ltd, 1997.
35. Guerrini R, Parmeggiani L, Berta E, Munari C. Occipital lobe seizures. In: Oxbury JM, Polkey CE, Duchowny MS (eds) *Intractable focal epilepsy: medical and surgical treatment*, pp. 77–88. London: Saunders & Co, 2000.
36. Williamson PD, Thadani VM, Darcey TM, Spencer DD, Spencer SS, Mattson RH. Occipital lobe epilepsy: Clinical characteristics, seizure spread patterns, and results of surgery. *Ann Neurol* 1992; 31:3–13.
37. Verity CM, Hosking G, Easter DJ. A multicentre comparative trial of sodium valproate and carbamazepine in paediatric epilepsy. The paeditric EPITEG collaborative Group. *Dev Med Child Neurol* 1995; 37: 97–108.
38. de Silva M, MacArdle B, McGowan M, Hughes E, Stewart J, Neville BG, *et al.* Randomised comparative monotherapy trial of phenobarbitone, phenytoin, carbamazepine, or sodium valproate for newly diagnosed childhood epilepsy. *Lancet* 1996; 347:709–13.
39. Gobbi G, Pini A, Bertani G, Menegati E, Tiberti A, Valseriati D, *et al.* Prospective study of first-line vigabatrin monotherapy in childhood partial epilepsies. *Epilepsy Res* 1999; 35:29–37.
40. Zamponi N, Cardinali C. Open comparative long-term study of vigabatrin vs carbamazepine in newly diagnosed partial seizures in children. *Arch Neurol* 1999; 56:605–7.
41. Kälviäinen R, Nousiainen I, Mantyjarvi M, Nikoskelainen E, Partanen J, Partanen K, *et al.* Vigabatrin, a GABAergic antiepileptic drug, causes concentric visual field defects. *Neurology* 1999; 53:922–6.
42. French JA, Kanner AM, Bautista J, Abou-Khalil B, Browne T, Harden CL, *et al.* Efficacy and tolerability of the new antiepileptic drugs I: treatment of new onset epilepsy: report of the Therapeutics and Technology Assessment Subcommittee and Quality Standards Subcommittee of the American Academy of Neurology and the American Epilepsy Society. *Neurology* 2004; 62:1252–60.
43. Gilliam FG, Veloso F, Bomhof MA, Gazda SK, Biton V, Ter Bruggen JP, *et al.* A dose-comparison trial of topiramate as monotherapy in recently diagnosed partial epilepsy. *Neurology* 2003; 60:196–202.
44. Privitera MD, Brodie MJ, Mattson RH, Chadwick DW, Neto W, Wang S; EPMN 105 Study Group. Topiramate, carbamazepine and valproate monotherapy: double-blind comparison in newly diagnosed epilepsy. *Acta Neurol Scand* 2003; 107:165–75.
45. Guerreiro MM, Vigonius U, Pohlmann H, de Manreza ML, Fejerman N, Antoniuk SA, *et al.* A double-blind controlled clinical trial of oxcarbazepine versus phenytoin in children and adolescents with epilepsy. *Epilepsy Res* 1997; 27:205–13.
46. Elterman RD, Glauser TA, Wyllie E, Reife R, Wu SC, Pledger G. A double-blind, randomized trial of topiramate as adjunctive therapy for partial-onset seizures in children. Topiramate YP Study Group. *Neurology* 1999; 52:1338–44.
47. Duchowny M, Pellock JM, Graf WD, Billard C, Gilman J, Casale E, *et al.* A placebo-controlled trial of lamotrigine add-on therapy for partial seizures in children. Lamictal Pediatric Partial Seizure Study Group. *Neurology* 1999; 53:1724–31.
48. Glauser TA, Nigro M, Sachdeo R, Pasteris LA, Weinstein S, Abou-Khalil B, *et al.* Adjunctive therapy with oxcarbazepine in children with partial seizures. The Oxcarbazepine Pediatric Study Group. *Neurology* 2000; 54: 2237–44.
49. Appleton R, Fichtner K, LaMoreaux L, Alexander J, Maton S, Murray G, Garofalo E. Gabapentin as add-on therapy in children with refractory partial seizures: a 24-week, multicentre, open-label study. *Dev Med Child Neurol* 2001; 43:269–73.
50. Allen JW, Oxley J, Robertson MM, Trimble MR, Richens A, Jawad SS. Clobazam adjunctive treatment in refractory epilepsy. *Brit Med J* 1983; 286:1246–7.

51. Keene DL, Whiting S, Humphreys P. Clobazam as an add-on drug in the treatment of refractory epilepsy of childhood. *Can J Neurol Sci* 1990; 17:317–19.
52. Berg AT, Langfitt J, Shinnar S, Vickrey BG, Sperling MR, Walczak T, *et al.* How long does it take for partial epilepsy to become intractable? *Neurology* 2003; 60:186–90.
53. Engel J Jr. International League Against Epilepsy (ILAE). A proposed diagnostic scheme for people with epileptic seizures and with epilepsy: report of the ILAE Task Force on Classification and Terminology. *Epilepsia* 2001; 42: 796–803.
54. Engel J Jr. Report of the ILAE classification core group. *Epilepsia* 2006; 47:1558–68.
55. Dravet C, Bureau M. Benign myoclonic epilepsy in infancy. *Adv Neurol* 2005; 95:127–37.
56. Guerrini R, Aicardi J. Epileptic encephalopathies with myoclonic seizures in infants and children (severe myoclonic epilepsy and myoclonic-astatic epilepsy). *J Clin Neurophysiol* 2003; 20:449–61.
57. Berg AT, Shinnar S, Levy SR, Testa FM. Newly diagnosed epilepsy in children: presentation at diagnosis. *Epilepsia* 1999; 40:445–52.
58. Guiwer J, Valenti MP, Bourazza A, Hirsch, E., Loiseau, P. Prognosis of idiopathic absence epilepsies. In: Jallon P, Berg A, Dulac O, Hauser A (eds) *Prognosis of Epilepsies*, pp. 249–57. Paris: John Libbey, 2003.
59. Caraballo RH, Darra F, Fontana E, Garcia R, Monese E, Dalla Bernardina B. Absence seizures in the first 3 years of life: an electroclinical study of 46 cases. *Epilepsia* 2011; 52:393–400.
60. Guerrini R, Sanchez-Carpintero R, Deonna T, Santucci M, Bhatia KP, Moreno T, *et al.* Early-onset absence epilepsy and paroxysmal dyskinesia. *Epilepsia* 2002; 43:1224–9.
61. Suls A, Mullen SA, Weber YG, Verhaert K, Ceulemans B, Guerrini R, *et al.* Early-onset absence epilepsy caused by mutations in the glucose transporter GLUT1. *Ann Neurol* 2009; 66:415–19.
62. Wang D, Pascual JM, Yang H, Engelstad K, Jhung S, Sun RP, De Vivo DC. Glut-1 deficiency syndrome: clinical, genetic, and therapeutic aspects. *Ann Neurol* 2005; 57:111–18.
63. Wolf P, Inoue Y. Juvenile absence epilepsy. In: Roger J, Bureau M, Dravet C, Genton P, Tassinari CA, Wolf P (eds) *Epileptic Syndromes in Infancy, Childhood and Adolescence* (3rd edn), pp. 331–4. London: John Libbey, 2002.
64. Wolf P, Gooses R. Relation of photosensitivity to epileptic syndromes. *J Neurol Neurosurg Psychiatry* 1986; 49:1386–91.
65. Sato W, White BG, Penry JK, Dreifuss FE, Sackellares JC, Kupferberg HJ. Valproic acid versus ethosuximide in the treatment of absence seizures. *Neurology* 1982; 32:157–63.
66. Callaghan N, O'Hare J, O'Driscoll D, O'Neill B, Daly M. Comparative study of ethosuximide and sodium valproate in the treatment of typical absence seizures (Petit Mal). *Dev Med Child Neurol* 1982; 24:830–6.
67. Frank LM, Enlow T, Holmes GL, Manasco P, Concannon S, Chen C, *et al.* Lamictal (lamotrigine) monotherapy for typical absence seizures in children. *Epilepsia* 1999; 40:973–9.
68. Besag FM, Wallace SJ, Dulac O, Alving J, Spencer SC, Hosking G. Lamotrigine for the treatment of epilepsy in childhood. *J Pediatr* 1995; 127:991–7.
69. Posner EB, Mohamed K, Marson AG. Ethosuximide, sodium valproate or lamotrigine for absence seizures in children and adolescents. *Cochrane Database Syst Rev* 2003; 4:CD003032.
70. Glauser TA, Cnaan A, Shinnar S, Hirtz DG, Dlugos D, Masur D, *et al.* Childhood Absence Epilepsy Study Group. Ethosuximide, valproic acid, and lamotrigine in childhood absence epilepsy. *N Engl J Med* 2010; 362:790–9.
71. Bureau M, Tassinari CA. Epilepsy with myoclonic absences. In: Roger J, Bureau M, Dravet C, Genton P, Tassinari CA, Wolf P (eds) *Epileptic Syndromes in Infancy, Childhood and Adolescence* (3rd edn), pp. 305–12. London: John Libbey, 2002.
72. Bureau M, Tassinari CA. Epilepsy with myoclonic absences. *Brain Dev* 2005; 27(3):178–84.
73. Thomas P, Genton P, Gelisse P, Wolf P. Juvenile myoclonic epilepsy. In: Roger J, Bureau M, Dravet C, Genton P, Tassinari CA, Wolf P (eds) *Epileptic syndromes in infancy childhood and adolescence* (3rd edn), pp. 335–56. London:John Libbey, 2002.
74. Fittipaldi F, Curra A, Fusco L, Ruggieri S, Manfredi M. EEG discharges on awakening: a marker of idiopathic generalized epilepsy. *Neurology* 2001; 56:123–6.
75. Nicolson A, Appleton RE, Chadwick DW, Smith DF. The relationship between treatment with valproate, lamotrigine, and topiramate and the prognosis of the idiopathic generalised epilepsies. *J Neurol Neurosurg Psychiatry* 2004; 75(1):75–9.
76. Noachtar S, Andermann E, Meyvisch P, Andermann F, Gough WB, Schiemann-Delgado J. N166 Levetiracetam Study Group. Levetiracetam for the treatment of idiopathic generalized epilepsy with myoclonic seizures. *Neurology* 2008; 70:607–16.
77. Biraben A, Allain H, Scarabin JM, Schück S, Edan G. Exacerbation of juvenile myoclonic epilepsy with lamotrigine. *Neurology* 2000; 55(11):1758.
78. Genton P, Gelisse P, Thomas P, Dravet C. Do carbamazepine and phenytoin aggravate juvenile myoclonic epilepsy? *Neurology* 2000; 55:1106–9.
79. Kasteleijn-Nolst Trenite DG, Guerrini R, Binnie CD, Genton P. Visual sensitivity and epilepsy: a proposed terminology and classification for clinical and EEG phenomenology. *Epilepsia* 2001; 42:692–701.
80. Porciatti V, Bonanni P, Fiorentini A, Guerrini R. Lack of cortical contrast gain control in human photosensitive epilepsy. *Nature Neuroscience* 2000; 3:259–63.
81. Guerrini R, Genton P. Epileptic syndromes and visually induced seizures. *Epilepsia* 2004; 45(Suppl1):14–18.
82. Guerrini R, Dravet C, Genton P, Bureau M, Bonanni P, Ferrari AR, *et al.* Idiopathic photosensitive occipital lobe epilepsy. *Epilepsia* 1995; 36:883–91.
83. Ishiguro Y, Takada H, Watanabe K, Okumura A, Aso K, Ishikawa T. A follow-up survey on seizures induced by animated cartoon TV program 'Pocket Monster'. *Epilepsia* 2004; 45:377–83.
84. Ricci S, Vigevano F, Manfredi M, Kasteleijn-Nolst Trenité DG. Epilepsy provoked by television and video games: Safety of 100 Hz screens. *Neurology* 1998; 50:790–3.
85. Covanis A, Stodieck SR, Wilkins AJ. Treatment of photosensitivity. *Epilepsia* 2004; 45(Suppl 1):40–5.
86. Kasteleijn-Nolst Trenité DG, Marescaux C, Stodieck S, Edelbroek PM, Oosting J. Photosensitive epilepsy: a model to study the effects of antiepileptic drugs. Evaluation of the piracetam analogue, levetiracetam. *Epilepsy Res* 1996; 25(3):225–30.
87. Takahashi Y, Sato Y, Goto K, Fujino M, Fujiwara T, Yamaga M, Isono H, Kondo N. Optical filters inhibiting television-induced photosensitive seizures. *Neurology* 2001; 57:1707–73.
88. Kepecs MR, Boro A, Haut S, Kepecs G, Moshé SL. A novel nonpharmacologic treatment for photosensitive epilepsy: a report of three patients tested with blue cross-polarized glasses. *Epilepsia* 2004; 45:1158–62.
89. Cross JH, Neal EG. The ketogenic diet—update on recent clinical trials. *Epilepsia* 2008; 49(Suppl 8):6–10.
90. Neal EG, Chaffe H, Schwartz RH, Lawson MS, Edwards N, Fitzsimmons G, *et al.* A randomized trial of classical and medium-chain triglyceride ketogenic diets in the treatment of childhood epilepsy. *Epilepsia* 2009; 50:1109–17.
91. Best TH, Franz DN, Gilbert DL, Nelson DP, Epstein MR. Cardiac complications in pediatric patients on the ketogenic diet. *Neurology* 2000; 54:2328–30.
92. Duchowny M. Pediatric epilepsy surgery: the widening spectrum of surgical candidacy. *Epileptic Disord* 1999; 1:143–51.

93. Lüders, H.O., Engel, J., Munari, C. General principles. In: Engel J (ed) *Surgical Treatment of the Epilepsies* (2nd edn), pp. 137–53. New York: Raven Press, 1993.
94. Bourgeois M, Sainte-Rose C, Lellouch-Tubiana A, Malucci C, Brunelle F, Maixner W, *et al.* Surgery of epilepsy associated with focal lesions in childhood. *J Neurosurg* 1999; 90:833–42.
95. Barbier EL, Lamalle L, Decorps M. Methodology of brain perfusion imaging. *J Magn Res Imag* 2001; 13:496–520.
96. Wyllie E. Catastrophic epilepsy in infants and children: identification of surgical candidates. *Epileptic Disord* 1999; 1(4):261–4.
97. Devlin AM, Cross JH, Harkness W, Chong WK, Harding B, Vargha-Khadem F, *et al.* Clinical outcomes of hemispherectomy for epilepsy in childhood and adolescence. *Brain* 2003; 126:556–66.
98. Oguni H, Olivier H, Andermann F, Comair J. Anterior callosotomy in the treatment of medically intractable epilepsies: A study of 43 patients with a mean follow-up of 39 months. *Ann Neurol.* 1991; 30:357–64.
99. Crumrine PK. Vagal nerve stimulation in children. *Semin Pediatr Neurol* 2000; 7:216–23.

CHAPTER 17

Epilepsy in Learning Disability

Tom Berney and Shoumitro Deb

Introduction

This chapter sets out what it is about people with learning disability (LD) and their services that affects their experience of epilepsy and its diagnosis and management.

1. What is it that distinguishes this group from the wider population and, in many countries, has led to the development of specialist psychiatric and social services?
2. How does this affect the diagnosis and management of epilepsy?

The nature of learning disability

The generic needs of people with LD and the services that developed in response have encouraged us to think of a discrete population. However, although cognitive ability (assessed by intelligence quotient (IQ)) has become the most widely used administrative characteristic, other qualities contribute to defining the group, particularly the person's ability to function and cope with everyday life (measured by scales such as the Vineland Adaptive Behaviour Scales) and this will vary with their circumstances, personality, and motivation. For example, someone with a mild degree of generalized LD may be unable to meet the academic demands of school but thereafter cope well enough with marriage and employment. Of those with LD, about 75–90% will have it in a mild degree (IQ = 55–70), about 1.1–1.6% of the general population, the exact figure depending on the age and circumstances of the group (1). A much smaller proportion, about 0.14% of the population, will have a severe/profound LD (IQ <35). Their aetiology is known for 70–90% of those with severe LD (2) but for only about 50% of those with mild LD.

The group is far from coherent, encompassing not only a wide range of age and ability but also a collection of developmental disabilities of varied form and intensity, giving great individual variation. In common, though, are problems with communication and dependency as well as atypical emotional and behavioural responses. These may form a characteristic pattern associated with the underlying cause of the LD as its behavioural phenotype.

Communication can be very idiosyncratic with large discrepancies between verbal and non-verbal as well as between receptive and expressive abilities. The patient is likely to have difficulty in reporting any adverse effects from treatment as well as a limited capacity to understand its implications. This gives the parent or carer unusual importance in the clinical assessment; they may be the only people who understand what is going on. It also gives doctors an unusual responsibility in making decisions so that they need to ensure that, as far as possible, they have consulted all those concerned.

Comorbidity

The greater the degree of LD, the more likely there are to be other disabilities (including motor and sensory components) and other developmental disabilities, notably autism and attention deficit disorder. It means that a person with LD is likely to have a complex porridge of psychopathology that may extend to include any of the psychiatric disorders found in the general population. Limited communication blocks descriptions of internal, subjective experiences and perceptions making it difficult to diagnose disorders such as schizophrenia or obsessive–compulsive disorder. There is a consequent risk of turning tentative inference and therapeutic trial into firm diagnosis and unjustified treatment.

Rather than a clear, defined psychiatric disorder, the result is often disturbed behaviour, amplified by anxiety or discomfort, which can become sufficiently intense, frequent, or severe as to threaten the physical safety of the individual or those around. At the least, the restrictive or aversive responses affect the quality of their life. All this is summed up in the term 'challenging behaviour' (3).

The prevalence of psychiatric disorder relates to LD and, indeed, is less frequent where epilepsy is present (4–6) although limited studies and variations in methodology make this hard to tease out. For example, where there is both LD and epilepsy, the prevalence of a schizophreniform psychosis ranges from 24% (7) to only 4.4% (5) (as against 6% in those with epilepsy but of normal ability). The range may reflect an additional factor however, the level of seizure control rather than simply the presence of epilepsy; psychosis being more frequent in those who have been seizure free for a period (8). There is also the suggestion that, in these circumstances, psychosis might be associated with mild LD and depression with severe LD.

Prevalence

In the community the prevalence of epilepsy in adults with LD is about 16–26% compared with 0.4–1% in the general population

(9–11). The risk of epilepsy increases with the degree of LD (10) and the presence of other disorders but the effects of age and genetic syndrome are more variable (9, 12). Adults with severe LD are 3–4 times as likely to have epilepsy as those with mild/moderate LD and, similarly, in childhood, 67% of those with severe LD have epilepsy compared to 7% of those with mild to moderate LD (13).

The association means that any overall figure will depend on the distribution of disability in the population surveyed, let alone those of age, aetiology, and accompanying neurological disorders. For example, the presence of cerebral palsy in addition to LD, increases the prevalence 10-fold (14).

Seizures begin before 5 years of age for 65% of people with an LD and before 20 years for a further 30% (15). Thereafter, the prevalence of epilepsy remains relatively constant and, although increased mortality is related to seizure type and frequency, the cause of death seldom relates directly to the seizures (16, 17). The epilepsies in LD tend to be refractory, only a minority becoming seizure free. However, a retrospective study in a specialist epilepsy centre found significant improvement over time with, as might be expected, the greatest shift in those who started with greatest seizure frequency. This found, in contrast with a Finnish study (18), 84% remained seizure free, possibly because of a more cautious approach to weaning people off their medication (19). One recurrent lesson is that successful treatment, particularly in this population, depends on the clinicians' degree of expertise in epilepsy (16, 19).

Tonic–clonic seizures are experienced by 60%, absences by 37%, and myoclonic jerks by 21%; drop attacks and complex partial seizures occurred in only 7% and 6% respectively and nearly half the group had only one type of seizure (15). In adults, however, there is likely to be a much higher prevalence of complex partial seizures (sometimes with secondary generalization) and a lower occurrence of absence seizures and myoclonic jerks. However, certain disorders bring their own characteristic patterns of epilepsy:

- *Tuberous sclerosis*: epilepsy, often intractable, occurs in up to 80–90% of patients, the relationship being summarized in a report by the Tuberous Sclerosis Study group (20).
- *Down syndrome*: at about 0.067% of the general population in the UK, this accounts for about 10–15% of the population with LD. The incidence of epilepsy is increased with a clear bimodal distribution; early-onset epilepsy occurring in about 10% and late-onset epilepsy, starting in adulthood, being associated with dementia (21–24). Of those with dementia, up to 90% have seizures, a higher prevalence than in the comparable non-Down population. Most frequently generalized tonic–clonic seizures, they are accompanied in about 10% of cases by partial complex and myoclonic seizures. Occasionally late-onset progressive myoclonic epilepsy may develop (25); of interest as the gene for Unverricht–Lundborg myoclonic epilepsy has been identified adjacent to the critical site for Down syndrome on chromosome 21 (26). The density of neurofibrillary tangles correlates closely with the presence of seizures and with dementia (27) and, although seizures may start in any phase of Alzheimer's disease, they are a poor prognostic sign, death following within 3–5 years (28).
- *Fragile X syndrome*: occurring in 0.5–4.2% of those with LD, this is the most frequent cause of *inherited* LD. Seizures begin in childhood in about 20% of cases but start in adulthood in a small subgroup raising the question as to whether their emergence may be a complication of later life (29)
- *Prader Willi syndrome*: the result of a failure to express (paternal) genes at 15q11–q13. Seizures occur in up to a quarter of those with this syndrome and may be associated particularly with a deletion genotype (as against uniparental disomy) (30).
- *Angelman syndrome*: seizures start in the first 3 years of life are varied, multiple, and difficult to control (31, 32)
- *Autism*:
  - Epilepsy can certainly make the symptoms of autism worse. The question became whether epilepsy might mimic autism, opening the way to therapeutic trials of antiepileptics for autistic symptomatology. These were unsuccessful and the present perception is that the two disorders may have common causation.
  - A meta-analysis, although hampered by the variable methodology and limited number of cases, confirmed that the prevalence of epilepsy in autism was associated with the degree of LD and was probably more frequent in females (9). However, even after allowing for LD, epilepsy is more frequent in autism compared to the general population.
  - Two categories of autism may be discerned; 80–90% of people have primary/essential autism where there is a greater heritability with a higher incidence in close relatives, no significant dysmorphology, and a higher degree of ability. The other group, secondary/complex/syndromal autism, comprises 10–20% and is associated with underlying medical disorders, dysmorphology, and lower levels of ability; this group is more likely to have epilepsy and, then, a higher seizure frequency.
  - The prevalence of epilepsy in the essential group ranges from 1.3% (33) to 7.4% (34) depending on the population studied. There is a sustained debate about the relationship of autistic regression to the epilepsies although supportive evidence is thin (35, 36).
- *Other disorders*: epilepsy occurs in about 75% of people with Rett syndrome, 50% with Lesch–Nyhan syndrome, 30% with Lowe syndrome, 25% with Rubenstein–Taybi syndrome, and is linked to callosal agenesis in Aicardi syndrome (37).

Behavioural disturbance

Physical discomfort, often the result of an ailment as simple as hay fever, toothache, or tonsillitis, can manifest as an increase in habitual symptomatology, irritability, or aggression and should be excluded at the start in the assessment of disturbed behaviour. Poorly controlled epilepsy can amplify symptomatology and there is the temptation to ascribe every unwanted symptom to it.

The relatively high prevalence of epilepsy and aggression leads to the suspicion that the one may lead to the other and the use of antiepileptic drugs (AEDs) to treat both.

- Ictal aggression is rare in practice and, when it occurs, is usually a defensive automatism directed reflexly at anyone seen as intrusive or threatening (38).
- Episodic dyscontrol syndrome (or intermittent explosive disorder, categorized as an impulse control disorder, 312.34 in the Diagnostic and Statistical Manual of Mental Disorders, 4th edition) is quite separate. That the recurrent, brief changes of state might be seen as analogous to the symptoms of a seizure coupled with a response to AEDs (39, 40) does not mean that this is

epilepsy and, indeed, treatment of associated anxiety and depression may be more fruitful (41). It is reputed to be more frequent in LD although limited communication blocks the subjective account necessary to disentangle this from other mechanisms producing rage.

- Postictal aggression may be a component of the confusional state of someone emerging from a seizure. This twilight state can be overshadowed by the characteristics of LD and those around may assume a greater awareness than is actually present. Their response to disturbed behaviour, applying restraint, for example, becomes inappropriate and unwittingly inflammatory.
- Interictal aggression and irritability probably are part of a wider range of dysphoria that also includes depression, anxiety, and even euphoria (42). While this may represent a prodromal or postictal state, it may become sustained in chronic epilepsy and, at this point, should be treated appropriately. Certain antiepileptic medications are also known anecdotally to cause problem behaviours in people with LD.

Services

LD implies a degree of lifelong dependency requiring varying levels of special education and support which ranges from supplementary input through to outright full-time specialist care in a residential placement. LD services are geared to habilitation that includes not just teaching, training, and supporting the individual but also their family as they come to terms both with their child's disability and then with the process of increasing autonomy. At some stage, the primary responsibility should shift from family to the individual, carers, and specialist services; the arrival of epilepsy compounds the disability, making it doubly difficult for a family to trust others to share the load.

A well-developed service will be a coordinate network of various agencies and disciplines that takes a holistic view of the individual's problems, promoting their independence and ability to take part in decision-making. While encouraging the use of mainstream resources, the emphasis shifts towards domiciliary services, taking them to individuals and those around them rather than being clinic-centred. It is also focused on long-term work rather than discrete episodes of care or treatment; factors that can provide a sound basis for the inclusion of an integrated epilepsy service. The frequency and familiarity of epilepsy in LD means that the services should be well adapted to its day-to-day management.

Service models have changed with the move from institutional to community care. In some areas the initial assessment and ongoing support of epilepsy has passed to neurology in a model of shared care that varies with the expertise and resources of different localities. However, in others, the result has been a detrimental detachment from specialist epilepsy resources (16, 19) that highlight the importance for hospital and community services to establish a clear, formal protocol for the management of people with LD and epilepsy (43).

The impact of epilepsy on people with learning disability

The last 30 years have seen substantial development in the measurement of the quality of life—the social and economic well-being of people with LD, their families and carers in coping with dependency and disturbance. On top of this comes epilepsy, often intractable, with its pervasive impact on both physical and psychosocial well-being; Kerr et al. (44) give a useful overview of the issues and instruments.

Management

Consensus guidelines have been produced by a working group using an evidence-based, modified Delphi process (45).

Diagnosis and misdiagnosis

Epilepsy is both under- and overdiagnosed. A review of misdiagnosis identified five categories of events which may be misidentified as epileptic (46):

1. Behavioural: tics, repetitive stereotypies, habitual smiles or grimaces, staring into space, catatonic freezing, and episodic inattentiveness.
2. Physiological: tics, dyskinetic movements, ataxic falls.
3. Syndromal:
   - Gastro-oesophageal reflux is frequent in people with severe LD, affecting as many as 50% in severe LD and even more for those on AEDs or with particular syndromes (notably Cornelia de Lange) or symptoms such as regurgitation (47). In early childhood it presents as Sandifer syndrome with sudden distress, abnormal postures or spasms, and eye deviation (48). This is beginning to be recognized in adults though limited communication together with a lack of characteristic symptomatology mean that diagnosis depends on a high level of suspicion (49).
   - Symptoms associated with Rett syndrome include breath holding, hand-wringing, and unresponsiveness.
4. Medication: the effects of AEDs.
5. Psychological: simulated seizures, (interictal) irritability, sudden aggressive bouts (episodic dyscontrol syndrome).

On the other hand, non-convulsive or even partial seizures are particularly prone to pass unnoticed or misinterpreted, especially if the symptoms are attributed to LD, autism or attention deficit disorder.

An eyewitness account is essential. Ideally this is supported by video, made possible by the growth of mobile phone technology.

While epilepsy is a clinical diagnosis, the electroencephalogram (EEG) can be helpful in teasing out the differential diagnosis, particularly in conjunction with video and as prolonged ambulatory recordings. However, the paroxysmal patterns that frequently accompany autism or language disorders are so misleading (50) as to make it unwise to carry out routine recording; the EEG should be used where there are sound clinical grounds for the diagnosis of epilepsy.

Neuroimaging has a particular importance because of the frequency of malformation in severe LD. At the same time anxiety and poor communication make it more likely that sedation (or even general anaesthesia) will be needed and its attendant risks taken into account.

Treatment

The main thrust of treatment must be on helping individuals and their families/carers find the best accommodation to the epilepsy.

Box 17.1 Special issues in the assessment of people with LD (53)

- Diagnosis can be overshadowed both by the characteristics and by the comorbidity of intellectual disability.
- These lead to diagnoses that are:
  - False positives—episodic behavioural and stereotypical disturbance mimic seizures.
  - False negatives—partial, absence and sensory seizures are easily missed.
- Definitive diagnosis requires a detailed eye-witness account—ideally supported by video recording.
- An assessment of the person's communication skills may help their inclusion in decisions about their management.
- A useful EEG may not be attainable.
- Abnormal EEGs are frequent in LD and autism, ranging from an increase in background slow activity through to epileptiform discharge; they do not necessarily indicate epilepsy.
- Epilepsy is a clinical diagnosis (neurophysiological findings are only supportive).

This means balancing the risk of seizure against restrictions on the person's autonomy. A checklist specific to LD has been developed to help specialist epilepsy nurses (51).

There is little evidence as to how LD affects drug efficacy or adverse effect although there is the suspicion that anomalous or paradoxical responses are more frequent; 'expect the unexpected' being the rule. Polypharmacy is a recurrent issue the more so as, besides AEDs, the individual is often taking other drugs, including psychotropics and medical remedies. Together with the effects of drug interactions, pre-existing cognitive impairment and poor communication make it difficult to judge which drug is having what impact on an individual. Consequently, although they do not diminish the need for careful clinical assessment, the measurement of drug levels may be of more value than in the general population.

LD is no bar to a neurosurgical approach to epilepsy provided the usual requirements have been met (52). Some of the specific issues related to the assessment and management of epilepsy in people with LD that clinicians need to consider are summarized in Boxes 17.1 and 17.2 (53).

Box 17.2 Special issues in the management of epilepsy in people with LD (53)

- Their epilepsy, (often with multiple seizure types, an earlier onset, and longer established) is more likely to be resistant to treatment.
- Its management can be grouped broadly into antiepileptic medication, neurosurgery, and psychosocial intervention.
- Many people with LD are on psychotropic drugs. These may interact with AEDs.
- AEDs can have adverse cognitive and behavioural effects that, in LD, are more difficult to discern.
- There should be a comprehensive care plan that includes therapeutic options, risk assessments, carer education and training, the activities of daily living (bathing, food preparation etc.), arrangements for independent living and the management of emergencies (prolonged seizures). This care plan should be reviewed regularly but at least annually.
- In addition to doctors, the multidisciplinary team (which may include community nurses, school nurses, respite carers, physiotherapists, speech and language therapists, clinical and educational psychologists, occupational therapists, and social workers) plays an important part in the care of these patients.
- AEDs—'start low, go slow'. Start at a dose lower than usually recommended and titrate the dose up more slowly than recommended in the datasheet until either there is an improvement or it is outweighed by adverse effects or a theoretical maximum is reached.
- If a second AED is introduced, again it should be introduced at a low dose and slowly increased. When an optimum is reached, the first AED should be slowly weaned.
- The aim should be to use monopharmacy whenever possible. However, the frequency of resistant epilepsy means that polypharmacy is common.

References

1. Leonard H, Petterson B, Bower C, Sanders R. Prevalence of intellectual disability in Western Australia. *Paediatr Perinat Epidemiol* 2003; 17(1):58–67.
2. Arvio M, Sillanpää M. Prevalence, aetiology and comorbidity of severe and profound intellectual disability in Finland. *J Intellect Disabil Res* 2003; 47(2):108–12.
3. Royal College of Psychiatrists. *Challenging behaviour: a unified approach. Clinical and service guidelines for supporting people with learning disabilities who are at risk of receiving abusive or restrictive practices.* Report No.: CR114. London: Royal College of Psychiatrists, 2007.
4. Arshad S, Winterhalder R, Underwood L, Kelesidi K, Chaplin E, Kravariti E, *et al.* Epilepsy and intellectual disability: Does epilepsy increase the likelihood of co-morbid psychopathology? *Res Dev Disabil* 2011; 32(1):353–7.
5. Deb S, Hunter D. Psychopathology of people with mental handicap and epilepsy: II. Psychiatric illness. *Br J Psychiatry* 1991; 159:826–30.
6. Espie CA, Watkins J, Curtice L, Espie A, Duncan R, Ryan JA, *et al.* Psychopathology in people with epilepsy and intellectual disability; an investigation of potential explanatory variables. *J Neurol, Neurosurg, Psychiatry* 2003; 74(11):1485–92.
7. Matsuura M, Adachi N, Muramatsu R, Kato M, Onuma T, Okubo Y, *et al.* Intellectual disability and psychotic disorders of adult epilepsy. *Epilepsia* 2005; 46:11–14.
8. Ring H, Zia A, Lindeman S, Himlok K. Interactions between seizure frequency, psychopathology, and severity of intellectual disability in a population with epilepsy and a learning disability. *Epilepsy Behav* 2007; 11(1):92–7.
9. Amiet C, Gourfinkel-An I, Bouzamondo A, Tordjman S, Baulac M, Lechat P, *et al.* Epilepsy in autism is associated with intellectual disability and gender: Evidence from a meta-analysis. *Biol Psychiatry* 2008; 64(7):577–82.

10. McGrother CW, Bhaumik S, Thorp CF, Hauck A, Branford D, Watson JM. Epilepsy in adults with intellectual disabilities: Prevalence, associations and service implications. *Seizure* 2006; 15(6):376–86.
11. Morgan CL, Baxter H, Kerr MP. Prevalence of epilepsy and associated health service utilization and mortality among patients with intellectual disability. *Am J Ment Retard* 2003; 108(5):293–300.
12. McDermott S, Moran R, Platt T, Wood H, Isaac T, Dasari S. Prevalence of epilepsy in adults with mental retardation and related disabilities in primary care. *Am J Ment Retard* 2005; 110(1):48–56.
13. Shepherd C, Hosking G. Epilepsy in school children with intellectual impairments in Sheffield: the size and nature of the problem and the implications for service provision. *J Intellect Disabil Res* 1989; 33(6):511–14.
14. Goulden KJ, Shinnar S, Koller H, Katz M, Richardson SA. Epilepsy in children with mental retardation: A cohort study. *Epilepsia* 1991; 32(5):690–7.
15. Branford D, Bhaumik S, Duncan F. Epilepsy in adults with learning disabilities. *Seizure* 1998; 7(6):473–7.
16. Branford D, Bhaumik S, Duncan F, Collacott RA. A follow-up study of adults with learning disabilities and epilepsy. *Seizure* 1998; 7(6):469–72.
17. Forsgren L, Edvinsson SO, Nystrom L, Blomquist HK. Influence of epilepsy on mortality in mental retardation: an epidemiologic study. *Epilepsia* 1996; 37(10):956–63.
18. Sillanpää M. Learning disability: occurrence and long-term consequences in childhood-onset epilepsy. *Epilepsy Behav* 2004; 5(6):937–44.
19. Huber B, Hauser I, Horstmann V, Jokeit G, Liem S, May T, *et al*. Long-term course of epilepsy in a large cohort of intellectually disabled patients. *Seizure* 2007; 16(1):35–42.
20. Holmes GL, Stafstrom CE. Tuberous sclerosis complex and epilepsy: recent developments and future challenges. *Epilepsia* 2007; 48(4): 617–30.
21. Collacott RA. Epilepsy, dementia and adaptive behavior in Down's syndrome. *J Intellect Disabil Res* 1993; 37:153–60.
22. Johannsen P, Christensen JEJ, Goldstein H, Kamp Nielsen V, Mai J. Epilepsy in Down syndrome—prevalence in three age groups. *Seizure* 1996; 5(2):121–5.
23. McVicker RW, Shanks OE, McClelland RJ. Prevalence and associated features of epilepsy in adults with Down's syndrome. *Br J Psychiatry* 1994; 164(4):528–32.
24. Prasher V. Age-specific prevalence, thyroid dysfunction and depressive symptomatology in adults with Down syndrome and dementia. *Int J Geriatr Psychiatry* 1995; 10(1):25–31.
25. Moller JC, Hamer HM, Oertel WH, Rosenow F. Late-onset myoclonic epilepsy in Down's syndrome (LOMEDS). *Seizure* 2001; 10(4):303–6.
26. Stafstrom CE. Epilepsy in Down syndrome: Clinical aspects and possible mechanisms. *Am J Ment Retard* 1993; 98:12–26.
27. Raghavan R, Khin-Nu C, Brown AG, Day KA, Tyrer SP, Ince PG, *et al*. Gender differences in the phenotypic expression of Alzheimer's disease in Down's syndrome (trisomy 21). *Neuroreport* 1994; 5(11):1393–6.
28. Prasher VP, Corbett JA. Onset of seizures as a poor indicator of longevity in people with Down syndrome and dementia. *Int J Geriatr Psychiatry* 1993; 8(11):923–7.
29. Hagerman PJ, Stafstrom CE. Origins of epilepsy in fragile X syndrome. *Epilepsy Curr* 2009; 9(4):108–12.
30. Fan Z, Greenwood R, Fisher A, Pendyal S, Powell CM. Characteristics and frequency of seizure disorder in 56 patients with Prader–Willi syndrome. *Am J Med Genet A* 2009; 149A(7):1581–4.
31. Dan B. Angelman syndrome: Current understanding and research prospects. *Epilepsia* 2009; 50(11):2331–9.
32. Fiumara A, PittalÃ A, Cocuzza M, Sorge G. Epilepsy in patients with Angelman syndrome. *Ital J Pediatr* 2010; 36:31.
33. Miles JH, Takahashi TN, Bagby S, Sahota PK, Vaslow DF, Wang CH, *et al*. Essential versus complex autism: definition of fundamental prognostic subtypes. *Am J Med Genet A* 2005; 135(2):171–80.
34. Pavone P, Incorpora G, Fiumara A, Parano E, Trifiletti RR, Ruggieri M. Epilepsy is not a prominent feature of primary autism. *Neuropediatrics* 2004; 35(4):207–10.
35. Deonna T, Roulet-Perez E. Early-onset acquired epileptic aphasia (Landau–Kleffner syndrome, LKS) and regressive autistic disorders with epileptic EEG abnormalities: the continuing debate. *Brain Dev* 2010; 32(9):746–52.
36. Parmeggiani A, Barcia G, Posar A, Raimondi E, Santucci M, Scaduto MC. Epilepsy and EEG paroxysmal abnormalities in autism spectrum disorders. *Brain Dev* 2010; 32(9):783–9.
37. Clarke DJ, Deb S. Syndromes causing intellectual disability. In: Gelder MG, Andreasen N, López-Ibor Jr JJ, Geddes JR (eds) *New Oxford Textbook of Psychiatry*, pp. 1838–48. Oxford: Oxford University Press, 2009.
38. Fessler AJ, Treiman DM. Epilepsy and aggression. *Neurology* 2009; 73(21):1720–1.
39. Ruedrich S, Swales TP, Fossaceca C, Toliver J, Rutkowski A. Effect of divalproex sodium on aggression and self-injurious behaviour in adults with intellectual disability: a retrospective review. *J Intellect Disabil Res* 1999; 43(2):105–11.
40. Stone JL, McDaniel KD, Hughes JR, Hermann BP. Episodic dyscontrol disorder and paroxysmal EEG abnormalities: successful treatment with carbamazepine. *Biol Psychiatry* 1986; 21(2):208–12.
41. van Elst LT, Woermann FG, Lemieux L, Thompson PJ, Trimble MR. Affective aggression in patients with temporal lobe epilepsy: A quantitative MRI study of the amygdala. *Brain* 2000; 123(2): 234–43.
42. Blumer D, Montouris G, Davies K. The interictal dysphoric disorder: recognition, pathogenesis, and treatment of the major psychiatric disorder of epilepsy. *Epilepsy Behav* 2004; 5(6):826–40.
43. Ring H, Zia A, Bateman N, Williams E, Lindeman S, Himlok K. How is epilepsy treated in people with a learning disability? A retrospective observational study of 183 individuals. *Seizure* 2009; 18(4):264–8.
44. Kerr MP, Turky A, Huber B. The psychosocial impact of epilepsy in adults with an intellectual disability. *Epilepsy Behav* 2009; 15 (2, Suppl 1):S26–30.
45. Kerr M; Guidelines Working Group, Scheepers M, Arvio M, Beavis J, Brandt C, *et al*. Consensus guidelines into the management of epilepsy in adults with an intellectual disability. *J Intellect Disabil Res* 2009; 53:687–94.
46. Chapman M, Iddon P, Atkinson K, Brodie C, Mitchell D, Parvin G, *et al*. The misdiagnosis of epilepsy in people with intellectual disabilities: A systematic review. *Seizure* 2011; 20(2):101–6.
47. de Veer AJ, Bos JT, Niezen-de Boer RC, Bohmer CJ, Francke AL. Symptoms of gastroesophageal reflux disease in severely mentally retarded people: a systematic review. *BMC Gastroenterol* 2008; 8:23.
48. Nanayakkara CS, Paton JY. Sandifer syndrome an overlooked diagnosis? *Dev Med Child Neurol* 1985; 27(6):816–19.
49. Somjit S, Lee Y, Berkovic SF, Harvey AS. Sandifer syndrome misdiagnosed as refractory partial seizures in an adult. *Epileptic Disord* 2004; 6(1):49–50.
50. Deonna T, Roulet E. Autistic spectrum disorder: Evaluating a possible contributing or causal role of epilepsy. *Epilepsia* 2006; 47:79–82.
51. Cole C, Pointu A, Wellsted DM, Angus-Leppan H. A pilot study of the epilepsy risk awareness checklist (ERAC) in people with epilepsy and learning disabilities. *Seizure* 2010; 19(9):592–6.
52. Henriksen O, Bjørnaes H, Røste GK. Epilepsy surgery in mental retardation: the role of surgery. In: Sillanpää M, Gram L, Johannessen SI, Tomson T (eds) *Epilepsy and Mental Retardation*, pp. 105–113. Philadelphia, PA: Biomedical Publishing Limited, 1999.
53. Deb S. Epilepsy in people with mental retardation. In: Jacobson JW, Mulick JA (eds) *Handbook of Mental Retardation and Developmental Disabilities*, pp. 81–96. New York: Kluwer Academic Publishers, 2007.

CHAPTER 18

Epilepsy in the Elderly

Trevor T.-J. Chong and Wendyl D'Souza

Introduction

Epilepsy has traditionally been thought of as a disease of the young, primarily affecting infants, children, and adolescents. Increasingly, however, epilepsy is becoming recognized as a common disorder of the elderly (1).[1] Within that population, it is the third most common neurological disease, after cerebrovascular disease and the dementias. Epilepsy today is therefore more a disease of old age, and our aging population will see it evolve into an increasingly important public health issue. Furthermore, although the phenomenon of population ageing is evident for high-income countries, the changing global economic landscape will also see it become an important consideration for low- and middle-income countries (LAMICs). In this chapter, we aim to provide a concise and practical reference to guide the treatment of the elderly patient with epilepsy.

Epidemiology

Any cerebral insult can predispose an individual to developing seizures. It is therefore unsurprising that seizures and epilepsy are so common in the elderly, who have a high incidence of stroke and neurodegenerative disorders. The prevalence of unprovoked seizures in those aged over 60 is at least 1%. This rate rises to 1.5% in those aged over 75, which is approximately twice that of younger adults (2, 3). Predictably, the prevalence is even higher (3–9%) in populations such as nursing home residents, who are more likely to suffer from cerebrovascular disease and dementia (4–6).

The high prevalence of seizures in the elderly (Fig. 18.1) is commensurate with the higher incidence of epilepsy in this population. Indeed, the incidence of epilepsy is greatest in those over the age of 65 (Fig. 18.2) (8–10). Above that age, the incidence continues to rise, with an annual incidence of 85.9 per 100,000 in those aged 65–69, to more than 135 per 100 000 in those aged older than 80 (11). This is compared to an overall incidence of 80.8 per 100,000 people across all age groups.

1 In most high-income countries, the definition of an 'elderly' person is held to be one who has exceeded a chronological age of 65 years. Of course, the situation is different in low- and middle-income countries and, although the United Nations does not have a standard numerical criterion for the 'elderly', it has accepted a cutoff of 60+ years.

Epilepsy in the elderly is associated with a significant morbidity and mortality. Old age is a significant predictor of seizure recurrence (9, 10, 13), and patients with a first unprovoked seizure have an overall risk of recurrence beyond 2 years of 25–52% (14–17). Similar to other age groups, this risk is increased in the presence of an abnormal electroencephalogram (EEG) and/or an identifiable epileptogenic substrate (15). Status epilepticus becomes more common with age, with a 2- to 10-fold increase in incidence in those older than 60 relative to younger adults (18–20). This increase is accompanied by a rise in mortality associated with status epilepticus, with a rate of 38% in those over 60 to nearly 50% in those over 80 (21, 22). Overall, the mortality in elderly patients with epilepsy is two to three times greater than that of the general population (23), which is likely due to their greater susceptibility to systemic illnesses, comorbidities, and the underlying aetiology of their epilepsy. Together, these findings underline the importance of optimizing the total care of the elderly patient with epilepsy.

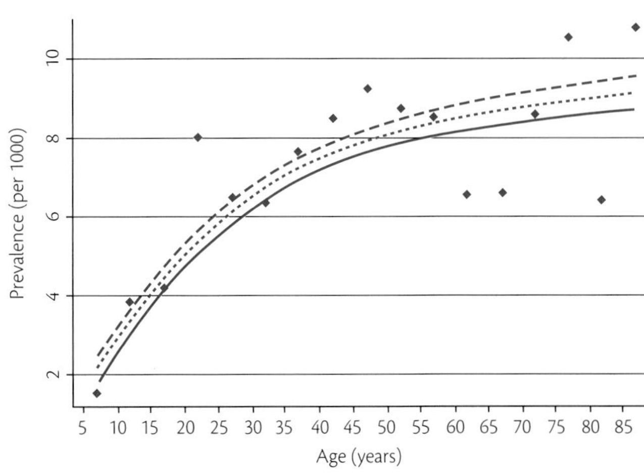

Fig. 18.1 The prevalence of treated epilepsy across age groups in Tasmania, Australia (7) Imputed prevalence reported (middle curve) with smoother and 95% confidence intervals also shown (top and bottom curve). The smoother and 95% confidence interval was obtained from a log binomial regression model with age modelled as $1/\sqrt{\text{age}}$.

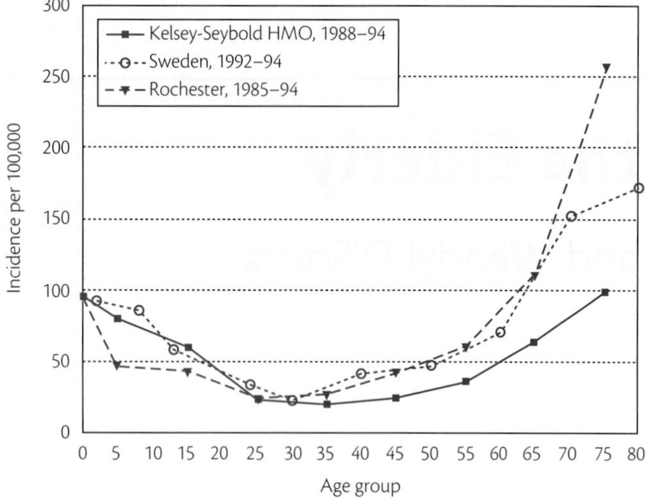

Fig. 18.2 The incidence of epilepsy across age groups. Reproduced from Annegers, J.F., et al. The incidence of epilepsy and unprovoked seizures in multiethnic, urban health maintenance organizations. *Epilepsia* 1999; 40(4):502–6.

Table 18.1 Identifiable aetiologies of symptomatic seizures in the elderly

Aetiology	Symptomatic seizures
Structural causes	**60–80%**
◆ Cerebrovascular disease (8, 25, 29–33)	(40–50%)
◆ Head trauma (8, 25, 29, 34, 35)	(4–17%)
◆ CNS infections (8, 25, 29)	(5–10%)
Drugs and metabolic disturbances (36–39)	**10–40%**
◆ Drugs[a], toxins, alcohol	(5–10%)
◆ Metabolic disturbances[b]	(6–30%)

[a] Drugs including: psychotropic agents, theophylline, narcotics, antimicrobials (high-dose penicillins and cephalosporins, imipenem, isoniazid, antimalarials), chemotherapeutic agents (methotrexate, chlorambucil, cyclosporin), anaesthetic agents (ketamine, toxic doses of lignocaine, disopyramide, bupivacaine), anti-arrhythmics (overdose of verapamil, propranolol), diphenhydramine, baclofen, chlorpromazine

[b] Metabolic insults including: hypo-/hypernatraemia, hypomagnesaemia, hypocalcaemia, hypoglycaemia/non-ketotic hyperglycaemia, uraemia, hypoxia, hyperthyroidism, porphyria, dialysis disequilibrium syndrome. Note that the rate of change of the respective metabolites, rather than their absolute value, predicts seizures.

Aetiology

Symptomatic seizures

An 'acute' symptomatic seizure is one that occurs shortly after a recent epileptogenic insult (e.g. strokes, metabolic disturbances, drug withdrawal), in contrast to a 'remote' symptomatic seizure which is one that occurs in the days to weeks following such an insult. In practice, the distinction between acute and remote symptomatic seizures is often blurred, particularly in the elderly. This is due to the inherent imprecision of the circumstances surrounding events, and the varying definitions for the acute period, from 48 hours to up to 3 months depending on the underlying aetiology (24). For example, the period for acute symptomatic seizures secondary to alcohol withdrawal is 48 hours, but that secondary to a head injury is up to 14 days. Therefore, a more pragmatic approach is to consider symptomatic seizures in the elderly in relation to their underlying structural or metabolic causes (Table 18.1).

In the elderly, symptomatic seizures are most often precipitated by cerebrovascular disease (40–50%), which includes haemorrhagic, ischaemic, and embolic strokes, as well as subarachnoid haemorrhages (8, 25, 26). Other structural insults, such as head trauma and central nervous system (CNS) infection, may also precipitate seizures and obviously increase the risk for epilepsy (although epilepsy is not an inevitable consequence). Drugs and metabolic insults also account for a significant proportion of symptomatic seizures. However, such seizures are eminently treatable by withdrawing the offending agent or correcting the metabolic abnormality. Finally, it is worth noting that the incidence of non-epileptic seizures in the elderly is not insignificant, with an incidence roughly similar to that seen in younger populations (27, 28).

Epilepsy

With regards to epilepsy itself, descriptions of its aetiology vary depending on the population studied, the definition of the elderly, and methodological factors (9, 40–43) (Table 18.2). In high-income countries, the most common identifiable antecedents include cerebrovascular disease, neurodegenerative disorders, intracerebral tumours, traumatic head injury, and CNS infections (44). However, in 33–50% of elderly patients, the aetiology remains unclear (9, 25, 34).

Cerebrovascular disease is the most common cause of epilepsy in the elderly, accounting for 30–40% of new cases (1, 26, 43). In fact population-based studies have shown that stroke increases the risk of a seizure by a factor of 23 and the risk of epilepsy in the first year after stroke by a factor of 17 (45). The risk of epilepsy can be further stratified depending on the type of stroke, with the risk being greatest in those that are haemorrhagic, cortical, large, multiple, and/or that present with acute symptomatic seizures (46).

The association between epilepsy and stroke is not always obvious and seizures may be the first presentation of previously unrecognized cerebrovascular disease. In one large study of patients with new-onset seizures over the age of 60, none of whom had any known history of cerebrovascular disease, tumour, trauma, dementia, or alcohol abuse, the 5-year risk of stroke was 2.89 times higher than that of control subjects without seizures (47). One may speculate that this is because such seizures reflect the presence of subclinical cortical lesions in patients with predisposing vascular risk factors. Indeed, hypertension itself has been identified as a risk factor for seizures, perhaps because of its association with progressive arterial changes (48).

Table 18.2 Identifiable aetiologies of epilepsy in the elderly

Aetiology	Symptomatic seizures
Cerebrovascular disease	30–50%
Neurodegenerative	10–20%
Neoplastic	10–30%
Trauma	10–20%

The second most common antecedent of epilepsy in the elderly is neurodegenerative disease, which is associated with a 5- to 10-fold increase in epilepsy relative to the general population (26, 49, 50). Alzheimer disease, Creutzfeldt–Jakob disease, and the adult form of Huntington disease have all been associated with epilepsy. Interestingly, however, it is rarely seen in dementia with Lewy bodies. Amongst patients with Alzheimer dementia, the incidence of epilepsy is approximately 8–20% (49, 51, 52). The risk of a patient with dementia developing epilepsy can be further stratified based on the earlier age of onset of the dementia, the stage of disease, and the presence of epileptiform changes on the EEG (51). Although seizure control does not appear to be more difficult as the disease progresses, the long-term effect of epilepsy on cognition and subsequent neurodegeneration is unknown (53).

In some studies, head trauma, usually secondary to falls, can account for up to 20% of epilepsy in the elderly (54). The severity of the injury can predict the risk of subsequent epilepsy, with a loss of consciousness increasing the risk of subsequent epilepsy threefold (26). Similar to other age-groups, other risk factors include sustaining a brain contusion with subdural haematoma, skull fracture, and loss of consciousness or amnesia for more than 1 day (55).

Of the remaining causes of epilepsy in the elderly, tumours account for between 10–30% of seizures, and are typically meningiomas, gliomas, or brain metastases (41, 56). Epilepsy is more common with primary relative to secondary tumours, and with low-grade tumours rather than high grade (57). Finally, CNS infections carry a threefold increase in risk of developing epilepsy (56).

Box 18.1 Reasons for difficulties in diagnosing epilepsy in the elderly

- Lack of medical awareness:
  - Lack of awareness of the high incidence of seizures in the elderly.
  - Nuances of seizure semiology, especially the presence of automatisms, not appreciated or systematically sought.
  - Inappropriate diagnostic expectation and interpretation of interictal EEG.
  - Failure to involve a specialist with expertise early in the diagnostic process.
- Limited, vague, or incomplete history:
  - Under-reporting of events (68).
  - Absence of a witness—imprecise semiology.
  - Cognitive impairment affecting patient and/or witness.
- Clinical features of complex partial seizures are more subtle:
  - Lack of auras and recognized automatisms (69).
  - Seizures may manifest as confusion and staring rather than convulsive events.
- Non-epileptic paroxysmal phenomena ('seizure mimickers') may be misattributed to, or be misdiagnosed as, epilepsy (see Box 18.2).

Presentation and diagnostic evaluation

The preceding considerations imply that epilepsy in the elderly is almost always focal, and indeed complex partial seizures are the most common seizure type (34, 43, 58). In fact, it is highly unusual for idiopathic generalized epilepsy to present in this demographic and, therefore, even apparently generalized tonic–clonic seizures rarely have a truly generalized onset.

Making the diagnosis of epilepsy in the elderly can be difficult. In fact, in the Veterans' Administration cooperative study of new-onset epilepsy in a community-dwelling cohort, 27% of patients with epilepsy had been initially misdiagnosed (43). Some elderly patients with epilepsy may remain undiagnosed altogether (59), and several factors contribute to making the diagnosis difficult (Box 18.1). A principal problem relates to the fact that epileptogenic lesions in the elderly appear to produce symptoms that may be atypical to those found in younger patients, and may be as non-specific as confusion or simply a sensation of feeling or appearing vague. Conversely, more typical epileptic phenomena that are seen in younger patients (e.g. auras, automatisms) may be less common in the elderly. Given the atypical nature of epileptiform symptoms in the elderly, such symptoms are often misattributed to non-epileptic paroxysmal phenomena, or 'seizure mimickers' (Box 18.2). The difficulty in making a diagnosis of epilepsy in the elderly is further compounded by the issues of cognitive impairment and social isolation.

When epilepsy is suspected a detailed seizure history should be acquired, with the broad aim of distinguishing seizures arising from brain pathology from seizure mimickers. The key step in reaching an accurate diagnosis is taking a detailed history from a witness. In fact, in the authors' experience, the diagnosis of epilepsy in an elderly patient is most difficult when such witnesses are unavailable or unreliable and remains accurate when present (60). Taking a corroborative history often takes time and patience, and sometimes requires a number of consultations if a precise record of the events cannot be gleaned.

After performing a neurological examination, with particular emphasis on establishing the presence of any cortical deficits, dedicated magnetic resonance imaging (MRI) is the critical investigation in establishing the presence of any structural lesions that may predispose to epilepsy. Computed tomography is useful only as an initial screening study (or when MRI is unavailable) for intracerebral haemorrhage, tumours and encephalomalacia, and should be followed by a MRI if any obvious pathology is not detected in a patient with definite epilepsy (61).

Generally, EEG has an important role in providing information pertinent to the activity and localization of the epilepsy. There is also data to suggest that the EEG may aid prognostication—for example, patients who experience focal spikes or periodic lateralized epileptiform discharges (PLEDs) after a stroke are at greater risk for developing seizures in the future (62). Furthermore, EEG is useful in patients who present with prolonged confusional states or unexplained coma due to non-convulsive status epilepticus (63–66). As an extension of routine EEG monitoring, video telemetry, is useful in uncertain cases, in which patients present with recurrent and frequent atypical events (28, 67), and to distinguish epileptic seizures from sleep disorders. In spite of its utility, however, one should also be aware that the interictal EEG is of relatively less

Box 18.2 Seizure mimickers in the elderly

- Syncope.
- Psychogenic non-epileptic attacks.
- Falls—multifactorial aetiologies.
- Confusional states (especially in cognitively vulnerable patients) secondary to systemic causes (e.g. electrolyte imbalance, infection, medications).
- Transient ischaemic attacks.
- Simple forgetfulness.
- Sleep disorders—periodic limb movements in sleep; REM sleep behaviour disorder.
- Stereotyped repetitive behaviours associated with dementia and other cognitive problems.
- Movement disorders (tremors, paroxysmal dyskinesias).
- Transient global amnesia.
- Hallucinations.
- Vertigo.

Box 18.3 Key principles in the treatment of the elderly patient with epilepsy

- Document previous drug reactions—idiosyncratic skin reactions and cross-reactivity is common (70).
- Attempt to use single, non-enzyme inducing, anticonvulsant drugs (71).
- Titrate AEDs cautiously with lower dose at onset, increment, and target.
- Screen for and manage the underlying aetiological disorder (e.g. cerebrovascular risk factors, neurodegenerative disorders).
- Consider surgical work-up and intervention if seizures remain refractory and the underlying pathological substrate is known (72).

utility in the elderly due to the high occurrence of non-specific abnormalities. In one study, for example, video-EEG monitoring detected interictal epileptiform discharges in 26% of those with non-epileptic events, and in 75% of those with epilepsy (28).

Treatment

The overarching goals in treating any patient with epilepsy are to improve overall quality of life, with good seizure control, while minimizing adverse pharmacological side effects. In the elderly, however, this can be challenging, as treatment is complicated by three main issues: (1) their comorbid medical conditions; (2) polypharmacy and drug–drug interactions; and (3) altered homeostatic mechanisms, which may render patients more susceptible to drug side effects. Key principles in treating the elderly patient with epilepsy are summarized in Box 18.3. However, no published guidelines, systematic reviews, or meta-analyses are currently available to formally guide management.

Pharmacology in the elderly

Pharmacokinetic changes

For otherwise healthy elderly patients who are not frail or malnourished, the main pharmacokinetic issue is that of a progressive decline in renal function. Thus, care must be given to those drugs that are excreted unchanged by the kidneys, and such drugs should be administered at lower doses in patients with moderate-to-severe renal impairment. Table 18.3 lists the other changes that occur during ageing and precautions one should take in prescribing the corresponding drugs.

Pharmacodynamic changes

Ageing is accompanied by a progressive decline in homeostatic mechanisms, which leads to a rise in the rate and severity of adverse drug reactions. Due to these impaired mechanisms, elderly patients may be more susceptible to drugs which lower the seizure threshold (e.g. antidepressants, antipsychotics, certain antibiotics (77)). However, these medications may be required for improved morbidity, mortality, and quality of life, thus necessitating their continued use. From a practical perspective, the impaired regulatory mechanisms imply that side effects can be seen at lower drug doses and, in the elderly, these adverse effects (e.g. falls) can be more devastating than in a younger adult. Thus, any anticonvulsant medication should be started at a lower dose and titrated cautiously to a lower target level. The patient, spouse, and family should be counselled regarding common and important side effects.

Choice of antiepileptic drug

Because old age is a significant predictor for seizure recurrence (13), patients should be carefully counselled about the risks and benefits of delaying treatment. In general, the older-generation antiepileptic drugs (AEDs), which include phenytoin, phenobarbital, carbamazepine, and valproate, have been effective in the treatment of focal epilepsies (Table 18.4). However, most of these drugs are subject to multiple interactions, and are poorly tolerated in the elderly (in particular carbamazepine). Of the older-generation drugs, valproate is notable in that it lacks the side effects of sedation and motor slowing, and does not induce hepatic enzymes—and can be a useful first treatment option when used in low dose (400–800 mg/day) in the elderly.

Overall, there has been a trend away from the use of older drugs, as the newer-generation AEDs are less sedating and offer more favourable side effect profiles particularly drug–drug interactions (Table 18.4). However, when used in lower doses the older drugs still have a role in this group. The reader is also referred to the 2004 AAN Guidelines on the efficacy and tolerability of the newer generation drugs (78). Unfortunately, due to the difficulty in conducting well-controlled trials in this population, there is limited evidence to guide treatment decisions.

The only class I or II evidence for the treatment of epilepsy in the elderly comes from three randomized, double-blind comparative clinical trials, which suggest lamotrigine to be the best tolerated AED. Brodie et al. (79) showed that lamotrigine is as effective as carbamazepine, but better tolerated, with a lower incidence of rash (3% vs. 19%) and somnolence (12% vs. 29%), resulting in an

Table 18.3 Pharmacokinetic changes in the elderly and the antiepileptic drugs (AEDs) most affected

Pharmacokinetic parameter	Change in the elderly	AEDs affected
Absorption	Variable and unpredictable, but overall reduction in bioavailability: ◆ Reduced gastric acid secretion ◆ Slowed gastric emptying ◆ Increased intestinal transit time ◆ Decreased mesenteric blood flow ◆ Decreased intestinal absorptive area (73, 74)	◆ PHT ◆ GBP (75)
Protein binding	Minimally reduced, unless frail or malnourished: ◆ Reduced serum albumin results in higher free fraction of protein-bound drugs. Causes more prominent side effects despite little change in the total serum level	Highly protein-bound AEDs (76): ◆ PHT ◆ CBZ ◆ VPA ◆ Benzodiazepines
Hepatic clearance	Variable and unpredictable, but overall reduction in clearance: ◆ Reduction in hepatic mass and blood flow ◆ Reduced function of CYP 450 ◆ Glucuronidation is less affected	Hepatically metabolized drugs: ◆ Primarily CYP450: PHT, PB, CBZ, OXC ◆ Partially CYP450: TPM, VPA, ZNS, LAC ◆ Glucuronidation: LTG, VPA, ZNS
Renal clearance	Most consistent age-related change	Renally excreted drugs ◆ Primarily GBP, LEV, LAC

AED, antiepileptic drug; CBZ, carbamazepine; GBP, gabapentin; LAC, lacosamide; LEV, levetiracetam; LTG, lamotrigine; OXC, oxcarbazepine; PB, phenobarbitone; PHT, phenytoin; TPM, topiramate; VPA, valproate; ZNS, zonisamide.

overall lower dropout rate (18% vs. 42%). The flexible dosing design used a low daily maintenance dose of 400 mg of carbamazepine and 100 mg of lamotrigine. A second study with an identical design actually showed no difference between lamotrigine and carbamazepine if a controlled-release formulation of carbamazepine was used, with a target dose of 400 mg daily (80). Finally, the Veterans' Administration Study compared lamotrigine, gabapentin, and carbamazepine (standard release) in a randomized double-blind design (81). The authors found that seizure control was similar across all groups, but that carbamazepine was significantly less well tolerated (discontinuation rates: lamotrigine 12%, gabapentin 22%, carbamazepine 31%).

Other than lamotrigine, levetiracetam has been suggested as an alternative first-line agent for several reasons (82). First, it is not metabolized by the liver, implying that it is free of non-linear elimination kinetics, auto-induction kinetics, and drug interactions. Second, it is not protein-bound, and therefore does not displace protein-bound drugs. Finally, it is largely well tolerated, and has favourable efficacy as indicated by one prospective Phase IV study (83). Furthermore, several open studies have supported its use (82, 84, 85), although a randomized controlled trial is yet to be conducted in the elderly. In addition to levetiracetam, there are also data from open studies in support of oxcarbazepine (86) and topiramate (87).

The elderly are more sensitive to the central and systemic side effects of AEDs (88). Almost all AEDs are associated with neurotoxicity, resulting in ataxia, dizziness, tremor, and cognitive side effects. Such toxicity may be even more problematic in the presence of comorbid conditions affecting balance, coexistent dementia, or previous cerebrovascular disease. In addition, unpleasant sedation is another side effect, which may be exacerbated in patients already on psychoactive drugs (e.g. benzodiazepines, antidepressants, antipsychotics). Lowering the dose of AED may reduce the number of side effects experienced by the patient while preserving their anticonvulsant effect. One study on elderly patients showed that both good seizure control and minimal side effects could be achieved with serum concentrations of valproate or carbamazepine that were at, or well below, the 'therapeutic range' (89). In general, therefore, we suggest halving the target dose of most AEDs, and titrating these drugs at dosage increments half that for younger adults, and over intervals twice as long (90). For example, carbamazepine may be started at a dose of 100 mg twice a day, and increased in 1 month's time to a maximum of 200 mg twice a day if the drug is tolerated and the patient continues to experience seizures (Table 18.4).

A further issue that arises in managing the elderly is that of polypharmacy. In one study, 25% of older patients with epilepsy were taking 15 or more drugs (mean of seven) (43). Such findings have two important implications. First, they raise the obvious issue of drug interactions, which one must consider prior to commencing patients on anticonvulsant therapy. Second, the need to administer multiple medications on a daily basis can very easily result in the omission of medications, uncertainty regarding their necessity, and confusion regarding the dosing regimes. Such potential problems with adherence are further amplified by the cognitive decline and visual impairment that are more prevalent amongst this cohort. Overall, therefore, we advocate starting patients on single agents with as simplified a regimen as possible.

To summarize, valproate, lamotrigine, levetiracetam, or pregabalin are useful as initial anticonvulsant therapy, as these drugs have the least potential for interaction with commonly used medications and are largely well tolerated. Lamotrigine has the strongest evidence in support of its use in the elderly, and should be titrated slowly to a target dose of 100 mg/day. An alternative is lower-dose oxcarbazepine if cerebrovascular risk management with warfarin is not anticipated. Zonisamide and topiramate also have relatively few drug–drug interactions, but are more likely to produce cognitive side effects and increase the risk of nephrolithiasis.

Table 18.4 The pharmacokinetics, pharmacodynamics, adverse effects, and recommended practical dosing regimens of commonly prescribed antiepileptic drugs (AEDs) in the elderly

AED	$T_{1/2}$ (hr)	Protein-binding (%)	Main route of elimination (enzyme)	Effect of other drugs on (AED)	Effect of AED on (other drugs)	Common side effects	Comments
Carbamazepine (CBZ)	5–26	75–85	Hepatic oxidation and glucuronidation (CYP 3A4/5)	↑ (CBZ) by drugs that inhibit CYP 3A4 (SSRIs, erythromycin, azoles, ritonavir, cimetidine, Ca^{2+} channel blockers, grapefruit juice) ↓ (CBZ) by drugs that induce CYP 3A4 (St John's wort)	↓ levels of VPA, LTG, TPM, ZNS, LEV, BZD and drugs metabolized by CYP 3A4 (Table 18.5)	*Notable*: hyponatraemia, sedation, neurotoxicity (gait/ataxia, dizziness, tremor, nystagmus), arrhythmias, bone loss *Other*: cognitive and behavioural, headache, gastrointestinal	*Advantages*: gold standard for partial seizures. Studied in elderly. Cheap. As effective as, and better tolerated than, PHT, PB, VPA *Disadvantages*: allergic reactions. Side effects. Multiple interactions as protein bound and enzyme inducer. Multiple interactions. As effective as LTG, but more side effects *Caution*: salt-restriction/diuretics (94), conduction defects, dose adjust with renal failure *Pragmatic dosing*: 100 mg bd ➡ 200 mg bd
Phenobarbital (PB)	77–128	55	Hepatic oxidation and glucuronidation (CYP 2C9)	↑ (PB) by chloramphenicol, dextropropoxyphene	↓ levels of VPA, LTG, TPM, ZNS, LEV, BZD and drugs metabolized by CYP 3A4 (Table 18.5)	*Notable*: sedation, cognitive, depression, bone loss	*Advantages*: broad spectrum. Once daily. Cheap *Disadvantages*: side effects. Enzyme inducer. Poorly tolerated relative to CBZ or PHT *Pragmatic dosing*: 15 mg bd ➡ 30 mg bd
Phenytoin (PHT)	7–42	90	Hepatic glucuronidation and oxidation (CYP 2C9, CYP 2C19)	↑ (PHT) by VPA, OXC, TPM; and drugs that inhibit CYP 3A4 (SSRIs, chloramphenicol, azoles, tamoxifen, allopurinol, omeprazole) ↓ (PHT) by CBZ	↓ levels of VPA, LTG, TPM, ZNS, LEV, BZD, and drugs metabolized by CYP 3A4 (Table 18.5)	*Notable*: sedation, cognition, imbalance/ataxia (even at modest doses), arrhythmias, bone loss	*Advantages*: once daily. No titration. Cheap *Disadvantages*: allergic reactions. Narrow therapeutic range. Saturation kinetics. Enzyme inducer. Multiple interactions *Caution*: conduction defects *Pragmatic dosing*: 200 mg/day ➡ 230 mg/day ➡ 260 mg/day
Valproate (VPA)	9–15	90	Hepatic glucuronidation (UGT 2B7) and oxidation	↑ (VPA) by sertraline, isoniazid, cimetiidine ↓ (VPA) by CBZ, PHT	VPA increases levels of LTG	*Notable*: hyperammonaemic encephalopathy, weight gain, tremor, parkinsonism and cognitive decline, bone loss *Other*: headache, fatigue, dizziness, diplopia, hair loss, reduced platelet function	*Advantages*: gold standard for generalized seizures. Broad spectrum. Rapid titration. Few interactions. Lack of sedating and motor slowing effects. No hepatic enzyme induction. Relatively cheap *Disadvantages*: side effects. Enzyme inhibition *Pragmatic dosing*: 200 mg bd ➡ 400 mg bd
Gabapentin (GBP)	5–7	<3	Renal	Nil	Nil	*Notable*: sedation, dizziness, weight gain *Other*: cognitive, gait/ataxia, affect, tremor	*Advantages*: therapeutic efficacy at starting dose. No interactions. Studied in elderly *Disadvantages*: thrice-daily dosing. Weak effect *Caution*: dose adjust with renal failure *Pragmatic dosing*: 400 mg bd ➡ 400 mg tds ➡ 600 mg tds ➡ 800 mg tds
Lamotrigine (LTG)	30	55	Hepatic glucuronidation (UGT 1A4)	↑ (LTG) by VPA, sertraline ↓ (LTG) by inducers of CYP 450 enzymes (CBZ, PHT, PB, hormone replacement therapy)	Minimal	Generally well-tolerated. *Notable*: allergic skin reactions. Insomnia (morning dosing)	*Advantages*: broad spectrum. Well tolerated. Few interactions. Studied in elderly. Single daily dosing tolerated *Disadvantages*: needs slow titration due to dose-associated rash *Caution*: interaction with VPA *Pragmatic dosing*: 25mg/d ➡ 50mg/d ➡ 75mg/d ➡ 100mg/d ➡ 150mg/d ➡ 200mg/d (fortnightly, halve dose with concomitant sodium valproate)

Levetiracetam (LEV)	6–8	< 10	Renal (75%), hepatic hydrolysis (hydrolase)	Nil	Nil	Generally well-tolerated. *Notable*: sedation early, neurobehavioural	*Advantages*: therapeutic efficacy at starting doses. No interactions *Disadvantages*: irritability, sedation at onset, mood disturbance uncommon but can be profound *Pragmatic dosing*: 250 mg bd ➡ 500 mg bd (monthly increments)
Oxcarbazepine (active metabolite MHD)	9 (MHD)	40 (MHD)	First-pass ⟶ MHD (aldoketo-reductase; CYP 3A4); then glucuronidation + renal excretion	↓ (MHD) by inducers of CYP 450 enzymes (i.e. CBZ, PHT, PB)	MHD increases levels of PHT ↓ drugs metabolized by CYP 3A4 (Table 18.5)	*Notable*: neurotoxicity (dizziness, ataxia, diplopia), fatigue, hyponatraemia (95) *Other*: tremor, rash	*Advantages*: well tolerated. *Disadvantages*: can induce CYP3A4 *Caution*: hyponatraemia especially with diuretics although clinically relevant when <124 (94) *Pragmatic dosing*: 150 mg bd ➡ 300 mg bd ➡ 450 mg bd ➡ 600mg/d (monthly increments; may need reduction if concomitant PHT)
Pregabalin	6	<1	Renal (>90%)	Nil	Nil	*Notable*: dizziness, weight gain. Constipation	*Advantages*: no interactions. *Disadvantages*: few data in elderly *Pragmatic dosing*: 75mg bd ➡ 150 mg bd (monthly increments)
Topiramate (TPM)	18–23	15	Hepatic (CYP 2C19) + unchanged renal excretion	↓ (TPM) by inducing agents	TPM increases PHT	Generally well-tolerated. *Notable*: cognitive, nephrolithiasis, word-finding difficulties (weak carbonic anhydrase inhibitor) *Other*: headache, fatigue, dizziness, paraesthesiae, affect, gait/ataxia, weight loss	*Advantages*: broad spectrum *Disadvantages*: slow titration. Nephrolithiasis. Cognitive slowing. *Caution*: clearance may decrease with age. Ensure adequate hydration. May need reduction if concomitant PHT *Pragmatic dosing*: 12.5 mg bd ➡ 25 mg bd ➡ 37.5 mg bd ➡ 50 mg bd (monthly increments)
Zonisamide (ZNS)	63	40	Hepatic (CYP 3A4)	Nil	Nil	Generally well-tolerated. *Notable*: cognitive and behavioural, rash, sedation, nephrolithiasis (weak carbonic anhydrase inhibitor). *Other*: somnolence, dizziness, weight loss	*Advantages*: broad spectrum; once daily; no interactions *Disadvantages*: slow titration. Nephrolithiasis *Caution*: ensure adequate hydration *Pragmatic dosing*: 50 mg/day ➡ 100 mg/day ➡ 150 mg/day (monthly increments)
Lacosamide (LAC)	13	15	Renal (95%) + some hepatic	Nil	Nil	Generally well-tolerated. *Notable*: sedation, ataxia, nausea *Other*: potentiates side effects of concomitant Na^+ channel-blocking AEDs. Potential AV block	*Advantages*: no drug levels *Disadvantages*: slow titration *Caution*: theoretical caution in comorbid cardiac dysfunction and rhythm disturbances. Warn patient and family that small decrement in other AEDs may be required (pharmacodynamics interaction?). Reduce dose in severe renal impairment (creatinine clearance ≤80 mL/min). *Target dose*: 25 mg bd ➡ 50 mg bd ➡ 75 mg bd ➡ 100 mg bd (monthly to bimonthly increments)

bd, twice a day. See Table 18.3 for drug abbreviations.

Table 18.5 Drugs whose serum concentrations are lowered by enzyme-inducing drugs (phenytoin, carbamazepine, phenobarbital)

Antidepressants	Amitriptyline, bupropion, citalopram, clomipramine, desipramine, doxepin, imipramine, mianserin, mirtazapine, nefazodone, nortriptyline, paroxetine
Antimicrobials	Albendazole, doxycycline, griseofulvin, indinavir, itraconazole, metronidazole, praziquantel
Antineoplastics	Busulfan, cyclophosphamide, etoposide, irinotecan, methotrexate, nitroureas, paclitaxel, procarbazine, tamoxifen, tenoposide, vinca alkaloids
Antipsychotics	Chlorpromazine, clozapine, haloperidol, olanazapine, quetiapine, risperidone, ziprasidone
Benzodiazepines	Alprazolam, clobazam, clonazepam, diazepam, midazolam
Cardiovascular	Amiodarone, atorvastatin, warfarin, digoxin, felodipine, metoprolol, mexiletine, nifedipine, nimodipine, propranolol, quinidine, simvastatin, verapamil
Immunosuppressants	Cyclosporine, sirolimus, tacrolimus
Steroids	Cortisol, dexamethasone, hydrocortisone, methylprednisolone, prednisolone, oral contraceptives
Miscellaneous	Fentanyl, methadone, paracetamol, pethidine, theophylline, thyroxine, vecuronium

Other management issues

In addition to the epilepsy itself, bone health is an important management issue. In the elderly, not only is the incidence of osteoporosis increased, but lack of exercise, inadequate nutrition, and poor mobility can contribute to impaired balance. Epilepsy increases the risk for falls and fractures by two- to sixfold. In addition, AEDs themselves pose two potential problems: first, neurotoxic side effects can predispose patients to falls; and, second, certain AEDs (most notably valproate and phenytoin) have been associated with bone loss which can increase the likelihood of fractures. It is therefore critical to monitor elderly patients for the development of such side effects, and to reduce the dose to the minimum. Vitamin D supplementation should be considered.

It is also worth recalling the association between seizures and stroke as described earlier. Because late-onset seizures are a predictor of subsequent stroke (91), those who have their first unprovoked seizure above age 60 should have their vascular risk evaluated, and their risk factors managed appropriately.

In the two-thirds in whom no aetiology is found, it is prudent to remain vigilant and monitor for the possibility of seizures as the sentinel event of an emerging neurodegenerative disorder.

Finally, for those patients who have had a severe traumatic brain injury (92) or cerebral neoplasm (93), there is no evidence for long-term seizure prophylaxis with anticonvulsant therapy.

Lifestyle factors

Against the background of having to manage the epilepsy itself is the patient's own complex psychosocial milieu. Few studies have been conducted on the impact of epilepsy on the morbidity of elderly patients. However, it is clear that the effect of epilepsy and the medications used to treat it can pose a threat to the independence of the elderly patient. There is significant potential for social isolation caused by falls, confusion, and amnesia, which can be further enhanced by the driving restrictions that are imposed following a seizure. Furthermore, there is a higher prevalence of depression, anxiety, and poor sleep compared to age-matched controls (96), which may be worsened by the stigma towards the disease. Together, these issues have the potential to contribute to a poorer overall quality of life, and the physician needs to be vigilant to advocate for independence with spouses, family, and regulating bodies.

Conclusions

Overall, the care of the elderly patient with epilepsy poses special challenges to the modern neurologist. Similar to other age groups, the cornerstone of management remains diagnostic rigor, especially as seizures present commonly, and sometimes atypically, in this population. However, this must always be balanced against the alternative likelihood of seizure 'mimickers'. Comorbidities, including cerebrovascular risk factors and cognitive impairment should be sought, as the impact of treatment should not risk overall morbidity and mortality. Close attention to anticonvulsant impact on patient's physical status, comorbidities, and concomitant medications is critical if these ideals are to be realized. It is important for physicians to have an understanding of the patient's social environment and the potential impact of any future seizures on individual safety and independence, which may require a more multidisciplinary perspective.

References

1. Hauser W, Hesdorffer D. *Epilepsy, Frequency, Causes and Consequences*. New York: Demos Publications, 1990.
2. de la Court A, Breteler MM, Meinardi H, Hauser WA, Hofman A. Prevalence of epilepsy in the elderly: the Rotterdam Study. *Epilepsia* 1996; 37(2):141–7.
3. Hauser W, Annegers J, Kurland L. Prevalence of epilepsy in Rochester, Minnesota: 1940–1980. *Epilepsia* 1991; 32(4):429–45.
4. Galimberti CA, Magri F, Magnani B, Arbasino C, Cravello L, Marchioni E, *et al.* Antiepileptic drug use and epileptic seizures in elderly nursing home residents: a survey in the province of Pavia, Northern Italy. *Epilepsy Res* 2006; 68(1):1–8.
5. Garrard J, Cloyd J, Gross C, Hardie N, Thomas L, Lackner T, *et al.* Factors associated with antiepileptic drug use among elderly nursing home residents. *J Gerontol A Biol Sci Med Sci* 2000; 55(7):M384–92.
6. Schachter SC, Cramer GW, Thompson GD, Chaponis RJ, Mendelson MA, Lawhorne L. An evaluation of antiepileptic drug therapy in nursing facilities. *J Am Geriatr Soc* 1998; 46(9):1137–41.
7. D'Souza WJ, Quinn SJ, Fryer JL, Taylor BV, Ficker DM, O'Brien TJ, *et al.* The prevalence and demographic distribution of treated epilepsy: A community-based study in Tasmania, Australia. *Acta Neurol Scand* 2012; 125(2):96–104.
8. Annegers JF, Hauser WA, Lee JR, Rocca WA. Incidence of acute symptomatic seizures in Rochester, Minnesota, 1935–1984. *Epilepsia* 1995; 36(4):327–33.
9. Hauser W, Annegers J, Kurland L. Incidence of epilepsy and unprovoked seizures in Rochester, Minnesota: 1935–1984. *Epilepsia* 1993; 34(3):453–68.
10. Olafsson E, Ludvigsson P, Gudmundsson G, Hesdorffer D, Kjartansson O, Hauser WA. Incidence of unprovoked seizures and epilepsy in Iceland and assessment of the epilepsy syndrome classification: a prospective study. *Lancet Neurol* 2005; 4(10):627–34.

11. Wallace H, Shorvon S, Tallis R. Age-specific incidence and prevalence rates of treated epilepsy in an unselected population of 2,052,922 and age-specific fertility rates of women with epilepsy. *Lancet* 1998; 352:1970–3.
12. Annegers JF, Dubinsky S, Coan SP, Newmark ME, Roht L. The incidence of epilepsy and unprovoked seizures in multiethnic, urban health maintenance organizations. *Epilepsia* 1999; 40(4):502–6.
13. Musicco M, Beghi E, Solari A, for the First Seizure Trial Group. Treatment of first tonic-clonic seizure does not improve the prognosis of epilepsy. *Neurology* 1997; 49:991–8.
14. First Seizure Trial Group (FIR.S.T. Group). Randomized clinical trial on the efficacy of antiepileptic drugs in reducing the risk of relapse after a first unprovoked tonic-clonic seizure. *Neurology* 1993; 43(3 (Part 1)):478–83.
15. Berg A, Shinnar S. The risk of seizure recurrence following a first unprovoked seizure: a quantitative review. *Neurology*, 1991; 41(7): 965–72.
16. Hart YM, Sander JW, Johnson AL, Shorvon SD. National General Practice Study of Epilepsy: recurrence after a first seizure. *Lancet* 1990; 336(8726):1271–4.
17. Hauser W, Rich SS, Annegers JF, Anderson VE. Seizure recurrence after a 1st unprovoked seizure: an extended follow-up. *Neurology* 1990; 40(8):1163–70.
18. DeLorenzo RJ, Hauser WA, Towne AR, Boggs JG, Pellock JM, Penberthy L, *et al.* A prospective population-based epidemiologic study of status epilepticus in Richmond Virginia. *Neurology* 1996; 46:1029–35.
19. Knake S, Rosenow F, Vescovi M, Oertel WH, Mueller HH, Wirbatz A, *et al.* Incidence of status epilepticus in adults in Germany: a prospective, population-based study. *Epilepsia* 2001; 42(6):714–18.
20. Vignatelli L, Tonon C, D'Alessandro R. Incidence and short-term prognosis of status epilepticus in adults in Bologna, Italy. *Epilepsia* 2003; 44(7):964–8.
21. DeLorenzo RJ, Pellock JM, Towne AR, Boggs JG. Epidemiology of status epilepticus. *J Clin Neurophysiol* 1995; 12(4):316–25.
22. Delorenzo R. *Clinical and epidemiologic study of status epilepticus in the elderly*. In: Rowan A, Ramsay R (eds) *Seizures and Epilepsy in the Elderly*, pp. 191–205. Boston, MA: Butterworth-Heineman, 1997.
23. Lhatoo SD, Johnson AL, Goodridge DM, MacDonald BK, Sander JW, Shorvon SD. Mortality in epilepsy in the first 11 to 14 years after diagnosis: multivariate analysis of a long-term, prospective, population-based cohort. *Ann Neurol* 2001; 49:336–44.
24. Hauser WA, Annegers JF, Kurland LT. Prevalence of epilepsy in Rochester Minnesota: 1940–1980. *Epilepsia* 1991; 42(4):429–45.
25. Loiseau J, Loiseau P, Duché B, Guyot M, Dartigues JF, Aublet B. A survey of epileptic disorders in southwest France: seizures in elderly patients. *Ann Neurol* 1990; 27(3):232–7.
26. Hauser W. Epidemiology of seizures and epilepsy in the elderly. In: Rowan A, Ramsay R (eds) *Seizures and Epilepsy in the Elderly*, pp. 7–20. Boston, MA: Butterworth-Heineman, 1997.
27. Kellinghaus C, Loddenkemper T, Dinner DS, Lachhwani D, Lüders HO. Non-epileptic seizures of the elderly. *J Neurol* 2004; 251:704–9.
28. McBride A, Shih T, Hirsch I. Video-EEG monitoring in the elderly: a review of 93 patients. *Epilepsia* 2002; 43(2):165–9.
29. Stephen L, Brodie M. Epilepsy in elderly people. *Lancet* 2000; 355(9213):1441–6.
30. Giroud M, Gras P, Fayolle H, André N, Soichot P, Dumas R. Early seizures after acute stroke: a study of 1,640 cases. *Epilepsia* 1994; 35(5):959–64.
31. Sung C, Chu N. Epileptic seizures in thrombotic stroke. *J Neurol* 1990; 237(3):166–70.
32. Bladin CF, Alexandrov AV, Bellavance A, Bornstein N, Chambers B, Coté R, *et al.* Seizures after stroke: a prospective multicenter study. *Arch Neurol* 2000; 57(11):1617–22.
33. Lancman ME, Golimstok A, Norscini J, Granillo R. Risk factors for developing seizures after a stroke. *Epilepsia* 1993; 34(1):141–3.
34. Hauser W. Seizure disorders: the changes with age. *Epilepsia* 1992; 33(Suppl 4):S6–S14.
35. Bruns JJ, Hauser W. The epidemiology of traumatic brain injury: a review. *Epilepsia* 2003; 44(Suppl 10):2–10.
36. Messing R, Closson R, Simon R. Drug-induced seizures: a 10-year experience. *Neurology* 1984; 34:1582.
37. Kearney TE, Dyer JE, Benowitz NL, Blanc PD. Seizures associated with poisoning and drug overdose. *Am J Emerg Med* 1994; 12:392.
38. Shorvon S, Tallis R, Wallace H. Antiepileptic drugs: coprescription of proconvulsant drugs and oral contraceptives: a national study of antiepileptic drug prescribing practice. *J Neurol Neurosurg Psychiatry* 2002; 72:114.
39. Gilmore R. Seizures associated with non-neurological medical conditions. In: Wyllie E (ed) *The treatment of epilepsy: principles and practice*, pp. 657–69. Baltimore, MA: Williams and Wilkins, 2001.
40. Luhdorf K, Jensen L, Plesner A. Etiology of seizures in the elderly. *Epilepsia* 1986; 27:458–63.
41. Roberts M, Godfrey J, Caird F. Epileptic seizures in the elderly: I. Aetiology and type of seizure. *Age Ageing* 1982; 11:24–8.
42. Sander JW, Hart YM, Johnson AL, Shorvon SD. National General Practice Study of Epilepsy: newly diagnosed epileptic seizures in a general population. *Lancet* 1990; 336(8726):1267–71.
43. Ramsay RE, Rowan A, Pryor F. Special considerations in treating the elderly patient with epilepsy. *Neurology* 2004; 62:S24–9.
44. Pugh MJ, Knoefel JE, Mortensen EM, Amuan ME, Berlowitz DR, Van Cott AC. New-onset epilepsy risk factors in older veterans. *J Am Geriatr Soc* 2009; 57:237–42.
45. So EL, Annegers JF, Hauser WA, O'Brien PC, Whisnant JP. Population-based study of seizure disorders after cerebral infarction. *Neurology* 1996; 46(2):350–5.
46. Lancman ME, Golimstok A, Norscini J, Granillo R. Risk factors for developing seizures after a stroke. *Epilepsia* 1993; 34:141–43.
47. Cleary P, Shorvon S, Tallis R. Late-onset seizures as a predictor of subsequent stroke. *Lancet* 2004; 363:1184–6.
48. Ng SK, Hauser WA, Brust JC, Susser M. Hypertension and the risk of new-onset unprovoked seizures. *Neurology* 1993; 43(2):425–8.
49. Hesdorffer DC, Hauser WA, Annegers JF, Kokmen E, Rocca WA. Dementia and adult-onset unprovoked seizures. *Neurology* 1996; 46(3):727–30.
50. McAreavey M, Ballinger B, Fenton G. Epileptic seizures in elderly patients with dementia. *Epilepsia* 1992; 33:657–60.
51. Amatniek JC, Hauser WA, DelCastillo-Castaneda C, Jacobs DM, Marder K, Bell K, Albert M, *et al.* Incidence and predictors of seizures in patients with Alzheimer's disease. *Epilepsia* 2006; 47:867–72.
52. Hommet C, Mondon K, Camus V, De Toffol B, Constans T. Epilepsy and dementia in the elderly. *Dement Geriatr Cogn Disord* 2008; 25:293–300.
53. Rao SC, Dove G, Cascino GD, Petersen RC. Recurrent seizures in patients with dementia: frequency, seizure types, and treatment outcome. *Epilepsy Behav* 2009; 14:118–20.
54. Hiyoshi T, Yagi K. Epilepsy in the elderly. *Epilepsia* 2004; 41 (Suppl 9):31–5.
55. Annegers JF, Hauser WA, Coan SP, Rocca WA. A population-based study of seizures after traumatic brain injuries. *N Engl J Med* 1998; 338:20–4.
56. Annegers JF, Hauser WA, Beghi E, Nicolosi A, Kurland LT. The risk of unprovoked seizures after encephalitis and meningitis. *Neurology* 1988; 38(9):1407–10.
57. Lote K, Stenwig AE, Skullerud K, Hirschberg H. Prevalence and prognostic significance of epilepsy in patients with gliomas. *Eur J Cancer* 1998; 34:98–102.
58. Dam AM, Fuglsang-Frederiksen A, Svarre-Olsen U, Dam M. Late-onset epilepsy: etiologies, types of seizure, and value of clinical

investigation, EEG, and computerized tomography scan. *Epilepsia* 1985; 26(3):227–31.

59. Chadwick D, Smith D. The misdiagnosis of epilepsy. *Br Med J* 2002; 324:495–6.
60. D'Souza WJ, Stankovich J, O'Brien TJ, Bower S, Pearce N, Cook MJ. The use of computer-assisted-telephone-interviewing to diagnose seizures, epilepsy and idiopathic generalized epilepsy. *Epilepsy Res* 2010; 91(1):20–7.
61. Duncan JS, Sander JW, Sisodiya SM, Walker MC. Adult epilepsy. *Lancet* 2006; 367:1087–100.
62. Holmes G. The electroencephalogram as a predictor of seizures following cerebral infarction. *Clin Electroencephalogr* 1980; 11(2): 83–86.
63. Towne AR, Waterhouse EJ, Boggs JG, Garnett LK, Brown AJ, Smith JR Jr, *et al.* Prevalence of nonconvulsive status epilepticus in comatose patients. *Neurology* 2000; 54:340–5.
64. Sheth RD, Drazkowski JF, Sirven JI, Gidal BE, Hermann BP. Protracted ictal confusion in elderly patients. *Arch Neurol* 2006; 60:529–32.
65. Beyenburg S, Elger C, Rueber M. Acute confusion or altered mental state: consider nonconvulsive status epilepticus. *Gerontology* 2007; 53:388–96.
66. Bottaro FJ, Martinez OA, Pardal MM, Bruetman JE, Reisin RC. Nonconvulsive status epilepticus in the elderly: a case-control study. *Epilepsia* 2007; 48:966–72.
67. Drury I, Selwa LM, Schuh LA, Kapur J, Varma N, Beydoun A, *et al.* Value of inpatient diagnostic CCTV-EEG monitoring in the elderly. *Epilepsia* 1999; 40:1100–2.
68. Detoledo J. Changing presentation of seizures with ageing: clinical and aetiological factors. *Gerontology* 1999; 45:329–35.
69. Ramsay RE, Pryor F. Epilepsy in the elderly. *Neurology* 2000; 55 (Suppl 1):S9–14.
70. Hirsch LJ, Arif H, Nahm EA, Buchsbaum R, Resor SR Jr, Bazil CW. Cross-sensitivity of skin rashes with antiepileptic drug use. *Neurology* 2008; 71:1527–34.
71. Vecht CJ. Optimizing therapy of seizures in patients with brain tumors. *Neurology* 2006; 67(12, Suppl 4):S10–13.
72. Grivas A, Schramm J, Kral T. Surgical treatment for refractory temporal lobe epilepsy in the elderly: seizure outcome and neuropsychological sequels compared with a younger cohort. *Epilepsia*; 2006; 47:1364–72.
73. Schmucker D. Aging and drug disposition: an update. *Pharmacol Rev* 1985; 37(2):133–48.
74. Schwartz J. The current state of knowledge on age, sex, and their interactions on clinical pharmacology. *Clin Pharmacol Ther* 2007; 82(1):87–96.
75. Goa K, Sorkin E. Gabapentin. A review of its pharmacological properties and clinical potential in epilepsy. *Drugs* 1993; 46(3):409–27.
76. Perucca E. *Pharmacokinetics*. In: Engel J Jr, Pedley T (eds) *Epilepsy: A Comprehensive Textbook*, pp. 1131–44. Philadelphia, PA: Lippincott-Raven Publishers, 1997.
77. Granger A. Ginkgo biloba precipitating epileptic seizures. *Age Ageing* 2001; 30:523–5.
78. French JA, Kanner AM, Bautista J, Abou-Khalil B, Browne T, Harden CL, *et al.* Efficacy and tolerability of the new antiepileptic drugs. II: treatment of refractory epilepsy: report of the Therapeutics and Technology Assessment Subcommittee and Quality Standards Subcommittee of the American Academy of Neurology and the American Epilepsy Society. *Neurology* 2004; 62(8):1261–73.
79. Brodie MJ, Overstall PW, Giorgi L. Multicentre, double-blind, randomised comparison between lamotrigine and carbamazepine in elderly patients with newly diagnosed epilepsy. *Epilepsy Res* 1999; 37:81–7.
80. Saetre E, Perucca E, Isojärvi J, Gjerstad L; LAM 40089 Study Group. An international multicenter randomised double-blind controlled trial of lamotrigine and sustained-release carbamazepine in the treatment of newly diagnosed epilepsy. *Epilepsia* 2007; 48:1292–302.
81. Rowan AJ, Ramsay RE, Collins JF, Pryor F, Boardman KD, Uthman BM, *et al.* New onset geriatric epilepsy: a randomised study of gabapentin, lamotrigine and carbamazepine. *Neurology* 2005; 64: 1868–73.
82. Alsaadi TM, Koopmans S, Apperson M, Farias S. Levetiracetam monotherapy for elderly patients with epilepsy. *Seizure* 2004; 13: 58–60.
83. Morrell MJ, Leppik I, French J, Ferrendelli J, Han J, Magnus L. The KEEPER(TM) trial: levetiracetam adjunctive treatment of partial-onset seizures in an open-label community-based study. *Epilepsy Res* 2003; 43:153–61.
84. Ferrendelli JA, French J, Leppik I, Morrell MJ, Herbeuval A, Han J, *et al.* Use of levetiracetam in a population of patients aged 65 years and older: a subset analysis of the KEEPER trial. *Epilepsy Behav*2003; 4:702–9.
85. Garcia-Escriva A, Lopez-Hernandez N. The use of levetiracetam in monotherapy in post stroke seizures in the elderly population. *Rev Neurol* 2007; 45:523–5.
86. Kutluay E, McCague K, D'Souza J, Beydoun A. Safety and tolerability of oxcarbazepine in elderly patients with epilepsy. *Epilepsy Behav* 2003; 4:175–80.
87. Ramsay RE, Uthman B, Pryor FM, Rowan AJ, Bainbridge J, Spitz M, *et al.* Topiramate in older patients with partial-onset seizures: a pilot double-blind, dose-comparison study. *Epilepsia* 2008; 49:1180–5.
88. Read CL, Stephen LJ, Stolarek IH, Paul A, Sills GJ, Brodie MJ. Cognitive effects of anticonvulsant monotherapy in elderly patients: a placebo-controlled study. *Seizure* 1998; 7:159–62.
89. Cameron H, Macphee G. Anticonvulsant therapy in the elderly—a need for placebo controlled trials. *Epilepsy Res* 1995; 21:149–57.
90. Leppik IE, Birnbaum AK. Epilepsy in the elderly. *Semin Neurol* 2002; 22:309–20.
91. Cleary P, Shorvon S, Tallis R. Late onset seizures as a predictor of subsequent stroke. *Lancet* 2004; 363:1184–6.
92. Chang B, Lowenstein D. Practice parameter: antiepileptic drug prophylaxis in severe traumatic brain injury: report of the Quality Standards Subcommittee of the American Academy of Neurology. *Neurology* 2003; 60:10–16.
93. Glantz MJ, Cole BF, Forsyth PA, Recht LD, Wen PY, Chamberlain MC, *et al.* Practice parameter: anticonvulsant prophylaxis in patients with newly diagnosed brain tumours: report of the Quality Standards Subcommittee of the American Academy of Neurology. *Neurology* 2000; 54:1886–93.
94. Ranta A,Wooten G. Hyponatraemia due to an additive effect of carbamazepine and thiazide diuretics. *Epilepsia* 2004; 45:879.
95. Dong X, Leppik IE, White J, Rarick J. Hyponatraemia from oxcarbazepine and carbamazepine. *Neurology* 2005; 65:1976–8.
96. Haut SR, Katz M, Masur J, Lipton RB. Seizures in the elderly: impact on mental status, mood and sleep. *Epilepsy Behav* 2009; 14: 540–4.

CHAPTER 19

Psychiatric Comorbidity in Epilepsy

Marco Mula

Introduction

Prevalence rates of psychiatric disorders are higher in people with seizures as compared with the general population, predominantly in patients with refractory epilepsy. Depression occurs in about 30%, anxiety disorders in 10–25%, and psychosis in 2–7% (1). However, such comorbidity frequently goes unrecognized and untreated while it should represent a major concern in the assessment of patients with epilepsy, as there are important reciprocal interactions between the disorders, not only in their clinical manifestations, but also in the effects of their treatments. In fact, antiepileptic drugs (AEDs), as well as other treatments for epilepsy, may exert various psychotropic effects, which can be negative as well as positive (2, 3). Conversely, psychotropic drugs may influence the propensity to have seizures.

The first step in the management of these patients should be an attempt to analyse and identify the various elements that may contribute to psychiatric symptoms, such as psychosocial issues, adverse treatment effects, or neurobiological factors directly related to the seizures or the epileptic disorder. Patients with epilepsy may experience a number of psychiatric manifestations around the ictus that have to be clearly differentiated from true psychiatric comorbidities. The practicality of classifying such symptoms according to their temporal relation to seizure occurrence (peri-ictal/paraictal symptoms vs. interictal symptoms) is well established (Table 19.1). Peri-ictal phenomena have been well described by Gowers (4) and Jackson (5) but also by Kraepelin (6) and Bleuler (7). The differentiation between peri-ictal and interictal psychiatric symptoms has relevant implications in terms of prognosis and treatment.

In this chapter, major psychiatric syndromes are discussed in the context of the management of epilepsy.

Mood and anxiety disorders

Mood and anxiety disorders represent the most frequent psychiatric comorbidity in patients with epilepsy and reasons for such a close link are both biological and psychosocial (8). On the one hand, epilepsy is a chronic disorder that brings about a number of social limitations (e.g. driving licence, job opportunities, etc,) and social discriminations leading to demoralization, poor self-esteem, and phobic avoidance. On the other hand, the biological contri bution to this association is given by neuroanatomical and neurochemical principles such as the involvement of the temporal lobes (9) and the psychotropic effects of AEDs (10). Mood disorders are one of the most important predictors of quality of life (11), and people with epilepsy and depression are more likely to experience side effects of AEDs (12), are more often drug-refractory (13), and have a poorer outcome after epilepsy surgery (14).

Peri-ictal mood and anxiety symptoms

Around one-third of patients with partial seizures report premonitory symptoms, usually before secondary generalized tonic–clonic seizures (1). Prodromal moods of depression or irritability may occur hours to days before a seizure and are often relieved by the convulsion (15). Among pre-ictal symptoms, behavioural changes are those most frequently reported (16). In our case series, around 13% of patients experience irritability, dysphoria, or depressed mood preceding seizures (17). Such feelings are almost indistinguishable from interictal ones, apart from duration and close relation with seizure occurrence. It seems, therefore, important for clinicians to enquire about these phenomena, because they cannot be detected by rating scales or questionnaires (18).

Ictal fear or ictal panic is the most frequently reported ictal psychiatric manifestation and it usually represents a partial seizure originating in right mesial temporal lobe structures (19). It seems to be reported by 10–15% patients with partial seizures (1), is more common in women than men (20, 21), and seems to have a poor prognostic value for surgery (22).

Ictal depression is the second most frequently reported ictal psychiatric manifestation. Such mood changes include anhedonia, feelings of guilt and intense suicidal ideation. It is reported in 1% of patients with temporal lobe epilepsy (1).

Table 19.1 Classification of psychiatric symptoms according to their temporal relation with seizures

Peri-ictal	Preictal Ictal Postictal
Paraictal	Alternative
Interictal	No relation

Postictal mood changes are less recognized in clinical practice. However, they are frequently reported by patients and relatives. A case series in a monitoring unit reported 18% of patients having at least five symptoms of depression lasting more than 24 hours (23). A comparison of seizure-related variables between these subjects and patients without any postictal psychiatric symptom failed to reveal any differences, although patients with postictal depression seem to be more likely to have a previous history of psychiatric disorders (24).

Manic/hypomanic symptoms are reported postictally in 22% of patients, often with associated psychotic phenomenology (23). It seems that postictal mania has a distinct position among psychiatric manifestations observed in the postictal period. Such manic episodes last for a longer period and have a higher frequency of recurrence than postictal psychoses, being associated with an older age at onset, electroencephalographic (EEG) frontal discharges, and non-dominant hemisphere involvement (25).

Postictal anxiety is reported by 45% patients (23). The median duration of symptoms ranges from 6–24 hours. In one-third of cases, postictal anxiety may last 24 hours or longer. In about 33% of cases postictal anxiety is reported by patients with a previous history of an anxiety disorder.

Interictal depressive and anxiety disorders

Data from community-based studies report prevalence rates for depressive disorders in the order of 20–22% (26, 27). In selected populations, such as tertiary referral centres or surgery programmes, the prevalence is even higher and ranges between 30–50% (28, 29). Such differences partially reflect the severity of the seizure disorder; in fact depression seems to occur in only 4% of seizure-free patients (30). Data on anxiety disorders are limited mainly because they are commonly comorbid with mood disorders but they are believed to have prevalence rates comparable to those of depression.

An interesting point, coming from epidemiological data, relates to the observation that the relationship between epilepsy and depression is not necessarily unidirectional, namely that some patients may present a mood disorder before the emergence of the seizure disorder (31). Although it is tempting to speculate that common pathogenetic mechanisms may be operant in both conditions, it has to be stated that such a bidirectional relationship has been noted in a number of chronic conditions such as Parkinson's disease (32), stroke (33), dementia (34), diabetes (35), cardiovascular disease (36), suggesting that depression is probably interlinked with a number of chronic conditions.

The issue of phenomenology of depression has been matter of debate having a number of implications in terms of diagnosis, treatment and prognosis. A number of authors have pointed out that depression in epilepsy is more often than not characterized by atypical features that are poorly reflected by conventional classificatory systems such as DSM (Diagnostic and Statistical Manual of Mental Disorders)-IV and ICD (International Statistical Classification of Diseases and Related Health Problems)-10 (37–39). However, other studies clearly suggest that it is possible to apply standardized criteria of DSM in a not negligible proportion of patients (40, 41). In general terms, the psychopathological spectrum of depression in epilepsy is likely to be large. On one hand, it is reasonable to hypothesize that patients with epilepsy can experience forms of mood disorders identical to those of patients without epilepsy. However, it is equally reasonable to assume that the underlying brain pathology can influence the expression of mood disorder symptoms making less evident some aspects or emphasizing others. A number of variables may account for such atypical features such as peri-ictal symptoms, the high comorbidity between mood and anxiety disorders (up to 73%), the underlying neurological condition, and the psychotropic effect of AEDs.

Pre-modern psychiatrists, such as Kraepelin and Bleuler, observed that patients with epilepsy may develop a pleomorphic pattern of depressive symptoms intermixed with euphoric moods, irritability, fear, and anxiety as well as anergia, pain and insomnia (42, 43). This concept has been revitalized during the 20th century by Blumer who coined the term interictal dysphoric disorder (IDD) to refer to this type of somatoform-depressive disorder claimed as typical of patients with epilepsy (44). Studies of our group pointed out that such a condition is a mood disorder probably not specific of epilepsy, being diagnosed also in patients with migraine, which is usually diagnosed during the depressive phase with a significant comorbid anxiety (social phobia and/or generalized anxiety disorder) and a relevant component of mood instability (45). Moreover, further studies demonstrated that a number of atypical and pheomorphic features of the so-called IDD are related to peri-ictal symptoms (17). These issues have relevant implications in terms of prognosis and treatment. On one hand, it emphasizes the need to dissect out peri-ictal manifestations from interictal ones being the former related to the prognosis and treatment of the epileptic syndrome. On the other hand, the presence of mood instability as an essential element of IDD suggest the need to prescribe mood stabilizing AED as preferred treatment and the utility of antipsychotic drugs in selective cases.

Psychoses

Psychoses and thought disorders are relatively rare in patients with epilepsy but represent serious complications affecting prognosis, morbidity, and mortality. Epidemiological evidence pointed out that the incidence of non-organic, non-affective psychoses, including schizophrenia and related disorders, is generally overrepresented (around 4–5%) in epilepsy as compared to the general population or other chronic medical conditions (46, 47). Higher prevalence rates have been found in selected samples such as hospital case series (48, 49). Interestingly, a family history of psychoses and a family history of epilepsy seem to be significant risk factors for psychosis suggesting strong neurobiological underpinnings between the two disorders (47).

Peri-ictal psychotic symptoms

The so-called ictal psychosis usually represents a complex partial status of temporal lobe origin and less frequently an extratemporal partial status (i.e. the frontal lobe) (50). Very rarely it has been reported as the manifestation of an absence status but studies are lacking. Simple focal status or aura continua may determine complex hallucinations resembling a thought disorder but insight is usually maintained making the differential diagnosis quite straightforward.

Among peri-ictal psychoses, postictal ones represent the most common type, accounting for approximately 25% of psychoses of epilepsy. They are usually precipitated by a series of secondary generalized tonic–clonic seizures (51, 52). Kanemoto and co-authors gave detailed description of the phenomenology and clinical features of patients with postictal psychoses (53, 54). Essentially, they seem to occur with later age of onset of epilepsy and at a later age than interictal psychoses. They are significantly associated with temporal lobe epilepsy, complex partial seizures, and magnetic resonance imaging (MRI) temporal plus extratemporal structural lesions. Patients are less likely to have learning disability, are less likely to have generalized spike wave abnormalities at the EEG. An association with déjà vu auras or ictal fear has been described (55). The lucid interval (i.e. a period of normal mental state preceding the onset of the psychotic episode) is another typical feature described in almost all patients, lasting from 1–6 days (52, 56). Failure to appreciate the presence of this lucid interval can lead to a misdiagnosis of this condition. The psychopathology of postictal psychosis is polymorphic, but most patients present with abnormal mood and paranoid delusions (52). Some patients are confused throughout the episode; others present with fluctuating impairment of consciousness and orientation; sometimes there is no confusion at all. Delusions of grandiosity and religiosity, often associated with an elevated mood, are dominant features. Patients may also be anxious and a typical symptom is fear of impending death. Because patients often have a clear sensorium and may receive command hallucinations if the latter relate to violence or suicide, it is during such states that violent attacks on the self or others may occur (57). The psychotic symptoms usually remit spontaneously within days or weeks, often without need for psychotropic drug treatment. However, in some cases, chronic psychoses develop from recurrent and even a single postictal psychosis (58). This is estimated to occur in about 25% of cases.

Interictal psychoses

Psychoses without a clear relationship to seizures are less frequent than peri-ictal psychoses (59). However, they are clinically more significant in terms of severity and duration than peri-ictal ones, being usually chronic disorders. Interictal psychoses may develop after several years of active temporal lobe epilepsy (60). The link between mesial-temporal structures and psychosis is supported by clinical and neuroimaging findings (61, 62). Neuropathology studies of resected temporal lobes from patients with interictal psychoses have suggested a link with the presence of cerebral malformations such as hamartomas and gangliogliomas as compared with mesial temporal sclerosis (63) but gross abnormalities such as enlarged ventricles or periventricular gliosis have also been noted (64). Left lateralization of temporal lobe dysfunction or temporal lobe pathology as a risk factor was originally suggested by Flor-Henry (65). Studies supporting the laterality hypothesis have been made using surface EEG, depth electrode recordings, computed tomography, neuropathology, neuropsychology, and positron emission tomography (PET), and more recently with MRI (66, 67).

Although the underlying pathology may be different, the absence of gliosis in the hippocampus and related structures characterizing schizophrenia, the site of the pathology, the timing of the lesions, and the consequent functional changes in the brain may all be crucial to the later development of any behaviour changes in both epilepsy and schizophrenia. Thus, the behaviour changes should be viewed as an integral part of the process of epilepsy that is manifest in some patients.

There have been persistent arguments as to the phenomenology of the interictal psychoses. Slater emphasized the presence of first-rank Schneiderian symptoms with religious mystical experiences and the preservation of affect (51). Other authors have stressed the rarity of negative symptoms and the absence of formal thought disorders and catatonic states (68). Nonetheless, there have been other authors who denied any clear psychopathologic differences between epileptic psychoses and schizophrenia. Phenomenology apart, the long-term prognosis of interictal psychosis seems to be better than that in process schizophrenia with less reported long-term institutionalization (51, 69, 70). This is probably due to the tendency of psychotic symptoms to attenuate and the rarity of personality deterioration.

Epilepsy and suicide

In the general population, suicide represents the 11th cause of death and the second in the group aged 25 to 34 years (71). It seems to be common in men, particularly in developed countries, while attempted suicide is more represented in women (72). In patients with epilepsy, the overall risk of committing suicide is about three times higher than that of the general population (73–75). Several studies have attempted to identify reasons for such an increased risk. In the general population, about 90% of people who successfully commit suicide have at least one psychiatric disorder at that time (76). Epilepsy is frequently associated with psychiatric comorbidity, but it is unlikely that such comorbidity is the only element responsible. A Danish study pointed out that the rate ratio of suicide in people with epilepsy is still doubled even after excluding people with psychiatric comorbidity and adjusting for various factors. Some have suggested a link with temporal lobe epilepsy (73). However, a recent study, using retrospective and prospective methods, found no epilepsy-related factors (77). Thus, the issue of epilepsy and suicide is still far from being elucidated but it is likely to be multifactorial with biological, constitutional, and psychosocial variables being implicated. At any rate, it seems evident that suicide prevention represents a relevant issue in epilepsy and careful attention need to be paid in selected cases.

In 2008, the US Food and Drug Administration (FDA) issued an alert to healthcare professionals about an increased risk of suicidal ideation and behaviour in people taking ADEs (78, 79). Drug companies had previously been asked to submit data from placebo-controlled trials, regardless of indication, when at least 30 people were enrolled. Eleven compounds were involved in 199 placebo-controlled trials, with over 27,000 people taking AEDs and 16,000 on placebo. The overall odds ratio (OR) for spontaneously reported suicidal behaviour or ideation in those taking active drugs was 1.8 (95% confidence interval (CI) 1.24–2.66). It has been suggested that the concern of the FDA might have been excessive, and the methodology of using only spontaneously reported suicidality events has been questioned (80). Others commented that analysing the data by indication, the OR was significantly raised in people with epilepsy (OR 3.53, 95% CI 1.28–12.10) but not for those taking AEDs for psychiatric conditions (OR 1.51, 95% CI 0.95–2.45) or other medical problems (OR 1.87, 95% CI 0.81–4.76), thus reflecting only the known increased risk of suicide in people with epilepsy (81). In general terms, the risk of stopping or not even taking AEDs might well be in excess of the so-called risk of suicide (82, 83). During the last year, a number of retrospective cohort and case–control studies have been published trying to examine the question raised by the FDA meta-analysis using observational study methodology (84–91). Such publications generated inconsistent results, attributable to a number of methodological limitations. The FDA will be requiring standardized assessment of suicidality at regular intervals during follow-up in future AED clinical trials and such data will probably shed light into this problem.

Postsurgery psychiatric problems

Temporal lobectomy is an established treatment for patients with intractable epilepsy. Ever since the early series, the possibility that surgery may be associated with the development of psychiatric disorders, in particular psychoses, has been discussed (63, 64). Most centres have stopped operating on floridly psychotic patients, based on the observation that psychoses generally do not improve with the operation. A few centres, however, regularly include psychiatric screening as part of their preoperative assessment, but postoperative psychiatric follow-up is often excluded. Assessment of psychosocial adjustment is rarely performed, in contrast to the often scrupulous recording of neuropsychological deficits.

Bruton suggested that the development of postoperative psychoses may be more common with certain pathologies (gangliogliomas) (92) and possibly in right-sided temporal resections (50). In some cases, the sudden relief of seizures that occurs following surgery may suggest a mechanism similar to forced normalization, although no persistent clear relationship emerges between success of operation and the development of psychotic postoperative states. In recent times, there have been several small series reported of patients with psychoses who have been successfully operated on, without worsening of their seizures but with marked improvement in seizure control (93). Data on *de novo* psychiatric disorders after surgery are still very limited. In general terms, they are often resistant to conventional psychotropic drugs but specific guidance of treatment is not available.

Antiepileptic drug-related psychiatric problems

AEDs have a number of mechanisms of action which are likely to be responsible for their antiseizure activity but also for their effect on mood and behaviour. A number of studies suggest that treatment with some AEDs is associated with the occurrence of depressive symptoms while other compounds are probably antidepressants. In general terms, the link between depression and barbiturates (94), vigabatrin (95), tiagabine (96), and topiramate (97) seems to be firmly established, as well as the beneficial properties of mood stabilizers such as carbamazepine, oxcarbazepine, lamotrigine, and valproate (3). In the majority of cases, a rapid titration of the drug (98) in patients with refractory epilepsy, a past history of depression (99) and limbic system dysfunction represent major determinants. In fact, it has been pointed out that a subgroup of patients with refractory epilepsy seems to be particularly vulnerable to the psychotropic effect of AEDs independently of the specific mechanism of action of the drug (99).

AED-related psychoses are usually toxic or in the context of the so-called forced normalization phenomenon. This concept refers to the publications of Heinrich Landolt who reported a group of patients who had florid psychotic episodes with 'forced normalization' of the EEG (100). Subsequently, Tellenbach (101) introduced the term 'alternative psychosis' for the clinical phenomenon of the reciprocal relationship between abnormal mental states and seizures, which did not, as Landolt's term did, rely on EEG findings. Since the early observations of Landolt, a sufficient number of patients with alternative psychosis have been reported (102). The clinical presentation doesn't need to be necessarily a psychosis but this is probably the most common. The disturbed behaviour may last days or weeks and it is often self-limiting with the reappearance of seizures. Landolt originally associated this phenomenon with focal epilepsies but subsequent studies suggested an association with generalized epilepsies. In any case, what seems to be striking is the association with neurobiological mechanisms underlying seizure control. In fact, forced normalization has been reported not only with AEDs but also with vagus nerve stimulation (103) and may probably be implicated in psychoses following surgery.

The use of psychotropic drugs in patients with epilepsy

Treatment of mood disorders and the use of antidepressant drugs

Data on treatment strategies of mood disorders in epilepsy are still limited. There is only one properly controlled trial of antidepressant drugs in epilepsy (107), and the evidence for treatment strategies relies heavily on clinical experience. An expert US panel comprising members from the Epilepsy Foundation's Mood Disorders Initiative have composed a Consensus Statement (108). In general terms, widely used guidelines for treatment of primary psychiatric disorders outside epilepsy are valuable (109, 110) taking into account a number of recommendations regarding the underlying neurological condition (Table 19.2).

Firstly, it has to be stated that full remission is the final goal of the treatment of a major depressive episode. Selective serotonin reuptake inhibitors (SSRIs) (e.g. citalopram 20 mg) can be reasonably considered first choice, bearing in mind that drug doses need to be adjusted according to clinical response, especially if AEDs with inducing properties are co-prescribed (111, 112). Fluvoxamine and nefazodone are the only difficult to use compounds. In fact, they are enzyme inhibitors and may potentially increase plasma levels of a number of AEDs (especially carbamazepine, phenytoin) (112). In psychiatric practice, approximately 50% of patients with a major depressive episode will reach remission within the first 6 months of treatment and approximately 66% within 2 years (113). When remission has lasted for 6–12 months, the patient can be considered in a recovery state. However, it is estimated that approximately 15–20% of patients will fail to respond to any antidepressant trial. In this regard, it is important to point out that it is still unclear whether patients with epilepsy respond equally to antidepressant drug treatment or they have different remission rates. The general impression is that depression in epilepsy is usually mild to moderate in severity with excellent response rates to adequate treatments.

Adverse effects of SSRIs include hyponatraemia, sexual dysfunction, antiplatelet properties with increased risk of bleeding, and extrapyramidal symptoms (114). In cases of malaise or confusion electrolytes need to be tested, and particular attention is required when SSRIs are prescribed in combination with oxcarbazepine or carbamazepine that are both associated with hyponatraemia.

Table 19.2 Classification of major psychotropic medications

Antidepressant drugs	
Reversible inhibitors of monoamine oxidase A (RIMAs)	Moclobemide
Tricyclic antidepressant drugs (TCAs)	Amitriptyline, clomipramine, desipramine, imipramine, maprotiline, nortriptyline, protriptyline, trimipramine
Selective serotonin reuptake inhibitors (SSRIs)	Citalopram, escitalopram, fluoxetine, fluvoxamine, paroxetine, sertraline
Selective noradrenergic reuptake inhibitors (NRIs)	Reboxetine
Noradrenaline and dopamine reuptake blockers (NDRIs)	Bupropion
Dual serotonin and noradrenaline reuptake inhibitors (SNRIs)	Duloxetine, venlafaxine
Noradrenergic and specific serotoninergic Antidepressants (NaSSAs)	Mianserine, mirtazapine
Dual serotonin 2 antagonists/ serotonin reuptake inhibitors (SARIs)	Nefazodone, trazodone
Antipsychotic drugs	
Typical	Chlorpromazine, fluphenazine, thioridazine, mesoridazine, thiothixene, zuclopenthixol, prochlorperazine, droperidol, haloperidol
Atypical	Clozapine, risperidone, olanzapine, quetiapine, iloperidone, ziprasidone, aripiprazole

Sexual dysfunction has been reported in up to 70% of patients taking SSRIs (115). Therefore, in young males, the use of SSRIs should be carefully considered and other compounds such as bupropion or duloxetine can be considered. Bleeding may represent a concern especially in elderly patients.

The issue of seizure worsening with antidepressants represents a special concern for clinicians. However, it has to be acknowledged that, for the majority of compounds prescribed at dosages within the therapeutic range, the incidence of seizures is less than 0.5% when other risk factors are excluded (116). In fact, the proconvulsive effect is likely to be dose-dependent, becoming significant for dosages other than those prescribed in the treatment of depression. SSRIs can be considered reasonably safe while clomipramine and maprotiline the only drugs that may represent a concern (117). Bupropion seems to be proconvulsant when administered in the immediate release formulation while the extended release one is similar to SSRIs (118). In this regard, it has to be acknowledged that available information come from psychiatric samples and it is not known whether such data are applicable to patients with epilepsy.

Electroconvulsive therapy is not contraindicated in patients with epilepsy, it is well tolerated and worth considering in patients with very severe and treatment-resistant mood episodes (119, 120).

Finally, clinicians must always bear in mind that the use of antidepressant drugs in subjects with bipolar disorder can cause manic/hypomanic symptoms. The diagnosis of bipolar disorder can be challenging even for experienced psychiatrists. A family history of bipolar disorder or a mood disorder not otherwise specified, or a previous history of postpartum depression (for female patients) may be helpful to identify those subjects that need to be referred to a psychiatrist for a more in-depth consultation.

Treatment of psychotic disorders and the use of antipsychotic drugs

In general terms, the treatment of peri-ictal and paraictal psychoses is connected with the treatment of the epilepsy. Neuroleptics can be used for a short period of time as symptomatic therapies to reduce morbidity and mortality. Interictal psychoses may require long-lasting antipsychotic drug treatment. In such cases, patients need to be followed-up in a psychiatric setting. Neurologists have to be aware that the dose of neuroleptics has to be always tailored to the patient's response because in almost all cases enzyme inducers reduce the plasma levels of these drugs (118). In particular, the use of clozapine has to be carefully monitored because its metabolism has a high interindividual and intraindividual variability and, especially in combination with valproate, interactions are difficult to predict (121) (Table 19.3).

Among possible adverse effects of antipsychotic drugs, it has to be acknowledged that weight gain and sedation could be emphasized by some AED combinations (e.g. valproate, barbiturates). The association of clozapine with AED characterized by bone marrow suppression (e.g. carbamazepine, oxcarbazepine, and so on) is highly contraindicated.

Traditional antipsychotics have long been recognized as a class of drugs that can increase the risk of seizures. As for antidepressant drugs, clinical data usually come from psychiatric samples, thus limiting the applicability of such findings to the population of patients with epilepsy. In particular it is still unknown whether different epileptic syndromes have different risks for psychotropic induced seizures.

Generally, chlorpromazine and clozapine are considered proconvulsant in epileptic patients. The former only at high doses (1000 mg/daily) and the latter at medium and high doses (>600 mg/daily) (122). Clozapine may cause epileptiform EEG changes and seizures even at therapeutic doses. Such effects seem to be dose-dependent and titration-dependent (123). EEG abnormalities have been reported in 1%, 2.7%, and 4.4% of patients for doses less than 300 mg, 300–600 mg, or 600–900 mg/daily respectively (124). However, the prevalence of seizures, in subjects without a previous history of epilepsy, seems to be much lower and in the region of 0.9%, 0.8%, and 1.5% for the same range of doses of the previous study (125). Seizures are often myoclonic but also generalized tonic–clonic or partial depending on the individual patient.

New antipsychotic drugs such are usually well tolerated and can be considered reasonably safe as compared to clozapine and chlorpromazine. In particular, olanzapine and quetiapine showed a seizure rate of 0.9% and risperidone an even lower risk of seizures (about 0.3%) (116).

Special treatments: the use of lithium

The use of lithium in epilepsy is very rarely considered. In case it is needed, it has to be considered that some combinations should be preferred.

Table 19.3 CYP enzymes and major psychotropic drugs: metabolism, induction and inhibition

Enzymes	Substrates	Inhibitors	Inducers	Enzymes	Substrates	Inhibitors	Inducers
CYP 1A2	**Antidepressants** TCAs Fluvoxamine Mirtazapine Duloxetine **Antipsychotics** Chlorpromazine Haloperidol Clozapine Olanzapine Ziprasidone	**Antidepressants** Fluvoxamine Fluoxetine Paroxetine Sertraline	St John's wort	**CYP2D6**	**Antidepressants** Fluoxetine Fluvoxamine Citalopram Escitalopram Duloxetine Paroxetine Mianserine Venlafaxine Trazodone Nefazodone Maprotiline Mirtazapine TCAs **Antispychotics** Chlorpromazine Thioridazine Haloperidol Olanzapine Risperidone Iloperidone	**Antidepressants** Fluoxetine Paroxetine Sertraline Bupropion Duloxetine Clomipramine **Antipsychotics** Thioridazine Haloperidol Clozapine Olanzapine Risperidone	
CYP2C9/10/19	**Antidepressants** Sertraline Fluoxetine Amitriptyline Bupropion Citalopram Escitalopram Clomipramine Imipramine Moclobemide **Antipsychotics** Thioridazine Olanzapine **Anticonvulsants** Phenytoin Mephenytoin Esobarbital Mephobarbital Phenobarbitone Primidone	**Antidepressants** Fluoxetine Sertraline Fluvoxamine **Antipsychotics** Thioridazine Clozapine	Phenobarbital Carbamazepine	**CYP3A4**	**Antidepressants** Nefazodone Sertraline Venlafaxine Reboxetine Escitalopram Mirtazapine Trazodone TCAs **Antipsychotics** Haloperidol Clozapine Risperidone Ziprasidone Iloperidone Quetiapine Aripiprazole **Anticonvulsants** Carbamazepine Zonisamide Tiagabine	**Antidepressants** Norfluoxetine Nefazodone Fluvoxamine **Antipsychotics** Chlorpromazine Thioridazine Haloperidol Risperidone	Carbamazepine Barbiturates Phenytoin St John's wort

The concomitant prescription of lithium carbonate and carbamazepine, though possibly associated with a favourable pharmacodynamic interaction on mood stabilization, may increase lithium toxicity with the potential occurrence of severe hyponatraemia when lithium alone is stopped (126) and a significant modification in thyroid function with decrease in T4 and free T4 (127). Conversely, the combination of lithium and valproate has a higher tolerability but side effects, such as weight gain, sedation, and tremor may be prominent. The combination with lamotrigine seems to be very well tolerated (128), while co-therapy with topiramate may reduce lithium clearance, leading to toxic lithium plasma levels (129).

Lithium may have proconvulsant properties especially plasma concentrations exceeding 3.0 mEq/L. At therapeutic levels, the effect of lithium on seizure frequency in individuals with epilepsy is inconsistent (130). If the prescription of lithium is needed and indicated, vigilant monitoring of lithium blood levels and careful clinical follow-up are warranted.

References

1. Gaitatzis A, Trimble MR, Sander JW. The psychiatric comorbidity of epilepsy. *Acta Neurol Scand* 2004; 110(4):207–20.
2. Mula M, Monaco F. Antiepileptic drugs and psychopathology of epilepsy: an update. *Epileptic Disord* 2009; 11(1):1–9.
3. Ettinger AB. Psychotropic effects of antiepileptic drugs. *Neurology* 2006; 67(11):1916–25.
4. Gowers WRS.. *Epilepsy, and other chronic convulsive diseases: their causes, symptoms & treatment:* pp. xiv, 309. London: J.&A. Churchill, 1881.

5. Jackson JMD. *On Epilepsy; in answer to the question-What is the nature of the internal commotion which takes place during an epileptic paroxysm?* London, 1850.
6. Kraepelin E, Johnstone T. *Lectures on clinical psychiatry* (3rd rev edn, Johnstone T (ed)). London: Bailliere Tindall and Cox, 1912.
7. Bleuler E. *Lehrbuch der Psychiatrie*, pp. viii, 518. Berlin, 1916.
8. Kanner AM, Balabanov A. Depression and epilepsy: how closely related are they? *Neurology* 2002; 58(8 Suppl 5):S27–39.
9. Quiske A, Helmstaedter C, Lux S, Elger CE. Depression in patients with temporal lobe epilepsy is related to mesial temporal sclerosis. *Epilepsy Res* 2000; 39(2):121–5.
10. Mula M, Sander JW. Negative effects of antiepileptic drugs on mood in patients with epilepsy. *Drug Saf* 2007; 30(7):555–67.
11. Boylan LS, Flint LA, Labovitz DL, Jackson SC, Starner K, Devinsky O. Depression but not seizure frequency predicts quality of life in treatment-resistant epilepsy. *Neurology* 2004; 62(2):258–61.
12. Cramer JA, Blum D, Reed M, Fanning K. The influence of comorbid depression on seizure severity. *Epilepsia* 2003; 44(12):1578–84.
13. Hitiris N, Mohanraj R, Norrie J, Brodie MJ. Mortality in epilepsy. *Epilepsy Behav* 2007; 10(3):363–76.
14. Kanner AM. Depression in epilepsy: a complex relation with unexpected consequences. *Curr Opin Neurol* 2008; 21(2):190–4.
15. Blanchet P, Frommer GP. Mood change preceding epileptic seizures. *J Nerv Ment Dis* 1986; 174(8):471–6.
16. Scaramelli A, Braga P, Avellanal A, Bogacz A, Camejo C, Rega I, *et al.* Prodromal symptoms in epileptic patients: clinical characterization of the pre-ictal phase. *Seizure* 2009; 18(4):246–50.
17. Mula M, Jauch R, Cavanna A, Gaus V, Kretz R, Collimedaglia L, *et al.* Interictal dysphoric disorder and periictal dysphoric symptoms in patients with epilepsy. *Epilepsia* 2010; 51(7):1139–45.
18. Mula M, Schmitz B, Jauch R, Cavanna A, Cantello R, Monaco F, *et al.* On the prevalence of bipolar disorder in epilepsy. *Epilepsy Behav* 2008; 13(4):658–61.
19. Guimond A, Braun CM, Belanger E, Rouleau I. Ictal fear depends on the cerebral laterality of the epileptic activity. *Epileptic Disord* 2008; 10(2):101–12.
20. Chiesa V, Gardella E, Tassi L, Canger R, Lo Russo G, Piazzini A, *et al.* Age-related gender differences in reporting ictal fear: analysis of case histories and review of the literature. *Epilepsia* 2007; 48(12): 2361–4.
21. Toth V, Fogarasi A, Karadi K, Kovacs N, Ebner A, Janszky J. Ictal affective symptoms in temporal lobe epilepsy are related to gender and age. *Epilepsia* 2010; 51(7):1126–32.
22. Feichtinger M, Pauli E, Schafer I, Eberhardt KW, Tomandl B, Huk J, *et al.* Ictal fear in temporal lobe epilepsy: surgical outcome and focal hippocampal changes revealed by proton magnetic resonance spectroscopy imaging. *Arch Neurol* 2001; 58(5):771–7.
23. Kanner AM, Soto A, Gross-Kanner H. Prevalence and clinical characteristics of postictal psychiatric symptoms in partial epilepsy. *Neurology* 2004; 62(5):708–13.
24. Kanner AM, Schachter SC. *Psychiatric controversies in epilepsy*. San Diego, CA: Elsevier/Academic Press, 2008.
25. Nishida T, Kudo T, Inoue Y, Nakamura F, Yoshimura M, Matsuda K, *et al.* Postictal mania versus postictal psychosis: differences in clinical features, epileptogenic zone, and brain functional changes during postictal period. *Epilepsia* 2006; 47(12):2104–14.
26. Edeh J, Toone BK. Antiepileptic therapy, folate deficiency, and psychiatric morbidity: a general practice survey. *Epilepsia* 1985; 26(5):434–40.
27. Tellez-Zenteno JF, Patten SB, Jette N, Williams J, Wiebe S. Psychiatric comorbidity in epilepsy: a population-based analysis. *Epilepsia* 2007; 48(12):2336–44.
28. Victoroff JI, Benson F, Grafton ST, Engel J, Jr., Mazziotta JC. Depression in complex partial seizures. Electroencephalography and cerebral metabolic correlates. *Arch Neurol* 1994; 51(2):155–63.
29. Ring HA, Moriarty J, Trimble MR. A prospective study of the early postsurgical psychiatric associations of epilepsy surgery. *J Neurol Neurosurg Psychiatry* 1998; 64(5):601–4.
30. Jacoby A, Baker GA, Steen N, Potts P, Chadwick DW. The clinical course of epilepsy and its psychosocial correlates: findings from a U.K. Community study. *Epilepsia* 1996; 37(2):148–61.
31. Hesdorffer DC, Hauser WA, Annegers JF, Cascino G. Major depression is a risk factor for seizures in older adults. *Ann Neurol* 2000; 47(2):246–9.
32. Menza M, Dobkin RD, Marin H, Mark MH, Gara M, Buyske S, *et al.* The impact of treatment of depression on quality of life, disability and relapse in patients with Parkinson's disease. *Mov Disord* 2009; 24(9):1325–32.
33. Thomas AJ, Kalaria RN, O'Brien JT. Depression and vascular disease: what is the relationship? *J Affect Disord* 2004; 79(1-3):81–95.
34. Panza F, D'Introno A, Colacicco AM, Capurso C, Del Parigi A, Caselli RJ, *et al.* Temporal relationship between depressive symptoms and cognitive impairment: the Italian Longitudinal Study on Aging. *J Alzheimers Dis* 2009; 17(4):899–911.
35. Pan A, Lucas M, Sun Q, van Dam RM, Franco OH, Manson JE, *et al.* Bidirectional association between depression and type 2 diabetes mellitus in women. *Arch Intern Med* 2010; 170(21):1884–91.
36. Lippi G, Montagnana M, Favaloro EJ, Franchini M. Mental depression and cardiovascular disease: a multifaceted, bidirectional association. *Semin Thromb Hemost* 2009; 35(3):325–36.
37. Kanner AM, Kozak AM, Frey M. The use of sertraline in patients with epilepsy: Is It Safe? *Epilepsy Behav* 2000; 1(2):100–5.
38. Mendez MF, Cummings JL, Benson DF. Depression in epilepsy. Significance and phenomenology. *Arch Neurol* 1986; 43(8):766–70.
39. Krishnamoorthy ES, Trimble MR, Blumer D. The classification of neuropsychiatric disorders in epilepsy: a proposal by the ILAE Commission on Psychobiology of Epilepsy. *Epilepsy Behav* 2007; 10(3):349–53.
40. Jones JE, Bell B, Fine J, Rutecki P, Seidenberg M, Hermann B. A controlled prospective investigation of psychiatric comorbidity in temporal lobe epilepsy. *Epilepsia* 2007; 48(12):2357–60.
41. Jones JE, Hermann BP, Barry JJ, Gilliam F, Kanner AM, Meador KJ. Clinical assessment of Axis I psychiatric morbidity in chronic epilepsy: a multicenter investigation. *J Neuropsychiatry Clin Neurosci* 2005; 17(2):172–9.
42. Kraepelin E, Diefendorf AR. *Clinical psychiatry (1907)*. Delmar, NY: Scholars' Facsimiles and Reprints, 1981.
43. Bleuler E. *Textbook of psychiatry*. New York: The Macmillan Co, 1924.
44. Blumer D. Dysphoric disorders and paroxysmal affects: recognition and treatment of epilepsy-related psychiatric disorders. *Harv Rev Psychiatry* 2000; 8(1):8–17.
45. Mula M, Jauch R, Cavanna A, Collimedaglia L, Barbagli D, Gaus V, *et al.* Clinical and psychopathological definition of the interictal dysphoric disorder of epilepsy. *Epilepsia* 2008; 49(4):650–6.
46. Bredkjaer SR, Mortensen PB, Parnas J. Epilepsy and non-organic non-affective psychosis. National epidemiologic study. *Br J Psychiatry* 1998; 172:235–8.
47. Qin P, Xu H, Laursen TM, Vestergaard M, Mortensen PB. Risk for schizophrenia and schizophrenia-like psychosis among patients with epilepsy: population based cohort study. *Br Med J* 2005; 331(7507):23.
48. Gureje O. Interictal psychopathology in epilepsy. Prevalence and pattern in a Nigerian clinic. *Br J Psychiatry* 1991; 158:700–5.
49. Mendez MF, Grau R, Doss RC, Taylor JL. Schizophrenia in epilepsy: seizure and psychosis variables. *Neurology* 1993; 43(6):1073–7.
50. Trimble MR. *The psychoses of epilepsy*. New York: Raven Press, 1991.
51. Slater E, Beard AW. The schizophrenia-like psychoses of epilepsy, V: Discussion and conclusions. 1963. *J Neuropsychiatry Clin Neurosci* 1995; 7(3):372–8; discussion 1-2.
52. Logsdail SJ, Toone BK. Post-ictal psychoses. A clinical and phenomenological description. *Br J Psychiatry* 1988; 152:246–52.

53. Kanemoto K, Kawasaki J, Kawai I. Postictal psychosis: a comparison with acute interictal and chronic psychoses. *Epilepsia* 1996; 37(6): 551–6.
54. Kanemoto K, Takeuchi J, Kawasaki J, Kawai I. Characteristics of temporal lobe epilepsy with mesial temporal sclerosis, with special reference to psychotic episodes. *Neurology* 1996; 47(5):1199–203.
55. Savard G, Andermann F, Olivier A, Remillard GM. Postictal psychosis after partial complex seizures: a multiple case study. *Epilepsia* 1991; 32(2):225–31.
56. Adachi N, Ito M, Kanemoto K, Akanuma N, Okazaki M, Ishida S, *et al.* Duration of postictal psychotic episodes. *Epilepsia* 2007; 48(8): 1531–7.
57. Kanemoto K, Kawasaki J, Mori E. Violence and epilepsy: a close relation between violence and postictal psychosis. *Epilepsia* 1999; 40(1):107–9.
58. Falip M, Carreno M, Donaire A, Maestro I, Pintor L, Bargallo N, *et al.* Postictal psychosis: a retrospective study in patients with refractory temporal lobe epilepsy. *Seizure* 2009; 18(2):145–9.
59. Schmitz EB, Robertson MM, Trimble MR. Depression and schizophrenia in epilepsy: social and biological risk factors. *Epilepsy Res* 1999; 35(1):59–68.
60. Adachi N, Matsuura M, Okubo Y, Oana Y, Takei N, Kato M, *et al.* Predictive variables of interictal psychosis in epilepsy. *Neurology* 2000; 55(9):1310–4.
61. Tebartz Van Elst L, Baeumer D, Lemieux L, Woermann FG, Koepp M, Krishnamoorthy S, *et al.* Amygdala pathology in psychosis of epilepsy: A magnetic resonance imaging study in patients with temporal lobe epilepsy. *Brain* 2002; 125(Pt 1):140–9.
62. Mula M, Cavanna A, Collimedaglia L, Viana M, Barbagli D, Tota G, *et al.* Clinical correlates of schizotypy in patients with epilepsy. *J Neuropsychiatry Clin Neurosci* 2008; 20(4):441–6.
63. Taylor DC. Ontogenesis of chronic epileptic psychoses: a reanalysis. *Psychol Med* 1971; 1(3):247–53.
64. Bruton CJ, Stevens JR, Frith CD. Epilepsy, psychosis, and schizophrenia: clinical and neuropathologic correlations. *Neurology* 1994; 44(1):34–42.
65. Flor-Henry P. Determinants of psychosis in epilepsy: laterality and forced normalization. *Biol Psychiatry* 1983; 18(9):1045–57.
66. Maier M, Mellers J, Toone B, Trimble M, Ron MA. Schizophrenia, temporal lobe epilepsy and psychosis: an in vivo magnetic resonance spectroscopy and imaging study of the hippocampus/amygdala complex. *Psychol Med* 2000; 30(3):571–81.
67. Flugel D, Cercignani M, Symms MR, Koepp MJ, Foong J. A magnetization transfer imaging study in patients with temporal lobe epilepsy and interictal psychosis. *Biol Psychiatry* 2006; 59(6):560–7.
68. Getz K, Hermann B, Seidenberg M, Bell B, Dow C, Jones J, *et al.* Negative symptoms in temporal lobe epilepsy. *Am J Psychiatry* 2002; 159(4):644–51.
69. Ashidate N. [Clinical study on epilepsy and psychosis]. *Seishin Shinkeigaku Zasshi* 2006; 108(3):260–5.
70. Fisekovic S, Burnazovic L. Epileptic psychoses—evaluation of clinical aspects. *Bosn J Basic Med Sci* 2007; 7(2):140–3.
71. Gelder MG, Andreasen NC, Lopez-Ibor JJ, Geddes JR (eds). *New Oxford Textbook of Psychiatry* (2nd edn). Oxford: Oxford University Press, 2009.
72. Sadock BJ, Sadock VA, Ruiz P (eds). *Kaplan and Sadock's comprehensive textbook of psychiatry* (9th edn). Philadelphia, PA: Wolters Kluwer Health/Lippincott Williams & Wilkins, 2009.
73. Harris EC, Barraclough B. Suicide as an outcome for mental disorders. A meta-analysis. *Br J Psychiatry* 1997; 170:205–28.
74. Bell GS, Gaitatzis A, Bell CL, Johnson AL, Sander JW. Suicide in people with epilepsy: how great is the risk? *Epilepsia* 2009; 50(8): 1933–42.
75. Christensen J, Vestergaard M, Mortensen PB, Sidenius P, Agerbo E. Epilepsy and risk of suicide: a population-based case-control study. *Lancet Neurol* 2007; 6(8):693–8.
76. Barraclough BM. The suicide rate of epilepsy. *Acta Psychiatr Scand* 1987; 76(4):339–45.
77. Hara E, Akanuma N, Adachi N, Hara K, Koutroumanidis M. Suicide attempts in adult patients with idiopathic generalized epilepsy. *Psychiatry Clin Neurosci* 2009; 63(2):225–9.
78. US Food and Drug Administration. *Antiepileptic drugs and suicidality.* FDA Alert, 2008.
79. US Food and Drug Administration. *Information for Healthcare Professionals: Suicidal Behavior and Ideation and Antiepileptic Drugs.* FDA Alert, 2008.
80. Hesdorffer DC, Kanner AM. The FDA alert on suicidality and antiepileptic drugs: Fire or false alarm? *Epilepsia* 2009; 50(5):978–86.
81. Bell GS, Mula M, Sander JW. Suicidality in people taking antiepileptic drugs: What is the evidence? *CNS Drugs* 2009; 23(4):281–92.
82. Mula M, Sander JW. Antiepileptic drugs and suicidality. Much ado about very little? *Neurology* 2010; 75(4):300–1.
83. Mula M, Sander JW. Antiepileptic drugs and suicide risk: could stopping medications pose a greater hazard? *Expert Rev Neurother* 2010; 10(12):1775–6.
84. Arana A, Wentworth CE, Ayuso-Mateos JL, Arellano FM. Suicide-related events in patients treated with antiepileptic drugs. *N Engl J Med* 2010; 363(6):542–51.
85. Gibbons R, Hur K, Brown CH, Mann JJ. Relationship between antiepileptic drugs and suicide attempts in patients with bipolar disorder. *Arch Gen Psychiatry* 2009; 66:1354–60.
86. Olesen JB, Hansen PR, Erdal J, Abildstrom SZ, Weeke P, Fosbol EL, *et al.* Antiepileptic drugs and risk of suicide: a nationwide study. *Pharmacoepidemiol Drug Saf* 2010; 19(5):518–24.
87. VanCott AC, Cramer JA, Copeland LA, Zeber JE, Steinman MA, Dersh JJ, *et al.* Suicide-related behaviors in older patients with new anti-epileptic drug use: data from the VA hospital system. *BMC Med* 2010; 8:4.
88. Patorno E, Bohn RL, Wahl PM, Avorn J, Patrick AR, Liu J, *et al.* Anticonvulsant medications and the risk of suicide, attempted suicide, or violent death. *JAMA* 2010; 303(14):1401–9.
89. Andersohn F, Schade R, Willich SN, Garbe E. Use of antiepileptic drugs in epilepsy and the risk of self-harm or suicidal behavior. *Neurology* 2010; 75(4):335–40.
90. Gibbons RD, Hur K, Brown CH, Mann JJ. Gabapentin and suicide attempts. *Pharmacoepidemiol Drug Saf* 2010 Dec; 19(12):1241–7.
91. Redden L, Pritchett Y, Robieson W, Kovacs X, Garofalo M, Tracy K, *et al.* Suicidality and divalproex sodium: analysis of controlled studies in multiple indications. *Ann Gen Psychiatry* 2011; 10(1):1.
92. Bruton CJ. *The neuropathology of temporal lobe epilepsy*. Oxford: Oxford University Press, 1988.
93. Reutens DC, Savard G, Andermann F, Dubeau F, Olivier A. Results of surgical treatment in temporal lobe epilepsy with chronic psychosis. *Brain* 1997; 120(Pt 11):1929–36.
94. Robertson MM, Trimble MR, Townsend HR. Phenomenology of depression in epilepsy. *Epilepsia* 1987; 28(4):364–72.
95. Levinson DF, Devinsky O. Psychiatric adverse events during vigabatrin therapy. *Neurology* 1999; 53(7):1503–11.
96. Trimble MR, Rusch N, Betts T, Crawford PM. Psychiatric symptoms after therapy with new antiepileptic drugs: psychopathological and seizure related variables. *Seizure* 2000; 9(4):249–54.
97. Mula M, Trimble MR, Lhatoo SD, Sander JW. Topiramate and psychiatric adverse events in patients with epilepsy. *Epilepsia* 2003; 44(5):659–63.
98. Mula M, Hesdorffer DC, Trimble M, Sander JW. The role of titration schedule of topiramate for the development of depression in patients with epilepsy. *Epilepsia* 2009; 50(5):1072–6.

99. Mula M, Trimble MR, Sander JW. Are psychiatric adverse events of antiepileptic drugs a unique entity? A study on topiramate and levetiracetam. *Epilepsia* 2007; 48(12):2322–6.
100. Landolt H. [Psychic disorders in epilepsy. Clinical and electroencephalographic research.]. *Dtsch Med Wochenschr* 1962; 87:446–52.
101. Tellenbach H. [Epilepsy as a Convulsive Disorder and as a Psychosis. On Alternative Psychoses of Paranoid Nature in "Forced Normalization" (Landolt) of the Electroencephalogram of Epileptics.]. *Nervenarzt* 1965; 36:190–202.
102. Trimble MR, Schmitz B. *Forced normalization and alternative psychoses of epilepsy*. Petersfield: Wrightson Biomedical Publising Ltd.; 1998.
103. Gatzonis SD, Stamboulis E, Siafakas, Angelopoulos E, Georgaculias N, Sigounas E, *et al*. Acute psychosis and EEG normalisation after vagus nerve stimulation. *J Neurol Neurosurg Psychiatry* 2000; 69(2):278–9.
104. Mula M. The Landolt's phenomenon: an update. *Epileptologia* 2010; 18(1):39–44.
105. Pakalnis A, Drake ME, Jr., John K, Kellum JB. Forced normalization. Acute psychosis after seizure control in seven patients. *Arch Neurol* 1987; 44(3):289–92.
106. Sachdev PS. Alternating and postictal psychoses: review and a unifying hypothesis. *Schizophr Bull* 2007; 33(4):1029–37.
107. Robertson MM, Trimble MR. The treatment of depression in patients with epilepsy. A double-blind trial. *J Affect Disord* 1985; 9(2):127–36.
108. Barry JJ, Ettinger AB, Friel P, Gilliam FG, Harden CL, Hermann B, *et al*. Consensus statement: the evaluation and treatment of people with epilepsy and affective disorders. *Epilepsy Behav* 2008; 13(Suppl 1):S1–29.
109. Bauer M, Whybrow PC, Angst J, Versiani M, Moller HJ. World Federation of Societies of Biological Psychiatry (WFSBP) Guidelines for Biological Treatment of Unipolar Depressive Disorders, Part 2: Maintenance treatment of major depressive disorder and treatment of chronic depressive disorders and subthreshold depressions. *World J Biol Psychiatry* 2002; 3(2):69–86.
110. Grunze H, Vieta E, Goodwin GM, Bowden C, Licht RW, Moller HJ, *et al*. The World Federation of Societies of Biological Psychiatry (WFSBP) Guidelines for the Biological Treatment of Bipolar Disorders: Update 2010 on the treatment of acute bipolar depression. *World J Biol Psychiatry* 2010; 11(2):81–109.
111. Schmitz B. Antidepressant drugs: indications and guidelines for use in epilepsy. *Epilepsia* 2002; 43(Suppl 2):14–8.
112. Mula M. Anticonvulsants—antidepressants pharmacokinetic drug interactions: the role of the CYP450 system in psychopharmacology. *Curr Drug Metab* 2008; 9(8):730–7.
113. Warden D, Rush AJ, Trivedi MH, Fava M, Wisniewski SR. The STAR*D Project results: a comprehensive review of findings. *Curr Psychiatry Rep* 2007; 9(6):449–59.
114. Stahl SM. *Stahl's essential psychopharmacology: neuroscientific basis and practical applications* (3rd edn, Fully rev. and expanded. edn). Cambridge: Cambridge University Press, 2008.
115. Settle EC Jr. Antidepressant drugs: disturbing and potentially dangerous adverse effects. *J Clin Psychiatry* 1998; 59(Suppl 16):25–30; discussion 40–2.
116. Alper K, Schwartz KA, Kolts RL, Khan A. Seizure incidence in psychopharmacological clinical trials: an analysis of Food and Drug Administration (FDA) summary basis of approval reports. *Biol Psychiatry* 2007; 62(4):345–54.
117. Mula M, Schmitz B, Sander JW. The pharmacological treatment of depression in adults with epilepsy. *Expert Opin Pharmacother* 2008; 9(18):3159–68.
118. Mula M, Monaco F, Trimble MR. Use of psychotropic drugs in patients with epilepsy: interactions and seizure risk. *Expert Rev Neurother* 2004; 4(6):953–64.
119. Shin HW, O'Donovan CA, Boggs JG, Grefe A, Harper A, Bell WL, *et al*. Successful ECT treatment for medically refractory nonconvulsive status epilepticus in pediatric patient. *Seizure* 2011; 20(5):433–6.
120. Aksoy-Poyraz C, Ozdemir A, Ozmen M, Arikan K, Ozkara C. Electroconvulsive therapy for bipolar depressive and mixed episode with high suicide risk after epilepsy surgery. *Epilepsy Behav* 2008; 13(4):707–9.
121. Mula M, Monaco F. Antiepileptic-antipsychotic drug interactions: a critical review of the evidence. *Clin Neuropharmacol* 2002; 25(5):280–9.
122. Alldredge BK. Seizure risk associated with psychotropic drugs: clinical and pharmacokinetic considerations. *Neurology* 1999; 53(5 Suppl 2): S68–75.
123. Langosch JM, Trimble MR. Epilepsy, psychosis and clozapine. *Hum Psychopharmacol* 2002; 17(2):115–19.
124. Devinsky O, Honigfeld G, Patin J. Clozapine-related seizures. *Neurology* 1991; 41(3):369–71.
125. Pacia SV, Devinsky O. Clozapine-related seizures: experience with 5,629 patients. *Neurology* 1994; 44(12):2247–9.
126. Vieweg V, Shutty M, Hundley P, Leadbetter R. Combined treatment with lithium and carbamazepine. *Am J Psychiatry* 1991; 148(3):398–9.
127. Kramlinger KG, Post RM. Addition of lithium carbonate to carbamazepine: hematological and thyroid effects. *Am J Psychiatry* 1990; 147(5):615–20.
128. Chen C, Veronese L, Yin Y. The effects of lamotrigine on the pharmacokinetics of lithium. *Br J Clin Pharmacol* 2000 Sep; 50(3):193–5.
129. Abraham G, Owen J. Topiramate can cause lithium toxicity. *J Clin Psychopharmacol* 2004; 24(5):565–7.
130. Erwin CW, Gerber CJ, Morrison SD, James JF. Lithium carbonate and convulsive disorders. *Arch Gen Psychiatry* 1973; 28(5):646–8.

MEDICAL LIBRARY
WESTERN INFIRMARY
GLASGOW

CHAPTER 20

Epilepsy due to Traumatic Brain Injury, Cerebrovascular Disease, Central Nervous System Infections, and Brain Tumours

Gagandeep Singh, J.M.K. Murthy, and Ashalatha Radhakrishnan

Introduction

Together, epilepsy due to traumatic brain injury (TBI), brain tumours, cerebrovascular disease (CVD), and central nervous system (CNS) infections comprise over one-fifth (20%) of cases of newly-diagnosed epilepsy (1). This estimate is based on data from a single community of Rochester, Minnesota in the United States. Although, this estimate might be different for other communities across the world, it provides sufficient justification to review the characteristics and management of epilepsy associated with each of these risk factors. In this chapter, each of the risk factors is discussed with respect to the following: classification and criteria, epidemiology, measurement and stratification of risk of epilepsy, clinical characteristics, outcome, and specific management of epilepsy associated with each of the conditions.

Traumatic brain injury

It has been predicted that TBIs would surpass any other cause for death and disability by the year 2020 (2). In the US, TBI affects about 1.4 million people, and leaves 50,000 dead and 80,000 with long-term disability each year (3). The figures might be an underestimate as many cases of mild TBI either do not present to hospital or are discharged from the Emergency Department and as a result, remain undocumented. Moreover, definitions of various categories of TBI vary between studies and hence it is not possible to provide reliable estimates from the available studies. The figures cannot be extrapolated to other countries and regions of the world on account of differences in socioeconomic, ethnic, and perhaps genetic compositions. If anything, the incidence of TBI appears to be higher in low- and middle-income countries of the world (4, 5). In all, 5 million deaths worldwide might perhaps be a result of TBI each year (6).

Classification and criteria

The term, 'traumatic brain injury' is preferred to head injury as the latter is somewhat ambiguous and might include other craniofacial injuries. Generally, TBI occurs in three different scenarios: road traffic accidents, falls, and violence. It is customary to classify TBI according to its severity and the anatomical extent of damage (Table 20.1). Classification of severity is traditionally based on the Glasgow Coma Scale and the durations of loss of consciousness and post-traumatic amnesia. The mildest form of TBI is concussion, which is a form of diffuse injury in the absence of contact damage and leads to transient impairment of consciousness only. A more serious form of diffuse injury is 'diffuse axonal injury', which represents severe angular or rotational injury. Focal injuries

Table 20.1 Classification of types of traumatic brain injury

Classification	Type of injury
1	Diffuse:
A	Concussion
B	Diffuse axonal injury
2	Focal:
A	Contusion
B	Intracranial haemorrhage:
(i)	Epidural haematoma
(ii)	Subarachnoid haemorrhage
(iii)	Subdural haematoma
(iv)	Intracerebral haematoma

might be classified as either contusions (comprised of subpial swelling and collection of blood) or intracranial haemorrhage (including epidural haematoma, subdural haematoma, subarachnoid haemorrhage, and intracerebral haemorrhage). Other injury-related terms include *coup* injury in which the contusion is located below the site of impact and *countre coup*, in which the injury is located opposite to the site of impact. Another term, laceration, refers to a tear in the pia matter.

The American Congress of Rehabilitation Medicine (ACRM) defines mild TBI as any period of transient confusion, disorientation, impairment (or loss) of consciousness, or amnesia lasting for less than 30 minutes with or without other neurological symptoms and signs such as seizures, headache and focal neurological deficits (7). 'More severe TBI' is defined as either loss of consciousness for more than 30 minutes or duration of amnesia more than 24 hours or penetrating cerebral injury. According to these definitions, the presence of focal neurological deficit (implying focal brain lesions such as either contusion or haemorrhage) or the demonstration of intracranial lesion/s on neuroimaging studies can occur in mild TBI and does not necessarily qualify for 'more severe TBI'. However, from the standpoint of risk stratification with regard to the incidence of post-traumatic epilepsy, the criteria for severity of TBI used in various epidemiological studies of TBI and epilepsy are somewhat different from the ACRM recommended definitions (8–10). In these studies, much importance has been accorded to the presence of cerebral contusions, focal neurological deficits, depressed skull fractures, and intracerebral haematomas as predictive factors for post-traumatic epilepsy.

Immediate, early, and late seizures and epilepsy in relation to TBI

Seizures may occur immediately after, or early (within 7 days) or later (after 7 days) following TBI. Immediate seizures (also known as impact convulsions or concussive convulsions) occur at the time of injury and consist of few focal or generalized myoclonic jerks or sometimes frank generalized tonic–clonic convulsions. They are generally regarded as non-epileptic as they are probably the result of transient loss of cortical inhibition at the time of injury or due to brainstem activation and do not carry any increased risk of late seizures. Early seizures (within 7 days of TBI) occur in about 2% of all TBIs. The risk of early seizures in 'more severe TBI' is 10–30%. The risk of late unprovoked seizures (beyond 7 days) is about 2%, though estimates in the literature vary on account of differences in criteria for selection of TBI samples and for definition of late seizures. Nearly two-thirds of late post-traumatic seizures evolve in to epilepsy (defined as two or more unprovoked seizures). Some of late seizures after TBI might be provoked and in this context, ethanol-withdrawal seizures are significant, having accounted for nearly 10% of all late post-traumatic seizures in one series (8). An increased incidence of ethanol-withdrawal seizures might simply be a reflection of the association between ethanol use and TBI.

Risk stratification for post-traumatic epilepsy

The risk of epilepsy following TBI depends on several factors, many of which have been dealt with in considerable detail in available studies (8–13). The most important determinant of the incidence of post-traumatic epilepsy appears to be the severity of TBI. The risk of epilepsy is marginally increased following mild TBI for at least 5 years, although in some studies, the risk has been shown to be elevated beyond 5 years also (10). Following more severe TBI, the risk is elevated considerably and might remain elevated for a period much beyond 10 years of follow-up. In the Vietnam Head Injury Study, which is a prospective longitudinal follow-up study of over 35 years of US war veterans, the risk was highest in the first year after penetrating TBI and decreased exponentially thereafter, but remained elevated up to 15 years after head injury (11, 12). The observations led the authors of the study to propose mathematical formulas to calculate the risk of epilepsy at any given period of time following penetrating TBI (13). The overall incidence of post-traumatic epilepsy in the Vietnam Head Injury cohort was 53%. Thus, a clear distinction in terms of the risk of post-traumatic epilepsy can be drawn in literature between civilian and military injuries. The high incidence of epilepsy following military injuries is probably due to more frequent penetrating injuries and haematomas, haematoma-products or retained metal fragments in the cerebral parenchyma. In civilian injuries, the risk is proportional to the severity of TBI and in follow-up studies of severe TBI, the risk over the first 1–2 years is 15–30%, regardless of whether antiepileptic drug (AED) treatment is prescribed to the patient or not (14, 15). In most follow-up studies, subjects with cerebral contusions and intracranial haematomas have been included in the category of severe TBI and this practice differs from the ACRM criteria for grading of severity of TBI (see 'Classification and criteria' section). The risk appears to be highest among those with focal neurological deficits, demonstrable brain contusions, and intracranial haemorrhage (including subdural haematoma). The risk of post-traumatic epilepsy following mild TBI was not found to be related to the occurrence of early post-traumatic seizures in the Olmsted County studies and none of the subjects with mild TBI who had early seizures, went on to have late seizures or epilepsy in this cohort (8, 9). In other studies however, those with early seizures particularly in relation to severe TBI were found to be at increased risk of developing epilepsy (16, 17). These differences might reflect the disparate mechanisms underlying seizures following mild and more severe TBI (16). Age, gender and family history of epilepsy also appear to influence the risk of developing late post-traumatic seizures and epilepsy (10). The risk possibly appears to be lesser in children and increases beyond the age of 65 years (8–10). Female gender and a family history of epilepsy are risk factors identified in some of the population studies of post-traumatic epilepsy (9, 10).

Course and outcome of post-traumatic epilepsy

The cumulative risk of a second seizure following an unprovoked, late post-traumatic seizure is about 75% (18). A follow-up study estimated that roughly 30% of individuals with a late post-traumatic seizure would experience at least 10 seizures over the next 10 years (18). In the Vietnam Head Injury Study, roughly half of the individuals with a late post-traumatic seizure following penetrating TBI continued to have seizures 15 years after the injury (11, 12). Precisely what proportion of those with a first late post-traumatic seizure eventually develops intractable epilepsy and what proportion goes into long-term remission are not known as only very few long-term follow-up studies of post-traumatic epilepsy are available.

Early post-traumatic seizures are often of the focal motor or generalized, tonic–clonic type. However, late post-traumatic epilepsy manifests with complex partial seizures in as many as 30% of cases (12). Few small series of patients who underwent surgical treatment for intractable epilepsy in relation to TBI are available but nothing conclusive can be gathered from these studies as these are descriptions of highly-selected patients mostly from tertiary-care centres (19–21). Limited data available also suggests that people with post-traumatic epilepsy experience increased mortality rates in comparison to the general population (22).

Traumatic brain injury: association with mesial temporal sclerosis

Data from highly-selected series of intractable epilepsy have shown that there is a proportion of patients with radiologically- and often pathologically-verified mesial temporal sclerosis (MTS) in whom there is no identifiable initial precipitating illness other than TBI (19–21). In one such report, all patients with MTS had sustained head injuries before the age of 5 years, while in other reports, the age at which the TBI was sustained was well beyond 10 years of age (19, 20, 23). It remains a matter of speculation, whether in the individuals with later-life TBI and MTS, the association is causal or merely coincidental (i.e. TBI was antedated by the MTS and it merely heralded the seizure disorder). In the Olmsted County community, TBI (in addition to other antecedents such as childhood febrile seizures, viral encephalitis, and a family history of epilepsy) was identified as an important risk factor for complex partial seizures, although the strength of association was not as strong as childhood febrile seizures (24). In this community, 12% of complex partial seizures were attributable to TBI and 20% to childhood febrile seizures. In clinical practice, there is a proportion of cases with MTS that have no other identifiable antecedent risk factor other than TBI, suggesting a cause–effect relationship between TBI and MTS.

The pathophysiological events that might lead to development of MTS after TBI are unclear. It is unlikely that the hippocampus gets involved directly during TBI episodes because it is located deeply and is hence well protected. Hippocampal involvement is more likely to be due to secondary damage during or after TBI, e.g. the effect of early seizures and status epilepticus, hypoxia, intracranial hypertension, cerebral circulatory impairment, and excitotoxic damage. Indeed, autopsy studies of fatal TBI, corroborated by experimental studies in animals have documented bilateral hippocampal pathology in the form of selective necrosis and loss of neurons in the CA1 subfield of the hippocampus in majority of the cases (25–28). In the rat fluid percussion model, which is used to study TBI-related epileptogenesis, the electrical disinhibition is preferentially located in the hilar region of the dentate gyrus in comparison to the CA1 subfield (29). Pathological studies have also shown preferential loss of neurons in the hilar region in the rat fluid percussion model. Likewise, an elegant study of human temporal lobectomy specimens obtained from surgery for intractable epilepsy in relation to TBI showed preferential loss of neurons in the hilar region as opposed to the CA1 subfield, which is typically found to be involved in pathological studies of hippocampal sclerosis in relation to childhood febrile seizures (23). The histological findings in TBI are thus more or less similar to end folium sclerosis. Elsewhere, however, preferential loss of neurons in the CA1 subfield in has been reported in TBI-related MTS (21).

Post-traumatic epilepsy: other pathological substrates

Other than MTS, pathological examination of resected specimens of the brain obtained after surgery for medically-refractory post-traumatic epilepsy have mostly shown gliosis and haemosiderin deposition either in the mesial temporal or neocortical location. How haemosiderin contributes to epileptogenicity is unclear but peroxidation reactions are likely to be involved in the process (23). The finding of heterotopic neurons in brain specimens resected during surgery for medically-refractory post-traumatic epilepsy remains controversial as microscopic dysplasia might pre-exist and be detected incidentally. It has been conjectured that these pre-existing heterotopias might contribute to the epileptogenicity of the post-traumatic lesions in the brain.

Non-epileptic seizures and TBI

Antecedent TBI has been reported in one-third of cases of non-epileptic seizures (NES) (30). The injury is most often mild as opposed to the relationship between TBI and epileptic seizures, for which the strength of the association increases with severity of TBI. Another characteristic feature is that individuals reporting NES following head injury are mostly males as opposed to NES in relation to physical and sexual abuse, which are commonly encountered among women. In individuals with prior TBI, NES represent a means of obtaining enduring disability benefits or financial compensation for the injury at workplace or otherwise. The mechanisms underlying the occurrence of NES following TBI are unclear but might include susceptibility of the injured brain to behavioural disorders.

Post-traumatic epilepsy: treatment considerations

The practice of administering anticonvulsants to patients with head injury regardless of whether they have seizures or not at any stage is widespread. The Quality Standards Subcommittee of the American Academy of Neurology and others have reviewed available studies of AED administration following TBI (31, 32). Pooled evidence from four trials of AED prophylaxis in severe TBI (two class I studies of phenytoin, one class II study of carbamazepine and one class III study of phenytoin) showed a significantly reduced rate of early (<7 days) seizures in the treated group versus the control group (relative risk: 0.37; 95% confidence interval (CI) 0.18–0.74) (32). There was no difference in the incidence of adverse effects in the treatment and control groups. In the same meta-analysis, pooled data from eight trials of AED treatment for the prevention of late post-traumatic seizures (including two class I studies of phenytoin, three class II studies—one each of phenytoin, carbamazepine, and valproate, and three class III studies—of phenytoin and phenobarbital), showed no difference in the incidence of late post-traumatic seizures between the treated and control groups (32). It is recommended that for adults with severe TBI, prophylactic treatment should begin with a loading dose of phenytoin as soon as possible after injury in order to decrease the risk of early seizures (in the first 7 days). Further treatment beyond 7 days does not reduce the incidence of late post-traumatic seizures and is not recommended. These recommendations do not apply for mild TBI in which case, AED prophylaxis might be considered on a case-by-case basis, largely determined by the occurrence of early post-traumatic seizures. Since the risk of seizure recurrence following a late unprovoked post-traumatic seizure is higher than 75%, AED treatment is generally indicated after a single late unprovoked post-traumatic seizure (18). The choice of AED largely depends upon the patient characteristics and side-effect profile of the AED used.

These recommendations are based on studies performed with the conventional AEDs (including phenytoin, phenobarbital, carbamazepine, and valproate). The role of the newer AEDs (particularly levetiracetam) in preventing unprovoked late post-traumatic seizures is worth considering especially in light of its demonstrated antiepileptogenic effects in animal experiments. Two small, preliminary controlled trials demonstrated that its administration in TBI is safe and of equivalent efficacy in comparison to phenytoin for the prevention of early seizures (33, 34).

An undetermined proportion of individuals with post-traumatic epilepsy continue to experience seizures that might be refractory to medical treatment. Presurgical evaluation and surgical treatment should be considered in such individuals. When imaging studies in such individuals unequivocally demonstrate unilateral MTS, the chances of seizure remission following surgery are excellent, though some authors have described slightly less favourable surgical outcome in MTS with TBI as an antecedent (19–21, 35). When MTS is not demonstrated, the surgical outcome is less favourable; it is comparatively better with focal, discrete lesions amenable to resection in comparison to extensive or multifocal lesions (20).

Cerebrovascular disease

The occurrence of epileptic seizures in the aftermath of stroke has a devastating impact on patient outcome and might lead to hospitalization, an increased cost of treatment, falls, and fractures, and very rarely even death. Besides the occurrence of epileptic seizures impacts the quality of life in general, which compounds upon the already compromised quality of life due to stroke.

Classification

As in the case of seizures in relation to TBI, post-stroke seizures are classified as 'early' and 'late'. However, unlike TBI, the time criteria for distinction between early and late epilepsy are not uniform. In different published studies, seizures occurring within 24 hours, 1 week, 2 weeks, or even 30 days of stroke have all been labelled as early seizures. As a result, the estimates of the incidence of early *versus* late seizures following stroke vary.

Epidemiology

The causal association between CVD and epileptic seizures is well known. Five per cent of all new-onset epilepsies and 30% of all epilepsies in the elderly (>60 years) can be attributed to stroke (1, 36). In the Olmsted County study, most of the epilepsies related to stroke occurred after the age of 70 years and none before the age of 50 years (1).

The incidence of seizures and epilepsy appears to be increased both in the period preceding and that following stroke. In the Oxfordshire Community project, 1% of the subjects with stroke had a seizure in the preceding 1 year (37). The occurrence of seizures preceding stroke can be explained if one considers seizures to be a manifestation of occult CVD, i.e. silent or asymptomatic cerebral infarcts or haemorrhages. Indeed, seizures and epilepsy have been documented to be presenting features of otherwise asymptomatic CVD (38). A small case–control study found significantly higher frequency of preceding seizures among stroke patients in comparison to controls (39). Another study concluded that elderly people (>60 years) with newly-diagnosed epilepsy were nearly three times more likely to have a stroke in comparison to the general population (40). These findings have led some authors to conclude that seizures might presage the usual manifestations of stroke in the elderly and that elderly people with newly-diagnosed epilepsy should be investigated for vascular risk factors for stroke (40, 41).

As alluded to earlier, estimates of the incidence of early seizures following stroke vary. In the Oxfordshire Community project, the incidence of onset seizures (within 24 hours) was 2% (37). The incidence was higher in other studies as the time criteria for early seizures was up to 1–2 weeks and many of the other studies were hospital-based and hence had a bias towards more severe stroke (42–44). One report stated an incidence of 43% but this was perhaps due to the highly-selected nature of the patient population (45). Over 90% of early seizures and 40% of all stroke-related seizures occur within the first 24 hours (43, 44).

The 5-year cumulative probability of a late stroke-related seizure varies from 7–12% (37, 43). Half of the late seizures can be expected to occur within the first year after stroke. The incidence of epilepsy following stroke is about 2–4% (37, 43, 46, 47).

Risk factors for stroke-related epilepsy include the type, location and size of the brain lesion/s. Although stroke-related epilepsy occurs mostly in the elderly, within this elderly group age appears to have no effect on the incidence of epilepsy (37, 43). In one study, however, younger age was identified as a significant risk factor for epilepsy (47). The risk of stroke-related epilepsy appears to be higher following intracerebral haemorrhage and subarachnoid haemorrhage (37, 43, 48). Epilepsy after subarachnoid haemorrhage appears to be more frequent among individuals with subdural haematoma and/or focal cerebral infarcts (49). Regardless of the type of stroke, i.e. whether intracerebral haemorrhage or ischaemic stroke, the risk of stroke-related epilepsy is elevated mainly in those with cortically-located lesions. The size of the lesion also determines the propensity to epilepsy; in the Oxfordshire Community Stroke project, the risk was highest in total anterior circulation occlusions, followed by partial anterior circulation occlusions, lacunar occlusions, and posterior circulation occlusions in that order (37). It has not been determined whether among all posterior circulation strokes, the risk is different for cerebral cortical infarcts and brainstem/cerebellar infarcts. In most studies, stroke survivors who were independent at discharge from hospital or at 1 or 6 months did not appear to have an increased risk of late seizures or epilepsy (37, 44). Lacunar infarcts and basal ganglionic haemorrhages do not appear to increase the risk of epilepsy; however there have been documented cases of late seizures in both conditions; these are probably due to concomitant cortical vascular lesions (37). In most studies, early stroke-related seizures or onset seizures were found to increase the risk of late seizures or epilepsy (43). A study examined the effect of treatment setting, between a specialized stroke unit and a general medical ward and found no effect of this variable on the incidence of epilepsy (47). Another study found that the cumulative risk of late seizures in subjects with recurrent strokes was higher after but not before 10 years when compared to those with a single stroke episode suggesting that recurrent stroke increases the risk of epilepsy over the long term (43). A post-stroke epilepsy risk scale has been proposed but needs further validation (50). Perhaps the effects of more variables such as haemorrhagic conversion of cerebral infarcts and magnetic resonance imaging (MRI) characteristics of the vascular lesion and the effect of interventions such as thrombolysis need to be examined in the evaluation of the risk of epilepsy. Finally, the occurrence of venous infarcts due to cerebral venous thrombosis also appears to increase the risk of epilepsy but the magnitude of risk cannot be determined due to the small number of reported cases (51).

Course and outcome of stroke-related epilepsy

One-half to two-thirds of those with a late unprovoked stroke-related seizure would have another unprovoked seizure, but this risk is probably less than the risk following an unprovoked late post-traumatic seizure (37, 43). Frequent seizures amounting to intractability appears to be uncommon; in the Oxfordshire Community Stroke project, 17% of those with stroke-related epilepsy had seizures more frequently than once a month (37). From the standpoint of semiology, both early and late stroke-related seizures are either simple partial or secondary-generalized seizures; complex partial seizures appear to be uncommon. Interesting but yet unanswered questions include whether the occurrence of late unprovoked stroke-related seizures independently alter the risk of subsequent stroke or long-term mortality. A Norwegian study found increased mortality due to stroke in those with stroke-related epilepsy but the size of this cohort was small (46).

Stroke-related epilepsy: treatment considerations

Early seizures

The European Stroke Initiative and the American Stroke Association/American Heart Association recommend that routine primary prophylaxis with AEDs is generally not indicated in intracerebral haemorrhage but might be considered in selected patients with lobar haemorrhage (52, 53). If instituted, the AED treatment should be given for 1 week. Otherwise, AED treatment is indicated only if early seizures occur and in such instances, the AEDs might be given for 4 weeks (53). There is no role for primary prophylaxis with AEDs in ischaemic stroke. When AEDs are indicated, intravenously administered AEDs including benzodiazepines and phenytoin or fos-phenytoin should be preferred. Some of the newer AEDs (e.g. levetiracetam) might have neuroprotective effects by counteracting excitatory neurotransmitters that are highly active during acute stroke (54). There is preliminary evidence of the usefulness of levetiracetam in preventing stroke-related seizures but clearly, this is an area for future research (55).

Effect of seizures and AEDs on stroke outcome and functional status

It is unclear whether the occurrence of early seizures independently influences functional status following stroke as measured by the modified Rankin's Scale upon discharge from hospital or later. Some hospital-based studies of selected patients have shown that early seizures increase mortality or the likelihood of poor functional outcome but have not adjusted outcome measures for stroke severity (39, 44). Hence, it is possible that the higher mortality rates or the poorer functional outcome in stroke patients with early seizures might be a reflection of stroke severity as more severe strokes are associated with an increased likelihood of occurrence of seizures. Likewise, it remains unclear whether status epilepticus has an independent effect on mortality and outcome of stroke as small studies of selected patients have shown contrasting effects on short-term mortality (56–58). While expectedly, late unprovoked stroke-related seizures might adversely impact quality of life in general as well the rehabilitation process following stroke by leading to potential hospitalization and falls and fractures as well as a temporary decline in functional status postictally, at least one follow-up study demonstrated that the occurrence of late seizures did not have any impact on the long-term functional outcome (59, 60).

There has been concern that the administration of some of the conventional AEDs, particularly phenobarbital, benzodiazepines, and phenytoin might negatively influence motor and perhaps cognitive recovery following stroke (61). Indeed, small studies of patents with intracerebral and sub-arachnoid haemorrhage have shown that administration of a short course of phenytoin was associated with poor motor and cognitive recovery during or after hospitalization (62, 63). The newer anticonvulsants, some of which are neuroprotective (e.g. levetiracetam) might be theoretically advantageous but little is known about their efficacy, safety, and their effect on long-term motor and cognitive outcomes.

Choice of AEDs following late unprovoked stroke-related seizures

There are no large randomized-controlled trials of AEDs in stroke-related epilepsy. A limited number of small, uncontrolled, and open-labelled studies (of levetiracetam and gabapentin) have shown that seizures are well-controlled over follow-up periods of 12–30 months in stroke-related epilepsy (64, 65). Randomized-controlled trials of AEDs in stroke-related epilepsy are not available. Since stroke is an important risk factor for epilepsy in the elderly, it is pertinent to review randomized trials of AEDs in elderly people with epilepsy. A randomized, parallel trial comparing monotherapy with gabapentin (1500 mg/day), lamotrigine (150 mg/day), and carbamazepine (600 mg/day) in which cerebral infarction was the most common aetiology of seizures found significantly higher retention rates in the lamotrigine and gabapentin groups in comparison to the carbamazepine group at 1 year (66). Efficacy (seizure control) was similar in all three groups, implying that both lamotrigine and gabapentin had superior tolerability profiles. The UK Lamotrigine Elderly Study compared lamotrigine (100 mg/day) with carbamazepine (400 mg/day) and reported greater drop-out rates due to adverse effects with carbamazepine (42%) in comparison to lamotrigine (18%) (67). Another small, open-labelled trial compared lamotrigine with sustained-release carbamazepine in patients with a first post-stroke seizure (excluding the first 24 hours) and found better seizure control rates and lesser adverse effects with lamotrigine (68). Finally, a fourth randomized trial compared lamotrigine (target dose: 100 mg/day) with sustained-release carbamazepine (target dose: 400 mg/day) and found no significant difference in efficacy and tolerability of the two AEDs (69). From the available controlled and uncontrolled trials of various AEDs in elderly people with epilepsy, it appears that good seizure control is achieved with the usual AEDs in approximately 80% of stroke-related epilepsies; however, since seizure control is not very difficult, tolerability becomes an important issue. With regard to tolerability, lamotrigine (100–150 mg/day), gabapentin (up to 1500 mg/day) and sustained-release (400 mg/day) (but not immediate-release) carbamazepine appear to be well-tolerated in the elderly.

Among the newer AEDs, topiramate is best avoided in view of its propensity to cause cognitive impairments, worsening of speech disorder in aphasic subjects and sometimes also motor deficit in hemiplegics (70, 71). There is no data available regarding the use of other newer AEDs, including levetiracetam and lacosamide in stroke-related epilepsy. Theoretically, these drugs do not have any known pharmacokinetic interactions with other medications. This might represent a significant advantage for many people with stroke-related epilepsy, who are often on multiple drugs with potential for drug interactions with AEDs.

Central nervous system infections

Seizures and status epilepticus can occur during the active phase of infectious disorders of the CNS and recurrent unprovoked seizures (or epilepsy) can be a long-term consequence of CNS infections. The interpretation of the association between CNS infections and epilepsy is complicated by the variety of known acute and chronic infectious disorders.

Epidemiology

The risk of an unprovoked seizures increases 11-fold after an episode of CNS infection (72). In population-based cohorts of survivors of all CNS infections, the reported risk of developing an unprovoked seizure is 6.8–8.3%, corresponding to an observed:expected ratio of 6.9 (72, 73). The increased incidence of unprovoked seizures is highest during the initial 5 years after the infection episode but remains elevated over the next 15 years (72).

In the general population of high-income countries, about 1–5% of incident cases of epilepsy might be presumed to be related to prior CNS infection (74–76). CNS infections have been cited as one of the reasons for the higher incidence of epilepsy observed in low- and middle-income countries of the world (77–80). In an Ecuadorian study, CNS infections were the antecedent events in 4.5% of cases of epilepsy (81); in sub-Saharan Africa, they accounted for 26% of putative risk factors for epilepsy (78); and finally, in a hospital-based study from south India, these accounted for 24.5% of established remote symptomatic aetiologies of focal epilepsies (82).

Specific CNS infections

The nature of epileptic complication depends on the type of the infectious illness, its duration, characteristics, and extent of CNS damage.

Bacterial meningitis

Epilepsy can be a long-term consequence of bacterial meningitis (83). In the Olmsted County cohort of survivors of bacterial meningitis, the 20-year risk of developing unprovoked seizures was 13% in those with early seizures and 2% in those without an early seizure (72). A meta-analysis of the 19 prospective cohorts of bacterial meningitis in children aged between 2 months and 19 years from developed countries found that the mean probability of developing an unprovoked seizure was 4.2%. In cohorts that were either retrospectively assembled or from developing countries, the mean probability was 5% (84).

The likelihood of developing unprovoked seizures probably varies according to the aetiological agent responsible for meningitis; it appears to be highest for meningitis caused by *Streptococcus pneumoniae* (14.8%) and is comparatively lower following *Haemophilus influenzae* (6.1%) and *Neisseria meningitides* meningitis (1.4%) (84). The risk factors for late epilepsy include early seizures during acute phase and persistent neurological deficits other than sensorineural hearing loss (83).

Encephalitis

For patients with viral encephalitis, the risk of epilepsy is increased 16-fold and the increased risk persists for at least 15 years after the episode. In the Olmsted County study, the 20-year risk of unprovoked seizures was 22% in those with early seizures and 10% in those without early seizures (72). Epilepsy is one of the common consequences of herpes simplex encephalitis (HSE) (Fig. 20.1A–D). In the Swedish nationwide retrospective study of HSE, the most frequent diagnosis upon readmission following an episode of HSE was epilepsy. A diagnosis of epilepsy on follow-up was documented in 21% of the entire cohort and 24% of survivors, with a median onset of 9 months after the diagnosis of HSE (85). Factors associated with a high risk of epilepsy include early seizures, anatomical involvement of hippocampal regions and associated changes in hippocampal excitability, and chronic, persistent herpes simplex virus infection or immunoreactivity in the CNS during HSE (86–88).

Malaria

Malaria is the most common parasitic disease and is a major public health problem in much of the sub-Saharan Africa and parts of South and Southeast Asia and South America. The estimated number of cases across the world each is 225 million with approximately 800,000 deaths thereof every year. Cerebral malaria, the neurological form of malaria, is a potential cause of epilepsy in the countries endemic to malaria. In sub-Saharan Africa, cerebral malaria is estimated to affect 600,000 children (<5 years of age) each year (89). Studies that have examined the association between cerebral malaria and epilepsy suggest a modestly-strong association between the two (90).

Neurocysticercosis (including calcific neurocysticercosis)

Cerebral infestation with the larval form of the pork tapeworm, *Taenia solium*, is endemic in many regions of the world including South and Central America and South and Southeast Asia and Africa. Cerebral calcifications, essentially constituting presumptive evidence of brain parenchymal involvement by cysticerci, are common findings on imaging studies in people with epilepsy in *T. solium*-endemic populations in these regions (Fig. 20.2). Accumulating evidence implicates calcific neurocysticercosis in the development and maintenance of seizures and epilepsy (91). In rural Guatemalan communities, calcifications alone were more frequent in those with epileptic seizures compared to matched controls without history of seizures (35–36% versus 9–15%) (92). Epilepsy was etiologically related to calcific neurocysticercosis in 8% of cases in a hospital-based study in south India, and in 9.6% of new-onset epilepsy cases in Ecuador (82, 93). The prevalence of epilepsy associated with calcific neurocysticercosis was 0.9–1.0 per 1000 in a population-based survey in south India (94, 95). There is evidence to suggest that calcific neurocysticercosis can be the focus of seizure activity. Electroclinical activity correlates with the location of brain calcifications in 26–55% of the cases (96-98). The other evidence implicating calcifications as foci of seizure activity is the episodic appearance of perilesional oedema often associated with seizures (91, 99).

Three possible scenarios exist with regard to the relationship between calcific neurocysticercosis and epilepsy: (1) a non-causal relationship, i.e. simple coincidence of two unrelated diseases in the same individual; (2) a causal relationship; and (3) dual pathology. However, calcific neurocysticercosis does not appear to be a risk factor for medically-intractable epilepsy. In a cross-sectional study of the 512 patients with intractable epilepsy, calcific neurocysticercosis was found in eight (1.6%) patients, but a clear relationship between calcified cysticercotic lesions and intractable epilepsy was confirmed in only two (0.4%) patients (100). In one small series, perilesional gliosis in relation to a calcific neurocysticercus lesion was associated with medically-intractable epilepsy (K. Radhakrishnan, personal communication).

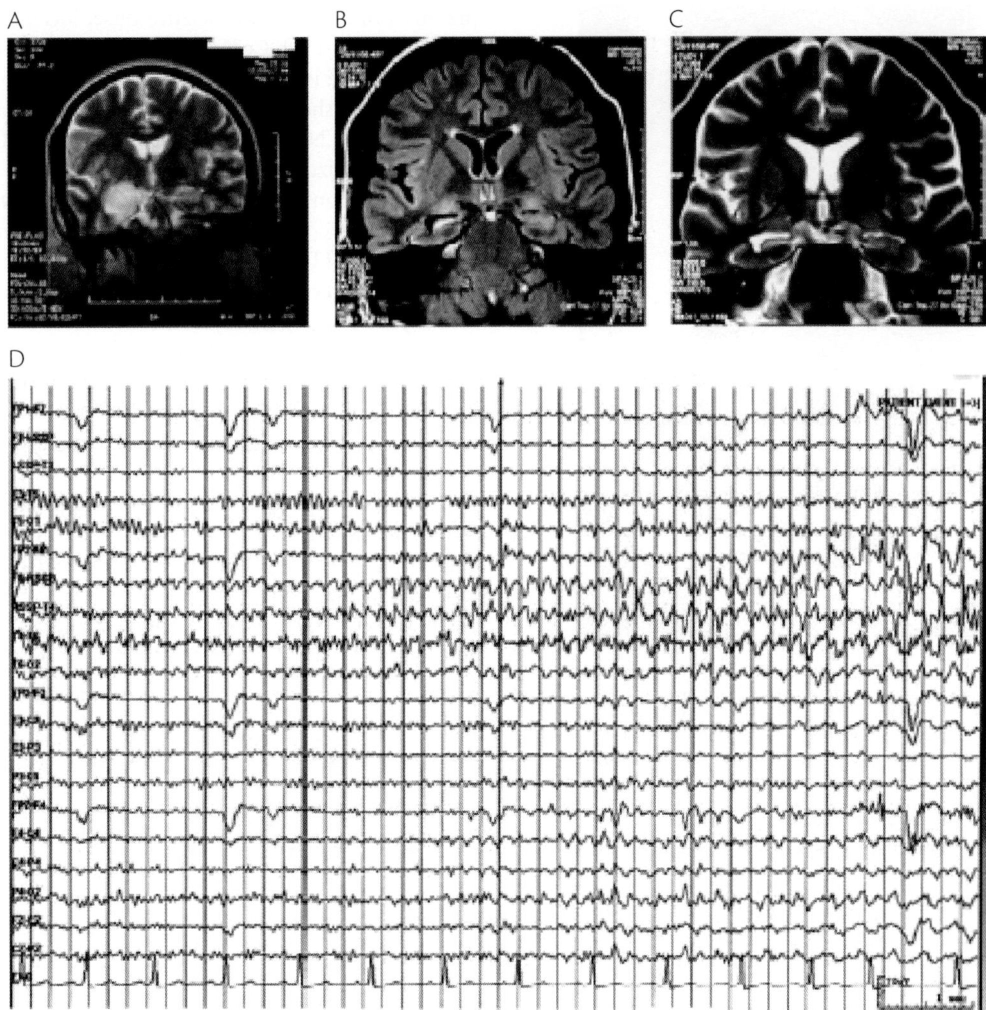

Fig. 20.1 A–D) Serial MRIs in an individual with presumed herpes simplex encephalitis showing (A) bilateral mesial temporal hyperintensities (more on the right side) on a coronal T2-weighted image during the acute encephalitic illness and follow-up fluid attenuated inversion recovery (FLAIR) (B) and T2-weighted (C) images obtained 3 years later demonstrating right-sided hippocampal atrophy and sclerosis. Following the encephalitic episode, this individual developed medically-refractory complex partial seizures that were demonstrated to be of right anterior temporal origin on EEG telemetry (D). She remains seizure free after standard right antero-mesial temporal lobe resection. Courtesy: *Epilepsia* with permission.

Seizure type and semiology

Epileptic seizures following CNS infections can be both focal-onset and generalized (72, 101, 102). In the Olmsted County study, the risk of focal-onset seizures after any CNS infection was increased by 12-fold, while that of generalized-onset seizures was increased by 3-fold (72). Myoclonic seizures might also occur (101). The seizure semiology includes automotor seizures, complex motor/hypermotor seizures, dialeptic seizures, tonic seizures and bilateral asymmetric tonic-clonic seizures. In patients with MTS in relation to CNS infection, the seizure semiology is similar to mesial temporal lobe epilepsy associated with other antecedents (103).

Medical treatment

The choice of antiepileptic drugs (AEDs) for people with epilepsy related to CNS infections depends on the seizure type and epilepsy syndrome and also takes into consideration the mechanism of action and the side-effect and interaction profiles of the drug. Tolerability is as important as efficacy in determining overall effectiveness of the AED. Broad-spectrum AEDs with least cognitive side-effects should be the initial choice; such an approach will be very useful in situations where the seizure type or the epilepsy syndrome is uncertain.

Initial treatment should be with monotherapy and treatment with two or three but not more AEDs may be a useful therapeutic option for patients not responding to monotherapy. Patients who do not attain long-term seizure freedom with the first three treatment schedules are likely to have refractory epilepsy and such patients are potential candidates for epilepsy surgery (104, 105).

There are virtually no data on the long-term prognosis of epilepsy related to CNS infections. Remission rates following AED therapy are perhaps similar to other symptomatic epilepsies. The remission rate in patients with epilepsy related to bacterial meningitis is about 50% (101). Remission rates for epilepsy associated

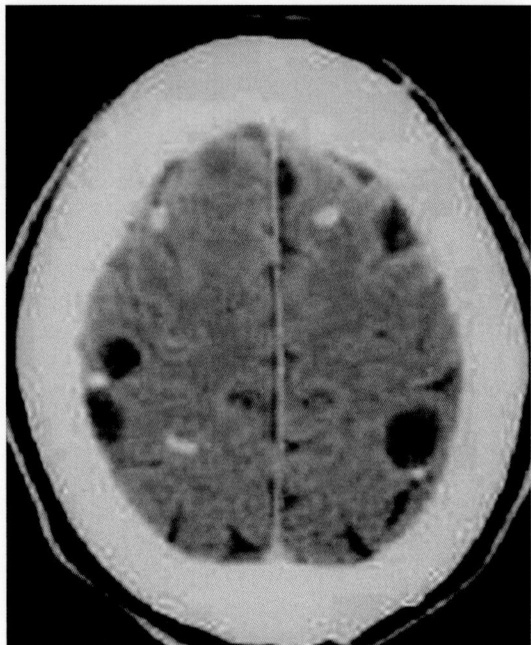

Fig. 20.2 Computed tomography image showing multiple calcifications as well as cystic lesions in a patient with neurocysticercosis.

with calcific neurocysticercosis is about 72% (95% CI 53.7–85.4) at 3 years and 66% at 5 years (95% CI 32.4–88.2) (96). As with other symptomatic epilepsies, prior CNS infection reduces the chance of successful AED withdrawal following a period of remission in people with epilepsy (106). High seizure relapse rates in patients with epilepsy related to calcified neurocysticercosis have been reported (96).

Epilepsy surgery

Surgery is a good option in selected patients with medically-refractory epilepsy related to prior CNS infections, especially in those with discrete, resectable lesions. Common surgical substrates in epilepsy related to CNS infections include hippocampal sclerosis, calcific neurocysticercosis and neocortical gliosis (72, 107–113) (K. Radhakrishnan, personal communication).

Neurocysticercosis (including calcific neurocysticercosis) by itself is rarely associated with medically-refractory epilepsy that might require surgical treatment. However, limited experience with surgical excision of cysticercal lesions has identified residual perilesional gliosis as the dominant pathological feature in the small number of cases in which epilepsy associated with a calcific cysticercus was truly refractory to medical treatment.

Mesial temporal sclerosis

Among various CNS infections, bacterial meningitis and viral encephalitis and possibly neurocysticercosis constitute antecedent events for the development of MTS. In patients with MTS in relation to prior CNS infection, factors associated with good post-surgical seizure outcome (Engel's Class 1a–2) include the occurrence of CNS infection before the age of 4 years, remote history of meningitis (in comparison to viral encephalitis, for which the surgical prognosis appears less favourable), documentation of unilateral MTS in the preoperative MRI, longer latent period to the onset of epilepsy, and seizure-onset localized to one temporal lobe (103, 107–111). Conversely, postoperative seizure outcome is not favourable in those without a demonstrable focal lesion on MRI, having a short latency period to epilepsy, later age (>5 years) at the time of CNS infection, history of encephalitis, or a neocortical origin of seizures (72, 107–111).

An association of calcific neurocysticercosis with MTS has been reported by several authors (100, 113). When compared to patients with isolated MTS, those with calcific neurocysticercosis and ipsilateral MTS have a lower incidence of febrile seizures, older age at initial precipitating injury or first seizure, older age at onset of complex partial seizures, higher rates of seizure clustering, and extratemporal/bitemporal interictal discharges. Although preliminary, these observations suggest that MTS associated with calcific neurocysticercosis might have a different pathophysiological basis than isolated MTS. The hypothesis needs to be proven with longitudinal follow-up studies. The surgical approach to a patient with MTS and calcific neurocysticercosis is unclear. In one study, patients underwent anteromesial temporal lobectomy, without resection of the cysticercotic lesion and were rendered seizure free (113). Others, however, have reported better outcomes following anteromesial temporal lobe resections combined with resection of the calcific lesion (K. Radhakrishnan, personal communication).

Brain tumours

Epilepsy is one of the most characteristic manifestations of brain tumours and it can significantly affect the quality of life of patients with brain tumours. Tumoural epilepsy is considered to be symptomatic, localization-related and manifests as focal or partial seizures with or without alteration of consciousness and/or secondary generalization.

Epidemiology of tumoural epilepsy

The incidence of epilepsy in patients with brain tumours is about 30% (114). This incidence depends largely on the tumour type (see 'Tumour type' section) (Table 20.2). Epilepsy is often the sole presenting manifestation of low-grade benign tumours. In contrast, high-grade malignant tumours present with a mixture of symptoms and signs including focal neurological deficits, raised intracranial pressure, and seizures. In population-based samples, brain tumours are the cause of about 4% of all new-onset epilepsies (115, 116). From a different perspective, seizures are the presenting manifestation in about one-third of the cases of brain tumours (117, 118).

Risk stratification and mechanisms of epileptogenesis

Various factors and mechanisms are known to be involved in the development of seizures in tumoural epilepsy. These include tumour type (Table 20.2) and its location, peritumoural tissue changes, intrinsic epileptogenic properties of certain tumour cells, and alterations in neurotransmitters and amino acids.

Tumour type

The overall incidence of seizures in individuals with low-grade gliomas (including dysembryoplastic neuroepithelial tumour (DNET), ganglioglioma and low-grade astrocytomas/oligodendrogliomas) is 75–100% in comparison to an incidence of 40–60% in those with glioblastoma multiforme (114, 115, 118). Thus, low-grade, slow-growing tumours appear to be highly epileptogenic

Table 20.2 Tumour types associated with epilepsy[a]

Low-grade tumours
Neuronal and glial neoplasms:
Dysembryoplastic neuroepithelial tumour Ganglioglioma
Glial neoplasms:
Pilocytic astrocytoma Low-grade astrocytoma Pleomorphic xanthoastrocytoma Oligodendroglioma Oligoastrocytoma
High-grade tumours
Meningioma Glioblastoma multiforme Metastasis Leptomeningeal tumour Primary central nervous system lymphoma

[a] According to the frequency of occurrence of seizures.

(Table 20.2) (119, 120). The precise reasons for this are unclear. Perhaps, a longer survival period in people with low-grade gliomas might be the reason for the greater number of seizures experienced by them (117, 118). A greater propensity to seizures might also be on account of the association of developmental tumours with cortical dysplasia, as well as the presence of specialized cells within the tumours, which release neurotransmitters capable of inducing seizures and epilepsy (120–123). In addition, the tumour slowly deafferents the neighbouring cerebral cortex, which in due course of time develops intrinsic epileptogenic properties.

Tumour location

Although more commonly observed with intra-axial tumours, seizures can also be the manifestation of extra-axial tumours such as meningiomas. Extra-axial tumours manifest with seizures as a result of compression of adjacent brain tissue (124, 125). Supratentorial tumours, particularly those involving the highly-epileptogenic rolandic/perirolandic cortex and the mesial temporal lobes have particular propensity to manifest with seizures and epilepsy. Those located in the occipital and parietal lobes, sellar region, and infratentorial compartment are less likely to manifest with seizures (124).

Alterations in peritumoural homeostasis

The potentially epileptogenic cerebral cortex is rendered hyperexcitable as a result of several factors including deranged blood–brain barrier integrity leading to alterations in peritumoural microenvironment, enzymatic changes, and impaired intercellular connections between adjacent glial cells via connexin gap junction proteins (126). Brain tumours also have a relatively higher metabolic rate than normal tissue which creates a relatively hypoxic environment with interstitial acidosis (127). Marked vasogenic oedema and an increase in the concentrations of sodium, calcium, and serum proteins are noted in the peritumoural tissue (127). Hence, several mechanisms are thought to contribute to the development of seizures and epilepsy.

Neurotransmitters and amino acids

An altered expression of neurotransmitter receptors (mainly inotropic and metabotropic glutamate receptors) has been noted in brain tumours (128). Besides abnormal receptor expression, alterations in levels of gamma aminobutyric acid have also been documented. Both mechanisms might be involved in the generation of seizures and epilepsy (129).

Secondary epileptogenesis and dual pathology

Secondary epileptogenesis refers to the development of a new epileptogenic lesion that is distinct from the initial or primary epileptogenic lesion. The occurrence of recurrent, often prolonged seizures before a certain age (usually 5 years but might be later) is thought to be critical to the development of secondary epileptogenesis (130). Of the various cortical structures, the hippocampus is most susceptible to be involved during secondary epileptogenesis. Dual pathology is the presence of additional or concomitant potentially-epileptogenic lesion/s distinct from the primary lesion (131, 132). The primary lesion can be either neoplastic, dysplastic, vascular, or infective and the secondary pathology most often is hippocampal sclerosis. Dual pathology is noted in 15–30% of surgical series of patients with medically-intractable epilepsy.

Treatment

Comprehensive management of epilepsy in patients with brain tumours is often neglected as epileptologists and neurologists are seldom actively involved in the care of such patients and oncologists devote their time mostly to the treatment of the tumours (133). Therefore, only limited data regarding medical treatment of tumoural epilepsy is available in published literature. On the other hand, a little more than a handful of series of cases describing results of surgical treatment of epilepsy associated with low-grade gliomas are available (see 'Surgical treatment' section).

Medical treatment

Conventional AEDs

Carbamazepine, phenytoin, and phenobarbital are effective AEDs for treatment of localization-related, partial epilepsy. However, these are all potent inducers of the hepatic P450 enzyme system. Many of the cancer chemotherapeutic agents used in the treatment of brain tumours are metabolized by the P450 enzyme system. Hence, there are concerns that the metabolism of the cancer chemotherapeutic agents might be increased as a result of the concurrent administration of enzyme-inducing AEDs, thereby potentially compromising their efficacy and reducing the survival of patients with brain tumours (134). The cancer chemotherapeutic agents most commonly used in treatment of brain tumours are lomustine (CCNU), temozolomide, vinblastin, and procarbazine. In addition, methotrexate and carmustine (BCNU) can be delivered directly to the brain tissue through the intrathecal route and via implantable gliadil wafers, respectively. The enzyme-inducing AEDs reduce the area under curve and maximally-tolerated doses of lomustine. There are no known interactions between enzyme-inducing AEDs and temozolomide or directly administered methotrexate and carmustine. The clinical relevance of drug interactions between enzyme-inducing AEDs and cancer-chemotherapeutic agents has not been adequately studied. A retrospective study in patients with glioblastoma multiforme found that median survival in patients who received enzyme-inducing AEDs (mostly carbamazepine) was considerably shorter than in those who received sodium valproate (135).

Valproate is a broad-spectrum AED with demonstrated efficacy in tumoural epilepsy. A retrospective study compared seizure control in brain tumour patients with valproate, carbamazepine, and phenytoin and found better remission rates with valproate (136). The doses of valproate can be titrated rapidly to achieve therapeutic levels. Although, it is known to reduce temozolomide clearance, the clinical significance of this interaction is uncertain. The drug has been demonstrated to inhibit histone-deacetylase activity both *in vitro* and *in vivo* leading to apoptosis of cancer cells (137, 138). This action can be potentially exploited to improve survival in brain tumours. Valproate is also known to inhibit the multidrug-resistance gene (*MDR1*), which is responsible for AED refractoriness in patients with brain tumours (139). Although, it can cause hepatotoxicity and abnormal coagulation profiles, the clinical impact of these side effects has been found to be negligible (135).

Newer AEDs

Among various newer AEDs, levetiracetam, gabapentin, and lacosamide have no known drug interactions with any of the cancer chemotherapeutic agents and hence are potentially useful drugs in the management of tumoural epilepsy and seizures. Experience with the newer AEDs, particularly levetiracetam in tumoural epilepsy is restricted to a handful of uncontrolled trials and very few small, controlled trials. At least six prospective or retrospective trials of levetiracetam demonstrated efficacy of the drug as add-on treatment in tumoural epilepsy (140–145). In one such trial, it was demonstrated that addition of levetiracetam led to more than 50% reduction in seizure frequency in two-thirds of the patients and that about half of these could be eventually converted to levetiracetam monotherapy (141). Other trials, albeit small and with many limitations, likewise demonstrated the efficacy of add-on levetiracetam in tumoural epilepsy. In these trials, the side effects of the drug were found to be insignificant, and were limited to fatigue, dizziness, mood changes, and somnolence (143). Monotherapy with levetiracetam in the treatment of seizures associated with brain tumours has also been evaluated in few small, uncontrolled and controlled trials. In these trials, the drug has been found to be safe and efficacious (146, 147). The drug has also been compared with phenytoin for use as an agent to prevent seizures immediately following craniotomy for brain tumours (up to 7 days postoperatively) and found to be safe and equally efficacious (148). In the perioperative period, levetiracetam might be preferable over phenytoin as it is suitable for intravenous administration, equally efficacious and is not associated with serious side effects observed with phenytoin, such as the Stevens–Johnson syndrome and purple glove syndrome. Moreover, psychiatric adverse effects do not appear to be an issue when levetiracetam is given for short periods (<7 days) in craniotomy patients. The advantages of levetiracetam in the long-term management of tumoural epilepsy are its lack of side effects apart from psychiatric disturbances and any known interactions with cancer chemotherapeutic agents used in the treatment of brain tumours. There is perhaps no experience with levetiracetam use in the primary prophylaxis of seizures in patients with brain tumours.

Other than the preliminary studies with levetiracetam, there is scanty data regarding the use of the newer AEDs in treatment or prevention of seizures associated with brain tumours. Limited data exists regarding the use of oxcarbazepine in the prevention of perioperative and late seizures and of gabapentin in the management of refractory tumoural epilepsy, but clearly more experience with the newer AEDs is desirable (149, 150).

Practical issues in the treatment of tumoural epilepsy with AEDs

Use of AEDs in the primary prophylaxis of seizures in individuals with brain tumours: a meta-analysis of trials available till 2004 found no significant benefit of administration of phenobarbital, phenytoin, and valproate in terms of seizure control at 1 week or 6 months in patients with brain tumours who had never experienced seizures (151). An American Academy of Neurology practice parameter recommended that AEDs should not be routinely used in patients with newly-diagnosed brain tumours (118). The recommendation is based on an independent meta-analysis of several studies that concluded that although seizures are common in patients with brain tumours, there is no evidence to suggest that AEDs reduce the seizure risk in those who do not have prior seizures. Rather, the routine use of AEDs is frequently associated with side effects, some of which can be potentially life-threatening (e.g. anticonvulsant hypersensitivity syndrome). Despite this, the practice of administering prophylactic AEDs, particularly covering the perioperative period in patients undergoing craniotomy for supratentorial tumours remains unchecked. When used purely for perioperative prophylaxis, the AED should be withdrawn within 7 days of craniotomy. The use of levetiracetam in this situation appears to be gaining favour, although robust evidence supporting its use is still lacking.

Choice of AED in individuals with brain tumours with seizures: when patients with brain tumours present with seizures, long-term use of AEDs for prevention of further seizures is recommended (Fig. 20.3). Besides the usual issues that dictate the choice of AED, certain considerations specific to brain tumours also influence the selection of AEDs in such situations. One consideration is the range of interactions between AEDs and cancer-chemotherapeutic agents. Besides the aforementioned interactions between enzyme-inducing AEDs (phenobarbital, phenytoin, and carbamazepine and also to some extent, oxcarbazepine and topiramate) and cancer-chemotherapeutic agents, reduction in the serum levels of several AEDs has been clearly documented largely due to impaired absorption of the latter across the gastrointestinal mucosa that might be damaged by chemotherapeutic agents (152). Another consideration is the potential lack of effectiveness of certain AEDs due to expression of multidrug-resistance proteins, which appears to be high in individuals with brain tumours (153). Insufficient concentration of AEDs in the brain might be due to the effect of multidrug-resistance gene *MDR1 (ABCB1*, P-glycoprotein) polymorphisms. Among various AEDs, phenytoin, phenobarbital, carbamazepine, and lamotrigine have been shown to be substrates for these gene effects (147). Levetiracetam appears not to be a substrate for these gene effects and valproate has been shown to induce apoptosis in tumour cells expressing *MDR1*; hence the use of either levetiracetam or valproate might be advantageous from this standpoint (141, 153).

Withdrawal of AEDs in tumoural epilepsy: no guidelines exist regarding when and how to withdraw AEDs in patients with tumoural epilepsy who enter a period of remission. In a retrospective study of 62 children with brain tumours and epilepsy in whom AEDs were withdrawn, one-third had seizure recurrence within 10 months (154). AED withdrawal might be a consideration in

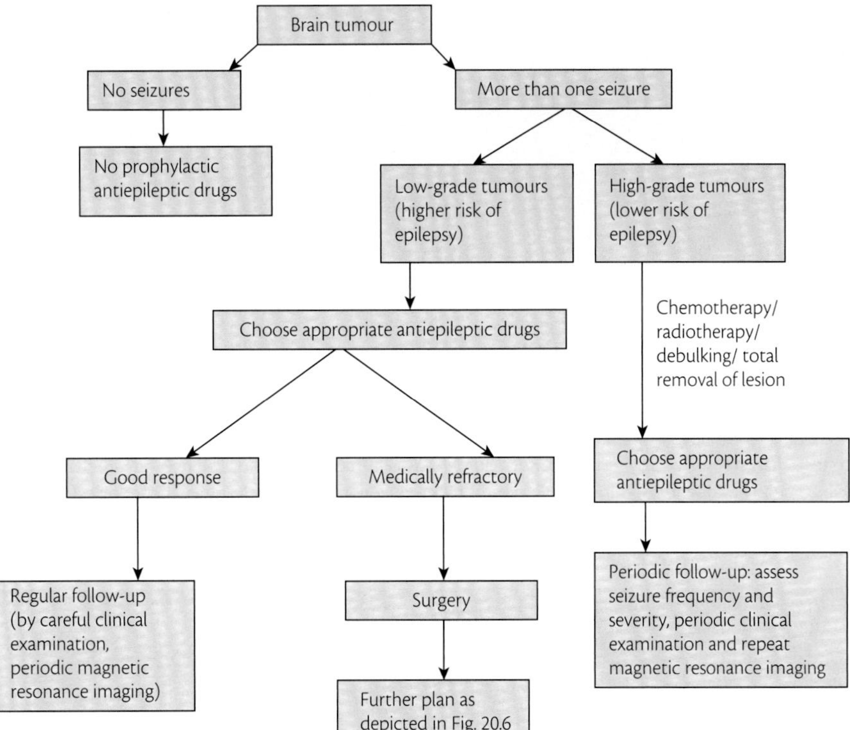

Fig. 20.3 A pragmatic approach to patients with epilepsy due to brain tumours.

patients who enter a period of remission following complete resection of low-grade brain tumours but in all the other situations it would perhaps be prudent to continue AED treatment for prolonged periods of time.

Effects of other forms of treatment on epilepsy: an interesting question is whether primary oncological treatment offers any benefits in terms of seizure control in patients with brain tumours. The role of surgery in the management of refractory tumoural epilepsy is discussed in the 'Surgical treatment' section. In small controlled and uncontrolled studies, both cranial irradiation and administration of chemotherapeutic agents, specifically temozolomide have been shown to improve seizure control to some extent (155, 156). This is an area that requires further study.

Surgical treatment

Over two-thirds of patients with medically refractory tumoural epilepsy experience complete seizure freedom or substantial reduction in seizure frequency following tumour excision (157, 158). Brain neoplasms comprise 10–30% of the lesions in various surgical series of refractory focal epilepsies (157, 158). Two low-grade tumours, DNET and ganglioglioma, are noteworthy in context of their association with medically refractory epilepsy. Thus, although these tumours constitute only a small proportion of primary brain neoplasms overall, they are well represented in surgical series of patients with refractory epilepsy (157, 158).

DNET: This tumour accounts for 10–20% of brain tumours in surgical series of refractory epilepsy from centres undertaking epilepsy surgery (120, 157). The tumour is cortically-located, most frequently in the temporal lobe but might also be located in the frontal lobe in one-third of the cases (120). Very characteristically, it presents in young people (typically <20 years of age) with chronic, medically-refractory epilepsy with complex partial seizures. Cranial computed tomography (CT) demonstrates a pseudocystic, cortically-based lesion, sometimes with overlying bone changes in the cranial vault. Likewise, MRI demonstrates a cortical lesion with no mass effect or surrounding oedema but might enhance following injection of gadolinium contrast and might rarely be partially calcified (Fig. 20.4A–C). The histological hallmark of the tumour is its glioneuronal element comprising of columns lined by glial cells with interspersed floating neuronal cells (Fig. 20.4D). Its association with cortical dysplasia is now well recognized (157). The pathological diagnosis may sometimes be handicapped by the absence of an adequate volume of tissue, as a result of which the typical disarray of the neuronal and glial elements might be missed.

Ganglioglioma: this tumour is the most commonly identified tumour in many surgical series of medically refractory tumoural epilepsy (157, 158). It is typically diagnosed in young individuals (<30 years of age) presenting with protracted medically refractory epilepsy with complex partial seizures. Magnetic resonance imaging is exquisitely sensitive in determining the location and characteristics of ganglioglioma (Fig. 20.5A–C). The temporal lobe is the most frequent location, but the tumour can be found at any site within the neuraxis. Both solid and cystic components can be identified and gadolinium enhancement is noted in two-thirds of the cases on MRI. Calcification is noted in one-third of cases and surrounding cerebral oedema is very rare. Upon histology, the tumour can be shown to comprise neoplastic astrocytic elements and dysplastic neuronal cells (Fig. 20.5D). The astrocytic elements are GFAP (+) and synaptophysin (+).

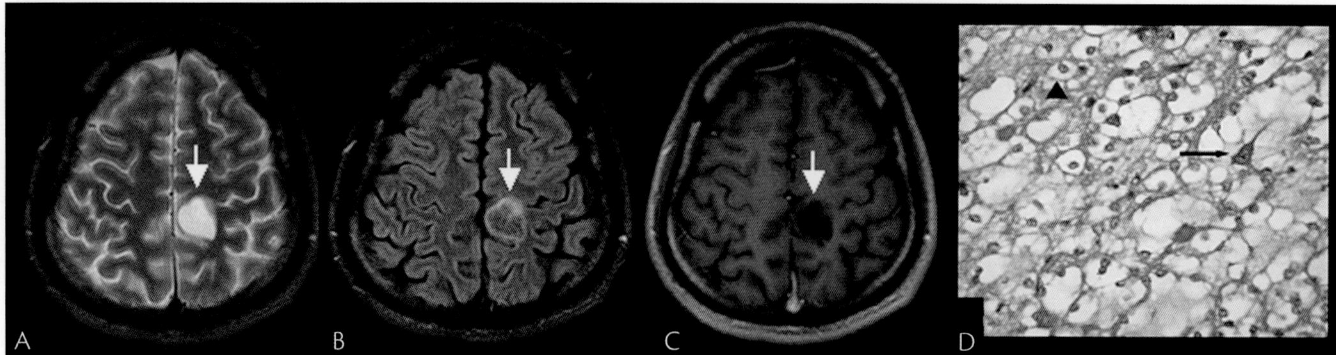

Fig. 20.4 Imaging and histopathological data of a 12-year-old boy with complex partial seizures since 2 years of age. A) Axial T2-weighted MRI showing a well-defined lesion occupying the left frontal lobe in the paracentral lobule (white arrow). B) Axial FLAIR sequence shows that the lesion is predominantly hypointense with a hyper intense rim. C) Axial T1-weighted postcontrast sequence did not show any contrast enhancement. D) Photomicrograph showing classical floating neurons (black arrow) and oligodendrocyte-like cells (black arrow heads), characteristic of a dysembryoplastic neuroepithelial tumour. These floating neurons are seen in microcystic spaces with mucoid material (haematoxylin and eosin × 400). The patient is seizure-free 18 months following lesionectomy without any neurological deficits.

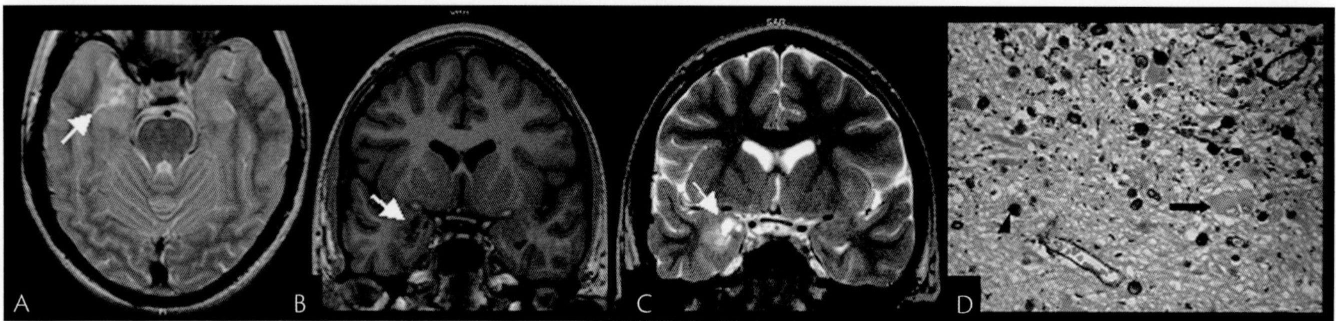

Fig. 20.5 Imaging and histopathological appearance of ganglioglioma in a 22-year-old female with complex partial seizures since 9 years of age. A) MRI axial T2-weighted sequence, B) coronal T1-weighted sequence and (C) Coronal T2 weighted sequence showing a mass lesion (white arrow) in the mesial temporal lobe (amygdala and head of hippocampus). The lesion had small cystic areas within it. There was no contrast enhancement. D) Photomicrograph showing an admixture of neoplastic ganglion cells (black arrow) scattered in between astrocytes, characteristic of ganglioglioma. Multiple calcified spherules are seen (black arrow head) (haematoxylin and eosin × 400).

Surgical excision is the recommended treatment for ganglioglioma in individuals with medically refractory epilepsy. Good seizure outcome is the rule (80% cases being seizure-free at 6 months) but the outcome perhaps depends on the extent of resection and duration of epilepsy. The oncological prognosis is also generally good and plausibly depends on the extent of resection. Malignant transformation has been described.

Low-grade glial neoplasms: low-grade glioma, pilocytic astrocytoma, pleomorphic xanthoastrocytoma, and oligodendroglioma are other low-grade neoplasms frequently associated with tumoural epilepsy (157, 159). More than two-thirds of the low-grade glial neoplasms associated with medically refractory epilepsy are located in the temporal lobe. In contrast to DNET and ganglioglioma, malignant transformation invariably occurs after a period of time in other low-grade glial tumours. Hence, total excision of these lesions is an important goal of management.

Presurgical evaluation and surgical strategies

Surgical excision of low-grade glial neoplasms might be undertaken for control of medically refractory epilepsy, for pathological verification of the lesion prior to planning radiotherapy or chemotherapy, and to preclude the risks of malignant transformation or haemorrhage into the tumour. All patients with medically refractory epilepsy and an MRI-identified lesion should proceed through standard presurgical evaluation (Fig. 20.6). The objective of epilepsy surgery is to render the patient seizure-free without producing unacceptable sequelae. The decision for proceeding to surgery for control of seizures is undertaken by a multidisciplinary team comprising of an epileptologist, neurosurgeon, neuroradiologist, and a neuropsychologist. The various surgical approaches include:

Lesionectomy: this refers to the complete removal of the MRI-identified lesion. The resection might be anatomically guided by visual impression of the neurosurgeon during operation but increasingly so by modern neuronavigation and image-guidance tools.

Extended lesionectomy: many of the developmental, low grade glial tumours are associated with cortical dysplasia. Excision of the dysplastic cortex perhaps becomes critical for optimal seizure control in such circumstances. Extended lesionectomy involves

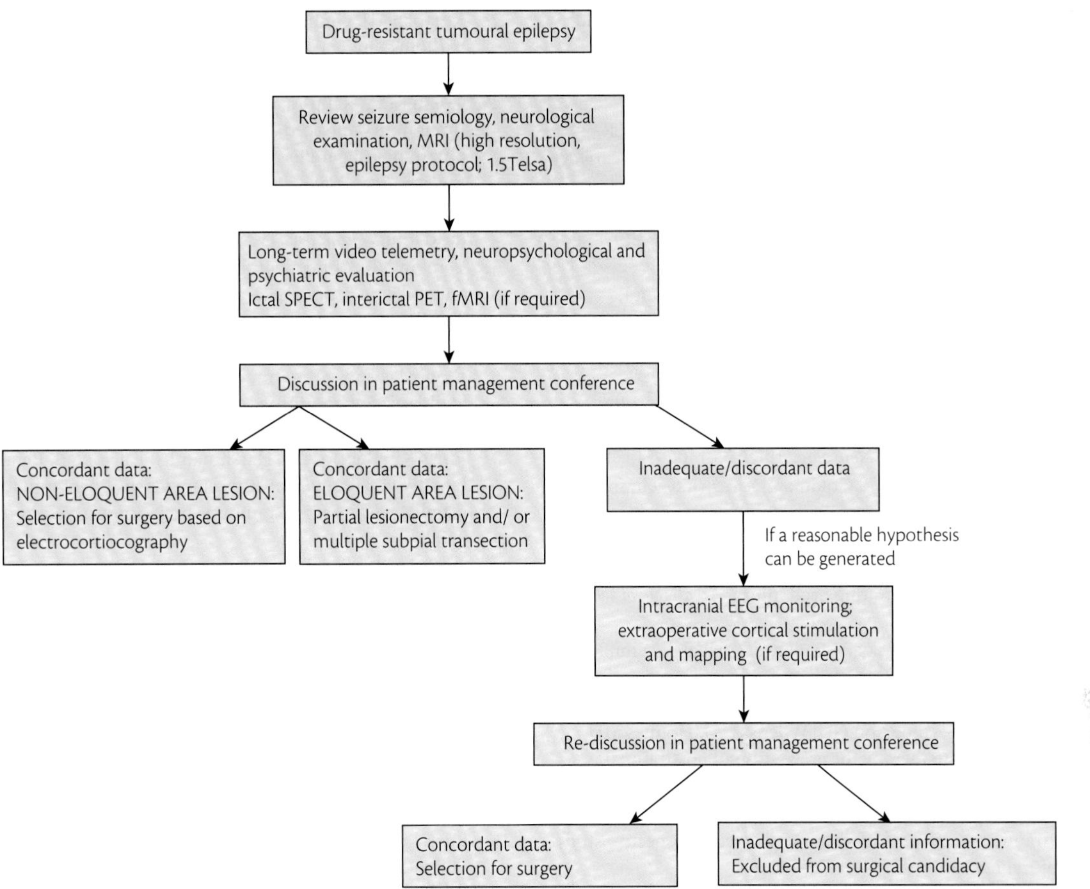

Fig. 20.6 Steps in presurgical evaluation of drug-resistant tumoural epilepsy. EEG, electroencephalography; fMRI, functional magnetic resonance imaging; HR, high-resolution; PET, positron emission tomography; SPECT, single-photon emission computed tomography.

excision of the lesion with an adjoining rim of tissue around the lesion which is apparently normal on MRI. It is achieved with the aid of either prior long-term intracranial electroencephalogram monitoring or intraoperative electrocorticography. It remains a matter of controversy whether lesionectomy alone or lesionectomy with excision of the surrounding epileptogenic zone is superior in terms of seizure outcome. In one series of surgical excisions guided by implanted subdural electrodes, it was observed that the epileptogenic zone frequently extended beyond the confines of lesion and at many times involved non-contiguous regions remote from the lesion. However, the postoperative seizure outcome appeared to depend on the completeness of resection of the lesion rather than the epileptogenic zone identified by mapping. When complete resection of the lesion was achieved in these patients, the extent of resection of the epileptogenic zone did not appear to affect postoperative seizure outcome (160). In certain situations, however, partial lesionectomy with a more complete epileptogenic zone resection might offer better postoperative seizure control. Therefore, complete resection of the lesion provides the maximal likelihood of complete seizure control following surgery but clearly, there are instances in which, carefully-planned resection of the lesion and of the epileptogenic zone might be advantageous. Extended lesionectomy might be limited at times due to close proximity of the lesion or epileptogenic zone to eloquent cortex, which can be delineated by functional mapping (either, electrical stimulation during or before surgery or prior functional MRI). When eloquent area hinders further resection of the lesion and epileptogenic zone, multiple subpial transection might be undertaken as an ancillary procedure along with lesionectomy.

Tackling dual pathology: whenever possible removal of both the lesion and the hippocampus affords superior seizure outcome when compared with resection of either lesion alone or the hippocampus alone in patients with demonstrated dual pathology (161). However, the ultimate decision to include both the lesion and hippocampus should be individualized and depends on the electroclinical and imaging data.

References

1. Annegers JF, Rocca WA, Hauser WA. Causes of epilepsy: contributions of the Rochester epidemiology project. *Mayo Clin Proc* 1996; 71:570–5.
2. WHO. *Projections of Mortality and Burden of Disease to 2030: Deaths by Income* Group. Geneva: World Health Organization, 2002.
3. Langlois JA, Rutland-Brown W, Wald MM. The epidemiology and impact of traumatic brain injury: a brief overview. *J Head Trauma Rehabil* 2006; 21:375–8.
4. Puvanachandra P, Hyder AA. The burden of tarumatic brain injury in Asia: A call for research. *Pak J Neurol Sci* 2009; 4:27–32.
5. Gururaj G. Epidemiology of traumatic brain injuries: Indian scenario. *Neurol Res* 2002; 24:24–8.

6. WHO. *World health report. 2003. Shaping the future*. Geneva: World Health Organization, 2003.
7. Medicine ACoR. Definition of mild traumatic brain injury. *J Head Trauma Rehabil* 1993; 8:86–8.
8. Annegers JF, Grabow JD, Groover RV, Laws ER, Jr., Elveback LR, Kurland LT. Seizures after head trauma: a population study. *Neurology* 1980; 30:683–9.
9. Annegers JF, Hauser WA, Coan SP, Rocca WA. A population-based study of seizures after traumatic brain injuries. *N Engl J Med* 1998; 338:20–4.
10. Christensen J, Pedersen MG, Pedersen CB, Sidenius P, Olsen J, Vestergaard M. Long-term risk of epilepsy after traumatic brain injury in children and young adults: a population-based cohort study. *Lancet* 2009; 373:1105–10.
11. Salazar AM, Jabbari B, Vance SC, Grafman J, Amin D, Dillon JD. Epilepsy after penetrating head injury. I. Clinical correlates: a report of the Vietnam Head Injury Study. *Neurology* 1985; 35:1406–14.
12. Raymont V, Salazar AM, Lipsky R, Goldman D, Tasick G, Grafman J. Correlates of posttraumatic epilepsy 35 years following combat brain injury. *Neurology*; 75:224–9.
13. Weiss GH, Salazar AM, Vance SC, Grafman JH, Jabbari B. Predicting posttraumatic epilepsy in penetrating head injury. *Arch Neurol* 1986; 43:771–3.
14. Temkin NR, Dikmen SS, Wilensky AJ, Keihm J, Chabal S, Winn HR. A randomized, double-blind study of phenytoin for the prevention of post-traumatic seizures. *N Engl J Med* 1990; 323:497–502.
15. Temkin NR, Dikmen SS, Anderson GD, Wilensky AJ, Holmes MD, Cohen W, *et al.* Valproate therapy for prevention of posttraumatic seizures: a randomized trial. *J Neurosurg* 1999; 91:593–600.
16. Angeleri F, Majkowski J, Cacchio G, Sobieszek A, D'Acunto S, Gesuita R, *et al.* Posttraumatic epilepsy risk factors: one-year prospective study after head injury. *Epilepsia* 1999; 40:1222–30.
17. Ferguson PL, Smith GM, Wannamaker BB, Thurman DJ, Pickelsimer EE, Selassie AW. A population-based study of risk of epilepsy after hospitalization for traumatic brain injury. *Epilepsia*; 51:891–8.
18. Haltiner AM, Temkin NR, Dikmen SS. Risk of seizure recurrence after the first late posttraumatic seizure. *Arch Phys Med Rehabil* 1997; 78:835–40.
19. Mathern GW, Babb TL, Vickrey BG, Melendez M, Pretorius JK. Traumatic compared to non-traumatic clinical-pathologic associations in temporal lobe epilepsy. *Epilepsy Res* 1994; 19:129–39.
20. Marks DA, Kim J, Spencer DD, Spencer SS. Seizure localization and pathology following head injury in patients with uncontrolled epilepsy. *Neurology* 1995; 45:2051–7.
21. Diaz-Arrastia R, Agostini MA, Frol AB, Mickey B, Fleckenstein J, Bigio E, *et al.* Neurophysiologic and neuroradiologic features of intractable epilepsy after traumatic brain injury in adults. *Arch Neurol* 2000; 57:1611–16.
22. Englander J, Bushnik T, Wright JM, Jamison L, Duong TT. Mortality in late post-traumatic seizures. *J Neurotrauma* 2009; 26:1471–7.
23. Swartz BE, Houser CR, Tomiyasu U, Walsh GO, DeSalles A, Rich JR, *et al.* Hippocampal cell loss in posttraumatic human epilepsy. *Epilepsia* 2006; 47:1373–82.
24. Rocca WA, Sharbrough FW, Hauser WA, Annegers JF, Schoenberg BS. Risk factors for complex partial seizures: a population-based case-control study. *Ann Neurol* 1987; 21:22–31.
25. Kotapka MJ, Gennarelli TA, Graham DI, Adams JH, Thibault LE, Ross DT, *et al.* Selective vulnerability of hippocampal neurons in acceleration-induced experimental head injury. *J Neurotrauma* 1991; 8:247–58.
26. Kotapka MJ, Graham DI, Adams JH, Doyle D, Gennarelli TA. Hippocampal damage in fatal paediatric head injury. *Neuropathol Appl Neurobiol* 1993; 19:128–33.
27. Kotapka MJ, Graham DI, Adams JH, Gennarelli TA. Hippocampal pathology in fatal non-missile human head injury. *Acta Neuropathol* 1992; 83:530–4.
28. Kotapka MJ, Graham DI, Adams JH, Gennarelli TA. Hippocampal pathology in fatal human head injury without high intracranial pressure. *J Neurotrauma* 1994; 11:317–24.
29. Coulter DA, Rafiq A, Shumate M, Gong QZ, DeLorenzo RJ, Lyeth BG. Brain injury-induced enhanced limbic epileptogenesis: anatomical and physiological parallels to an animal model of temporal lobe epilepsy. *Epilepsy Res* 1996; 26:81–91.
30. Westbrook LE, Devinsky O, Geocadin R. Nonepileptic seizures after head injury. *Epilepsia* 1998; 39:978–82.
31. Temkin NR. Antiepileptogenesis and seizure prevention trials with antiepileptic drugs: meta-analysis of controlled trials. *Epilepsia* 2001; 42:515–24.
32. Chang BS, Lowenstein DH. Practice parameter: antiepileptic drug prophylaxis in severe traumatic brain injury: report of the Quality Standards Subcommittee of the American Academy of Neurology. *Neurology* 2003; 60:10–16.
33. Jones KE, Puccio AM, Harshman KJ, Falcione B, Benedict N, Jankowitz BT, *et al.* Levetiracetam versus phenytoin for seizure prophylaxis in severe traumatic brain injury. *Neurosurg Focus* 2008; 25:E3.
34. Szaflarski JP, Sangha KS, Lindsell CJ, Shutter LA. Prospective, randomized, single-blinded comparative trial of intravenous levetiracetam versus phenytoin for seizure prophylaxis. *Neurocrit Care*; 12:165–72.
35. Schuh LA, Henry TR, Fromes G, Blaivas M, Ross DA, Drury I. Influence of head trauma on outcome following anterior temporal lobectomy. *Arch Neurol* 1998; 55:1325–8.
36. Forsgren L, Bucht G, Eriksson S, Bergmark L. Incidence and clinical characterization of unprovoked seizures in adults: a prospective population-based study. *Epilepsia* 1996; 37:224–9.
37. Burn J, Dennis M, Bamford J, Sandercock P, Wade D, Warlow C. Epileptic seizures after a first stroke: the Oxfordshire Community Stroke Project. *BMJ* 1997; 315:1582–7.
38. Roberts RC, Shorvon SD, Cox TC, Gilliatt RW. Clinically unsuspected cerebral infarction revealed by computed tomography scanning in late onset epilepsy. *Epilepsia* 1988; 29:190–4.
39. Shinton RA, Gill JS, Zezulka AV, Beevers DG. The frequency of epilepsy preceding stroke. Case-control study in 230 patients. *Lancet* 1987; 1:11–13.
40. Cleary P, Shorvon S, Tallis R. Late-onset seizures as a predictor of subsequent stroke. *Lancet* 2004; 363:1184–6.
41. Gibson LM, Allan SM, Parkes LM, Emsley HC. Occult cerebrovascular disease and late-onset epilepsy: could loss of neurovascular unit integrity be a viable model? *Cardiovasc Psychiatry Neurol* 2011; 2011:130406.
42. Kilpatrick CJ, Davis SM, Tress BM, Rossiter SC, Hopper JL, Vandendriesen ML. Epileptic seizures in acute stroke. *Arch Neurol* 1990; 47:157–60.
43. So EL, Annegers JF, Hauser WA, O'Brien PC, Whisnant JP. Population-based study of seizure disorders after cerebral infarction. *Neurology* 1996; 46:350–55.
44. Bladin CF, Alexandrov AV, Bellavance A, Bornstein N, Chambers B, Coté R, *et al.* Seizures after stroke: a prospective multicenter study. *Arch Neurol* 2000; 57:1617–22.
45. Meyer JS, Charney JZ, Rivera VM, Mathew NT. Cerebral embolization: prospective clinical analysis of 42 cases. *Stroke* 1971; 2:541–54.
46. Lossius MI, Ronning OM, Slapo GD, Mowinckel P, Gjerstad L. Poststroke epilepsy: occurrence and predictors—a long-term prospective controlled study (Akershus Stroke Study). *Epilepsia* 2005; 46:1246–51.
47. Kammersgaard LP, Olsen TS. Poststroke epilepsy in the Copenhagen stroke study: incidence and predictors. *J Stroke Cerebrovasc Dis* 2005; 14:210–14.
48. Olafsson E, Gudmundsson G, Hauser WA. Risk of epilepsy in long-term survivors of surgery for aneurysmal subarachnoid hemorrhage: a population-based study in Iceland. *Epilepsia* 2000; 41:1201–5.

49. Claassen J, Peery S, Kreiter KT, Hirsch LJ, Du EY, Connolly ES, *et al.* Predictors and clinical impact of epilepsy after subarachnoid hemorrhage. *Neurology* 2003; 60:208–14.
50. Strzelczyk A, Haag A, Raupach H, Herrendorf G, Hamer HM, Rosenow F. Prospective evaluation of a post-stroke epilepsy risk scale. *J Neurol*; 257:1322–6.
51. Benbir G, Ince B, Bozluolcay M. The epidemiology of post-stroke epilepsy according to stroke subtypes. *Acta Neurol Scand* 2006; 114:8–12.
52. Olsen TS, Langhorne P, Diener HC, Hennerici M, Ferro J, Sivenius J, *et al.* European Stroke Initiative Recommendations for Stroke Management-update 2003. *Cerebrovasc Dis* 2003; 16:311–37.
53. Broderick J, Connolly S, Feldmann E, Hanley D, Kase C, Krieger D, *et al.* Guidelines for the management of spontaneous intracerebral hemorrhage in adults: 2007 update: a guideline from the American Heart Association/American Stroke Association Stroke Council, High Blood Pressure Research Council, and the Quality of Care and Outcomes in Research Interdisciplinary Working Group. *Circulation* 2007; 116:e391–413.
54. Calabresi P, Cupini LM, Centonze D, Pisani F, Bernardi G. Antiepileptic drugs as a possible neuroprotective strategy in brain ischemia. *Ann Neurol* 2003; 53:693–702.
55. Kutlu G, Gomceli YB, Unal Y, Inan LE. Levetiracetam monotherapy for late poststroke seizures in the elderly. *Epilepsy Behav* 2008; 13:542–4.
56. Waterhouse EJ, Vaughan JK, Barnes TY, Boggs JG, Towne AR, Kopec-Garnett L, *et al.* Synergistic effect of status epilepticus and ischemic brain injury on mortality. *Epilepsy Res* 1998; 29:175–83.
57. Velioglu SK, Ozmenoglu M, Boz C, Alioglu Z. Status epilepticus after stroke. *Stroke* 2001; 32:1169–72.
58. Rumbach L, Sablot D, Berger E, Tatu L, Vuillier F, Moulin T. Status epilepticus in stroke: report on a hospital-based stroke cohort. *Neurology* 2000; 54:350–4.
59. Bogousslavsky J, Martin R, Regli F, Despland PA, Bolyn S. Persistent worsening of stroke sequelae after delayed seizures. *Arch Neurol* 1992; 49:385–8.
60. Paolucci S, Silvestri G, Lubich S, Pratesi L, Traballesi M, Gigli GL. Poststroke late seizures and their role in rehabilitation of inpatients. *Epilepsia* 1997; 38:266–70.
61. Goldstein LB. Common drugs may influence motor recovery after stroke. The Sygen In Acute Stroke Study Investigators. *Neurology* 1995; 45:865–71.
62. Naidech AM, Garg RK, Liebling S, Levasseur K, Macken MP, Schuele SU, *et al.* Anticonvulsant use and outcomes after intracerebral hemorrhage. *Stroke* 2009; 40:3810–15.
63. Naidech AM, Kreiter KT, Janjua N, Ostapkovich N, Parra A, Commichau C, *et al.* Phenytoin exposure is associated with functional and cognitive disability after subarachnoid hemorrhage. *Stroke* 2005; 36:583–7.
64. Alvarez-Sabin J, Montaner J, Padro L, Molina CA, Rovira R, Codina A, *et al.* Gabapentin in late-onset poststroke seizures. *Neurology* 2002; 59:1991–3.
65. Kwan J, Wood E. Antiepileptic drugs for the primary and secondary prevention of seizures after stroke. *Cochrane Database Syst Rev* 2010; 1:CD005398.
66. Rowan AJ, Ramsay RE, Collins JF, Pryor F, Boardman KD, Uthman BM, *et al.* New onset geriatric epilepsy: a randomized study of gabapentin, lamotrigine, and carbamazepine. *Neurology* 2005; 64:1868–73.
67. Brodie MJ, Overstall PW, Giorgi L. Multicentre, double-blind, randomised comparison between lamotrigine and carbamazepine in elderly patients with newly diagnosed epilepsy. The UK Lamotrigine Elderly Study Group. *Epilepsy Res* 1999; 37:81–7.
68. Gilad R, Sadeh M, Rapoport A, Dabby R, Boaz M, Lampl Y. Monotherapy of lamotrigine versus carbamazepine in patients with poststroke seizure. *Clin Neuropharmacol* 2007; 30:189–95.
69. Saetre E, Perucca E, Isojarvi J, Gjerstad L. An international multicenter randomized double-blind controlled trial of lamotrigine and sustained-release carbamazepine in the treatment of newly diagnosed epilepsy in the elderly. *Epilepsia* 2007; 48:1292–302.
70. Mula M, Trimble MR, Thompson P, Sander JW. Topiramate and word-finding difficulties in patients with epilepsy. *Neurology* 2003; 60:1104–7.
71. Stephen LJ, Maxwell JE, Brodie MJ. Transient hemiparesis with topiramate. *BMJ* 1999; 318:845.
72. Annegers JF, Hauser WA, Beghi E, Nicolosi A, Kurland LT. The risk of unprovoked seizures after encephalitis and meningitis. *Neurology* 1988; 38:1407–10.
73. Rantakallio P, Leskinen M, von Wendt L. Incidence and prognosis of central nervous system infections in a birth cohort of 12,000 children. *Scand J Infect Dis* 1986; 18:287–94.
74. de Graaf AS. Epidemiological aspects of epilepsy in northern Norway. *Epilepsia* 1974; 15:291–9.
75. Bergamini L, Bergamasco B, Benna P, Gilli M. Acquired etiological factors in 1,785 epileptic subjects: clinical-anamnestic research. *Epilepsia* 1977; 18:437–44.
76. Hauser WA, Kurland LT. The epidemiology of epilepsy in Rochester, Minnesota, 1935 through 1967. *Epilepsia* 1975; 16:1–66.
77. Murthy JM, Yangala R, Srinivas M. The syndromic classification of the International League Against Epilepsy: a hospital-based study from South India. *Epilepsia* 1998; 39:48–54.
78. Preux PM, Druet-Cabanac M. Epidemiology and aetiology of epilepsy in sub-Saharan Africa. *Lancet Neurol* 2005; 4:21–31.
79. Mac TL, Tran DS, Quet F, Odermatt P, Preux PM, Tan CT. Epidemiology, aetiology, and clinical management of epilepsy in Asia: a systematic review. *Lancet Neurol* 2007; 6:533–43.
80. Carpio A, Hauser WA. Epilepsy in the developing world. *Curr Neurol Neurosci Rep* 2009; 9:319–26.
81. Carpio A, Hauser WA, Lisanti N, Aguirre R, Roman M, Pesantez M, *et al.* Etiology of epilepsy in Ecuador. *Epilepsia* 2001; 42(Suppl 2):122.
82. Murthy JM, Yangala R. Etiological spectrum of symptomatic localization related epilepsies: a study from South India. *J Neurol Sci* 1998; 158:65–70.
83. Murthy JM, Prabhakar S. Bacterial meningitis and epilepsy. *Epilepsia* 2008; 49(Suppl 6):8–12.
84. Baraff LJ, Lee SI, Schriger DL. Outcomes of bacterial meningitis in children: a meta-analysis. *Pediatr Infect Dis* J 1993; 12:389–94.
85. Hjalmarsson A, Blomqvist P, Skoldenberg B. Herpes simplex encephalitis in Sweden, 1990–2001: incidence, morbidity, and mortality. *Clin Infect Dis* 2007; 45:875–80.
86. Whitley RJ, Soong SJ, Linneman C, Jr., Liu C, Pazin G, Alford CA. Herpes simplex encephalitis. *Clinical Assessment. JAMA* 1982; 247:317–20.
87. Skoldenberg B, Aurelius E, Hjalmarsson A, Sabri F, Forsgren M, Andersson B, *et al.* Incidence and pathogenesis of clinical relapse after herpes simplex encephalitis in adults. *J Neurol* 2006; 253:163–70.
88. Solbrig MV, Adrian R, Chang DY, Perng GC. Viral risk factor for seizures: pathobiology of dynorphin in herpes simplex viral (HSV-1) seizures in an animal model. *Neurobiol Dis* 2006; 23:612–20.
89. Murphy SC, Breman JG. Gaps in the childhood malaria burden in Africa: cerebral malaria, neurological sequelae, anemia, respiratory distress, hypoglycemia, and complications of pregnancy. *Am J Trop Med Hyg* 2001; 64:57–67.
90. Ngoungou EB, Preux PM. Cerebral malaria and epilepsy. *Epilepsia* 2008; 49(Suppl 6):19–24.
91. Nash TE, Del Brutto OH, Butman JA, Corona T, Delgado-Escueta A, Duron RM, *et al.* Calcific neurocysticercosis and epileptogenesis. *Neurology* 2004; 62:1934–8.
92. Garcia-Noval J, Moreno E, de Mata F, Soto de Alfaro H, Fletes C, Craig PS, *et al.* An epidemiological study of epilepsy and epileptic seizures in two rural Guatemalan communities. *Ann Trop Med Parasitol* 2001; 95:167–75.
93. Carpio A, Hauser, A.W. Prognosis of epilepsy in Ecuador: a preliminary report. *Epilepsia* 2001; 40:110.

94. Murthy JMK, Vijay, S., Ravi Raju, C., Thomas, J. Acute symptomatic seizures associated with neurocysticercosis: a community-based prevalence study and comprehensive rural epilepsy study in south India (CRESSI). *Neurology Asia* 2004; 9:86.
95. Rajshekhar V, Raghava MV, Prabhakaran V, Oommen A, Muliyil J. Active epilepsy as an index of burden of neurocysticercosis in Vellore district, India. *Neurology* 2006; 67:2135–9.
96. Murthy JM, Subba Reddy YV. Prognosis of epilepsy associated with single CT enhancing lesion: a long term follow up study. *J Neurol Sci* 1998; 159:151–5.
97. Cukiert A, Puglia P, Scapolan HB, Vilela MM, Marino Junior R. Congruence of the topography of intracranial calcifications and epileptic foci. *Arq Neuropsiquiatr* 1994; 52:289–94.
98. Singh G, Sachdev MS, Tirath A, Gupta AK, Avasthi G. Focal cortical-subcortical calcifications (FCSCs) and epilepsy in the Indian subcontinent. *Epilepsia* 2000; 41:718–26.
99. Nash TE, Pretell EJ, Lescano AG, Bustos JA, Gilman RH, Gonzalez AE, *et al.* Perilesional brain oedema and seizure activity in patients with calcified neurocysticercosis: a prospective cohort and nested case-control study. *Lancet Neurol* 2008; 7:1099–105.
100. Velasco TR, Zanello PA, Dalmagro CL, Araújo D Jr, Santos AC, Bianchin MM, *et al.* Calcified cysticercotic lesions and intractable epilepsy: a cross sectional study of 512 patients. *J Neurol, Neurosurger, Psychiatry* 2006; 77:485–8.
101. Pomeroy SL, Holmes SJ, Dodge PR, Feigin RD. Seizures and other neurologic sequelae of bacterial meningitis in children. *N Engl J Med* 1990; 323:1651–57.
102. Rosman NP, Peterson DB, Kaye EM, Colton T. Seizures in bacterial meningitis: prevalence, patterns, pathogenesis, and prognosis. *Pediatr Neurol* 1985; 1:278–85.
103. Donaire A, Carreno M, Agudo R, Delgado P, Bargalló N, Setoaín X, *et al.* Presurgical evaluation in refractory epilepsy secondary to meningitis or encephalitis: bilateral memory deficits often preclude surgery. *Epileptic Disord* 2007; 9:127–33.
104. Stephen LJ, Brodie MJ. Seizure freedom with more than one antiepileptic drug. *Seizure* 2002; 11:349–51.
105. Mohanraj R, Brodie MJ. Diagnosing refractory epilepsy: response to sequential treatment schedules. *Eur J Neurol* 2006; 13:277–82.
106. Britton JW. Antiepileptic drug withdrawal: literature review. *Mayo Clin Proc* 2002; 77:1378–88.
107. Lancman ME, Morris HH, 3rd. Epilepsy after central nervous system infection: clinical characteristics and outcome after epilepsy surgery. *Epilepsy Res* 1996; 25:285–90.
108. Lee JH, Lee BI, Park SC, Kim WJ, Kim JY, Park SA, *et al.* Experiences of epilepsy surgery in intractable seizures with past history of CNS infection. *Yonsei Med J* 1997; 38:73–8.
109. Marks DA, Kim J, Spencer DD, Spencer SS. Characteristics of intractable seizures following meningitis and encephalitis. *Neurology* 1992; 42:1513–18.
110. O'Brien TJ, Moses H, Cambier D, Cascino GD. Age of meningitis or encephalitis is independently predictive of outcome from anterior temporal lobectomy. *Neurology* 2002; 58:104–9.
111. Trinka E, Dubeau F, Andermann F, Hui A, Bastos A, Li LM, Köhler S, *et al.* Successful epilepsy surgery in catastrophic postencephalitic epilepsy. *Neurology* 2000; 54:2170–3.
112. Chandra PS, Bal C, Garg A, Gaikwad S, Prasad K, Sharma BS, *et al.* Surgery for medically intractable epilepsy due to postinfectious etiologies. *Epilepsia*; 51:1097–100.
113. Leite JP, Terra-Bustamante VC, Fernandes RM, Santos AC, Chimelli L, Sakamoto AC, *et al.* Calcified neurocysticercotic lesions and postsurgery seizure control in temporal lobe epilepsy. *Neurology* 2000; 55:1485–91.
114. Hauser WA, Annegers JF, Kurland LT. Incidence of epilepsy and unprovoked seizures in Rochester, Minnesota: 1935-1984. *Epilepsia* 1993; 34:453–68.
115. Herman ST. Epilepsy after brain insult: targeting epileptogenesis. *Neurology* 2002; 59:S21–6.
116. Olafsson E, Ludvigsson P, Gudmundsson G, Hesdorffer D, Kjartansson O, Hauser WA. Incidence of unprovoked seizures and epilepsy in Iceland and assessment of the epilepsy syndrome classification: a prospective study. *Lancet Neurol* 2005; 4:627–34.
117. Wen PY, Marks PW. Medical management of patients with brain tumors. *Curr Opin Oncol* 2002; 14:299–307.
118. Glantz MJ, Cole BF, Forsyth PA, Recht LD, Wen PY, Chamberlain MC, *et al.* Practice parameter: anticonvulsant prophylaxis in patients with newly diagnosed brain tumors. Report of the Quality Standards Subcommittee of the American Academy of Neurology. *Neurology* 2000; 54:1886–93.
119. Luyken C, Blumcke I, Fimmers R, Urbach H, Wiestler OD, Schramm J. Supratentorial gangliogliomas: histopathologic grading and tumor recurrence in 184 patients with a median follow-up of 8 years. *Cancer* 2004; 101:146–55.
120. Daumas-Duport C, Scheithauer BW, Chodkiewicz JP, Laws ER, Jr., Vedrenne C. Dysembryoplastic neuroepithelial tumor: a surgically curable tumor of young patients with intractable partial seizures. Report of thirty-nine cases. *Neurosurgery* 1988; 23:545–56.
121. Wolf HK, Birkholz T, Wellmer J, Blumcke I, Pietsch T, Wiestler OD. Neurochemical profile of glioneuronal lesions from patients with pharmacoresistant focal epilepsies. *J Neuropathol Exp Neurol* 1995; 54:689–97.
122. Wolf HK, Roos D, Blumcke I, Pietsch T, Wiestler OD. Perilesional neurochemical changes in focal epilepsies. *Acta Neuropathol* 1996; 91:376–84.
123. Schick V, Majores M, Koch A, Elger CE, Schramm J, Urbach H, *et al.* Alterations of phosphatidylinositol 3-kinase pathway components in epilepsy-associated glioneuronal lesions. *Epilepsia* 2007; 48(Suppl 5):65–73.
124. Liigant A, Haldre S, Oun A, Linnamägi U, Saar A, Asser T, *et al.* Seizure disorders in patients with brain tumors. *Eur Neurol* 2001; 45:46–51.
125. Lynam LM, Lyons MK, Drazkowski JF, Sirven JI, Noe KH, Zimmerman RS, *et al.* Frequency of seizures in patients with newly diagnosed brain tumors: a retrospective review. *Clin Neurol Neurosurg* 2007; 109:634–8.
126. Aronica E, Gorter JA, Jansen GH, Leenstra S, Yankaya B, Troost D. Expression of connexin 43 and connexin 32 gap-junction proteins in epilepsy-associated brain tumors and in the perilesional epileptic cortex. *Acta Neuropathol* 2001; 101:449–59.
127. Schwartzkroin PA, Baraban SC, Hochman DW. Osmolarity, ionic flux, and changes in brain excitability. *Epilepsy Res* 1998; 32:275–85.
128. Mody I, Heinemann U. NMDA receptors of dentate gyrus granule cells participate in synaptic transmission following kindling. *Nature* 1987; 326:701–4.
129. Palma E, Amici M, Sobrero F, Spinelli G, Di Angelantonio S, Ragozzino D, *et al.* Anomalous levels of Cl- transporters in the hippocampal subiculum from temporal lobe epilepsy patients make GABA excitatory. *Proc Natl Acad Sci U S A* 2006; 103:8465–8.
130. Morrell F. Secondary epileptogenesis in man. *Arch Neurol* 1985; 42:318–35.
131. Fried I, Kim JH, Spencer DD. Hippocampal pathology in patients with intractable seizures and temporal lobe masses. *J Neurosurg* 1992; 76:735–40.
132. Levesque MF, Nakasato N, Vinters HV, Babb TL. Surgical treatment of limbic epilepsy associated with extrahippocampal lesions: the problem of dual pathology. *J Neurosurg* 1991; 75:364–70.
133. van Breemen MS, Wilms EB, Vecht CJ. Epilepsy in patients with brain tumours: epidemiology, mechanisms, and management. *Lancet Neurol* 2007; 6:421–30.
134. Vecht CJ, Wagner GL, Wilms EB. Interactions between antiepileptic and chemotherapeutic drugs. *Lancet Neurol* 2003; 2:404–9.

135. Oberndorfer S, Piribauer M, Marosi C, Lahrmann H, Hitzenberger P, Grisold W. P450 enzyme inducing and non-enzyme inducing antiepileptics in glioblastoma patients treated with standard chemotherapy. *J Neurooncol* 2005; 72:255–60.
136. Wick W, Menn O, Meisner C, Steinbach J, Hermisson M, Tatagiba M, *et al.* Pharmacotherapy of epileptic seizures in glioma patients: who, when, why and how long? *Onkologie* 2005; 28:391–6.
137. Eyal S, Yagen B, Sobol E, Altschuler Y, Shmuel M, Bialer M. The activity of antiepileptic drugs as histone deacetylase inhibitors. *Epilepsia* 2004; 45:737–44.
138. Singh G, Driever PH, Sander JW. Cancer risk in people with epilepsy: the role of antiepileptic drugs. *Brain* 2005; 128:7–17.
139. Tang R, Faussat AM, Majdak P, Perrot JY, Chaoui D, Legrand O, *et al.* Valproic acid inhibits proliferation and induces apoptosis in acute myeloid leukemia cells expressing P-gp and MRP1. *Leukemia* 2004; 18:1246–51.
140. Hildebrand J, Lecaille C, Perennes J, Delattre JY. Epileptic seizures during follow-up of patients treated for primary brain tumors. *Neurology* 2005; 65:212–15.
141. Wagner GL, Wilms EB, Van Donselaar CA, Vecht Ch J. Levetiracetam: preliminary experience in patients with primary brain tumours. *Seizure* 2003; 12:585–6.
142. Maschio M, Albani F, Baruzzi A, Zarabla A, Dinapoli L, Pace A, *et al.* Levetiracetam therapy in patients with brain tumour and epilepsy. *J Neurooncol* 2006; 80:97–100.
143. Newton HB, Goldlust SA, Pearl D. Retrospective analysis of the efficacy and tolerability of levetiracetam in brain tumor patients. *J Neurooncol* 2006; 78:99–102.
144. van Breemen MS, Rijsman RM, Taphoorn MJ, Walchenbach R, Zwinkels H, Vecht CJ. Efficacy of anti-epileptic drugs in patients with gliomas and seizures. *J Neurol* 2009; 256:1519–26.
145. Newton HB, Dalton J, Goldlust S, Pearl D. Retrospective analysis of the efficacy and tolerability of levetiracetam in patients with metastatic brain tumors. *J Neurooncol* 2007; 84:293–6.
146. Maschio M, Dinapoli L, Sperati F, Pace A, Fabi A, Vidiri A, *et al.* Levetiracetam monotherapy in patients with brain tumor-related epilepsy: seizure control, safety, and quality of life. *J Neurooncol* 2011; 104:205–14.
147. Usery JB, Michael LM, 2nd, Sills AK, Finch CK. A prospective evaluation and literature review of levetiracetam use in patients with brain tumors and seizures. *J Neurooncol* 2010; 99:251–60.
148. Milligan TA, Hurwitz S, Bromfield EB. Efficacy and tolerability of levetiracetam versus phenytoin after supratentorial neurosurgery. *Neurology* 2008; 71:665–9.
149. Perry JR, Sawka C. Add-on gabapentin for refractory seizures in patients with brain tumours. *Can J Neurol Sci* 1996; 23:128–31.
150. Maschio M, Dinapoli L, Sperati F, Fabi A, Pace A, Vidiri A, *et al.* Oxcarbazepine monotherapy in patients with brain tumor-related epilepsy: open-label pilot study for assessing the efficacy, tolerability and impact on quality of life. *J Neurooncol* 2012; 106(3):651–6.
151. Sirven JI, Wingerchuk DM, Drazkowski JF, Lyons MK, Zimmerman RS. Seizure prophylaxis in patients with brain tumors: a meta-analysis. *Mayo Clin Proc* 2004; 79:1489–94.
152. Neef C, de Voogd-van der Straaten I. An interaction between cytostatic and anticonvulsant drugs. *Clin Pharmacol Ther* 1988; 43:372–5.
153. Calatozzolo C, Gelati M, Ciusani E, Sciacca FL, Pollo B, Cajola L, *et al.* Expression of drug resistance proteins Pgp, MRP1, MRP3, MRP5 and GST-pi in human glioma. *J Neurooncol* 2005; 74:113–21.
154. Khan RB, Onar A. Seizure recurrence and risk factors after antiepilepsy drug withdrawal in children with brain tumors. *Epilepsia* 2006;
47:375–9.
155. Frenay MP, Fontaine D, Vandenbos F, Lebrun C. First-line nitrosourea-based chemotherapy in symptomatic non-resectable supratentorial pure low-grade astrocytomas. *Eur J Neurol* 2005; 12:685–90.
156. Brada M, Viviers L, Abson C, Hines F, Britton J, Ashley S, *et al.* Phase II study of primary temozolomide chemotherapy in patients with WHO grade II gliomas. *Ann Oncol* 2003; 14:1715–21.
157. Panda S, Radhakrishnan VV, Radhakrishnan K, Rao RM, Sarma SP. Electro-clinical characteristics and postoperative outcome of medically refractory tumoral temporal lobe epilepsy. *Neurol India* 2005; 53:66–71; discussion 71-62.
158. Radhakrishnan A, Abraham M, Radhakrishnan VV, Sarma SP, Radhakrishnan K. Medically refractory epilepsy associated with temporal lobe ganglioglioma: characteristics and postoperative outcome. *Clin Neurol Neurosurg* 2006; 108:648–54.
159. Cascino GD. Epilepsy and brain tumors: implications for treatment. *Epilepsia* 1990; 31(Suppl 3):S37–44.
160. Awad IA, Rosenfeld J, Ahl J, Hahn JF, Luders H. Intractable epilepsy and structural lesions of the brain: mapping, resection strategies, and seizure outcome. *Epilepsia* 1991; 32:179–86.
161. Cascino GD, Jack CR, Jr., Parisi JE, Sharbrough FW, Schreiber CP, Kelly PJ, *et al.* Operative strategy in patients with MRI-identified dual pathology and temporal lobe epilepsy. *Epilepsy Res* 1993; 14:175–82.

CHAPTER 21

Epilepsy in Renal, Hepatic, and Other Conditions

Aidan Neligan

Aetiology is an important determinant of prognosis in epilepsy yet is largely ignored in the International League Against Epilepsy classifications of seizures (1) and epileptic syndromes (2). This is of particular relevance when discussing seizures occurring in the context of systemic diseases and where they should fit in such a classification. Seizures in systemic diseases are not an inconsiderable problem, especially in the critically ill. The currently used terms, acute and remote symptomatic seizures (as differentiated by the temporal relationship to the provoking factor), are confusing and probably too simplistic as most seizures occurring in systematic disease are likely to be multifactorial, even if one cause predominates. In a recently proposed aetiological classification of epilepsy (3), epilepsy is divided into four broad categories: idiopathic, symptomatic, provoked, or cryptogenic epilepsy. The term 'provoked seizures' seems more appropriate for seizures in the context of systematic disease which may occur as a direct consequence of the underlying condition, its predisposing factors, its treatment, or a combination of all three.

Estimating the true frequency of seizures in people with primarily non-neurological conditions is difficult as this has rarely been subject to systematic examination. Nevertheless it does seem that seizures are one of the more common neurological manifestations of systemic disease. In a prospective study of all admissions to a medical ITU over a 2-year period, 1850 people were identified, of whom 92 were admitted with a primary neurological condition. Of the remaining 1758 people, 217 (12.3%) developed neurological complications of which 61 (28%) were seizures (4).

Seizures arising as a consequence of systemic disease can be convulsive or non-convulsive, focal or generalized (either primary or secondary generalized), and particularly status epilepticus (convulsive and non-convulsive), the majority of which occurs in people with no prior history of epilepsy (5). A high index of suspicion for the possibility of subtle convulsive or non-convulsive status epilepticus as well as the possibility of non-epileptic seizures needs to be maintained in the critical care setting.

In this chapter, we will primarily deal with what are termed situation-related seizures and as such the seizures can be explained by the provoking circumstances. We shall not deal further with epileptic syndromes in which systemic disease features prominently such as the progressive myoclonus epilepsies, action-myoclonus renal syndrome or metabolic conditions such as glucose transporter type 1 (GLUT-1) deficiency syndrome in which seizures frequently occur.

Pathophysiology of seizures in systemic diseases

Any critically ill person can develop seizures if the provoking stimulus is severe enough to lower their seizure threshold sufficiently, much the same as people with epilepsy may experience an exacerbation in their seizure control in the context of concurrent illness. Nevertheless, the systemic insult required to provoke seizures is much greater in people without a prior history of epilepsy. Conditions in which seizures can occur, listed by system, are shown in Table 21.1.

Electrolyte imbalances such as sodium, glucose, calcium, magnesium, and, rarely, low levels of potassium, can affect neuronal excitability and are important precipitants of seizures in the critically ill. Seizures as a consequence of electrolyte disturbances typically occur in the context of encephalopathy, drowsiness, headache, stupor, and other neurological symptoms (6). Similarly, disturbances in the balance of neurotransmitters can predispose to seizures such as depletion of the inhibitory neurotransmitter gamma-aminobutyric acid or accumulation of excitatory amino acids such as glutamate and aspartate which occurs after hypoxic-ischaemic brain injury, leading to increased neuronal excitability and neuronal damage (7).

Table 21.1 Systematic conditions in which seizures are a feature

Renal disease	**Hepatic disease**
Uraemic encephalopathy	Hepatic encephalopathy
Haemodialysis associated seizures	Wilson's disease
Haemolytic uraemic syndrome	Liver transplants
Renal transplants	Porphyrias
Dialysis disequilibrium syndrome	**Respiratory conditions**
Endocrine conditions	Neurosarcoidosis
Hypothyroidism	**Rheumatological conditions**
Thyrotoxicosis	Systemic lupus erythematosus
GLUT-1 deficiency	Vasculitis
Hashimoto's encephalopathy (SREAT)	Cancer
Malignant hypertension/hypertensive encephalopathy	

It is also possible that some people who do not normally have seizures may have molecular genetic or mitochondrial DNA defects which predispose them to having seizures in the context of critical illness (7).

Seizures in renal disease

Seizures are one of the most common manifestations of neurological dysfunction in uraemic encephalopathy which can occur in either acute or untreated chronic renal failure, either as a direct consequence of the condition itself or as a complication of its treatment, or both.

Depending on the rapidity of the onset and degree of renal failure, people with uraemic encephalopathy present with headaches, irritability, fluctuating levels of consciousness, seizures (epilepsia partialis continua, convulsive and non-convulsive status epilepticus), coma and death (8). The precise pathophysiology of uraemic encephalopathy is poorly understood but an accumulation of metabolites, hormonal disturbance, imbalance in inhibitory and excitatory neurotransmitters and disturbance of the intermediary metabolism have all been postulated as potential contributing factors (8).

It has been estimated that one-third of people presenting with uraemic encephalopathy have seizures, sometimes as the initial symptom (9, 10). A significant cause of seizures is hypocalcaemia which be can be exacerbated by shifting towards alkalosis by bicarbonate treatment in people with metabolic acidosis (11).

Seizures also occur during haemodialysis, although the tendency to initiate dialysis early in uraemic patients has reduced the incidence of dialysis-associated seizures (DAS). In a retrospective review of 180 children and adolescents receiving dialysis over a 14-year period, 7.2% (13/180) experienced DAS, with a significantly increasing risk of DAS in people receiving haemodialysis (HD) only (9%, 7/78) compared with people receiving peritoneal dialysis (PD) only (0%, 0/79) (chi-squared = 5.5, 1 degree of freedom (df), P = 0.02). In the 101 people receiving HD (78 HD only, 23 HD and PD), the risk of DSA was significantly higher in those with a prior history of seizures (29%, 6/21) compared with those without a history of seizures (8%, 6/80) (chi-squared = 5.2, 1 df, P = 0.02). A prior history of seizures did not increase the risk of DAS in people having PD (12).

Seizures can also occur in people who develop chronic dialysis encephalopathy or dialysis dementia, a subacute progressive condition with personality changes, apraxia, seizures, myoclonus, and dementia (8). This was linked to the use of aluminium-containing dialysate and aluminium-based phosphate binders and is now a rare condition since the cessation of the use of aluminium (8, 9).

Seizures are also associated with the dialysis disequilibrium syndrome (DDS), which occurs during or immediately after dialysis with symptoms of muscle cramps, anorexia, nausea, and headache in mild cases and confusion, seizures, coma, and death in more severe cases (13). Risk factors include rapid dialysis (particularly if the serum urea is >60 mmol/L), severe metabolic acidosis, young or old age, central nervous system (CNS) disease, and previous seizures (13). Different theories explaining the pathogenesis of DDS exist in the literature which is due to the rapid removal of urea during HD. The 'reverse urea hypothesis' proposes that urea is more rapidly removed from plasma than the brain, thus creating an osmotic gradient leading to a net flow of water into the brain with resultant transient cerebral oedema (8, 13). Awareness of the condition and slow initial HD in people with high serum urea has decreased the incidence of DDS.

Seizures also occur in PD in the particular context of non-ketotic hyperosmolar coma as a result of glucose fast exchanges. Such seizures are best prevented by monitoring the dialysis glucose content (9).

The administration of erythropoietin (EPO) for the treatment of renal anaemia may result in a rapid rise in blood pressure with hypertension in 35% and a hypertensive encephalopathy, which can result in seizures, in about 5%. The reported incidence of seizures with EPO ranges from 2–17% with higher rates typically observed in the early years of treatment and with supratherapeutic doses. There is little evidence of an increased risk of seizures with EPO in people with normal blood pressures (8, 14–16).

In a phase III trial of the use of EPO for the treatment of anaemia in people, 5.4% of those receiving EPO had seizures (14). Similarly in a meta-analysis of randomized control trials of the use of EPO for the treatment of renal anaemia, the risk of seizures in EPO treatment versus non-EPO treatment groups was assessed. There was a higher risk of seizures in the non-EPO group (lower haemoglobin) (four trials, 219 patients; relative risk (RR) 5.25; 95% confidence interval (CI) 1.13, 24.3; p = 0.03) compared with the group treated with EPO (15).

People with chronic renal failure are at increased risk of cerebrovascular disease (both ischaemic and haemorrhagic strokes), which is a significant risk for the development of subsequent seizures particularly in the elderly. The risk of cerebrovascular disease for people with end-stage renal disease (ESRD) on dialysis is estimated to be 4–10 times higher than the general population in part due to accelerated atherosclerosis and anaemia in people with ESRD (17, 18).

Seizures are a relatively common occurrence after renal transplants (19, 20). In a series of 154 children who underwent 207 renal transplants for ESRD, 48 (31%) had convulsive seizures before, during, or after transplantation (17), although this is likely to be an underestimate of the true incidence as non-convulsive seizures are rarely recognized (10).

Sixty per cent of seizures were single seizures with few of the remaining children developing long-term seizures. The main aetiological factor was hypertension with seizures often heralding onset of hepatic encephalopathy. The majority of people with seizures did not a recurrence of seizures following control of hypertension (19). In a series of 119 renal transplants in 109 children over a 10-year period, 20 children (17.6%) (21 transplants) had seizures. Seizures occurred within 8 weeks of transplantation in 13 (62%) and within 6 months in 18 (85.7%) with seizures significantly more common in younger children (ages 5–10 years) (p = 0.03). Of the seizures in the 21 transplant patients, 13 (62%) were single seizures, nine children experienced multiple seizures, and one child had status epilepticus. Twenty-one children had a prior history of epilepsy (two were on antiepileptic drugs (AEDs) at the time of transplantation), five (23.8%) of whom had further seizures. Of the remaining 88 children, 15 (17.0%) developed seizures. The risk of seizures post transplant was not significantly different between the two groups (p = 0.69). The most commonly identified aetiology for the development of seizures was hypertension (15 (71.4%)) either alone or in combination with other factors (fever, graft rejection, cyclosporine A toxicity, hypomagnesaemia). Overall the long-term prognosis was very good with only five children requiring long-term

AED treatment (two of whom developed seizures as a consequence of significant intracranial pathology) (20).

Haemolytic uraemic syndrome (HUS), characterized by the clinical triad of micro-angiopathic haemolytic anaemia, thrombocytopenia, and acute renal injury, is one of the main causes of acute renal injury in young children. It is typically caused by a shiga-toxin-producing *Escherichia coli* (usually *E. coli* 0157) (90% of cases occur in children) with a typical prodrome of abdominal pain, diarrhoea, and vomiting immediately followed by the typical symptoms (21–24). Seizures are the most common neurological manifestation affecting up to 25% of children with HUS (21) and may be the presenting symptom in 15% (22). Most seizures are short, single, generalized seizures which are well controlled with AEDs (21, 22, 24). Children with CNS manifestations including seizures have a poorer prognosis with increased mortality and development of long-tem ESRD (23). Children with generalized seizures in association with HUS have a better prognosis than children with focal-onset seizures who are more likely to have structural lesions particularly stroke, have neurological sequelae and develop epilepsy (24).

The management of seizures in renal disease

Renal failure alters the pharmacokinetics of many AEDs necessitating changes in doses.

Proteinuria (albuminuria) and metabolic acidosis which occur in renal failure reduce serum albumin levels and its protein binding affinity, thus increasing the free active levels of AEDs. Small changes in serum albumin can lead to marked increases in the free fraction of AEDs. Similarly, reduced glomerular filtration and tubular secretion increase drug elimination half-lives (25, 26). The newer AEDs such as gabapentin, topiramate, levetiracetam, vigabatrin, and the older drug ethosuximide are highly water soluble, have a low volume of distribution, and have lower protein-binding affinity and therefore accumulate in renal disease. They are largely removed by HD and therefore postdialysis dose supplementation is required (25, 26). In contrast, HD has little impact on the dosages of the older highly lipophilic protein-bound AEDs like carbamazepine, phenytoin, benzodiazepines, and valproate. These AEDs are therefore preferable in patients with seizures and ESRD (26). The effect of PD on AEDs levels is unpredictable. The dose of phenytoin may need to be adjusted in people with severe hypoalbuminaemia (either due to renal or hepatic disease); free (biologically active) phenytoin levels can accumulate leading to toxicity and paradoxical seizures despite a low or low-therapeutic total phenytoin level (10–20 mg/L). Phenytoin should be monitored by therapeutic free phenytoin levels (maintaining levels between 1–2 mg/L) (26, 27). Gabapentin has been reported to cause multifocal myoclonus and altered mental states in people with ESRD without a history of epilepsy and should therefore be used cautiously in renal failure (28).

Seizures in hepatic disease

Fulminant liver failure can occur as a consequence of many different causes including viral or drug-induced hepatitis, alcohol-induced cirrhosis, sepsis, haemorrhage of oesophageal varices, hypoxia, hypovolaemia, and infections, including subacute bacterial peritonitis. People with hepatic encephalopathy typically present with psychiatric symptoms, such as euphoria, sleep disturbance and depression in the early stages (I–II), with neurological symptoms predominating in the latter stages (III–IV). Neurological symptoms include ataxia, somnolence, confusion, seizures (both generalized and non-convulsive), and coma (29). Seizures occurring in the context of hepatic encephalopathy are often refractory to standard AEDs but may respond to specific treatment for the hepatic dysfunction including correction of the ammonia levels with lactulose, phosphate enemas for constipation, and antibiotic therapy for concurrent infections (25, 29).

Based on the premise that subclinical seizures are common in patients with acute liver failure and therefore influences prognosis, a randomized controlled trial of prophylactic phenytoin in patients with acute liver failure was performed. Twenty people were randomized to receive phenytoin and 22 to placebo control. There was no difference between the two groups in the number developing cerebral oedema (12 (60%) in the phenytoin group versus 10 (45%), $p = 0.35$), the number requiring mechanical ventilation (10 (50%) versus 12 (55%), $p = 0.77$), the number developing seizures (all generalized: 5 (25%) versus 5 (22.7%), $p = 0.86$) or mortality (14 (70%) versus 15 (68.2%), $p = 0.89$). Overall there was no evidence for the benefit of prophylactic AEDs in people with acute liver failure (30).

Wilson disease

Seizures are reputedly rare in Wilson disease (WD) with isolated reports of seizures and status epilepticus occurring with treatment with D-penicillamine (which can cause pyridoxine deficiency with resultant seizures). When seizures occur in such a context, treatment with copper chelators such as trientine, or replacement with pyridoxine, is recommended (25).

Two large cohort studies of patients with WD followed over 30 years, suggest that the prevalence of epilepsy is significantly higher than that of the general population.

In a case series from Cambridge, UK of 200 cases the prevalence of epilepsy was 6.2% (10/161 cases surviving) (estimated incidence 430 per 100,000/year) while in a review of the literature, 47/856 (5.5%) of people with WD had seizures (31). Prior to the availability of treatment with D-penicillamine in 1955, seizures typically occurred late in the course of the condition and were a prelude of death, with a median survival of 1 year following onset of seizures. Thirteen of 200 people (6.5%) with WD had epilepsy of whom five had focal-onset seizures and eight had generalized seizures. Two people had at least one episode of generalized convulsive status epilepticus. In almost half of cases, seizures started before the start of copper chelating therapy, with the majority of seizures felt not to be related to D-penicillamine. Seven had no further seizures following commencement of AED treatment with 75% seizure free for 2 years or more at last follow-up (32).

In a cohort of 490 patients with WD seen in a tertiary centre in India, 41(8.3%) had seizures. The predominant seizure types were simple partial (8), complex partial (6), secondary generalized (2), generalized tonic–clonic (29), and periodic myoclonus (1). The onset of seizures varied with seizures (along with other symptoms of WD) noted before diagnosis in 19 (46.3%) and were part of a terminal event in two. Overall, seizures occurred before other symptoms of WD in seven (17.1%), concomitant with other symptoms in 17 (41.5%), and during treatment in 14 (34.1%). Overall seizure prognosis was good with complete seizure control obtained in 28 (68.3%), intermittent breakthrough seizures in seven (17.1%), and poor seizure control in four (9.7%) (two patients were lost to follow-up). All were treated with D-penicillamine and AEDs with no therapeutic or demographic factors predictive of seizure prognosis (31).

Overall it appears that the prevalence of epilepsy in people with WD is not as rare as previously claimed with the vast majority of seizures not occurring as a result of D-penicillamine induced pyridoxine deficiency. The prognosis of seizures often mirrors that of the underlying condition with worsening seizure control heralding the terminal stage of WD. Successful treatment of seizures in WD requires treatment with AEDs and chelating agents.

Liver transplantation

Neurological complications are common after liver transplantation with seizures being the second most common neurological complication after encephalopathy. In a retrospective study of all liver transplantations carried out at a single specialist centre over a 12-year period, 630 people who underwent liver transplantation were identified. Of these 28 (4%) developed seizures all of which were generalized (four secondary generalized) with the majority occurring in the perioperative period. None had a previous history of epilepsy and there were no episodes of status epilepticus. The principal aetiologies of seizures were CNS neurotoxicity with immunosuppression agents in 17 (FK506 (6), cyclosporine (11)), CNS infections (listeria, aspergillus, nocardia) in three, and catastrophic CNS insults (intracranial haemorrhage, cerebral oedema with fulminant liver failure and hypovolaemic shock with postanoxic ischaemic encephalopathy) in three. Seizure onset was a terminal event in seven. All were treated with intravenous phenytoin with seizures recurring in five. Phenytoin was successfully discontinued in all patients who survived, by 3 months with no seizure recurrence noted after a median follow-up of 2 years (33).

In a series of 427 consecutive liver transplantations in 391 patients, seizures occurred in 12 (3.1%) and all neurological complications were more common in adults (nine adults (3.3%), three children (0.03%)). The causes of seizures were cyclosporine toxicity in four, primary graft non-function in three, cerebrovascular accidents (two), CNS infection (one), fever (one) and unknown (one). Three people with seizures post transplant died (34).

Overall the prognosis of people with seizures after liver transplantation, in which the seizures do not represent part of an agonal process, is excellent with little evidence of a long-term propensity for further seizures. The most common causes of seizures are CNS neurotoxicity (cyclosporine, FK506) and CNS infections.

Management of seizures in hepatic disease

AED metabolism is affected by hepatic dysfunction. As with renal disease, hepatic disease results in hypoalbuminaemia increasing the levels of free unbound AEDs (diazepam, phenytoin, and valproate). AEDs with sedating side effects such as the benzodiazepines and phenobarbital may precipitate or worsen pre-existing hepatic encephalopathy. Many of the AEDs (such as phenytoin, carbamazepine, and phenobarbital) are potent hepatic CYP450 enzyme inducers, which increase the metabolic rate. Valproate should be used with extreme caution in people with hepatic disease as it can cause idiosyncratic hepatotoxicity. Lamotrigine is extensively metabolized by the liver with the potential for toxicity in people with hepatic disease (25).

Newer AEDs with low protein-bound profiles which are not metabolized by the liver should be used for the treatment of seizures in hepatic disease. Preferred AEDs include levetiracetam, zonisamide, gabapentin, vigabatrin, and tiagabine which have no effect on the CYP450 isoenzymes (35).

Management of people with hepatic porphyria-induced generalized seizures is difficult as many AEDs are hepatic enzyme P-450 system inducers increasing haeme and porphyrin synthesis with worsening seizures (phenobarbital, phenytoin, carbamazepine, valproate, clonazepam, lamotrigine). Treatment with non-enzyme-inducing AEDs such as levetiracetam or gabapentin is recommended. Oxcarbazepine, which has a low level of hepatic enzyme induction, has also been shown to be effective in the management of seizures with hepatic porphyria (36).

Seizures in other conditions

In this section we will briefly discuss other conditions in which seizures feature prominently. A list of conditions categorized by system in which seizures can occur is shown in Table 21.2.

Systemic lupus erythematosus (SLE)

Neurological symptoms are common in SLE, occurring in 10–80% of people and form part of the diagnostic criteria for SLE. Seizures, which can be partial or more usually generalized, are a common feature occurring in 10–20% of people with SLE, the majority of which are single seizures (37, 38).

Seizures can be the first manifestation of the condition and usually occur early in the course of the condition with younger age and more severe disease activity at onset (39). Factors found to confer an increased risk of seizures include previous history of stroke, male gender, the presence of immunoglobulin G (IgG) antiphospholipid antibodies, anti-cardiolipin IgG antibodies, anti-Smith antibodies, a history of psychosis, and abnormal neuroimaging (37–39). In contrast the presence of anti-La autoantibodies is associated with a lower risk of developing seizures (and lupus nephritis) (40). Other factors reported to be associated with a lower risk

Table 21.2 Potential causes of seizures in systemic disease

Electrolyte disturbances	**Metabolic disturbances**
Hypoglycaemia	Hyperammonaemia
Hyperglycaemia	Pyridoxine/folate/thiamine deficiency
Hypocalcaemia	
Hypercalcaemia (rare)	**Immunosuppressive therapy**
Hypermagnesaemia	Opportunistic Infections
Hyponatraemia	Graft rejection
Hypernatraemia	**Miscellaneous**
Hypokalaemia (very rare)	Fever
Organ failure	Infections
Ischaemia, hypnoxia	Alcohol
Hypertensive encephalopathy	Sleep deprivation
Postoperative	
Anaesthetic related	
Medication related	

of seizures are mucocutaneous involvement, photosensitivity, and hydroxychloroquine use (39, 40).

Posterior reversible encephalopathy syndrome

Posterior reversible encephalopathy syndrome (PRES) or hyperperfusion encephalopathy is a clinical radiological syndrome of heterogeneous aetiologies which typically presents with headache, altered mental functioning, visual disturbances, and seizures (41). The exact pathophysiology of the condition remains uncertain but appears to be related to loss of cerebral autoregulation of blood pressure and endothelial dysfunction (41). Conditions which may give rise to PRES include eclampsia, hypertensive encephalopathy (16), renal disease, immunosuppressive, immunomodulatory and chemotherapy medications (e.g. cyclosporine A, intravenous immunoglobulins, tacrolimus) and vasculitis among others. Seizures are a prominent feature of the condition (87% in one large series (42)) and may be the presenting symptom (41). Seizures are usually generalized tonic–clonic seizures (either primary or secondary generalized), often with involvement of the occipital lobes and visual hallucinations. Some people can present with status epilepticus as the initial manifestation of PRES (43). Management involves the rapid lowering of the blood pressure with the use of parental antihypertensive agents like labetalol and sodium nitroprusside and dose reduction or withdrawal of the suspected precipitating drug. Seizures are typically managed with IV phenytoin (except in the case of suspected eclampsia). Overall PRES has a good short-term prognosis with rapid resolution in the majority (with slower radiological resolution). Similarly long-term seizure prognosis is favourable with only 2/25 having a recurrence after a mean follow-up of 2250 days (44).

Autoimmune encephalitis

Seizures are a common feature of the newly described CNS autoimmune diseases presenting with limbic or more diffuse encephalitis or encephalopathy (45). Seizures occur in almost all cases of limbic encephalitis and three-quarters of cases of anti-NMDA receptor encephalitis (45, 46). Voltage-gated potassium channel (VGKC)-complex/Lgi1 antibodies can present with a distinctive seizure semiology typically involving the face and ipsilateral arm (faciobrachial dystonic seizures). These seizures may occur prior to the onset of the typical limbic encephalitis (47). In a study of the causes of encephalitis in 203 patients in England, seizures were much more common with antibody associated causes compared to other causes of encephalitis ((14/16 (88%); 95% CI 62–98) versus (24/38 (63%); 95% CI 46–78, p <0.001) for herpes simplex virus encephalitis) (48).

Seizures are often refractory to standard antiepileptic medication and often progress to status epilepticus. Effective management of the seizures involves immunotherapy (corticosteroids, intravenous immunoglobulin, or plasma exchange), tumour removal (in cases of confirmed paraneoplastic immune mediated encephalitis), and antiepileptic medication. Overall more than three-quarters of people with anti-NMDAR encephalitis will respond to treatment although many are left with significant cognitive dysfunction and a long-term potential for seizures persists (45, 46).

In summary, seizures can occur in the context of many systemic conditions particularly renal and hepatic dysfunction. In the majority of cases, seizures are single seizures (less than half having a recurrence) or a short-lived period of recurrent seizures, which occur in the context of a clear precipitant (e.g. infection, fever). AED dosages may need to be adjusted in renal and hepatic dysfunction. The long-term prognosis is excellent with few (<10%) developing persistent seizures.

References

1. Commission on Classification and Terminology of the International League Against Epilepsy. Proposal for revised clinical and electrographic classification of epileptic seizures. *Epilepsia* 1981; **22**(4):489–501.
2. Commission on Classification and Terminology of the International League Against Epilepsy. Proposal for revised classification of epilepsies and epileptic syndromes. *Epilepsia* 1989; **30**(4):389–99.
3. Shorvon SD. The etiologic classification of epilepsy. *Epilepsia* 2011; **52**(6):1052–7.
4. Bleck TP, Smith MC, Pierre-Louis SJ, Jares JJ, Murray J, Hansen CA. Neurologic complications of critical medical illnesses. *Crit Care Med* 1993; **21**(1):98–103.
5. Neligan A, Shorvon SD. Frequency and prognosis of status epilepticus of different causes: a systematic review. *Arch Neurol* 2010; **67**(8):931–40.
6. Menon B, Shorvon SD. Electrolyte and sugar disturbances. In: Shorvon SD, Andermann F, Guerrini R (eds) *The Causes of Epilepsy*, pp. 655–63. Cambridge: Cambridge University Press, 2011.
7. Delanty N, Vaughan CJ, French JA. Medical causes of seizures. *Lancet* 1998; **352**(9125):383–90.
8. Brouns R, De Deyn PP. Neurological complications in renal review: a review. *Clin Neurol Neurosurg* 2004; **107**(1):1–16.
9. Palmer CA. Neurologic manifestations of renal disease. *Neurol Clin* 2002; **20**(1):23–34.
10. Danlami ZT, Obeid T, Awada A, Huraib S, Iqbal A. Absence status; an overlooked cause of acute confusion in haemodialysis patients. *J Nephrol* 1998; **11**(3):146–7.
11. Canavese C, Morellini V, Lazzarich E, Brustia M, Quaglia M, Stratta P. Seizures and renal failure: is there a link? *Nephrol Dial Transplant* 2005; **20**(12):2855–7.
12. Glenn CM, Astley SJ, Watkins SL. Dialysis-associated seizures in children and adolescents. *Pediatr Nephrol* 1992; **6**(2):182–6.
13. Arieff AI. Dialysis disequilibrium syndrome: Current concepts on pathogenesis and prevention. *Kidney Int* 1944; **45**(3):629–45.
14. Eschbach JW, Abdulhadi MH, Browne JK, Delano BG, Downing MR, Egrie JC, *et al.* Recombinant human erythropoietin in anemic patients with end-stage renal disease. *Ann Intern Med* 1989; **111**(12):992–1000.
15. Strippoli GFM, Craig JC, Manno C, Schena FP. Hemoglobin targets for the anemia of chronic kidney disease: A meta-analysis of randomised, controlled trials. *J Am Soc Nephrol* 2004; **15**(12):3154–65.
16. Delanty N, Vaughan C, Frucht S, Stubgen P. Erythropoietin-associated hypertensive posterior leukoencephalopathy. *Neurology* 1997; **49**(3):686–9.
17. Seliger SL, Gillen DL, Longstreth WT, Kestenbaum B, Stehman-Breen CO. Elevated risk of stroke among patients with end-stage renal disease. *Kidney Int* 2003; **64**(2):603–9.
18. Abramson JL, Jurkovitz CT, Vaccarino V, Weinstraub WS, McClellan W. Chronic kidney disease, anaemia, and incident stroke in a middle-aged, community-based population: The ARIC Study. *Kidney Int* 2003; **64**(2):610–5.
19. McEnery PT, Nathan J, Bates SR, Daniels SR. Convulsions in children undergoing transplantation. *J Pediatr* 1989; **115**(4):532–6.
20. Awan AQ, Lewis MA, Postlethwaite RJ, Webb NA. Seizures following renal transplantation in childhood. *Pediatr Nephrol* 1999; **13**(4):275–7.
21. Gerber A, Karch H, Allerberger F, Verweyen HM, Zimmerhackl LB. Clinical course and role of shiga toxin-producing Escherichia coli infection in the haemolytic-uraemic syndrome in paediatric patients,

1997-2000, in Germany and Austria: a prospective study. *J Infect Dis* 2002; **186**(4):493–500.

22. Bale JF Jr, Brasher C, Siegler RL. CNS manifestations of the haemolytic-uraemic syndrome. Relationship to metabolic alterations and prognosis. *Am J Dis Child* 1980; **134**(9):869–72.
23. Garg AX, Suri RS, Barrowman N, Rehman F, Matsell D, Rosas-Arellano MP, *et al.* Long-term renal prognosis of diarrhoea-associated haemolytic uraemic syndrome: A systematic review, meta-analysis, and meta-regression. *JAMA* 2003; **290**(10):1360–70.
24. Dhuna A, Pascual-Leone A, Talwar D, Torres F. EEG and seizures in children with haemolytic–uraemic syndrome. *Epilepsia* 1992; **33**(3):482–6.
25. Lacerda G, Krummel T, Sabourdy C, Ryvlin P, Hirsch E. Optimising therapy of seizures in patients with renal or hepatic dysfunction. *Neurology* 2006; **67**(12, Suppl 4):S28–33.
26. Israni RK, Kasbekar N, Haynes K, Berns JS. Use of antiepileptic drugs in patients with kidney disease. *Semin Dial* 2006; **19**(5):408–16.
27. De Schoenmakere G, De Waele J, Terryn W, Deweweire M, Verstraete A, Hoste E, *et al.* Phenytoin intoxication in critically ill patients. *Am J Kid Dis* 2005; **45**(1):189–92.
28. Zhang C, Glenn DG, Bell WL, O'Donovan CA. Gabapentin-induced myoclonus in end-stage renal disease. *Epilepsia* 2005; **46**(1):156–8.
29. Eleftheriadis N, Fourla E, Eleftheriadis D, Karlovasitou A. Status epilepticus as a manifestation of hepatic encephalopathy. *Acta Neurol Scand* 2003; **107**(2):142–4.
30. Bhatia V, Batra Y, Acharya SK. Prophylactic phenytoin does not improve cerebral oedema or survival in acute liver failure—a controlled clinical trail. *J Hepatol* 2004; **41**(1):89–96.
31. Dening TR, Berrios GE, Walshe M. Wilson's disease and epilepsy. *Brain* 1988; **111**(5):1139–55.
32. Prashanth LK, Sinha S, Tally AB, Mahadevan A, Shankar SK. Spectrum of epilepsy in Wilson's disease with electroencephalographic, MR imaging and pathological correlates. *J Neurol Sci* 2010; **291**(1–2):44–51.
33. Wijdicks EFM, Plevak DJ, Wiesner RH, Steers JL. Causes and outcome of seizures in liver transplant recipients. *Neurology* 1996; **47**(6):1523–5.
34. Menegaux F, Keeffe EB, Andrews BT, Egawa H, Monge H, Concepcion W, *et al.* Neurological complications of liver transplantation in adult versus paediatric patients. *Transplantation* 1994; **58**(4):447–50.
35. Anderson GD. Pharmacogenetics and enzyme induction/inhibition properties of antiepileptic drugs. *Neurology* 2004; **63**(10, Suppl 4):S3–8.
36. Gaida-Hommernick B, Rieck K, Runge U. Oxcarbazepine in focal epilepsy and hepatic porphyria: A case report. *Epilepsia* 2001; **42**(6):793–5.
37. Mikdashi J, Krumholz A, Handwerger H. Factors at diagnosis predict subsequent occurrence of seizures in systemic lupus erythematosus. *Neurology* 2005; **64**(12):2102–7.
38. Appenzeller S, Cendes F, Costallat LTL. Epileptic seizures in systemic lupus erythematosus. *Neurology* 2004; **63**(10):1808–12.
39. Andrade RM, Alarcón GS, González LA, Fernández M, Apte M, Vilá LM, *et al.* Seizures in patients with systemic lupus erythematosus: data from LUMINA, a multiethnic cohort (LUMINA LIV). *Ann Rheum Dis* 2008; **67**(6):829–34.
40. Malik S, Bruner GR, Williams-Weese C, Feo L, Scofield RH, Reichlin M, *et al.* Presence of anti-La autoantibody is associated with a lower risk of nephritis and seizures in lupus patients. *Lupus* 2007; **16**(11):863–6.
41. Hinchey J, Chaves C, Appignani B, Breen J, Pao L, Wang A, *et al.* A reversible posterior leukoencephalopathy syndrome. *New Eng J Med* 1996; **334**(8):494–500.
42. Lee VH, Wijdicks EF, Manno EM, Rabinstein AA. Clinical spectrum of reversible posterior leukoencephalopathy syndrome. *Arch Neurol* 2007; **65**(2):205–10.
43. Kozak OS, Wijdicks EF, Manno EM, Miley JT, Rabinstein AA. Status epilepticus as initial manifestation of posterior reversible encephalopathy syndrome. *Neurology* 2007; **69**(9):894–7.
44. Roth C, Ferbert A. Posterior reversible encephalopathy syndrome: long-term follow-up. *J Neurol Neurosurg Psychiatry* 2010; **81**(7):773–7.
45. Lunn MPT. Inflammatory and immunological diseases of the nervous system. In: Shorvon SD, Andermann F, Guerrini R (eds) *The Causes of Epilepsy*, pp.585–92. Cambridge: Cambridge University Press, 2011
46. Dalmau J, Lancaster E, Martinez-Hernandez E, Rosenfeld MR, Balice-Gordon R. Clinical experience and laboratory investigations in patients with anti-NMDAR encephalitis. *Lancet Neurol* 2011; **10**(1):63–74.
47. Irani SR, Mitchell A, Lang B, Pettingill P, Waters P, Johnson MR, *et al.* Faciobrachial dystonic seizures precede Lgi1 antibody limbic encephalitis. *Ann Neurol* 2011; **69**(5):892–900.
48. Granerod J, Ambrose HE, Davies NW, Clewley JP, Walsh AL, Morgan D, *et al.* Causes of encephalitis and differences in their clinical presentations in England: a multicentre, population-based prospective study. *Lancet Infect Dis* 2010; **10**(12), 835–44.

CHAPTER 22

Management of Patients with First Seizure and Early Epilepsy

Zachary Grinspan and Shlomo Shinnar

Introduction

Clinical and epidemiological research over the past 30 years has established a rational approach to the evaluation and treatment for an individual presenting with seizures. For patients with single seizures and early epilepsy (excluding epileptic encephalopathy), antiepileptic drug (AED) therapy reduces seizure recurrence risk, but it does not alter the underlying disease process, overturning Gower's idea that in epilepsy 'the tendency of the disease is to self-perpetuation' (1), i.e. seizures beget seizures. In most cases, treatment with AEDs can be safely deferred after a single unprovoked seizure. For patients with early epilepsy (i.e. those with two or more unprovoked seizures), treatment is usually indicated, given the morbidity of recurrent seizures. This chapter will review the rationale for withholding treatment in children and adults with a single unprovoked seizure as well as the approach to treating an individual with early epilepsy. Treatment of epileptic encephalopathy (which requires aggressive management from onset) and medically refractory epilepsy are covered elsewhere in this volume.

Single seizure

Overview and natural history

Patients with a single unprovoked seizure make up one-third to one-half of initial office visits for seizure (2). They form a distinct group with a lower risk of recurrence than those who initially present with multiple seizures, i.e. with new onset epilepsy. The definition of one seizure in this case includes a single seizure or a flurry of seizures in 24 hours in patients older than 1 month without prior unprovoked seizures (3, 4).

Review of the natural history after one unprovoked seizure guides both evaluation and treatment (5–19). Carefully excluding patients with prior seizures from studies before 1991 (5) and integrating recent studies (7, 13, 17) suggest a recurrence risk of 27–54%. If seizures recur, most recur early, with approximately 50% within 6 months of the initial seizure, and 80% within 2 years of the initial seizure (5, 13, 14). Later recurrences are unusual, but may occur up to 10 years after the initial event (14, 16).

Risk factors for recurrence

Only three factors consistently predict increased risk for seizure recurrence after a single unprovoked seizure: remote symptomatic aetiology, abnormal electroencephalogram (EEG), and seizure while asleep. The data are less consistent on the effect of other factors, such as age of onset, number of seizures in 24 hours, duration of seizure, type of seizure, family history, and prior history of febrile seizures. These should not be considered to confer additional risk (16, 20, 21).

The aetiology of unprovoked seizures is classified as remote symptomatic (i.e. due to an underlying structural or metabolic abnormality), idiopathic (i.e. probably genetic), or cryptogenic (i.e. unknown cause) (22, 23). Unsurprisingly, most studies find patients with a remote symptomatic aetiology have increased risk for recurrence. A meta-analysis of studies prior to 1991 found a relative risk of 1.8 (95% confidence interval (CI) 1.5–2.1) suggesting a 57% recurrence risk for patients with a remote symptomatic aetiology and 32% for those without (5). Except for the FIR.S.T. (First Seizure Trial Group) trial (7), subsequent multivariable analyses have repeatedly confirmed the increased risk in this group (13, 14, 17, 24).

Most studies report that an abnormal EEG predicts increased risk for recurrence (5, 8, 9, 11, 14, 24). The effect is uniformly found in children and is more pronounced in patients with idiopathic or cryptogenic aetiology (5, 11, 12, 14–17, 21). Epileptiform abnormalities are probably more important than slow wave abnormalities (8, 17, 19, 25), but any EEG abnormality predicts increased risk (5, 14, 21, 24).

Studies investigating sleep state find that individuals who have a first seizure while asleep are more likely to have recurrences (12, 14). This finding appears independent of the association of certain epilepsy syndromes with seizures in sleep. For example, even children with centrotemporal spikes meeting criteria for benign rolandic epilepsy (26) have a higher risk of recurrence if their first seizure occurred in sleep (14). However, seizures that occur during sleep tend to recur in sleep (14) and are thus less likely to cause injury.

Risks and benefits of treatment

The decision to treat after a single seizure rests on weighing the risk of further seizures, estimated by the epidemiological and trial data, against the risks of treatment, and typically favours watchful waiting as an initial strategy (Table 22.1).

Starting treatment after a first seizure reduces the risk of recurrence, as demonstrated in several trials comparing treatment with

Table 22.1 Balancing the risks of antiepileptic therapy versus seizures

Risk of antiepileptic drug therapy	Risk of seizures
Toxicity/injury	
Dose-related toxicity (i.e. ataxia)	Falls
Chronic toxicity (i.e. osteoporosis)	Burns (bathing or cooking)
Idiosyncratic toxicity (i.e. drug rash)	Drowning
Teratogenicity	Driving accidents
Reduced fertility	Fractures (especially in the elderly)
	SUDEP
Higher cortical functioning	
Cognitive impairment	Postictal confusion
Behavioural dyscontrol (including aggression)	Postictal aggression/psychosis
Suicidality (especially with premorbid depression)	
Psychosocial	
Need for daily medication	Fear of more seizures
Stigma of chronic illness	Stigma of seizures
	Restrictions on school/social activities
	Loss of driving privileges
	Difficulty providing childcare
Economic/time	
Cost of medications	Time lost from seizure and recovery
Cost/time of medical testing	Discrimination in employment
Cost/time of physician visits	

Adapted from Shinnar and O'Dell, 2008 (59).

watchful waiting (6, 7, 13, 27). In the most recent and largest study from the UK, the MESS trial (Multicenter Trial for Early Epilepsy and Single Seizures), immediate treatment reduced seizure recurrence from 26% to 18% at 6 months and from 39% to 32% at 2 years (13). An older Italian study, the FIR.S.T. trial, focused only on generalized tonic–clonic seizures and reported a 50% reduction of recurrence risk associated with treatment (7). Of critical importance, early treatment did not change long-term outcome (i.e. remission rate) in either of these studies (13, 28).

Starting AED therapy entails several potential risks, primarily from medication side effects. Like all medications, AEDs have dose related, idiosyncratic, and chronic side effects. The chronic toxicities are particularly important to consider given the tendency for patients to stay on AEDs for several years. Many AEDs have adverse cognitive and behavioural side effects, which may affect school performance, speech fluency, and memory (29–31). Women of childbearing age face issues of teratogenicity and negative reproductive and endocrine consequences from AED therapy. Long-term use of AEDs may decrease bone density, particularly in women and in the elderly (32–36). Patients with comorbid depression may be at increased risk of self-harm and suicidal behaviour, in particular with some of the newer AEDs (37, 38).

In the MESS trial, more patients complained of at least one adverse effect in the immediate treatment group than the delayed treatment group (39% versus 31%). Furthermore, at 5 years, 60% in the immediate treatment group were still taking AEDs versus 41% in delayed group, suggesting patients who begin treatment early are more likely to remain on treatment, and are therefore at greater risk for chronic medication toxicities (13).

The economic impact of AED therapy should also be considered, including both the cost of the medication and time lost to doctor's visits and diagnostic testing.

Finally, there is the hidden side effect of being labelled. People who had a single seizure but do not take medication are considered healthy by themselves and society, whereas those taking a daily medication are considered to have a chronic disease, even if they have not had a seizure for many years. This concern is particularly important in children and adolescents, as the perception of chronic illness may negatively affect psychosocial development (39, 40).

Risks and benefits of deferring treatment

The major risk of deferring medication after a first seizure or in early epilepsy is seizure recurrence. However, for patients with a single seizure, several observations temper the potential harm from a second seizure.

Of key importance, delaying treatment after a first seizure does not lead to chronic epilepsy (13, 18, 28, 29, 41–46). In the MESS trial, for example, among the patients who presented with a single seizure, the percent seizure free between years 1–3 was not statistically different between the immediate and deferred treatment groups (74% vs. 71%), and the percentage seizure free for 2 years by year 5 was identical at 92% (13). In other words, delayed treatment did not affect remission. Additional evidence comes from the developing world, where limited availability of medications and poor access to care leads to treatment delays. Patients who receive medication after prolonged untreated epilepsy have the same response rates as patients treated shortly after the seizures begin (44, 45).

There is no convincing evidence that brief seizures cause brain damage (29, 43, 47, 48). While there is substantial risk of injury in patients having many seizures, the risk from a single seizure is low (49, 50). Interestingly, scalds and injuries were more common in the early treatment group of the MESS trial than in the deferred treatment group (13). In the elderly, increased risk for fractures with seizures should be considered in treatment decisions (51).

Although 10–12% of initial seizures present as status epilepticus (4, 14, 52) (defined as seizures lasting longer than 30 minutes, or recurrent seizures over more than 30 minutes without return to neurological baseline between seizures), these patients do not have a higher risk of recurrence (53). However, should their seizures recur, these individuals are at increased risk for a prolonged seizure (53). Therefore, while the authors recommend abortive therapy rather than chronic AED therapy in most cases, it is legitimate to consider that these patients require a somewhat different risk:benefit assessment (29).

The risk of status epilepticus is often cited as a reason to treat individuals with a single seizure. However, for patients whose first seizure was self-limited, the risk of status epilepticus is low. For example, in a prospective study of 407 children with a first unprovoked seizure, a subgroup of 137 children had a brief initial seizure and then recurred. Of these 137 second seizures, only 2 were status epilepticus

(29). Similarly, in the MESS trial, only 2 of the 721 patients in the deferred treatment group experienced an episode of status epilepticus after enrolment (13). Furthermore, the morbidity of status epilepticus is largely a function of aetiology, and is usually low in patients with only a single unprovoked seizure (47, 54–56).

The effect of treatment on quality of life is mixed. In adults, loss of driving privileges is the most salient disadvantage of deferred treatment (57). In the MESS trial, more patients in the delayed treatment group did not hold a driver's licence because of seizures (17% vs. 10%) (58). However, other quality of life indicators, including general health, anxiety, depression, social restriction, feeling stigmatized, and paid work were not statistically different between the two groups (58).

For children and adolescents, we generally do not treat individuals with a single unprovoked seizure, even for patients with remote symptomatic aetiology and an abnormal routine EEG. For some patients with a single seizure presenting as status epilepticus, an acceptable strategy is to provide an abortive medication, such as rectal diazepam, and defer daily AED therapy. In all cases, the risks and benefits of early treatment versus deferred treatment must be considered and tailored to the specific patient. In select patients the risk benefit assessment may favour treatment after even a single seizure, e.g. to reduce the risk of fractures in the elderly.

Second seizure

After a second unprovoked seizure, the balance of risks and benefits shifts towards treatment. In both adults and children, the recurrence risk jumps to approximately 70% (10, 13, 16). Remote symptomatic aetiology confers additional risk after two seizures and is also associated with an increased risk of developing intractable epilepsy (16). Interestingly, after two unprovoked seizures, abnormal EEG and sleep state no longer affect the rate of recurrence (16).

Although most patients should be treated after two unprovoked seizures, at least two potential exceptions deserve mention.

It is common to defer treatment in school-aged children with idiopathic epilepsy syndromes who have infrequent and brief seizures, especially if at night (e.g. benign rolandic epilepsy). The morbidity of AED treatment in this group may outweigh the benefits. Furthermore, the recurrence risk is often age dependent and fades in adolescence (42, 48, 59). Although these children may have significant psychosocial difficulties (60, 61), there are insufficient data to support the concept that treatment with conventional AEDs alters these comorbidities.

Women of childbearing age who wish to conceive in the near future and who have only brief non-convulsive events need to consider potential teratogenicity to the fetus from AEDs. However, seizures are more dangerous for the fetus and the mother than the AEDs (62), and treatment is generally offered in this setting. Many of the new AEDs have fewer teratogenic effects (63), easing the decision to start treatment.

Principles of antiepileptic drug therapy in early epilepsy

Once the decision to treat has been made, several factors guide the appropriate medication choice from among the many currently available AEDs.

The majority of patients with early epilepsy who are starting their first drug will achieve seizure freedom. Given that these patients may need years of treatment, medication selection should prioritize safety and tolerability from within the spectrum of appropriate AEDs for the seizure type. For example, although phenobarbital and topiramate are both effective agents in a variety of circumstances, neither is widely used as first line therapy because of adverse cognitive effects (31, 64).

In selecting the proper AED, seizure type is the most important factor to consider. The epilepsy syndrome is next in importance, in that it predicts the expected length of therapy, as well as the expected seizure types. Age, gender, comorbidities, and genetic background each merit additional consideration, as they will influence the tolerability and safety of the medication chosen. Cost also needs thought, as many people with epilepsy need years of therapy, which may financially burden those who are uninsured or under-insured.

Many early epilepsy patients will respond to AEDs at a relatively low dose (65). Therefore, one should choose a reasonable target dose and increase it only if ineffective. A slow titration schedule may delay achieving complete seizure freedom, but will minimize toxicity and often result in better outcomes.

Several formal literature reviews, consensus guidelines, and surveys of expert opinion have been published with specific medication recommendations for patients with new onset seizures (66–71). As clinical experience grows with recently approved medications, and as new medications and formulations become available, these recommendations will evolve.

Seizure type and epilepsy syndrome

Both seizure type and epilepsy syndrome are important in choosing an AED, but the primary consideration should be seizure type. There are no strong data indicating that a given seizure type will be more responsive to a particular drug in one syndrome than another. For example, focal seizures in rolandic epilepsy are more likely to respond to treatment than those in cortical dysplasia, but there are no compelling data to choose a different medication as first line in these two syndromes. Knowledge of the epilepsy syndrome provides insight into the expected course of the disorder, including the length of treatment, and the range of seizure types. For example, a patient with benign rolandic epilepsy may need medication only for a few years, whereas a patient with juvenile myoclonic epilepsy may need decades. A 10-year-old with juvenile absence epilepsy is more likely to have a tonic clonic convulsion than a 7-year-old with childhood absence epilepsy.

For focal seizures, carbamazepine and oxcarbazepine are the most widely used first-line medications in both children and adults with newly diagnosed epilepsy, followed by lamotrigine, because of their efficacy and tolerability, based on clinical experience and well designed clinical trials (72–74).

For generalized seizures, the choices depend on the seizure type and the syndrome. Valproate remains the choice for the symptomatic generalized epilepsies due to its efficacy (84), but is a problematic drug in women of childbearing age. For these women, lamotrigine is an attractive alternative, as is levetiracetam, which has been shown effective for juvenile myoclonic epilepsy (75–77). In childhood absence epilepsy, ethosuximide has superior efficacy and tolerability compared with lamotrigine and valproic acid in a double blind randomized head-to-head trial, and should be the first line therapy for these children (78). For other syndromes, the data are less clear.

As more experience is gained with the newer drugs, some have moved from add-on therapy to first-line treatment. Levetiracetam, for example, is increasingly used as a first-line medication in focal and generalized epilepsies.

Several medications may worsen seizures in patients with generalized epilepsy. Carbamazepine, oxcarbazepine, tiagabine, vigabatrin, and gabapentin may exacerbate generalized seizures, occasionally causing absence or myoclonic status epilepticus (79–81), and should be avoided as first line for generalized epilepsy. Lamotrigine, while effective in generalized seizures, may worsen myoclonic jerks (82, 83).

Age

Children, adolescents, and the elderly each require special consideration in choosing a medication.

Children often have age-related syndromes, and may require medication only for a few years. Therefore, bone health and teratogenicity are less of a concern in this population. Behavioural and cognitive abnormalities in children with epilepsy may be caused either as a comorbidity of the underlying epilepsy syndrome or as a side effect of an AED (60, 61, 84); clinically disentangling these can be challenging. Therefore, there is particular attention to choose drugs that have as few adverse effects on cognition and behaviour as possible (31, 85). Choosing a medication available in liquid, sprinkle, or chewable formulations may also help with compliance.

Adolescents, as they progress towards independence, may fail to take medication, experiment with drugs and alcohol, or become sleep deprived when socializing or studying (86, 87). There is a need to enable adolescents to be compliant without overly disrupting their lives. Long acting formulations or an AED with a long half-life may help in this regard. Adolescents may have a low tolerance for any adverse effects of a newly started medication, which can be partly mitigated with slow titration schedules and lower goal doses. Since sexual activity often begins in adolescence, adolescent females should be considered as women of childbearing age. Valproic acid should be avoided as first-line therapy in women with epilepsy when less potentially teratogenic options are available, and folic acid supplementation should accompany any AED choice (62, 88, 89).

The elderly may have more susceptibility to side effects, more medical comorbidities, polypharmacy, and altered pharmacokinetics and central nervous system pharmacodynamics (90–92). New-onset epilepsy in the elderly is almost always focal and often occurs in individuals with prior stroke or dementia (92). Preferred medications will have few drug–drug interactions, little protein binding, minimal induction or inhibition of liver enzymes, and minimal cognitive side effects. Slow titration to lower goal doses may help reduce side effects. At present, trial data indicate that lamotrigine (90, 93), gabapentin (90), and an extended release formulation of carbamazepine (94) are effective and well tolerated in the elderly.

Gender and implications for pregnancy

Women with epilepsy require special attention to reproductive and endocrine function. Unlike some other neurological disorders such as stroke or Parkinson's, which occur after the childbearing years, epilepsy tends to occur in young people and persist through the childbearing years. Treatment with AEDs, particularly with valproic acid, increases risk of birth defects and poor cognitive outcomes in children exposed *in utero* (88, 95). However, seizures during pregnancy, particularly convulsive seizures, are also associated with adverse pregnancy outcomes (62). The American Academy of Neurology recommends folate supplementation for all women with epilepsy (88, 89), though folate does not guarantee favourable pregnancy outcomes. As young women are likely to remain on AEDs for many years, it is important to consider these issues in all women of childbearing age, including adolescents, even if there are no immediate plans for having children. Most of the serious teratogenic effects occur early in pregnancy and so it is prudent to utilize medications that, if effective, will be appropriate to continue during pregnancy. Fortunately, the majority of women with epilepsy are able to have successful pregnancies with good outcomes (62).

Contraception is also an important issue for women with epilepsy. For women on oral contraception, enzyme-inducing drugs may reduce efficacy of oral contraception pills; higher doses or a change in birth control method may be required (36, 96). Pregnancy decreases the concentration of several AEDs, including lamotrigine, carbamazepine, phenytoin, and possibly levetiracetam and oxcarbazepine (89).

Comorbidities and concurrent medical problems

A significant proportion of individuals with epilepsy have comorbid conditions, particularly the elderly and those with symptomatic epilepsy. In these individuals, initial choice of medication must take into account potential interactions with other medications as well as potential effects on the comorbidities themselves. Hepatic and renal impairment may affect clearance of medications, leading to higher than expected blood levels. Many of the older AEDs are hepatic enzyme inducers (phenytoin, carbamazepine, phenobarbital, oxcarbazepine) and may impact the efficacy of other medications. Others, such as valproic acid, are strongly protein bound and may displace other medications, potentially causing acute toxicity. In addition, valproic acid inhibits the metabolism of other drugs, which may also cause toxicity.

Zonisamide and topiramate increase the risk of renal calculi and should be used with caution in individuals predisposed to kidney stones. Carbamazepine and oxcarbazepine each may cause hyponatraemia and should be used cautiously in patients with hyponatraemia from other causes. Weight gain (mild with carbamazepine and gabapentin, moderate with valproic acid and pregabalin) and loss (topiramate, zonisamide, felbamate) should be considered in overweight and underweight patients (97, 98).

Long-term AED therapy is associated with decreased bone health and fractures. Enzyme inducing agents such as phenytoin, phenobarbital, and primidone are most consistently implicated, whereas the data are mixed on carbamazepine, oxcarbazepine, and valproic acid. Topiramate and acetazolamide may lead to increased bone turnover via acidosis. Data on newer, non-enzyme-inducing drugs are limited but not exculpatory (99).

Genetics

Advances in epilepsy genetics have increased our understanding of the underlying pathophysiology and may eventually lead to targeted treatments. However, at present, specific genetic mutations do not alter first-line therapy for newly diagnosed epilepsy. Instead, clinical phenotype guides treatment. Even in the rare circumstances where a genetic diagnosis will lead to a specific AED, such as vigabatrin for infantile spasms in tuberous sclerosis (100), it is the clinical diagnosis (i.e. tuberous sclerosis) rather than the specific mutation that informs treatment.

The field of pharmacogenomics, however, is rapidly assuming clinical importance by identifying individuals at increased risk for dangerous side effects of AEDs (101). For example, the HLA-B*1502 allele places some East Asians, particularly Han Chinese, at higher risk for Stevens–Johnson syndrome or toxic epidermal necrolysis when taking carbamazepine (102), and screening may reduce the risk (103). Similarly, the HLA-B*3101 allele may increase the risk in people of Northern European descent, though the risks are lower and the cost benefit of this screening remains somewhat controversial (104). It is expected that within a decade, screening tools will identify additional genetic susceptibilities to adverse events, and help guide clinicians on which medications to avoid in individual patients. This susceptibility information may eventually guide medication choice in newly diagnosed epilepsy.

Affordability

All of the potential first-line medications discussed in this chapter are available generically, and are thus increasingly affordable to uninsured or underinsured patients. In patients with newly diagnosed epilepsy, the controversial issue of brand versus generic is less important than in refractory patients or in those with prior adverse events. In regions with limited resources for medical care, the older AEDs, such as phenobarbital or phenytoin, are often significantly cheaper than newer medications. These drugs provide similar efficacy, though a higher rate of adverse side effects, and may be considered when cost is an over-riding concern (105, 106).

Counselling

After a first seizure or the diagnosis of epilepsy, ideally after the results of the initial EEG and neuroimaging are available, dedicate sufficient time with the patient (or family) to provide counselling and answer questions. Tailor the discussion to balance the need to convey critical advice with the ability of the patient (or family) to absorb the information. For patients starting medication, there are likely to be opportunities at future office visits to reinforce counselling and raise additional issues not covered in the first encounter. These patients have just recently been diagnosed and therefore need discussion of the issues common to all AEDs and seizure disorders as well as the specifics related to their particular diagnosis and treatment regimen.

Patients may be reassured that the risk of brain damage, serious injury, or death from an individual seizure is low; however, they will need to take certain precautions. Patients should not swim alone due to the risk of drowning after a seizure. Burns sustained while cooking are a common cause of injury in patients with epilepsy, and supervision and extra care should be taken when cooking (50). The possibility of a change in employment may need to be discussed with adults who drive, operate heavy machinery, or work at heights if they are not seizure free.

Adults and adolescents should stop driving after a seizure; the time period depends on the municipality. In the UK, driving is forbidden for 1 year after the last seizure, and patients are required to notify the Department for Transportation of their status (107). In the US and Canada, the length of driving prohibition and reporting requirements vary by state or province.

Prognosis

Several factors help predict the prognosis for seizure control, including initial presentation (one seizure versus multiple seizures), aetiology, number of seizures at onset and in the first 6 months after diagnosis, response to initial AED, and epilepsy syndrome. Individuals who initially present with a single unprovoked seizure have a greater than 90% chance of remission at 5 years, irrespective of drug therapy (13, 16). For newly diagnosed epilepsy, about half will respond to the first trial of monotherapy, and another 15% will respond to a second trial of monotherapy or a two-drug combination (65). More than 80% of patients with focal and generalized epilepsies may expect a 1-year remission within 5 years of diagnosis (74, 108). Remote symptomatic aetiology (61, 109–111), failure to respond to the initial AED (61, 109–111), and many seizures at onset (65) or in the first 6 months after treatment (112) each suggest a poorer prognosis for remission.

Identifying the epilepsy syndrome greatly helps understand the prognosis. For example, the seizures in children with self-limited syndromes, such as benign rolandic epilepsy, will remit with or without treatment; whereas fewer than 50% of individuals with temporal lobe epilepsy will attain full remission (113). While there is clearly a need for better epilepsy treatments, as well as improved early identification of those with refractory epilepsy who may be candidates for more aggressive therapy, the majority of patients with early epilepsy will attain seizure remission.

References

1. Gowers WR. *Epilepsy and Other Chronic Convulsive Diseases*. London: J&A Churchill, New Burlington Street, 1881.
2. Sander JW, Hart YM, Johnson AL, Shorvon SD. National General Practice Study of Epilepsy: newly diagnosed epileptic seizures in a general population. *Lancet* 1990; 336(8726):1267–71.
3. Guidelines for epidemiologic studies on epilepsy. Commission on Epidemiology and Prognosis, International League Against Epilepsy. *Epilepsia* 1993; 34(4):592–6.
4. Kho LK, Lawn ND, Dunne JW, Linto J. First seizure presentation: do multiple seizures within 24 hours predict recurrence? *Neurology* 2006; 67(6):1047–9.
5. Berg AT, Shinnar S. The risk of seizure recurrence following a first unprovoked seizure: a quantitative review. *Neurology* 1991; 41(7): 965–72.
6. Camfield P, Camfield C, Dooley J, Smith E, Garner B. A randomized study of carbamazepine versus no medication after a first unprovoked seizure in childhood. *Neurology* 1989; 39(6):851–2.
7. Randomized clinical trial on the efficacy of antiepileptic drugs in reducing the risk of relapse after a first unprovoked tonic-clonic seizure. First Seizure Trial Group (FIR.S.T. Group.) *Neurology* 1993; 43(3 Pt 1):478–83.
8. Hauser WA, Anderson VE, Loewenson RB, McRoberts SM. Seizure recurrence after a first unprovoked seizure. *N Engl J Med* 1982; 307(9):522–8.
9. Hauser WA, Rich SS, Annegers JF, Anderson VE. Seizure recurrence after a 1st unprovoked seizure: an extended follow-up. *Neurology* 1990; 40(8):1163–70.
10. Hauser WA, Rich SS, Lee JR, Annegers JF, Anderson VE. Risk of recurrent seizures after two unprovoked seizures. *N Engl J Med* 1998; 338(7):429–34.

11. Hirtz D, Ashwal S, Berg A, Bettis D, Camfield C, Camfield P, *et al.* Practice parameter: evaluating a first nonfebrile seizure in children: report of the quality standards subcommittee of the American Academy of Neurology, The Child Neurology Society, and The American Epilepsy Society. *Neurology* 2000; 55(5):616–23.
12. Hopkins A, Garman A, Clarke C. The first seizure in adult life. Value of clinical features, electroencephalography, and computerised tomographic scanning in prediction of seizure recurrence. *Lancet* 1988; 1(8588):721–6.
13. Marson A, Jacoby A, Johnson A, Kim L, Gamble C, Chadwick D. Immediate versus deferred antiepileptic drug treatment for early epilepsy and single seizures: a randomised controlled trial. *Lancet* 2005; 365(9476):2007–13.
14. Shinnar S, Berg AT, Moshe SL, O'Dell C, Alemany M, Newstein D, *et al.* The risk of seizure recurrence after a first unprovoked afebrile seizure in childhood: an extended follow-up. *Pediatrics* 1996; 98 (2 Pt 1):216–25.
15. Shinnar S, Berg AT, Moshe SL, Petix M, Maytal J, Kang H, *et al.* Risk of seizure recurrence following a first unprovoked seizure in childhood: a prospective study. *Pediatrics* 1990; 85(6):1076–85.
16. Shinnar S, Berg AT, O'Dell C, Newstein D, Moshe SL, Hauser WA. Predictors of multiple seizures in a cohort of children prospectively followed from the time of their first unprovoked seizure. *Ann Neurol* 2000; 48(2):140–7.
17. Stroink H, Brouwer OF, Arts WF, Geerts AT, Peters AC, van Donselaar CA. The first unprovoked, untreated seizure in childhood: a hospital based study of the accuracy of the diagnosis, rate of recurrence, and long term outcome after recurrence. Dutch study of epilepsy in childhood. *J Neurol Neurosurg Psychiatry* 1998; 64(5):595–600.
18. van Donselaar CA, Brouwer OF, Geerts AT, Arts WF, Stroink H, Peters AC. Clinical course of untreated tonic-clonic seizures in childhood: prospective, hospital based study. *BMJ* 1997; 314(7078):401–4.
19. van Donselaar CA, Schimsheimer RJ, Geerts AT, Declerck AC. Value of the electroencephalogram in adult patients with untreated idiopathic first seizures. *Arch Neurol* 1992; 49(3):231–7.
20. Berg AT. Risk of recurrence after a first unprovoked seizure. *Epilepsia* 2008; 49(Suppl 1):13–8.
21. Haut SR, Shinnar S. Considerations in the treatment of a first unprovoked seizure. *Semin Neurol* 2008; 28(3):289–96.
22. Proposal for revised classification of epilepsies and epileptic syndromes. Commission on Classification and Terminology of the International League Against Epilepsy. *Epilepsia* 1989; 30(4):389–99.
23. Berg AT, Berkovic SF, Brodie MJ, Buchhalter J, Cross JH, van Emde Boas W, *et al.* Revised terminology and concepts for organization of seizures and epilepsies: report of the ILAE Commission on Classification and Terminology, 2005–2009. *Epilepsia* 2010; 51(4):676–85.
24. Kim LG, Johnson TL, Marson AG, Chadwick DW. Prediction of risk of seizure recurrence after a single seizure and early epilepsy: further results from the MESS trial. *Lancet Neurol* 2006; 5(4):317–22.
25. Camfield PR, Camfield CS, Dooley JM, Tibbles JA, Fung T, Garner B. Epilepsy after a first unprovoked seizure in childhood. *Neurology* 1985; 35(11):1657–60.
26. J Roger MB, Ch Dravet, P Genton, CA Tassinari, P Wolf. *Epileptic Syndromes in Infancy, Childhood, and Adolescence* (4th edn). Montrouge: John Libbey Eurotext, 2005.
27. Gilad R, Lampl Y, Gabbay U, Eshel Y, Sarova-Pinhas I. Early treatment of a single generalized tonic-clonic seizure to prevent recurrence. *Arch Neurol* 1996; 53(11):1149–52.
28. Musicco M, Beghi E, Solari A, Viani F. Treatment of first tonic-clonic seizure does not improve the prognosis of epilepsy. First Seizure Trial Group (FIRST Group). *Neurology* 1997; 49(4):991–8.
29. Hirtz D, Berg A, Bettis D, Camfield C, Camfield P, Crumrine P, *et al.* Practice parameter: treatment of the child with a first unprovoked seizure: Report of the Quality Standards Subcommittee of the American Academy of Neurology and the Practice Committee of the Child Neurology Society. *Neurology* 2003; 60(2):166–75.
30. Loring DW, Marino S, Meador KJ. Neuropsychological and behavioral effects of antiepilepsy drugs. *Neuropsychol Rev* 2007; 17(4):413–25.
31. Mula M, Trimble MR, Thompson P, Sander JW. Topiramate and word-finding difficulties in patients with epilepsy. *Neurology* 2003; 60(7):1104–7.
32. Pack A. Bone health in people with epilepsy: is it impaired and what are the risk factors? *Seizure* 2008; 17(2):181–6.
33. Petty SJ, Paton LM, O'Brien TJ, Makovey J, Erbas B, Sambrook P, *et al.* Effect of antiepileptic medication on bone mineral measures. *Neurology* 2005; 65(9):1358–65.
34. Ensrud KE, Walczak TS, Blackwell T, Ensrud ER, Bowman PJ, Stone KL. Antiepileptic drug use increases rates of bone loss in older woman: a prospective study. *Neurology* 2004; 62(11):2051–7.
35. Ensrud KE, Walczak TS, Blackwell TL, Ensrud ER, Barrett-Connor E, Orwoll ES, *et al.* Antiepileptic drug use and rates of hip bone loss in older men: a prospective study. *Neurology* 2008; 71(10):723–30.
36. Crawford P. Best practice guidelines for the management of women with epilepsy. *Epilepsia* 2005; 46(Suppl 9):117–24.
37. Arana A, Wentworth CE, Ayuso-Mateos JL, Arellano FM. Suicide-related events in patients treated with antiepileptic drugs. *N Engl J Med* 2010; 363(6):542–51.
38. Andersohn F, Schade R, Willich SN, Garbe E. Use of antiepileptic drugs in epilepsy and the risk of self-harm or suicidal behavior. *Neurology* 2010; 75(4):335–40.
39. Jacoby A, Johnson A, Chadwick D. Psychosocial outcomes of antiepileptic drug discontinuation. The Medical Research Council Antiepileptic Drug Withdrawal Study Group. *Epilepsia* 1992; 33(6):1123–31.
40. Hoare P. Does illness foster dependency? A study of epileptic and diabetic children. *Dev Med Child Neurol* 1984; 26(1):20–4.
41. van Donselaar CA, Geerts AT, Schimsheimer RJ. Idiopathic first seizure in adult life: who should be treated? *BMJ* 1991; 302(6777): 620–3.
42. Ambrosetto G, Tassinari CA. Antiepileptic drug treatment of benign childhood epilepsy with rolandic spikes: is it necessary? *Epilepsia* 1990; 31(6):802–5.
43. Berg AT, Shinnar S. Do seizures beget seizures? An assessment of the clinical evidence in humans. *J Clin Neurophysiol* 1997; 14(2):102–10.
44. Sander JW. Some aspects of prognosis in the epilepsies: a review. *Epilepsia* 1993; 34(6):1007 16.
45. Shinnar S, Berg AT. Does antiepileptic drug therapy prevent the development of 'chronic' epilepsy? *Epilepsia* 1996; 37(8):701–8.
46. Camfield P, Camfield C, Smith S, Dooley J, Smith E. Long-term outcome is unchanged by antiepileptic drug treatment after a first seizure: a 15-year follow-up from a randomized trial in childhood. *Epilepsia* 2002; 43(6):662–3.
47. Shinnar S, Babb TL, Moshé SL, Wasterlain CG. Long-term sequelae of status epilepsticus. In: Engel J Jr, Pedley TA (ed) *Epilepsy, A Comprehensive Textbook*, pp. 751–9. Philadelphia, PA: Lippincott Williams & Williams, 2008.
48. Freeman JM, Tibbles J, Camfield C, Camfield P. Benign epilepsy of childhood: a speculation and its ramifications. *Pediatrics* 1987; 79(6):864–8.
49. Neufeld MY, Vishne T, Chistik V, Korczyn AD. Life-long history of injuries related to seizures. *Epilepsy Res* 1999; 34(2–3):123–7.
50. Spitz MC. Injuries and death as a consequence of seizures in people with epilepsy. *Epilepsia* 1998; 39(8):904–7.
51. Lees A. Retrospective study of seizure-related injuries in older people: a 10-year observation. *Epilepsy Behav* 2010; 19(3):441–4.
52. Ramos Lizana J, Cassinello Garcia E, Carrasco Marina LL, Vazquez Lopez M, Martin Gonzalez M, Munoz Hoyos A. Seizure recurrence after a first unprovoked seizure in childhood: a prospective study. *Epilepsia* 2000; 41(8):1005–13.

53. Shinnar S, Berg AT, Moshe SL, Shinnar R. How long do new-onset seizures in children last? *Ann Neurol* 2001; 49(5):659–64.
54. DeLorenzo RJ, Hauser WA, Towne AR, Boggs JG, Pellock JM, Penberthy L, *et al.* A prospective, population-based epidemiologic study of status epilepticus in Richmond, Virginia. *Neurology* 1996; 46(4):1029–35.
55. Treatment of convulsive status epilepticus. Recommendations of the Epilepsy Foundation of America's Working Group on Status Epilepticus. *JAMA* 1993; 270(7):854–9.
56. Maytal J, Shinnar S, Moshe SL, Alvarez LA. Low morbidity and mortality of status epilepticus in children. *Pediatrics* 1989; 83(3): 323–31.
57. Jacoby A, Baker G, Chadwick D, Johnson A. The impact of counselling with a practical statistical model on patients' decision-making about treatment for epilepsy: findings from a pilot study. *Epilepsy Res* 1993; 16(3):207–14.
58. Jacoby A, Gamble C, Doughty J, Marson A, Chadwick D. Quality of life outcomes of immediate or delayed treatment of early epilepsy and single seizures. *Neurology* 2007; 68(15):1188–96.
59. Shinnar S, O'Dell C. Treatment decisions in childhood seizures. In: Pellock JM, Bourgeois B, Dodson WE (eds) *Pediatric Epilepsy* (3rd edn), pp. 401–12. New York: Demos Medical Publishing, 2008.
60. Fastenau PS, Johnson CS, Perkins SM, Byars AW, deGrauw TJ, Austin JK, *et al.* Neuropsychological status at seizure onset in children: risk factors for early cognitive deficits. *Neurology* 2009; 73(7):526–34.
61. Sillanpaa M, Jalava M, Kaleva O, Shinnar S. Long-term prognosis of seizures with onset in childhood. *N Engl J Med* 1998; 338(24):1715–22.
62. Harden CL, Hopp J, Ting TY, Pennell PB, French JA, Hauser WA, *et al.* Practice parameter update: management issues for women with epilepsy—focus on pregnancy (an evidence-based review): obstetrical complications and change in seizure frequency: report of the Quality Standards Subcommittee and Therapeutics and Technology Assessment Subcommittee of the American Academy of Neurology and American Epilepsy Society. *Neurology* 2009; 73(2):126–32.
63. Molgaard-Nielsen D, Hviid A. Newer-generation antiepileptic drugs and the risk of major birth defects. *JAMA* 2011; 305(19):1996–2002.
64. Vining EP, Mellitis ED, Dorsen MM, Cataldo MF, Quaskey SA, Spielberg SP, *et al.* Psychologic and behavioral effects of antiepileptic drugs in children: a double-blind comparison between phenobarbital and valproic acid. *Pediatrics* 1987; 80(2):165–74.
65. Kwan P, Brodie MJ. Early identification of refractory epilepsy. *N Engl J Med* 2000; 342(5):314–9.
66. French JA, Kanner AM, Bautista J, Abou-Khalil B, Browne T, Harden CL, *et al.* Efficacy and tolerability of the new antiepileptic drugs I: treatment of new onset epilepsy: report of the Therapeutics and Technology Assessment Subcommittee and Quality Standards Subcommittee of the American Academy of Neurology and the American Epilepsy Society. *Neurology* 2004; 62(8):1252–60.
67. Glauser T, Ben-Menachem E, Bourgeois B, Cnaan A, Chadwick D, Guerreiro C, *et al.* ILAE treatment guidelines: evidence-based analysis of antiepileptic drug efficacy and effectiveness as initial monotherapy for epileptic seizures and syndromes. *Epilepsia* 2006; 47(7):1094–120.
68. Care NCCfP. *Clinical Guideline 20. The epilesies: the diagnosis and management of the epilepsies in adults and children in primary and secondary care.* London: The National Institute for Health and Clinical Excellence, 2004.
69. Semah F, Picot MC, Derambure P, Dupont S, Vercueil L, Chassagnon S, *et al.* The choice of antiepileptic drugs in newly diagnosed epilepsy: a national French survey. *Epileptic Disord* 2004; 6(4):255–65.
70. Wheless JW, Clarke DF, Arzimanoglou A, Carpenter D. Treatment of pediatric epilepsy: European expert opinion, 2007. *Epileptic Disord* 2007; 9(4):353–412.
71. Karceski S, Morrell MJ, Carpenter D. Treatment of epilepsy in adults: expert opinion, 2005. *Epilepsy Behav* 2005; 7(Suppl 1):S1–64; quiz S5–7.
72. Mattson RH, Cramer JA, Collins JF. A comparison of valproate with carbamazepine for the treatment of complex partial seizures and secondarily generalized tonic-clonic seizures in adults. The Department of Veterans Affairs Epilepsy Cooperative Study No. 264 Group. *N Engl J* Med 1992; 327(11):765–71.
73. Mattson RH, Cramer JA, Collins JF, Smith DB, Delgado-Escueta AV, Browne TR, *et al.* Comparison of carbamazepine, phenobarbital, phenytoin, and primidone in partial and secondarily generalized tonic-clonic seizures. *N Engl J Med* 1985; 313(3):145–51.
74. Marson AG, Al-Kharusi AM, Alwaidh M, Appleton R, Baker GA, Chadwick DW, *et al.* The SANAD study of effectiveness of carbamazepine, gabapentin, lamotrigine, oxcarbazepine, or topiramate for treatment of partial epilepsy: an unblinded randomised controlled trial. *Lancet* 2007; 369(9566):1000–15.
75. Rosenfeld WE, Benbadis S, Edrich P, Tassinari CA, Hirsch E. Levetiracetam as add-on therapy for idiopathic generalized epilepsy syndromes with onset during adolescence: analysis of two randomized, double-blind, placebo-controlled studies. *Epilepsy Res* 2009; 85(1): 72–80.
76. Berkovic SF, Knowlton RC, Leroy RF, Schiemann J, Falter U. Placebo-controlled study of levetiracetam in idiopathic generalized epilepsy. *Neurology* 2007; 69(18):1751–60.
77. Noachtar S, Andermann E, Meyvisch P, Andermann F, Gough WB, Schiemann-Delgado J. Levetiracetam for the treatment of idiopathic generalized epilepsy with myoclonic seizures. *Neurology* 2008; 70(8):607–16.
78. Glauser TA, Cnaan A, Shinnar S, Hirtz DG, Dlugos D, Masur D, *et al.* Ethosuximide, valproic acid, and lamotrigine in childhood absence epilepsy. *N Engl J Med* 2010; 362(9):790–9.
79. Perucca E, Gram L, Avanzini G, Dulac O. Antiepileptic drugs as a cause of worsening seizures. *Epilepsia* 1998; 39(1):5–17.
80. Thomas P, Valton L, Genton P. Absence and myoclonic status epilepticus precipitated by antiepileptic drugs in idiopathic generalized epilepsy. *Brain* 2006; 129(Pt 5):1281–92.
81. Vendrame M, Khurana DS, Cruz M, Melvin J, Valencia I, Legido A, *et al.* Aggravation of seizures and/or EEG features in children treated with oxcarbazepine monotherapy. *Epilepsia* 2007; 48(11):2116–20.
82. Biraben A, Allain H, Scarabin JM, Schuck S, Edan G. Exacerbation of juvenile myoclonic epilepsy with lamotrigine. *Neurology* 2000; 55(11):1758.
83. Carrazana EJ, Wheeler SD. Exacerbation of juvenile myoclonic epilepsy with lamotrigine. *Neurology* 2001; 56(10):1424–5.
84. Berg AT, Smith SN, Frobish D, Levy SR, Testa FM, Beckerman B, *et al.* Special education needs of children with newly diagnosed epilepsy. *Dev Med Child Neurol* 2005; 47(11):749–53.
85. Loring DW, Meador KJ. Cognitive side effects of antiepileptic drugs in children. *Neurology* 2004; 62(6):872–7.
86. Snodgrass SR, Vedanarayanan VV, Parker CC, Parks BR. Pediatric patients with undetectable anticonvulsant blood levels: comparison with compliant patients. *J Child Neurol* 2001; 16(3):164–8.
87. Nordli DR, Jr. Special needs of the adolescent with epilepsy. *Epilepsia* 2001; 42(Suppl 8):10–7.
88. Harden CL, Meador KJ, Pennell PB, Hauser WA, Gronseth GS, French JA, *et al.* Practice parameter update: management issues for women with epilepsy—focus on pregnancy (an evidence-based review): teratogenesis and perinatal outcomes: report of the Quality Standards Subcommittee and Therapeutics and Technology Assessment Subcommittee of the American Academy of Neurology and American Epilepsy Society. *Neurology* 2009; 73(2):133–41.
89. Harden CL, Pennell PB, Koppel BS, Hovinga CA, Gidal B, Meador KJ, *et al.* Practice parameter update: management issues for women with epilepsy—focus on pregnancy (an evidence-based review): vitamin K, folic acid, blood levels, and breastfeeding: report of the Quality Standards Subcommittee and Therapeutics and Technology

Assessment Subcommittee of the American Academy of Neurology and American Epilepsy Society. *Neurology* 2009; 73(2):142–9.

90. Rowan AJ, Ramsay RE, Collins JF, Pryor F, Boardman KD, Uthman BM, *et al.* New onset geriatric epilepsy: a randomized study of gabapentin, lamotrigine, and carbamazepine. *Neurology* 2005; 64(11):1868–73.
91. Ramsay RE, Rowan AJ, Pryor FM. Special considerations in treating the elderly patient with epilepsy. *Neurology* 2004; 62(5 Suppl 2):S24–9.
92. Brodie MJ, Elder AT, Kwan P. Epilepsy in later life. *Lancet Neurol* 2009; 8(11):1019–30.
93. Brodie MJ, Overstall PW, Giorgi L. Multicentre, double-blind, randomised comparison between lamotrigine and carbamazepine in elderly patients with newly diagnosed epilepsy. The UK Lamotrigine Elderly Study Group. *Epilepsy Res* 1999; 37(1):81–7.
94. Saetre E, Perucca E, Isojarvi J, Gjerstad L. An international multicenter randomized double-blind controlled trial of lamotrigine and sustained-release carbamazepine in the treatment of newly diagnosed epilepsy in the elderly. *Epilepsia* 2007; 48(7):1292–302.
95. Meador KJ, Baker GA, Browning N, Clayton-Smith J, Combs-Cantrell DT, Cohen M, *et al.* Cognitive function at 3 years of age after fetal exposure to antiepileptic drugs. *N Engl J Med* 2009; 360(16):1597–605.
96. Herzog A. Disorders of Reproduction and Fertility. In: Engel J, Pedley T (eds) *Epilepsy, A Comprehensive Textbook*, pp. 2053–9. Philadelphia, PA: Lippincott Williams & Wilkins, 2008.
97. Ben-Menachem E. Weight issues for people with epilepsy—a review. *Epilepsia* 2007; 48(Suppl 9):42–5.
98. Biton V. Weight change and antiepileptic drugs: health issues and criteria for appropriate selection of an antiepileptic agent. *Neurologist* 2006; 12(3):163–7.
99. Pack AM. Treatment of Epilepsy to Optimize Bone Health. *Curr Treat Options Neurol* 2011; 13(4):346–54.
100. Pellock JM, Hrachovy R, Shinnar S, Baram TZ, Bettis D, Dlugos DJ, *et al.* Infantile spasms: a U.S. consensus report. *Epilepsia* 2010; 51(10):2175–89.
101. Loscher W, Klotz U, Zimprich F, Schmidt D. The clinical impact of pharmacogenetics on the treatment of epilepsy. *Epilepsia* 2009; 50(1):1–23.
102. Chung WH, Hung SI, Hong HS, Hsih MS, Yang LC, Ho HC, *et al.* Medical genetics: a marker for Stevens-Johnson syndrome. *Nature* 2004; 428(6982):486.
103. Chen P, Lin JJ, Lu CS, Ong CT, Hsieh PF, Yang CC, *et al.* Carbamazepine-induced toxic effects and HLA-B*1502 screening in Taiwan. *N Engl J Med* 2011; 364(12):1126–33.
104. McCormack M, Alfirevic A, Bourgeois S, Farrell JJ, Kasperaviciute D, Carrington M, *et al.* HLA-A*3101 and carbamazepine-induced hypersensitivity reactions in Europeans. *N Engl J Med* 2011; 364(12):1134–43.
105. Ding D, Hong Z, Chen GS, Dai XY, Wu JZ, Wang WZ, *et al.* Primary care treatment of epilepsy with phenobarbital in rural China: cost-outcome analysis from the WHO/ILAE/IBE global campaign against epilepsy demonstration project. *Epilepsia* 2008; 49(3):535–9.
106. Wang WZ, Wu JZ, Ma GY, Dai XY, Yang B, Wang TP, *et al.* Efficacy assessment of phenobarbital in epilepsy: a large community-based intervention trial in rural China. *Lancet Neurol* 2006; 5(1):46–52.
107. Carter T. *Fitness to Drive: A Guide for Health Professionals.* London: Royal Society of Medicine Press Ltd, 2006.
108. Marson AG, Al-Kharusi AM, Alwaidh M, Appleton R, Baker GA, Chadwick DW, *et al.* The SANAD study of effectiveness of valproate, lamotrigine, or topiramate for generalised and unclassifiable epilepsy: an unblinded randomised controlled trial. *Lancet* 2007; 369(9566):1016–26.
109. Berg AT, Shinnar S, Levy SR, Testa FM, Smith-Rapaport S, Beckerman B. Early development of intractable epilepsy in children: a prospective study. *Neurology* 2001; 56(11):1445–52.
110. Cockerell OC, Johnson AL, Sander JW, Shorvon SD. Prognosis of epilepsy: a review and further analysis of the first nine years of the British National General Practice Study of Epilepsy, a prospective population-based study. *Epilepsia* 1997; 38(1):31–46.
111. Geerts A, Arts WF, Stroink H, Peeters E, Brouwer O, Peters B, *et al.* Course and outcome of childhood epilepsy: a 15-year follow-up of the Dutch Study of Epilepsy in Childhood. *Epilepsia* 2010; 51(7):1189–97.
112. MacDonald BK, Johnson AL, Goodridge DM, Cockerell OC, Sander JW, Shorvon SD. Factors predicting prognosis of epilepsy after presentation with seizures. *Ann Neurol* 2000; 48(6):833–41.
113. Stephen LJ, Kwan P, Brodie MJ. Does the cause of localisation-related epilepsy influence the response to antiepileptic drug treatment? *Epilepsia* 2001; 42(3):357–62.

CHAPTER 23

The Medical Treatment of Chronic Active Epilepsy

Simon Shorvon

Chronic epilepsy can be defined as epilepsy in which seizures are still occurring 5 or more years after the initiation of therapy (1). Therapy in this situation is less likely to be successful than in newly diagnosed epilepsy, and there are several alternative theories about why this might be so. It has been suggested, for instance, that the longer epilepsy remains active, the more resistant it becomes to treatment due to the many molecular changes that occur in ongoing epilepsy. Alternatively, it is possible that the difference is due simply to selection and that patients with chronic epilepsy comprise the inherently more severe forms of the condition which is unresponsive to therapy from the very start of therapy when compared to the milder epilepsies where seizures are controlled at the onset of therapy.

The goal of drug therapy in newly diagnosed cases is the complete control of seizures, and this occurs in about 60–70% of patients within a few years of the onset of the condition (2–6). This leaves 30–40% of patients who continue to have seizures, and thus develop chronic epilepsy. Treatment in chronic epilepsy is more complex and more difficult than in the newly diagnosed epilepsy. However, long-term seizure control in patients with chronic epilepsy can be obtained, with skilful treatment, in about 30%, and it should be further possible to greatly lessen the frequency or severity of seizures in many of those in whom complete control is not possible. There remain about 10% of all those developing epilepsy in whom seizures remain severe, frequent, or intractable. Although small in number, these patients require a high level of medical input. Factors associated with chronicity include: high seizure density prior to commencing treatment, certain epileptic syndromes, certain aetiologies, the presence of additional learning disability, neuropsychological signs, or neurological signs, psychological disturbance (6–8). The additional learning disability, psychosocial problems, or other neurological handicaps which coexist with chronic epilepsy can complicate medical therapy further. Chronic epilepsy can have a major impact on an individual, impacting on personal and domestic life, employment, and education (9).

This chapter focuses on the principles of drug therapy in chronic epilepsy, although it must be emphasized that drug therapy is only part of a treatment strategy which should also include counselling, lifestyle manipulation and avoidance of provoking factors, and non-pharmacological therapy. These are discussed elsewhere in this volume (Chapter 12). The chapter also focuses on the therapy of adults in an outpatient setting. The special aspects of therapy in children, persons with learning disability, and in the elderly are covered elsewhere (Chapters 16–18).

Choice of antiepileptic drug therapy in chronic epilepsy

In chronic epilepsy, the choice of drug will be usually largely independent of the cause of epilepsy. This lack of specificity is a striking feature of most adult epilepsies and perhaps is because the antiepileptic drugs (AEDs) act mechanistically on the final physiological pathways of epileptogenesis, which are similar in many cases whatever the cause (a concept proposed by John Russell Reynolds and Hughlings Jackson in the 19th century (10)). The overall chance of effecting seizure control is similar for individual drugs, at least in the generality of partial and secondarily generalized epilepsy, but side effects vary more, and the choice of drugs is often more influenced by relative tolerability than efficacy (11). This lack of specificity applies to tonic–clonic and partial-onset seizures, which are the most common forms of epilepsy in adults, but not to other seizure types, which are much less common, nor to the specific childhood syndromes discussed in Chapter 16.

Seizure type and the choice of antiepileptic drugs

The usual choices of drugs in different seizure types can be summarized under four categories (Table 23.1).

Generalized tonic–clonic and partial onset seizures

A wide range of drugs are licensed for use in tonic–clonic or partial-onset seizures in chronic epilepsy, whether primarily or secondarily generalized (12–14). In almost all randomized controlled studies, the available AEDs show similar comparative efficacy (11).

A number of drugs are licensed for use in monotherapy, including: carbamazepine (best used in its slow-release formulation), lamotrigine, valproate, levetiracetam, oxcarbazepine, or topiramate (15, 16). These drugs are often used as first-line drugs also in chronic epilepsy. The other drugs, which are licensed as add-on therapy, are used as second-line therapy. The older drugs, phenobarbital and phenytoin, are also used as first-line therapy in some countries. A number of comparative studies have been carried out, but no one first- or second-line drug has been found to be consistently

Table 23.1 Antiepileptic drugs in different seizure types

Seizure type	Drugs which show efficacy	Drugs which may worsen seizures
Partial seizures, secondarily generalized tonic–clonic seizures, primary generalized tonic–clonic seizures	First-line AEDs: carbamazepine (best used in its slow-release formulation), lamotrigine, valproate, levetiracetam, oxcarbazepine, topiramate Second-line AEDs: acetazolamide, clobazam, clonazepam, gabapentin, lacosamide, oxcarbazepine, phenobarbital, phenytoin, pregabalin, primidone, tiagabine, vigabatrin, zonisamide	
Absence seizures (typical absence)	First-line AEDs: ethosuximide, lamotrigine, levetiracetam, valproate Second-line AEDs: acetazolamide, clobazam, clonazepam, phenobarbital, topiramate,	Carbamazepine, gabapentin, oxcarbazepine, tiagabine, vigabatrin
Myoclonic seizures	First-line AEDs: lamotrigine, levetiracetam, valproate Second-line AEDs: clobazam, clonazepam, phenobarbital, piracetam, topiramate	Carbamazepine, gabapentin, oxcarbazepine, phenytoin, tiagabine, vigabatrin
Atypical absence, tonic and atonic seizures	First-line AEDs: lamotrigine, levetiracetam, topiramate, rufinamide, valproate. Zonisamide. Second-line AEDs: acetazolamide, clobazam, clonazepam, phenobarbital, phenytoin, primidone	Carbamazepine, gabapentin, oxcarbazepine, phenytoin, tiagabine, vigabatrin

(List based on author's preference.)

superior or inferior in terms of seizure control. The most striking finding from all these studies is the similarity, not the difference, in responder rates on treatment with the various AEDs. However, the similarity in overall antiepileptic effects hides important individual differences, both in side-effects and in efficacy, and there are many patients who fail to respond to one drug but who do respond to another. It is therefore usual, and indeed logical, to rotate a patient through trials of treatment with all appropriate therapies (17).

In idiopathic generalized epilepsy (IGE) there is a clinical impression that valproate is a better choice than carbamazepine for first-line therapy of tonic–clonic seizures (18). However, there is little, if any, conclusive evidence to support this proposition; and indeed most well-conducted studies show little difference in efficacy between any of the major AEDs. However, myoclonus and/or absence seizures which often coexist with tonic–clonic seizures in IGE do respond well to valproate or levetiracetam, and are frequently worsened by carbamazepine or oxcarbazepine. In partial-onset seizures, it is also frequently stated that carbamazepine is more effective than valproate, but again there is little or no definitive evidence of such a difference, and in chronic epilepsy, either drug can be highly effective.

Generalized absence seizures

Generalized absence seizures occur only in the syndrome of IGE. Valproate is the commonest first choice AED. Other drugs which can be used as first-line therapy, but which have less reliable effects are levetiracetam, lamotrigine, topiramate, zonisamide, and the benzodiazepines. Ethosuximide is another highly effective drug but is largely ineffective in controlling generalized tonic–clonic seizures, which often coexist with absence seizures.

Myoclonic seizures

Myoclonus occurs in various clinical settings (Table 23.2). The myoclonus in IGE is generally well controlled on single drug therapy with valproate which is the drug of first choice. Where valproate is inappropriate or ineffective, other agents which can be used are levetiracetam, lamotrigine, topiramate, zonisamide, and the benzodiazepines. The myoclonus in the symptomatic generalized, progressive myoclonic epilepsy or in the focal epilepsies is more difficult to treat, and drug combinations may be necessary.

Piracetam is an unusual drug which is uniquely effective in myoclonus and which has no effect in other types of epilepsy. High doses are required, but the drug is well tolerated. It is most used in the treatment of myoclonus in the progressive myoclonic epilepsy syndromes.

Some drugs exacerbate absence or myoclonic seizures in the generalized epilepsies, or indeed precipitate myoclonus for the first time in susceptible patients. Phenytoin has been reported to worsen the myoclonus in the Lafora body disease, and carbamazepine, oxcarbazepine, and phenytoin can aggravate myoclonus in juvenile myoclonic epilepsy.

Atypical absence, atonic, and tonic seizures

These seizure types occur in the context of the Lennox–Gastaut syndrome or the other severe epileptic encephalopathies. The drug treatment is essentially similar for each, although full control of seizures is usually not possible. Valproate or lamotrigine are recommended by most as first-choice drugs. Traditional alternatives are the benzodiazepine drugs (e.g. clobazam or clonazepam), acetazolamide, phenobarbital, or primidone. Levetiracetam has promise in these types of epilepsy on an anecdotal level but formal studies are limited. Phenytoin may be useful for tonic seizures, but may exacerbate atonic seizures. Topiramate and zonisamide have been shown to be effective in various open and controlled studies.

Table 23.2 Epilepsies in which myoclonus is part of the phenotype

- Idiopathic generalized epilepsy (IGE)
- Benign myoclonic epilepsy syndromes of childhood
- Severe epilepsy syndromes of childhood and epileptic encephalopathies
- Progressive myoclonic epilepsies (PMEs)
- Focal epilepsies in the central cortex
- Symptomatic focal epilepsies (particularly those due to mitochondrial disease, inherited or acquired metabolic disease, infections, drug and toxins)

Derived from Shorvon (14).

Felbamate also has a powerful effect in atypical absence, tonic, and atonic seizures, and the drug still has a useful place in refractory cases where other medication has failed. Rufinamide is also useful in the various seizure types in the Lennox–Gastaut syndrome and is licensed only for this indication.

Drugs which exacerbate seizures

Carbamazepine and oxcarbazepine are frequently reported to exacerbate atypical absence and tonic seizures. Tiagabine can dramatically worsen atypical absence seizures, resulting sometimes in a rather characteristic non-convulsive status epilepticus. It is probable that gabapentin, pregabalin, and vigabatrin have similar effects. Benzodiazepine can exacerbate tonic seizures, and occasionally precipitate tonic status epilepticus. All drugs can occasionally worsen seizures, emphasizing the individual nature of response.

Tailoring drugs to different patient profiles

In spite of the lack of differentiation between drugs in the regulatory trials, it is clear in routine clinical practice that there are qualitative differences, in their antiepileptic potency, their side effects, and their tolerability. The art of good epilepsy therapy is to tailor a drug to individual patient needs. People differ, for instance, in their willingness to risk specific side effects (e.g. weight gain). Preferences will depend on age, gender, comorbidity, co-medication and dosing frequencies, cost, and such factors as risks in pregnancy In Table 23.3 are some examples of factors which commonly influence the use of some drugs.

Although large fortunes have been sunk into pharmacogenetics, no genetic predisposition has been identified in any situation which helps predict who will respond and who will not to any specific drug. Given the heterogeneity of epilepsy and the importance of environmental factors, this is perhaps not surprising. Prescribing patterns also vary depending on other factors such marketing pressures, the medical system, teaching, and information sources and there are surprisingly large differences in the relative use of drugs in different countries.

Side effects

The side effects of AEDs are a major factor influencing drug choice, not least because the efficacy of different drugs, in population terms shows little difference (19). Each drug has a specific side-effect profile and these are outlined in more detail in Chapter 26. However, the following side effects are those which are most frequently influence drug choice:

1. Weight gain—and those who are overweight might be keener to try topiramate or zonisamide which both typically result in weight loss, rather than gabapentin, pregabalin or valproate which typically result in weight gain.

Table 23.3 Tailoring antiepileptic drugs in partial-onset epilepsy to patient characteristics (based on preferences from the author's clinical practice)

Patient characteristics	Drugs that are particularly suitable	Drugs that should be particularly avoided
Patients with severe partial-onset seizures	Clobazam, carbamazepine, lacosamide, levetiracetam, oxcarbazepine, phenytoin, topiramate, zonisamide	Gabapentin, lamotrigine, valproate
Patients who wish particularly to avoid cosmetic effects		Phenobarbital, phenytoin, primidone, valproate (for its effects on hair)
Patients with prominent anxiety	Clobazam (and other benzodiazepines), carbamazepine, gabapentin, phenobarbital, pregabalin, valproate	Levetiracetam
Patients with prominent depression	Carbamazepine, lamotrigine, valproate	Levetiracetam, vigabatrin, phenobarbital
Patients with renal stones		Acetazolamide topiramate, zonisamide,
Patients with migraine	Topiramate, valproate	
Patients with the need to lose weight (or not to gain weight)	Topiramate, zonisamide	Gabapentin, pregabalin, valproate
Patients with foreign tissue lesional epilepsy (e.g. tumour)	Carbamazepine, clobazam, levetiracetam, oxcarbazepine, phenytoin, tiagabine	
Patients with hyponatraemia		Carbamazepine, oxcarbazepine,
Patients at particular risk from allergy	Clobazam, gabapentin, lacosamide, levetiracetam, pregabalin, topiramate, vigabatrin	Acetazolamide, carbamazepine, felbamate, lamotrigine, oxcarbazepine, phenytoin, zonisamide
Patients at particular risk of heart disease		Carbamazepine, lacosamide, lamotrigine, oxcarbazepine
Patients at risk from osteoporosis	Gabapentin, levetiracetam, pregabalin	Phenobarbital, phenytoin
Patients in whom the risk of hepatic enzyme interactions have to be avoided (e.g. those co-mediated with antibiotics, immunosuppressive drugs, oncological drugs, antipsychotics, etc.)	Clobazam, gabapentin, lacosamide, levetiracetam, pregabalin, topiramate, vigabatrin	

Derived from Shorvon (14).

2. Psychological effects the patient's affective and psychological states are important considerations in drug choice. Some drugs, notably valproate and carbamazepine tend to stabilize mood. Levetiracetam tends to cause anxiety and agitation, and particularly so in patients already anxious or agitated. Phenobarbital and the benzodiazepines tend to exacerbate depression and sedation.
3. Teratogenicity—in women planning to embark on pregnancy, valproate is relatively contraindicated and only carbamazepine and lamotrigine, and possibly levetiracetam, have proven relative safety.
4. Cosmetic effects—phenytoin and barbiturate are associated with long-term cosmetic effects not shared with other antiepileptics. Valproate can cause hair loss.
5. Cognitive impairment—some drugs, notably topiramate, zonisamide, pregabalin, and phenobarbital, have reputations for being more likely to result in sedation or cognitive impairment than other drugs.
6. Comorbidities—these may influence drug choice, depending on the system involved and the therapies employed.

Pharmacokinetics and drug interactions

The pharmacokinetics of individual drugs influences choice. Parameters such as the T_{max}, the half life, the absorption, the mode of metabolism and excretion, the diurnal variation of levels, and the effect of comorbid conditions such as renal or hepatic disease can be clinically important. Drug interactions can have a strong influence of drug choice (20, 21).

Evidence for comparative efficacy in chronic epilepsy—meta-analysis of regulatory drug trials

The US Food and Drug Administration has mandated that all new candidate AEDs must demonstrate superior efficacy to a comparator in a clinical trial, not just simple equivalence. From the clinical (in contrast to the regulatory) perspective, this has had one serious disadvantage—all new drugs have been compared, in the randomized clinical trials, primarily with placebo, rather than with each other. Thus, the trials do not individually give much information to the clinician about the *relative* benefits of individual drugs. One way around this problem has been to perform meta-analyses of trials, and to use meta-analytical statistical methods to compare and contrast the effectiveness of individual drugs trialled against placebo (13). Such analyses have obvious and well-known disadvantages, but potentially provide the best information available for making drug choice. However, in the published meta-analyses all licensed drugs were found to be statistically superior to placebo (and indeed it is on this basis that they are licensed), and although there were sometimes nearly twofold differences between the mean odds ratios of seizure control for different drugs, the confidence intervals were wide and overlap, and thus these differences between drugs were not statistically significant. One criticism of this method of analysis is that drugs are being compared at the dosages used in the clinical trials, and that higher doses of the seemingly less effective drugs might produce better results, and it remains true that the regulatory trials and the meta-analysis provide only very limited information about the true utility of a licensed drug in routine clinical practice.

Drug resistance

The concept has recently arisen that some epilepsy is inherently 'drug resistant'. Indeed, the International League Against Epilepsy has even proposed a standardized definition of drug-resistant epilepsy—epilepsy which remains active despite trials of at least two appropriately selected antiepileptic drugs (23). Two predominant theories have been cited to explain resistance: that this is due to genetic changes in enzymes which transport drugs across the blood–brain barrier (notably p-glycoprotein coded by the *ABCB1* gene) or in drug-target proteins (for instance, the gamma-aminobutyric acid (GABA) receptor). However, as not all drugs are transported by the same enzymes, or indeed any transporter enzymes at all, and as different drugs act at different targets or multiple targets, the concept of universal drug resistance due to such genetic variation is untenable. Furthermore, other factors are associated with resistance, including the nature of the underlying aetiology, the cerebral position and size of a structural aetiology such as a tumour, the syndrome, the severity, or duration of epilepsy, presence of associated handicap, environmental and provoking factors, hepatic enzyme induction, drug dosage, receptor upregulation, and so on. Also, as discussed in the following section, many patients attain good periods of remission after more than two drugs have proved ineffective. For all these reasons, a unitary concept of drug-resistance, at least to this author, seems an illusory one. Epilepsy is too heterogenous a condition, and its treatment also too various, for this concept to have any meaningful validity.

A treatment protocol in chronic epilepsy

Recent studies have shown that a systematic approach to the AED therapy of chronic patients can result in seizure freedom in about 30% of cases and significant improvement in a further 50%. Taking a nihilistic view (that nothing can be done to improve seizure control in chronic epilepsy) is a common mistake which consigns many patients to lifelong disability. When first seeing a patient with chronic uncontrolled epilepsy, a two-stage procedure should be adopted: first, assessment and second, a treatment plan should be devised (14, 24) (Table 23.4).

Table 23.4 Two-stage approach to therapy in chronic active epilepsy

Assessment
◆ Review diagnosis and aetiology (history, EEG, imaging) ◆ Classify seizures and syndrome ◆ Review compliance ◆ Review drug history (including dose, length of therapy, and reasons for discontinuation): ▪ Which drugs were useful in the past? ▪ Which drugs were not useful in the past? ▪ Which drugs have not been used in the past? ◆ Review precipitants and non-pharmacological factors
Treatment plan
◆ Document proposed sequence of AEDs to 'trial' ◆ Decide the duration of drug 'trials' ◆ Decide which background medication to continue and to withdraw ◆ Consider non-pharmacological measures (lifestyle, alternative therapy, etc.) ◆ Consider surgical therapy ◆ Recognize the limitations of therapy ◆ Provide information on these to patient

Assessment

The assessment of all patients presenting with chronic epilepsy should consider the following points:

Review the diagnosis of epilepsy

In up to 20% of patients referred to specialized clinics because of apparent chronic epilepsy, the seizures are not predominately epileptic in origin. Misdiagnosis arises most commonly in relation to psychogenic seizures, reflex syncope, and cardiac arrhythmia. A detailed eye-witness account of the attacks therefore should be obtained and will usually be diagnostic. A series of normal electroencephalogram (EEG) results should alert one to the possibility that the attacks are non-epileptic, although this is not an infallible rule. An invaluable aid to diagnosis can be the viewing of a recording of the attack made by home video or on a mobile phone.

Establish aetiology

The cause of the epilepsy must be established. This is important as specific cerebral conditions may require therapy in their own right, and also because prognosis and response to therapy are strongly influenced by the underlying cause. This may require MRI scanning and/or other investigations. A high-quality MRI scan is a mandatory test in a patient with chronic epilepsy without a known cause.

Classify seizure type and syndrome

Knowledge of the syndrome and seizure type guides the choice of medication and other therapies. Accurate seizure and syndrome classification requires a detailed clinical history and EEG.

Review previous treatment history

The response to an AED is, generally speaking, relatively consistent over time. A knowledge of the previous treatment history is therefore vital to the formulation of a rational treatment plan. This part of the history is often overlooked.

Review compliance

Erratic compliance can be a reason for poor seizure control. A drug wallet, filled up for the whole week, can be of great assistance for patients who often forget to take the medication.

Treatment plan

A key step in the successful treatment of chronic epilepsy is the development of a prospective treatment plan. This should be based on the assessment, and the plan should be documented in medical records and discussed with the patient.

Although, as mentioned earlier, none of the currently available first- and second-line drugs have been shown conclusively significantly more efficacious than any other in population terms, individual patients who have failed to respond to one drug may well respond to an alternative (17, 25–28). It follows from this that the only logical approach to approach AED treatment, in a patient in whom improvements in seizure control are desired, is to try one suitable drug after another. The treatment plan therefore should comprise, at its heart, a sequence of what are in effect n = 1 treatment trials, each to be tried in turn if the previous trial fails to meet the targeted level of seizure control.

Such a sequence of drug changes can take months to complete and requires patience and tenacity. The procedure should be explained in advance to the patient to maintain confidence and compliance. Ideally, each antiepileptic should be tried in a reasonable dose added to a baseline drug regimen—usually one or two other AEDs—and as the drug is added, withdrawal or change in dose of other drugs may be needed. Thus decisions have to be made about: which drugs to trial and in what sequence, and which drugs to retain as a baseline regime; which drugs to withdraw; the duration of each treatment trial.

The treatment plan can take a number of months to complete, requiring patience and tenacity, and the procedure should be explained in advance to the patient to maintain confidence and compliance. This needs the expenditure of time and effort by the doctor, who should be available throughout for guidance and reassurance. Perseverance brings rewards, however, and the resolute will, following this protocol, become established on effective long-term therapy.

The effectiveness of this approach was shown in one study in which a total of 265 drug additions were studied in 155 adult patients with chronic epilepsy (defined as epilepsy active at least 5 years after and initiation of therapy) (17). Other therapy was varied (and some drugs withdrawn) according to normal clinic practice. If one drug addition was ineffective, another would be tried. Of the 155 patients, the study found that after one, two, or three drug additions, 28% overall were rendered seizure free by this protocol of active medication change. Sixteen per cent of all drug additions resulted in seizure freedom (defined as seizure freedom at last follow-up for 12 months or longer), and a 50–99% seizure reduction occurred in a further 21%.

Choice of drug to trial and to retain as the baseline regimen

The drugs should be selected from those which have either not been previously used in optimal doses or which have been used and did prove helpful. Rational choices therefore depend on a well-documented history of previous drug therapy. A most important element of the treatment plan is to decide the 'batting order' of drug trials and this will depend on seizure type, side effects, interactions, the patient profile, personal preference and other factors.

The new drugs added to a regimen should be introduced slowly. This results in better tolerability. It is usual to aim initially for a low maintenance dose and then to titrate upwards depending on response, but in severe epilepsy, higher doses are often required right away.

Choice of drugs to withdraw and the drug withdrawal process

Drugs which should be considered for withdrawal are those which have been given in the past in an adequate trial at optimal doses and which were either ineffective or caused unacceptable side effects. Drug withdrawal needs care, and should be carried out in a gradual step-wise fashion. The sudden reduction in dose of an AED can result in a severe worsening of seizures or in status epilepticus. Only one drug should be withdrawn at a time. If the withdrawal period is likely to be difficult, the dangers can be reduced by covering withdrawal with a benzodiazepine drug (usually clobazam 10 mg at day), given during the phase of active withdrawal. A benzodiazepine can also be given in clustering of seizures following withdrawal. If seizures dramatically worsen during the period of withdrawal, the drug should usually be rapidly reinstated. The patient should have access to immediate specialist advice during a withdrawal period.

Duration of treatment trial

This will depend on the baseline seizure rate. The trial should be long enough to have differentiated the effect of therapy from that of chance fluctuations in seizures. If the seizures are very frequent, it will take only a few weeks to ascertain whether or not the new drug is having any effect.

Serum level monitoring and drug interactions

For drugs where effectiveness and/or side effects are closely linked to serum level—notably phenytoin, carbamazepine, and phenobarbital—measurement of the serum level can be helpful in deciding dosage. Monitoring serum level is particularly important for phenytoin which has a non-linear relationship between dose and serum level.

Intractability and the limits of drug therapy

Drug therapy will fail to control seizures completely in about 10–30% of patients with epilepsy. In this situation, the epilepsy can be categorized as 'intractable' and therapy should provide in these patients the best compromise between inadequate seizure control and drug induced side effects. Individual patients will take very different view about where to strike this balance. Intractability is inevitably an arbitrary decision.

Lifestyle measures

Although this chapter is focused primarily on drug treatment, it must be emphasized that this is only part of an approach to therapy. Many seizures are provoked by factors such as stress, tiredness, emotional disturbance, circadian rhythms, the menstrual cycle, alcohol, and lack of sleep. Avoiding provoking factors can be extremely important. Such 'lifestyle' manipulation can assist drug therapy and render a previously refractory epilepsy completely controlled. These factors should not be overlooked. Their importance varies according to the type of epilepsy. In IGE, especially in adolescence, the avoidance of sleep deprivation or excessive alcohol intake can be very beneficial. Many patients learn to recognize dangerous times, and take individual avoidance measures. Photosensitive patients should be counselled to avoid relevant stimuli. Occasionally, patients with established mild epilepsy can avoid drug treatment altogether with these simple measures. Alternative or complementary medicine can be a useful adjunct to therapy (22).

Surgical and dietary therapy

Resective surgical therapy for epilepsy should be considered in all patients with chronic epilepsy, both adults and children (28) although it will be possible or appropriate in only a small minority (perhaps 5%). In adults, surgery is most effective in lesional and in mesial temporal lobe epilepsy, where surgical therapy can result in seizure freedom in about 50% of cases and significant improvement in a further 30% (29, 30, 31). In other clinical situations, the outcome of surgery is less good. The assessment of a patient for suitability for epilepsy surgery should be carried out in experienced centres, where the necessary experience and resources are available. Surgical therapy is considered further in Chapters 27–29.

Vagal nerve stimulation is another option for intractable epilepsy, but must be considered palliative only, and very few patients become seizure-free using this technique and few benefit in the longer term.

The ketogenic diet is the only dietary therapy shown in randomized studies to be effective in epilepsy, but its use is restricted to children with severe epilepsy and in status epilepticus (33) (see Chapter 12).

Prognosis of chronic epilepsy—patterns of remission and relapse

It has been long recognized that the majority of people with epilepsy who enter seizure remission do so early in the course of the condition (2, 3, 5–7, 34, 35). The related proposition that, if early treatment is unsuccessful, then the patient is likely to develop chronic epilepsy resistant to any treatment (7) is unduly pessimistic. It is clear that patients enter remission after several years of continuous activity and after trials of more than two drugs (3, 17, 25–28, 34–38).

At a population level, the patterns of remission and relapse during the course of their epilepsy in people with chronic epilepsy have been investigated in a recent study, in which a model of prognosis was proposed (Fig. 23.1) (39). According to this model, about 60% of people developing epilepsy will go into long-term (probably permanent) remission within 5 years of diagnosis (pathway a). To what extent this good prognosis simply represents the natural history of benign epilepsy or is a treatment effect is not known—but probably both play a part. The other people (40%) still have active epilepsy at 5 years after onset (i.e. are classified as 'chronic' epilepsy; pathway b). About 10% of these patients will enter subsequent long-term remission (pathway c) and included in this group are some of the age-specific epilepsy syndromes. About 20% of persons have continuous epilepsy, with no periods of remission (pathway d), and about 10% epilepsy with an intermittent pattern of relapse and remission (pathway e).

Of course, it needs to be emphasized that seizure freedom is not the only good outcome, and therapy will often reduce the severity, timing, or frequency of seizures in beneficial ways which are not represented in this model.

Acknowledgements

This chapter is partly derived from Shorvon S. *Handbook of Epilepsy Treatment* (3rd edn). Oxford: Wiley Blackwell, 2009. This work

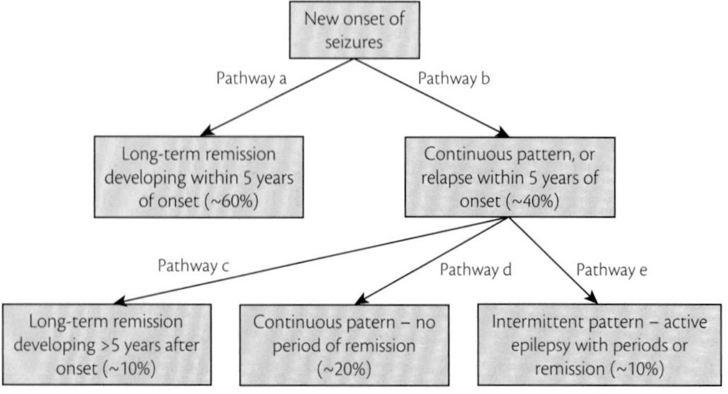

Fig. 23.1 Patterns of epilepsy over time. Neligan A, Bell G, Sander S, Shorvon S. How refractory is refractory epilepsy? Patterns of relapse and remission in refractory epilepsy. *Epilepsy Res* 2011; 96 (3):225–30.

was undertaken at UCLH/UCL who received a proportion of funding from the Department of Health's NIHR Biomedical Research Centres funding scheme.

References

1. Shorvon S. The treatment of chronic epilepsy: a review of recent studies of clinical efficacy and side effects. *Curr Opin Neurol* 2007; 20: 159–63.
2. Shorvon SD. The temporal aspects of prognosis in epilepsy. *J Neurol Neurosurg Psychiatry* 1984; 47: 1157–65.
3. Annegers JF, Hauser WA, Elveback LR. Remission of seizures and relapse in patients with epilepsy. *Epilepsia* 1979; 20: 729–37.
4. Geerts A, Arts WF, Stroink H, Peeters E, Brouwer O, Peters B, *et al.* Course and outcome of childhood epilepsy: a 15-year follow-up of the Dutch Study of Epilepsy in Childhood. *Epilepsia* 2010; 51: 1189–97.
5. Lindsten H, Stenlund H, Forsgren L. Remission of seizures in a population-based adult cohort with a newly diagnosed unprovoked epileptic seizure. *Epilepsia* 2001; 42: 1025–30.
6. MacDonald BK, Johnson AL, Goodridge DM, Cockerell OC, Sander JW, Shorvon SD. Factors predicting prognosis of epilepsy after presentation with seizures. *Ann Neurol* 2000; 48: 833–41.
7. Kwan P, Brodie MJ. Early identification of refractory epilepsy. *N Engl J Med* 2000; 342: 314–19.
8. Semah F, Picot MC, Adam C, Broglin D, Arzimanoglou A, Bazin B, *et al.* Is the underlying cause of epilepsy a major prognostic factor for recurrence? *Neurology* 1998; 51: 1256–62.
9. Moran NF, Poole K, Bell G, Solomon J, Kendall S, McCarthy M, *et al.* Epilepsy in the United Kingdom: seizure frequency and severity, anti-epileptic drug utilization and impact on life in 1652 people with epilepsy. *Seizure* 2004; 13: 425–33.
10. Shorvon SD. Historical introduction: The causes of epilepsy in the pre-molecular era (1860–1960). In: Shorvon SD, Andermann F, Guerrini R (eds) *The Causes of Epilepsy Common and Uncommon Causes in Adults and Children*, pp. 1–20. Cambridge: Cambridge University Press, 2011.
11. French JA, Kanner AM, Bautista J, Abou-Khalil B, Browne T, Harden CL, *et al.* Efficacy and tolerability of the new antiepileptic drugs II: treatment of refractory epilepsy: report of the Therapeutics and Technology Assessment Subcommittee and Quality Standards Subcommittee of the American Academy of Neurology and the American Epilepsy Society. *Neurology* 2004; 62: 1261–73.
12. Levy RH, Mattson RH, Meldrum B, Perucca E. *Antiepileptic drugs* (5th edn). Philadelphia, PA: Lippincott, Williams & Wilkins, 2002.
13. Shorvon SD. Management of chronic epilepsy. In: Shorvon SD, Perucca E, Engel J (eds) *Treatment of epilepsy* (3rd edn), pp. 153–62. Oxford: Blackwell Science, 2009.
14. Shorvon SD. *Handbook of the treatment of epilepsy* (3rd edn). Oxford: Wiley-Blackwell, 2010.
15. Glauser T, Ben-Menachem E, Bourgeois B, Cnaan A, Chadwick D, Guerreiro C, *et al.* ILAE treatment guidelines: evidence-based analysis of antiepileptic drug efficacy and effectiveness as initial monotherapy for epileptic seizures and syndromes. *Epilepsia* 2006; 47: 1094–120.
16. Marson AG, Al-Kharusi AM, Alwaidh M, Appleton R, Baker GA, Chadwick DW; SANAD Study group. The SANAD study of effectiveness of carbamazepine, gabapentin, lamotrigine, oxcarbazepine, or topiramate for treatment of partial epilepsy: an unblended randomized controlled trial. *Lancet* 2007; 369: 1000–15.
17. Luciano AL, Shorvon SD. Results of treatment changes in patients with apparently drug- resistant chronic epilepsy. *Ann Neurol* 2007; 62: 375–81.
18. Genton P, Gelisse P, Thomas P. Juvenile myoclonic epilepsy today: Current definitions and limits. In: Schmitz B, Sander T (eds) *Juvenile Myoclonic Epilepsy: The Janz Syndrome*, pp. 11–32. Stroud: Wrightson Biomedical Publishing Ltd, 2000.
19. Zaccara G, Franciotta D, Perucca E. Idiosyncratic adverse reactions to antiepileptic drugs. *Epilepsia* 2007; 48: 1223–44.
20. Patsalos PN, Perucca E. Clinically important drug interactions in epilepsy: interactions between antiepileptic drugs and other drugs. *Lancet Neurol* 2003; 2: 473–81.
21. Patsalos PN, Perucca E. Clinically important drug interactions in epilepsy: general features and interactions between antiepileptic drugs. *Lancet Neurol* 2003; **2**: 347–56.
22. Ricotti V, Delanty N. Use of complementary and alternative medicine in epilepsy. *Curr Neurol Neurosci Rep* 2006; 6: 347–53.
23. Kwan P, Arzimanoglou A, Berg AT, Brodie MJ, Allen Hauser W, Mathern G, *et al.* Definition of drug resistant epilepsy: consensus proposal by the AD hoc Task Force of the ILAE Commission on Therapeutic Strategies. *Epilepsia* 2010; 51: 1069–77.
24. Shorvon SD. Medical assessment and treatment of chronic epilepsy. *Br Med J* 1991; 302: 363–6.
25. Schiller Y. Seizure relapse and development of drug resistance following long-term seizure remission. *Arch Neurol* 2009; 66: 1233–9.
26. Berg AT, Levy SR, Testa FM, D'Souza R. Remission of epilepsy after two drug failures in children: a prospective study. *Ann Neurol* 2009; 65: 510–19.
27. Callaghan BC, Anand K, Hesdorffer D, Hauser WA, French JA. Likelihood of seizure remission in an adult population with refractory epilepsy. *Ann Neurol* 2007; 62: 382–9.
28. Choi H, Heiman G, Pandis D, Cantero J, Resor SR, Gilliam FG, *et al.* Seizure remission and relapse in adults with intractable epilepsy: a cohort study. *Epilepsia* 2008; 49: 1440–5.
29. Jeha LE, Najm IM, Bingaman WE, Khandwala F, Widdess-Walsh P, Morris HH, *et al.* Predictors of outcome after temporal lobectomy for the treatment of intractable epilepsy. *Neurology* 2006; 66:1938–40.
30. de Tisi J, Bell GS, Peacock JL, McEvoy AW, Harkness WF, Sander JW, *et al.* The long-term outcome of adult epilepsy surgery, patterns of seizure remission, and relapse: a cohort study. *Lancet* 2011; 378(9800):1388–95.
31. Cross JH, Jayakar P, Nordli D, Delalande O, Duchowny M, Wieser HG, *et al.* International League against Epilepsy, Subcommission for Paediatric Epilepsy Surgery; Commissions of Neurosurgery and Paediatrics. Proposed criteria for referral and evaluation of children for epilepsy surgery: recommendations of the Subcommission for Pediatric Epilepsy Surgery. *Epilepsia.* 2006; 47:952–9.
32. Cohen-Gadol AA, Wilhelmi BG, Collignon F, White JB, Britton JW, Cambier DM, *et al.* Long-term outcome of epilepsy surgery among 399 patients with nonlesional seizure foci including mesial temporal lobe sclerosis. *J Neurosurg* 2006; 104:513–24.
33. Keene DL. A systematic review of the use of the ketogenic diet in childhood epilepsy. *Pediatr Neurol* 2006; 35:1–5.
34. Goodridge DM, Shorvon SD. Epileptic seizures in a population of 6000. II: Treatment and prognosis. *Br Med J* 1983; 287: 645–7.
35. Shorvon S, Luciano AL. Prognosis of chronic and newly diagnosed epilepsy: revisiting temporal aspects. *Curr Opin Neurol* 2007b; 20: 208–12.
36. Del Felice A, Beghi E, Boero G *et al.* Early versus late remission in a cohort of patients with newly diagnosed epilepsy. *Epilepsia* 2010; 51: 37–42.
37. Shorvon SD, Sander JW. Temporal patterns of remission and relapse in patients with epilepsy. Schmidt D, Morceli P. (eds) *Intractable Epilepsy: experimental and clinical aspects*, pp. 13–23. New York: Raven Press, 1986.
38. Sillanpaa M, Schmidt D. Natural history of treated childhood-onset epilepsy: prospective, long-term population-based study. *Brain* 2006; 129: 617–24.
39. Neligan A, Bell G, Sander S, Shorvon S. How refractory is refractory epilepsy? Patterns of relapse and remission in refractory epilepsy. *Epilepsy Res* 2011; 96(3):225–30.

CHAPTER 24

Epilepsy in Remission

Jerry J. Shih

Introduction

The question of whether an epileptic condition is likely to go into remission is arguably the single most important question patients have for their treating physicians. When seizures go into remission there is a dramatic increase in quality of life (1, 2) and sense of well-being, as well as the opening up of avenues for employment and greater personal freedoms such as driving (3). Together with being side effect-free on seizure treatment, seizure freedom constitutes one of the major goals of successful epilepsy management.

This topic has been the subject of numerous studies over the past 50 years. However, it is important to note that this extensive literature is not homogenous. Methodologies differ, and research design varies greatly based on the specific questions asked. Many of the earlier studies on seizure remission rates were drawn from select populations seen at tertiary medical centres (4). Some more recent studies are retrospective, population-based, and derived from rural populations (5, 6), but may lack the rigorous data collection seen in earlier single centre studies. Studies also differ in terms of when their populations were evaluated vis-à-vis the disease and then remission process. Some studies specifically evaluated patients with newly diagnosed or untreated epilepsy; others recruited only patients who were deemed medically intractable and have failed at least several anticonvulsant medications. Patients with new-onset seizures represent a different epilepsy population than patients who have been refractory to multiple treatment approaches (7). Elderly patients suffering from post-stroke epilepsy have differing outcomes compared to children with familial epilepsies. Thus, in terms of clinical usefulness, any discussion on seizure remission needs to take into account patient demographics and the aetiology of the seizure disorder.

Population-based studies have fairly consistently shown that 60–80% of patients diagnosed with a new-onset seizure disorder will achieve seizure remission in their lifetime (4, 8, 9). We routinely teach neurology trainees the dictum that 'you can make about two-thirds of your epilepsy patients seizure free with antiseizure medication treatment' (Table 24.1). However, depending on the clinical history and epilepsy syndrome, individual patients can expect varying chances of seizure remission. In general, the idiopathic generalized epilepsies have a higher seizure remission rate than partial-onset epilepsy or symptomatic epilepsy (9–11). Certain epilepsy syndromes have a poor prognosis for seizure control. This chapter will review seizure remission rates by age group, epilepsy syndromes, and the specific clinical circumstance of medically refractory epilepsy. Favourable and unfavourable factors affecting outcome will be discussed.

New-onset seizures

By definition, epilepsy is diagnosed after a patient has two or more unprovoked seizures. A person who presents with a single

Table 24.1 Terminal remission data from selected studies (7)

Reference	Study setting	Special study features	No. of patients	Median follow-up (years)	Years in remission	% in remission at median follow-up
Elwes et al. (10)	Hospital		106	5.5	2	79
Shafer et al. (11)	Community		432	17	5	66
Collaborative Group (12)	Hospital		280	4	1	70
Cockerell et al. (13)	Community	Definite epilepsy	564	7	5	68
Sillanpaa et al. (14)	Hospital	Children only	176	28	1	80
Lindsten et al. (15)	Community	≥1 baseline seizure	107	9	5	64
		≥2 baseline seizures	89	9	5	58

Reprinted with permission from Kwan P, Sander JW. *J Neurol Neurosurg Psychiatry* 2004; 75:1376–81.

unprovoked seizure does not carry the epilepsy diagnosis, but by virtue of having the seizure, differs from the general population as far as the risk of developing epilepsy. Population-based studies place the general risk of a person developing epilepsy in her lifetime at 1–3% (12, 13). Prospective studies in the paediatric age group and general population of patients identified after a first unprovoked seizure estimate that about 25% will go on to have a second unprovoked seizure and be classified as epileptic (14, 15). In looking at this from a different perspective, 75% of patients with a single unprovoked seizure will achieve 'remission' without any treatment.

In patients with new-onset epilepsy, several seminal studies over the past 35 years have established the 'two-thirds' dictum. A meta-analysis by Berg and Shinnar (16) of pre-1990 prospective observational studies found that on average, 60% of patients achieve remission as defined by seizure freedom for at least 2 years. In a longitudinal study of patients with epilepsy in Rochester, Minnesota, the probability of being in remission (at least 5 consecutive years seizure free, and continuing) at 20 years after diagnosis was 70% (4) (Fig. 24.1). A large prospective population-based British study enrolling from 275 general practices found a 5-year seizure remission rate of 68% in patients with a 'definite' diagnosis of epilepsy (17). In a prospective single-centre study of newly diagnosed and mostly untreated epilepsy patients, Kwan and Brodie found 63% achieved at least a 1-year seizure remission after anticonvulsant treatment (18). These studies have shown consistently similar results over the last several decades, despite advances in therapy and changes to the classification of seizures and epilepsy (19). This has led to a belief amongst many epileptologists that a majority of patients will achieve seizure remission regardless of the specific form of treatment.

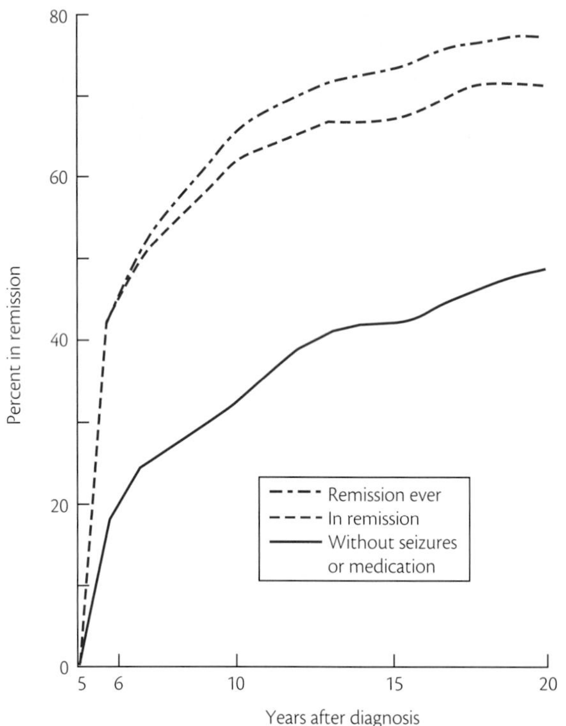

Fig. 24.1 Remission of seizures in epilepsy patients followed in Rochester, MN from 1935–1974. From Annegers et al. *Epilepsia* 1979; 20:729–37, with permission.

An interesting corollary to the question of epilepsy remission with treatment is the issue of *spontaneous* remission of seizures after a diagnosis of epilepsy is made. Because effective drug treatments have been in existence for almost 100 years, there are minimal data regarding the natural history of the untreated disease state. There are no prospective longitudinal studies of untreated epilepsy and the prospect of future studies of this kind is unlikely on ethical grounds. However, data do exist from developing or resource-poor countries (7). Nicoletti et al. (6) conducted an epidemiological survey of an untreated or undertreated population of chronic epileptics in rural Bolivia. At the 10-year point of follow-up, 'adequate' seizure information was obtained from 71 of the 118 people originally identified as having 'active epilepsy'. Of these 71 people, 31 (44%) were in seizure remission defined as seizure free for greater than 5 years. A household survey in Ecuador identified 1029 people with 'probable or definite' epilepsy who were untreated or undertreated, and 31% were in remission for greater than 1 year (5). A retrospective Finnish study of 33 people with untreated epilepsy found a 2-year remission rate of 42% (20). It is important to point out that these studies suffer from methodological limitations which reduce the level of scientific confidence in the results. However, there is no doubt that a small population of persons with epilepsy, whether it be 10%, 20%, or higher, will achieve long-term spontaneous remission of their seizures.

Age and remission rates

The general perception is that seizures beginning in childhood are more likely to go into remission than seizures that start in adulthood, although evidence to that effect is sparse. Some of the earliest data on childhood epilepsy remission rates were derived from a population-based study in Nova Scotia which followed 504 children for an average of 7 years (21). Even though children with absence epilepsy and minor motor seizures were excluded from the analysis, 55% of the cohort was in remission at the end of the follow-up period. A prospective long-term population-based study in Finland followed 144 patients with seizure onset before age 16, an average of 37 years. At the end of follow-up, 67% of 144 patients were in terminal remission, on or off antiepileptic drugs (22). About one-third (31%) had remission from first treatment, while 50% of those in terminal remission did so with a mean delay of 9 years. In a 15-year Dutch follow-up study of patients diagnosed with childhood new-onset epilepsy, 5-year seizure remission was reached by 71% of the cohort (23). Berg and colleagues (11) prospectively followed 613 children with newly diagnosed epilepsy in the US and found a 2-year remission rate of 74%. Age of onset between 5–9 years old was associated with a substantially increased remission rate.

There are far fewer studies evaluating the natural history of adult-onset epilepsy. Elwes et al. (24) prospectively assessed the prognosis for seizure control in 106 patients referred to an adult neurology clinic with previously untreated tonic–clonic, partial, or mixed seizures. After treatment, 73% had at least a 2-year remission period at the end of 4 years. However, only 51 of the 106 patients remained seizure free at the termination of the study. Lindsten et al. (25) followed an adult population-based cohort of 107 patients with newly diagnosed epilepsy for approximately

10 years. One-year, 3-year, and 5-year seizure remission rates were 68%, 64%, and 58%, respectively. Thus, when one compares population-based studies of purely childhood epilepsy versus adult-onset epilepsy, there is no clear difference in seizure remission rate. The perception that childhood onset seizures have a higher remission rate likely stems from some studies with high numbers of patients diagnosed with childhood syndromes associated with excellent long-term prognosis.

Remission rate and epilepsy syndrome

Although the recent International League Against Epilepsy (ILAE) Commission on Classifications recommended changes to terminology and concepts, no changes or revisions were made to the epilepsy syndromes recognized in previous ILAE classifications (19). An epilepsy syndrome is defined as 'a complex of signs and symptoms that define a unique epilepsy condition' (26). The groups of syndromes are: idiopathic focal epilepsies of infancy and childhood, familial (autosomal dominant) focal epilepsies, symptomatic (or probably symptomatic) focal epilepsies, idiopathic generalized epilepsies, reflex epilepsies, epileptic encephalopathies, progressive myoclonus epilepsies, and seizures not necessarily requiring a diagnosis of epilepsy. There are over 25 specific syndromes in the 1989 ILAE report. Many syndromes have been extensively studied, and outcome and prognosis data are available.

Childhood absence epilepsy

Childhood absence epilepsy (CAE) is a distinct syndrome in the ILAE Classification System (19, 27). CAE typically begins between 6–8 years of age. Patients often have multiple absence seizures daily, but are developmentally and cognitively normal. Absence seizures are associated with a generalized 3–4 Hz spike and wave pattern on the electroencephalogram (EEG), and may be provoked by hyperventilation or photic stimulation. An early meta-analysis of the outcome of CAE found widely varying remission rates ranging between 21–89% (28). These differing remission rates stem mainly from methodological differences in classifying CAE, length of follow-up, and the definition of remission. Some studies defined remission as seizure freedom off anticonvulsant treatment for more than 1 year (29, 30). Others used terminal remission defined as seizure freedom for more than 1 year at the end of follow-up (31). The highest remission rate was found in the Dutch Study of Epilepsy in Childhood at 93% being seizure free for greater than 1 year at the end of at least 12 years of follow-up (31). The authors also noted that 67% of the children were free of seizures for over 10 years at study termination. In a further subanalysis, the remission rate was 77% if the criterion of 1-year seizure remission off medication was applied. A North American study of 75 children with CAE found a 2-year remission rate of 88% (11). A study in Nova Scotia followed 82 children with typical CAE a mean of 14 years with the goal of determining the proportion and characteristics of children who were seizure-free for longer than 1 year at the last year of long-term follow-up and who were off of anticonvulsant medications (29). Their remission rate was 65%, and the development of generalized tonic–clonic seizures and myoclonic seizures were poor prognostic signs for remission. Grosso and colleagues retrospectively analysed 119 children who fulfilled the criteria for CAE according to the ILAE classification system (30). The children were further subdivided into two groups depending on whether their histories showed inclusion/exclusion characteristics of 'typical' absence as initially proposed by Panayiotopoulos (32). Children fulfilling the criteria for 'typical absence' had seizure remission rate of 95% versus 77% for the non-Panayiotopoulos group, and terminal remission rates of 82% versus 51%. While this study suffers from the limitations of a retrospective study, it does highlight the fact that there may be subgroups within the broad CAE syndrome with slightly different remission outcomes. Nevertheless, the likelihood of seizure remission for children with CAE is clearly higher than patients in a general population-based study.

Juvenile absence epilepsy

Juvenile absence epilepsy (JAE) is classified as an idiopathic generalized epilepsy. The age of onset is typically at or after puberty between the ages of 10–17. Unlike in CAE where absence seizures can occur many times per day, absence seizures in JAE may only occur sporadically. There is less impairment of consciousness with absence seizures in JAE compared to absences in CAE. Patients with JAE can have generalized tonic–clonic seizures (usually upon awakening), myoclonic seizures, and even absence status epilepticus. There is a strong genetic component with linkage to chromosomes 5, 8, 18, and 21. The response to antiepileptic medication is usually excellent (33). Some of the same longitudinal studies which recruited children with CAE also recruited subjects diagnosed with JAE. The Dutch Study of Epilepsy in Childhood documented a remission rate of 75% in their eight subjects around the 15-year follow-up mark (23). The North American study showed 82% of their 17 JAE patients achieved a 2-year remission; however, three of the 14 (21%) adolescents relapsed when followed for longer periods (11). Therefore, like CAE, JAE is associated with a high likelihood of seizure remission. However, the number of JAE patients in these longitudinal studies is usually smaller, and caution must be used when interpreting these data.

Juvenile myoclonic epilepsy

Juvenile myoclonic epilepsy (JME) is also classified as an idiopathic generalized epilepsy. The age of onset is usually mid teens. Patients may present with myoclonic jerks upon awakening in the morning. The myoclonus usually involves the neck, shoulders, arms, or legs with the upper extremities being more frequently affected. Consciousness is usually not impaired during the myoclonic seizures. Generalized tonic–clonic and absence seizures are also seen. The interictal EEG consists of generalized polyspike and wave discharges greater than 3 Hz (34). There is a strong genetic component with linkage to chromosomes 2, 3, 5, 6, and 15. The North American cohort included 15 patients with JME, eight (53%) of whom achieved a 2-year remission. However, five of the eight patients experienced a relapse during extended follow-up (11). The Dutch cohort had only seven JME patients, and 57% achieved seizure remission (23). Penry et al. retrospectively analysed the data of 50 patients with JME to determine long-term seizure control and relapse rates in response to treatment with valproate (35). Follow-up ranged from 2 months to 9 years. Forty-three patients (86%) were seizure-free for over 1 year, but over half of this group experienced at least one relapse. Most of the relapses consisted of myoclonic seizures. Thus, the response to AED treatment is often good, but there is a high rate of relapse, especially if drug therapy is subtherapeutic or discontinued (33).

Benign childhood epilepsy with centrotemporal spikes

Benign childhood epilepsy with centrotemporal spikes (BECTS) is a common focal onset epilepsy syndrome with an age of onset peaking between 7–10 years of age (36). BECTS is characterized by sensorimotor seizures affecting the facial and oropharyngeal muscles, with clinical manifestations of drooling, dysarthria or anarthria, facial paraesthesias, and twitching of the lower face. Seizures may occasionally evolve to upper extremity clonic shaking or secondarily generalized tonic–clonic seizures. The classic interictal EEG shows high amplitude diphasic spikes in the centrotemporal region(s) with a transverse dipole (37). As the name implies, BECTS is associated with an excellent outcome and high remission rates. The Dutch Study of Epilepsy in Childhood (38) followed 29 children diagnosed with BECTS according to the ILAE classification. After a follow-up period of 12–17 years, 96% had a terminal remission greater than 5 years and 89% greater than 10 years. In a meta-analysis encompassing 13 cohort groups and 794 patients, Bouma et al. (39) found a remission rate of 81–100%, with 99.8% of patients over age 18 being seizure free. These data support the fact that the seizures associated with BECTS are easy to control and will almost always remit by adulthood.

Lennox–Gastaut syndrome

Lennox–Gastaut syndrome (LGS) is classified as an epileptic encephalopathy. The age of onset is usually before age 8 with a peak age of onset between 3–5 years of age. The syndrome is characterized by a triad of multiple seizure types (tonic and atypical absence are the most common), slow spike and wave on EEG (1–2.5 Hz), and some degree of mental retardation. The aetiology can be symptomatic or cryptogenic, and is often a sequelae of infants diagnosed with infantile spasms or West syndrome. Tonic seizures are considered a prerequisite for the diagnosis. The interictal EEG is characterized by slow spike and wave complexes (<2.5 Hz) and activation of generalized paroxysmal fast activity during sleep. The seizures in LGS are typically refractory to medical treatment (40). The North American study (11) found only one of 19 children (5%) diagnosed with LGS achieved a 2-year remission (Table 24.2). That subject went on to relapse on later follow-up. None of the five children with LGS in the Dutch study (23) achieved remission.

Mesial temporal lobe epilepsy with hippocampal sclerosis

Mesial temporal lobe epilepsy with hippocampal sclerosis (MTLE-HS) is a symptomatic focal epilepsy and subcategorized as a limbic epilepsy. The age of onset is typically between late childhood to mid adolescence. Most patients report an aura, which consists of an epigastric sensation (a rising sensation, butterflies, nausea), fear, olfactory hallucinations, lightheadedness, or déjà vu (41). Seizure semiology often involve impairment of cognition and awareness as well as ipsilateral upper extremity automatisms, contralateral dystonic posturing, Todd's paralysis, and late forced head turning prior to secondary generalization.

MTLE-HS is often refractory to anticonvulsant drug treatment and one of the most common types of epilepsy referred for epilepsy surgery. Kim et al. (42) followed 104 patients with MRI evidence of mesial temporal sclerosis for more than 2 years. Only 25% of this cohort entered into a 1-year seizure remission period. In a large hospital-based survey of over 2200 adult patients with varying epilepsy diagnoses, only 11% with hippocampal sclerosis were seizure-free with medical treatment (10). Because surgery is considered superior to medications for the treatment of mesial temporal lobe epilepsy (43), most of the seizure remission data for MTLE-HS come from the surgical literature. The majority of patients who undergo surgical resection for MTLE-HS become seizure free (44, 45), with the accepted rate of remission around 70–80%.

Remission rate in medically refractory epilepsy

Epileptologists have long recognized that a subpopulation of persons with epilepsy continues to have recurrent seizures despite multiple medication trials. Terms that have been used to describe these patients include chronic epilepsy, pharmacoresistant, medication resistant, medically intractable, and medically refractory. For our purposes, the term medically refractory will be used. The current definition of medically refractory epilepsy that is accepted by most epileptologists encompasses: (1) failure to achieve seizure freedom after at least two appropriate medication trials, (2) at least one seizure per month for at least the past 3 months. The Glasgow study gave us an indication that seizure remission rates diminished significantly after two medication trials (18). While 47% of the initial Glasgow cohort became seizure free with the first medication tried and an additional 13% went into seizure remission with the second drug, only 4% became seizure free with further medication trials. Callaghan and colleagues identified 246 patients in a single medical centre with medically refractory epilepsy in 2003 and prospectively followed them for up to 7 years (46, 47). The 12-month seizure remission rate was 5% per year, but 71% of these patients experienced a breakthrough seizure within 5 years. A retrospective single centre cohort of 187 medically refractory epilepsy patients was followed for a mean of almost 6 years (48, 49). Using Kaplan–Meier analysis, the investigators found the probability of attaining 1-year seizure remission to be 3–4% per year. However, of those achieving remission, the cumulative probability of seizure relapse was 81%. A population-based cohort of 128 children who failed two drugs was prospectively followed for at least 1 year (50). Seventy-three children (57%) had a remission period of greater than 1 year. However, of the 124 children followed for 3 years, only 28 (23%) achieved a greater than 3-year remission rate at last contact, leading the authors to conclude that remission after two-drug failure in children was common but often temporary. The overall data for seizure control in medically refractory epilepsy demonstrate the chances for seizure remission to be low, with the added unfortunate factor of a fairly high relapse rate. Children have a better prognosis than adults.

Prognostic factors for seizure remission

Different studies have used different methodologies, and prognostic factors which were analysed varied between studies, making strong conclusions untenable. In addition, there are only a few papers with multivariate analysis, and the potential interaction between prognostic factors is not well studied. Nevertheless, a few consistent factors emerge for both positive and negative prognosis for seizure remission. Positive predictors for seizure remission include the diagnosis of one of the benign idiopathic epilepsies such as BECTS, CAE, and JAE. Young age of seizure onset, a normal

Table 24.2 Remission rates by syndromes (11)

Syndrome grouping[a]	No. total after 2-year reassessment of syndromes and aetiology	No. (%) achieving 2-year remission	No. (%) relapse
Total	594	441 (74)	107 (24)
Partial epilepsies	354	274 (77)	65 (24)
Idiopathic partial:	62	55 (93)	4 (7)
Benign rolandic	59	52 (88)	3 (6)
Benign occipital	3	3 (100)	1 (33)
Symptomatic partial:	205	147 (72)	44 (30)
Cryptogenic partial	87	72 (83)	7 (24)
Generalized epilepsies	191	132 (69)	32 (24)
Idiopathic generalized (IGE):	133	111 (83)	28 (25)
Benign myoclonic epilepsy in infancy	2	2 (100)	0 (0)
Childhood absence	75	66 (88)	15 (23)
Juvenile absence	17	14 (82)	3 (21)
Juvenile myoclonic	15	8 (53)	5 (63)
With generalized tonic–clonic seizure on awakening	2	1 (50)	1 (100)
Other IGE/unclassified IGE	18	17 (94)	3 (19)
With specific modes of precipitation	4	3 (75)	1 (33)
Symptomatic/cryptogenic generalized:	49	20 (41)	4 (20)
Not further classified	3	1 (33)	—
West	17	9 (53)	1 (11)
Lennox–Gastaut	19	1 (5)	1 (100)
Doose	8	7 (88)	1 (14)
With myoclonic absence	2	2 (100)	1 (50)
Symptomatic generalized:	9	1 (11)	0 (0)
With non-specific aetiology	3	0 (0)	—
With specific aetiology	6	1 (17)	0 (0)
Epilepsies of undetermined onset	49	36 (73)	10 (28)
Undetermined with both focal and generalized features	2	1 (50)	1 (100)
Undetermined without unequivocal focal or generalized features	47	35 (74)	9 (26)

[a]A few syndromes with only a single individual were not shown but included in the more general category under which they fell.
From Berg AT et al. *Epilepsia* 2001; 42:1553–62, with permission.

neurological examination, and generalized onset seizures all portend a higher likelihood for seizure remission (8, 51, 52). As shown earlier in this chapter, continued seizure activity after adequate trials of two to three first-line anticonvulsant drugs portends a lower possibility of sustained seizure remission. In addition, the duration of active seizure activity is inversely correlated to the chances of becoming seizure free. Annegers et al. (4) demonstrated that only around 10% of their initial cohort entered remission if the period of active epilepsy was greater than 4 years, with less than 5% achieving seizure freedom if their seizures were uncontrolled for greater than 10 years. Frequent generalized tonic–clonic seizures, the presence of multiple seizure types, epileptiform abnormalities on the EEG, structural abnormalities on brain imaging, and the presence of mental retardation also are poor prognostic factors for seizure remission (51, 53–57). Frequent seizures ('high density') after initial diagnosis was also found to be a negative predictor (58).

Conclusion

The prognosis for persons with epilepsy to enter remission is generally favourable. Data from resource-poor countries indicate that even some untreated or undertreated patients will spontaneously become seizure free. With appropriate treatment, about two-thirds of people will achieve seizure remission. Certain syndromes such as BECTS, CAE, and JAE are associated with a high likelihood of seizure control. Other syndromes such as LGS and MTLE-HS are associated with a poor overall prognosis (LGS) or poor prognosis with medication treatment (MTLE-HS). Clearly, there is a minority of epilepsy patients who become medically refractory, and currently are unlikely to achieve any prolonged period of seizure remission. It is for this population of patients that newer treatment options can make the most dramatic impact.

References

1. Tellez-Zenteno JF, Dhar R, Wiebe S. Long-term seizure outcomes following epilepsy surgery: a systematic review and meta-analysis. *Brain* 2005; 128(Pt 5):1188–98.
2. Spencer SS, Berg AT, Vickrey BG, Sperling MR, Bazil CW, Haut S, *et al.* Health-related quality of life over time since resective epilepsy surgery. *Ann Neurol* 2007; 62(4):327–34.
3. Shih JJ, Ochoa JG. A systematic review of antiepileptic drug initiation and withdrawal. *Neurologist.* 2009; 15(3):122–31.
4. Annegers JF, Hauser WA, Elveback LR. Remission of seizures and relapse in patients with epilepsy. *Epilepsia* 1979; 20(6):729–37.
5. Placencia M, Sander JW, Roman M, Madera A, Crespo F, Cascante S, *et al.* The characteristics of epilepsy in a largely untreated population in rural Ecuador. *J Neurol Neurosurg Psychiatry* 1994; 57(3):320–5.
6. Nicoletti A, Sofia V, Vitale G, Bonelli SI, Bejarano V, Bartalesi F, *et al.* Natural history and mortality of chronic epilepsy in an untreated population of rural Bolivia: a follow-up after 10 years. *Epilepsia* 2009; 50(10):2199–206.
7. Kwan P, Sander JW. The natural history of epilepsy: an epidemiological view. *J Neurol Neurosurg Psychiatry* 2004; 75(10):1376–81.
8. Goodridge DM, Shorvon SD. Epileptic seizures in a population of 6000. II: Treatment and prognosis. *Br Med J (Clin Res Ed)* 1983; 287(6393):645–7.
9. Sillanpaa M, Jalava M, Kaleva O, Shinnar S. Long-term prognosis of seizures with onset in childhood. *N Engl J Med* 1998; 338(24):1715–22.
10. Semah F, Picot MC, Adam C, Broglin D, Arzimanoglou A, Bazin B, *et al.* Is the underlying cause of epilepsy a major prognostic factor for recurrence? *Neurology* 1998; 51(5):1256–62.
11. Berg AT, Shinnar S, Levy SR, Testa FM, Smith-Rapaport S, Beckerman B, *et al.* Two-year remission and subsequent relapse in children with newly diagnosed epilepsy. *Epilepsia* 2001; 42(12):1553–62.
12. Hauser WA, Kurland LT. The epidemiology of epilepsy in Rochester, Minnesota, 1935 through 1967. *Epilepsia* 1975; 16(1):1–66.
13. Juul-Jensen P, Foldspang A. Natural history of epileptic seizures. *Epilepsia* 1983; 24(3):297–312.
14. Hauser WA, Rich SS, Annegers JF, Anderson VE. Seizure recurrence after a 1st unprovoked seizure: an extended follow-up. *Neurology* 1990; 40(8):1163–70.
15. Shinnar S, Berg AT, Moshe SL, Petix M, Maytal J, Kang H, *et al.* Risk of seizure recurrence following a first unprovoked seizure in childhood: a prospective study. *Pediatrics* 1990; 85(6):1076–85.
16. Berg AT, Shinnar S. The risk of seizure recurrence following a first unprovoked seizure: a quantitative review. *Neurology* 1991; 41(7): 965–72.
17. Cockerell OC, Johnson AL, Sander JW, Hart YM, Shorvon SD. Remission of epilepsy: results from the National General Practice Study of Epilepsy. *Lancet* 1995; 346(8968):140–4.
18. Kwan P, Brodie MJ. Early identification of refractory epilepsy. *N Engl J Med* 2000; 342(5):314–19.
19. Berg AT, Berkovic SF, Brodie MJ, Buchhalter J, Cross JH, van Emde Boas W, *et al.* Revised terminology and concepts for organization of seizures and epilepsies: report of the ILAE Commission on Classification and Terminology, 2005-2009. *Epilepsia* 2010; 51(4): 676–85.
20. Keranen T, Riekkinen PJ. Remission of seizures in untreated epilepsy. *BMJ* 1993; 307(6902):483.
21. Camfield C, Camfield P, Gordon K, Smith B, Dooley J. Outcome of childhood epilepsy: a population-based study with a simple predictive scoring system for those treated with medication. *J Pediatr* 1993; 122(6):861–8.
22. Sillanpaa M, Schmidt D. Natural history of treated childhood-onset epilepsy: prospective, long-term population-based study. *Brain* 2006; 129(Pt 3):617–24.
23. Geerts A, Arts WF, Stroink H, Peeters E, Brouwer O, Peters B, *et al.* Course and outcome of childhood epilepsy: a 15-year follow-up of the Dutch Study of Epilepsy in Childhood. *Epilepsia* 2010; 51(7):1189–97.
24. Elwes RD, Johnson AL, Shorvon SD, Reynolds EH. The prognosis for seizure control in newly diagnosed epilepsy. *N Engl J Med* 1984; 311(15):944–7.
25. Lindsten H, Stenlund H, Forsgren L. Remission of seizures in a population-based adult cohort with a newly diagnosed unprovoked epileptic seizure. *Epilepsia* 2001; 42(8):1025–30.
26. Engel J, Jr. A proposed diagnostic scheme for people with epileptic seizures and with epilepsy: report of the ILAE Task Force on Classification and Terminology. *Epilepsia* 2001; 42(6):796–803.
27. Proposal for revised classification of epilepsies and epileptic syndromes. Commission on Classification and Terminology of the International League Against Epilepsy. *Epilepsia* 1989; 30(4):389–99.
28. Bouma PA, Westendorp RG, van Dijk JG, Peters AC, Brouwer OF. The outcome of absence epilepsy: a meta-analysis. *Neurology* 1996; 47(3):802–8.
29. Wirrell EC, Camfield CS, Camfield PR, Gordon KE, Dooley JM. Long-term prognosis of typical childhood absence epilepsy: remission or progression to juvenile myoclonic epilepsy. *Neurology* 1996; 47(4):912–18.
30. Grosso S, Galimberti D, Vezzosi P, Farnetani M, Di Bartolo RM, Bazzotti S, *et al.* Childhood absence epilepsy: evolution and prognostic factors. *Epilepsia* 2005; 46(11):1796–801.
31. Callenbach PM, Bouma PA, Geerts AT, Arts WF, Stroink H, Peeters EA, *et al.* Long-term outcome of childhood absence epilepsy: Dutch Study of Epilepsy in Childhood. *Epilepsy Res* 2009; 83(2-3):249–56.
32. Panayiotopoulos CP, Obeid T, Waheed G. Differentiation of typical absence seizures in epileptic syndromes. A video EEG study of 224 seizures in 20 patients. *Brain* 1989; 112 (Pt 4):1039–56.
33. Beghi M, Beghi E, Cornaggia CM, Gobbi G. Idiopathic generalized epilepsies of adolescence. *Epilepsia* 2006; 47(Suppl 2):107–10.
34. Grunewald RA, Panayiotopoulos CP. Juvenile myoclonic epilepsy. A review. *Arch Neurol* 1993; 50(6):594–8.
35. Penry JK, Dean JC, Riela AR. Juvenile myoclonic epilepsy: long-term response to therapy. *Epilepsia* 1989; 30(Suppl 4):S19–23; discussion S4–7.
36. Panayiotopoulos CP, Michael M, Sanders S, Valeta T, Koutroumanidis M. Benign childhood focal epilepsies: assessment of established and newly recognized syndromes. *Brain* 2008; 131(Pt 9):2264–86.
37. Medeiros LL, Yasuda C, Schmutzler KM, Guerreiro MM. Rolandic discharges: clinico-neurophysiological correlation. *Clin Neurophysiol* 2010; 121(10):1740–3.
38. Callenbach PM, Bouma PA, Geerts AT, Arts WF, Stroink H, Peeters EA, *et al.* Long term outcome of benign childhood epilepsy with centrotemporal spikes: Dutch Study of Epilepsy in Childhood. *Seizure* 2010; 19(8):501–6.
39. Bouma PA, Bovenkerk AC, Westendorp RG, Brouwer OF. The course of benign partial epilepsy of childhood with centrotemporal spikes: a meta-analysis. *Neurology* 1997; 48(2):430–7.
40. Arzimanoglou A, French J, Blume WT, Cross JH, Ernst JP, Feucht M, *et al.* Lennox-Gastaut syndrome: a consensus approach on diagnosis, assessment, management, and trial methodology. *Lancet Neurol* 2009; 8(1):82–93.
41. French JA, Williamson PD, Thadani VM, Darcey TM, Mattson RH, Spencer SS, *et al.* Characteristics of medial temporal lobe epilepsy: I. Results of history and physical examination. *Ann Neurol* 1993; 34(6):774–80.
42. Kim WJ, Park SC, Lee SJ, Lee JH, Kim JY, Lee BI, *et al.* The prognosis for control of seizures with medications in patients with MRI evidence for mesial temporal sclerosis. *Epilepsia* 1999; 40(3):290–3.

43. Wiebe S, Blume WT, Girvin JP, Eliasziw M. A randomized, controlled trial of surgery for temporal-lobe epilepsy. *N Engl J Med* 2001; 345(5):311–18.
44. Thom M, Mathern GW, Cross JH, Bertram EH. Mesial temporal lobe epilepsy: How do we improve surgical outcome? *Ann Neurol* 2010; 68(4):424–34.
45. Ozkara C, Uzan M, Benbir G, Yeni N, Oz B, Hanoglu L, *et al.* Surgical outcome of patients with mesial temporal lobe epilepsy related to hippocampal sclerosis. *Epilepsia* 2008; 49(4):696–9.
46. Callaghan B, Schlesinger M, Rodemer W, Pollard J, Hesdorffer D, Allen Hauser W, *et al.* Remission and relapse in a drug-resistant epilepsy population followed prospectively. *Epilepsia* 2011; 52(3): 619–26.
47. Callaghan BC, Anand K, Hesdorffer D, Hauser WA, French JA. Likelihood of seizure remission in an adult population with refractory epilepsy. *Ann Neurol* 2007; 62(4):382–9.
48. Choi H, Heiman GA, Munger Clary H, Etienne M, Resor SR, Hauser WA. Seizure remission in adults with long-standing intractable epilepsy: an extended follow-up. *Epilepsy Res* 2011; 93(2-3):115–19.
49. Choi H, Heiman G, Pandis D, Cantero J, Resor SR, Gilliam FG, *et al.* Seizure remission and relapse in adults with intractable epilepsy: a cohort study. *Epilepsia* 2008; 49(8):1440–5.
50. Berg AT, Levy SR, Testa FM, D'Souza R. Remission of epilepsy after two drug failures in children: a prospective study. *Ann Neurol* 2009; 65(5):510–19.
51. Annegers JF, Shirts SB, Hauser WA, Kurland LT. Risk of recurrence after an initial unprovoked seizure. *Epilepsia* 1986; 27(1):43–50.
52. Arts WF, Geerts AT, Brouwer OF, Boudewyn Peters AC, Stroink H, van Donselaar CA. The early prognosis of epilepsy in childhood: the prediction of a poor outcome. The Dutch study of epilepsy in childhood. *Epilepsia* 1999; 40(6):726–34.
53. Camfield PR, Camfield CS, Gordon K, Dooley JM. If a first antiepileptic drug fails to control a child's epilepsy, what are the chances of success with the next drug? *J Pediatr* 1997; 131(6): 821–4.
54. Reynolds EH. The prevention of chronic epilepsy. *Epilepsia* 1988; 29(Suppl 1):S25–8.
55. Schmidt D, Tsai JJ, Janz D. Generalized tonic-clonic seizures in patients with complex-partial seizures: natural history and prognostic relevance. *Epilepsia* 1983; 24(1):43–8.
56. Liimatainen SP, Raitanen JA, Ylinen AM, Peltola MA, Peltola JT. The benefit of active drug trials is dependent on aetiology in refractory focal epilepsy. *J Neurol Neurosurg Psychiatry* 2008; 79(7):808–12.
57. Wirrell EC. Prognostic significance of interictal epileptiform discharges in newly diagnosed seizure disorders. *J Clin Neurophysiol* 2010; 27(4):239–48.
58. MacDonald BK, Johnson AL, Goodridge DM, Cockerell OC, Sander JW, Shorvon SD. Factors predicting prognosis of epilepsy after presentation with seizures. *Ann Neurol* 2000; 48(6):833–41.

CHAPTER 25

Drug Interactions

Philip N. Patsalos

Introduction

Antiepileptic drugs (AEDs) are the mainstay of epilepsy treatment and the treatment goal is seizure freedom. Indeed, monotherapy AEDs can render approximately 65% of newly diagnosed patients seizure-free (1). However, for the remaining 35% of patients it is common practice to prescribe AEDs in combination so as to achieve optimal seizure control. When AED combinations are used there is an increased risk of pharmacokinetic and/or pharmacodynamic interactions which in turn can result in adverse clinical consequences. For newly licensed AEDs, which can only be prescribed as adjunctive therapy in the first instance, combination therapy is the only option and therefore their propensity to interact is a major consideration.

For patients with epilepsy, AEDs are administered for prolonged periods comprising of many years and often for a lifetime and therefore increasing the probability of prescribing polytherapies, particularly for those patients that inevitably develop intercurrent or associated conditions which will require AEDs to be combined with non-AED drugs. Even those patients that respond to monotherapy may similarly experience the consequences of AED interactions as AEDs are added and withdrawn during the optimization of their monotherapy drug regimen. Furthermore, polytherapy AED regimens are often required to treat patients with multiple seizure types.

That AEDs are commonly associated with clinically relevant drug interactions can be attributed to their various characteristics: (1) most AEDs have a narrow therapeutic index so that even small changes in their plasma drug concentration can result in seizure exacerbation or increased adverse effects; (2) the most widely used AEDs (carbamazepine, phenobarbital, phenytoin, and valproic acid) have a substantial ability to induce and/or inhibit hepatic metabolism; (3) additionally these AEDs, along with some of the newer AEDs (e.g. eslicarbazepine acetate, felbamate, lamotrigine, oxcarbazepine, retigabine, tiagabine, topiramate, and zonisamide), are susceptible to inhibition and induction of their own metabolism (2–4).

This chapter will review those interactions that are most frequently encountered clinically and those interactions which because of their magnitude are particularly likely to result in adverse clinical consequences.

Mechanisms of drug interactions

There are two types of interaction, pharmacokinetic interactions and pharmacodynamic interactions.

Pharmacokinetic interactions

The vast majority (>99%) of clinically significant identifiable AED interactions are the consequence of pharmacokinetic interactions and are associated with a change in drug plasma concentration and are therefore more readily detectable and quantifiable and their time course is often well characterized. Induction or inhibition of drug metabolizing enzymes are the principal mechanisms of these interactions whilst pharmacokinetic interactions at the level of absorption, protein binding, and excretion are rare.

Drug absorption interactions

AED absorption interactions are rare but include the impairment of absorption of carbamazepine, gabapentin, phenobarbital, and phenytoin by antacids (3, 4). More recently it has been observed that drugs that modulate the expression of gastrointestinal drug transporters such as P-glycoprotein and multiple drug resistance proteins 2 and 3 can reduce drug absorption and it is via this mechanism that carbamazepine reduces talinolol absorption (5).

Protein binding interactions

The best documented plasma protein binding displacement interaction involving AEDs is that of phenytoin by valproic acid (6). This results, in some patients, in a modest rise in free phenytoin concentration occurring due to a concomitant inhibition of phenytoin metabolism by valproic acid and occasionally in phenytoin toxicity. For these displacement interactions to be significant, protein binding needs to be 90% or higher and only phenytoin, valproic acid, diazepam, tiagabine, lacosamide, and stiripentol have this characteristic (6–8). However, unless additional mechanisms occur, although a fall in total drug concentration (as the displaced drug redistributes rapidly into tissues and undergoes compensatory elimination) occurs, the free drug concentration remains practically unchanged and therefore the pharmacological consequence of such interactions is negligible. Nevertheless, the interpretation of plasma drug concentration measurements requires the appreciation that therapeutic and toxic effects will occur at total drug concentrations lower than usual and that patient management may best be guided by monitoring free unbound drug concentrations (9).

Renal excretion interactions

Despite numerous AEDs undergoing primarily renal excretion (e.g. gabapentin, levetiracetam, pregabalin, and vigabatrin) there are no documented AED interactions involving a change in renal excretion processes.

Metabolic drug interactions

The metabolic characteristics of the various AEDs and their propensity to undergo metabolic interactions is summarized in Table 25.1. Metabolic interactions are subdivided into induction interactions in which drug metabolism is increased and inhibition interactions in which drug metabolism is decreased (10, 11). AEDs that undergo metabolism by cytochrome P450s (CYPs) (e.g. carbamazepine, phenytoin, phenobarbital, ethosuximide, primidone, tiagabine, topiramate, zonisamide) or uridine diphosphate glucuronyltransferases (UGTs) (e.g. lamotrigine, valproic acid, oxcarbazepine, eslicarbazepine acetate) are susceptible to these types of interactions (12, 13). In contrast, AEDs that are renally eliminated (e.g. gabapentin, levetiracetam, pregabalin, vigabatrin), or undergo non-CYP or non-UGT metabolism (e.g. lacosamide) or whose metabolism is non-hepatic (e.g. levetiracetam) are devoid of such interactions (13, 14).

Inhibition mechanisms

Enzyme inhibition occurs when a drug or its metabolite(s) blocks the activity of one or more drug metabolizing enzymes. This results in a decrease in the rate of metabolism of the affected drug leading to increased plasma concentrations and, possibly, clinical toxicity.

Table 25.1 Metabolic characteristics of antiepileptic drugs and their propensity to interact

AED	Hepatic metabolism	Enzymes involved in metabolism	Elimination by renal excretion	Propensity to interact
Carbamazepine	Substantial (98%)	CYP1A2, CYP2C8, CYP3A4	Minimal (2%)	Substantial
Phenytoin	Substantial (95%)	CYP2C9, CYP2C19	Minimal (2%)	Substantial
Phenobarbital	Substantial (80%)	CYP2E1, CYP2C19	Minimal (20%)	Substantial
Primidone	Minimal (35%)	CYP2E1, CYP2C9, CYP2C19	Moderate (65%)	Substantial
Stiripentol	Substantial (73%)	CYP1A2, CYP2C19, CYP3A4	Minimal (27%)	Substantial
Valproic acid	Substantial (97%)	CYP2A6, CYP2C9, CYP2C19, CYP2B6, UGT1A3, UGT2B7	Minimal (3%)	Substantial
Lamotrigine	Substantial (90%)	UGT1A4, UGT1A1, UGT2B7	Minimal (10%)	Moderate
Topiramate	Moderate (50%)	Not identified but involve CYP isoenzymes	Moderate (50%)	Moderate
Clobazam	Substantial (100%)	CYP3A4	None (0%)	Minimal
Clonazepam	Substantial (99%)	CYP3A4	Minimal (1%)	Minimal
Eslicarbazepine acetate	Substantial (>99%)	Not identified but UGTs are involved	Minimal (1%)	Minimal
Ethosuximide	Substantial (80%)	CYP2B, CYP2E1, CYP3A4	Minimal (20%)	Minimal
Felbamate	Moderate (50%)	CYP3A4, CYP2E1	Moderate (50%)	Minimal
Retigabine	Moderate (50–65%)	UGT1A1, UGT1A3, UGT1A4, UGT1A9	Minimal (20–30%)	Minimal
Rufinamide	Substantial (96%)	Unknown (but not CYP-dependent)	Minimal (4%)	Minimal
Oxcarbazepine	Substantial (>99%)	Not identified but UGTs are involved	Minimal (<1%)	Minimal
Tiagabine	Substantial (98%)	CYP3A4	Minimal (<2%)	Minimal
Zonisamide	Moderate (65%)	CYP3A4	Minimal (35%)	Minimal
Gabapentin	Not metabolized	None	Substantial (100%)	Insignificant/non-interacting
Lacosamide	Moderate (60%)	Demethylation	Minimal (40%)	Insignificant/non-interacting
Levetiracetam	Minimal (30%)—non-hepatic occurs in whole blood	Type-B esterase	Moderate (66%)	Insignificant/non-interacting
Pregabalin	Not metabolized	None	Substantial (98%)	Insignificant/non-interacting
Vigabatrin	Not metabolized	None	Substantial (100%)	Insignificant/non-interacting

Inhibition is usually competitive in nature and dose-dependent, and tends to begin as soon as sufficient concentrations of the inhibitor are achieved, with significant inhibition being often observed within 24 hours after addition of the inhibitor (10). The time to maximal inhibition will depend on the elimination half-life of the affected drug and the inhibiting agent which will now have a more prolonged half-life, to achieve steady-state (Table 25.2). Thus, AEDs with short half-lives will achieve maximum increase in blood concentrations sooner than those with longer half-lives (e.g. rufinamide versus phenobarbital; Table 25.2). The time course of de-inhibition, when the inhibitor is withdrawn, is dependent on the elimination half-life of the inhibitor.

Induction mechanisms

Induction of drug metabolizing enzymes in the liver results in an increase in enzyme activity which in turn results in an increase in the rate of metabolism of drugs which are substrates of those enzymes, leading to a decrease in plasma concentration of the affected drug. If the affected drug has an active metabolite, induction leads to increased metabolite concentration and a possible increase in drug toxicity. As enzyme induction requires synthesis of new enzymes, the time course of induction (and its reversal upon removal of the inducer) is dependent on the rate of enzyme synthesis and degradation and the time to reach steady-state concentrations of the inducing drug. Consequently, induction is usually gradual and dose-dependent and differs between the different enzyme-inducing AEDs. For phenobarbital, induction starts after approximately 1 week, with maximal induction occurring after 2–3 weeks following its initiation. Phenytoin induction is maximal by 1–2 weeks after phenytoin initiation and carbamazepine is associated with autoinduction (induces its own metabolism) which is complete within 3–5 weeks (11, 15, 16). In contrast to the other enzyme-inducing AEDs, the process of de-induction, upon cessation of carbamazepine, is rapid with greater than 68% de-induction occurring within 6 days (17).

Table 25.2 Time to steady-state and therefore maximum therapeutic outcome consequent to an inhibitory interaction of those antiepileptic drugs (AEDs) which are known to be affected by inhibitory interactions

Affected AED	Half-life (hours)[a]	Steady-state (days) achieved after 5 half-lives (values are rounded up or down for clarity)
Carbamazepine	8–20	2–4
Clobazam	10–30	2–7 (7–10)[b]
Ethosuximide	40–60	8–12
Felbamate	16–22	3–5
Lamotrigine	15–35	3–7
Phenobarbitone	70–140	15–29
Phenytoin	30–100	6–21
Rufinamide	6–10	1–2
Valproic acid	11–20	2–4

[a] Values are in the absence of interacting medication (9).
[b] Includes time to steady-state for pharmacologically active metabolite N-desmethyl-clobazam.

Interactions between AEDs

Inhibition interactions resulting in increased AED concentration

Of the AEDs, valproic acid, topiramate, oxcarbazepine, stiripentol, and felbamate are inhibitors of hepatic metabolism and thus elevate the plasma concentrations of other AEDs. By far the most potent and broad ranging inhibitor of drug metabolism is valproic acid. Topiramate is a modest inhibitor and oxcarbazepine a weak inhibitor. In contrast, stiripentol and felbamate are potent inhibitors, resulting in clinically important interactions, but these AEDs are rarely used in epilepsy. Felbamate can cause serious liver and bone marrow toxicity and stiripentol has a limited licence for the adjunctive treatment of seizures in children with severe myoclonic epilepsy in infancy (Dravet syndrome). Sulthiame is another potent inhibitor of hepatic metabolism (e.g. increases phenytoin and phenobarbital blood concentration several-fold) but is rarely used clinically (12).

Valproic acid is a potent inhibitor of CYP2C9, UGT1A4, and epoxide hydrolase activity and a weak inhibitor of CYP2C19 and CYP3A4 activity and this results in major interactions with carbamazepine, phenobarbital, and lamotrigine and two moderate interactions with felbamate and rufinamide. Plasma concentrations of the pharmacologically active metabolite of carbamazepine, carbamazepine-10,11- epoxide, are increased in patients treated with carbamazepine and valproic acid in combination. This is the consequence of inhibition of the enzyme epoxide hydrolase which is responsible for the metabolism of carbamazepine-10,11- epoxide and can occur without any significant changes in carbamazepine concentrations and result in toxicity (18). The interaction with phenobarbital is the result of inhibition of CYP2C9 and CYP2C19 by valproic acid and this results in a 30–50% increase in plasma phenobarbital concentration and a reduction in phenobarbital (or primidone) dosage by up to 80% may be required to avoid side effects (particularly sedation and cognitive impairment) (19). The interaction with lamotrigine is the result of inhibition of the UGT1A4 enzyme responsible for the glucuronide conjugation of lamotrigine and results in an approximate 2-fold increase in plasma lamotrigine concentrations (20). Indeed this potent interaction is already optimum at relatively low valproate doses (≥500mg/day in an adult) (21). Because lamotrigine administration can be associated with a cutaneous rash, which is particularly prevalent when a fast increment in plasma lamotrigine concentration occurs, the introduction of lamotrigine in a patient already taking valproic acid should be undertaken with caution, using a low starting dose and a slow dose escalation rate. However, it should be noted that there is no risk of rash if valproic acid is introduced in a patient already stabilized on lamotrigine. Valproic acid may inhibit the metabolism of other AEDs including ethosuximide, felbamate, phenytoin, and rufinamide. A particularly complex interaction is that with phenytoin in which valproic acid inhibition occurs along with a concurrent displacement of phenytoin from plasma protein binding sites. This results in an increase in free plasma phenytoin concentration which may not be apparent when a patient is monitored by use of total phenytoin concentrations and thus free phenytoin concentrations should be used to guide patient management in this situation (9).

Stiripentol inhibits CYP1A2, CYP2C19, and CYP3A4 and consequently can decrease the clearance of carbamazepine, clobazam, phenobarbital, phenytoin, primidone, and valproic acid (7). The inhibition of clobazam metabolism is associated with a concurrent and even more potent inhibition of the pharmacologically active metabolite, N-desmethylclobazam, so that stiripentol increases clobazam plasma levels and N-desmethylclobazam plasma levels severalfold (22). Felbamate inhibits CYP2C19 and epoxide hydrolase so that plasma concentration of carbamazepine-10,11-epoxide, N-desmethyl-clobazam, phenobarbital, phenytoin and valproic acid are increased.

Oxcarbazepine is a weak inhibitor and topiramate is a modest inhibitor of CYP2C19. Consequently, oxcarbazepine, particularly when used at high dosages (>1800 mg/day), can increase plasma phenytoin concentrations by up to 40% and to a lesser extent phenobarbital (23). Topiramate can increase plasma phenytoin concentrations in a small subset of patients by 25%. Rufinamide can decrease the clearance of phenobarbital and phenytoin by less than 20% and increase their plasma concentrations (24). Other inhibitory drug interactions caused by AEDs also occur but these are less common and are usually of modest clinical significance.

Induction interactions resulting in decreased AED concentration

Most AEDs (e.g. gabapentin, lacosamide, lamotrigine, levetiracetam, pregabalin, stiripentol, tiagabine, topiramate, vigabatrin, and zonisamide) are not associated with enzyme-inducing effects on the metabolism of concurrently administered AEDs. In contrast, carbamazepine, phenytoin, phenobarbital, and primidone are potent inducers of various CYP isoenzymes and they also induce UGT and epoxide hydrolases (3). Consequently, these AEDs stimulate the metabolism and decrease the plasma concentrations of numerous AEDs, including clobazam, clonazepam, ethosuximide, felbamate, lamotrigine, oxcarbazepine and its active monohydroxy-metabolite, rufinamide, stiripentol, tiagabine, topiramate, valproic acid, and zonisamide. Rufinamide can decrease plasma concentrations of carbamazepine and lamotrigine, probably via hepatic induction of metabolism (24). In addition, phenobarbital, phenytoin, and primidone can markedly induce the metabolism of carbamazepine so that mean plasma carbamazepine concentrations are decreased by 33%, 44%, and 25% respectively (25). Co-medication of valproic acid with carbamazepine, phenobarbital, or phenytoin can reduce mean plasma valproic acid concentrations by 66%, 76%, and 49% respectively (26). In addition, the metabolism of lamotrigine is significantly enhanced by oxcarbazepine (27) and methsuximide (28).

In some patients, these interactions have modest clinical consequences because the loss of efficacy resulting from the decreased concentration of the affected drug is compensated for by the independent anticonvulsant effect of the enzyme-inducing AED. In other patients, however, the decrease in plasma concentration of the affected drug impacts adversely on seizure control, and an increase in dosage is then required. Drugs whose dosage requirements are most significantly increased in the presence of enzyme-inducing AEDs include carbamazepine, valproic acid, tiagabine, and lamotrigine.

The consequence of enzyme induction is complicated when AEDs are associated with pharmacologically active metabolites (e.g. carbamazepine-epoxide of carbamazepine, various metabolites of valproic acid, phenobarbital of primidone, and N-desmethyl-clobazam of clobazam). There can be a paradoxical outcome and a good example of this effect is that of primidone when phenytoin or carbamazepine are co-prescribed. Because primidone is metabolized partly to phenobarbital, stimulation of metabolism may actually result in enhanced production of the phenobarbital metabolite and therefore an increased pharmacological effect. Another example relates to valproic acid the metabolism of which is typically enhanced by carbamazepine, phenytoin, and phenobarbital resulting in decreased plasma concentrations and decreased effectiveness of valproic acid However, this interaction may also lead to increased formation of hepatotoxic metabolites and may explain why patients taking these AEDs are more susceptible to valproate-induced liver toxicity (25).

An interesting interaction is that between phenytoin and the angiotensin-receptor blocker losartan. While phenytoin increases plasma concentrations of losartan by 17%, it decreases the plasma concentrations of the active carboxylic acid metabolite E3174 by 63% through inhibition of its CYP2C9-mediated formation clearance. Therefore, a reduced antihypertensive effect may be anticipated (29).

Pharmacodynamic interactions

Pharmacodynamic interactions are less well described because they occur at the site of action in the brain and are usually inferred by default when a change in the clinical status of a patient cannot be attributable to a pharmacokinetic change in plasma concentrations. These interactions, which can be additive (when they equal the sum of the effects of the individual drugs), synergistic (when the combined effects are greater than expected from the sum of individual drugs) or antagonistic (when the combined effects are less than additive), are more common than previously thought and in order that a rational approach to the use of AED combinations in the management of epilepsy can occur we must enhance our understanding of this type of interaction.

A mechanistic approach, in which combinations of drugs acting via different mechanisms could be co-prescribed and thus facilitate the use of rational AED polytherapy is highly desirable (30). Indeed, although our current knowledge of AED pharmacology is insufficient universally to take this approach, there is some evidence that certain AED combinations (e.g. valproate plus lamotrigine and valproate plus ethosuximide) are associated with beneficial interactions at the pharmacodynamic level (31, 32). Such AED combinations act synergistically and are associated with seizure control in patients previously unresponsive to the highest tolerated dose of either drug given alone. Unfortunately, additive neurotoxicity can also occur when AEDs that share a common mechanism of action (e.g. blockage of voltage-dependent sodium channels) are co-prescribed (33). These effects have been more commonly associated with the combinations of lamotrigine plus carbamazepine, lamotrigine plus valproate and oxcarbazepine plus carbamazepine (23, 28, 34).

Interactions between AEDs and other drugs

Inhibition interactions resulting in increased AED concentration

There are many drugs that are used to treat other conditions in patients with epilepsy that are potent inhibitors of CYP isoenzymes resulting in elevated plasma AED concentrations and toxicity. Most such interactions have been reported for carbamazepine, phenytoin and phenobarbital, and new AEDs appear to be rarely affected. This can be attributed in part to the fact that many new AEDs undergo little or no hepatic metabolism but also because there is limited clinical experience with the newer AEDs.

Many antimicrobial agents are potent inhibitors of CYP isoenzymes. The imidazole antifungals ketoconazole and fluconazole can inhibit CYP3A4 and, if co-prescribed in patients taking carbamazepine, significant increases in plasma carbamazepine concentration (up to 29%) can occur resulting in carbamazepine intoxication. Likewise, the CYP2C9 inhibitors miconazole and fluconazole can significantly increase plasma phenytoin concentrations 2–4-fold. In contrast, itraconazole increases phenytoin levels by only 10% (25). Isoniazid, used as an antituberculosis agent, inhibits the metabolism of carbamazepine, ethosuximide, phenytoin, and valproic acid, resulting in increased plasma concentrations and associated toxicity.

Some macrolide antibiotics are potent inhibitors of CYP3A4 and can significantly increase plasma carbamazepine concentrations (35). Particularly potent inhibitors are erythromycin and troleandomycin, with some patients experiencing serious carbamazepine toxicity consequent to up to 2–4-fold increases in plasma carbamazepine concentrations.

The antiulcer drugs cimetidine and omeprazole can inhibit CYP2C19 and thus decrease the metabolic clearance of phenytoin so that phenytoin plasma concentrations are increased by 20% and 25%, respectively (36, 37). Similarly cimetidine and omeprazole can increase plasma carbamazepine concentrations through an action on CYP3A4. Danazol, a synthetic oestrogen used in the management of endometriosis, is a potent inhibitor of carbamazepine metabolism and has been observed to increase plasma carbamazepine concentrations by 50–100% (38).

Psychotropic drugs are frequently co-prescribed to patients with epilepsy and thus several clinically important drug interactions have been described with these drugs. Some antidepressants including fluoxetine, fluvoxamine, sertraline, trazodone, viloxazine and, possibly, imipramine exert an inhibitory effect on the metabolism of phenytoin (25). Carbamazepine metabolism can be inhibited by viloxazine, trazodone, nefazodone and, possibly, fluoxetine and fluvoxamine so that plasma carbamazepine concentrations are increased. The concentrations of valproic acid and lamotrigine may be increased by sertraline. In contrast, carbamazepine plasma concentrations are unaffected by paroxetine and sertraline and in addition plasma concentrations of valproic acid and phenytoin are unaffected by paroxetine. Some antipsychotic drugs, for example risperidone can increase plasma carbamazepine concentrations by 20% whilst co-medication with thioridazine and chlorpromazine has been associated with precipitating signs of phenytoin toxicity (39).

Special care is needed when AEDs are co-prescribed with antineoplastic and antiviral agents because many of these drugs inhibit drug metabolizing enzymes and increase plasma AED concentrations. Indeed the antineoplastic agents doxifluridine, 5-fluorouracil, tamoxifen, and UFT (a mixture of uracil and the 5-fluorouracil prodrug tegafur) can inhibit phenytoin metabolism and cause phenytoin intoxication whilst ritonavir, an antiviral agent, profoundly inhibits carbamazepine metabolism resulting in a 2–3-fold increase in plasma carbamazepine concentrations (4, 40). Therefore, for patients treated with antineoplastic or antiviral agents, it would be best to select AEDs (e.g. gabapentin, lacosamide, levetiracetam, pregabalin, or vigabatrin), which are not metabolized by CYP isoenzymes or have CYP enzyme inhibiting effects and thus have an insignificant propensity to interact at the metabolic level (Table 25.1) (2).

Induction interactions resulting in decreased AED concentration

Oral hormonal contraceptive steroids can induce the metabolism of UGT1A4 and enhance the metabolism of lamotrigine and decrease plasma lamotrigine concentrations by 50% (41). This is considered to be the consequence of the oestrogen component of the combined contraceptive pill and in some women a reduction in seizure control occurs (42). Valproic acid, which is in part metabolized via UGT1A3 and UGT2B7 isoenzymes, is also affected by intake of contraceptive steroids so that the mean clearance of total and unbound plasma valproic acid concentrations increased by 21.5% and 45.2% respectively (43). Similar induction of metabolism may occur with oxcarbazepine and eslicarbazepine acetate, both of which undergo metabolism via UGT isoenzymes.

There are various additional interactions resulting in clinically important decreases in plasma AED concentrations. For example, the antineoplastic agent cisplatin and methotrexate decrease plasma valproic acid concentrations, whilst cisplatin, in addition decreases plasma carbamazepine concentrations. Also, the antituberculosis agent rifampicin acts as a potent enzyme inducer and can significantly decrease phenytoin, carbamazepine, valproic acid, ethosuximide, and lamotrigine plasma concentrations (4). The use of carbapenem antibiotics (e.g. meropenem and ertapenem) in combination with valproic acid is contraindicated because plasma valproic acid concentrations are decreased by more than 80% as a result of induction of valproic acid glucuronidation (44).

Inhibition interactions resulting in increased concentration of the other drug

Inhibition interactions in which AEDs increase the plasma concentrations of drugs used for other conditions are rare and primarily involve valproic acid. Valproic acid can inhibit the metabolism of a variety of drugs including amitriptyline, aripiprazole clomipramine, chlorpromazine, etoposide, lorazepam, nortriptyline, nitrosurea, paroxetine, and zidovudine. With regards to amitriptyline and nortriptyline, their plasma concentrations can increase by 50–60% and lead to symptoms of toxicity, including worsening or precipitation of seizures. Topiramate can increase plasma haloperidol concentration by 28% and its pharmacologically active metabolite by 50% (45).

Induction interactions resulting in decreased concentration of the other drug

Because enzyme-inducing AEDs (carbamazepine, phenytoin, phenobarbital, and primidone) are extensively prescribed there are many interactions described in which decreases in drug plasma concentrations occur and most can be of clinical significance (Table 25.3). Of particular concern are those involving drugs that undergo extensive first-pass metabolism since their plasma concentrations are decreased to such an extent that treatment failure is common. Examples of such drugs include the antifungals itraconazole and ketoconazole; the antimicrobials metronidazole and doxycycline; the antihelmintics albendazole and praziquantel (46); the antiviral agents nevirapine, efavirenz, delaverdine, indinavir, ritonavir, and saquinavir. In one report, the plasma concentration

Table 25.3 Enzyme-inducing AEDs (carbamazepine, phenobarbital, phenytoin, and primidone) and their enhancement of metabolism resulting in decreased plasma concentrations of various drugs

Antimicrobials
Phenytoin:
Albendazole, delaverdine, doxycycline, efavirenz, erythromycin, indinavir, itraconazole, ketoconazole, mebendazole, nelfinavir, nevirapine, praziquantel, ritonavir, saquinavir, voriconazole, zidovudine
Carbamazepine:
Albendazole, delaverdine, doxycycline, efavirenz, erythromycin, indinavir, isoniazid, itraconazole, ketoconazole, mebendazole, nelfinavir, nevirapine, praziquantel, ritonavir, saquinavir, zidovudine
Phenobarbital:
Albendazole, chloramphenicol, delaverdine, doxycycline, efavirenz, indinavir, itraconazole, ketoconazole, metronidazole, nelfinavir, nevirapine, praziquantel, ritonavir, saquinavir, zidovudine
Primidone:
Delaverdine, efavirenz, indinavir, nelfinavir, nevirapine, ritonavir, saquinavir, zidovudine
Antineoplastic agents
Phenytoin:
9-aminocampthotecin, busulphan, cyclophosphamide, docetaxel, etoposide, ifofosfamide, irinotecan, methotrexate, paclitaxel, procarbazine, teniposide, topotecan, vincristine
Carbamazepine:
9-aminocampthotecin, docetaxel, methotrexate, paclitaxel, procarbazine, teniposide, vincristine
Phenobarbital:
9-aminocampthotecin, docetaxel, etoposide, ifofosfamide, methotrexate, paclitaxel, procarbazine, teniposide, vincristine
Cardiovascular drugs
Phenytoin:
Amiodarone, dicoumarol, digoxin, disopyramide, felodipine, losartan[a], mexiletine, nimodipine, nisoldipine, quinidine, verapamil, warfarin[b]
Carbamazepine:
Amiodarone, dicoumarol, felodipine, nimodipine, nivadipine, phenprocoumon, warfarin
Phenobarbital:
Alprenalol, dicoumarol, felodipine, nifedipine, nimodipine, propranolol, quinidine, verapamil, warfarin
Primidone:
Dicoumarol
Immunosuppressants
Phenytoin:
Cyclosporine A, sirolimus, tacrolimus
Carbamazepine:
Cyclosporine A
Phenobarbital:
Cyclosporine A
Primidone:
Cyclosporine A
Psychotropic drugs
Phenytoin:
Alprozolam, amitriptyline, citalopram, clobazam, clomipramine, clonazepam, clozapine, desipramine, desmethylclomipramine, diazepam, fluphenazine, haloperidol, imipramine, mianserin, midazolam, mirtazapine, nefazodone, nortriptyline, olanzapine, paroxetine, protriptyline, quetiapine, risperidone, thioridazine, ziprasidone
Carbamazepine:
Alprozolam, amitriptyline, citalopram, clobazam, clomipramine, clonazepam, clozapine, desipramine, desmethylclomipramine, diazepam, doxepin, fluphenazine, haloperidol, imipramine, mianserin, midazolam, mirtazapine, nefazodone, nortriptyline, olanzapine, paroxetine, protriptyline, quetiapine, risperidone, sertraline, thioridazine, ziprasidone
Phenobarbital:
Alprozolam, amitriptyline, citalopram, clobazam, clomipramine, clonazepam, chlorpromazine, clozapine, desipramine, desmethylclomipramine, diazepam, fluphenazine, haloperidol, imipramine, mianserin, midazolam, nefazodone, nortriptyline, olanzapine, paroxetine, protriptyline, quetiapine, risperidone, ziprasidone
Primidone:
Alprozolam, amitriptyline, citalopram, clobazam, clomipramine, clonazepam, desipramine, desmethylclomipramine, diazepam, fluphenazine, haloperidol, imipramine, midazolam, nefazodone, nortriptyline, olanzapine, paroxetine, protriptyline, quetiapine, risperidone, ziprasidone

[a] Only pharmacologically active carboxylic acid metabolite (E3174) is affected.

[b] A biphasic interaction occurs whereby initially phenytoin acts as an inhibitor and subsequently induction prevails.

of indinavir was decreased to insignificant levels upon addition of carbamazepine (47).

Enzyme inducing AEDs increase the metabolism of many antineoplastic agents including busulfan, cyclophosphamide, etoposide, ifosfamide, methotrexate paclitaxel, and teniposide and some vinca alkaloids. Overall, these interactions would be expected to result in decreased efficacy of the affected drug, even though for drugs that have active metabolites (e.g. ifofosfamide and cyclophosphamide) enzyme induction could theoretically potentiate drug effects. Other examples, whereby the increased formation of a pharmacologically active metabolite can complicate the therapeutic outcome of an induction interaction, include amiodarone, disopyramide and bupropion.

Enzyme inducing AEDs can increase the metabolism of hypotensive agents such as β-adrenoceptor blockers (e.g. propranolol, metoprolol), alprenolol, dihydropyridine calcium antagonists (e.g. nifedipine, felodipine, nimodipine and nisoldipine), and other such agents (e.g. verapamil). In the case of most dihydropyridine calcium antagonists, the magnitude of the interaction and its high inter-patient variability practically negate the use of these agents in patients co-medicated with enzyme inducing AEDs (48).

Phenytoin can induce the metabolism of numerous lipid lowering agents (e.g. atorvastatin, lovastatin, simvastatin), via an action on CYP3A4, and reduces their effectiveness. A similarly interaction occurs between carbamazepine and simvastatin and in these settings higher statin doses need to be prescribed (49).

The anticoagulant effects of dicoumarol and warfarin can be reduced by carbamazepine and other enzyme-inducing AEDs, possibly via an induction of CYP2C9 (50). The interaction between phenytoin and warfarin, however, is more complex and initially inhibition of CYP2C9 occurs (with enhancement in anticoagulant action) followed after 1–2 weeks by induction of CYP2C9 (with decreased anticoagulant action) (51). Because anticoagulants have a narrow therapeutic index, it is advisable to always monitor the INR whenever a significant change in AED dosage or therapy occurs.

Patients that require immunosuppression with cyclosporine A, tacrolimus or sirolimus and have seizures their seizures are best treated with AEDs devoid of CYP enzyme inducing activity, such as gabapentin, lacosamide, lamotrigine, levetiracetam, tiagabine, or vigabatrin. The metabolism of cyclosporine A, a substrate of CYP3A4, is enhanced by carbamazepine, phenobarbital, phenytoin and primidone so that plasma cyclosporine A concentrations are decreased and an increase in the dosage of the immunosuppressant is usually required to prevent therapeutic failure (52). A similar effect can occur with oxcarbazepine whereby plasma cyclosporine A concentrations are decreased. Tacrolimus, which is also primarily metabolized by CYP3A, is also susceptible to induction interactions by phenytoin and carbamazepine and typically tacrolimus dose increments of up to 1.4-fold can be needed in order to maintain adequate therapeutic tacrolimus blood concentrations. Finally, phenytoin can enhance the metabolism of sirolimus by up to 4-fold via an action on CYP3A4/5.

Because psychiatric disorders are commonly associated with epilepsy, the concomitant administration of AEDs and psychotropic drugs can result in several clinically important drug interactions (39, 53). Indeed, plasma concentration of many tricyclic antidepressants (e.g. amitriptyline, nortriptyline, imipramine, desipramine, clomipramine, desmethylclomipramine, protriptyline, and doxepin), and of many newer generation antidepressants (e.g. mianserin, nomifensine, bupropion, nefazodone, citalopram and paroxetine) are readily decreased by enzyme inducing AEDs. Higher dosages of these antidepressants may be required for clinical efficacy. The interactions between antipsychotics (chlorpromazine, clozapine, haloperidol, olanzapine, risperidone, quetiapine and ziprasidone) and enzyme-inducing AEDs are similar to those described for antidepressants and are often of clinical significance.

There are nine AEDs (carbamazepine, phenytoin, phenobarbital, primidone, felbamate, oxcarbazepine, rufinamide, eslicarbazepine acetate, and topiramate) which enhance the metabolism of oestrogen component of the contraceptive pill so as to decrease oestrogen blood concentrations and therefore decrease the efficacy of steroid oral contraceptives (Table 25.4) (54, 55). With regards to topiramate, the interaction appears to be minimal or absent at topiramate daily dosages of 200 mg or less. Women taking these AEDs should be prescribed an oral contraceptive containing 50 micrograms of ethinyloestradiol and if breakthrough bleeding occurs, ethinyloestradiol doses may need to be increased to 75 or 100 micrograms. In contrast, there are 12 AEDs which do not affect the metabolism of oral contraceptives (Table 25.4). With lamotrigine the interaction occurs in reverse and oral contraceptives induce the metabolism of lamotrigine and decrease its plasma concentration by 40–65%, potentially leading to worsened seizure control or signs of toxicity when the contraceptive is discontinued (41). Oxcarbazepine and valproic acid plasma concentrations are similarly decreased (by ~20%) due to induction of glucuronidation.

Pharmacodynamic interactions

Most pharmacodynamic interactions between AEDs and other drugs relate to increased toxicity. For example, the combination

Table 25.4 Oral contraceptive steroids and interactions with antiepileptic drugs (AEDs)

AEDs that do not interfere with the metabolism of oral contraceptives	AEDs that enhance the metabolism of oral contraceptives and compromise contraception control
Clobazam	Carbamazepine
Clonazepam	Eslicarbazepine acetate
Ethosuximide	Felbamate
Gabapentin	Oxcarbazepine
Lacosamide	Phenobarbital
Lamotrigine[a]	Phenytoin
Levetiracetam	Primidone
Pregabalin	Rufinamide
Retigabine	Topiramate (>200 mg/day)
Tiagabine	
Vigabatrin	
Zonisamide	

[a] Although lamotrigine is without effect overall, it does enhance the progesterone component of the pill so that blood concentrations are reduced by ~10% and this effect may be clinically significant in patients taking the progesterone-only contraceptive pill. The interaction between stiripentol and oral contraceptive steroids is not known. However, its clinical indication is such that it is unlikely that it would be prescribed to women of childbearing potential.

of nitroso-urea-cisplatinum-based chemotherapy with valproic acid has been associated with increased haematological toxicity whilst the concurrent use of lithium and valproic acid has been associated with additive adverse reactions such as weight gain, sedation, gastrointestinal complaints, and tremor. The increased incidence of neurotoxicity when lithium and carbamazepine are used concurrently may also be the consequence of a pharmacodynamic interaction. The combination of carbamazepine with clozapine is generally contraindicated due to a pharmacodynamic interaction which results in additive adverse haematological adverse effects (25).

Acknowledgements

This work was undertaken at UCLH/UCL who received a proportion of funding from the Department of Health's NIHR Biomedical Research Centres funding scheme.

References

1. Kwan P, Brodie MJ. Early identification of refractory epilepsy. *New Eng J Medicine* 2000; 342:314–19.
2. Patsalos PN, Froscher W, Pisani F, van Rijn C. The importance of drug interactions in epilepsy therapy. *Epilepsia* 2002; 43:365–5.
3. Patsalos PN, Perucca E. Clinically important interactions in epilepsy: General features and interactions between antiepileptic drugs. *Lancet Neurol* 2003; 2:347–56.
4. Patsalos PN, Perucca E. Clinically important interactions in epilepsy: Interactions between antiepileptic drugs and other drugs. *Lancet Neurol* 2003; 2:473–81.
5. Giessmann T, May K, Modess C, Wegner D, Hecker U, Zschiesche M, *et al.* Carbamazepine regulates intestinal P-glycoprotein and multidrug resistance protein MRP2 and influences disposition of talinolol in humans. *Clin Pharmacol Ther* 2004; 76:182–200.
6. Perucca E, Hebdige S, Frigo GM, Gatti G, Lecchini S, Crema A. Interaction between phenytoin and valproic acid: Plasma protein binding and metabolic effects. *Clin Pharmacol Ther* 1980; 28:779–89.
7. Chiron C. Stiripentol. *Neurotherapeutics* 2007; 4:123–5.
8. Greenaway C, Ratnaraj N, Sander JW, Patsalos PN. Saliva and serum lacosamide concentrations in patients with epilepsy. *Epilepsia* 2011; 52:258–63.
9. Patsalos PN, Berry DJ, Bourgeois BFD, Cloyd JC, Glauser TA, Johannessen SI, *et al.* Antiepileptic drugs—Best practice guidelines for therapeutic drug monitoring: A position paper by the Subcommission on Therapeutic Drug Monitoring, ILAE Commission on Therapeutic Strategies. *Epilepsia* 2008; 49:1239–76.
10. Anderson GD. A mechanistic approach to antiepileptic drug interactions. *Ann Pharmacother* 1998; 32:554–63.
11. Perucca E, Hedges A, Makki KA, Ruprah M, Wilson JF, Richens A. A comparative study of the enzyme inducing properties of anticonvulsant drugs in epileptic patients. *Br J Clin Pharmacol* 1984; 18:401–10.
12. Patsalos PN, Bourgeois BFD. *The epilepsy prescribers guide to antiepileptic drugs*. Cambridge: Cambridge University Press, 2010.
13. Johannessen Landmark C, Patsalos PN. Drug interactions involving the new second- and third-generation antiepileptic drugs. *Exp Rev Neurotherapeut* 2010; 10:119–40.
14. Patsalos PN, Ghattaura S, Ratnaraj N, Sander JW. In situ metabolism of levetiracetam in blood of patients with epilepsy. *Epilepsia* 2006; 47:1818–21.
15. Perucca E. Clinical implications of hepatic microsomal enzyme induction by antiepileptic drugs. *Pharmacol Ther* 1987; 33:139–44.
16. Patsalos PN, Duncan JS, Shorvon SD. Effect of the removal of antiepileptic drugs on antipyrine kinetics in patients taking polytherapy. *Br J Clin Pharmacol* 1988; 26:253–9.
17. Schaffler L, Bourgeois BFD, Luders HO. Rapid reversibility of autoinduction of carbamazepine metabolism upon temporary discontinuation. *Epilepsia* 1994; 35:195–8.
18. Pisani F, Fazio A, Oteri G, Ruello C, Gitto C, Russo F, Perucca E. Sodium valproate and valpromide: Differential interactions with carbamazepine in epileptic patients. *Epilepsia* 1986; 27:548–52.
19. Kapetanovic IM, Kupferberg HJ, Porter RJ, Theodore W, Schulman E, Penry JK. Mechanism of valproate–phenobarbital interaction in epileptic patients. *Clin Pharmacol Ther* 1981; 29:480–6.
20. Yuen AWC, Land G, Weatherley B, Peck AW. Sodium valproate inhibits lamotrigine metabolism. *Br J Clin Pharmacol* 1992; 33:511–13.
21. Gidal BE, Anderson GD, Rutecki PR, Shaw R, Lanning A. Lack of an effect of valproate concentration on lamotrigine pharmacokinetics in developmentally disabled patients with epilepsy. *Epilepsy Res* 2000; 42:23–31.
22. Levy RH, Loiseau P, Guyot M, Blehaut H, Tor J, Moreland TA. Stiripentol kinetics in epilepsy: Nonlinearity and interactions. *Clin Pharmacol Ther* 1984; 36:661–9.
23. Barcs G, Walker EB, Elger CE, Scaramelli A, Stefan H, Sturm Y, *et al.* Oxcarbazepine placebo-controlled, dose-ranging trial in refractory partial epilepsy. *Epilepsia* 2000; 41:1597–607.
24. Perucca E, Cloyd J, Critchley D, Fuseau E. Rufinamide: Clinical pharmacokinetics and concentration-response relationships in patients with epilepsy. *Epilepsia* 2008; 49:1123–41.
25. Patsalos PN. *Anti-epileptic drug interactions: A clinical guide*. Guildford: Clarius Press, 2005.
26. May T, Rambeck B. Serum concentrations of valproic acid: influence of dose and comedication. *Ther Drug Monit* 1985; 7:387–90.
27. May TW, Rambeck B, Jurgens U. Serum concentrations of lamotrigine in epileptic patients: the influence of dose and comedication. *Ther Drug Monit* 1996; 18:523–31.
28. Besag FMC, Berry DJ, Pool F, Newbery JE, Subel B. Carbamazepine toxicity with lamotrigine: pharmacokinetic or pharmacodynamic interaction? *Epilepsia* 1998; 39:183–7.
29. Fischer TL, Pieper JA, Graff SW, Rodgers JE, Fischer JD, Parnell KJ, *et al.* Evaluation of potential losartan-phenytoin drug interactions in healthy volunteers. *Clin Pharmacol Ther* 2002; 72:238–46.
30. Deckers CLP, Czucwar SJ, Hekster YA, Keyser A, Kubova H, Meinardi H, *et al.* Selection of antiepileptic drug polytherapy based on mechanisms of action: The evidence reviewed. *Epilepsia* 2000; 41:1364–74.
31. Pisani F, Otero G, Russo MF, Di Perri R, Perucca, E, Richens A. The efficacy of valproate-lamotrigine comedication in refractory complex partial seizures: evidence for a pharmacodynamic interaction. *Epilepsia* 1999; 402:1141–6.
32. Rowan AJ, Meijer JWA, de Beer-Pawlikowski N, van der Geest P, Meinardi H. Valproate-ethosuximide combination therapy for refractory absence seizures. *Arch Neurol* 1983; 40:797–802.
33. Novy J, Patsalos PN, Sander JW, Sisodiya SM. Lacosamide neurotoxicity associated with concomitant use of sodium channel-blocking antiepileptic drugs: A pharmacodynamic interaction? *Epilepsy Behav* 2011; 20:20–3.
34. Reutens DC, Duncan JS, Patsalos PN. Disabling tremor after lamotrigine with sodium valproate. *Lancet* 1993; 342:185–6.
35. Babany G, Larrey D, Pessayre D. Macrolide antibiotics as inducers and inhibitors of cytochrome P450 in experimental animals and man. *Prog Drug Metab* 1988; 11:61–98.
36. Frigo GM, Lecchini S, Caravaggi M, Gatti G, Tonini M, S'Angelo L, *et al.* Reduction in phenytoin clearance caused by cimetidine. *Eur* J Clin Pharmacol 1983; 25:135–7.
37. Levine M, Jones MW, Sheppard I. Differential effect of cimetidine on serum concentrations of carbamazepine and phenytoin. *Neurology* 1985; 35:562–5.
38. Zielinski JJ, Lichten EM, Haidukewych D. Clinically significant danazol-carbamazepine interaction. *Ther Drug Monit* 1987; 9:24–7.

39. Spina E, Perucca E. Clinical significance of pharmacokinetic interactions between antiepileptic and psychotropic drugs. *Epilepsia* 2002; 43(Suppl. 2):37–44.
40. Garcia AB, Ibara AL, Etessam JP, Salio AM, Martinez DP, Diaz RS, *et al.* Protease inhibitor-induced carbamazepine toxicity. *Clin Neuropharmacol* 2000; 23:216–8.
41. Sabers A, Ohman I, Christensen J, Tomson T. Oral contraceptives reduce lamotrigine plasma levels. *Neuro*logy 2003; 61:570–1.
42. Reimers A, Helde G, Brodtkorb E. Ethinyl estradiol, not progesterone, reduces lamotrigine serum concentrations. *Epilepsia* 2005; 46:1414–17.
43. Galimberti CA, Mazzucchelli I, Arbasino C, Canevini MP, Fattore C, Perucca E. Increased apparent oral clearance of valproic acid during intake of combined contraceptive steroids in women with epilepsy. *Epilepsia* 2006; 47:1569–72.
44. Haroutiunian S, Ratz Y, Rabinovich B, Adam M, Hoffman A. Valproic acid plasma concentration decreases in a dose-independent manner following administration of meropenem: A retrospective study. *J Clin Pharmavol* 2009; 49:1363–9.
45. Doose DR, Kohl KA, Desai-Krieger D. No clinically significant effect of topiramate on haloperidol plasma concentration. *Eur Neuropsychopharmacol* 1999; 9:S357.
46. Bittencourt PRM, Gracia CM, Martins R, Fernandes AG, Diekmann HW, Jung W. Phenytoin and carbamazepine decrease oral bioavailability or praziquentel. *Neurology* 1992; 42:492–6.
47. Hugen PW, Burger DM, Brinkman K.Ter Hofstede HJ, Schuurman R, Koopmans PP, *et al.* Carbamazepine-indinavir interaction causes antiretroviral therapy failure. *Ann Pharmacother* 2000; 34:465–70.
48. Michelucci R, Cipolla G, Passarelli D, Gatti G, Ochan M, Heinig R, *et al.* Reduced plasma nisoldipine concentrations in phenytoin-treated patients with epilepsy. *Epilepsia* 1996; 37:1107–10.
49. Murphy M, Dominiczak M. Efficacy of statin therapy: possible effect of phenytoin. *Postgrad Med* 1999; 75:359–60.
50. Freedman MD, Olatidoye AG. Clinically significant drug interactions with the oral anticoagulants. *Drug Saf* 1994; 10:381–94.
51. Levine M, Sheppard I. Biphasic interaction of phenytoin and warfarin. *Clin Pharm* 1984; 3:200–3.
52. Campana C, Regazi MB, Buggia I, Molinaro M. Clinically significant drug interactions with cyclosporin. *An update. Clin Pharmacokin* 1996; 30:141–79.
53. Mula M. Anticonvulsants—antidepressants pharmacokinetic drug interactions: the role of CYP450 system in psychopharmacology. *Curr Drug Metab* 2008; 9:730–7.
54. Crawford P. Interactions between antiepileptic drugs and hormonal contraception. *CNS Drugs* 2002; 16:263–72.
55. Sabers A. Pharmacokinetic interactions between contraceptives and antiepileptic drugs. *Seizure* 2008; 17:141–4.

CHAPTER 26

The Pharmacokinetics and Clinical Therapeutics of the Antiepileptic Drugs

Mark Cook and Simon Shorvon

Pharmacokinetics of antiepileptic drugs

Pharmacokinetics is the study of drug absorption, distribution, metabolism, and elimination. A working knowledge of the pharmacology, pharmacokinetics, indications, and common and serious side effects are important for appropriate use of the anticonvulsant medications, which are summarized in this chapter.

Between 1989–2011, 15 new antiepileptic drugs (AEDs) were licensed (1, 2). These are eslicarbazepine felbamate, gabapentin, lacosamide lamotrigine, levetiracetam, oxcarbazepine, pregabalin, retigabine, rufinamide, stiripentol, tiagabine, topiramate, vigabatrin, and zonisamide (3). Generally these new AEDs are licensed as 'add-on' therapies, at least for initial use, after which there may be scope for conversion to monotherapy. Because they are used in combination, pharmacokinetic interactions can be of importance. Such interactions include those relating to protein-binding displacement from albumin in blood, and metabolic inhibitory and induction interactions occurring in the liver. Overall, the newer AEDs are less prone to be involved in interactions because their pharmacokinetics are more favourable and many are minimally or not bound to blood albumin (eslicarbazepine, felbamate, gabapentin, lacosamide levetiracetam, rufinamide, topiramate, and vigabatrin) and are primarily renally excreted or metabolized by non-cytochrome P450 or uridine glucoronyl transferases (e.g. gabapentin, lacosamide levetiracetam, rufinamide, topiramate, and vigabatrin). Gabapentin, lacosamide, levetiracetam, pregabalin, retigabine, and vigabatrin have few clinically significant pharmacokinetic interactions. Of the new AEDs, lamotrigine and topiramate have the greatest range of significant interactions (4–6).

Metabolism of retigabine, topiramate, tiagabine, zonisamide, and felbamate can be induced by enzyme-inducing AEDs. These agents are less susceptible to the enzyme inhibition induced by valproate, however.

Of the newer agents, only five may significantly impair the efficacy of oral contraceptives: eslicarbazepine, felbamate, oxcarbazepine, rufinamide, and topiramate.

The most clinically significant pharmacodynamic interaction relates to the synergism of valproate and lamotrigine. This interaction can be quite complex when these together are used in conjunction with enzyme inducing agents, such as carbamazepine, when unexpected toxicities may result paradoxically through reduction of the enzyme-inducing agent.

Other drugs are more rarely given including acetazolamide, piracetam, and adrenocorticotropic hormone (ACTH), and these agents are not discussed here.

Basic pharmacokinetic parameters are shown in Tables 26.1 and 26.2.

The pharmacokinetics of the various agents may be significantly altered by metabolic dysfunction, age, and pregnancy. The reader is directed to the relevant chapters of this book for the specific details of these situations.

Pharmacology and clinical therapeutics of antiepileptic drugs

Carbamazepine

This is an important and very well-established drug (it has been used in clinical practice since the late 1960s) and is widely recommended as first-line therapy for partial and secondarily generalized epilepsy. It has for many years been amongst the most widely prescribed drugs worldwide. It acts by inhibiting voltage-dependent sodium conductance, with other less significant actions on monoamine, acetylcholine, and N-methyl-D-aspartate (NMDA) receptors.

The pharmacokinetics of the drug are not optimal. It is variably and poorly absorbed. Although it has linear kinetics, there is an active metabolite (carbamazepine 10,11 epoxide). Carbamazepine is metabolized in the liver by the CYP3A4 isoform of the P450 enzyme system. Drugs that induce or inhibit CYP3A4 can have marked effects on carbamazepine levels and as carbamazepine is a potent inducer of drug metabolizing enzymes, and so is involved in many drug interactions. Amongst these are decrease of carbamazepine levels by concomitant therapy with phenytoin and barbiturates. Increase in carbamazepine-10,11-epoxide levels by valproate. Carbamazepine levels can be increased by verapamil, erythromycin, dextropropoxyphene, and many other drugs. Carbamazepine significantly lowers levels of many other antiepileptic drugs and other medications. It also autoinduces its own

Table 26.1 Pharmacokinetic parameters of commonly used antiepileptics

Drug	Oral bio-availability (%)	Time to peak level (h)	Metabolism	Half -life (h)
Carbamazepine	75–85	4–8	Hepatic	5–26
Clobazam	90	1–4	Hepatic	10–77 (50)
Clonazepam	80	1–4	Hepatic	20–80
Elsicarbazepine	~90	2	Hepatic	13–20
Ethosuximide	~100	<4	Hepatic	30–60
Gabapentin	~65	2–3	None	5–7
Lacosamide	~100	1–4	Hepatic	13
Lamotrigine	~100	1–3	Hepatic	12–60
Levetiracetam	~100	1–2	Non-hepatic	6–8
Oxcarbazepine	<100	4–6	Hepatic	8–10
Phenobarbital	80–100	1–3	Hepatic	75–120
Phenytoin	95	4–12	Hepatic	7–42
Pregabalin	90	1	None	6
Primidone	~100	3	Hepatic	5–18 (75–120)
Retigabine	60%	1–2	Hepatic	6–10
Tiagabine	~96	1–2	Hepatic	5–9
Topiramate	~100	2–4	Hepatic	19–25
Valproate	~100	0.5–8	Hepatic	12–17
Vigabatrin	~100	0.5–2	None	4–7
Zonisamide	~100	2–4	Hepatic	50–70

Table 26.2 Pharmacokinetic parameters of commonly used antiepileptics

Drug	Protein binding (%)	Active metabolite	Drug interactions
Carbamazepine	75	CBZ-epoxide	**
Clobazam	83	N-desmethyl clobazam	*
Clonazepam	86	None	*
Ethosuximide	<10	None	**
Gabapentin	None	None	None
Lacosamide	<15	None	*
Lamotrigine	55	None	**
Levetiracetam	None	None	*
Oxcarbazepine	60	MHD	**
Phenobarbital	45–60	None	**
Phenytoin	85–95	None	**
Pregabalin	None	None	None
Primidone	25	Phenobarbital	**
Retigabine	80	None	*
Tiagabine	96	None	**
Topiramate	15	None	*
Valproate	85–95	None	**
Vigabatrin	None	None	None
Zonisamide	30–60	None	**

** = Many interactions, frequently of clinical relevance and many require dose modification.
* = Minor interactions which can be common, but are not usually of much clinical relevance.

metabolism. Its interactions with the oral contraceptive and warfarin are particularly noteworthy.

Common or important side effects include drowsiness, fatigue, dizziness, ataxia, diplopia, blurring of vision, sedation, headache, insomnia, nausea, loss of appetite, gastrointestinal disturbance, tremor, weight gain, impotence, effects on behaviour and mood, other psychiatric and psychological effects, hepatic disturbance, rash and other skin reactions, bone marrow dyscrasia, changes in blood parameters especially leucopenia, hyponatraemia, water retention, hepatic, renal and endocrine effects, cardiorespiratory effects.

About 5% of patients develop a rash on initiation of therapy and all should be warned about this. Stevens–Johnson syndrome and the related disease toxic epidermal necrolysis are serious and potentially life-threatening reactions to the use of carbamazepine, which have been shown in certain ethnic groups, particularly Han Chinese, to be associated with a genetic marker, HLA-B*1502 (7). The FDA has recently recommended that patients with ancestry from areas in which HLA-B*1502 is present (Asia and South East Asia) should be screened for the HLA-B*1502 allele before starting treatment with carbamazepine. This is a rapidly evolving area of knowledge, and other HLA types have been associated with rash in European populations (8). Therapy should be immediately stopped if rash develops. Other side effects are generally worse on initiation of therapy, and this is why the initial dose should be low and then slowly incremented.

It is a highly effective drug, and indeed is the gold standard still against which other drugs are compared—and this after nearly 50 years of usage. The usual indication for use, in adults and children, is first-line therapy in partial and generalized tonic–clonic seizures (not absence and myoclonus), and also in childhood epilepsy syndromes.

Preparations included tablets in a range of doses, slow-release preparations, liquid and suppositories. The usual starting dosage for adults is 100–200 mg/day, and increased every 2–3 weeks by 100/200 mg. Maintenance dosages are usually in the range of 400–1600 mg/day. For slow-release formulations, a 30% higher dosage should be given as plasma levels are lower for these slightly less bioavailable compounds.

Usual dosage in children: less than 1 year, 100–200mg/day; 1–5 years, 200–400mg/day; 5–10 years, 400–600mg/day;10–15 years, 600–1000mg. Again, for the slow-release formulations, higher dosages are required.

Dosing interval is usually 2 times/day, but 2–4 times/day may be better tolerated at higher doses or in children.

Blood level monitoring can be useful; the usually quoted target range is 17–51 μmol/L (4–12 micrograms/mL). Good effect may be achieved at lower levels however, and high levels may be very well tolerated. As with other AEDs, clinical parameters are generally more useful when monitoring the effects and tolerability of the drug.

Clobazam

Clobazam is an interesting and valuable second-line therapy and has been in clinical use since 1979. It acts as a gamma aminobutyric acid A ($GABA_A$) receptor agonist. Popular in Europe for many years, trials of clobazam in Lennox–Gastaut syndrome have rekindled interest in this agent recently (9), and it has been approved in the US only since late 2011. It is the only commonly used 1,5-benzodiazepine and perhaps as a result of this has distinctive properties that set it apart from the others.

Drug interactions are generally minor, but clobazam clearance is increased by enzyme-inducing agents, and occasionally clobazam may result in an increase in the plasma levels of other antiepileptic drugs.

Common or important side effects include sedation, dizziness, weakness, blurring of vision, restlessness, ataxia, hypotonia, behavioural disturbance, withdrawal symptoms and paradoxical agitation, particularly in children.

Clobazam is widely felt to be the most useful benzodiazepine in chronic treatment. It has a broad-spectrum activity; relatively high response rates in refractory epilepsy, and is generally very well tolerated. It is also used as a one-off therapy for periods of seizure exacerbation (or seizure clusters) and also taken on a single day as prophylaxis on days when the occurrence of a seizure needs to be particularly avoided (e.g. travel, exams, etc.). The development of tolerance is its main problem. It is easy to use, without the need for starting at a low dose or dosage incrementation. As with the other benzodiazepines, tolerance is prone to develop with prolonged use, particularly with large doses. Accumulation of the active metabolite desmethylclobazam, which has a half-life of about 50 hours can be an important factor.

Indications are as second-line therapy for partial and generalized tonic–clonic seizures, for both adults and children. Clobazam is also used for intermittent therapy, and one-off prophylactic therapy. A tablet is the only available preparation.

The usual adult dosage is 10–20 mg/day (adults), but higher doses can be used depending on tolerability. The usual dosage in children 3–12 years is 5–10mg/daily 1–2 times/daily. Blood level monitoring is not generally useful.

Clonazepam

Introduced into clinical practice in 1963, Clonazepam is now only occasionally used in routine therapy in adults. It has a greater place in severe childhood epilepsies. It can be useful as monotherapy occasionally, particularly when seizures occur at a predictable time such as in sleep. Myoclonus is sometimes dramatically suppressed by clonazepam. It has a broad-spectrum action but tolerance and withdrawal seizures limit its value in routine therapy in chronic epilepsy. It is widely used as an effective intravenous therapy in status epilepticus. Like the other benzodiazepine drugs, its main action is as an agonist at the $GABA_A$ receptor.

Clonazepam levels can be lowered by co-medication with enzyme inducing drugs.

Important or common side effects include sedation, which is common and may be severe, cognitive impairment, drowsiness, ataxia, personality and behavioural changes, hyperactivity (typically in children), restlessness, aggressiveness, psychotic reaction, seizure exacerbations, drooling and excessive saliva production (especially in children), leucopenia, and withdrawal symptoms

Usual indications for use are as second-line therapy in partial and generalized seizures, including absence and myoclonus, in both adults and children. Clonazepam is also used in Lennox–Gastaut syndrome, neonatal seizures, infantile spasms, and status epilepticus.

Available preparations include tablets and liquid formulations. Usual adult dosage is initially 0.25 mg at night, with maintenance doses of 0.5–4 mg/day. The usual dosage in children: under 1 year, 1mg/day; 1–5 years: 1–2mg/day; and above 5 years: 1–3mg/day. The dosing interval is 1–2 times/day. Blood level monitoring is not useful.

Eslicarbazepine acetate

Eslicarbazepine acetate was licensed for clinical use in Europe in 2009. It is a derivative of carbamazepine and acts as a prodrug to the pharmacologically active eslicarbazepine (S–licarbazepine). Eslicarbazepine acetate is rapidly absorbed after oral ingestion. Its minor metabolites (R-licarbazepine and oxcarbazepine) are pharmacologically active. The bioavailability of eslicarbazepine is 90% and it is 30% protein bound in serum. It is eliminated chiefly through glucuronic acid, as are its metabolites, and excreted renally. As with carbamazepine and oxcarbazepine, it acts on the voltage-gated sodium channel.

Phenytoin can decrease eslicarbazepine serum levels significantly as may carbamazepine, phenobarbital, and primidone. Eslicarbazepine can decrease the clearance of phenytoin and increase phenytoin serum levels. Eslicarbazepine can increase the clearance of lamotrigine and topiramate. Eslicarbazepine can decrease the level of levonorgestrel and ethinyloestradial and so impair the efficacy of the oral contraceptive. It can significantly decrease warfarin blood levels. Co-administration with carbamazepine can aggravate neurotoxic side effects such as diplopia, abnormal coordination, and dizziness.

Side effects are as for carbamazepine and oxcarbazepine. The most common side effects observed are dizziness, somnolence, headache, nausea, vomiting, diarrhoea, blurred vision and vertigo. These side effects are dose-dependent. Hyponatraemia has been observed in 0.6–1.3% of patients treated with Eslicarbazepine during the pre-marketing clinical trials. Dose should be adjusted in patients with renal or hepatic impairment.

Its licensed indication is as adjunctive therapy in adults with partial-onset seizures with or without secondary generalization.

The preparations available are as liquid suspension or tablet form of 400, 600, and 800 mg sizes. The drugs should be started at a dose of 400 mg/day for 1–2 weeks before reaching the maintenance dose of 800–1200 mg/day.

Plasma levels are of uncertain value as yet, and a therapeutic range has not been established.

Ethosuximide

Ethosuximide was introduced into practice in 1958, and was first-line therapy of generalized absence seizures for many years.

It has been only occasionally used in recent years, but demonstration of superiority to lamotrigine in the therapy of absence has recently been demonstrated and rekindled interest in the use of this agent (10). It acts by blocking conduction in low voltage (LVA) T type calcium channels.

Ethosuximide is well absorbed, has linear kinetics, and is metabolized in the liver (cytochrome CYP3A4), and is only 10% protein bound. Its clearance is reduced by co-medication with valproate. Ethosuximide has a number of important interactions, levels are reduced by co-administration of carbamazepine, phenytoin, phenobarbital, and other drugs such as rifampicin. Serum valproic acid levels may be decreased by ethosuximide. Ethosuximide levels are increased by some drugs (e.g. isoniazid). Co-medication with ethosuximide does not generally interfere with levels of other AEDs.

Side effects can be problematic and serious, and include idiosyncratic blood reactions and the induction of behavioural and psychiatric symptoms. Headache, drowsiness and sedation are common effects. Gastrointestinal symptoms are common, and can be prominent. Other effects include lethargy, ataxia, diplopia, dizziness, hiccups, behavioural disturbances including aggression and irritability, hyperexcitibility in children, acute psychotic reactions and other psychiatric side effects especially depression. Extrapyramidal symptoms, insomnia, blood dyscrasias of various sorts that can be severe, rash, lupus-like syndrome, and other severe idiosyncratic reactions can be occasionally seen.

The usual indication is generalized absence seizures, in adults and children. Ethosuximide is available as either capsules or syrup.

The starting dose is 250 mg daily. Maintenance doses are 750–2000 mg/day. The usual dosage in children initially is 10–15 mg/kg/day, and maintenance 20–40 mg/kg/day. Dosing is 2–3 times daily.

Blood level monitoring is of limited practical value, and is increasingly difficult to obtain in many countries. The stated therapeutic range is 40–100 mg/L.

Felbamate

Felbamate was licensed in 1993, but its use now is very limited due to the risk of serious idiosyncratic liver failure and bone marrow toxicity. Felbamate is recommended only in patients who have not responded to other AED treatments.

Felbamate has a bioavailability of 90–95%, and is minimally protein bound. Metabolism is hepatic with renal excretion of metabolites. Felbamate is an inhibitor of hepatic enzymes and can increase concentrations of phenobarbital, phenytoin, valproic acid, carbamazepine and clobazam. The metabolism of felbamate is increased by enzyme-inducing agents such as carbamazepine, phenobarbital, phenytoin, and primidone, resulting in reduced serum half-life. A novel mode of interaction is with gabapentin, which can reduce the elimination half-life of felbamate and clearance significantly due to an interaction at the level of renal excretion. Felbamate inhibits the metabolism of warfarin and may reduce the effectiveness of oral contraceptives.

Adverse reactions include decreased appetite, vomiting, insomnia, nausea, dizziness, somnolence, and headache. Aplastic anaemia and hepatic (liver) failure are rare but serious effects. The risk of aplastic anaemia has been estimated between 1:3600 and 1:5000. Of these 30% of cases are fatal. The risk of hepatic failure is between 1:24,000 to 1:34,000, and 40% of cases are fatal.

Indications for use are as monotherapy or adjunctive therapy in the treatment of partial seizures, with and without generalization in adults, and in children as adjunctive therapy in the treatment of partial and generalized seizures associated with Lennox–Gastaut syndrome.

Felbamate is available in tablets of 400 and 600 mg size, and as a oral suspension (600 mg/5 mL). The dosage in adults is 1200 mg daily, and in children 2–14 years 15–45 mg/kg/day. Dosing interval is 3–4 times daily.

Gabapentin

Gabapentin was designed to be an analogue of GABA, but in fact its antiepileptic effects are probably due to its binding to the $\alpha 2\delta$ subunit of the neuronal voltage-dependent calcium channel. It has been used mainly in neurogenic pain, and its epilepsy usage is confined to adjunctive therapy in refractory partial epilepsy. Its place in the therapy of both pain and epilepsy has been to some extent superseded by the newer drug pregabalin, which has the same mechanism of action but is more potent.

It has variable absorption, and is poorly absorbed at high doses, but has otherwise excellent pharmacokinetics and is excreted unchanged. Gabapentin has no important drug interactions.

Significant side effects include drowsiness, dizziness, weight gain, seizure exacerbation, ataxia, headache, tremor, psychiatric disturbance especially depression and anxiety, cognitive blunting, concentration and memory difficulties, impotence, diplopia, nausea, vomiting, flatulence and other gastrointestinal effects, rhinitis, peripheral oedema (which can be painful), joint and muscle pains, cough, dyspnoea, itching, pancreatic and hepatic disturbance. However, generally gabapentin is a well-tolerated drug, but has a reputation of having rather modest efficacy. It has a role particularly in the treatment of mild epilepsy, in children or in the elderly where the excellent pharmacokinetics and lack of interactions are a useful feature.

The usual indications for use are partial or secondarily generalized epilepsy, in adults and children. It is available in tablet and capsule preparations of 100, 300, 400, 600, and 800 mg. The usual adult dosage initially is 300 mg/day, aiming for a maintenance dose of 900–3600 mg/day. In children, the initial dose is 10–15 mg/kg/day, and maintenance 40 mg/kg/day in children aged 3–4 years, and 25–35 mg/kg/day in children 5–12 years of age. Dosing intervals are typically 2–3 times/day. Blood level monitoring is not useful.

Lacosamide

This agent has a relatively novel action on the slow inactivation current of the neuronal sodium channel, an action which differs in a minor way from that of other conventional AEDs acting on the sodium channel such as carbamazepine, phenytoin, or lamotrigine. It also has unique binding site to the CMRP-2 protein, though the significance of this is uncertain. It shows efficacy in a broad range of experimental epilepsy models.

Lacosamide has excellent pharmacokinetics—complete absorption, linear kinetics, a plasma half-life of about 13 hours, dose-level proportionality, low protein bindings, and 95% of the dose is excreted in the urine as drug and metabolites. There are no clinical important drug interactions. It has no effect on the plasma levels of other drugs. Co-medication with other enzyme-inducing drugs may reduce the lacosamide level slightly.

Reported side effects include: dizziness, headache, nausea, fatigue and blurring of vision. Angioneurotic oedema has been reported. Aggravation of side effects of the common neurotoxic side effects of other sodium channel blockers, particularly carbamazepine and phenytoin is well recognized, and reduction in the doses of these agents may significantly improve tolerability. It is a generally well-tolerated medication.

Clinical trials show the drug to have good efficacy and the long-term retention rate in the open extension of the trials was also very good. It is newly licensed for use as add-on therapy for partial onset seizures in adults, and its place in routine therapy has not yet been established.

The usual indication for use is therapy of partial-onset seizures with or without secondary generalization in adults. Preparations include tablets of 50, 100, 150, 200 mg strengths; IV solution (10 mg/mL), and oral syrup (15 mg/mL).

The usual initial adult dosage is 50 mg/day, aiming for a maintenance dose of 200–400 mg/day. The dosing interval is 2 times/day. Blood level monitoring is not useful.

Lamotrigine

This drug was first licensed for use in 1991. It has since established a place as a useful first- and second-line therapy in a broad spectrum of epilepsies. It acts by a variety of mechanisms, most important being sodium channel conduction blockade, like phenytoin and carbamazepine.

It has complex pharmacokinetics, is metabolized in the liver, and has drug interactions, which complicate its use. The most important interaction is with valproate, co-medication with which can result in a very marked elevation of lamotrigine levels. Serum lamotrigine levels are reduced by many drugs including enzyme inducing antiepileptic drugs (e.g. carbamazepine, phenytoin, phenobarbital), rifampicin, combined steroid contraceptives. Lamotrigine may reduce the serum levels of levonorgestrel. In the later stages of pregnancy, the levels of lamotrigine can fall greatly.

Important or common side effects include rash and hypersensitivity reaction involving fever, hepatic dysfunction, blood dyscrasias, disseminated intravascular coagulation, and multiorgan failure. A troublesome side effect is an allergic rash which can be occasionally severe or progress to a Stevens–Johnson syndrome. The frequency of skin rash is higher in children than in adults. Early reports suggested that 1 in 50 children developed a potentially life-threatening rash, but the incidence has fallen since the recognition that slow incrementation—particularly in patients co-medicated with valproate—greatly reduces the risk. Headache can be marked, and aseptic meningitis is recognized (11). Ataxia, asthenia, fatigue, diplopia, nausea, vomiting, dizziness, somnolence, insomnia, depression, psychosis, tremor, movement disorder, other neurological and psychiatric effects, arthralgia, lupus-like syndrome, and photosensitivity have all been reported.

In spite of all this, the impact of side effects in routine practice is generally low and the drug is generally well tolerated, although some side effects such as insomnia can limit its use.

Its main disadvantages relate to the need to individualize dose according to co-medication and the need for a slow introduction of therapy. Its main advantages are its broad spectrum and relatively good tolerability. There is some uncertainty as to whether lamotrigine aggravates myoclonus in all idiopathic generalized syndromes, but it is recognized to aggravate severe myoclonic epilepsy of infancy (12), and there are case reports aggravation of other seizure types. Lamotrigine is nevertheless a useful agent in most patients with idiopathic generalized epilepsies, and concerns over myoclonus aggravation are perhaps overemphasized.

The usual indications for use are therapy of partial and generalized epilepsy, Lennox–Gastaut syndrome, and other generalized epilepsy syndromes, in both adults and children.

It is available as tablets in 5, 25, 50, 100, 150, and 200 mg size, and in dispersible forms. The usual adult dose is initially 12.5–25 mg/day, the lower dose being appropriate when co-administered with valproate.

The usual maintenance dose in combination therapy without valproic acid and without enzyme-inducing agents is 200–400 mg/day. As initial monotherapy the dose is typically 100–400 mg/day. When given as combination therapy with valproic acid, without enzyme inducing agents, 100–400 mg/day. As combination therapy with enzyme inducing agents without valproic acid: 300–500 mg/day.

The usual dosage in children when used as part of combination therapy without valproic acid, and without enzyme inducing agents, children 2–12 years of age: 2.5–7.5 mg/kg/day. As combination therapy with valproic acid without enzyme inducing agents in children 2–12 years of age: 1–3 mg/kg/day. As combination therapy with enzyme inducing agents without valproic acid for children 2–12 years of age: 5–15 mg/kg/day.

Given the very long serum half-life, particularly with co-administration of valproate, the dosing interval is 1–2 times/day.

Blood level monitoring is of limited usefulness, it may have particular utility in establishing an effective target range prior to pregnancy, when the dose may need to be increased 50–100% in the last trimester through increased clearance (13). The usual target range is generally considered 2.5–15 mg/L, but much higher levels are often tolerated very well.

Levetiracetam

The drug was licensed in 1999/2000 in the USA/Europe and is a powerful antiepileptic compound, which has rapidly gained an important place in clinical practice both in monotherapy and polytherapy. It acts by binding to the synaptic vesicle (SV2A) protein and this is a unique mode of action not shared by other widely used antiepileptics (14).

It has excellent pharmacokinetics and is metabolized largely by hydrolysis and only 24% of the drug is metabolized in the liver. Co-medication with levetiracetam does not affect levels of other drugs. Levetiracetam levels can fall by up to 20–30% on co-medication with enzyme-inducing AEDs.

It is generally very well tolerated without the usual sedative effects of other AEDs or the typical central nervous system side effects of the sodium channel-blocking antiepileptics. Its main drawback is its tendency in susceptible individuals to cause marked irritability and occasionally aggressive or psychotic behaviour (15, 16). It can paradoxically increase seizure frequency in occasional patients especially at high doses. Other important or common side effects include behavioural change, irritability, aggression, mood change, depression, anxiety, and psychosis. Other side effects include headache, unsteadiness, tremor and hyperkinesis, memory and attention disturbance, somnolence, asthenia, visual disturbance, gastrointestinal disturbance, infection, itching, rash, alopecia, blood dyscrasia, myalgia, pancreatic and hepatic disturbance, and cough.

It is easy to use in clinical practice and has a broad-spectrum activity in epilepsy, controlling generalized and partial seizures.

Its current licensing is as adjunctive therapy for partial seizures in adults and children from 4 years of age; adjunctive therapy for myoclonic seizures in adults and adolescents with juvenile myoclonic epilepsy from 12 years of age; as adjunctive therapy for primary generalized tonic–clonic seizures in adults and adolescents with idiopathic generalized epilepsy from 12 years of age in Europe and from 6 years of age in the US; initial monotherapy for partial seizures in adults, in Europe but not the US.

The usual indication for use is as first line and adjunctive therapy of partial-onset seizures and of generalized tonic–clonic seizures and myoclonic seizures in IGE. Levetiracetam may also be useful for other generalized seizure types.

Usual preparations include tablets of 250, 500, 750, 1000 mg size, oral solution (100 mg/mL), and an IV preparation (500 mg/5mL)

The usual adult dosage is initially 125–250 mg/day, with increments of 125–250 mg every 2 weeks. Maintenance doses are typically 750–3000 mg/day. Dosage needs to be reduced in renal disease.

In children the initial dosage is 10–20 mg/kg/day with increments of 10–20 mg/kg/day every 2 weeks, and maintenance of 20–60 mg/kg/day.

The dosing interval is 2 times/day

Serum level monitoring is not routinely available in most centres, and only occasionally useful. The target range is 12–46 mg/L.

Oxcarbazepine

Oxcarbazepine is the 10-keto analogue of carbamazepine. It was introduced into clinical practice in Denmark in 1990, but licensed in other EU countries in 1999 and in the US in 2000. Oxcarbazepine is metabolized first by reduction, avoiding the oxidative step that carbamazepine undergoes and thus the production of the oxidative metabolite of carbamazepine (CBZ-epoxide), which is responsible for some carbamazepine side effects. The pharmacological action of oxcarbazepine is exerted almost exclusively through its active 10-monohydroxy derivative metabolite (MHD). Its antiepileptic effects are very similar to those of carbamazepine, and its mode of action is identical

It has generally fewer and less marked drug interactions than carbamazepine. Other enzyme inducing antiepileptic drugs reduce the serum levels of the active metabolite MHD. Oxcarbazepine comedication increases serum levels of phenytoin and phenobarbital, and reduces serum levels of oral contraceptives.

Side effects are also similar to those of carbamazepine. It has however a more marked propensity to cause hyponatraemia, which can be severe. Although the risk of serious rash is lower that with carbamazepine, a mild skin rash is relatively common (about 5–10% of all patients). About 25–30% of those experiencing a serious rash or hypersensitivity on carbamazepine will also experience similar symptoms on oxcarbazepine. It may share the link described earlier with the HLA-B*1502 and carbamazepine (17). Other side effects are dizziness, unsteadiness, diplopia, ataxia, somnolence, headache, fatigue, nausea, and gastrointestinal disturbances. Other side effects include anorexia, alopecia, pancreatic disturbance, lupus-like syndrome, cardiorespiratory disturbance, and other cognitive and neurological symptoms.

Its usual indication is as a first- or second-line treatment in partial and secondarily generalized seizures, in both adults and children.

Available preparations are tablets of 150, 300, 600 mg size, and oral suspension. The usual adult dosage initially is 600 mg/day, with maintenance doses of 900–2400 mg/day. In children the usual dosage is initially 4–5 mg/kg/day, increased by increments of 5 mg/kg/day weekly, with a maintenance dose of 20–45 mg/kg/day.

Dosing intervals are 2 times/day.

Serum level monitoring may be useful in some cases. The target range 3–35 mg/L.

Phenobarbital

Phenobarbital is a remarkable compound, introduced into practice in 1912, and still, in volume terms, the most commonly prescribed AED in the world. It is by far the cheapest of the AEDs commonly available. It is highly effective with an efficacy that generally speaking has not been bettered by any subsequent drug. It is extensively metabolized in the liver and is involved in a number of drug interactions, although these are usually minor. It has a very long half-life and a tendency to accumulate. Its main disadvantages relate to its cerebral side effects and its tendency to cause sedation, but this is seldom a problem at low doses. In children, there is a strong tendency to cause hyperexcitibility and behavioural change, which often limits its use. Its main mechanism of action is enhancement of $GABA_A$ receptor activity, but it also depresses glutamate excitability and affects sodium, potassium, and calcium conductance.

Phenobarbital is a potent hepatic enzyme inducer and stimulates the metabolism of many other drugs including antiepileptics. Serum phenobarbital levels are also reduced due to induction by many other drugs, and increased due to inhibition by co-administration of drugs such as valproate.

Common and important adverse events include rash and other idiosyncratic reactions. Other side effects include sedation, lethargy, somnolence, headache, dizziness, diplopia, ataxia, rash, hyponatraemia, weight gain, alopecia, nausea, gastrointestinal disturbance. Neuropsychiatric side effects can occur including depression, aggressiveness, cognitive dysfunction, impotence, reduced libido, paradoxical hyperkinesis and behavioural change in children (which can be severe). Cognitive effects including memory and attentional disturbances, folate and vitamins D and K deficiency, Dupuytren's contracture, frozen shoulder, other connective tissue and cosmetic effects, osteopenia, and osteomalacia are also reported.

The primary indication is as first- or second-line therapy for partial or generalized seizures (including absence and myoclonus), Lennox–Gastaut syndrome, and other childhood epilepsy syndromes. It has also been extensively used in febrile convulsions and neonatal seizures.

Available preparations tablets of 15, 30, 50, 60, 100 mg strength, liquid (15 mg/5mL), and injection (200 mg/mL).

Usual dosage for adults is initially 30 mg/day, with increments of 30 mg every 2 weeks. Maintenance doses are typically 30–180 mg/day.

Usual dosage for neonates is 3–4 mg/kg/day, and for children 3–8 mg/kg/day.

Dosing interval is 1–2 times/day.

Serum level monitoring may be useful in some patients, with a target range of 10–40 mg/L.

Phenytoin

Phenytoin was introduced into clinical practice in 1938. Although no longer considered first-line therapy in Europe, it remains one of the most widely used AEDs in the world because of its low cost and strong antiepileptic effect.

It has difficult pharmacokinetic properties, with non-linear kinetics, extensive hepatic metabolism, and many drug interactions. Because of this, its use requires regular serum level monitoring especially when changing therapy. However, once a satisfactory phenytoin dosage regimen has been achieved in a particular patient, it will rarely be necessary to alter the regimen over many years. The list of side effects is long but most patients on chronic therapy do not experience marked side effects, and there is no strong evidence of any general difference in tolerability between phenytoin and other old (or new) drugs. It is now usually reserved as a drug of second choice in partial and secondarily generalized seizures, and also in primary generalized tonic–clonic seizures. Its major mechanism of action, as with carbamazepine, is mediated by inhibition of voltage-dependent sodium channels.

There are many common and important drug interactions. Phenytoin is a strong enzyme inducer and reduces the serum levels of many other drugs. Similarly, numerous drugs interfere with phenytoin absorption, plasma protein binding, and metabolism.

A hypersensitivity reaction to phenytoin is rare but can be severe and can take various forms including rash, fever, hepatic and renal disturbance, a lupus-like syndrome, lymphadenopathy or blood dyscrasias. Other side effects include: ataxia, dizziness, lethargy, sedation, psychiatric disturbance including depression and anxiety and psychosis, headache, dyskinesia, acute encephalopathy (phenytoin intoxication), insomnia, tremor, psychological changes including memory and attentional defects, connective tissue alterations, gingival hyperplasia, coarsened facies, hirsutism, osteopenia and osteomalacia, vitamins D and K and folate deficiency, megaloblastic anaemia, hypocalcaemia, hormonal dysfunction, loss of libido, pseudolymphoma, hepatitis, coagulation defects, bone marrow hypoplasia, gastrointestinal disturbance including nausea and vomiting and anorexia, weight change.

Primary indications for use are partial and primary and secondarily generalized seizures (excluding myoclonus and absence). Available preparations include capsules: 25, 30, 50, 100, 200 mg; chewtabs: 50 mg; liquid suspension (30 mg/5 mL, 125 mg/50 mL), and injection (250 mg/5 mL).

The usual adult dosage initially is 300 mg at night, with maintenance doses of 200–500 mg/day (higher doses can be used; guided by serum level monitoring). The non-linear kinetics of the drug mean 25–50 mg increments and decrements of the dose are usually appropriate when near the target range, and conversely that relatively small changes in the dose can cause large changes in serum levels.

In children the usual maintenance dose is 10 mg/kg/day. Again, higher doses can be used; guided by serum level monitoring.

Dosing interval is 1–2 times/day.

Serum level monitoring is mandatory when establishing therapy. Target range is 40–80 μmol/L (10–20 mg/L)

Pregabalin

Pregabalin was licensed as an antiepileptic drug in 2004 for adjunctive use in partial seizures in adults, both in the US and in Europe. In addition to its epilepsy indications, it is licensed as an analgesic for neuropathic pain. It is structurally similar to gabapentin and acts in the same way, by modulating neurotransmitter release by binding to the $\alpha 2\delta$ subunit of voltage-gated calcium channels. However, its binding is stronger and it has greater efficacy than gabapentin. It has excellent pharmacokinetics, with a low potential for drug interaction and is excreted largely unchanged. These are significant advantages in many clinical situations. It also has a mild anxiolytic effect. Its main side effects are weight gain and CNS effects such as sedation, and these tend to be dose-related and may be dose-limiting. It is a powerful antiepileptic and a useful addition to second-line therapy, though its most common use is in pain management.

Common or important side effects include dizziness, somnolence, ataxia, asthenia, increased appetite and weight gain, visual disturbances, tremor, memory and attentional deficit, confusion and other cognitive effects, psychiatric disturbance, change in sexual function, blurred vision, peripheral oedema, dry mouth, gastrointestinal disturbances (particularly constipation), flatulence, cardiorespiratory disturbance, myalgia, joint pains, hepatic and pancreatic disturbance. Rare cases of hypersensitivity have been reported including severe skin reactions and blood dyscrasia.

It has no important drug interactions.

Primary indications for use are as second-line therapy for partial seizures with or without secondary generalization in adults.

The preparations available are capsules: 25, 50, 75, 100, 150, and 300 mg size. The usual adult dosage is initially 50 mg/day, with increments of 50 mg every 2 weeks. Maintenance doses are 150–600 mg/day.

Dosing interval is 2 times/day.

Serum level monitoring is not routinely needed or useful.

Primidone

Primidone is a 'pro-drug' of phenobarbital, introduced into clinical practice in 1952, and its action is probably entirely due to the derived phenobarbital. It has no clinical advantage (and significant disadvantages) compared to phenobarbital, although it is not, like phenobarbital, a drug of abuse and therefore not subject to special controls. The side effects are the same as those of phenobarbital, with the additional problem of a propensity to intense dizziness, nausea and sedation at the onset of therapy (sometimes after only one tablet) if the dose started is too high. These effects are probably due to the initially high concentration of the parent drug and disappear after a week or so. Because of this reaction it is always advisable to start primidone at a very low dose. The drug interaction profile of primidone is that same as that of phenobarbital.

Usual indications are as for phenobarbital. The available preparations are a tablet, 250 mg, and suspension: 50 mg/mL. The usual adult dosage is initially 62.5–125 mg/day. Increasing by 125–250 mg increments every 2 weeks to a maintenance dose of 500–1500 mg/day.

The usual dosage in children initially is 50 mg increased gradually to a maintenance dose of 10–25 mg/kg/day.

Dosing interval is 2 times/day.

Serum level monitoring is useful to measure the derived phenobarbital levels.

Retigabine

Retigabine was licensed in Europe in 2011. It has a completely novel mechanism of action and thus its use in epilepsy was eagerly awaited. Retigabine acts primarily by opening neuronal potassium channels (KCNQ2 [Kv7.2] and KCNQ3 [Kv7.3]) and thus stabilizing the resting membrane potential and controlling the subthreshold electrical excitability in neurons (18). This seems to be its only action and this action is not shared by other antiepileptic drugs.

The drug is absorbed only to about 60%. It is approximately 80% bound to plasma protein over the concentration range of 0.1 to 2 micrograms/mL. It is extensively metabolized in the liver eventually to N-glucuronides, and is excreted largely via the kidney. It does not induce or block liver enzymes and retigabine does not significantly alter the levels of other AEDs, although phenytoin and carbamazepine can reduce retigabine systemic exposure by about one-third.

The most common side effects are dizziness, fatigue and somnolence. Other side effects are weight gain, confusion, psychotic disorders, hallucinations, disorientation and anxiety. The usual neurological side effects of antiepileptic drugs have been reported including: diplopia, blurred vision, memory disturbance, unsteadiness, vertigo, paraesthesia, tremor, speech disturbance and malaise. Gastrointestinal disturbance and peripheral oedema have been reported. Because of its mode of action, difficulty with micturition and even urinary retention have been reported as an unusual but troublesome side effect.

The drug has shown striking efficacy. The licensed indication currently is as adjunctive treatment for partial onset seizures with or without secondary generalization in adults aged 18 years and above.

The usual starting dose is 50 mg 3 times a day. This is increased every week or two by 50 mg, 3 times a day until an effective maintenance dose of between 600–1200 mg is reached. The maximum licensed dose currently is 400 mg, 3 times a day. In severe renal or hepatic failure the dose should be halved, but there is no requirement to change the dose in mild or moderate renal or hepatic failure.

Retigabine is available as 50, 100, 200, 300, and 400 mg tablets. The recommended dosing intervals are three times a day.

Serum level monitoring is not required

Rufinamide

Rufinamide was licensed in Europe in 2007 through the European Orphan Drug Program. It is a triazole derivative structurally unrelated to any other current antiepileptic drugs. Rufinamide's exact mechanism of action is unknown, though it is thought to modulate sodium channels and produce membrane stabilization.

The absorption is slow but complete, with bioavailability of 85%. It is 34% protein bound. Rufinamide is metabolized in the liver, primarily by hydrolysis, and the pharmacologically inactive metabolite is excreted in urine. The half-life is 6–12 hours.

Carbamazepine, phenobarbital, phenytoin, primidone and vigabatrin can significantly decrease rufinamide serum levels through increased clearance. Valproic acid can increase rufinamide serum levels through a decrease in hepatic metabolism. Rufinamide can decrease serum levels of carbamazepine and lamotrigine, and may increase serum levels of phenobarbital and phenytoin. Rufinamide may also increase the clearance of ethinyloestradiol and norethindrone and consequently impair the efficacy of the oral contraceptive. No dosage adjustment is needed in the presence of renal dysfunction, but it is not recommended for use in patients with hepatic impairment. Haemodialysis may reduce serum concentrations by approximately 30%.

The indication for use currently is as adjunctive treatment of seizures in Lennox–Gastaut syndrome in patients 4 years and older.

The recommended starting dose for adults is 400–800 mg/day. The dose may be increased by 400–800 mg/day increments every 2 days to a maximum dose of 3200 mg/day. The recommended starting dose in children is 10 mg/kg/day, increasing by 10 mg/kg every 2 days up to a dose of 45 mg/kg/day or 3200 mg/day.

Stiripentol

Stiripentol was licensed in Europe in 2008, again though the orphan drug programme. Its precise mechanism of action is unknown, other than that it enhances the effect of GABA (19). The drug is rapidly absorbed after oral ingestion, but its bioavailability has not yet been determined. It is 99% bound to serum proteins. Stiripentol is extensively metabolized, and only traces detectable unchanged in the urine.

Stiripentol is a potent hepatic enzyme inhibitor, and can increase serum levels of phenytoin, carbamazepine, phenobarbital, valproic acid, and clobazam. Enzyme-inducing agents such as carbamazepine, phenobarbital, phenytoin and primidone induce the metabolism of stiripentol, and may lower stiripentol serum levels. No significant interactions between stiripentol and other non-AEDs have been reported, but it is a potent inhibitor of hepatic enzymes and the potential exists for interactions with other medications metabolized by the liver. It is not currently known to have any significant effect on sex hormones or oral contraceptive agents.

The only current licensed indication for stiripentol is as adjunctive treatment of seizures in children with severe myoclonic epilepsy in infancy (Dravet syndrome)(20). Available preparations are a capsule, 250 and 500 mg size; and powder also 250 and 500 mg. The initial dose is 50 mg/kg/day, increasing up to 100 mg/kg per day, with a maximum of 4g.

The dosing interval is 2–3 times daily. Because of its potential for interactions, the doses of other anticonvulsants may have to be reduced, and potential interactions with other hepatically metabolized agents will need to be careful monitored.

Tiagabine

Tiagabine was introduced into clinical practice in 1998 as adjunctive therapy in refractory patients with partial or secondarily generalized seizures, in adults and in children over the age of 12 years. It is a GABA reuptake blocker, and acts by enhancing GABAergic transmission. This is a similar mechanism of action to that of vigabatrin, but tiagabine does not carry the risk of psychosis and depression, or visual field defects, which are major side effects of vigabatrin. It is metabolized by the hepatic cytochrome CYP3A4 enzymes, is 96% protein bound and has a half-life of 5–9 hours but which is reduced to 2–4 hours in co-medication with enzyme-inducing drugs. Its use however is complicated by the need to titrate slowly, the potential for drug interactions that result in the need for dose changes, and the frequent need for 3 or even 4 times a day dosing. It should always be taken with food, and preferably at the end of meals, to avoid rapid rises in plasma concentrations—and the giving with food will greatly improve tolerability. Individual dosing 4 times daily may also be helpful, at least with higher doses. Minor dose-related side effects are common but the frequency of idiosyncratic drug-related reactions, including cutaneous reactions, is very low. It has a tendency to exacerbate seizures in the generalized epilepsies, and to provoke non-convulsive status (21).

Most enzyme-inducing AEDs increase tiagabine clearance by stimulating its metabolism and dose changes are often needed under these circumstances.

It is often poorly tolerated, and common or adverse events include dizziness, tiredness, nervousness, tremor, diarrhoea, nausea, headache, ataxia, confusion, psychosis, depression, word-finding difficulties and other cognitive effects, emotional lability, flu-like symptoms, gastrointestinal disturbances, and exacerbation especially of myoclonic and absence seizures and the precipitation of non-convulsive status epilepticus.

The usual indications for use are as adjunctive therapy in partial and secondarily generalized seizures in patients over 12 years of age, but it has generally only a small role in contemporary therapy.

Usual preparations are tablets 2.5, 5, 10, 15 mg size in Europe: 2, 4, 12, 16, and 20 mg in the US and Canada. The usual adult dosage initially is 4–5 mg/day, then slow increase by increments of 4–5 mg/week. Maintenance doses are 15–35 mg/day (30–50 mg/day in co-medication with enzyme-inducing drugs).

Dosing interval is 3 times a day.

Serum level monitoring is not needed.

Topiramate

Topiramate was licensed in the UK in 1994, and subsequently in the US, Europe, and many countries worldwide. It is a sulfamate-substituted monosaccharide with multiple mechanisms of action, which include inhibition of voltage-gated sodium channels, potentiation of GABA-mediated inhibition at the $GABA_A$ receptor, reduction of AMPA receptor activity, inhibition of high voltage calcium channels and carbonic anhydrase activity. Its pharmacokinetic properties are generally favourable, although it is metabolized in the liver and can be involved in drug interactions, albeit usually of a minor nature. It has gained a reputation as a powerful antiepileptic drug, effective in some patients in whom all other medications have failed. It is effective in a broad spectrum of epilepsies, but has a particular place in the treatment of resistant focal seizures, and symptomatic generalized epilepsies. The early clinical trials were carried out at higher doses than are now currently recommended, and although these studies showed marked efficacy, the rate of neurological and cognitive side effects was also high. However, subsequent experience shows that lower doses are also effective and confer better tolerability, and in routine practice now, the rate of side effects is lower than initially feared. The risk of side effects can also be greatly reduced by starting the drug at a very low dose and titrating upwards slowly.

Drug interactions are generally slight. However, topiramate levels can be lowered by co-medication with carbamazepine, phenobarbital and phenytoin. Topiramate co-medication can increase phenytoin levels.

Common and important adverse events include dizziness, ataxia, headache, paraesthesia, tremor, somnolence, visual blurring, cognitive dysfunction (especially difficulties with memory, attention, language and word finding) confusion, agitation, amnesia, depression, anxiety, psychosis, emotional lability, diplopia, loss of appetite and weight loss (which can be marked), nausea, abdominal pain, taste disturbance, dyspepsia, acidosis, and alopecia. Open-angle glaucoma is rarely reported.

The usual indications for use are as adjunctive therapy or monotherapy in partial and secondarily generalized seizures. It is also useful for Lennox–Gastaut syndrome and primary generalized tonic–clonic seizures in adults and children over 2 years of age.

Preparations available include tablets: 25, 50, 100, 200 mg size and sprinkles of 15 and 25 mg size. The usual adult dosage is initially 25–50 mg/day, increasing in 25 mg increments every 2 weeks. Maintenance doses are 100–500 mg/day. Usual dosage in children initially is 0.5–1 mg/kg/day, and maintenance doses 2–9 mg/kg/day.

Dosing interval is 2 times/day.

Serum level monitoring can be helpful in occasional cases. The target level 5–20 mg/L.

Valproate

Valproate was licensed in Europe in the early 1960s and then in the US in 1978. It is marketed as a sodium, magnesium, or calcium salt, an acid, and also as sodium hydrogen divalproate. Its mechanisms of action have not been fully established, but it has effects on GABA and glutaminergic activity, calcium (T) conductance, and potassium conductance. Sodium valproate is the usual form in the UK and depakote in Europe. Valpromide (dipropylacetamide), a prodrug of valproate, is also marketed, as is a delayed release formulation of sodium valproate. The term valproate is usually adopted to refer to all these forms. Although properties vary to some extent, none of these formulations has been shown to confer any real superiority over the others. Valproate is still one of the most commonly used antiepileptics throughout the world. It is a drug of first choice in all seizure types (absence, myoclonus, tonic–clonic) in idiopathic generalized epilepsy and is strikingly more effective than lamotrigine, topiramate and barbiturate drugs in this syndrome. Whether levetiracetam can compete with its effectiveness is not yet clear. It is also a drug of first choice in the Lennox–Gastaut syndrome where it controls atypical absence and atonic seizures better than most other first line drugs. It is also a drug of first choice in the syndromes of myoclonic epilepsy and the progressive myoclonic epilepsies, and for epilepsies with photosensitivity and/or generalized spike wave electrographically. In partial and secondarily generalized epilepsy, carbamazepine is usually tried before valproate, although there is no real evidence that valproate is less effective in new or mild cases.

Side effects remain a problem. Weight gain is common and often problematic. Other side effects, such as the neurotoxic effects and effects on hair growth are also common, but often only slight and usually are not a reason for drug withdrawal. In female patients, the possibility that valproate increases the frequency of polycystic ovaries, cause menstrual irregularities and reduce fertility are enough for many to avoid its use although scientific evidence on these points is generally slight. Valproate teratogenicity is a major concern and is a further reason for avoiding valproate in female patients where pregnancy is an issue. Its use in young children, especially those under 2 years of age, carries a small but definite risk of hepatic failure and where other drugs are available, these tend now to be used. It is contraindicated in the presence of hepatic or pancreatic disease. Valproate pharmacokinetics are complex and there are many and varied interactions. It slightly inhibits the metabolism of other AEDs, usually without consequence, but does cause major rises in lamotrigine levels when given as co-medication. Imipenem antibiotics profoundly lower valproate levels and should not be used in co-medication. Valproate concentrations are lowered by co-medication with commonly used antineoplastic drugs and elevated by co-medication with commonly used antidepressant and psychotropic drugs. Other drugs, such as isoniazid, can increase valproic acid levels. Valproic acid inhibits the metabolism of a number of drugs, most notably phenobarbital, lamotrigine, and rufinamide. Valproic acid displaces phenytoin from plasma protein binding sites and can also inhibit phenytoin metabolism.

Common and important side effects include nausea, vomiting, hyperammonaemia and other metabolic effects, endocrine effects, weight gain, severe hepatic toxicity, gastrointestinal disturbance, pancreatitis, drowsiness, cognitive disturbance, aggressiveness, tremor, ataxia, weakness, encephalopathy, extrapyramidal symptoms, oedema, thrombocytopenia, neutropenia, platelet and coagulation dysfunction, aplastic anaemia, hair thinning and hair loss, polycystic ovarian syndrome, Fanconi syndrome, and hyponatraemia.

Vaproate is indicated in all forms of epilepsy at all age groups. The usual preparations are enteric-coated tablets: 200, 500 mg; crushable tablets: 100 mg; capsules: 150, 300, 500 mg; solution or syrup: 200 mg/5 mL, 250 mg/5 mL; sustained-release tablets: 200, 300 500 mg; sustained-release microspheres, sachets: 100, 250, 500, 750, 1000 mg; divalproex tablets: 125, 300, 500 mg (as valproic acid equivalents); divalproex tablets delayed release: 125, 250, 500 mg (as valproic acid equivalents); divalproex sprinkles, 125 mg (as valproic acid equivalents); divalproex tablets extended release: 250, 500 mg (as valproic acid equivalents); solution for intravenous injection: 100 mg/mL

The usual adult dosage initially is 200–500 mg/day increasing by 200–500mg increments every 2 weeks to maintenance doses of 600–2000 mg/day. The usual dosage in children initially is 15 mg/kg/day (children <20 kg); and 40 mg/kg/day (children >20 kg). Maintenance doses in children < 20kg: 20–40 mg/kg/day, and in children > 20 kg: 20–30 mg/kg/day.

Dosing intervals is 2 times/day.

Blood levels show marked diurnal variation, but serum level monitoring can be useful in occasional cases. The target range is 50–100 mg/L. It should be noted that the drug can be very effective at low serum levels, and as with other agents clinical parameters should be used to guide therapy wherever possible.

Vigabatrin

Vigabatrin is a GABA agonist, which was introduced in 1989 for the treatment of partial seizures. It was then discovered in 1997 to cause visual field constriction, a side effect which is now known to occur in over 40% of treated patients (22). Because of this, its use has become severely limited to a very small number of patients with partial epilepsy whose seizures are controlled with no other available AED. It also has other significant side effects, including depression and psychosis. It has a strong effect in infantile spasms, and is often effective in cases resistant to ACTH, and because of this has become a drug of first choice in this small indication. It is particularly effective in cases in which the infantile spasms are due to tuberous sclerosis.

Apart from the visual field restrictions and the psychiatric effects, other common and important side effects of vigabatrin include nausea, abdominal pain, drowsiness, dizziness, encephalopathy, stupor, confusion, visual field restriction, weight gain, headache, tremor, and paraesthesia.

Vigabatrin has no important or common drug interactions.

The usual indication for use is as adjunctive therapy in partial epilepsy, but only in exceptional circumstances and where supervised by a specialist, and infantile spasm. The available preparations are tablets 500 mg size, and powder 500 mg/sachet. The usual adult dosage is initially 500 mg, increasing by 500 mg increments to 2–3 g/day. The usual dosage in children is: 10–15 kg: 0.5–1 g/day; for children 15–30 kg: 1–1.5 g/day; and for children 30–50 kg: 1.5–3 g/day.

Dosing interval is 2 times/day.

Serum level monitoring is not useful.

Zonisamide

Zonisamide is a chemically distinctive sulfonamide drug, with striking effectiveness in a wide spectrum of partial and generalized seizures. It has been licensed in Japan for some years, although has become available in Europe only since 2002. It has multiple potential mechanisms of action, and inhibits the voltage-gated sodium channel and T-type calcium channel currents, acts to enhance the benzodiazepine $GABA_A$ receptor, is a carbonic anhydrase and also has actions on excitatory glutaminergic transmission. It is prone to cause various side effects and tolerability can be improved by slow introduction. The risk of renal stones has been a concern particularly in Europe and the US, but less so in Japan, and patients should be advised to remain well hydrated when taking this drug. It has about 50% protein binding, and a very long half life (50–70 hours) but this is significantly reduced (25–40 hours) by co-medication with enzyme-inducing AEDs and dose changes when co-medicating are appropriate.

Serum zonisamide levels are markedly lowered by carbamazepine, phenytoin, and barbiturates. Zonisamide co-medication does not usually significantly influence levels of other drugs.

Common and important adverse events are somnolence, ataxia, dizziness, insomnia, headache, attention and concentration difficulties, memory impairment, irritability, confusion, depression, impaired concentration, mental slowing, speech disturbance, fatigue, nausea, vomiting, weight loss, anorexia, itching, abdominal pain, hyperthermia, nephrolithiasis, acidosis, pyrexia, renal impairment, oligohidrosis and risk of heat stroke. Rash and other manifestations of a hypersensitivity are rare but can be serious.

Usual indications include adjunctive therapy in partial and generalized epilepsy, Lennox–Gastaut syndrome, West syndrome, and progressive myoclonic epilepsy. It is licensed in Europe, Japan and Asia in children and adults. It is licensed in the US only for refractory partial epilepsy in patients 16 or more years of age

The usual preparations are capsules 25, 50, 100 mg size, tablets 25 and 100 mg size, and powder: 20%. Initial dose in adults is

50 mg/day, increased by 50 mg increments each 2 weeks, to a maintenance dose of 200–500 mg/day. In children the initial dose is 2–4 mg/kg/day, and maintenance 4–8 mg/kg/day.

Dosing intervals are 1–2 times/day.

Serum level monitoring may be useful in some cases. The target range is 10–40 mg/L (30–120 μmol/L).

Acknowledgement

Some of the text is based on: Shorvon S. *Epilepsy* (Oxford Neurology Library Series). Oxford: Oxford University Press, 2009.

References

1. Prunetti P, Perucca E. New and forthcoming anti-epileptic drugs. *Curr Opin Neurol* 2011; 24(2):159–64.
2. Stephen LJ, Forsyth M, Kelly K, Brodie MJ. Antiepileptic drug combinations-Have newer agents altered clinical outcomes? *Epilepsy Res* 2012; 98(2–3):194–8.
3. Bialer M. Chemical properties of antiepileptic drugs (AEDs). *Adv Drug Deliv Rev* 2011; Nov 21. [Epub ahead of print]
4. Beghi E, Beghi M, Cornaggia CM. The use of recently approved antiepileptic drugs: use with caution, use in refractory patients or use as first-line indications? *Expert Rev Neurother* 2011; 11(12):1759–67.
5. Lasoń W, Dudra-Jastrzębska M, Rejdak K, Czuczwar SJ. Basic mechanisms of antiepileptic drugs and their pharmacokinetic/pharmacodynamic interactions: an update. *Pharmacol Rep* 2011; 63(2):271–92.
6. Johannessen Landmark C, Patsalos PN. Drug interactions involving the new second- and third-generation antiepileptic drugs. *Expert Rev Neurother* 2010; 10(1):119–40.
7. Chung W-H, Hung S-I, Hong H-S, Hsih M-S, Yang L-C, Ho H-C, *et al.* Medical genetics: a marker for Stevens-Johnson syndrome. *Nature* 2004; 428(6982):486.
8. McCormack M, Alfirevic A, Bourgeois S, Farrell JJ, Kasperavičiūtė D, Carrington M, *et al.* HLA-A*3101 and carbamazepine-induced hypersensitivity reactions in Europeans. *N Engl J Med* 2011; 364(12):1134–43.
9. Ng YT, Conry JA, Drummond R, Stolle J, Weinberg MA, OV-1012 Study Investigators. Randomized, phase III study results of clobazam in Lennox-Gastaut syndrome. *Neurology* 2011; 77(15):1473–81.
10. Glauser TA, Cnaan A, Shinnar S, Hirtz DG, Dlugos D, Masur D, *et al.* Ethosuximide, valproic acid, and lamotrigine in childhood absence epilepsy. *N Engl J Med* 2010; 362(9):790–99.
11. Simms KM, Kortepeter C, Avigan M. Lamotrigine and aseptic meningitis. *Neurology* 2012; 78(12):921–7.
12. Genton P. When antiepileptic drugs aggravate epilepsy. *Brain Dev* 2000; 22(2):75–80.
13. Pennell PB, Newport DJ, Stowe ZN, Helmers SL, Montgomery JQ, Henry TR. The impact of pregnancy and childbirth on the metabolism of lamotrigine. *Neurology* 2004; 62(2):292–95.
14. Nowack A, Malarkey EB, Yao J, Bleckert A, Hill J, Bajjalieh SM. Levetiracetam reverses synaptic deficits produced by overexpression of SV2A. *PLoS ONE* 2011; 6(12):e29560.
15. Delanty N, Jones J, Tonner F. Adjunctive levetiracetam in children, adolescents, and adults with primary generalized seizures: open-label, noncomparative, multicenter, long-term follow-up study. *Epilepsia* 2012; 53(1):111–19.
16. Kanner AM. Can antiepileptic drugs unmask a susceptibility to psychiatric disorders? *Nature clinical practice Neurology* 2009; 5(3):132–3.
17. Hu F-Y, Wu X-T, An D-M, Yan B, Stefan H, Zhou D. Pilot association study of oxcarbazepine-induced mild cutaneous adverse reactions with HLA-B*1502 allele in Chinese Han population. *Seizure* 2011; 20(2):160–2.
18. Gunthorpe MJ, Large CH, Sankar R. The mechanism of action of retigabine (ezogabine), a first-in-class K(+) channel opener for the treatment of epilepsy. *Epilepsia* 2012; 53(3):412–24.
19. Fisher JL. The anti-convulsant stiripentol acts directly on the GABA(A) receptor as a positive allosteric modulator. *Neuropharmacology* 2009; 56(1):190–7.
20. Chiron C, Dulac O. The pharmacologic treatment of Dravet syndrome. *Epilepsia* 2011; 52(Suppl 2):72–5.
21. Bauer J, Cooper-Mahkorn D. Tiagabine: efficacy and safety in partial seizures—current status. *Neuropsychiatr Dis Treat* 2008; 4(4):731–6.
22. Chiron C, Dulac O. Epilepsy: Vigabatrin treatment and visual field loss. *Nat Rev Neurol* 2011; 7:189–90.

MEDICAL LIBRARY
WESTERN INFIRMARY
GLASGOW

CHAPTER 27

Principles of Epilepsy Surgery

Samden D. Lhatoo

Epilepsy surgery is generally understood to mean resective surgery where the primary surgical imperative is the control of seizures rather than the underlying pathology causing seizures (e.g. brain tumour), although on occasion both epilepsy as well as its cause merit equal surgical attention. It is primarily used for refractory focal epilepsy syndromes and has no role in the primary generalized epilepsy syndromes (with the exception of vagal nerve or potentially, deep brain stimulation). Since up to a third of patients with epilepsy do not respond to medication, surgery becomes a viable treatment alternative in up to half of the patient population with refractory focal epilepsy, carrying with it the promise of seizure freedom, a reduction in seizure or medication-related morbidity, and a reduction in the risk of sudden unexpected death. Non-resective surgery, where brain tissue is not removed but where seizure control is the main indication, is now also a distinct category of epilepsy surgery (Table 27.1).

The era of modern epilepsy surgery can be said to have begun with Victor Horsley (Fig. 27.1) in 1886 when, as a young neurosurgeon newly appointed to the National Hospital for the Paralysed and the Epileptic at Queen Square, London, he operated on a 22-year-old man with focal motor seizures and a depressed skull fracture (1). This was followed a month later by surgery on a 20-year-old man with left-hand clonic seizures and postictal palsy caused by what turned out to be a tuberculoma in the predicted frontoparietal juncture. This prediction was made on the basis of the patient's seizure semiology, at that time the only available tool for the localization of the epileptogenic zone—the brain area critical to seizure generation and the resection of which renders a patient seizure free.

Since then, a number of sophisticated technologies, described in this and following chapters, have been developed to supplement semiological information in the direct or indirect identification of the epileptogenic zone as well as the identification of eloquent brain tissue. The latter is an important consideration as the surgical decision-making process has to account for the risk and probability of postsurgical deficits rendered by resections involving these areas. Modern epilepsy surgery is now therefore a highly complex, multimodal, and multidisciplinary process. Its fundamental principles however, are simple:

1. Firstly to conclusively identify the focus of the individual's medically refractory epilepsy.
2. Second, to remove this focus in order to render the individual seizure free.
3. Third, to avoid harm to the patient in doing so (e.g. permanent postoperative deficits).
4. Fourth, if principles 1–3 are not possible, to reduce the individual's seizure burden (palliate) as much as possible.

The manner in which these are achieved and the principles that guide the processes involved are described next and in subsequent chapters.

Table 27.1 Types of epilepsy surgery

Resective surgeries

- Lobar/sublobar resections[a]
  - Frontal
  - Temporal:
    - Standard resection (anterior temporal lobe + mesial structures)
    - Selective amygdalohippocampectomy
    - Tailored resections (variations of the above 2)
  - Parietal
  - Occipital
  - Other—insula, cingulate
- Multilobar resections
- Hemispherectomies:
  - Functional hemispherectomy/hemispherotomy
  - Anatomical hemispherectomy
- Corpus callosotomy[b]

Non-resective surgeries

- Multiple subpial transection[b]
- Hippocampal transection
- Gamma knife surgery
- Deep brain stimulation[b]
- Vagal nerve stimulation[b]

[a] Many 'lobectomies' are tailored to individual patients according to the presurgical investigation findings and range from small corticectomies to large subtotal or rarely, total lobectomies.

[b] These are generally considered to be primarily palliative procedures.

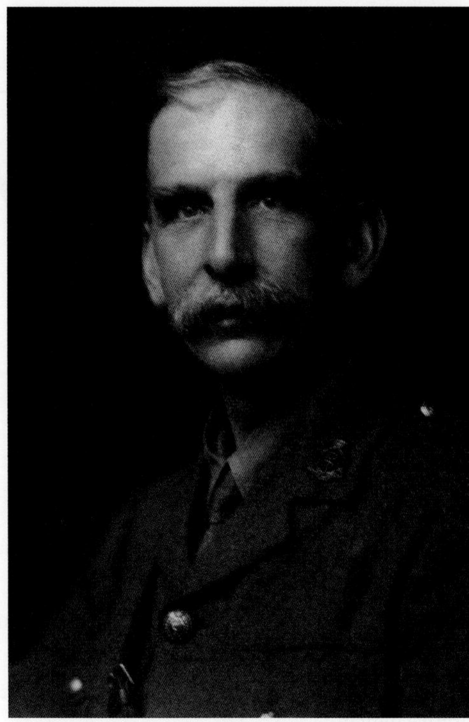

Fig. 27.1 Victor Horsley (14 April 1857–16 July 1916). Image courtesy of the Queen Square Library, Archive and Museum. Copyright National Hospital for Neurology & Neurosurgery.

The epileptogenic zone

The main purpose of epilepsy surgery is the removal of the seat of an individual's focal epilepsy—the epileptogenic zone. The epileptogenic zone has been defined as that 'area of cortex that is indispensable for the generation of epileptic seizures' (2). However, only after complete and lasting seizure freedom from surgical resection of a particular cortical area can that area be said to definitely represent the epileptogenic zone. The challenge of the presurgical work-up therefore lies in the identification of a number of other 'zones' that if consistently indicative of the same brain area as abnormal (i.e. 'concordant'), provide the best indication of where the true epileptogenic zone might lie (Fig. 27.2). 'Discordance' on the other hand, where there is poor congruity between zones, predicts poor seizure freedom outcomes with surgery. These zones are identified by different clinical and investigative tools.

1. The *symptomatogenic zone*. This is the part of the brain that gives rise to the clinical symptoms and signs (semiology) of the epilepsy. It may or may not be in close relation to the epileptogenic zone. For example, seizures arising from an epileptogenic zone in the left hippocampus may not be symptomatic until the seizure discharge reaches the left insular area (Fig. 27.2) where it may cause the patient to experience a rising epigastric sensation. This area is then the symptomatogenic zone, relatively distant from the epileptogenic zone. In such cases, information from other zones becomes mandatory in strengthening the case for surgery. In general, close attention to history of the patient's aura and video recordings of seizures provide excellent clues to the location of the symptomatogenic zone.
2. The *epileptic lesion zone*. Neuroimaging, namely high-resolution magnetic resonance imaging (MRI), best identifies the epileptic lesion. This area is usually in close relation to the epileptogenic zone and sometimes within the epileptogenic zone itself as in the case of hippocampal sclerosis (Fig. 27.2). On the other hand, in cases of tumoural epilepsy, for example, the epileptogenic zone often lies along the borders of the lesion zone.
3. The *irritative zone*. This is the area represented by epileptiform activity as evidenced by electroencephalography (EEG) or magnetoencephalography (MEG) in the form of spikes or sharp waves. In the case of hippocampal sclerosis, there is an extremely close relationship with the lesion zone and the epileptogenic zone is usually contained within it. However, with some close to midline, extratemporal epilepsies such as a mesial parietal epilepsy, for example, the sharp waves can appear elsewhere and thus provide 'discordant' information.
4. The *ictal-onset zone*. This area is identified by the initial seizure pattern and the EEG electrodes on surface or intracranial EEG where it is recorded. More recently, ictal single-positron emission computed tomography (SPECT) and, to a lesser extent, MEG are also used. It is usually in intimate relation to the epileptogenic zone and its identification is crucial to successful epilepsy surgery. The concept of the ictal onset zone can be expanded to include the actual seizure onset zone as recorded by the earlier mentioned investigations, and the potential seizure onset zone. If both are not included in the surgical resection, the patient may not become seizure free or will develop seizure recurrence at some time after surgery, perhaps even years later (Fig. 27.3).
5. The *functional deficit zone*. This is an area of dysfunctional brain identified in the interictal period, consequent to structural or functional abnormalities arising from a focal epilepsy. It is identified by a variety of means including physical examination (e.g. hemiparesis implies a functional deficit zone in the contralateral

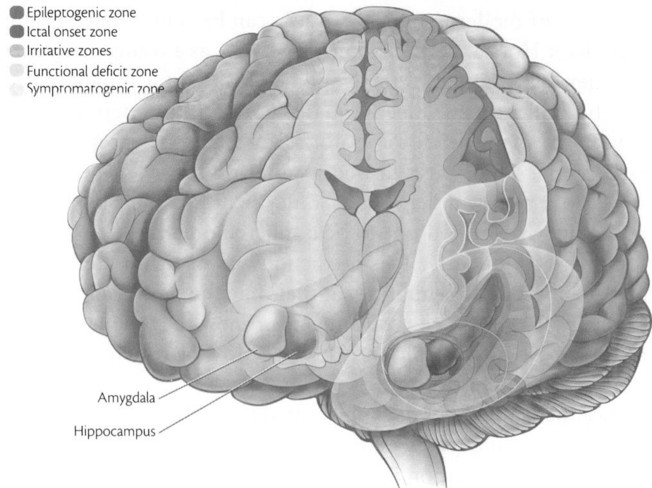

Fig. 27.2 (Also see Colour plate 13.) The epileptogenic zone and its relationship with related zones in a patient with left hippocampal sclerosis. These are: (1) Epileptogenic zone = left hippocampus and amygdala. (2) Epileptic lesion zone and ictal onset zone = left hippocampus. (3) Irritative zones = left and right hippocampus + adjacent temporal neocortex. (4) Functional deficit zone = left temporal lobe (reduced left temporal neuropsychological measures—e.g. verbal memory). (5) Symptomatogenic zone = left insula and lower motor strip (e.g. causing epigastric sensation followed by a right face clonic seizure). Copyright Samden D. Lhatoo.

frontal lobe), positron emission tomography (PET) imaging (regional hypometabolism), functional MRI, neuropsychological testing (verbal memory deficits in a right-handed individual may indicate a left mesial temporal functional deficit zone), the intracarotid amobarbital or Wada test (poor memory function in one hemisphere) evoked potentials (reduced amplitude or delay in appropriate cortex), and others. The functional deficit zone is often, but not always, large and in proximity to the epileptogenic zone.

Often, one or more zones may not be evident. For example, in a patient who has normal high-resolution brain MRI scans, the epileptic lesion zone is by definition unidentifiable. When several zones are poorly or not at all identifiable, the case for successful surgery is weakened and any such undertaking becomes extremely challenging. Equally, the presence of more than one ictal onset zone, several irritative zones and/or more than one epileptic lesion zone (dual or multiple pathology) render surgery a far from straightforward option.

Seizure semiology in epilepsy surgery

Stringent analysis of the seizure symptoms and signs is a crucial part of the presurgical work-up of the patient. This identifies the symptomatogenic zones which in turn can (1) lateralize the seizure to one hemisphere and (2) localize the seizure to a specific brain region in that hemisphere. This allows the clinician to focus attention on a specific area of interest.

Since the aura of the partial seizure constitutes its beginning, the cortical area producing the aura is likely to be closer to the seizure focus than the areas responsible for the later manifestations of the seizure. For example, in a seizure that begins with a simple auditory aura, progresses to a complex visual hallucination and then a secondary generalized tonic–clonic seizure, the epileptogenic zone is likely to lie closer to the primary auditory cortex in the superior temporal area (Heschl's gyrus) than to the visual association areas or motor areas which produce the later symptoms and signs. Hence the aura provides important information about the symptomatogenic zone (Table 27.2), information that can then be used to analyse the presence or absence of discordance with other investigations. Much of what we know of aura localization is derived from brain stimulation studies where electrical stimulation of specific brain areas using intracranial electrodes in epilepsy patients consistently reproduced a specific symptom relating to that patient's epileptic aura (3, 4).

Semiological analysis of the seizure does not end with the aura, however, and indeed, many patients either do not have or cannot remember their auras. Specific features of the seizures can point to the symptomatogenic zone. The twitching thumb (a thumb clonic

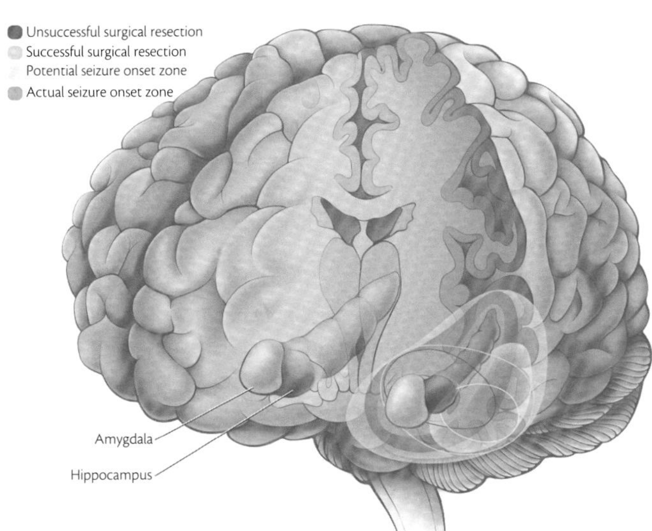

Fig. 27.3 (Also see Colour plate 14.) Surgical resection and the epileptogenic zone. Copyright Samden D. Lhatoo.

Table 27.2 Some auras and their usual symptomatogenic zones

Aura manifestation	Symptomatogenic zone
Unilateral sensory aura	Contralateral primary sensory area
Bilateral sensory aura	Secondary sensory area
	Supplementary sensorimotor area
Simple auditory aura	Primary auditory cortex
Complex auditory aura	Auditory association area
Simple hemifield visual hallucination	Contralateral primary visual cortex
Complex visual hallucination	Visual association area
Fear	Amygdala
Olfactory aura	Amygdala
Gustatory aura	Parietal opercular area
Abdominal aura	Insula
Déjà vu aura	Basal temporal area

Table 27.3 Some seizure features used in localization and lateralization in epilepsy surgery[a] (5)

Seizure manifestation	Localization/lateralization of seizure
Hypermotor movements	Frontal lobe
Bilateral asymmetric tonic posturing	Supplementary sensorimotor area
Dystonic hand posturing in a seizure with early automatisms	Contralateral temporal lobe
'Sign of four' posturing at onset of a secondary generalized seizure (one arm extends, one arm flexes over chest)	Hemisphere contralateral to extended arm
Forced head version at onset of a secondary generalized seizure	Hemisphere contralateral to side of version
Ictal speech	Non-dominant temporal lobe
Preserved consciousness and memory during a seizure with automatisms	Non-dominant temporal lobe
Ictal piloerection	Ipsilateral hemisphere
Unilateral eye blinking	Ipsilateral hemisphere
Postictal aphasia	Dominant hemisphere
Postictal limb weakness	Contralateral hemisphere
Postictal nose wiping	Ipsilateral hemisphere

[a] Sensitivities and specificities of individual manifestations vary.

Table 27.4 Neuroimaging investigations in epilepsy surgery

Technique	Zone identified
MRI	Epileptic lesion zone
fMRI	Eloquent cortex
EEG-fMRI	Irritative zone
PET	Functional deficit zone
SPECT/SISCOM[a]	Ictal onset zone

[a] SISCOM, subtraction Ictal SPECT co-registered to MRI

seizure) will be produced by epileptic activity in the contralateral thumb area of the motor strip. A sudden bilateral asymmetric tonic posturing of the upper limbs indicates seizure symptoms arising from one of the supplementary sensorimotor areas, located in the mesial aspect of the frontal lobe just anterior to the motor strip. A complex partial seizure with prominent, early oral and distal upper limb automatisms usually suggests a temporal lobe seizure. A hyper motor seizure suggests a frontal lobe seizure, usually arising from the mesial or orbitofrontal areas. The postictal period can also provide clues to seizure localization. Ictal and postictal localizing and lateralizing signs are detailed in Table 27.3.

Neuroimaging in epilepsy surgery

A variety of neuroimaging techniques are used in epilepsy surgery. These help define one or more zones and are extremely important to the presurgical work-up (Table 27.4).

MRI in epilepsy surgery

Focal structural brain abnormalities are the usual cause of focal epilepsies. Modern MRI techniques, vastly superior to CT scanning, have revolutionized epilepsy surgery where identification of a lesion renders the hunt for the epileptogenic zone much easier (6). There are several additional uses that further emphasize the importance of this tool (Table 27.5). 3 Tesla MRI scans have a distinct yield advantage over older 1 and 1.5 Tesla MRI scans; 7 Tesla machines which are now undergoing clinical evaluation may increase yield in previously 'lesion negative' cases. The use of surface coils, targeting brain regions identified as abnormal by other investigations, e.g. EEG, can also contribute in identifying abnormal brain areas previously thought normal on standard MRI or better defining characteristics and extent of known abnormalities. It is important that MRI scans are carried out according to specific epilepsy protocols. These usually involve fine cut (1–2 mm) images using volumetric T1-weighted sequences, proton density T2-weighted sequences, fluid attenuated inversion recovery (FLAIR) sequences, and gradient echo sequences in the oblique coronal and axial planes.

Voxel-based analysis of MRI scans can be helpful where visual analysis does not show abnormalities. Diffusion tensor imaging (DTI) can show abnormal diffusivity in areas known to be epileptogenic and so is a potential additional tool although it is not routinely used in clinical practice. Tractography is a technique used for imaging white matter tracts which standard MRI cannot. The direction of diffusion of water in each voxel determines the orientation of the white matter tracts. It potentially has substantial clinical utility in surgical planning where information on the optic

Table 27.5 MRI in epilepsy surgery

MRI techniques	Use
Standard epilepsy protocol MRI	Identification of structural abnormalities
Voxel-based analysis	Identification of structural abnormalities
Manual and automated hippocampal volumetry	Identification of hippocampal atrophy
DTI	Identification of structural abnormalities
Tractography	Identification of white matter tracts
fMRI	Identification of eloquent cortex
EEG-fMRI	Identification of the irritative zone
Pre and postsurgical image co-registration	Identifies positions of subdural and depth electrodes in patients undergoing epilepsy surgery

radiation, primary motor, primary sensory, and language tracts may make the difference between the presence or absence of major postoperative deficits.

Functional MRI (fMRI) is based on the principle of cerebral blood oxygen level-dependent (BOLD) signal changes in response to activation of specific brain areas. Language testing paradigms can provide a reliable, non-invasive means of lateralizing and localizing expressive language (Broca's area); identification of receptive language areas may not be as reliable. Motor activation fMRI and sensory activation fMRI can reliably identify motor and sensory cortices. EEG-fMRI is an investigation that combines the ability of EEG to provide information on electrophysiological changes very quickly (temporal resolution), in the millisecond range, and the ability of MRI to provide very detailed spatial information (in millimetres). When epileptiform spikes are analysed using this technique, information on the source of these spikes can be obtained. This has not yet achieved widespread clinical utility but holds promise.

An important function of MRI in epilepsy surgery is the co-registration of pre- and postoperative brain images in order to define the positions of electrodes in relation to brain structures. This is done through specialized commercially available software programs. Knowledge of the location of electrodes is important in identifying cortex from which seizures arise and in identifying cortex where specific brain functions are located.

PET in epilepsy surgery

The main utility of PET is in the identification of the functional deficit zone in patients in whom there is no demonstrable structural lesion. The standard PET ligand used is ^{18}F-fluorodeoxyglucose and imaging is carried out in the interictal state to identify areas of hypometabolism. The sensitivity and specificity of PET varies according to the brain region producing epilepsy. In temporal lobe epilepsy (see Chapter 28) in particular, there can be a close correlation between the areas of PET abnormality, the epileptogenic zone, and surgical outcome. In extratemporal epilepsies, it provides contributory information less often. In clinical practice, co-registering PET information with the patient's MRI scan can identify areas of abnormality previously missed when either investigation is used alone. Subtle gyral abnormalities due to malformations of cortical development can become more evident.

Table 27.6 Some common indications for intracranial electrode studies

High-resolution MRI does not show a lesion although other evidence suggests a single focus
MRI shows two or more potentially epileptogenic lesions
MRI shows large lesion and precise estimation of the ictal onset zone cannot be reliably made
Discordance between investigations, e.g. MRI shows left hippocampal sclerosis, EEG shows right temporal ictal onset zone
Identification of relationship between eloquent cortex and candidate epileptogenic zone

SPECT in epilepsy surgery

In contrast to PET, this investigation is carried out in the ictal stage and so provides information on the ictal onset zone although in common with PET, its greatest utility is in lesion-negative patients with focal epilepsy. Technetium 99-m is the radiolabelled tracer used to identify areas of increased cerebral blood flow or hyperperfusion. Testing has to be carried out under ideal conditions. A pre-ictal SPECT scan establishes baseline. The tracer is injected within seconds of seizure onset. Injection and focal tracer uptake within 10 seconds of the start of the seizure is much more likely to indicate the area of seizure onset than an injection 60 seconds later when spread of the seizure discharge makes the information much less meaningful. The seizure also has to be of sufficient duration and a very brief partial seizure of less than 10 seconds is unlikely to provide substantial information. Co-registration of the subtracted SPECT images to the patient's MRI (SISCOM) can provide further anatomical information on the location of the seizure focus. Neither PET nor SPECT information independently make the case for surgery in a particular brain area in lesion-negative epilepsy and it is usually advisable that information from these investigations is used together with clinical and EEG information.

EEG in epilepsy surgery

Information from EEG is critical to the presurgical process without which epilepsy surgery is usually inadvisable and the outcome much less predictable. EEG performs two crucial functions—identifying the irritative and ictal onset zones (Fig. 27.2). Some patients have two or more potentially epileptogenic lesions (dual or multifocal pathology). Identification of the true focus or both foci as epileptogenic can usually only be achieved through EEG. As described in Chapter 9, EEG information is derived from prolonged video-EEG monitoring where a patient is admitted for several days of continuous EEG recording under video surveillance in an epilepsy monitoring unit manned by trained nurses and EEG personnel. The assessment is carried out using the standard scalp or surface electrode array (10–20 electrode system) although a denser array with more electrodes (the 10–10 system) is required in many cases. In many centres, special electrodes such as deep sphenoidal electrodes are used. These sample EEG activity from the mesial and basal temporal lobes and are inserted under local anaesthesia through the lateral face into the proximity of the foramen ovale in the skull base.

EEG and the irritative zone

Sharp waves seen in the interictal record indicate the irritative zone (Fig. 27.4). There can be more than one irritative zone in unilateral hippocampal sclerosis (illustrative case in Fig. 27.3) where two irritative zones produce both left and right sharp waves although all the other information available is concordant with a left mesial temporal epileptogenic zone and surgical resection of this area renders the patient seizure free. Simultaneous recordings from depth electrodes inserted into both hippocampi confirm that both of these areas generate sharp waves independently and are not indicative of spread from one to the other. Surface recorded sharp waves from more than one brain region can indicate a multifocal, or tendency to multifocal, epilepsy. Sometimes, multiple irritative zones in the same hemisphere can indicate a unifocal epilepsy with

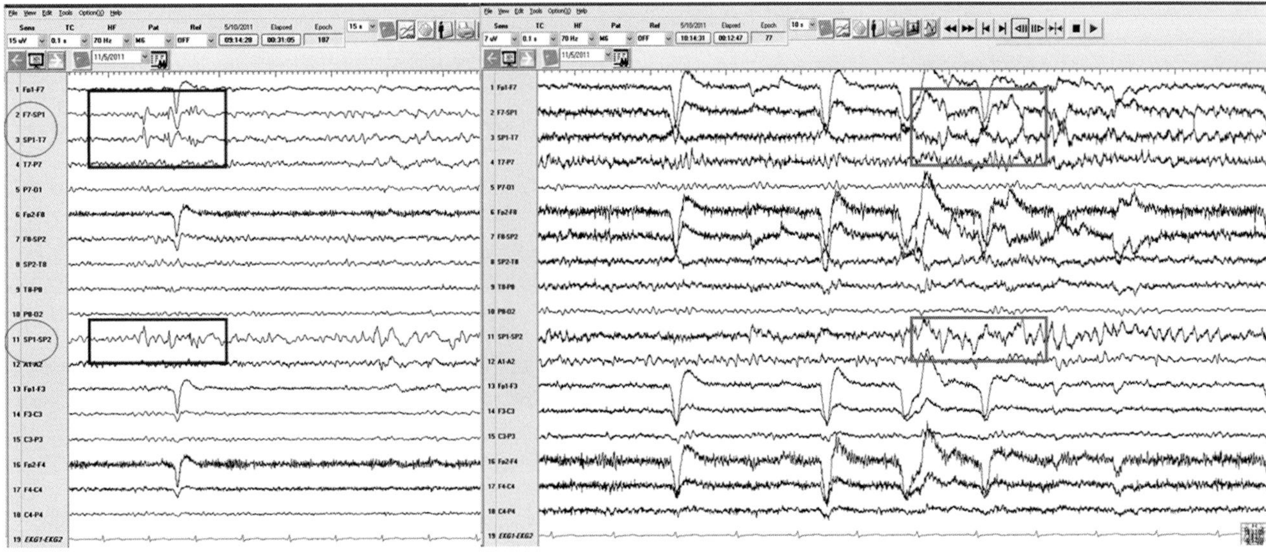

Fig. 27.4 Surface EEG of a patient with left hippocampal sclerosis showing interictal left mesial temporal sharp waves (two boxes on left), maximum in the left sphenoidal recording electrode (Sp1) and a seizure starting in the same region (two boxes on right), suggesting both irritative and ictal onset zones in the left mesial temporal lobe. Copyright Samden D. Lhatoo.

either propagation of sharp wave discharges from a single deeper focus in different directions at different times or a change in the orientation of the focus (dipole) that generates the sharp wave discharge which is then seen in different brain regions at different times. In general, a single irritative zone is a good indicator that the epileptogenic zone is within it.

The ictal onset zone

Seizures captured during video-EEG monitoring provide important semiological clues as described earlier but also allow close examination of the EEG seizure record. Analysis of the EEG onset often indicates the brain region that comprises the ictal onset zone which in turn is intimately related to the epileptogenic zone. The EEG onset can be focal (Fig. 27.4), more widespread but restricted to one hemisphere (lateralized), or generalized (non-lateralizable). In general, the more localized the EEG onset, the more precise the depiction of the ictal onset zone.

Intracranial EEG in epilepsy surgery

In some cases, for a variety of reasons (Table 27.6), despite extensive investigations, the case for surgery cannot be reliably made. In many instances, there is considerable discordance between investigations, hampering a strong candidate epileptogenic zone for resection. In others, the epileptogenic zone is suspected to be close to eloquent cortex and so a more accurate depiction of the ictal onset zone and mapping of cortical function close to this zone is necessary. In general, an extremely good hypothesis based on all the available information is necessary for the placement of electrodes in a targeted part of the brain. Invasive electrodes carry substantial risk of morbidity and mortality, directly proportional to the number of electrodes implanted. Studies of the entire brain or even one whole hemisphere—so-called 'fishing expeditions' are therefore inadvisable and unlikely to succeed.

There are two main approaches to intracranial EEG studies: (1) the use of depth electrodes which are stereotactically implanted into the brain (stereo-EEG) and (2) the use of subdural EEG electrodes which are placed on the brain surface, both targeting specific brain areas. Each has its advantages and disadvantages and so centres that have expertise in both can use either technique according to the clinical situation.

1. Stereo-EEG (Fig. 27.5). A hypothesis is formulated to identify the potential epileptogenic zone. The number and position of depths is determined in advance. The surgeon plans the trajectory of the depth electrodes, using very detailed preoperative MRI and conventional or MR angiogram information to avoid vital structures such as blood vessels. The patient then undergoes surgery, usually with frame-based stereotactic insertion of depth electrodes through multiple skull burr holes. The depth electrodes have multiple 'contacts' that are capable of recording electrical brain activity as well as stimulating the brain that they are in contact with when current is passed through them. The main advantage of this technique is that it allows access to very deep parts of the brain such as the cingulate regions and other mesial brain structures. They are also less likely to cause brain oedema, haemorrhage, headaches, infections, and other adverse effects that can limit the use of subdural electrodes. In the last few years, highly specialized robotic techniques have been used for stereo-EEG depth electrode insertion by some centres.
2. Subdural EEG (Fig. 27.6). Again, a suitable hypothesis for the insertion of subdural electrodes is mandatory. Under general

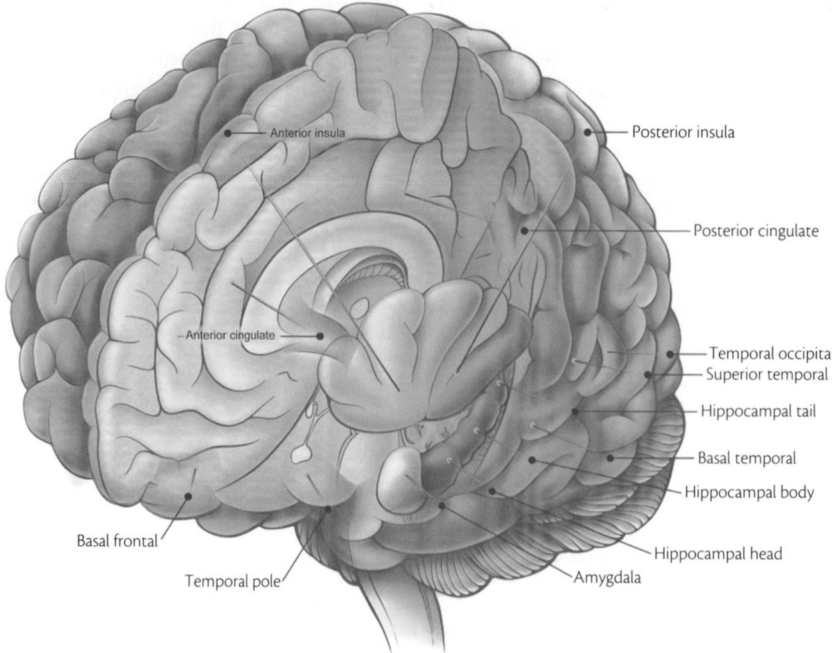

Fig. 27.5 (Also see Colour plate 15.) Diagrammatic representation of stereotactically implanted depth electrodes in a patient with lesion-negative temporal lobe epilepsy. Electrode labels denote the main anatomical structures targeted by the innermost electrode contacts. The outer contacts also sample cortex at or close to the point of electrode insertion. For example, the deep anterior insular contacts sample the anterior insular gyri whilst the superficial contacts of the same electrode sample the superior frontal gyrus where the electrode is inserted. Similarly, the deep contacts of the hippocampal body electrode sample the hippocampal body whilst the superficial contacts sample the lateral temporal neocortex in the middle temporal gyrus. Copyright Samden D. Lhatoo.

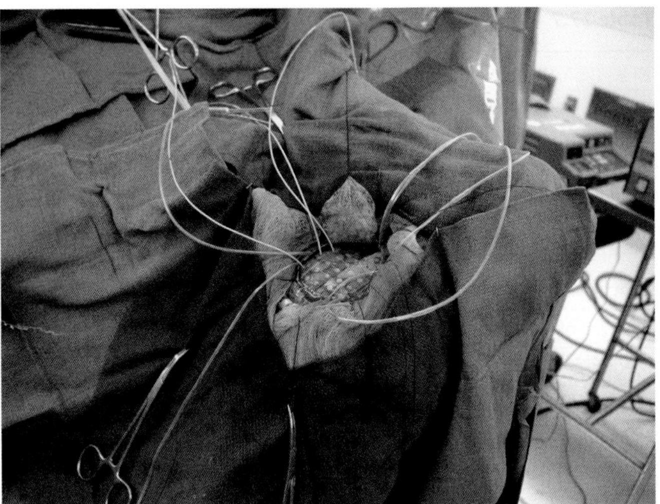

Fig. 27.6 (Also see Colour plate 16.) A right craniotomy with an 8 × 8 (64 electrode) grid covering the frontal and temporal areas of a patient with lesion negative right hemisphere epilepsy. Copyright Samden D. Lhatoo.

anaesthesia, the surgeon performs a large craniotomy and inserts electrode 'grids' or smaller 'strips' subdurally onto the surface of the brain. Each grid or strip usually contains between six and 64 'contacts'. These primarily record from the brain surface and can cover large areas of contiguous cortex. Stimulation of contacts (brain mapping) can therefore provide excellent information on eloquent cortex, identifying primary motor, sensory, supplementary sensorimotor, visual, auditory, and language cortices among other brain regions. The relative disadvantages are that these do not record well from deep sulci, are difficult to insert into the inferior or mesial aspects of the brain, and can cause significant morbidity.

With both techniques, postoperative CT scans or MRIs are merged with the preoperative scans using specialized software programs that then provide co-registered images of the implanted electrode positions superimposed on the MRI, each of which is identified and numbered. Patients are video-EEG monitored in the epilepsy monitoring unit for several days under close clinical observations for both seizures as well as potential complications. Note is made of interictal discharges and their electrode locations as well as the electrode locations where seizures begin (Fig. 27.7). The resection must include this ictal onset zone.

Brain mapping in epilepsy surgery

Brain mapping is essential if any resections are to be undertaken in the vicinity of functioning eloquent cortex. It is performed with the application of very small currents through intracranial electrodes on brain surface or within the brain to stimulate discrete cortical areas. This can be done either intraoperatively as an 'awake' operation or during the monitoring period in the epilepsy monitoring unit after electrode insertion. Stimulation protocols vary according to centres, the invasive electrode used, and the brain regions being

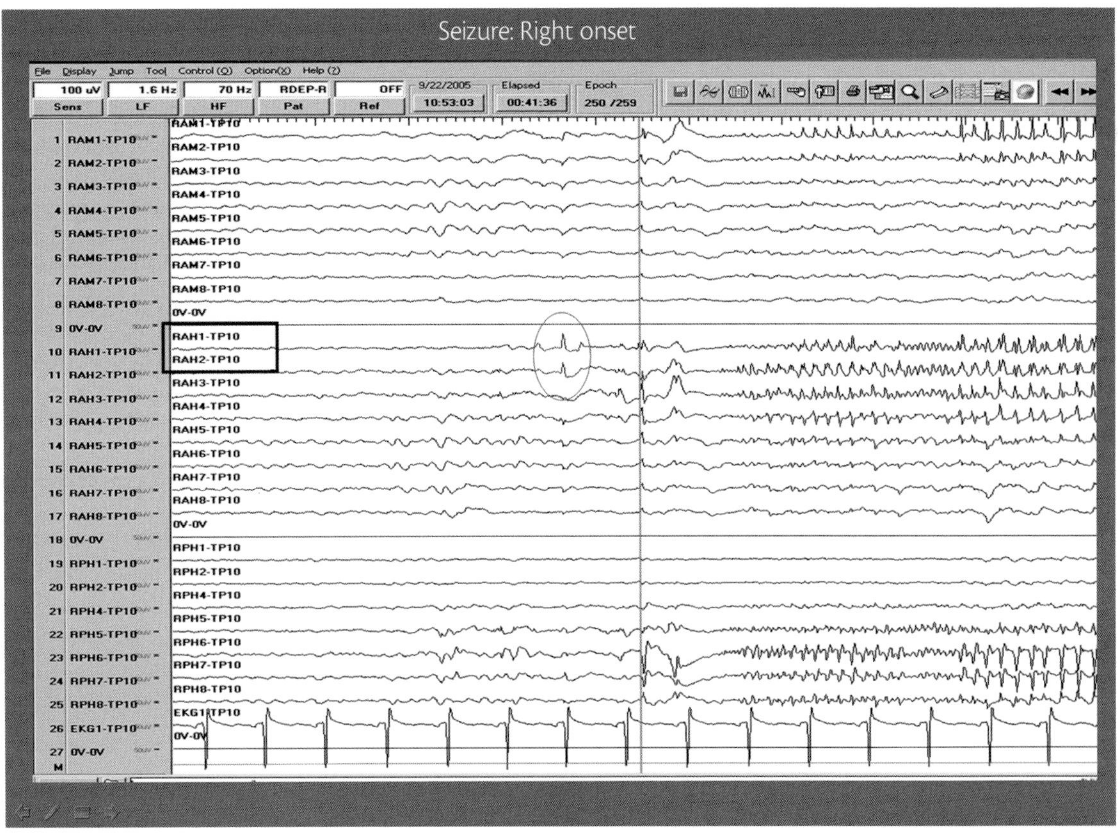

Fig. 27.7 Depth electrodes in a patient with lesion negative right temporal lobe epilepsy showing a seizure (circled) beginning in the right anterior hippocampus (electrodes RAH 1 and RAH 2) and spreading to the amygdala and posterior hippocampus. Copyright Samden D. Lhatoo.

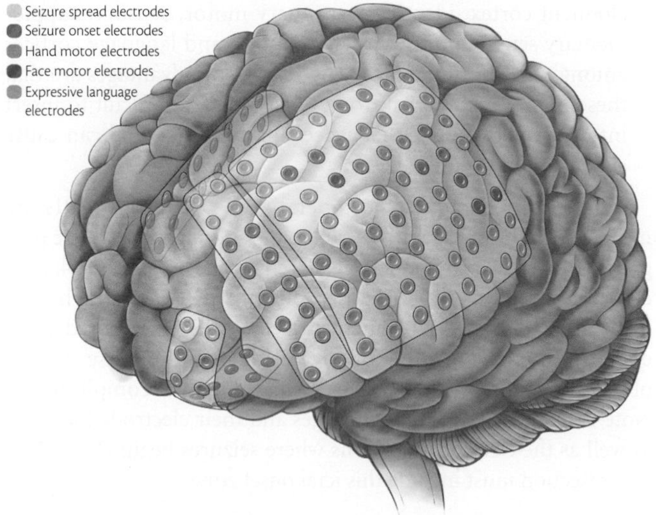

Fig. 27.8 (Also see Colour plate 17.) Brain map of a patient with left frontal lobe epilepsy showing the language, hand motor, and face motor areas with their relationship to the seizure onset (red) and seizure spread (yellow) electrodes. The ictal onset zone in this case therefore lies in the left superior frontal gyrus of the prefrontal cortex, is relatively distant from eloquent cortex and unlikely to cause deficits if resected. Copyright Samden D. Lhatoo.

studied. Stereo-EEG stimulation of primary motor cortex usually involves 1 hertz stimulation, using a 1 millisecond pulse width and 1–3 milliampere current for 40 seconds. Subdural EEG stimulation of the language areas is performed with a 50 hertz, 0.2 millisecond pulse width, 1–20 milliampere stimuli for 5 seconds. Stimulation of the primary cortex will produce twitching of the appropriate contralateral area whereas stimulation of the language areas will produce a temporary aphasia. Information derived from stimulation is mapped to depict cortical functions in different brain regions. Where these 'eloquent' regions lie in relation to the ictal onset zone as revealed by intracranial electrodes will determine whether surgery is possible without substantial risk of major deficits and if yes, how the surgeon tailors the extent and area of the resection (Fig. 27.8).

Surgical resection is then tailored according to the information provided. Resection of cortex underlying the ictal onset electrodes is usually necessary for achieving seizure freedom unless doing so is likely to produce unacceptable deficits. The epileptic lesion zone, if well identified by imaging, is also resected as far as possible. Whether the irritative zones and the areas to which the electrical seizure spreads should also be resected has not been systematically studied and practice varies according to centre.

Contraindications to epilepsy surgery

There are several relative as well as absolute contraindications to surgery (Table 27.7). These are mainly related to an increased likelihood of unacceptable postoperative deficits after surgery. The classical such situation is that of a global amnestic syndrome through removal of one temporal lobe when the remaining brain is incapable of supporting memory function. Neuropsychological testing and/or the intracarotid amobarbital test or Wada test in the preoperative phase usually identifies patients most at risk and surgery is an absolute contraindication then. Many other situations are relative and have to be weighed against potential benefit. Non-dominant hand weakness would be unacceptable in a classical guitarist, for example, but acceptable to another individual who placed great value in seizure freedom. The personal circumstances of the patient including family support in the postoperative period may be important considerations in some cases.

Table 27.7 Contraindications to epilepsy surgery

Ictal onset zone remains undefined
Temporal lobectomy where contralateral hemisphere is incapable of supporting memory
Primary motor area resection (particularly hand and foot areas)
Primary sensory area resection (particularly hand and foot areas)
Language area resection (Broca's, Wernicke's, or basal temporal language areas)
Primary visual cortex resection
Removal of homotopic areas in both hemispheres
Medical contra-indications (e.g. bleeding diathesis)
Untreated psychiatric comorbidity[a]
Complicating socioeconomic factors

[a] Psychogenic non-epileptic seizures are not a contraindication to surgery for epileptic seizures provided these are appropriately managed.

References

1. Horsley V. Brain surgery. *BMJ* 1886; 2:670–4.
2. Rosenow F, Luders H. Presurgical evaluation of epilepsy. *Brain* 2001; 124:1683–700.
3. Luders. HO, Noachtar. S, Burgess RC. Semiologic classification of epileptic seizures. In: Luders HO, Noachtar S (eds) *Epileptic Seizures: Pathophysiology and Clinical Semiology*, pp. 261–85. Philadelphia, PA: Churchill Livingstone, 2000.
4. Schulz. R, Luders. H. Auras elicited by electrical stimulation. In: Luders HO, Noachtar S (eds) *Epileptic Seizures: Pathophysiology and Clinical Semiology*, pp. 254–60. Philadelphia, PA: Churchill Livingstone, 2000.
5. Loddenkemper T, Kotagal P. Lateralizing signs during seizures in focal epilepsy. *Epilepsy Behav* 2005; 7(1):1–17.
6. Duncan JS. Imaging in the surgical treatment of epilepsy. *Nat Rev Neurol* 2010; 6(10):537–50.

CHAPTER 28

Resective Surgery of Temporal Lobe Epilepsy

Simon V. Liubinas, Andrew P. Morokoff, and Terence J. O'Brien

Introduction

Epilepsy has a prevalence of 5–10 per 1000 and temporal lobe epilepsy (TLE) accounts for 25–50% of epilepsy cases (1, 2). Approximately 15–20% of these patients suffer from epilepsy not adequately controlled with maximal medical management, i.e. drug-resistant epilepsy (1, 3). Epilepsy surgery is the only treatment option that offers a reasonable chance of seizure control in patients with chronic drug-resistant epilepsy. It is estimated that at least 4.5% of patients with epilepsy could potentially benefit from surgical resection of an epileptogenic zone (defined as the region of cortex responsible for seizure generation and whose complete resection or disconnection results in seizure freedom) (4, 5). The most common type of drug-resistant epilepsy to be treated surgically is TLE. However, despite the growing safety and efficacy of temporal lobe resection it is still seen by many clinicians and patients as a 'last resort' treatment option. The International League against Epilepsy (ILAE) defines drug-resistant epilepsy as: 'failure of adequate trails of two tolerated and appropriately chosen and used AED schedules (whether as monotherapies or in combination) to achieve sustained seizure freedom' (6). It is estimated that in the US alone only 1500 of the 100,000–200,000 potentially eligible patients undergo surgical resection each year (5, 7–9). Perhaps due to the growing number of new antiepileptic drugs (AEDs) available, it is estimated that the average interval between seizure onset and resective surgery has increased from an average of 12.5 years to 18 years. This is despite the established safety and efficacy of resective surgery (10).

The potential benefits of surgery for drug-resistant temporal lobe epilepsy

Drug-resistant seizures are associated with elevated rates of injury, death, psychiatric comorbidities, and psychosocial disability as well as significant personal and societal economic cost. The mortality rate of patients with epilepsy is overall 2–3 times that of the general population, and highest in those with drug-resistant seizures—in particular those who have had a generalized tonic–clonic seizure or status epilepticus in the past 12 months (11, 12). The incidence of sudden unexpected death in epilepsy (SUDEP) is 1 in 100–1000 per year, while the rate of seizure-related injuries, including burns or scalds, head injury, or dental injury, is significantly increased by seizure frequency and by having multiple seizure types (13).

Patients with drug-resistant epilepsy have significantly increased rates of psychiatric comorbidity and psychosocial disability. Clinically significant anxiety and depression are more common in those patients with drug-resistant epilepsy compared to those who are seizure-free, as are lower self-assessed scores of relationships, ability to perform social activities, work, overall health, plans for the future and self-fulfilment and higher perceptions of stigmatization (11, 13).

The economic cost of drug-resistant epilepsy is considerable. For example, a study performed in England, France, and Germany analysing direct, indirect, and hospital costs for patients with epilepsy showed that the cost per 3-month period was less than UK £500 for those who were seizure-free compared to more than UK £1300 for those with more than one seizure per day (11). Higher seizure frequency is also associated with reduced employment and more days lost to epilepsy (11). Using a decision tree analysis, our group found that there were significant direct cost-savings of performing epilepsy surgery for drug-resistant TLE surgery compared to continued medical therapy, even when the cost of presurgical evaluation, including a combination of video electroencephalography (EEG) monitoring (VEM), magnetic resonance imaging (MRI), 2-(^{18}F) fluro-2-deoxy-D-glucose positron emission tomography (FDG-PET), and single-positron emission computed tomography (SPECT), was taken into account (14).

A randomized controlled trial has confirmed the belief that surgery is superior to continued medical therapy only in patients with drug-resistant TLE with respect to rates of seizure freedom and quality of life (QOL) (2). Many authorities in the field now advocate that patients with potentially surgically remediable epilepsy be referred early for consideration for surgical therapy rather than waiting many years until multiple drugs have failed, as timely surgery may not only improve seizure control and disability, but may also prevent injury and death (2, 7, 15, 16).

The development of surgical approaches for temporal lobe epilepsy

Surgical resection for mostly post-traumatic epileptogenic foci was pioneered by Sir Victor Horsley at Queens Square, London, in

1886, using the clinical features of the seizures to guide the site of craniotomy and resection (17). In the 1930s, Penfield and Jasper at the Montreal Neurological Institute using intraoperative electrocorticography during awake craniotomy to map the epileptogenic zone, developed the techniques of resective surgery, including temporal lobectomy, as it is known today (18–20).

The preoperative evaluation and surgical techniques have been refined as technology, both diagnostic and surgical, have improved over the years. However the basic goal remains the same as discussed in Chapter 27, i.e. resection of the epileptogenic focus, to maximize the chance of post-surgical reduction in seizure frequency, while minimizing the impact on eloquent cortex, and therefore the chance of inducing a neurological deficit. There are a number of different surgical techniques and approaches which are collectively referred to as a 'temporal lobectomy'. Most approaches are based on that developed by Falconer and colleagues who in the 1960s first described mesial temporal sclerosis and the resection of the medial temporal lobe and temporal neocortex (17). Different centres and surgeons vary in the amounts of temporal neocortex, parahippocampal gyrus, hippocampus, and amygdala that they resect. The selective amygdalohippocampectomy, via a pterional craniotomy and trans-sylvian approach, was first described by Yaşargil in Zurich in 1973, as a method of resecting the mesial temporal lobe epileptogenic foci while minimizing the impact on anterior and lateral temporal structures, and thereby potentially decreasing the risk of inducing postoperative neurological or neurocognitive deficits (21). The Engel Surgical Outcome Classification is the most commonly used system to categorize the post-outcome with respect to seizures (22, 23) (see Table 28.1)

Preoperative evaluation

It is essential that all patients being considered for epilepsy surgery undergo a comprehensive, multidisciplinary presurgical evaluation in a centre that specializes in epilepsy surgery. The primary goals of this evaluation are twofold. First to localize the epileptogenic zone, which is the region of brain that needs to be resected to render the patient the maximal chance of being seizure free, and second to assess for, and minimize, the risks of postoperative problems.

Table 28.1 Classification of the outcome of epilepsy surgery ('Engel Classification' (23))

Class I	◆ Free of disabling seizures ◆ Completely seizure-free since surgery, non-disabling simple partial seizures only since surgery, some disabling seizures after surgery but completely seizure-free for at least 2 years, and convulsions only when medications are withdrawn
Class II	◆ Almost seizure-free ◆ Initially seizure-free but has disabling seizures now, rare disabling seizures since surgery, more than rare seizures after surgery but now rare seizures for at least 2 years, nocturnal seizures only
Class III	◆ Worthwhile improvement ◆ Worthwhile seizure reduction or prolonged seizure-free intervals amounting to half the follow-up period, but not less than 2 years
Class IV	◆ No worthwhile improvement ◆ No significant seizure reduction, no appreciable change, or seizures getting worse

Video-EEG monitoring and magnetic resonance imaging

VEM and structural MRI remain the standard first-line investigations in presurgical evaluation for TLE to localize the epileptogenic zone. VEM provides localizing information in approximately 62.2% of patients being evaluated for a potential temporal lobectomy. Similarly, MRI does so in approximately 50–60% of patients (14). It is critical that the MRI is performed using a dedicated epilepsy protocol, and interpreted by radiologists and neurologists who are experienced in interpreting scans in patients with epilepsy, as some of the subtle epileptogenic lesions can otherwise be missed, such as hippocampal sclerosis or focal cortical dysplasia (24). In many centres if a patient with drug-resistant TLE has a resectable lesion identified on MRI, concordant data on VEM, and there are no neuropsychological or neuropsychiatric contraindications, no further tests are required before offering a temporal lobectomy. Most such patients would be expected to have a good outcome (25). However if the MRI is non-localizing, functional imaging with FDG-PET and/or ictal blood flow SPECT are commonly used (26). Concordance between structural MRI and VEM, PET and ictal SPECT is reported as 58%, 68%, and 58% respectively (26). In patients with conflicting data, or in those when only one or none is localizing, surgically implanted intracranial electrodes may be required to localize the epileptogenic zone (27–29).

Discordant VEM and imaging results, such as an EEG seizure onset from the opposite side of the MRI lesion, presents a difficult dilemma. Discordance may represent a contralateral epileptogenic focus not seen on MRI, or may simply represent false EEG lateralization resulting from rapid ictal activity spread. Discordance may be associated with poorer postsurgical outcome and further investigation with ictal SPECT, FDG-PET, or invasive monitoring may be helpful (25, 29). In TLE patients with no lesion seen on MRI, with a localizing PET, SPECT, and/or intracranial EEG, seizure freedom is reported to be achieved in 29–85% of patients in different series (14, 29–35). Cortical dysplasia is found on histopathological examination in of the resected temporal lobe in these MRI non-lesional cases in 15–43% (27, 29–34).

Positron emission tomography

FDG-PET is the most commonly used functional imaging modality used in the presurgical evaluation of TLE (36). FDG-PET scans are performed in the interictal period and show hypometabolism in the epileptogenic temporal lobe in up to 80–95% of patients with drug-resistant TLE, including many patients with a non-lesional MRI (14, 34, 36–41). When PET hypometabolism and MRI identified hippocampal sclerosis are both present and concordant, the likelihood of successful resection may be higher (38). The pathophysiological mechanisms that result in this hypometabolism are unknown. The extent of the hypometabolism on FDG-PET is usually larger than the underlying epileptogenic lesion (if present) or the epileptogenic zone identified on intracranial EEG (36, 37). Using statistical parametric analysis of the FDG-PET images co-registered to a postoperative MRI, our group showed that patients rendered seizure free following a temporal lobectomy have on average only 25% of the region of hypometabolism resected (42). Therefore the decision regarding the extent of temporal neocortical resection should not be made on the basis of FDG-PET alone, but should be made in conjunction with MRI, EEG (including intracranial EEG if warranted), and other imaging modalities.

Both the presence of an MRI lesion and the presence of unilateral temporal hypometabolism have been shown to be independently predictive of a good surgical outcome with respect to seizures (14, 42). A meta-analysis of 46 studies performed by Willman et al. showed that ipsilateral PET hypometabolism had an 86% predictive values for good outcome (defined as Engel class I or II) (43). The predictive value of PET hypometabolism in those requiring intracranial EEG recording, and those with non-localizing EEG and MRI were 75%, 73%, and 80% respectively (43).

Single-positron emission computed tomography

Blood flow SPECT involves intravenous injection of a technetium-based radiotracer either during seizures, following or between seizures, and hence allows imaging of patterns of cerebral blood flow in the ictal, postictal, and interictal phases (36, 40, 44). Ictal SPECT is estimated to be 73–97% sensitive in TLE and is highly specific for the epileptogenic zone, while interictal SPECT has a lower sensitivity of approximately 50% and is less specific (40). Digital subtraction of an interictal from an ictal SPECT creates an image of the pattern of change during seizures from the baseline cerebral perfusion patterns, while co-registration with an anatomical MRI scan (computer-aided subtraction ictal SPECT co-registered to MRI, or SISCOM) provides anatomical localization of this region of perfusion change, improving the utility for surgical planning (27, 45, 46). True ictal SPECT (i.e. injection of the isotope within 45 seconds of stereotypical seizure onset) has been shown to be accurate in predicting localization, even when ictal EEG and MRI are non-localizing or non-concordant (47–50). Patients in whom SISCOM localization is concordant with site of resective surgery are more likely to have excellent postsurgical outcomes with respect to seizure frequency than those in whom SISCOM is non-localizing or non-concordant with surgical site (46, 47, 51).

In MRI-VEM concordant cases, SPECT shows unilateral increased blood flow in approximately 85% (25). If SPECT, MRI, and VEM are concordant, a 78% good outcome rate was shown (25).

Magnetoencephalography

Magnetoencephalography (MEG), usually co-registered with structural MRI (magnetic source imaging or MSI), is used in some centres as an ancillary test to localize the source of interictal epileptogenic discharges using magnetic fields rather than the electrical spikes seen in EEG. In a retrospective study of 455 drug-resistant TLE patients, MEG was shown to be concordant with the epileptogenic side of epilepsy surgery in 54–80% (depending on the method used). In 24% of cases, MEG provided localizing information not given by EEG or other methods, and in 11% altered or influenced surgical decision-making (52). In other studies, MEG was concordant with video-EEG in 32%, correctly lateralized the surgical site in 59% of those with non-localizing video-EEG (53) and was second only to subdural grid EEG recording in predicting surgical outcome (54). Although a potentially promising as non-invasive method of presurgical work-up, in practice the limited availability and expense of MEG means that its application is currently restricted to selected centres and cases.

Intracranial EEG in temporal lobe epilepsy

In modern epilepsy surgery centres, less than 10% of patients with drug-resistant TLE undergo intracranial EEG studies. The indications include: inconclusive or discordant results from video-EEG and other non-invasive investigations, when there appears to be bilateral seizure onsets on the scalp EEG, suspected extratemporal foci and epileptogenic foci adjacent to or overlapping with eloquent cortex requiring extraoperative functional stimulation mapping (55–58). The yield of intracranial EEG implantations, and of the respective surgery that follows, can be optimized by using imaging modalities such as SPECT or PET, identifying the regions most likely to be the seizure focus, to guide the site and extent of the electrode implantations (27, 29).

Subdural strips and grids for intracranial EEG recordings have long been used to assist with localization of the epileptogenic zone in patients with medically refractory focal epilepsy undergoing presurgical evaluation (56, 59–65). Invasive EEG monitoring has a reported concordance of 47% with structural MRI, 58% with PET and 56% with ictal SPECT (26). The advent of MRI saw a decrease in the use of invasive EEG techniques (28) as it was realized that resection of a focal lesion detected on MRI was highly predictive of a good outcome with respect to seizures following epilepsy surgery (5, 27). However over the last 5–10 years there has been a resurgence in the use of intracranial EEG recordings, as epilepsy centres have seen an increased proportion of patients in whom the MRI does not detect a lesion, or in whom the potential epileptogenic abnormalities on the MRI are extensive and not completely resectable. It is estimated that in approximately 30–50% of patients considered for surgical resection of medically refractory epilepsy, an epileptogenic focus cannot be localized on non-invasive functional and structural studies (65, 66). In such patients, invasive EEG monitoring with subdural electrodes may be helpful in localizing the epileptogenic zone, and its relationship to neighbouring eloquent cortex, allowing a resective procedure to be more safely and effectively performed.

However, the manner in which intracranial recordings is now being utilized by many epilepsy surgery programs is very different to how they have traditionally been used. In contrast to the previously common use of 'blind implantations', when non-invasive techniques were non-localizing, the strategy for the intracranial implantation now incorporates the results of modern neuroimaging. The intracranial EEG is used to test or refine the hypothesis for the localization of the epileptogenic zone put forward by the results of neuroimaging. Murphy and colleagues have described the use of MMIGS in the treatment of medically refractory epilepsy (27, 35). This technique involves the co-registration of functional imaging, in particular PET and SPECT, with MRI and subdural grid arrays allowing their incorporation into a frameless stereotactic neurosurgical navigation system (27, 35). In this manner, epileptogenic foci can be delineated and the eloquent cortex mapped, thus maximizing outcome with respect to seizure control whilst minimizing neurological complications.

Intracranial EEG recordings with surgically implanted subdural grids, strip, or depth electrodes utilize stainless steel or platinum electrodes embedded in a synthetic material which are implanted in proximity to the suspected epileptogenic zone via craniotomy or burr hole methods (4). Subdural grid arrays have the advantage over strip electrodes of allowing a greater cortical surface to be mapped and electrically stimulated (56). However, subdural strip electrodes can be introduced via a burr hole, instead of a large craniotomy which is required for depth electrodes, thereby decreasing the risk of postoperative complications (56). Depth electrodes are implanted into the brain, and therefore have the advantage of being able to record seizure foci deep to the cortical surface which may have not been detected with subdural electrodes (28). Risk of bleeding is reduced by the use of modern image guided surgical implantation techniques (28).

As with any invasive procedure, serious complications can occur with the use of intracranial EEG electrodes, but in experienced epilepsy surgery centres these are uncommon (27–29). Fountas and Smith presented a retrospective 20-year series of 185 patients who underwent subdural grid or strip implantation. They reported postoperative epidural haematoma in three patients (1.6%) and subdural haematoma in two patients (1.1%) (67). Significant brain oedema occurred in two patients (1.1%), while two developed infection and two developed transient aphasia. Two patients had fatal outcomes and five (2.7%) experienced non-habitual seizures (67). Such complications may mandate re-opening the craniotomy with or without removal of the grids.

It has been reported that 4–52% of patients with pathologically confirmed focal cortical dysplasia have normal MRI studies (68–70). This wide range may reflect the use of older generations of MRI machines and as advances are made in imaging technology it is expected that this range will decrease. However, invasive EEG monitoring remains an important investigation in pre-resection evaluation of patients with medically refractory epilepsy due to dysplasia. Similarly, complete resection of a lesion visible on MRI is not always adequate to predict seizure free outcome, supporting the use of invasive EEG monitoring to enable the surgeon to perform a tailored resection of the ictal onset zone as well as the MRI visible lesion in these patients (70). The ictal onset zone may include a variable extent of macroscopically normal brain surrounding a discrete epileptogenic lesion. There is evidence that the complete resection of both the ictal-onset zone and the MRI lesion is associated with an improved outcome with respect to seizures as opposed to resection of the lesion only (71–74). Therefore it is vital that subdural grid coverage of the cortical surface should be extensive enough to allow accurate mapping of the ictal onset zone and the neighbouring eloquent cortex. This approach maximizes long-term seizure freedom while minimizing damage to functional cortex (75, 76).

Surgical approaches

Temporal lobectomy or selective amygdalohippocampectomy is usually performed via a pterional craniotomy with the patient's head fixed in a 3-point Mayfield frame, with the head elevated 30 degrees above the chest and turned 30 degrees to the opposite side (21). Intraoperative frameless stereotactic navigation may be used. The two usual approaches comprise the standard anterior temporal resection or 'anterior temporal lobectomy' and the more selective removal of mesial temporal structures with sparing of the lateral temporal lobe called the selective amygdalohippocampectomy. Several approaches are used including the trans-sylvian (Yaşargil's method), subtemporal, and trans-gyral approaches. Using meticulous microneurosurgical technique, the anterior temporal neocortex and/or the mesial temporal structures are resected. For a standard temporal lobectomy up to 6.5 cm of anterolateral non-dominant, and up to 4.5 cm of dominant neocortex may be resected. The mesial resection includes the entire amygdala, and as much as possible of the hippocampus (2, 21, 56). The selective amygdalohippocampectomy, if deemed appropriate from preoperative evaluation, aims to avoid resection of, and trauma to, the overlying healthy temporal neocortex, deep white matter tracts, and vasculature, while still removing the amygdala and the anterior portion of the hippocampus (21, 77). The surgical procedure takes usually takes 3–5 hours (21).

Complications of temporal lobectomy

Complications of temporal lobectomy include: hemiparesis from infarctions in the internal capsule caused by damage to the deep perforators (1–5%), wound infection (2.5%), intracerebral haemorrhage, subdural haemorrhage (1.4%), neuropsychological or memory sequelae impairing QOL (1–5%), and death (<1%) (2, 21, 56, 78, 79). Depression occurs in approximately 18% of surgical patients, compared to 20% of medically treated patients, and is often most prominent in the first 3–6 months postoperatively (2). Superior quadrantanopia visual field deficits are an expected outcome following formal temporal lobectomy (although not selective amygdalohippocampectomy) occurring in 55% of patients, are largely asymptomatic and as such should not be classified as a complication of surgery (2, 21).

Early postoperative seizures in temporal lobe surgery

Up to 20% of patients will have seizures in the early postoperative period (80, 81). The significance of early postoperative seizures on likelihood of seizure recurrence has often been discounted because of possible association with perioperative factors. However, McIntosh et al. performed a retrospective review of 321 patients who underwent surgery for TLE. In the first week after surgery 30 (9.3%) had seizures, while 69 (21.5%) had seizures within the first 28 days. Kaplan–Meier analysis showed patients who have 'early seizures' (within the first 28 postoperative days), have a 23.2% probability of being seizure free at 1 year, compared to 71.8% for those who had no early seizures. At 2 years the probability of seizure freedom for those with and without early postoperative seizures was 20.3% and 65.8% respectively (80). Numerous seizure precipitants, including changes in AED dose, were identified, and it was found that although patients who had a precipitant to their early seizure had a risk of recurrence that was half that of those without a precipitant, the overall recurrence rate was higher than for those without early seizures (80). These authors found that the number, type and similarity of postoperative to preoperative seizure was not significant in predictor likelihood of recurrence (80). In contrast, another study found that patients whose seizures in the first week following a temporal lobectomy were similar to their preoperative habitual seizures had a lower rate of either an excellent or favourable outcome with respect to seizures than those whose postoperative seizures were auras, or were focal motor and/or generalized tonic–clonic seizures (14.3%, 77.8%, and 75.0% respectively) (81).

Outcome with respect to seizure control, AED use, and quality of life

Wiebe et al. performed a study in which 80 patients with TLE were randomly assigned to either surgery or medical therapy for 1 year. At 1 year, 58% of those in the surgery group were free of awareness impairing seizures, compared to 8% in the medical group (p <0.001), and had significantly better QOL (2). Thirty-eight per cent in the surgical group were free of all seizures, including auras, compared to 3% in the medical group (2). It is important to note that this was an intention to treat analysis and four of the patients in the 'surgical group' did not actually undergo surgery, and of the patients who did undergo surgery 64% were seizure free at 1 year. The numbers needed to treat to render one patient free of consciousness impairing seizures at 1 year, and of all seizures at 1 year were calculated at 2 and 3 respectively (2). Approximately 15% of those in the surgical group continued to have 1–4 seizures impairing consciousness per month (2). Residual seizure activity was similar in severity for both the surgical and medical groups. QOL measured by the QOLIE-89 score was better for the surgical group (P <0.001) although it improved in both groups over time (p = 0.003). A higher proportion in the surgical group were employed or attending school at 1 year (56.4% vs. 38.5%), this did not reach statistical significance (p = 0.11) (2). There was one unexpected death (SUDEP) in the medical group and none in the surgical group.

In a meta-analysis including 83 studies and over 3000 patients, Tellez-Zenteno showed that 66% of patients achieve long-term seizure freedom after temporal lobe resection and 14% of patients achieve long-term AED discontinuance (82, 83). Forty-one per cent remained on one medication and 31% remained on polytherapy. The paediatric population achieved better AED outcome than adults (82). Tonini et al. performed a meta-analysis of 47 articles involving 3511 patients and reported that febrile convulsions, mesial temporal sclerosis, tumours (most commonly low-grade, long-term epilepsy associated tumours such as ganglioglioma and dysembryoplastic neuroepithelial tumours), lesions on MRI, EEG/MRI concordance, and extensive resection were the strongest predictors of postoperative seizure freedom (84, 85). Postoperative discharges, and the need for intracranial monitoring were associated with poorer outcomes (85).

McIntosh et al. retrospectively reviewed 325 patients who had undergone surgery for TLE. Using survival analysis and multivariate regression, the probability of complete seizure freedom at 2, 5, and 10 years postoperatively was calculated as 55.3%, 47.7%, and 41% respectively (86). Patients with discrete MRI abnormalities were found to have a higher chance of seizure freedom postoperatively, while duration of seizures, age at seizure onset, and age at surgery had no effect on outcome (86).

Many studies have found that the presence of a MRI lesion (including mesial temporal sclerosis) that is able to be completely surgically excised is associated with an improved rate of long-term seizure control postoperatively as compared to those with a normal MRI (60–85% vs. 30–50%) (87–89). As may be expected, incomplete resection of the epileptogenic zone as demonstrated on MRI or by subdural EEG is more likely to result in seizure recurrence (31, 70, 90, 91). However, it is now clear that there are a group of patients with drug-resistant TLE without a definite lesion on the MRI scan who have prominent unilateral hypometabolism on FDG-PET and concordant seizure onset on video-EEG who have long-term outcomes that are similar to those with an MRI lesion (34, 92). A minority of these patients have focal cortical dysplasia on histopathological examination of the resected temporal lobe specimen, but in the majority only non-specific changes are seen. The underlying pathophysiology in these patients with surgical remedial non-lesional TLE remains uncertain.

Yaşargil et al. presented a series of 73 patients with medically refractory TLE who underwent selective amygdalohippocampectomy. Mean duration of seizure activity of 21.9 years. Preoperative MRI demonstrated MTS in 45.2%. Mean follow-up was 4.3 years. Seizure outcome was Engel class I, II, and III in 75.3%, 17.8%, and 6.8% respectively; 42.5% had ceased their AED. Histopathology showed sclerosis in 48%, gliosis in 41%, and no abnormality in 11%. Patients with MTS were more likely to have an Engel class I outcome. The best outcomes were seen in the group of patients in whom MRI, EEG and pathology were all abnormal (90% Engel class I). In contrast, in those with normal MRI and pathology, 42.9% achieved a good surgical result (21). There were no deaths in this series.

Many studies have shown that patients who achieve seizure freedom following epilepsy surgery overall have an improved QOL (2, 89, 93), although this improvement may take up to 2 years to establish (93). Good postoperative outcomes with respect to QOL are associated with good preoperative QOL, early surgical intervention, and with pathological findings of mesial temporal sclerosis, whereas TLE caused by tumours and in those with either presurgery psychopathology are more likely to have poorer QOL outcomes (93–97).

Cunha et al. prospectively followed 32 patients undergoing resection for TLE. Overall QOL increased after surgery until the 5th post-surgical year (p <0.05) (93). Cognitive function and social function were significantly enhanced postsurgery, and seizure related worry was significantly reduced (93). Previous psychopathology was found to have a significant impact on postoperative social function and seizure worry scores (93). Patients with right TLE had significantly better outcomes than those with left sided epilepsy in terms of postoperative cognitive function and overall QOL, consistent with the role played by the left hippocampus in verbal memory (93). There were no associations found between patient age or duration of disease prior to surgery and improved postoperative QOL (93). As a whole, patients had improved QOL if their seizure frequency decreased, even if they did not achieve complete seizure freedom, however those with Engel class I outcomes had a greater increase in QOL (93). Therefore even if surgery is not expected to achieve total freedom, the impact on QOL of decreased seizure burden should be taken into account when deciding on surgery.

What to do if surgery fails?

Approximately 20–30% of patients who undergo an temporal lobectomy for drug-resistant epilepsy do not achieve seizure control postoperatively (21, 86, 98–100). There are a number of small series reported of patients who failed to achieve seizure freedom post-initial temporal lobe resection who subsequently underwent repeat surgery. In those with ipsilateral temporal EEG findings, with or without residual mesial temporal structures, repeat operation extending the surgical resection is successful in achieving a good outcome (Engel class I or II) in approximately 34–60% of cases (99, 101–106). Invasive monitoring may be considered prior to repeat surgery and SISCOM also can help define the epileptogenic zone in these patients (107). Some patients may be diagnosed as having another, extratemporal, lesion and in these cases resection with or without invasive monitoring can be performed (99). Autopsy series suggest that 47–86% of patients with TLE have bitemporal hippocampal sclerosis (108). Therefore in some post-resection patients a new or previously dormant ictal focus may become active in the contralateral temporal lobe. Due to the cognitive, behavioural, and memory sequelae of bilateral mesial temporal resection, these patients are not suitable for further resective surgery and therapeutic options are limited to optimization of medical therapy and consideration of vagus nerve stimulator implantation (99).

What to do with medications if surgery succeeds?

While the primary goal of epilepsy surgery for drug-resistant TLE is seizure control, many patients also have the goal to be able to cease their AED therapy. Most centres have the practice of maintaining essentially the same AED regimen postoperatively as the patient was on prior to the surgery until the patient has been seizure free for a period of time—commonly 6–12 months. After this some of the drugs are weaned or reduced in dose, but most patients will be advised to continue to take at least a one AED at least 2 years postoperatively. It remains controversial whether patients who remain seizure free postoperatively should wean off AEDs after this time. Schiller and colleagues followed the outcomes of 210 patients who were seizure free for 1 or more years: in 84 the AEDs were ceased, in 90 the drugs were reduced, and in 30 the AEDs were kept unchanged (109). Approximately 40% of the patients in whom AEDs were discontinued experienced a return of seizures compared to approximately 20% in those who the drugs were reduced but not stopped and less than 10% of those in whom medications were not changed. Of the 22 patients with recurrent seizures post-medication reduction, in two the seizures continued despite restarting the AEDs (109).

Conclusions

Resective surgery, whether by selective amygdalohippocampectomy or including resection of the overlying anterior temporal neocortex, is a safe and effective method for treating drug-resistant TLE. A multidisciplinary comprehensive preoperative evaluation with a combination of MRI, VEM, neuropsychology, and neuropsychiatry, and in selected cases FDG-PET, ictal SPECT, and/or intracranial EEG monitoring, combined with advances in microneurosurgical and image-guided techniques, can provide excellent surgical results in terms of decreased seizure burden, decreased AED use, increased QOL, and economic cost-effectiveness. Early consideration of surgical treatment should be considered in cases of temporal lobe epilepsy who have failed to achieve seizure control after trials of two or more AEDs.

References

1. Engel J Jr. Intractable epilepsy: definition and neurobiology. *Epilepsia* 2001; 42(Suppl 6):3.
2. Wiebe S, Blume WT, Girvin JP, Eliasziw M. Effectiveness and Efficiency of Surgery for Temporal Lobe Epilepsy Study Group. A randomized, controlled trial of surgery for temporal-lobe epilepsy. *N Engl J Med* 2001; 345(5):311–18.
3. Hamer HM, Morris HH, Mascha EJ, Karafa MT, Bingaman WE, Bej MD, *et al.* Complications of invasive video-EEG monitoring with subdural grid electrodes. *Neurology* 2002; 58:97–103.
4. Najm IM, Bingaman WE, Lüders H. The use of subdural grids in the management of focal malformations due to abnormal cortical development. *Neurosurg Clin North Am* 2002; 37(1):87–92.
5. Rosenow F, Lüders H. Presurgical evaluation of epilepsy. *Brain* 2001; 124:1683–700.
6. Kwan P, Arzimanoglou A, Berg AT, Brodie MJ, Allen Hauser W, Mathern G, *et al.* Definition of drug resistant epilepsy: consensus proposal by the ad hoc Task Force of the ILAE Commission on Therapeutic Strategies. *Epilepsia* 2010; 51(6):1069–77.
7. Semah F, Picot M, Adam C. Is the underlying cause of epilepsy a major prognostic factor for recurrence? *Neurology* 1998; 51:1256–62.
8. Engel J, Van Ness P, Ramussen T. Overview: Who should be considered a surgical candidate? . In: Engel J (ed) *Surgical Treatment of the Epilepsies*, pp. 23–34. New York: Raven Press, 1993.
9. Engel J Jr, Wiebe S, French J, Sperling M, Williamson P, Spencer D, *et al.* Practice parameter: temporal lobe and localized neocortical resections for epilepsy: report of the Quality Standards Subcommittee of the American Academy of Neurology, in association with the American Epilepsy Society and the American Association of Neurological Surgeons. *Neurology* 2003; 60(4):538–47.
10. Engel J. A greater role for surgical treatment of epilepsy: Why and when? *Epilepsy Curr* 2003; 3(2):37–40.
11. Baker GA, Nashef L, van Hout BA. Current issues in the management of epilepsy: the impact of frequent seizures on cost of illness, quality of life, and mortality. *Epilepsia* 1997; 38(Suppl 1):S1–8.
12. Strauss DJ, Day SM, Shavelle RM, Wu YW. Remote symptomatic epilepsy: does seizure severity increase mortality? *Neurology* 2003; 60(3):395–9.
13. Baker GA, Jacoby A, Buck D, Stalgis C, Monnet D. Quality of life of people with epilepsy: a European study. *Epilepsia* 1997; 38(3): 353–62.
14. O'Brien TJ, Miles K, Ware R, Cook MJ, Binns DS, Hicks RJ. The cost-effective use of F-18-FDG PET in the presurgical evaluation of medically refractory focal epilepsy. *J Nucl Med* 2008; 49(6): 931–7.
15. Engel J Jr. The timing of surgical intervention for mesial temporal lobe epilepsy: a plan for a randomized controlled trial. *Arch Neurol* 1999; 56:1338–41.
16. Sperling MR, O'Connor MJ, Saykin AJ, Plummer C. Temporal lobectomy for refractory epilepsy. *JAMA* 1996; 276:470–5.
17. Falconer MA, Taylor DC. Surgical treatment of drug-resistant epilepsy due to mesial temporal sclerosis. *Arch Neurol* 1968; 19:353–61.
18. Foerster O, Penfield W. The structural basis of traumatuc epilepsy and results of radical operation. *Arch Neurol* 1930; 53(2):99–119.
19. Penfield W, Jasper H. *Epilepsy and the functional anatomy of the human brain.* Boston, MA: Little Brown & Co, 1954.
20. Feindel W, Leblanc R, Villemure J-G. History of the surgical treatment of epilepsy. In: Greenblatt SH (ed) *A History of Neurosurgery*, pp. 465–88. Park Ridge, IL: The American Association of Neurological Surgeons, 1997.
21. Yaşargil MG, Krayenbühl N, Roth P, Hsu SP, Yaşargil DC. The selective amygdalohippocampectomy for intractable temporal limbic seizures. *J Neurosurg* 2010; 112(1):168–85.
22. Engel J, Van Ness P, Ramussen T. Outcome in respect to epileptic seizures. In: Engel J (ed) *Surgical Treatment of the Epilepsies*, pp. 609–21. New York: Raven Press, 1993.
23. Engel J. Approaches to localization of the epileptogenic lesion. In: Engel J (ed) *Surgical Treatment of the Epilepsies*, pp. 75–96. New York: Raven Press, 1993.
24. Kilpatrick C, O'Brien T, Matkovic Z, Cook M, Kaye A. Preoperative evaluation for temporal lobe surgery. *J Clin Neurosci* 2002; 10(5): 535–9.
25. Castro LH, Serpa MH, Valério RM, Jorge CL, Ono CR, Arantes PR, *et al.* Good surgical outcome in discordant ictal EEG-MRI unilateral mesial temporal sclerosis patients. *Epilepsia* 2008; 49(8):1324–32.

26. Won HJ, Chang KH, Cheon JE, Kim HD, Lee DS, Han MH, *et al.* Comparison of MR Imaging with PET and ictal SPECT in 118 patients with intractable epilepsy. *Am J Neuroradiol* 1999; 20:593–9.
27. Murphy M, O'Brien TJ, Morris K, Cook MJ. Multimodality image-guided epilepsy surgery. *J Clin Neurosci* 2001; 8(6):534–8.
28. Murphy MA, O'Brien TJ, Cook MJ. Insertion of depth electrodes with or without subdural grids using frameless stereotactic guidance system- technique and outcome. *Br J Neurosurg* 2002; 16:119–25.
29. Liubinas SV, Cassidy D, Roten A, Kaye AH, O'Brien TJ. Tailored cortical resection following image guided subdural grid implantation for medically refractory epilepsy. *J Clin Neurosci* 2009; 16:1398–408.
30. Alarcón G, Valentín A, Watt C, Selway RP, Lacruz ME, Elwes RD, *et al.* Is it worth pursuing surgery for epilepsy in patients with normal neuroimaging? *J Neurol Neurosurg Psychiatry* 2006; 77:474–80.
31. Chapman K, Wyllie E, Najm I, Ruggieri P, Bingaman W, Lüders J, *et al.* Seizure outcome after epilepsy surgery in patients with normal preoperative MRI. *J Neurol Neurosurg Psychiatry* 2005; 76:710–13.
32. Siegel AM, Jobst BC, Thadani VM, Rhodes CH, Lewis PJ, Roberts DW, *et al.* Medically intractable, localization-related epilepsy with normal MRI: Presurgical evaluation and surgical outcome in 43 patients. *Epilepsia* 2001; 42(7):883–8.
33. Kuzniecky R, Burgard S, Faught E, Morawetz R, Bartolucci A. Predictive value of magnetic resonance imaging in temporal lobe epilepsy surgery. *Arch Neurol* 1993; 50(1):65–9.
34. Carne RP, O'Brien TJ, Kilpatrick CJ, MacGregor LR, Hicks RJ, Murphy MA, et *al.* MRI-negative PET-positive temporal lobe epilepsy: a distinct surgically remediable syndrome. *Brain* 2004; 127(Pt 10):2276–85.
35. Murphy MA, O'Brien TJ, Morris K, Cook MJ. Multimodality image-guided surgery for the treatment of medically refractory epilepsy. *J Neurosurg* 2004; 100:452–62.
36. Knowlton RC. The role of FDG-PET, ictal SPECT, and MEG in the epilepsy surgery evaluation. *Epilepsy Behav* 2006; 8(1):91–101.
37. Ryvlin P, Bouvard S, Le Bars D, De Lamérie G, Grégoire MC, Kahane P, *et al.* Clinical utility of flumazenil-PET versus 18F fluorodeoxyglucose-PET and MRI in refractory partial epilepsy. A prospective study in 100 patients. *Brain* 1998; 121(Pt 11):2067–81.
38. Gaillard WD, Bhatia S, Bookheimer SY, Fazilat S, Sato S, Theodore WH. FDG-PET and volumetric MRI in the evaluation of patients with partial epilepsy. *Neurology* 1995; 45(1):123–6.
39. Locharernkul C, Tepmongkol S, Limotai C, Loplumlert J. Positron emission tomography (PET) scan in epilepsy. *Asian Biomed* 2008; 2(1):3–17.
40. la Fougère C, Rominger A, Förster S, Geisler J, Bartenstein P. PET and SPECT in epilepsy: A critical review. *Epilepsy Behav* 2009; 15(1):50–5.
41. O'Brien TJ, Hicks RJ, Ware R, Binns DS, Murphy M, Cook MJ. The utility of a 3-dimensional, large-field-of-view, sodium iodide crystal-based PET scanner in the presurgical evaluation of partial epilepsy. *J Nucl Med* 2001; 42:1158–65.
42. Vinton AB, Carne R, Hicks RJ, Desmond PM, Kilpatrick C, Kaye AH, *et al.* The extent of resection of FDG-PET hypometabolism relates to outcome of temporal lobectomy. *Brain* 2007; 130(Pt 2):548–60.
43. Willmann O, Wennberg R, May T, Woermann FG, Pohlmann-Eden B. The contribution of 18F-FDG PET in preoperative epilepsy surgery evaluation for patients with temporal lobe epilepsy A meta-analysis. *Seizure* 2007: 16(6):509–20.
44. Rathore C, Kesavadas C, Ajith J, Sasikala A, Sarma SP, Radhakrishnan K. Cost-effective utilization of single photon emission computed tomography (SPECT) in decision making for epilepsy surgery. *Seizure* 2011: 20(2):107–14.
45. Zubal IG, Spencer SS, Imam K, Seibyl J, Smith EO, Wisniewski G, Hoffer PB. Difference images calculated from ictal and interictal technetium-99m-HMPAO SPECT scans of epilepsy. *J Nucl Med* 1995: 36(4):684–9.
46. O'Brien TJ, So EL, Mullan BP, Hauser MF, Brinkmann BH, Bohnen NI, *et al.* Subtraction ictal SPECT co-registered to MRI improves clinical usefulness of SPECT in localizing the surgical seizure focus. *Neurology* 1998: 50(2):445–54.
47. O'Brien TJ, So EL, Cascino GD, Hauser MF, Marsh WR, Meyer FB, *et al.* Subtraction SPECT coregistered to MRI in focal malformations of cortical development: localization of the epileptogenic zone in epilepsy surgery candidates. *Epilepsia* 2004: 45(4):367–76.
48. Véra P, Kaminska A, Cieuta C, Hollo A, Stiévenart JL, Gardin I, *et al.* Use of subtraction ictal SPECT co-registered to MRI for optimizing the localization of seizure foci in children. *J Nucl Med* 1999: 40(5):786–92.
49. Won HJ, Chang KH, Cheon JE, Kim HD, Lee DS, Han MH, *et al.* Comparison of MR imaging with PET and ictal SPECT in 118 patients with intractable epilepsy. *AJNR Am J Neuroradiol* 1999: 20(4):593–9.
50. Hong KS, Lee SK, Kim JY, Lee DS, Chung CK. Pre-surgical evaluation and surgical outcome of 41 patients with non-lesional neocortical epilepsy. *Seizure* 2002: 11(3):184–92.
51. Wichert-Ana L, de Azevedo-Marques PM, Oliveira LF, Terra-Bustamante VC, Fernandes RM, Santos AC, *et al.* Interictal hyperemia correlates with epileptogenicity in polymicrogyric cortex. *Epilepsy Res* 2008: 79(1):39–48.
52. Stefan H, Hummel C, Scheler G, Genow A, Druschky K, Tilz C, *et al.* Magnetic brain source imaging of focal epileptic activity: a synopsis of 455 cases. *Brain* 2003: 126(Pt 11):2396–405.
53. Pataraia E, Simos PG, Castillo EM, Billingsley RL, Sarkari S, Wheless JW, *et al.* Does magnetoencephalography add to scalp video-EEG as a diagnostic tool in epilepsy surgery? *Neurology* 2004: 62(6):943–8.
54. Wheless JW, Willmore LJ, Breier JI, Kataki M, Smith JR, King DW, *et al.* A comparison of magnetoencephalography, MRI, and V-EEG in patients evaluated for epilepsy surgery. *Epilepsia* 1999: 40(7):931–41.
55. Kral T, Clusmann H, Blümcke I, Fimmers R, Ostertun B, Kurthen M, *et al.* Outcome of epilepsy surgery in focal cortical dysplasia. *J Neurol Neurosurg Psychiatry* 2003: 74:183–8.
56. Fabinyi G. Operative diagnostic methods in the treatment of epilepsy. In: Kaye AH, Black PM (eds) *Operative Neurosurgery*, pp. 1251–8. London: Churchill Livingstone, 2000.
57. Jayakar P. Invasive EEG monitoring in children: When, where and what? *J Clin Neurophysiol* 1999; 16:408–18.
58. Bruce DA, Bizzi JWJ. Surgical technique for the insertion of grids and strips for invasive monitoring in children with intractable epilepsy. *Child's Nerv Syst* 2000; 16:724–30.
59. Risinger MW. Electroencephalographic strategies for determining the epileptogenic zone. In: Lüders H (ed) *Epilepsy Surgery*, pp. 337–47. New York: Raven Press, 1992.
60. Roper SN. Implantation of grid and strip electrodes. *Tech Neurosurg* 1995; 1:5–10.
61. Jennum P, Dhuna A, Davies K, Fiol M, Maxwell R. Outcome of resective surgery for intractable partial epilepsy guided by subdural electrode arrays. *Acta Neurol Scand* 1993; 87:434–7.
62. Wyler AR, Ojemann GA, Lettich E, Ward AA Jr. Subdural strip electrodes for localizing epileptogenic foci. *J Neurosurg* 1984; 60: 1195–200.
63. Hong SC, Kang KS, Seo DW, Hong SB, Lee M, Nam DH, *et al.* Surgical treatment of intractable epilepsy accompanying cortical dysplasia. *J Neurosurg* 2000; 93:766–73.
64. Spencer SS, Spencer DD, Williamson PD, Mattson R. Combined depth and subdural electrode investigation in uncontrolled epilepsy. *Neurology* 1990; 40:74–9.
65. Brekelmans GJ, van Emde Boas W, Velis DN, Lopes da Silva FH, van Rijen PC, van Veelen CW. Comparison of combined versus subdural or intracerebral electrodes alone in presurgical focus localization. *Epilepsia* 1998; 39(12):1290–301.
66. Engel J. Approaches to localization of the epileptogenic lesion. In: Engel J (ed) *Surgical Treatment of the Epilepsies*, pp.75–96. New York: Raven Press, 1987.

67. Fountas KN, Smith JR. Subdural electrode-associated complications: a 20-year experience. *Stereotact Funct Neurosurg*, 2007; 85:264–72.
68. Ruggieri PM, Najm I, Bronen R, Campos M, Cendes F, Duncan JS, *et al*. Neuroimaging of the cortical dysplasias. *Neurology* 2004; 62(Suppl 3):S27–9.
69. Widdess-Walsh P, Diehl B, Najm I. Neuroimaging of focal cortical dysplasia. *J Neuroimaging* 2006; 16:185–96.
70. Widdess-Walsh P, Jeha L, Nair D, Kotagal P, Bingaman W, Najm I. Subdural electrode analysis in focal cortical dysplasia. *Neurology* 2007; 69:660–7.
71. Drake J, Hoffman HJ, Kobayashi J, Hwang P, Becker LE. Surgical management of children with temporal lobe epilepsy and mass lesions. *Neurosurgery* 1987; 21:792–7.
72. Berger MS, Kincaid J, Ojemann GA. Brain mapping techniques to maximise resection, safety, and seizure control in children with brain tumours. *Neurosurgery* 1989; 25:786–92.
73. Yeh HS, Kashiwagi S, Tew JM Jr, Berger TS. Surgical management of epilepsy associated with cerebral arteriovenous malformations. *J Neurosurg* 1990; 72:216–23.
74. Weber JP, Silbergeld DL, Winn HR. Surgical resection of epileptogenic cortex associated with structural lesions. *Neurosurg Clin North Am* 1993; 4:327–36.
75. Morris K, O'Brien TJ, Cook MJ, Murphy M, Bowden SC. A Computer generated stereotactic 'virtual subdural grid' to guide resective epilepsy surgery. *Am J Neuroradiol* 2004; 25:77–83.
76. Cukiert A, Buratini JA, Machado E, Sousa A, Vieira JO, Argentoni M, *et al*. Results of surgery in patients with refractory extratemporal epilepsy with normal or nonlocalizing magnetic resonance findings investigated with subdural grids. *Epilepsia* 2001; 42(7):889–94.
77. Wieser HG, Yaşargil MG. Selective amygdalohippocampectomy as a surgical treatment of mesiobasal limbic epilepsy. *Surg Neurol* 1982; 17(6):445–57.
78. Popovic EA, Fabinyi GC, Brazenor GA, Berkovic SF, Bladin PF. Temporal lobectomy for epilepsy—complications in 200 patients. *J Clin Neurosci* 1995; 2:238–44.
79. Walczak TS, Radtke RA, McNamara JO, Lewis DV, Luther JS, Thompson E, *et al*. Anterior temporal lobectomy for complex partial seizures: evaluation, results, and long-term follow-up in 100 cases. *Neurology* 1990; 40(3 Pt 1):413–18.
80. McIntosh AM, Kalnins RM, Mitchell LA, Berkovic SF. Early seizures after temporal lobectomy predict subsequent seizure recurrence. *Ann Neurol* 2005; 57(2):283–8.
81. Malla BR, O'Brien TJ, Cascino GD, So EL, Radhakrishnan K, Silbert P, *et al*. Acute postoperative seizures following anterior temporal lobectomy for intractable partial epilepsy. *J Neurosurg* 1998; 89:177–82.
82. Téllez-Zenteno JF, Dhar R, Hernandez-Ronquillo L, Wiebe S. Long-term outcomes in epilepsy surgery: antiepileptic drugs, mortality, cognitive and psychosocial aspects. *Brain* 2007; 130(Pt 2):334–45.
83. Tellez-Zenteno JF, Dhar R, Wiebe S. Long-term seizure outcomes following epilepsy surgery: a systematic review and meta-analysis. *Brain* 2005; 128(Pt 5):1188–98.
84. Schramm J, Kral T, Grunwald T, Blümcke I. Surgical treatment for neocortical temporal lobe epilepsy: clinical and surgical aspects and seizure outcome. *J Neurosurg* 2001; 94(1):33–42.
85. Tonini C, Beghi E, Berg AT, Bogliun G, Giordano L, Newton RW, *et al*. Predictors of epilepsy surgery outcome: a meta-analysis. *Epilepsy Res* 2004; 62(1):75–87.
86. McIntosh AM, Kalnins RM, Mitchell LA, Fabinyi GC, Briellmann RS, Berkovic SF. Temporal lobectomy: long-term seizure outcome, late recurrence and risks for seizure recurrence. *Brain* 2004; 127(Pt 9):2018–30.
87. Paolicchi JM, Jayakar P, Dean P, Yaylali I, Morrison G, Prats A, *et al*. Predictors of outcome in pediatric epilepsy surgery. *Neurology* 2000; 54:642–7.
88. Rossi GF, Colicchio G, Scerrati M. Resection surgery for partial epilepsy: relation of surgical outcome with some aspects of the epileptogenic process and surgical approach. *Acta Neurochir (Wien)* 1994; 130(101–110):101.
89. Lowe AJ, David E, Kilpatrick CJ, Matkovic Z, Cook MJ, Kaye A, *et al*. Epilepsy surgery for pathologically proven hippocampal sclerosis provides long term seizure control and improved quality of life. *Epilepsia* 2004; 45:237–42.
90. Schiller Y, Cascino GD, Sharbrough FW. Chronic Intracranial EEG Monitoring for Localizing the Epileptogenic Zone: An Electroclinical Correlation. *Epilepsia* 1998; 39(12):1302–8.
91. Schulz R, Lüders HO, Tuxhorn I, Ebner A, Holthausen H, Hoppe M, *et al*. Localization of epileptic auras induced on stimulation by subdural electrodes. *Epilepsia* 1997. 38(12):1321–9.
92. Cohen-Gadol AA, Bradley CC, Williamson A, Kim JH, Westerveld M, Duckrow RB, *et al*. Normal magnetic resonance imaging and medial temporal lobe epilepsy: the clinical syndrome of paradoxical temporal lobe epilepsy. *J Neurosurg* 2005; 102:902–9.
93. Cunha I, Oliveira J. Quality of life after surgery for temporal lobe epilepsy: a 5-year follow-up. *Epilepsy Behav* 2010; 17(4):506–10.
94. Mihara T, Inoue Y, Matsuda K, Tottori T, Otsubo T, Watanabe Y, *et al*. Recommendation of early surgery from the viewpoint of daily quality of life. *Epilepsia* 1996; 37(Suppl 3):33–6.
95. Kellett MW, Smith DF, Baker GA, Chadwick DW. Quality of life after epilepsy surgery. *J Neurol Neurosurg Psychiatry* 1997; 63(1):52–8.
96. McLachlan RS, Rose KJ, Derry PA, Bonnar C, Blume WT, Girvin JP. Health-related quality of life and seizure control in temporal lobe epilepsy. *Ann Neurol* 1997; 41(4):482–9.
97. Spencer SS, Berg AT, Vickrey BG, Sperling MR, Bazil CW, Haut S, *et al*. Health-related quality of life over time since resective epilepsy surgery. *Ann Neurol* 2007; 62(4):327–34.
98. Jehi LE, Silveira DC, Bingaman W, Najm I. Temporal lobe epilepsy surgery failures: predictors of seizure recurrence, yield of reevaluation, and outcome following reoperation. *J Neurosurg* 2010; 113(6): 1186–94.
99. Ramos E, Benbadis S, Vale FL. Failure of temporal lobe resection for epilepsy in patients with mesial temporal sclerosis: results and treatment options. *J Neurosurg* 2009; 110(6):1127–34.
100. Lowe NM, Eldridge P, Varma T, Wieshmann UC. The duration of temporal lobe epilepsy and seizure outcome after epilepsy surgery. *Seizure* 2010; 19(5):261–3.
101. Abosch A, Bernasconi N, Boling W, Jones-Gotman M, Poulin N, Dubeau F, *et al*. Factors predictive of suboptimal seizure control following selective amygdalohippocampectomy. *J Neurosurg* 2002; 97(5):1142–51.
102. Awad IA, Nayel MH, Lüders H. Second operation after the failure of previous resection for epilepsy. *Neurosurgery* 1991; 28(4):510–18.
103. Germano IM, Poulin N, Olivier A. Reoperation for recurrent temporal lobe epilepsy. *J Neurosurg* 1994; 81(1):31–6.
104. González-Martínez JA, Srikijvilaikul T, Nair D, Bingaman WE. Long-term seizure outcome in reoperation after failure of epilepsy surgery. *Neurosurgery* 2007; 60(5):873–80; discussion 873–80.
105. Salanova V, Markand O, Worth R. Temporal lobe epilepsy: analysis of failures and the role of reoperation. *Acta Neurol Scand* 2005; 111(2):126–33.
106. Wyler AR, Hermann BP, Richey ET. Results of reoperation for failed epilepsy surgery. *J Neurosurg* 1989; 71(6):815–19.
107. Wetjen NM, Cascino GD, Fessler AJ, So EL, Buchhalter JR, Mullan BP, *et al*. Subtraction ictal single-photon emission computed tomography coregistered to magnetic resonance imaging in evaluating the need for repeated epilepsy surgery. *J Neurosurg* 2006; 105:71–6.
108. Margerison JH, Corsellis JA. Epilepsy and the temporal lobes. A clinical, electroencephalographic and neuropathological study of the brain in epilepsy, with particular reference to the temporal lobes. *Brain* 1966; 89(3):499–530.
109. Schiller Y, Cascino GD, So EL, Marsh WR. Discontinuation of antiepileptic drugs after successful epilepsy surgery. *Neurology* 2000; 54(2):346–9.

CHAPTER 29

Resective Surgery of Extratemporal Epilepsy

Shahram Amina and Hans O. Lüders

Introduction

Up to a third of patients have epilepsy that is intractable to medical treatment. Despite the availability of many new antiepileptic medications in recent decades, the percentage of medically intractable cases remains relatively unchanged (1). As discussed in Chapter 27, surgical treatment is an alternative option for drug-resistant focal epilepsies and in appropriately selected cases, resective surgery can result in either complete seizure freedom or significant seizure reduction. The availability of modern neuroimaging techniques, digital electroencephalogram (EEG), and advanced neurosurgical equipment in many epilepsy centres has now made surgical options available for a far greater number of patients than was previously feasible.

From a surgical perspective, epilepsies can be classified into two major categories, namely epilepsies arising from the temporal lobe (mainly anterior mesiotemporal region) and epilepsies of extratemporal origin. The main reasons for this classification are the high epileptogenicity of the mesiotemporal structures (hippocampus, amygdala, and parahippocampal gyri), the high frequency of mesial temporal sclerosis in the refractory population, and the relatively high representation of temporal lobe epilepsy in the surgically remediable epilepsies. In contrast, extratemporal lobe epilepsies consist of heterogeneous neuroanatomical regions with often ill-defined borders and more heterogeneous aetiologies which in general make identification of the epileptogenic zone more difficult (2). In particular with cases which are magnetic resonance imaging (MRI)-negative or 'non-lesional', localizing the epileptogenic zone can be quite challenging. Surgically, the structures that are usually resected in mesiotemporal epilepsies are 'standardized' (i.e. amygdala, hippocampus, parahippocampal gyri) whilst in extratemporal epilepsies, the epileptogenic structures vary for each case. Another challenge with surgical resections in extratemporal epilepsies is the possibility of the overlapping of the epileptogenic zone and eloquent cortices. In such cases, careful mapping of eloquent cortex is essential for the avoidance of significant and permanent neurological deficits. These factors are some of the main reasons why favourable outcomes are more common in the resective surgery of mesiotemporal epilepsies.

Although historically the first epilepsy surgeries were carried out in extratemporal cases, large published series from different epilepsy centres suggest that only 30–40% of surgical resections in the modern era are of extratemporal epilepsies (3). These surgeries range from lesionectomies to large multilobar resections and hemispherectomies. In this chapter we only discuss regional resections. Hemispherectomies and disconnection procedures are discussed in Chapter 31. The most common extratemporal surgeries are frontal resections followed by parietal and occipital resections. Most of these surgeries are carried out in 'lesional' cases with identifiable brain abnormalities on neuroimaging studies (2).

Classification of extratemporal epilepsies

We routinely use a classification system (the Cleveland classification) which has been in use for more than two decades in our institution and several other major epilepsy centres around the world. This system classifies epilepsy for each patient in four dimensions: (1) *location* of the epileptogenic zone, (2) *aetiology* of epileptic seizures, (3) *seizure symptomatology*, and (4) other *related medical conditions*. Based on the complexity of each case, different investigations may be needed to define these four dimensions of epilepsy with greater precision. For example, in pharmacoresponsive cases of epilepsy, a detailed history and physical exam, basic neuroimaging, and a routine EEG may usually suffice. However, in a complex case of drug-resistant epilepsy an extensive work-up (discussed in Chapter 27) may be needed to determine surgical candidacy based on these four dimensions. A full discussion of this classification system can be found elsewhere (4–6).

Extratemporal epilepsies are commonly classified according to the presumed anatomical localization of the epileptogenic zone. Such a classification can be based on lobar regions, i.e. into frontal, parietal, occipital, or insular. The anatomical localization can also be specified with more precision. For example, frontal lobe epilepsies can be subdivided into lateral frontal, mesial frontal, prefrontal, basal frontal, and orbitofrontal. One should also note that multiple lobar or sublobar territorial overlap may occur (Fig. 29.1).

Epileptogenic and symptomatogenic zones

In any discussion of surgical therapy in epilepsy, the important concepts of the epileptogenic zone, seizure onset zone, irritative zone, symptomatogenic zone, functional deficit zone, epileptogenic lesion zone, and their mutual spatial relationships need to be fully

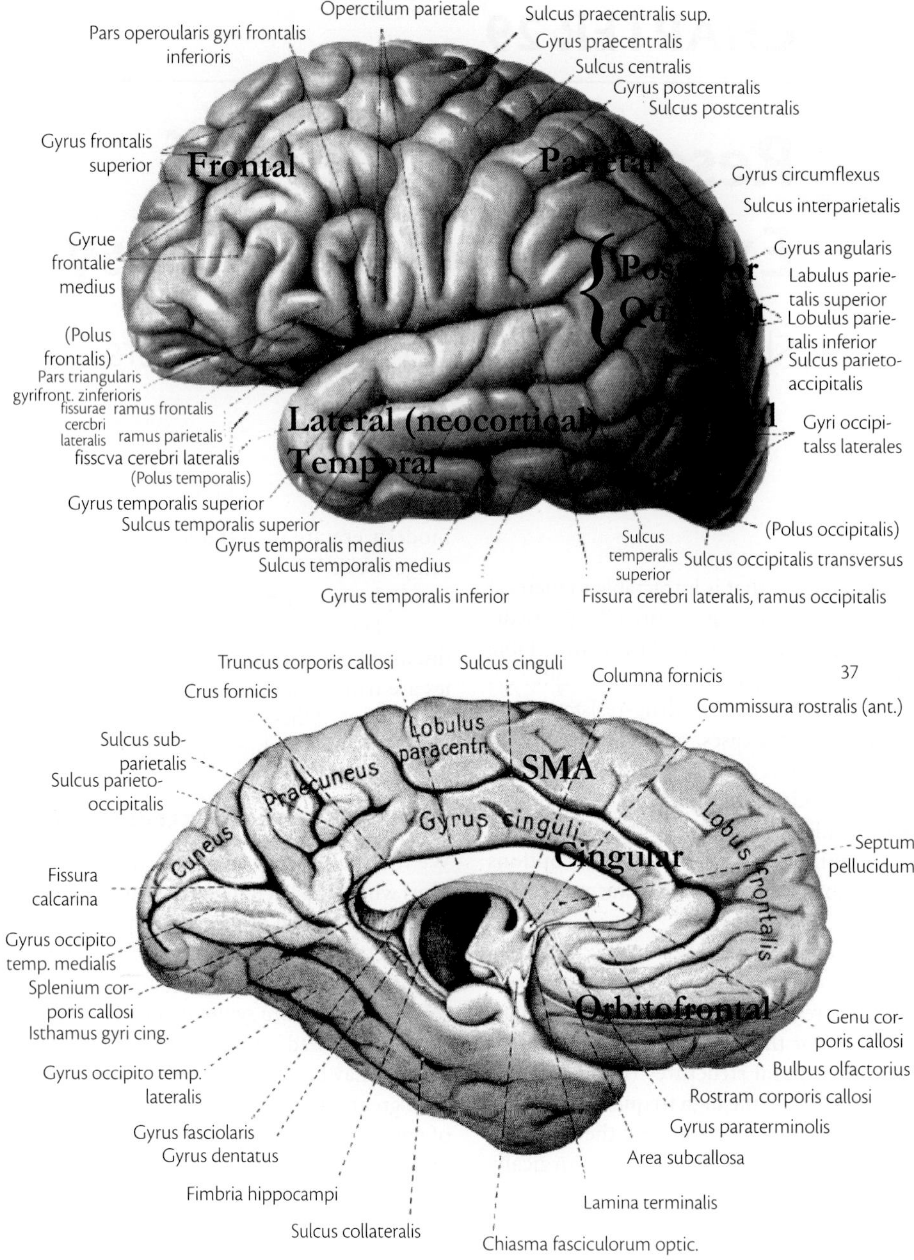

Fig. 29.1 Anatomical classification of the human brain.

appreciated (Chapter 27). By definition, the epileptogenic zone is the area of cortex that is indispensable for the generation of epileptic seizures and its total removal results in seizure freedom. In other words, if surgical resection renders complete seizure freedom, a conclusion can be made that the epileptogenic zone was included in the resected cortex (7). However, there is no direct method to measure the epileptogenic zone. Detailed surgical work-up allows more or less precise measurement of the other five zones mentioned (seizure onset zone, irritative zone, symptomatogenic zone, epileptogenic lesion, functional deficit zone), all of which have a close spatial relationship with the epileptogenic zone. Their analysis allows the epileptologist to establish a more or less reliable hypothesis regarding the location and extent of the epileptogenic zone.

The symptomatogenic zone is defined as an area of cortex whose ictal activation produces the initial ictal symptoms. Careful analysis of seizure semiology helps to identify this zone. Not uncommonly, seizures arise from a relatively silent region in the brain and do not become symptomatic until they propagate to eloquent cortex. In other words, seizure semiology points to the symptomatogenic zone which frequently does not overlap with the epileptogenic zone. Figs. 29.2–29.4 illustrate the symptomatogenic zones and seizure types (8). Some of these seizure semiologies are reproducible through direct cortical stimulation of the symptomatogenic cortex in patients with subdural and depth electrodes. The exact symptomatogenic regions of some seizure semiologies are less understood and remain controversial, perhaps due to involvement

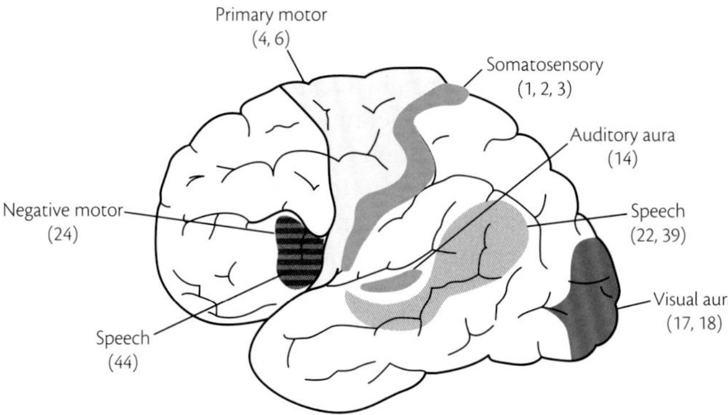

Fig. 29.2 Symptomatogenic zones in convexity regions identified by electrical stimulation. Reproduced from Hans O. Lüders, Soheyl Noachtar. *Atlas of Epileptic Seizures and Syndromes*. W.B. Saunders Company, 2001.

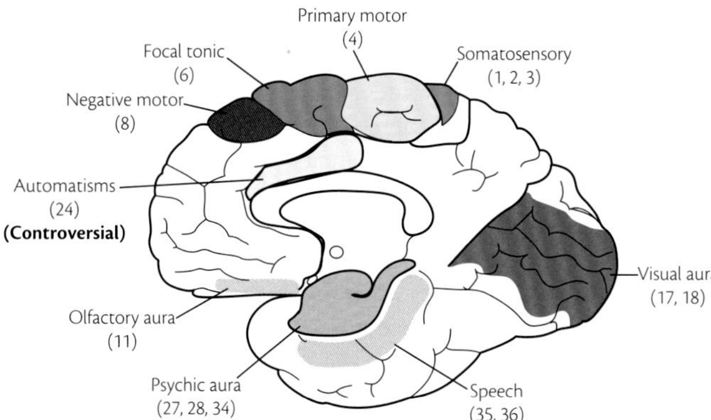

Fig. 29.3 Symptomatogenic zones in mesial cortices identified by electrical stimulation. Reproduced from Hans O. Lüders, Soheyl Noachtar. *Atlas of Epileptic Seizures and Syndromes*. W.B. Saunders Company, 2001.

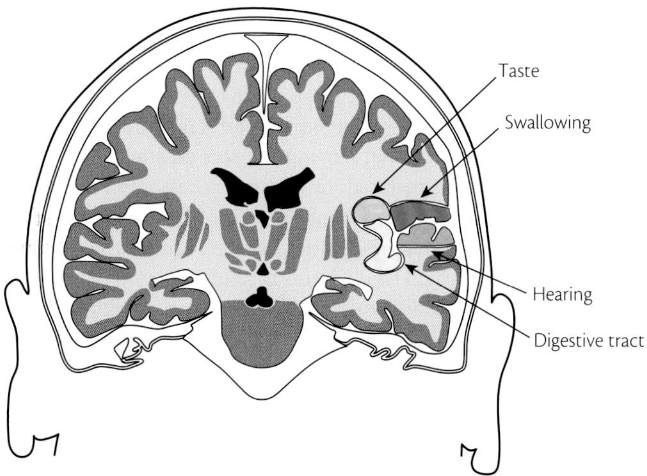

Fig. 29.4 Symptomatogenic zones in the insula and operculum identified by electrical stimulation. Reproduced from Hans O. Lüders, Soheyl Noachtar. *Atlas of Epileptic Seizures and Syndromes*. W.B. Saunders Company, 2001.

of more complex neural networks. In our institution we use a semiological classification of epileptic seizures to describe each seizure type and its topography. Often clinical seizures consist of more than one seizure type component and in this classification, evolution and propagation of seizures can be described by linking seizure components. Here we only discuss the seizure semiologies of particular interest in extratemporal epilepsies and a full discussion of epileptic seizures and semiological classification can be found in published references (4, 8).

Common seizure semiologies which can be seen in frontal lobe epilepsies include simple motor, hypermotor, complex motor, and dialeptic seizures. Because of the connectivity of the lateral orbitofrontal lobe to the anterior temporal lobe, epilepsies of these regions can mimic temporal lobe epilepsy. Seizures with brief duration, nocturnal predominance, minimal postictal confusion, and rapid generalization are more characteristic of frontal lobe epilepsies. While hypermotor and complex motor seizures are often indicative of frontal lobe involvement, the exact symptomatogenic zones of these seizures are not well known. Ictal activation of primary motor cortex often produces contralateral clonic activity in a topographical manner and marching of the clonic activity is indicative of seizure spread over the motor strip (Jacksonian march). Ictal activation of supplementary motor cortex (SMA) typically produces bilateral asymmetric tonic posturing with preserved consciousness. Often, a fencing posture, vocalization or speech arrest is seen in these seizures. Activation of the frontal eye field usually leads to contralateral versive movement of the eyes and head (versive seizure). Olfactory auras can occur when the orbitofrontal region and rectus gyrus are activated. Auditory auras occur with activation of Heschl's gyrus. Ictal activation of the operculum and insula are thought to produce salivation, mastication and swallowing movements, laryngeal constriction, unpleasant sensations in the pharyngolaryngeal region, and a feeling of strangulation. Because of the strong connectivity of the anterior insula and mesiotemporal structures, insular epilepsies can also mimic temporal lobe epilepsy. It has been proposed that ictal involvement of cingulate gyrus is responsible for automatisms (automotor seizures) but this has not been reproduced by conventional cortical stimulation methods and remains controversial. Seizures originating from the parietal lobe can be divided into those of post-central gyral origin and posterior parietal gyral origin. Post-central gyrus ictal activation often produces contralateral positive somatosensory symptoms such as tingling sensation. Less commonly these seizures are associated with numbness or pain. Posterior parietal activation can produce somatic or visual illusions. Seizures of the occipital lobe often result in primary visual phenomena of flashing or flickering white and coloured lights if the primary visual cortex is activated. Complex visual hallucinations can occur with activation of association visual cortex. One should keep in mind that epilepsies of a certain lobe can also spread to other lobes to produce symptoms and secondary generalized tonic–clonic seizures can occur in any focal epilepsy (4, 8, 9).

Aetiology

Whilst the aetiology of most epilepsies is likely to be multifactorial (i.e. susceptibility genes plus exogenous factors plus one or more neuropathological lesions), here we refer to aetiology mainly as an identifiable neuropathology. From an aetiological standpoint, focal epilepsies can be classified into two major groups, namely MRI negative or 'non-lesional' and MRI positive or 'lesional' epilepsies (10, 11). This distinction is particularly significant because most surgical series have shown that the presence of an identifiable pathology on MRI is associated with a more favourable surgical outcome (12–14). We prefer the term 'MRI negative' over the expression 'non-lesional' which can give the wrong impression of a complete absence of an identifiable pathology.

MRI positive aetiologies include neoplasms, vascular malformations (arteriovenous malformation (AVM), cavernous angioma), malformations of cortical development (MCDs), tuberous sclerosis, non-specific encephalomacias, and gliosis (from remote strokes, traumatic brain injuries, encephalitis, and anoxic brain injuries). Neoplasms and MCDs are the two major groups representing 30–70% of the aetiologies in reported surgical series. Neoplasms that are seen in patients with chronic epilepsy include low-grade astrocytic tumours, oligodendrogliomas, gangliogliomas, dysembryoplastic neuroepithelial tumours, and pleomorphic xanthoastrocytomas (14–17).

Focal cortical dysplasia without balloon cells is the aetiology in most cases with negative MRIs. Identification of the epileptogenic zone in these cases is challenging but surgical outcome can be excellent if neurophysiology and other presurgical techniques define a limited focus with clear borders located at a safe distance from eloquent cortex. Taylor type cortical dysplasia (with balloon cells) can usually be seen in high-resolution MRI and is classified under lesional epilepsies (18).

Presurgical work-up

The presurgical work-up of extratemporal epilepsies follows the same approach and rationale as temporal lobe epilepsies. Non-lesional cases and patients in whom the epileptogenic zone is in close proximity, or even overlaps with eloquent cortex, almost invariably require chronic invasive EEG recordings and detailed brain mapping by direct electrical stimulation. In general EEG plays a critical role in localizing the seizure onset and irritative zones. However, in extratemporal epilepsies, scalp EEG may not show any interictal abnormality. Besides, early ictal changes may not be detectable until seizure activity has spread to the brain convexity (19, 20). This is due to limitations of scalp EEG in detecting epileptiform activity from deeper brain regions which include a large portion of extratemporal cortex. The common problem areas for scalp EEG in detecting interictal and ictal discharges include mesial frontal cortex (i.e. the SMA), the orbitofrontal cortex (which can be semiologically indistinguishable from temporal lobe seizures), and also small foci in the primary motor or sensory cortex which can produce clinical seizures but remain undetected by scalp EEG because of the relatively restricted area of cortex involved. Ictal EEG changes may also be obscured by muscle artefact that, not infrequently, occurs simultaneously with EEG seizure onset in extratemporal lobe epilepsies.

MRI is the cornerstone of any search for structural neuropathologies and obtaining a high-resolution epilepsy protocol MRI is crucial in all surgical candidates. Focal cortical dysplasia can be very difficult to detect on routine MRI. High-resolution, 3 Tesla MRIs read by experienced neuroradiologists may not reveal a subsequently pathologically confirmed abnormality. Functional MRI (fMRI) is becoming more available in major epilepsy centres and can be helpful in the non-invasive mapping of eloquent cortex. While fMRI usually reliably localizes the primary motor cortex, its reliability in lateralization and localization of language areas depend on the subject's cooperation and the experience of the centres utilising this investigation (10, 11).

Interictal positron emission tomography (PET) scanning often plays an important role in non-lesional temporal lobe epilepsies but its role in extratemporal epilepsies is less clearly defined. More recently, it has been reported that the overlaying of MRI and PET images can be a powerful tool in the identification of abnormalities that are not visually detectable by either method used separately (30).

Ictal SPECT (single-positron emission computed tomography) with technetium 99-m has been found very useful in identifying seizure onset area in some centres (21, 22). SISCOM, is a statistical method expressing in z-values the difference of ictal from interictal SPECT and superimposing the z-values on an MRI. SISCOM is often used to identify areas of hypermetabolism during ictal activation of the cortex. One should be aware of technical and interpretational limitations of this method which may lead to false localization of the epileptogenic zone elucidating areas of seizure propagation instead of the seizure onset zone.

All surgical patients should also have a neuropsychological evaluation to determine their neurocognitive baseline and to identify possible preoperative deficits. Neuropsychological data can be helpful in predicting postoperative neurocognitive outcome. The Wada test is still the gold standard study in lateralizing the dominant hemisphere for language and may need to be done in extratemporal cases when there is concern for developing language deficits from resective surgery.

Invasive (intracranial) EEG is the gold standard for the precise identification of the ictal onset and irritative zones. Essentially, almost all cases with negative MRI and those cases in which the epileptogenic lesion is close to eloquent cortex will need invasive EEG (23–25). Careful planning of subdural or depth electrodes placement is essential, based on analysis of the information gathered from all non-invasive studies. A clear hypothesis with regard to the localization of the epileptogenic zone should be formulated and appropriate invasive studies capable of confirming the hypothesis as well as defining with precision the location and extent of the epileptogenic zone, should be planned. Invasive EEG studies should be carried out in experienced centres that benefit from modern neurophysiological and neurosurgical technologies with highly skilled epileptologists and neurosurgeons. In more challenging cases, invasive EEG studies may need to be staged into more than one implantation operation. During the second stage, more electrodes may need to be inserted for accurate localization of the epileptogenic zone based on information derived from the first stage.

Direct electrical stimulation of the cortex remains the gold standard for brain mapping. Detailed and careful mapping of eloquent cortex can be done extraoperatively in the epilepsy monitoring unit while patients are fully awake and cooperative. Cortical mapping needs to be performed by a trained and experienced neurophysiologist. Intraoperative mapping is more limited because of time constraints in the operative room and technical difficulties in performing craniotomies under awake conditions. However, mapping in the operative room can be done for patients who do not undergo chronic invasive EEG recordings or in order to confirm the results of extraoperative mapping.

Surgical methods and outcomes

Lesionectomy is the most common type of surgical resection in extratemporal epilepsy. In most cases, complete resection of the visible MRI lesion is necessary to achieve seizure freedom. However, in the majority of the patients, additional resection of the area surrounding the lesion is also necessary for a successful outcome. The extent of perilesional resection is determined by the pathology of the lesion and also the results of invasive ictal and interictal EEG recordings. Besides, mapping of possible adjacent eloquent cortex will also influence the extent of the cortical resection. In cases with no identifiable lesion on MRI the extent of the topectomy is defined primarily by functional data (ictal and interictal EEG,). Modern neurosurgical operating rooms benefit from neuronavigation and stereotactic systems that can aid surgery with more precise resection.

There has not been a prospective controlled study in extratemporal resective surgery and outcomes from published retrospective surgical series vary widely. This outcome variability is likely related to the heterogeneity of these cases, selection biases, different investigational approaches, and the variability of surgical methods amongst different epilepsy centres. Nevertheless, it is clear that in comparison to temporal lobectomies, seizure-free outcomes are lower in extratemporal resections (2). In a systemic review of outcome data in 298 neocortical resections from 24 published studies with more than 1-year follow-up, a seizure-free rate of 50% and an improvement rate of 79% were found (26). Another meta-analysis of surgical outcomes found long-term (more than 5 years follow-up) seizure-free rates of 34% for extratemporal resections (27). Results from a major epilepsy centre showed that the seizure-free rate for frontal lobe resections drops from 56% at 1-year follow-up to 30% at 5 years (28). So far, the existence of an identifiable structural lesion is the single most important factor for the prediction of a favourable surgical outcome in extratemporal resections. Cortical dysplasia and generalized ictal EEG patterns have been reported to be other predictors of poorer surgical outcomes in frontal epilepsy resections.

In large retrospective series, the occurrence of complications have been reported as 0.4% for perisurgical death, 5% for infection, 6% for neurological deficits (3% were transient), and 6% for behavioural and cognitive complications (26, 29).

Case studies

Case A A 59-year-old woman with a history of epilepsy since age 25. Her seizures consisted of stereotyped hypermotor movements of the right upper extremity with no alteration of awareness, occasionally followed by secondary generalized tonic–clonic seizures. Seizures occurred up to 20 times per day mostly during sleep. Her epilepsy remained intractable despite treatment with different antiepileptic medications. She had a surgical evaluation with invasive EEG recording more than 30 years ago, prior to availability of MRI as an investigational tool. At that time she underwent bifrontal depth electrode placement through burr holes. This evaluation failed to lateralize the origin of her seizures and no surgical resection was performed. She underwent another surgical evaluation more recently. A presurgical MRI showed bifrontal encephalomalacia and gliosis under the previous surgical burr holes. Due to lack of prior MRI for comparison, a differentiation between the possibilities of primary lesions versus postsurgical changes from prior depth electrodes placements could not be made. Scalp EEG was negative interictally and showed no changes during her habitual seizures. She underwent stereotactic placement of multiple depth electrodes in both frontal lobes in two stages. Perilesional, anterior cingulate, orbitofrontal, frontal pole, and lateral frontal areas were sampled bilaterally. After recording numerous seizures it was concluded that the seizures originated primarily in the right perilesional area and rapidly propagated to the contralateral frontal lobe. She underwent a partial right frontal lobectomy which included

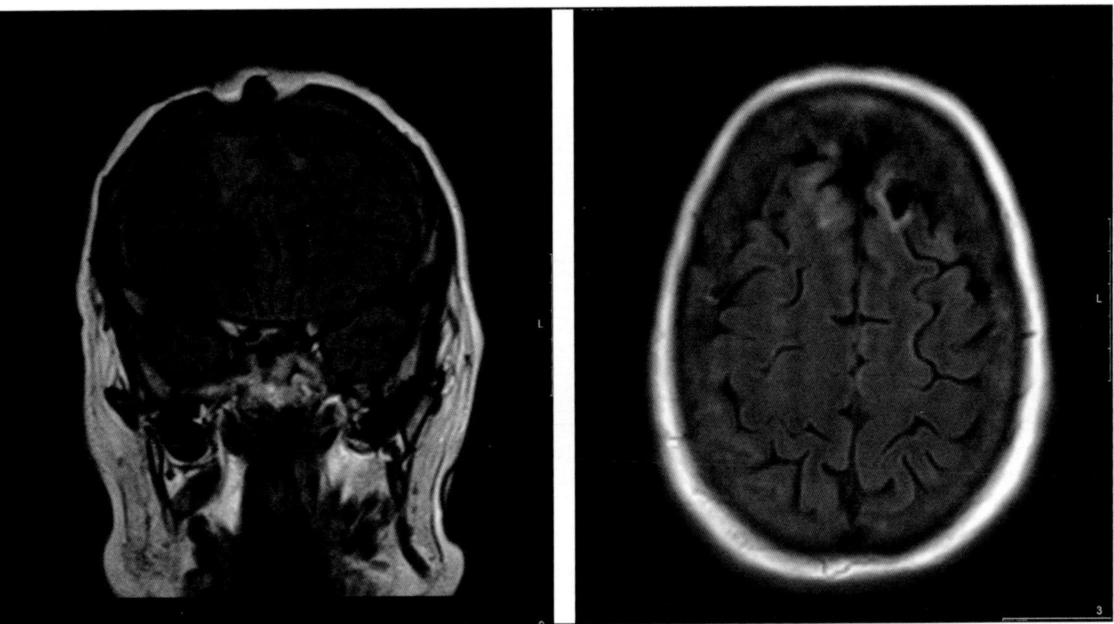

Fig. 29.5 Bifrontal lesions. Note the burr hole defects in the skull from previous surgery overlying the lesions.

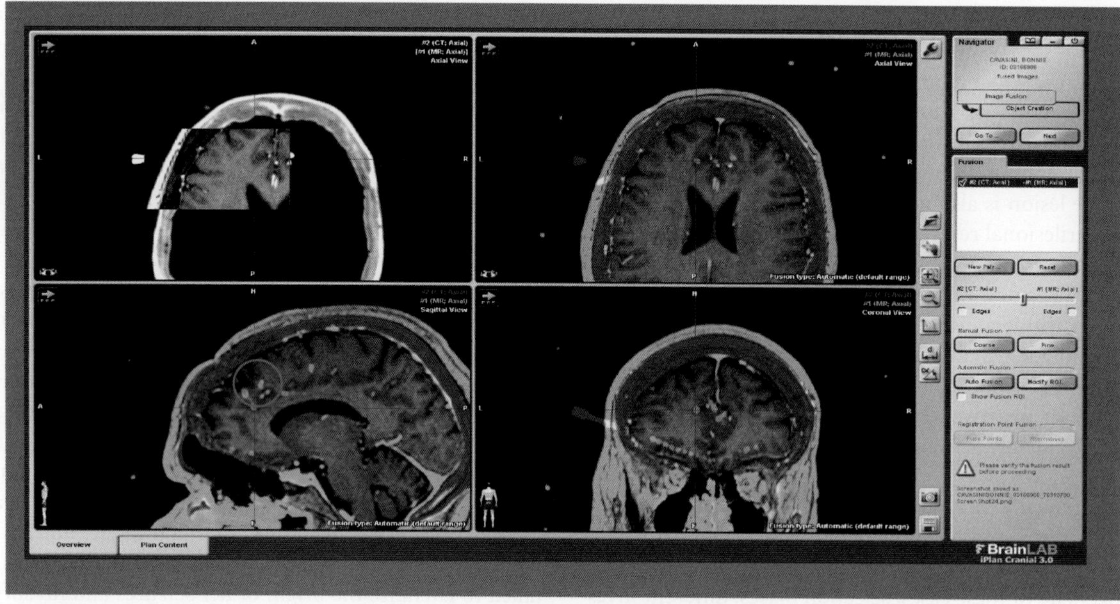

Fig. 29.6 (See also Colour plate 18.) Location of depth electrodes can be determined by the fusion of high-resolution computed tomography images (taken after placing the electrodes) with preoperative MRI. The red circle shows the area of seizure onset around the right mesiofrontal lesion.

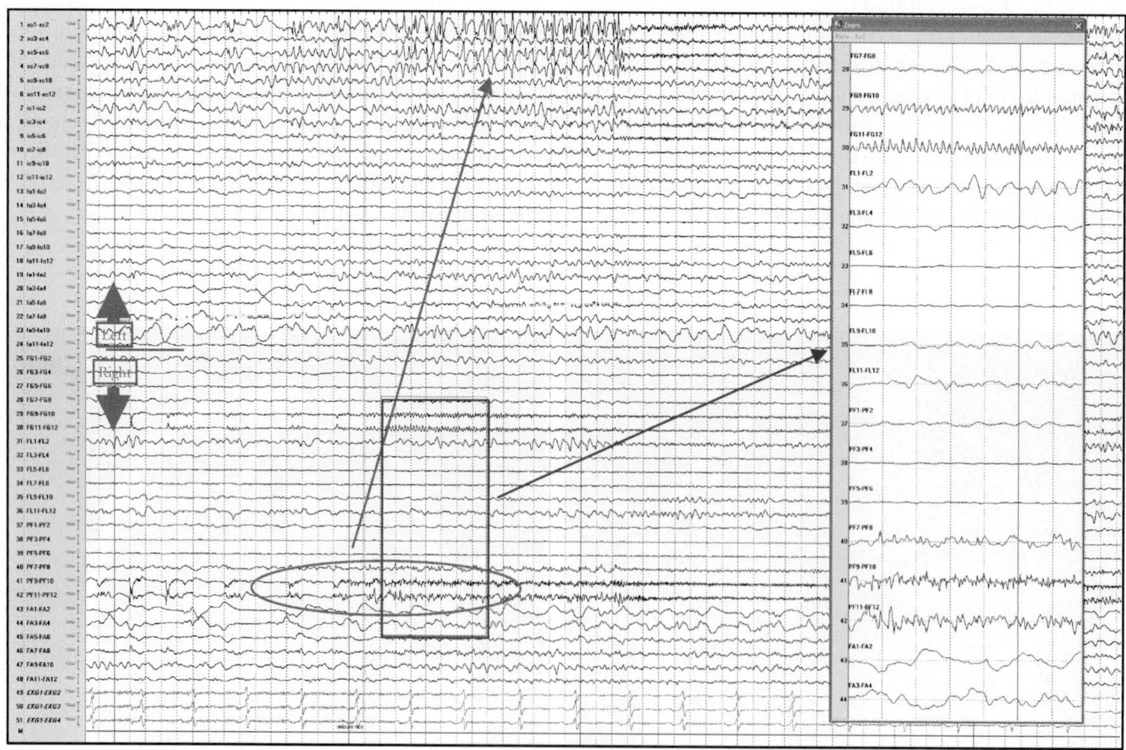

Fig. 29.7 Ictal EEG from depth electrodes showing seizure onset in the right mesial area (oval) with rapid propagation to the left mesial electrodes (arrow from oval), the boxed area is blown up to the right depicting selected channels from the right mesial area which show ictal onset characterized by appearance of fast frequencies.

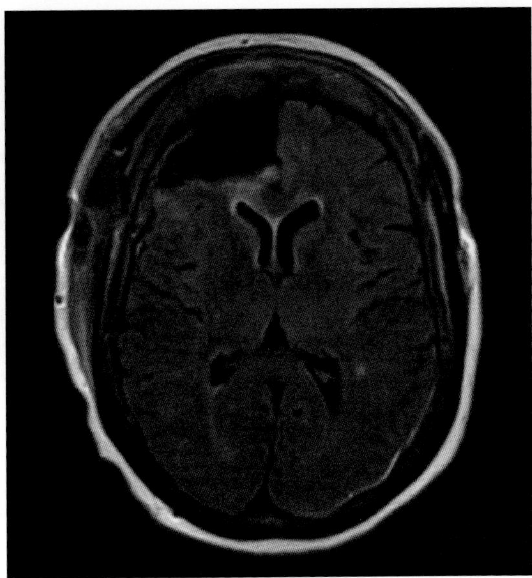

Fig. 29.8 Postoperative MRI of the right frontal resection.

the MRI lesion. Pathology examination confirmed cortical dysplasia with balloon cells. She was seizure free at the 6-month follow-up but has remained on antiepileptic medications (Figs. 29.5–29.8).

Case B A 20-year-old woman who had a left frontal intracerebral haemorrhage from a ruptured AVM 5 years previously which left her with right-hand weakness. At that time she underwent evacuation of the haematoma and resection of the AVM. She developed epilepsy 4 years later which rapidly became intractable even to high doses of antiepileptic medications. The seizures consisted of right arm tonic movements with secondary generalization. MRI revealed a large left frontal encephalomalacia and gliosis. Scalp EEG showed interictal generalized spikes maximally lateralized to the left. Invasive EEG recordings of the seizures and electrical stimulation of subdural electrodes were performed to identify the seizure onset zone and the motor strip. She then had a partial left frontal lobectomy which included the lesion but spared the motor strip. The patient was seizure free at 6-month follow-up and antiepileptic medications were safely lowered (Figs. 29.9–29.12).

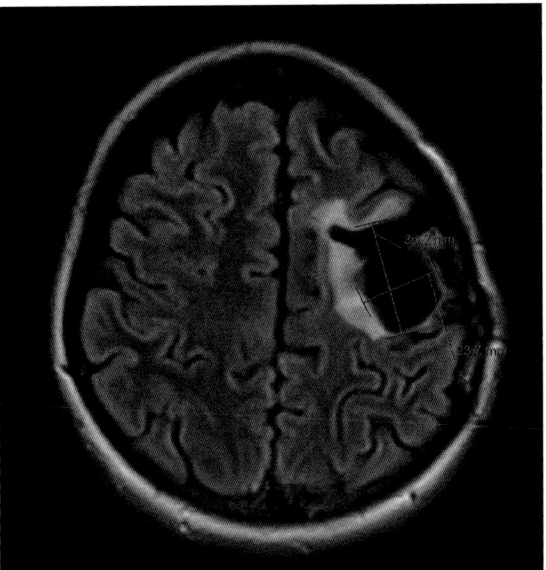

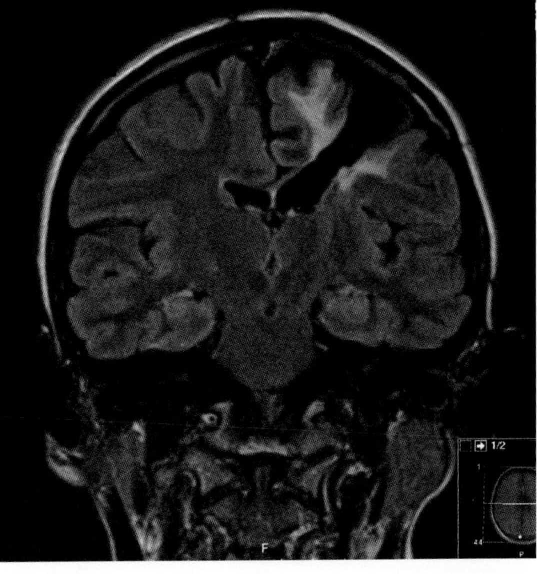

Fig. 29.9 Axial and coronal images of the left frontal lesion (residual encephalomalacia and gliosis from a previously ruptured arteriovenous malformation which was resected 5 years ago).

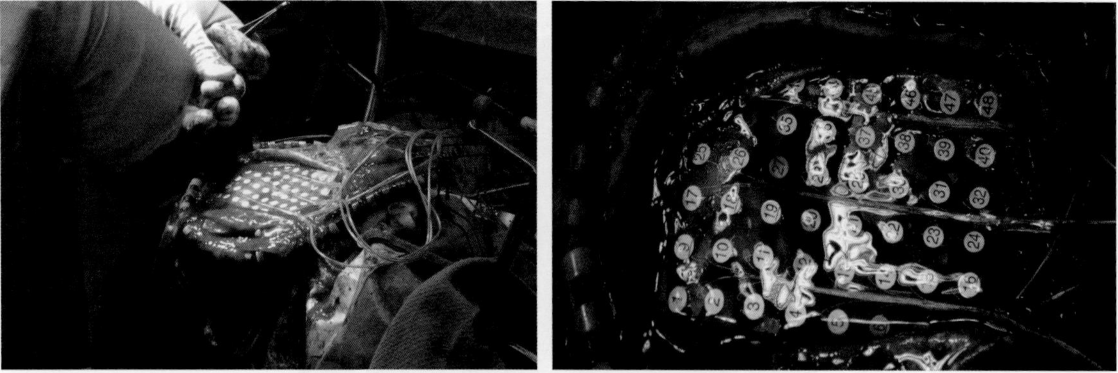

Fig. 29.10 Intraoperative photograph of subdural grid covering the lesion and surrounding normal cortex.

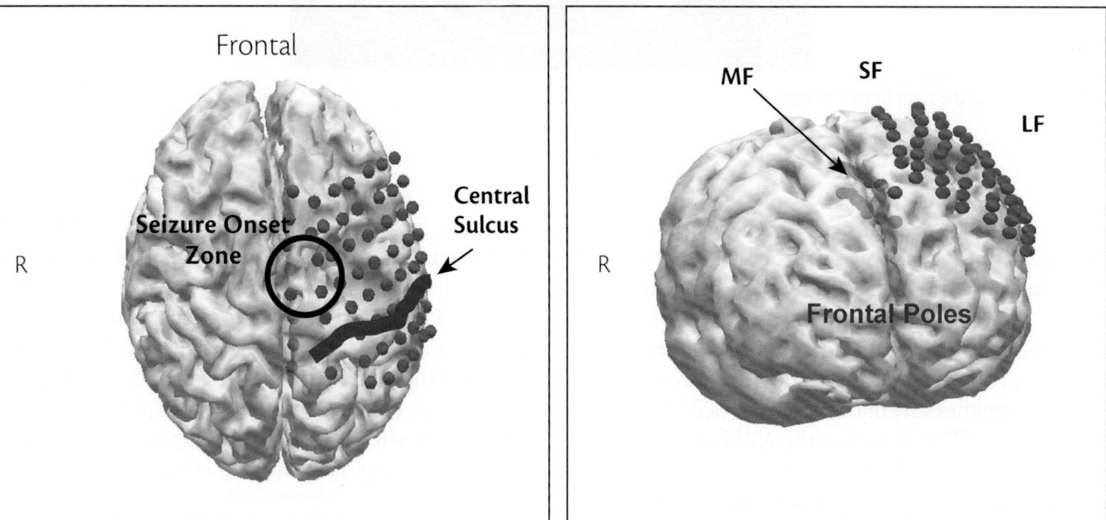

Fig. 29.11 Three-dimensional reconstruction of fused preoperative MRI and postoperative CT shows exact location of three subdural grids; lateral frontal (LF), superior frontal (SF), and mesiofrontal (MF). Subdural grids cover the left frontal lesion and surrounding normal cortex. Maps of the ictal onset zone (circle), and central sulcus (black line) are shown.

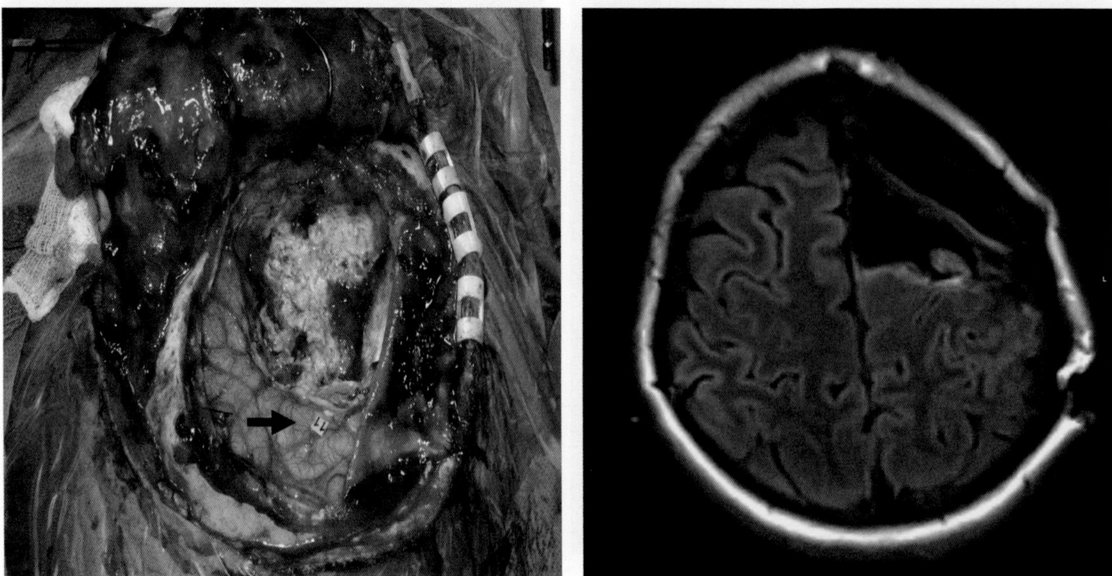

Fig. 29.12 Left frontal partial lobectomy anterior to the central sulcus (arrow shows the motor strip) and intraoperative MRI to confirm an adequate resection.

References

1. Mohanraj R, Brodie MJ. Outcomes in newly diagnosed localization-related epilepsies. *Seizure* 2005; 14(5):318–23.
2. Roper SN. Surgical treatment of the extratemporal epilepsies. *Epilepsia* 2009; 50(Suppl 8):69–74.
3. Williamson PD, Van Ness P, Wieser HG, Quesney LF. Surgically remediable extratemporal syndromes. In Engel J (ed) *Surgical Treatment of the Epilepsies* (2nd edn), pp. 65–76. New York: Raven Press, 1993.
4. Lüders H, Acharya J, Baumgartner C, Benbadis S, Bleasel A, Burgess R, *et al.* Semiological seizure classification. *Epilepsia* 1998; 39(9):1006–13.
5. Bautista JF, Lüders HO. Semiological seizure classification: relevance to pediatric epilepsy. *Epileptic Disord* 2000; 2(1):65–72; discussion 73.
6. Lüders HO, Amina S, Baumgartner C, Benbadis S, Bermeo-Ovalle A, Devereaux M, *et al.* Modern technology calls for a modern approach to classification of epileptic seizures and the epilepsies. *Epilepsia* 2012: 53(3):405–11.
7. Lüders HO, Najm I, Nair D, Widdess-Walsh P, Bingman W. The epileptogenic zone: general principles. *Epileptic Disord* 2006; 8(Suppl 2):S1–9.
8. Lüders, HO, Noachtar S. *Atlas of Epileptic Seizures and Syndromes.* Philadelphia, PA: W.B. Saunders Company, 2001.
9. VanGompel J, Worrel GA. Semiology of extratemporal lobe epilepsy (overview). In: Koubeissi MZ, Maciunas RJ (eds) *Extratemporal Lobe Epilepsy Surgery*. Paris: John Libbey Eurotext, in press.
10. Duncan JS. Imaging and epilepsy. *Brain* 1997; 120:339–77.
11. Duncan JS. Imaging in the surgical treatment of epilepsy. *Nat Rev Neurol* 2010; 6(10):537–50.
12. Talairach J, Bancaud J, Bonis A, Szikla G, Trottier S, Vignal JP, *et al.* Surgical therapy for frontal epilepsies. In: Chauvel P, Delgado-Escueta AV, Halgren E, Bancaud J (eds) *Frontal lobe seizures and epilepsies*, pp. 707–32. New York: Raven Press, 1992.
13. Van Ness PC. Surgical outcome for neocortical (extrahippocampal) focal epilepsy. In: Lüders H (ed) *Epilepsy surgery*, pp. 337–47. New York: Raven Press, 1992.
14. Zentner J, Hufnagel A, Ostertun B, Wolf HK, Behrens E, Campos MG, *et al.* Surgical treatment of extratemporal epilepsy: clinical, radiologic, and histopathologic findings in 60 patients. *Epilepsia* 1996; 37:1072–80.
15. Pasquier B, Bost F, Peoc'h M, Barnoud R, Pasquier D. Neuropathologic data in drug-resistant partial epilepsy. Report of a series of 195 cases. *Ann Pathol* 1996; 16:174–81.
16. Wolf HK, Zentner J, Hufnagel A, Campos MG, Schramm J, Elger CE, *et al.* Surgical pathology of chronic epileptic seizure disorders: experience with 63 specimens from extratemporal corticectomies, lobectomies and functional hemispherectomies. *Acta Neuropathol (Berlin)* 1993; 86:466–72.
17. Vital A, Rivel J, Loiseau H, Marchal C, Rougier A, Vital C. The histopathology of 110 cortical resections for drug-resistant epilepsy. *Rev Neurol (Paris)* 1994; 150:33–8.
18. Widdess-Walsh P, Diehl B, Najm I. Neuroimaging of focal cortical dysplasia. *J Neuroimaging* 2006; 16:185–96.
19. Quesney LF. Extratemporal epilepsy: clinical presentation, preoperative EEG localization and surgical outcome. *Acta Neurol Scand* 1992; 140(Suppl):81–94.
20. Kutsy RL. Focal extratemporal epilepsy: clinical features, EEG patterns, and surgical approach. *J Neurol Sci* 1999; 166:1–15.
21. O'Brien TJ, So EL, Mullan BP, Cascino GD, Hauser MF, Brinkmann BH, *et al.* Subtraction peri-ictal SPECT is predictive of extratemporal epilepsy surgery outcome. *Neurology* 2000; 55:1668–77.
22. O'Brien TJ, So EL, Cascino GD, Hauser MF, Marsh WR, Meyer FB, *et al.* Subtraction SPECT coregistered to MRI in focal malformations of cortical development: localization of the epileptogenic zone in epilepsy surgery candidates. *Epilepsia* 2004; 45:367–76.
23. Wetjen NM, Marsh WR, Meyer FB, Cascino GD, So E, Britton JW, *et al.* Intracranial electroencephalography seizure onset patterns and surgical outcomes in nonlesional extratemporal epilepsy. *J Neurosurg* 2009; 110:1147–52.
24. Munari C, Hoffmann D, Francione S, Kahane P, Tassi L, Lo Russo G, *et al.* Stereo-electroencephalography methodology: advantages and limits. *Acta Neurol Scand Suppl* 1994; 152:56–67, discussion 68–59.
25. Cossu M, Cardinale F, Colombo N, Mai R, Nobili L, Sartori I, *et al.* Stereoelectroencephalography in the presurgical evaluation of children with drug-resistant focal epilepsy. *J Neurosurg* 2005; 103:333–43.
26. Engel J Jr, Wiebe S, French J, Sperling M, Williamson P, Spencer D, *et al.* Practice parameter: temporal lobe and localized neocortical resections for epilepsy. *Epilepsia* 2003; 44:741–51.
27. Tellez-Zenteno JF, Dhar R, Wiebe S. Long-term seizure outcomes following epilepsy surgery: a systematic review and meta-analysis. *Brain* 2005; 128:1188–98.
28. Jeha LE, Najm I, Bingaman W, Dinner D, Widdess-Walsh P, Luders H. Surgical outcome and prognostic factors of frontal lobe epilepsy surgery. *Brain* 2007; 130:574–84.
29. Behrens E, Schramm J, Zentner J, Konig R. Surgical and neurological complications in a series of 708 epilepsy surgery procedures. *Neurosurgery* 1997; 41:1–9.
30. Chassoux F, Rodrigo S, Semah F, Beuvon F, Landre E, Devaux B, *et al.* FDG-PET improves surgical outcome in MRI negative Taylor-type focal cortical dysplasia. *Neurology* 2010; 75(24):2168–75.

CHAPTER 30

Vagal Nerve Stimulation and Deep Brain Stimulation in Epilepsy

Paul A. J. M. Boon and Kristl E. Vonck

Introduction

Although neurostimulation is not a new treatment modality, it is emerging for medical treatment-resistant neuropsychiatric disorders. Currently about 30% of patients with epilepsy are not seizure-free with the available pharmacological and surgical treatments (1).

Electrical stimulation of the 10th cranial nerve or vagus nerve stimulation (VNS) is an extracranial type of stimulation that is currently routinely available. Through an implanted device and electrode, electrical pulses are administered to the afferent fibres of the left vagus nerve in the neck. VNS is indicated in patients with refractory epilepsy who are unsuitable candidates for epilepsy surgery or who have had insufficient benefit from such a treatment (2).

Intracerebral neurostimulation requires access to the intracranial nervous system for the insertion of stimulation electrodes into specific targets for 'deep brain stimulation' (DBS) or placement over the cortical convexity for 'cortical stimulation' (CS). Recently trials with DBS in various intracerebral structures such as the thalamus, the subthalamic nucleus, the caudate nucleus, and medial temporal lobe structures have been performed (3–6). CS in a closed loop system (responsive neurostimulator system, RNS) has recently been investigated in a multicentre trial (7). It seems likely that neurostimulation for epilepsy will become a more practical and more frequently used treatment modality for patients with refractory epilepsy.

Vagus nerve stimulation

Electrical stimulation of the 10th cranial nerve or VNS has become a valuable treatment option for patients with refractory epilepsy and it is currently routinely available in epilepsy centres worldwide. Through an implanted device and electrode, electrical pulses are administered to the afferent fibres of the left vagus nerve in the neck. It is indicated in patients with refractory epilepsy who are unsuitable candidates for epilepsy surgery or who have had insufficient benefit from such a treatment (2).

Anatomical basis and mechanism of action

The vagus nerve is a mixed cranial nerve that consists of approximately 80% afferent fibres originating from the heart, aorta, lungs, and gastrointestinal tract and of approximately 20% efferent fibres that provide parasympathetic innervation of these structures and also innervate the voluntary striated muscles of the larynx and the pharynx (8–10). Afferent fibres that are targeted for therapeutic VNS, have their origin in the nodose ganglion and primarily project to the nucleus of the solitary tract. At the cervical level the vagus nerve mainly consists of small diameter unmyelinated C-fibres (65–80%) and of a smaller portion of intermediate-diameter myelinated B-fibres and large-diameter myelinated A-fibres. The nucleus of the solitary tract connects to other brainstem nuclei and has widespread projections to numerous areas in the forebrain including important areas for epilepsy such as the amygdala and the thalamus. Fig. 30.1 shows the main anatomical and functional connections of the vagus nerve in the central nervous system. The diffuse pathways of the vagus nerve mediate important visceral reflexes such as coughing, vomiting, swallowing, control of blood pressure, and heart rate (which is mostly influenced by the right vagus nerve) (11).

Following a limited number of animal experiments in dogs and monkeys, investigating safety and efficacy, the first human trial was performed (12). To date, the precise mechanism of action of VNS and how it suppresses seizures remains to be elucidated.

Research directed towards the identification of involved fibres, intracranial structures, and neurotransmitter systems has been performed. Animal experiments and research in humans treated with VNS have comprised electrophysiological studies (electroencephalography (EEG), electromyography, electrophysiology), functional anatomical brain imaging studies (positron emission tomography, single-positron emission computed tomography, functional magnetic resonance imaging, c-fos, densitometry), neuropsychological, and behavioural studies. Also from the extensive clinical experience with VNS interesting clues concerning the mechanism of action of VNS have arisen. More recently the role of the vagus nerve in the immune system has been investigated.

From the extensive body of research on the mechanism of action, it has become conceivable that effective stimulation in humans is primarily mediated by afferent vagal A- and B-fibres (13, 14). Unilateral stimulation influences both cerebral hemispheres, as shown in several functional imaging studies (15, 16). Crucial brainstem and

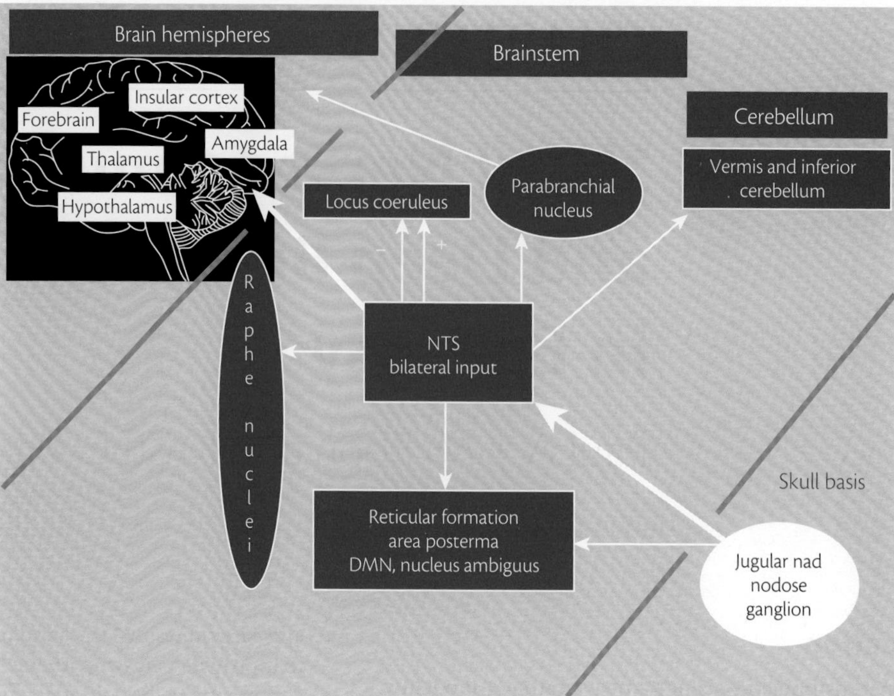

Fig. 30.1 Anatomical and functional connections in the central nervous system of the vagus nerve.

intracranial structures have been identified and include the locus coeruleus, the nucleus of the solitary tract, the thalamus, and limbic structures (17–19). Neurotransmitters playing a role may involve the major inhibitory neurotransmitter gamma-aminobutyric acid but also serotoninergic and adrenergic systems (20). Recent microdialysis experiments in pilocarpine-induced limbic seizures from our own group suggest that increased hippocampal noradrenaline may be a biomarker for the efficacy of VNS (Fig. 30.2) (21). An extensive overview on the mechanism of action of vagus nerve stimulation can be found in Vonck et al. (22).

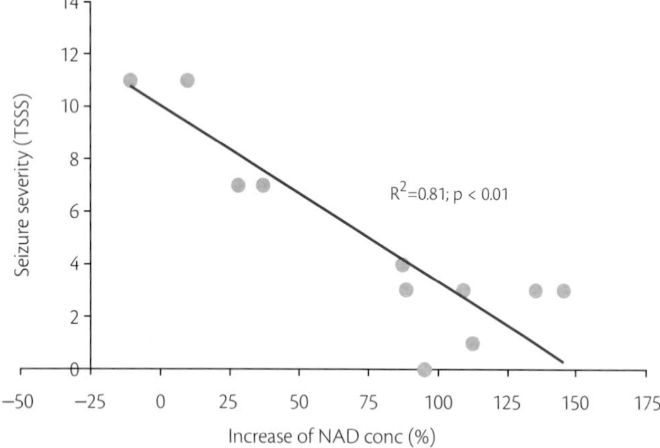

Fig. 30.2 VNS induces increases of noradrenaline in the hippocampus; the increase in noradrenaline is linearly related to the seizure suppressing effect of VNS; TSSS, total seizure severity score. Reproduced with permission *from J Neurochem* 117(3). Raedt R, Clinckers R, Mollet L, et al., Increased hippocampal noradrenaline is a biomarker for efficacy of vagus nerve stimulation in a limbic seizure model, 461–9. Copyright (2011), with permission from Wiley.

Clinical efficacy

The first descriptions of the implantable VNS Therapy™ system for electrical stimulation of the vagus nerve for epilepsy in humans appeared in the literature in the early 1990s (23, 24). At the same time initial results from two single-blinded pilot clinical trials (phase-1 trials EO1 and EO2) in a small group of patients with refractory complex partial seizures who were implanted since November 1988 in three epilepsy centres in the US were reported (12, 25–27). In nine out of 14 patients, treated for 3–22 months a reduction in seizure frequency of at least 50% was observed (24). Complex partial seizures, simple partial seizures, as well as secondary generalized seizures were affected (25). It was noticed that a reduction in frequency, duration, and intensity of seizures lagged 4–8 weeks after the initiation of treatment (12). In the meantime, two prospective multicentre (n = 17) double-blind randomized studies (EO3 and EO5) were started including patients from centres in the US (n = 12), Canada (n = 1), as well as in Europe (n = 4) (28–32). In these two studies patients over the age of 12 with partial seizures were randomized to a HIGH or LOW stimulation paradigm. The parameters in the HIGH stimulation group (output: gradual increase up to 3.5 mA, 30 Hz, 500 μs, 30 s on, 5 min off) were those believed to be efficacious based on animal data and the initial human pilot studies. Because patients can sense stimulation, the LOW stimulation parameters (output: single increase to point of patient perception, no further increase, 1 Hz, 130 μs, 30 s on, 3 hours off) were chosen to provide some sensation to the patient in order to protect the blinding of the study. LOW stimulation parameters were believed to be less efficacious and the patients in this group represented an active control group. The results of EO3 in 113 patients showed a decrease in seizures of 24% in the HIGH stimulation group versus 6% in the LOW stimulation group after 3 months of treatment (29–31). The number of patients was insufficient to achieve Food and Drug Administration (FDA) approval leading to the EO5 study in the US including 198 patients.

Ninety-four patients in the HIGH stimulation group had a 28% decrease in seizure frequency versus 15% in patients in the LOW stimulation group (32).

The controlled EO3 and EO5 studies had their primary efficacy end-point after 12 weeks of VNS. In all published reports on long-term results increased efficacy with longer treatment was found (33–37). The mean reduction in seizure frequency increased up to 35% at 1 year and up to 44% at 2 years of follow-up. After that improved seizure control reached a plateau (36).

In the following years, other large prospective clinical trials were conducted in different epilepsy centres worldwide. In Sweden, long-term follow-up in the largest patient series (n = 67) in one centre not belonging to the sponsored clinical trials at that time, reported similar efficacy rates with a mean decrease in seizure frequency of 44% in patients treated up to 5 years (38). A joint study of two epilepsy centres in Belgium and the US included 118 patients with a minimum follow-up duration of 6 months. They found a mean reduction in monthly seizure frequency of 55% (39). Only in a small minority of patients (7%) long-term seizure freedom was achieved. In China, a mean seizure reduction of 40% was found in 13 patients after 18 months of VNS (40). From a clinical point of view, prospective randomized trials investigating long-term efficacy in comparison to other therapeutic options for patients with refractory epilepsy are still lacking. A multicentre randomized trial called PulSE failed to recruit enough patients and was arrested prematurely. On the basis of currently available data the responder rate in patients treated with VNS is not substantially higher compared to recently marketed antiepileptic drugs (AEDs).

Children

There are no controlled studies of VNS in children, but many epilepsy centres have reported safety and efficacy results in patients less than 18 years of age in a prospective way. All these studies report similar efficacy and safety profiles compared to findings in adults (41–44). Rare adverse events, unique to this age group, included drooling and increased hyperactivity (45). In children with epileptic encephalopathies efficacy may become evident only after more than 12 months of treatment (46). A recent Korean multicentre study evaluated long-term efficacy in 28 children with intractable epilepsy. In half of the children there was a greater than 50% seizure reduction after a follow-up of at least 12 months (47). In our own prospective analysis of 118 patients, 13 children with a mean age of 12 years (range: 4–17 years) were included with similar efficacy rates and without specific side effects (39).

Elderly

A study of Sirven et al. included 45 patients who were 50 years of age and older. Thirty-one of 45 patients had a follow-up of 1 year, with a reported responder rate of 68%, good tolerance, and improvement of quality of life scores (48).

Seizure types and syndromes

The open label, longitudinal, multicentre EO4 study also included patients with generalized epilepsy (n = 24) (49, 50). In these patients overall seizure frequency reduction was 46%. Quintana et al. (51), Michael et al. (52), and Kostov et al. (53) described in a retrospective way that primary generalized seizures and generalized epilepsy syndromes responded equally well to VNS compared to partial epilepsy syndromes. A prospective study of Holmes et al. in 16 patients with generalized epilepsy syndromes and stable AED regimens showed an overall mean seizure frequency reduction of 43% after a follow-up of at least 12 months (54). Ben-Menachem et al. included nine patients with generalized seizures in a prospective long-term follow-up study. Especially the patients with absence epilepsy had a significant seizure reduction (38).

A few studies are available specifically describing the use of VNS in patients diagnosed with Lennox–Gastaut syndrome (LGS). One prospective study in 16 patients with LGS found that one-quarter of patients had a more than 50% reduction in seizure frequency after 6 months of follow-up which is comparable to the response rates in the controlled studies, that included few patients with LGS (55). Other prospective studies reported higher responder rates with a more than 50% seizure frequency reduction in half of the patients (n = 13, follow-up = 6 months) (56), in six of seven patients (follow-up = 6 months) (57) and in seven of nine patients (follow-up = 1–35 months) (58). A retrospective multicentre study in 46 patients with LGS reported responder rates of 43% (59).

There have been many reports on various other seizure types and syndromes such as seizures in patients with hypothalamic hamartomas (60), tuberous sclerosis (61, 62), progressive myoclonic epilepsy (63, 64), Landau–Kleffner syndrome (65), Asperger syndrome (66), epileptic encephalopathies (76), and syndromes with developmental disability and mental retardation (67–70) and infantile spasms (71). All these studies reported limited to reasonable efficacy with regard to controlling seizures as well as other disease-related symptoms such as cerebellar dysfunction, behavioural and mood disturbances. A recent report on the efficacy of VNS in five children with mitochondrial electron transport chain deficiencies described no significant seizure reduction in any of the children (72). Also a study in patients with previous resective epilepsy surgery showed a limited seizure suppressing effect of VNS (73) although another report described improved seizure control in this specific patient group (74).

Safety, side effects, and tolerability

The most prominent and consistent sensation in patients when the vagus nerve is stimulated for the first time, even at low output current levels, is a tingling sensation in the throat and hoarseness of the voice due to secondary stimulation of the superior laryngeal nerve (75–77).

With regard to side effects related to stimulation of vagal efferents, effect on heart rate and gastrointestinal digestion are of major concern. Stimulation of the efferent fibres may induce bradycardia and hypersecretion of gastric acid. The stimulation electrode is always implanted on the left vagus nerve, which is believed to contain fewer sinoatrial fibres than the right. It has been suggested that the electrode is implanted below the superior cardiac branch of the vagus nerve. No systematic side effects on heart functioning or other internal organ or cerebral functions were found. There was no effect on AED serum levels (12, 78).

In the long-term extension trials, the most frequent side effects were hoarseness in 19% of patients and coughing in 5% of patients at 2 years follow-up; shortness of breath in 3% of patients at 3 years (36). There was a clear trend towards diminishing side effects over the 3-year stimulation period. Ninety-eight per cent of the symptoms were rated mild or moderate by the patients and the investigators (78). Side effects can usually be resolved by decreasing stimulation parameters. Central nervous system side effects typically seen with AEDs were not reported. After 3 years of treatment, 72% of the patients were still on the treatment (36). The most frequent reason for discontinuation was lack of efficacy.

Initial studies on small patient groups treated for 6 months with VNS showed no negative effect on cognitive motor performance and balance (79–81). These findings were confirmed in larger patient groups with a follow-up of 2 years (82, 83). Hoppe et al. showed no changes in extensive neuropsychological testing in 36 patients treated for 6 months with VNS (84).

Vagus nerve stimulation electrodes can be safely revised and removed, when necessary (85).

Cardiac side effects

Despite the fact that the initial studies showed no clinical effect on heart rate, occurrence of bradycardia and ventricular asystole during intraoperative testing of the device (stimulation parameters: 1 mA, 20 Hz, 500 µs, ~17 s) have been reported in a small number of patients. None of the reported patients had a history of cardiac dysfunction, nor did they show abnormal cardiac testing after surgery. Tatum et al. reported on four patients who experienced ventricular asystole intraoperatively during device testing (86). In three patients, the implantation procedure was aborted. Asconape et al. reported on a single patient who developed asystole during intraoperative device testing. After removal of the device, the patient recovered completely (87). Ali et al. described three similar cases (88). Andriola et al. reported on three patients who experienced an asystole during intraoperative lead testing and who were subsequently chronically stimulated (89). Ardesch et al. reported on three patients with intraoperative bradycardia and subsequent uneventful stimulation (90). Possible hypotheses with regard to the underlying cause are inadvertent placement of the electrode on one of the cervical branches of the vagus nerve or indirect stimulation of these branches, reversal of the polarities of the electrodes which would lead to primary stimulation of efferents instead of afferents, indirect stimulation of cardiac branches, activation of afferent pathways affecting higher autonomic systems or of the parasympathetic pathway with an exaggerated effect on the atrioventricular node, technical malfunctioning of the device, or idiosyncratic reactions. The contributing role of specific AEDs should be further investigated. Very recently, one case report described a late-onset bradyarrhythmia after 2 years of vagus nerve stimulation (91).

Magnetic resonance imaging

Based on laboratory testing using a phantom to simulate a human body, the VNS TherapyTM system device is labelled magnetic resonance imaging (MRI) compatible when used with a send and receive head coil (92). In addition to the safety issues, there was no significant image distortion (93). A retrospective analysis of 27 MRI scans performed in 25 patients at 12 different centres using a 1.5 Tesla machine reported one patient with a mild voice change for several minutes; one child reported chest pain and claustrophobia. Twenty-three patients reported no discomfort around the lead or the generator. It was concluded that MRI is safe as long as guidelines stated in the physician's manual of the implanted device are followed (94). In these guidelines it is suggested to program the pulse generator output current to 0 mA. There have been several studies in patients treated with VNS for epilepsy as well as for depression showing that functional MRI is safe and feasible (95–99).

Deep brain stimulation

DBS is a relatively more recently explored treatment modality in epilepsy. Compared to VNS it is a more invasive treatment option. Parallel to VNS, the precise mechanism of action and the ideal candidates for this treatment option are currently unidentified. Moreover it is unknown which intracerebral structures should be targeted to achieve optimal clinical efficacy. Two major strategies for targeting have been followed. One approach is to target crucial central nervous systems structures that are assumed to have a 'pacemaker', 'triggering' or 'gating' role in the epileptogenic networks such as the thalamus or the subthalamic nucleus (100). Another approach is to interfere with the ictal onset zone itself. This implies the identification of the ictal onset zone, a process that sometimes requires implantation with intracranial electrodes.

Targets

The earliest reports on intracranial neurostimulation involved stimulation of cerebellar structures. In most instances electrical current was administered through electrodes bilaterally placed on the superior medial cerebellar cortex (101). Intermittent (1–8 min on, 1–8 min off) high-frequency (150–200 Hz) cerebellar stimulation was initially investigated for the treatment of spasticity due to cerebral palsy or stroke in several hundreds of patients with implantation duration times of up to 20 years. Some of these patients also had refractory seizures that were completely abolished in 60% of patients. Two controlled studies in small patient groups (n = 5, n = 12) did, however, not show significant effects (102, 103). In view of this controversy and with the advent of fully implantable and programmable pulse generators, Velasco et al. performed a re-evaluation double-blind study in five patients showing significant decreases in tonic–clonic seizures after 1–2 months of stimulation (104).

The selection of other targets for DBS in humans partially resulted from the progress in the identification of epileptogenic networks (100). Although the cortex plays an essential role in seizure origin, increasing evidence shows that subcortical structures may be involved in the clinical expression, propagation, control and sometimes initiation of seizures. Consequently, several subcortical nuclei have been targeted in pilot trials for different types of epilepsy. The suppressive effects of pharmacological or electrical inhibition of the subthalamic nucleus (STN) in different animal models for epilepsy and the extensive experience with STN DBS in patients with movement disorders led to a pilot trial with high-frequency (130 Hz) continuous STN DBS in five patients by the group from Grenoble (4, 105). Three patients with symptomatic partial seizures had a >60% reduction in seizure frequency. Four other centres have reported STN DBS results. In one patient with LGS, generalized seizures were fully suppressed and myoclonic and absence seizures reduced by more than 75% (106). Loddenkemper et al. reported seizure frequency reductions of more than 60% in two out of five patients treated with STN DBS (107). Handforth et al. reported on one patient with bitemporal seizures in whom half of the seizures were suppressed and on one patient with frontal lobe epilepsy who experienced a one-third reduction of seizures (108). Vesper et al. described a 50% reduction in myoclonic seizures in a patient with progressive myoclonic epilepsy in whom generalized seizures had been successfully treated with previous VNS (109).

Thalamocortical interactions are known to play an important role in several types of seizures. Since 1984, Velasco et al. have investigated a large patient series (n = 57) with different seizure types who underwent DBS of the centromedian (CM) nucleus, a structure that can be stereotactically targeted fairly easily due to its relatively large size, its spherical shape and location on each side of the third ventricle (110, 111). Intermittent (1 min on, 4 min off) high-frequency (60–130 Hz) stimulation that alternated between the left and right CM thalamic nucleus was most effective in children (n = 5) with epilepsia partialis continua in whom full seizure control was reached between 3–4 months after stimulation. Secondary generalized seizures in these children were the earliest to respond after 1 month of treatment. Atypical absences and generalized seizures responded significantly. Three out of 22 patients with LGS became seizure-free. Complex partial seizures responded less although after long-term stimulation over 1 year partial improvements were found and patients tended to be satisfied with the treatment that significantly decreased or abolished secondary generalized convulsions. In a separate report Velasco et al. report on 11 patients with LGS with an overall seizure reduction of 80% and two patients rendered seizure free (112).

In a double-blind cross-over protocol performed by Fisher et al., CM thalamic stimulation did not significantly improve generalized seizures in seven patients (113). Bilateral intermittent (1 min on, 5 min off during 2 h/day) high-frequency (60 Hz) stimulation was performed in blocks of 3 months alternating between on and off stimulation in a double-blinded manner. A reduction of 30% of tonic–clonic seizures had been observed during blocks with the stimulation on versus 8% in blocks with stimulation off. An open extension phase of the trial using 24-hour stimulation resulted in a 50% decrease in three out of six of the patients. It has become clear, especially from the experience with VNS, but also from other studies, that increased efficacy may be observed after longer duration of stimulation, possibly on the basis of neuromodulatory changes that take time to develop (111, 114).

There is sufficient evidence to suggest an equally important role of the anterior nucleus (AN) of the thalamus in the pathogenesis of seizure generalization. Hodaie et al. performed bilateral AN thalamic DBS (1 min on, 5 min off, 100 Hz, alternating between right and left AN) in five patients and showed a seizure frequency reduction between 24–89% (115). Andrade et al. reported on the long-term follow-up of six patients with AN DBS. After 7 years of follow-up five patients showed a more than 50% reduction in seizure frequency (116). Changes in stimulation parameters over the years did not further improve seizure control. Kerrigan et al. reported that four out of five patients who underwent high frequency AN DBS showed significant decreases in seizure severity and in the frequency of secondarily generalized seizures. Moreover, there was an immediate seizure recurrence when DBS was stopped (117). These studies all preceded a multicentre double-blind randomized trial of bilateral AN stimulation (SANTE trial) in patients with partial onset seizures with or without secondary generalization (3). One hundred and ten patients have been included at 17 medical centres in the USA. Half received stimulation and half did not receive stimulation during a 3-month blinded phase; then all received unblinded stimulation. In the last month of the blinded phase the stimulated group had a 29% greater reduction in seizures compared with the control group. Complex partial and 'most severe' seizures were significantly reduced by stimulation. By 2 years, there was a 56% median percent reduction in seizure frequency; 54% of patients had a seizure reduction of at least 50%, and 14 patients were seizure-free for at least 6 months. Cognition and mood showed no group differences, but participants in the stimulated group were more likely to report depression or memory problems as adverse events.

The medial temporal lobe region, more specifically the hippocampus is a rational target for DBS. This region often shows specific initial electroencephalographic epileptiform discharges that can be recorded with invasive EEG electrodes and represent the ictal onset zone. Temporal lobectomy and more specifically selective amygdalohippocampectomy are effective in reducing seizures with a well-defined mesiobasal limbic ictal onset (118). Basic research involving evoked potential excitability studies in humans and anatomical studies with tracer injections and single-unit recordings with histological studies in animals have also confirmed the involvement of the amygdala and the hippocampus in the epileptogenic network (119–121). Some studies have applied electrical fields to *in vitro* hippocampal slices with positive effects on epileptic activity (122, 123). Also our own *in vivo* studies in rats have shown that high-frequency stimulation affects seizures in the kindling model (Fig. 30.3) (124).

High-frequency stimulation is more efficacious than low-frequency stimulation and Poisson-distributed stimulation seems more efficacious compared to regular high-frequency stimulation (125, 126). Bragin et al. described repeated stimulation of the hippocampal perforant path in rats showing spontaneous seizures 4–8 months after intrahippocampal kainate injection (127). During perforant path stimulation spontaneous seizures were significantly reduced. In humans, preliminary short-term stimulation of hippocampal structures showed promising results on interictal epileptiform activity and seizure frequency (128). Not all patients with temporal lobe epilepsy who underwent resective epilepsy surgery remain seizure free in the long term. Moreover, temporal lobe resection, especially left-sided, may be associated with memory decline and temporal lobe resection is contraindicated in patients with bilateral ictal onset. In a pilot trial, 10 patients scheduled for invasive video-EEG monitoring of the medial temporal lobe were offered high-frequency medial temporal lobe DBS following ictal onset localization (6). Long-term follow-up in 10 of these patients showed that one stimulated patient was seizure-free (>1 year), one patient had a more than 90% reduction in seizure frequency; five patients had a seizure frequency reduction of 50% or more; two patients had a seizure frequency reduction of 30–49%; one patients was considered a non-responder. None of the patients reported side effects. In one patient MRI showed an asymptomatic intracranial haemorrhage at the occipital cortical entry of one of the DBS electrodes. None of the patients showed changes in clinical neurological testing. Fig. 30.4 shows the electrode positions in the hippocampus. A controlled randomized multicentre study (CoRaStiR—Controlled Randomised Stimulation versus Resection) is currently recruiting patients with unilateral hippocampal sclerosis and TLE to be randomized to amygdalohippocampal resection or medial temporal lobe DBS.

In four patients with complex partial seizures based on left-sided hippocampal sclerosis high-frequency stimulation was performed in a randomized, double-blind protocol with periods of 1 month off or on by Tellez-Zenteno et al. (129). During the stimulation on periods seizures decreased by 26% as compared to baseline. During the off periods seizures increased by 49%. Neuropsychological testing revealed no difference between on or off periods, not even in one patient who was stimulated left-sided following previous right-sided temporal lobectomy. Velasco et al. reported results in

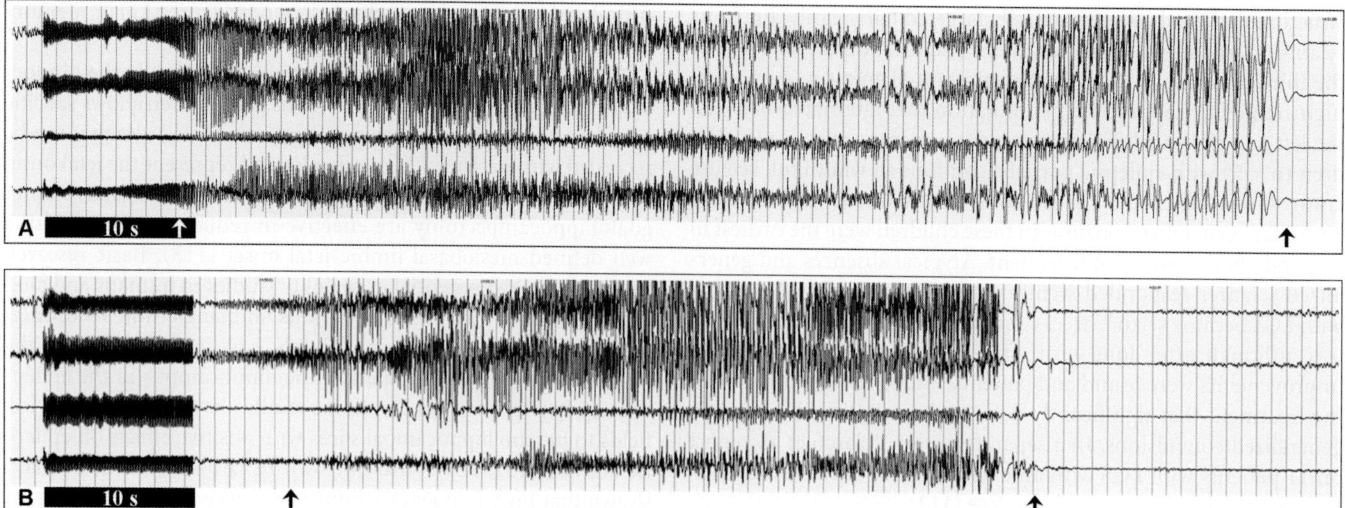

Fig. 30.3 Increase of afterdischarge latency and decrease of afterdischarge Rproduced from *Epilepsia* 48, Wyckhuys T, De Smedt T, Claeys P, et al. High frequency deep brain stimulation in the hippocampus modifies seizure characteristics in kindled rats, 1543–50. Copyright (2007), with permission from Wiley.

11 patients after 18 months of hippocampal high frequency stimulation (uni- or bilateral, with or without hippocampal sclerosis on MRI) (130). Patients with normal MRIs showed optimal outcome with four of them seizure-free after 1–2 months of stimulation. None of the patients showed neuropsychological decline with a trend towards improval.

An implanted responsive neurostimulator (the RNS system) has been evaluated for safety and efficacy in a multicentre trial. The device records cortical EEG signals by means of subdural electrodes and delivers responsive stimulation. Morrell reported 19 patients with partial onset epilepsy who were treated with the RNS system and showed a 37.9% reduction in seizure frequency in the stimulated group versus 17.3% in the SHAM group (p= 0.012) (7).

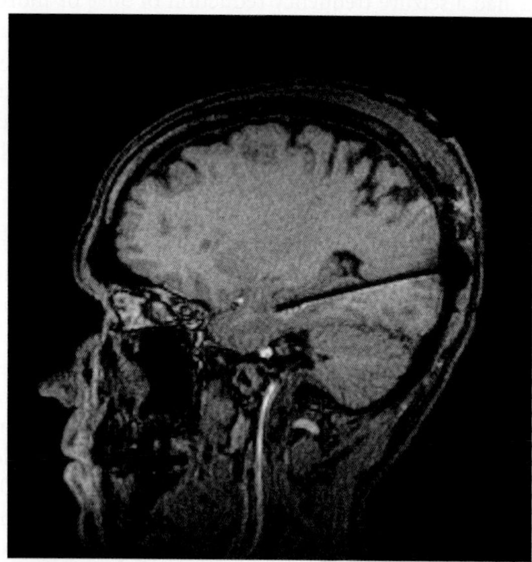

Fig. 30.4 Electrode positions in the hippocampus and amygdala; R, right-sided; L, left-sided; A, amygdala; H, hippocampus. From Boon et al. (6).

Conclusion

The lack of adequate treatments for all medically refractory epilepsy patients, the general search for less invasive treatments, and the progress in biotechnology have led to an renewed and increasing interest in neurostimulation as a therapeutic option.

For all types of neurostimulation currently being used and investigated, major issues remain unresolved. The ideal targets and stimulation parameters for a specific type of patient, seizure, or epilepsy syndrome are unknown. Long-term side effects need to be further investigated. The elucidation of the mechanism(s) of action of different neurostimulation techniques requires more basic research in order to demonstrate its potential to achieve long-term changes and true neuromodulation.

VNS is a moderately efficacious treatment for patients with refractory epilepsy; it is a broad-spectrum treatment; identification of specific responders on the basis of type of epilepsy or specific patient characteristics proves difficult. Large patient groups have been examined and identifying predictive factors for response may demand more complex investigations. VNS is a safe treatment and lacks the typical cognitive side effects associated with many other antiepileptic treatments. Moreover, many patients experience a positive effect of VNS on mood, alertness, and memory. In contrast to many pharmacological compounds, treatment tolerance does not develop in VNS. In contrast, efficacy tends to increase with longer treatment. However, on the basis of currently available data the responder rate in patients treated with VNS is not substantially higher compared to recently marketed AEDs. To increase efficacy, research towards the elucidation of the mechanism of action and optimization of stimulation parameters is crucial.

Deep brain stimulation is evolving from an experimental stage towards a reasonable treatment option for patients with refractory epilepsy. In addition to several pilot trials in different targets one randomized controlled trial of DBS in the anterior nucleus of the thalamus showed to be a feasible and safe treatment option, responder rate being slightly superior to the results of VNS. Results of randomized trials in hippocampal DBS are currently pending. The precise role of DBS in the treatment in refractory epilepsy remains to be determined.

Acknowledgements

Professor Boon and Professor Vonck are supported by grants from the Fund for Scientific Research Flanders, the Ghent University Research Fund and the European Union (6FP Imane). They have received support from Cyberonics and Medtronic in the form of consultancy fees, speaker fees and educational grants in favour of the Ghent University Hospital Clinical Epilepsy Grant.

References

1. Kwan P, Brodie M. Early identification of refractory epilepsy. *N Engl J Med* 2000; 342(5):314–9.
2. Ben-Menachem E. Vagus-nerve stimulation for the treatment of epilepsy. *Lancet Neurol* 2002; 1:477–82.
3. Fisher R, Salanova V, Witt T, Worth R, Henry T, Gross R, *et al.* Electrical stimulation of the anterior nucleus of the thalamus for treatment of refractory epilepsy. *Epilepsia* 2010; 51(5):899–908.
4. Chabardes S, Kahane P, Minotti L, Koudsie A, Hirsch E, Benabid AL. Deep brain stimulation in epilepsy with particular reference to the subthalamic nucleus. *Epil Disord* 2002; 4(S3):83–93.
5. Chkhenkeli SA, Chkhenkeli IS. Effects of therapeutic stimulation of nucleus caudatus on epileptic electrical activity of brain in patients with intractable epilepsy. *Stereotact Funct Neurosurg* 1997; 69:221–4.
6. Boon P, Vonck K, De Herdt V, Van Dycke A, Goethals M, Goossens L, *et al.* Deep brain stimulation in patients with refractory temporal lobe epilepsy. *Epilepsia* 2007; 48:1551–60.
7. Morrell MJ, RNS' system in Epilepsy Study Group, *Neurology* 2011; 77(13):1295–304.
8. Paintal AS. Vagal sensory receptors and their reflex effects. *Physiol Rev* 1997; 53:159–227.
9. Foley J, DuBois F. Quantitative studies of the vagus nerve in the cat. I. The ratio of sensory and motor fibers. *J Compr Neurol* 1937; 67:49–97.
10. Agostini E, Chinnock JE, Daly MD, Murray JG. Functional and histological studies of the vagus nerve and its branches to the heart, lungs and abdominal viscera in the cat. *J Physiol* 1957; 135:182–205.
11. Saper C, Kibbe M, Hurley K, Spencer S, Holmes HR, Leahy KM *et al.* Brain natriuretic peptide-like immunoreactive innervation of the cardiovascular and cerebrovascular systems in the rat. *Circ Res* 1990; 67:1345–54.
12. Uthman BM, Wilder BJ, Hammond EJ, Reid S. Efficacy and safety of vagus nerve stimulation in patients with complex partial seizures. *Epilepsia* 1990; 31:S44–50.
13. Zagon A, Kemeny A. Slow hyperpolarization in cortical neurons: a possible mechanism behind vagus nerve stimulation therapy for refractory epilepsy? *Epilepsia* 2000; 41:1382–9.
14. Evans MS, Verma-Ahuja S, Naritoku DK, Espinosa JA. Intraoperative human vagus nerve compound action potentials. *Acta Neurol Scand* 2004; 110:232–8.
15. Henry TR, Bakay RAE, Votaw JR, Pennell PB, Epstein CM, Faber TL, *et al.* Brain blood flow alterations induced by therapeutic vagus nerve stimulation in partial epilepsy: I. acute effects at high and low levels of stimulation. *Epilepsia* 1998; 39:983–90.
16. Van Laere K, Vonck K, Boon P, Versijpt J, Dierckx R. Perfusion SPECT changes after acute and chronic vagus nerve stimulation in relation to prestimulus condition and long-term clinical trial. *J Nucl Med* 2002; 43:733–44.
17. Naritoku D, Terry WJ, Helfert RH. Regional induction of fos immunoreactivity in the brain by anticonvulsant stimulation of the vagus nerve. *Epilepsy Res* 1995; 22:53–62.
18. Krahl SE, Clark KB, Smith DC, Browning RA. Locus coeruleus lesions suppress the seizure-attenuating effects of vagus nerve stimulation. *Epilepsia* 1998; 39(7):709–14.
19. Osharina V, Bagaev V, Wallois F, Larnicol N. Autonomic response and Fos expression in the NTS following intermittent vagal stimulation: importance of pulse frequency. *Auton Neurosci* 2006; 126–127:72–80.
20. Ben-Menachem E, Hamberger A, Hedner T, Hammond EJ, Uthman BM, Slater J, *et al.* Effects of vagus nerve stimulation on amino acids and other metabolites in the CSF of patients with partial seizures. *Epilepsy Res* 1995; 20:221–7.
21. Raedt R, Clinckers R, Mollet L, Vonck K, El Tahry R, Wyckhuys T, *et al.* Increased hippocampal noradrenaline is a biomarker for efficacy of vagus nerve stimulation in a limbic seizure model. *J Neurochem* 2011; 117(3):461–9.
22. Vonck K, Boon P, Van Roost D. Anatomical and physiological basis and mechanism of action of neurostimulation for epilepsy. *Acta Neurochir Suppl* 2007; 97(2):321–8.
23. Terry R, Tarver WB, Zabara J. An implantable neurocybernetic prosthesis system. *Epilepsia* 1990; 31:S33–7.
24. Terry RS, Tarver WB, Zabara J. The implantable neurocybernetic prosthesis system. *Pacing Clin Electrophysiol* 1991; 14:86–93.
25. Penry KJ, Dean C. Prevention of intractable partial seizures by intermittent vagal stimulation in humans: preliminary results. *Epilepsia* 1990; 31:S40–3.
26. Hammond EJ, Uthman BM, Reid SA, Wilder BJ, Ramsay RE. Vagus nerve stimulation in humans: neurophysiological studies and electrophysiological monitoring. *Epilepsia* 1990; 31:S51–9.
27. Wilder BJ, Uthman BM, Hammond EJ. Vagal stimulation for control of complex partial seizures in medically refractory epileptic patients. *Pacing Clin Electrophysiol* 1991; 14:108–15.
28. Holder LK, Wernicke JF, Tarver WB. Treatment of refractory partial seizures: preliminary results of a controlled study. *Pacing Clin Electrophyisol* 1992; 15(10):1557–71.
29. Ben-Menachem E, Manon-Espaillat R, Ristanovic R, Wilder BJ, Stefan H, Mirza W, *et al.* Vagus nerve stimulation for treatment of partial seizures: 1. A controlled study of effect on seizures. *Epilepsia* 1994; 35(3):616–26.
30. Ramsay RE, Uthman BM, Augustinsson LE, Upton AR, Naritoku D, Willis J, *et al.* Vagus nerve stimulation for treatment of partial seizures 2. Safety, side-effects and tolerability. *Epilepsia* 1994; 35:627–36.
31. The Vagus Nerve Stimulation Study Group. A randomized controlled trial of chronic vagus nerve stimulation for treatment of medically intractable seizures. *Neurology* 1995; 45:224–30.
32. Handforth A, DeGiorgio CM, Schachter SC, Uthman BM, Naritoku DK, Tecoma ES, *et al.* Vagus nerve stimulation therapy for partial onset seizures. A randomized, active control trial. *Neurology* 1998; 51:48–55.
33. Holder L, Wernicke JF, Tarver W. Long-term follow-up of 37 patients with refractory partial seizures treated with vagus nerve stimulation. *J Epilepsy* 1993; 6:206–14.
34. George R, Salinsky M, Kuzniecky R, Rosenfeld W, Bergen D, Tarver WB, *et al.* Vagus nerve stimulation for treatment of partial seizures: 3. Long-term follow-up on first 67 patients exiting a controlled study. *Epilepsia* 1994; 35(3):637–43.
35. Salinsky MC, Uthman BM, Ristanovic RK, Wernicke JF, Tarver WB. Vagus nerve stimulation for the treatment of medically intractable seizures. Results of a 1-year open-extension trial. *Arch Neurol* 1996; 53:1176–80.
36. Morris GL, Mueller WM. Long-term treatment with vagus nerve stimulation in patients with refractory epilepsy. *Neurology* 1999; 53:1731–5.
37. DeGiorgio CM, Schachter SC, Handforth A, Salinsky M, Thompson J, Uthman B, *et al.* Prospective long-term study of vagus nerve stimulation for the treatment of refractory seizures. *Epilepsia* 2000; 41(9):1195–200.

38. Ben-Menachem E, Hellstrom K, Waldton C, Augustinsson LE. Evaluation of refractory epilepsy treated with vagus nerve stimulation for up to 5 years. *Neurology* 1999; 52:1265–7.
39. Vonck K, Thadani V, Gilbert K, Dedeurwaerdere S, De Groote L, De Herdt V, *et al.* Vagus nerve stimulation for refractory epilepsy: a transatlantic experience. *J Clin Neurophysiol* 2004; 21:283–9.
40. Hui Che Fai A, Lam Man Kuen J, Ka Shing W, Kay R, Wai Sing P. Vagus nerve stimulation for refractory epilepsy: long-term efficacy and side-effects. *Chin Med J* 2004; 117(1):58–61.
41. Lundgren J, Amark P, Blennow G, Stromblad LG, Wallstedt L. Vagus nerve stimulation in 16 children with refractory epilepsy. *Epilepsia* 1998; 39:809–13.
42. Murphy JV, the Pediatric VNS Study group. Left vagal nerve stimulation in children with medically refractory epilepsy. *J Pediatr* 1999; 134:563–66.
43. Zamponi N, Rychicki F, Cardinali C, Luchetti A, Trignani R, Ducati A. Intermittent vagal nerve stimulation in paediatric patients: 1 year follow-up. *Child Nerv Syst* 2002; 18:61–6.
44. Buoni S, Mariottini A, Pieri S, Zalaffi A, Farnetani MA, Strambi M, *et al.* Vagus nerve stimulation for drug-resistant epilepsy in children and young adults. *Brain Dev* 2004; 26:158–63.
45. Helmers SL, Wheless JW, Frost M, Gates J, Levisohn P, Tardo C, *et al.* Vagus nerve stimulation therapy in pediatric patients with refractory epilepsy: retrospective study. *J Child Neurol* 2001; 16:843–8.
46. Parker APJ, Polkey CE, Binnie C, Madigan C, Ferrie C, Robinson O. Vagal nerve stimulation in epileptic encephalopathies. *Pediatrics* 1999; 103:778–82.
47. You SJ, Kang HC, Kim HD, Ko TS, Kim DS, Hwang YS, *et al.* Vagus nerve stimulation in intractable childhood epilepsy: a Korean multicenter experience. *J Korean Med Sci* 2007; 22:442–5.
48. Sirven JI, Sperling M, Naritoku D, Schachter S, Labar D, Holmes M, *et al.* Vagus nerve stimulation therapy for epilepsy in older adults. *Neurology* 2000; 54:1179–82.
49. Salinsky M. Results from an open label safety study: the EO4 experience. In: *Proceedings of the 1997 VNS Investigator meeting and Symposium*, pp. 33–4, 1997.
50. Labar D, Murphy J, Tecoma E. Vagus nerve stimulation for medication-resistant generalized epilepsy. *Neurology* 1999; 52: 1510–12.
51. Quintana C, Tecoma ES, Iragui VJ. Evidence that refractory partial onset and generalized epilepsy syndromes respond comparably to adjunctive vagus nerve stimulation therapy. *Epilepsia* 2002; 43(S7):344–5.
52. Michael NG and Devinsky O. Vagus nerve stimulation for refractory idiopathic generalised epilepsy. *Seizure* 2004; 13:176–8.
53. Kostov H, Larsson PG, Roste GK. Is vagus nerve stimulation a treatment option for patients with drug-resistant idiopathic generalized epilepsy? *Acta Neurol Scan Suppl* 2007; 187:55–8.
54. Holmes MD, Silbergeld DL, Drouhard D, Wilensky AJ, Ojemann LM. Effect of vagus nerve stimulation on adults with pharmacoresistant generalized epilepsy syndromes. *Seizure* 2004; 13:340–5.
55. Majoie HJM, Berfelo MW, Aldenkamp AP, Evers SMAA, Kessels AGH, Renier WO. Vagus nerve stimulation in children with therapy-resistant epilepsy diagnosed as Lennox-Gastaut syndrome. *J Clin Neurophysiol* 2001; 18:419–28.
56. Hosain S, Nikalov B, Harden C, Li M, Fraser R, Labar D. Vagus nerve stimulation treatment for Lennox-Gastaut syndrome. *J Child Neurol* 2000; 15:509–12.
57. Helmers S, Al-Jayyousi M, Madsen J. Adjunctive treatment in Lennox-Gastaut syndrome using vagal nerve stimulation. *Epilepsia* 1998; 39(S6):169.
58. Murphy J, Hornig G. Chronic intermittent stimulation of the left vagal nerve in nine children with Lennox-Gastaut syndrome. *Epilepsia* 1998; 39(S6):169.
59. Frost M, Gates J, Helmers S, Wheless JW, Levisohn P, Tardo C, *et al.* Vagus nerve stimulation in children with refractory seizures associated with Lennox-Gastaut syndrome. *Epilepsia* 2001; 42:1148–52.
60. Murphy JV, Wheless JW, Schmoll CM. Left vagal nerve stimulation in six patients with hypothalamic hamartomas. *Pediatr Neurol* 2000; 23:167–8.
61. Parain D, Delangre T, Piniello MJ, Freger P. Vagal nerve stimulation in refractory epilepsy with tuberous sclerosis. *Epilepsia* 1997; 38(S8):109.
62. Parain D, Peniello M, Berquen P, Delangre T, Billard C, Murphy JV. Vagal nerve stimulation in tuberous sclerosis patients. *Pediatr Neurol* 2001; 25:213–16.
63. Smith B, Shatz R, Elisevich K, Bespalova IN, Burmeister M. Effects of vagus nerve stimulation on progressive myoclonus epilepsy of Unverricht–Lundborg Type. *Epilepsia* 2000; 41:1046–8.
64. Silander HC, Runnerstam M, Ben-Menachem E. Use of vagus nerve stimulation in patients with Baltic myoclonic epilepsy (PME1). *Epilepsia* 2000; 41(S7):226.
65. Park YD. The effects of vagus nerve stimulation therapy on patients with intractable seizures and Landau-Kleffner syndrome or autism. *Epilepsy Behav* 2003; 4:286–90.
66. Warwick TC, Griffith J, Reyes B, Legesse B, Evans M. Effects of vagus nerve stimulation in a patient with temporal lobe epilepsy and Asperger syndrome: case report and review of the literature. *Epilepsy Behav* 2007; 10:344–7.
67. Andriola MR, Vitale SA. Vagus nerve stimulation in the developmentally disabled. *Epilepsy Behav* 2007; 2:129–34.
68. Gates J, Huf R, Frost M. Vagus nerve stimulation for patients in residential treatment facilities. *Epilepsy Behav* 2001; 2:563–7.
69. Huf RL, Mamelak A, Kneedy-Cayem K. Vagus nerve stimulation therapy: 2-year prospective open-label study of 40 subjects with refractory epilepsy and low IQ who are living in long-term care facilities. *Epilepsy Behav* 2005; 6:417–23.
70. Penovich PE, Korby B. Vagus nerve stimulation use in patients with epilepsy and mental retardation. Paper prepared for AES 2002, Seattle, USA.
71. Fohlen M, Jalin C, Pinard JM, Delalande O. Results of vagus nerve stimulation in 10 children with refractory infantile spasms. *Epilepsia* 1998; 39(S6):170.
72. Arthur TM, Saneto RP, Sotero de Menezes M, Devinsky O, LaJoie J, *et al.* Vagus nerve stimulation in children with mitochondrial electron transport chain deficiencies. *Mitochondrion* 2007; 7:279–83.
73. Koutroumanidis M, Binnie CD, Henessy MJ, Alarcon G, Elwes RDC, Toone BK, *et al.* VNS in patients with previous unsuccessful resective epilepsy surgery: antiepileptic and psychotropic effects. *Acta Neurol Scand* 2003; 107:117–21.
74. Frost MD, Hoskin C, Moriarty GL, Penovich PE, Ritter FJ, Gates J. Use of the vagus nerve stimulator in patients who have failed epilepsy surgery. *Epilepsia* 1998; 39(S6):192.
75. Claes J, Jaco P. The nervus vagus. *Acta Oto-Rhino-Laryngol Belg* 1986; 40:215–41.
76. Banzett RB, Guz A, Paydarfar D, Shea SA, Schachter SC, Lansing RW. Cardiorespiratory variables and sensation during stimulation of the left vagus in patients with epilepsy. *Epilepsy Res* 1999; 35:1–11.
77. Charous SJ, Kempster G, Manders E, Ristanovic R. The effect of vagal nerve stimulation on voice. *Laryngoscope* 2001; 111:2028–31.
78. Ben Menachem E. Vagus nerve stimulation, side effects and long-term safety. *J Clin Neurophysiol* 2001; 18:415–18.
79. Clarke BM, Upton ARM, Griffin HM. Cognitive motor function after electrical stimulation of the vagus nerve. *Pacing Clin Electrophysiol* 1992; 15:1603–7.
80. Clarke BM, Upton ARM, Kamath M, Griffin HM. Electrostimulation effects of the vagus nerve on balance in epilepsy. *Pacing Clin Electrophysiol* 1992; 15:1614–30.

81. Clarke BM, Upton ARM, Kamath M, Griffin HM. Acute effects of high frequency vagal nerve stimulation on balance and cognitive motor performance in epilepsy: three case study reports. *Pacing Clin Electrophyisol* 1992; 15:1608–13.
82. Clarke BM, Upton ARM, Griffin H, Fitzpatric D, DeNardis M. Chronic stimulation of the left vagus nerve in epilepsy: balance effects. *Can J Neurol Sci* 1997; 24:230–4.
83. Clarke BM, Upton ARM, Griffin H, Fitzpatric D, DeNardis M. Chronic stimulation of the left vagus nerve in epilepsy: cognitive motor effects. *Can J Neurol Sci* 1997; 24:226–9.
84. Hoppe C, Helmstaedter C, Scherrmann J, Elger CE. No evidence for cognitive side effects afer 6 months of vagus nerve stimulation in epilepsy patients. *Epilepsy Behav* 2001; 2:351–6.
85. Espinosa J, Aiello MT, Naritoku DK. Revision and removal of stimulating electrodes following long-term therapy with the vagus nerve stimulator. *Surg Neurol* 1999; 51:659–64.
86. Tatum WO, Moore DB, Stecker MM. Ventricular asystole during vagus nerve stimulation for epilepsy in humans. *Neurology* 2000; 52:1267–9.
87. Asconape JJ, Moore DD, Zipes DP, Hartman LM, Duffell WH. Bradycardia and asystole with the use of vagus nerve stimulation for the treatment of epilepsy: a rare complication of intraoperative device testing. *Epilepsia* 1998; 39:998–1000.
88. Ali I, Pirzada N, Kanjwal Y. Complete heart block with ventricular asystole during left vagus nerve stimulation for epilepsy. *Epilepsy Behav* 2004; 5:768–71.
89. Andriola MR, Rosenweig T, Vlay S, Brook S. Vagus nerve stimulator (VNS): induction of asystole during implantations with subsequent succesfull stimulation. *Epilepsia* 2000; 41(s7):223.
90. Ardesch JJ, Buschman HP, van der Burgh PH, Wagener-Schimmel LJ, van der Aa HA, Hageman G. Cardiac responses of vagus nerve stimulation: intraoperative bradycardia and subsequent chronic stimulation. *Clin Neurol Neurophysiol* 2007; 109:849–52.
91. Amark P. Stodberg T, Wallstedt L. Late onset bradyarrhythmia during vagus nerve stimulation. *Epilepsia* 2007; 48(5):1023–5.
92. Nyenhuis JA, Bourland JD, Foster KS, Graber GP, Terry RS, Adkins RA. Testing of MRI compatibility of the cyberonics model 100 NCP and model 300 series lead. *Epilepsia* 1997; 38(S8):140.
93. Benbadis SR, Nyhenhuis J, Tatum WO, Murtagh FR, Gieron M, Vale FL. MRI of the brain is safe in patients implanted with the vagus nerve stimulator. *Seizure* 2001; 10:512–15.
94. Duncan J. The current status of neuroimaging for epilepsy. *Curr Opin Neurol* 2003; 16:163–4.
95. Achten E, Jackson GD, Cameron JA, Abbott DF, Stella DL, Fabinyi GCA. Presurgical evaluation of the motor hand area with functional MR imaging in patients with tumors and dysplastic lesions. *Radiology* 1999; 210:529–38.
96. Sucholeiki R, Alsaadi TM, Morris GL, III, Ulmer JL, Biswal B, Mueller WM. fMRI in patients implanted with a vagal nerve stimulator. *Seizure* 2002; 11:157–62.
97. Bohning DE, Lomarev MP, Denslow S, Nahas Z, Shastri A, George MS. Feasibility of vagus nerve stimulation-synchronized blood oxygenation level-dependent functional MRI. *Invest Radiol* 2001; 36:470–9.
98. Narayanan JT, Watts R, Haddad N, Labar DR, Li PM, Filippi CG. Cerebral activation during vagus nerve stimulation: a functional MR study. *Epilepsia* 2002; 43:1509–14.
99. Lomarev M, Denslow S, Nahas Z, Chae JH, George MS, Bohning DE. Vagus nerve stimulation (VNS) synchronized BOLD fMRI suggests that VNS in depressed adults has frequency/dose dependent effects. *J Psychiatr Res* 2002; 36:219–27.
100. Proctor M, Gale K. Basal ganglia and brain stem anatomy and physiology. In: Engel J, Pedley TA (eds) *Epilepsy: The Comprehensive CD Rom*. Philadelphia, PA: Lippincot Williams and Wilkins, 1999.
101. Davis R. Cerebellar stimulation for cerebral palsy spasticity, function and seizures. *Arch Med Res* 2000; 31:290–9.
102. Wright GD, McLellan DL, Brice JC. A double-blind trial of chronic cerebellar stimulation in twelve patients with severe epilepsy. *J Neurol Neurosurg Psychiatry* 1984; 47:769–74.
103. Van Buren JM, Wood JH, Oakley J, Hambrecht F. Preliminary evaluation of cerebellar stimulation by double-blind stimulation and biological criteria in the treatment of epilepsy. *J Neurosurg* 1978; 48:407–16.
104. Velasco F, Carrillo-Ruiz JD, Brito F, Velasco M, Velasco A, Marquez I, Davis R. Double-blind, randomized controlled pilot study of bilateral cerebellar stimulation for the treatment of intractable motor seizures. *Epilepsia* 2005; 46(7):1071–81.
105. Benabid A, Minotti L, Koudsie A, de Saint Martin A, Hirsch E. Antiepileptic effects of high-frequency stimulation of the subthalamic nucleus (corpus Luysi) in a case of medically intractable epilepsy caused by focal dysplasia: a 30-month follow-up: technical case report. *Neurosurgery* 2002; 50:1385.
106. Alaraj A, Commair Y, Mikati M, Wakim J, Louak E, Atweh S. Subthalamic nucleus deep brain stimulation: a novel method for the treatment of non-focal intractable epilepsy. Neuromodulation: defining the future, poster presentation Cleveland Ohio 2001.
107. Loddenkemper T, Pan A, Neme S, Baker KB, Rezai AR, Dinner DS, *et al.* Deep brain stimulation in epilepsy. *J Clin Neurophysiol* 2001; 18:514–32.
108. Handforth A, DeSalles A, Krahl SE. Deep brain stimulation of the subthalamic nucleus as adjunct treatment for refractory epilepsy. *Epilepsia* 2006; 47(7):1239–41.
109. Vesper J, Steinhoff B, Rona S, Wille C, Bilic S, Nikkhah G, *et al.* Chronic high-frequency deep brain stimulation of the STN/SNr for progressive myoclonic epilepsy. *Epilepsia* 2007; 48(10):1984–9.
110. Velasco M, Velasco F, Velasco AL. Centromedian-thalamic and hippocampal electrical stimulation for the control of intractable epileptic seizures. *J Clin Neurophysiol* 2001; 18:495–513.
111. Velasco F, Velasco M, Jimenez F, Velasco AL, Rojas B, Perez ML. Centromedian nucleus stimulation for epilepsy. Clinical, electroencephalographic and behavioural observations. *Thal Syst* 2002; 1:387–98.
112. Velasco A, Velasco F, Jimenez F, Velasco M, Castro G, Carrillo-Ruiz JD, *et al.* Neuromodulation of the centromedian thalamic nuclei in the treatment of generalized seizures and the improvement of the quality of life in patients with Lennox-Gastaut syndrome. *Epilepsia* 2006; 47(7):1203–12.
113. Fisher RS, Uematsu S, Krauss GL, Cysyk BJ, McPherson R, Lesser RP, *et al.* Placebo-controlled pilot study of centromedian thalamic stimulation in treatment of intractable seizures. *Epilepsia* 1992; 33:841–51.
114. Parain D, Blondeau C, Peudenier S, Delangre T. Vagus nerve stimulation in refractory childhood absence epilepsy. *Epilepsia AES abstract*, 2003.
115. Hodaie M, Wennberg R, 102. Wright GD, McLellan DL, Brice JG. A double-blind trial of chronic cerebellar stimulation in twelve patients with severe epilepsy. *J Neurol Neurosurg Psychiatry* 1984; 47:769–74.
116. Andrade DM, Zumsteg D, Hamani C. Long-term follow-up (up to 7 years) of patients with thalamic deep brain stimulation for epilepsy. *Neurology* 2006; 66:1571–3.
117. Kerrigan JF, Litt B, Fisher RS, Cranstoun S, French JA, Blum DE, *et al.* Electrical stimulation of the anterior nucleus of the thalamus for the treatment of intractable seizures. *Epilepsia* 2004; 45:346–54.
118. Wiebe S, Blume WT, Girvin JP, Eliasziw M. A randomized, controlled trial of surgery for temporal lobe epilepsy. *N Engl J Med* 2001; 345:311–18.
119. Bragin A, Wilson CL, Engel J. Chronic epileptogenesis requires development of a network of pathologcially interconnected neuron clusters: a hypothesis. *Epilepsia* 2000; 41:S144–52.

120. Kemppainen S, Jolkkonen E, Pitkanen A. Projections from the posterior cortical nucleus of the amygdala to the hippocampal formation and parahippocampal region in rat. *Hippocampus* 2002; 12(6):735–55.
121. Wilson CL, Engel J: Electrical stimulation of the human epileptic limbic cortex. In: Devinsky O, Beric A, Dogali M (eds) *Electric and magnetic stimulation of the brain and spinal cord*, pp. 103–13. New York: Raven Press, 1993.
122. Lian J, Bikson M, Sciortino C, Stacey WC, Durand DM. Local suppression of epileptiform activity by electrical stimulation in rat hippocampus in vitro. *J Physiol* 2003; 547:427–34.
123. Su Y, Radman T, Vaynshteyn J, Parra LC, Bikson M. Effects of high-frequency stimulation on epileptiform activity in vitro: on/off control paradigm. *Epilepsia* 2008; 49(9):1586–93.
124. Wyckhuys T, De Smedt T, Claeys P, Raedt R, Waterschoot L, Vonck K, *et al.* High frequency deep brain stimulation in the hippocampus modifies seizure characteristics in kindled rats. *Epilepsia* 2007; 48:1543–50.
125. Wyckhuys T, Raedt R, Vonck K, Wadman W, Boon P. Comparison of hippocampal deep brain stimulation with high (130 Hz) and low (5 Hz) frequency on afterdischarges in kindled rats. *Epilepsy Res* 2010; 88(2–3):239–46.
126. Wyckhuys T, Boon P, Raedt R, Van Nieuwenhuyse B, Vonck K, Wadman W. Suppression of hippocampal epileptic seizures in the kainate rat by Poisson distributed stimulation. *Epilepsia* 2010; 51(11):2297–304.
127. Bragin A, Wilson CL, Engel J. Increased afterdischarge treshold during kindling in epileptic rats. *Exp Brain Res* 2002; 144:30–7.
128. Velasco M, Velasco F, Velasco AL, Boleaga B, Jimenez F, Brito F, *et al.* Subacute electrical stimulation of the hippocampus blocks intractable temporal lobe seizures and paroxysmal EEG activities. *Epilepsia* 2000; 41:158–69.
129. Tellez-Zenteno JF, McLachlan RS, Parrent A, Kubu CS, Wiebe S. Hippocampal electrical stimulation in mesial temporal lobe epilepsy. *Neurol* 2006; 66:1490–4.
130. Velasco A, Velasco F, Velasco M, Trejo D, Castro G, Carrillo-Ruiz JD. Electrical stimulation of the hippocampal epileptic foci for seizure control: a double-blind, long-term follow-up study. *Epilepsia* 2007; 48(10):1895–903.

CHAPTER 31

Other Surgeries for Epilepsy and New Approaches

Kitti Kaiboriboon and Samden D. Lhatoo

Introduction

In this chapter, we describe epilepsy surgeries at two ends of the spectrum in terms of the volume of brain tissue subjected to surgery. Hemispherectomies, at the one end, represent extensive, complex, unilateral resections and removal of close to entire hemispheres of epileptogenic brain whilst multiple hippocampal transections (a new surgical technique) at the other end, constitute discrete, limited transections of just one hippocampus. Although resection of the epileptogenic zone offers the most effective method of obtaining seizure freedom as detailed in previous chapters, this is not always possible. Unacceptable proximity of the epileptogenic zone to eloquent cortex can contraindicate wide resection as can multifocal epilepsy where multiple resections are impractical or dangerous. In the generalized epilepsy syndromes, resection is clearly not possible. In many of these situations, an attempt at seizure freedom or a substantial reduction in seizure burden can still be made through additional surgical techniques that do not involve removal of the epileptogenic zone or stimulator implantation.

Multiple subpial transection

The principle behind multiple subpial transection (MST) epitomizes the classical situation where resection of a brain region identified as the likely epileptogenic zone would probably result in significant and unacceptable neurological deficits and where resective surgery would therefore be impractical (Box 31.1). Morrell et al. (1) initially described MST for this particular scenario. The technique is based on the columnar organization of normal human cortex, the hypothesis that synchronization and propagation of epileptic spikes and/or seizures often occurs horizontally and that a critical mass of cortex is required to generate seizures. MST cuts horizontally oriented cortical fibres while preserving vertically oriented fibres as well as blood vessels (Fig. 31.1), thereby blocking the synchronization of epileptogenic neurons without causing functional deficit. The plan for MST (e.g. defining the cortical area that will be transected) is critical and the distance between cuts should be approximately 5 mm. Transections are made by passing a modified right-angled hook transector deep into the gyrus (Fig. 31.1) which is then swept forward perpendicular to the cortical surface towards the opposite sulci. The tip of the transector is raised and pulled backwards underneath the pia, creating a small track (2). This process is continued over the selected area until the abnormal discharges on simultaneous electrocorticography is minimized or abolished (Fig. 31.2).

The utility of MST in epilepsy can be measured by assessing postoperative functional deficits (if any) and seizure control. In general, it is accepted that MST leads to minimal long-term functional deficits. However, initial neurological deficits can be quite common (3–8). Recent functional magnetic resonance imaging (MRI) (9), positron emission tomography (PET) (10), and transcranial magnetic stimulation studies (11) confirm that MST does not interfere with the functioning of transected cortical regions.

On the other hand, the efficacy of MST in controlling seizures has been debated. Seizure freedom outcomes vary from study to study depending primarily on the indications for surgery and whether cortical resection is performed to supplement MST. In general, a combination of MST and resection has a higher rate of seizure freedom than pure MST (1, 5, 7, 8, 12–15). A meta-analysis evaluating 211 patients, most of whom underwent MST combined with cortical resection, demonstrated that MST with and without accompanying resection had a more than 95% reduction in seizure frequency (16). Interestingly, approximately 15–20% of patients had increased frequency of simple partial seizures after MST, presumably due to disconnection of inhibitory inputs from neighbouring cortex (16). Late seizure recurrence can occur in some patients who initially experience good seizure control and conversely, late improvement in patients with initial, relatively poor outcome has been observed (7, 17). The mechanisms of late seizure recurrence or late improvement of seizure control are unknown.

Box 31.1 Candidates for multiple subpial transection

- Intractable focal or multifocal epilepsy involving eloquent cortex
- Epilepsia partialis continua or refractory focal status epilepticus
- Landau–Kleffner syndrome
- Rasmussen's encephalitis with functional use of hand and/or language.

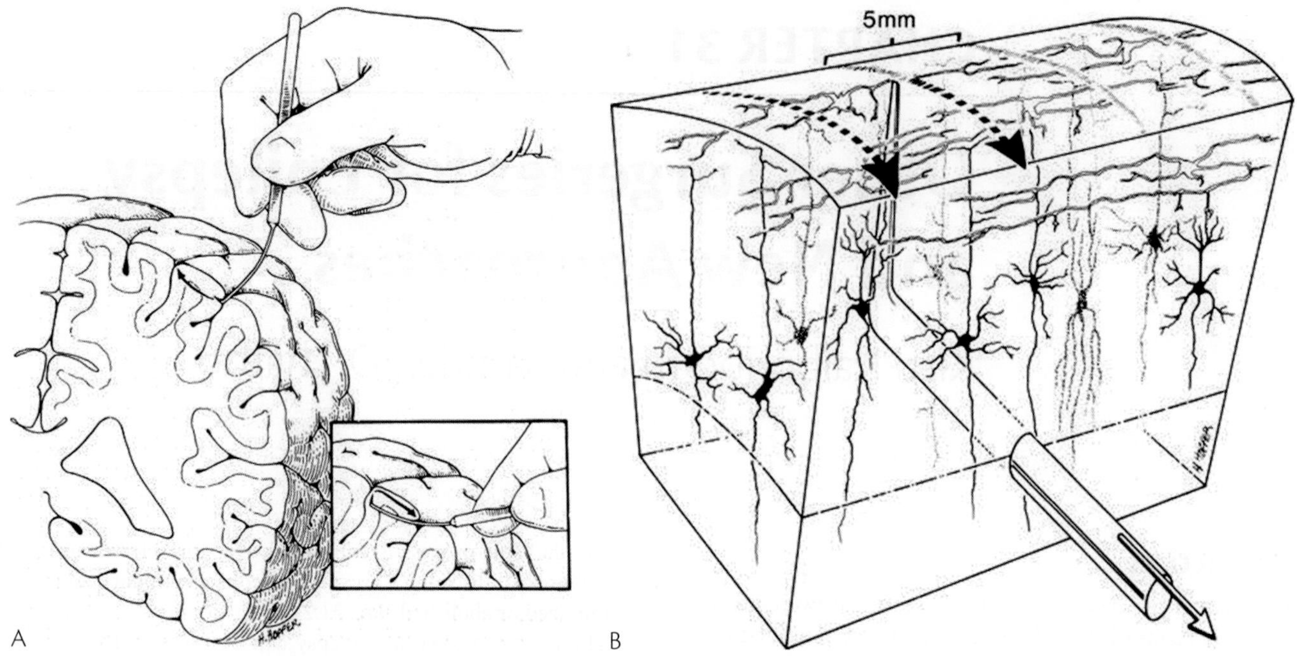

Fig. 31.1 Artist's drawings to illustrate the technique of insertion and movement of the subpial transector (A) and the anatomical principles involved in multiple subpial transection (B) where horizontally oriented nerve fibres are transected whilst vertically oriented fibres are spared. Reproduced permission of *Journal of Neurosurgery*, American Assn. of Neurosurgeons (1).

The application of MST in patients with multifocal epilepsy who are not candidates for conventional surgery has shown promising results. A study of 13 patients with independent multifocal epileptogenic foci demonstrated that cortical resection combined with MST in eloquent cortex improved seizure outcome in 77% (15). The best results were observed in patients with discrete epileptogenic foci limited to two lobes. Another study of 61 patients with multifocal epilepsy who underwent MST with and without cortical resection found no significant differences in seizure outcomes between the two groups (18). Approximately half of their patients were seizure free.

MST combined with cortical resection has also been used successfully in stopping seizures in patients with refractory focal status epilepticus or epilepsia partialis continua (19–24). In this situation, pure MST has been used in cortical dysplasia of the left motor cortex (25) and of the angular gyrus, superior temporal gyrus, and suprasylvian frontal lobe in another case (26).

MST has also been used in a variety of epilepsy syndromes including Landau–Kleffner syndrome (LKS), Rasmussen's encephalitis, Lennox–Gastaut syndrome, and infantile spasms (Box 31.1). However, no clear recommendations can be made for MST in these syndromes based on the very small number of patients reported. A few surgical series of patients with LKS have demonstrated significant improvement in language function after MST (27, 28) but this, however, has not been reproduced by others (8, 29, 30). Patient selection and resolution of the severe epileptiform abnormality are important factors in predicting good outcome (13). Incorrect diagnoses may contaminate some of the poorer reported results. In general, continued recovery of language function can be seen at least 6 months after surgery and adjunctive, intensive speech therapy is usually necessary. For patients with atypical LKS or autistic epileptiform regression, only a temporary response to MST has been demonstrated (31, 32).

Several MST series have contained patients with Rasmussen's encephalitis (3, 5, 6, 13, 33). Since Rasmussen's encephalitis is a progressive disease, most patients with this condition either did not have good outcome or achieved only temporary relief. In these patients, therefore, MST should be considered as a mainly palliative intervention to delay hemispherectomy in patients who have functional use of hand and/or language (13).

An improvement in seizure control after MST has been reported in a few patients with infantile spasms (18, 34). In a report of two patients with infantile spasms (34), one patient developed infantile spasms after meningoencephalitis with a resulting diffuse structural abnormality on MRI and focal metabolic abnormality on PET. The other patient had cortical dysplasia with focal metabolic abnormality on PET. Both patients had reduction of seizures frequency. In another report (18), two patients with infantile spasms underwent MST in both hemispheres. One patient became seizure free whereas the other patient did not show any improvement. In the same series (18), three patients with Lennox–Gastaut syndrome also improved after MST.

Multiple hippocampal transection

Approximately 30–60% of patients who undergo language dominant anterior temporal lobectomy experience a significant decline in verbal memory and visual naming postoperatively (35–38). Several studies suggest that patients with mild or moderate hippocampal neuronal loss have the greatest risk of postoperative memory decline (36, 39, 40). The severity of postoperative memory deterioration depends on the extent of removal of non-lesional hippocampus (41).

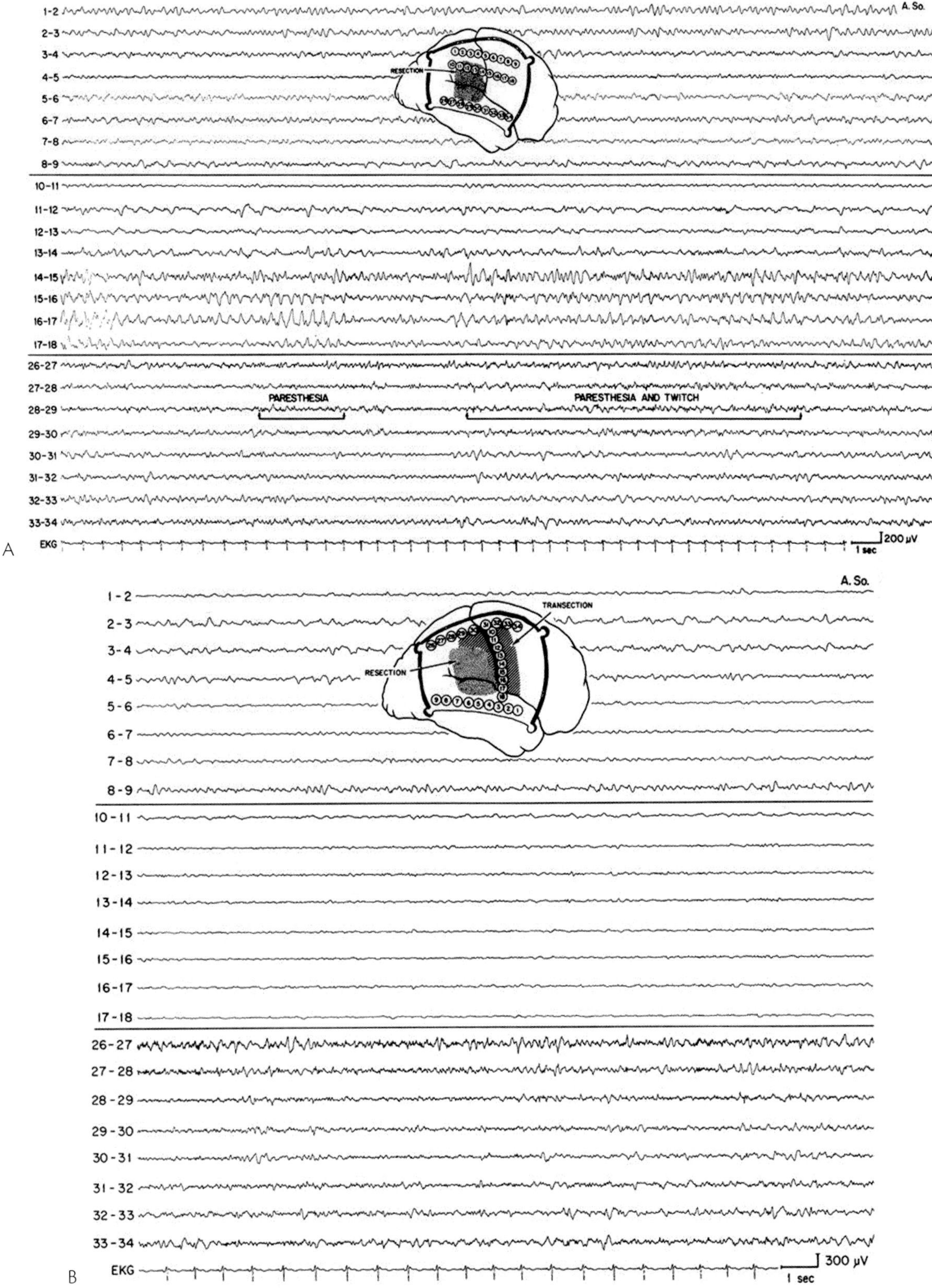

Fig. 31.2 A) Electrocorticographic recordings obtained following removal of a cystic meningocerebral scar from the right parietal cortex. Electrodes were placed as indicated on the superimposed diagram. Epileptiform potentials can be readily identified in the channels labelled with electrodes numbered 12, 13, 15, 16. Overt symptoms were reported by the patient during the time intervals marked by upturned arrows. The electrographic accompaniments of these symptoms may be discerned in derivations from electrodes 15 and 16. EKG = electrocardiographic tracing. Reproduced permission of *Journal of Neurosurgery*, American Assn. of Neurosurgeons (1). B) Electrocorticographic recordings obtained following multiple subpial transection (MST) of the precentral gyrus and a small portion of the postcentral gyrus superior to the ablation in the same patient. The ablated region is stippled; the zone subjected to MST is shown by diagonal lines. Electrode positions are shown on the superimposed diagram. The electrical records from derivations overlying the transected zone (channels 9 to 16) reveal no trace of the epileptiform abnormality so prominently shown in (A). Reproduced permission of *Journal of Neurosurgery*, American Assn. of Neurosurgeons (1).

In order to minimize the impact of adverse neuropsychological outcomes, more limited resections of the mesial temporal structures such as selective amygdalohippocampectomy or more restricted variants of anterior temporal lobectomy have been used. A recent review of different surgical approaches in mesial temporal lobe epilepsy demonstrated that more restricted or selective approaches provide good seizure outcome similar to standard or more extensive approaches (42). However, selective approaches yield better postoperative cognitive and memory outcomes (42–45). Nonetheless, left-sided hippocampectomy can still result in significant memory decline (41, 46).

Recently, the principle of MST has been applied to the hippocampus in patients with dominant mesial temporal lobe epilepsy in order to preserve verbal memory (47, 48). The technique of multiple hippocampal transection (MHT) (Fig. 31.3) was developed based on the hypothesis that disruption of horizontal connections in the pyramidal layer of the hippocampus can interrupt synchronization and spread of epileptic activity without interfering with memory function (48). To avoid the disruption of direct hippocampal pathways, the hippocampus is accessed via a small corticotomy on the anterior superior temporal gyrus along the sylvian veins (47). Intraoperative electrocorticography in the amygdala and hippocampus is necessary to determine the extent of transection. When the amygdala produces epileptic discharges, it is also resected. After the extent of MHT is determined, the pyramidal cell layer and the dentate gyrus are transected sequentially from anterior to posterior using small ring transectors (Fig. 31.3). The epileptic discharges in the hippocampus can completely disappear after transection is completed (Fig. 31.4). In some cases, resection of the anterior basal temporal and MST in the posterior basal temporal lobe may be required.

Shimizu et al. (47, 48) first reported MHT as an effective surgical approach with excellent seizure and memory outcomes for patients with unilateral mesial temporal lobe epilepsy. Between 2001 and 2006, 35 cases of intractable unilateral mesial temporal lobe epilepsy with normal MRI underwent this procedure at their centre. Twenty-two patients underwent left MHT and 23 patients had right MHT. Of the 23 patients who had more than 1 year follow-up postoperatively, 78% were seizure free and 17% had rare seizures. Verbal memory was evaluated in 13 patients who underwent left MHT. Twelve of these patients did not show verbal memory decline at 6 months after surgery. Besides unilateral temporal lobe epilepsy, bilateral MHT was performed in 10 patients with bilateral temporal lobe epilepsy. However, 60% of the patients had poor outcomes and one patient had severe memory deficits (48) suggesting that the procedure is best restricted to unilateral mesial temporal lobe epilepsy.

In a more recent report of 10 patients with unilateral mesial temporal lobe epilepsy (49), all patients had MHT with MST in the neocortex and some had resections of the temporal tip. The median follow-up was 21 months (range 10–34 months). Nine patients had excellent seizure outcomes, seven of whom were seizure free. Among patients who had pre- and postoperative memory testing, 62% had improvement of verbal memory, 37% had improvement of visual memory, and 37% had a slight decline in visual memory. At our centre, MHT is offered to patients with unilateral dominant, non-lesional mesial temporal lobe epilepsy and normal or excellent verbal memory indices. All such patients undergo intracranial monitoring to confirm mesial temporal epilepsy and MHT is carried out either as the sole procedure or with removal of the amygdala and temporal pole.

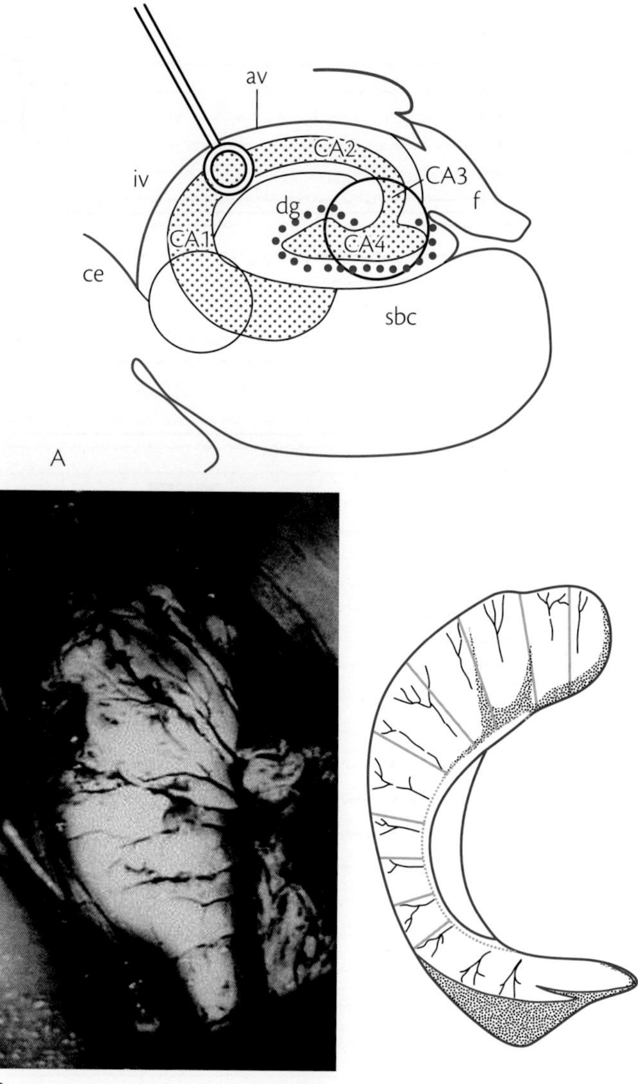

Fig. 31.3 A) A schematic drawing of hippocampal transection. After the alveus is incised with micro-scissors, the pyramidal cell layer and dentate gyrus are transected using ring transectors with 2 mm and 4 mm diameters. ce, collateral eminence; iv, inferior ventricle; av, alveus; f, fimbria; sbc, subiculum; dg, dentate gyrus. B) Intraoperative view of hippocampal transection is shown. Schematic drawing on the right illustrates transection lines (grey solid lines) being placed along the digitations marks at the hippocampal head and small surface vessels in the remaining area (47). Reproduced with permission from *Journal of Clinical Neuroscience*, Science Direct.

MHT appears a logical approach for patients with unilateral, non-lesional mesial temporal lobe epilepsy, particularly where chances of significant postoperative memory declines are otherwise high, and has a sound biological basis. The results from different groups so far are encouraging but short follow-up periods emphasize the requirement for larger series with long-term outcomes.

Corpus callosotomy

The rationale of surgical division of corpus callosum is to limit the propagation of epileptic activity to one hemisphere. This procedure

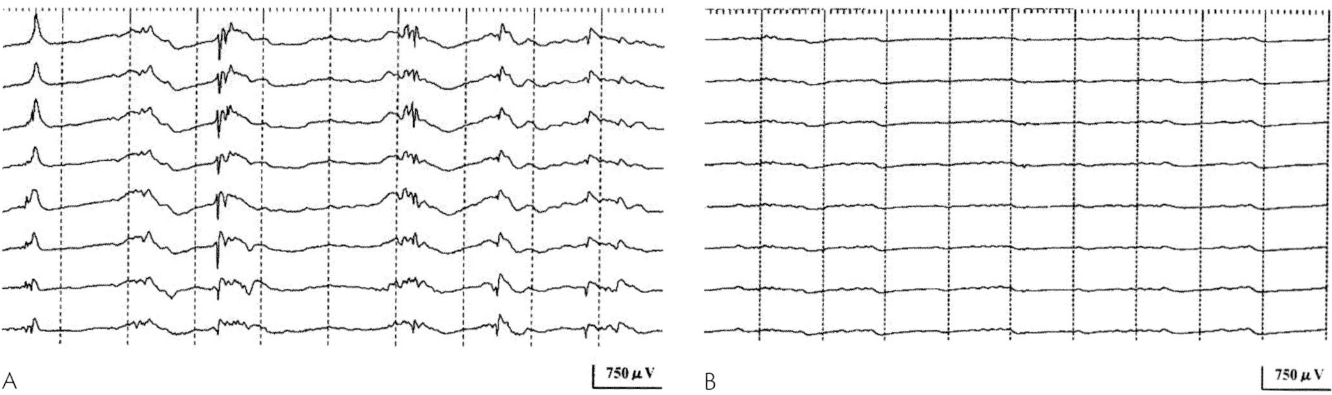

Fig. 31.4 Electrocorticography over the hippocampus is recorded to determine the extent of the epileptic areas (A). The upper four leads are recorded from the hippocampal head and the lower four from the hippocampal body and tail. After completion of hippocampal transection, active epileptic discharges over the hippocampus are abolished (B) (47) Reproduced with permission from *Journal of Clinical Neuroscience*, Science Direct.

was first performed in patients with epilepsy based on the observations that the corpus callosum was the major route of seizure propagation and that seizures usually improved after occurrence of stroke or tumour involving the corpus callosum (50). Corpus callosotomy is considered palliative surgery for patients with severe medically intractable epilepsy with major motor manifestations such as tonic, atonic, myoclonic, or generalized tonic–clonic seizures. Among these, drop attacks elicited by tonic or atonic seizures are most likely to improve (51). Patients with diffuse or multifocal pathologies who are not eligible for resective surgery such as infantile hemiplegia, Rasmussen's encephalitis, Lennox–Gastaux syndrome, Sturge–Weber syndrome, and tuberous sclerosis might receive some benefit. In general, patients with any debilitating non-resectable epilepsy should be considered for corpus callosotomy regardless of age or type of epilepsy (Box 31.2).

A variety of techniques of corpus callosotomy have been described over the years. The modern techniques are mainly restricted to division of the corpus callosum and the hippocampal commissure (52). However, how much of the structure is divided remains unclear. Some studies showed that the extent of callosal sections correlated with seizure outcome and, therefore, more extensive sections yielded better results (53–57). Other studies

Box 31.2 Candidates for corpus callosotomy

Intractable generalized seizures with:

- Drop attacks
- Generalized tonic–clonic seizures
- Myoclonic seizures
- Other major motor manifestations.

Patients with diffuse or multifocal pathologies, e.g.:

- Rasmussen's encephalitis
- Lennox–Gastaux syndrome
- Sturge–Weber syndrome
- Tuberous sclerosis.

report that anterior section is as effective as complete section (58, 59). Currently, many centres prefer sectioning of the anterior two-thirds or three-quarters initially and reserve the complete resection only for patients who do not have sufficient improvement following the initial procedure (53, 55, 60). Nevertheless, an upfront one-stage complete callosal section might be an optimal choice for patients with non-functional, severe global developmental delay (54, 57, 61).

Seizure improvement and reduction of bisynchronous discharges after corpus callosotomy has been well documented. Between 50–80% of the patients who underwent callosotomy have at least 50% seizure reduction (51, 55, 61–64). Atonic seizures usually respond best to callosotomy compared to other types of seizures (53) while focal motor seizures receive the least benefit. Partial seizures can be worsened and sometimes new types of seizures can emerge after callosotomy, especially in patients with independent bifrontal epileptogenic foci (60, 65, 66).

Several studies have investigated prognostic factors for callosotomy outcomes. The results from these studies, however, are conflicting. For example, a few studies did not find age at seizure onset or at the time of surgery to have prognostic significance (58, 59, 62) whereas other studies suggest that younger age at the time of surgery or earlier seizure onset have better outcomes including improvement in quality of life, family satisfaction, and fewer complications (67, 68). The presence of significant cognitive impairment and/or mixed cerebral dominance are associated with poor outcome in a few studies (58, 60, 67, 69). However, these findings have not been confirmed by others (59, 70, 71). Moreover, recent series of callosotomy in children with severe mental retardation demonstrate favourable results (61, 72). Ictal and interictal EEG have been found to be prognostically useful in some studies (59, 67, 70, 71, 73). Ictal patterns of generalized slow spike wave discharges, electrodecrement, and non-evolving low amplitude fast activity have been associated with excellent outcomes (71). A few studies have shown that bilateral independent spikes are indicative of poor outcomes after callosotomy (67, 73). Disruption of synchrony as well as reduction of generalized bilateral synchronous spikes in the intraoperative or postoperative electroencephalogram (EEG) recordings are good indicators for favourable outcomes (59, 70). Some studies, however, have not found clear relationships between EEG findings and outcomes after callosotomy (74, 75).

Corpus callosotomies can result in acute as well as chronic disconnection syndromes. In the acute setting, an apathetic mutism lasting days to weeks can occur, usually related to the extent of callosal section. Other deficits including hemiparesis and a variety of apraxias can also occur. In the chronic setting, deficits can be more subtle. Poor naming of objects in the dominant hemifield or of those held in the dominant hand can be observed. This is most likely due to a disruption of the pathways from the non-dominant hemisphere where sensation or vision is perceived, to the dominant hemisphere where language is necessary to express receipt of these inputs. Several other, more subtle deficits of motor, language and other functions may also exist.

Hemispherectomy

When seizures arise from multiple regions in one hemisphere, removal of the abnormal hemisphere seems a logical approach to getting rid of seizures. Drastic as this might seem, applied to the correct clinical situations and with the right expertise, it is a dramatically effective intervention in many, both in the short and long term. Seizure freedom and cognitive outcomes can be impressive with postoperative deficits that are acceptable enough to allow functionality.

Anatomical hemispherectomy, where the entire hemisphere is removed, was successfully performed with encouraging results in the late 1960s (76). However, severe late complications including hydrocephalus and superficial haemosiderosis occurred in up to one-third of the patients (77, 78). In order to reduce the risk of postoperative complications, several technical modifications of hemispherectomy have been introduced, variously referred to as functional hemispherectomy, hemispherotomy, hemicorticectomy, peri-insularhemispherotomy, and hemispheric deafferentation (79). In these, the anatomical cortical resection is subtotal rather than total but coupled with a physiological hemispherectomy where deafferentation or disconnection is carried out. This approach of 'functional' hemispherectomy is to minimize cortical resection and functionally isolate abnormal hemisphere by disrupting neuronal fibre connections (80). A large meta-analysis of data from 11 epilepsy centres demonstrated that the new techniques that focused on disconnection were as good or slightly better with a clear benefit in perisurgical morbidity compared to the old techniques involving large resections (79). Although anatomical hemispherectomies are now rare in epilepsy surgery practice, these are still used in patients who failed functional hemispherectomies where there is a strong case for epilepsy arising from remnant brain tissue.

Hemispherectomy is most often performed in the paediatric population and is indicated in medical refractory epilepsy with extensive or multiregional epileptogenic foci in a single hemisphere (Box 31.3). However, the criteria for patient selection are still in evolution (81). Studies have suggested that patients with asymmetric MRI abnormalities, where one abnormal side predominates over the other, might still be benefit from hemispherectomy (82). Nonetheless, patients without contralateral MRI lesions usually have better seizure outcome and cognitive development after surgery (83).

Functional hemispherectomy (Fig. 31.5) involves removal of the central part of the hemisphere (the frontal and parietal opercula, including the inferolateral frontal and parietal lobes) and the ipsilateral temporal lobe. The extent of the resection can vary to include the superolateral frontal and parietal lobes but the posterior quadrant and anterior frontal lobes are usually left intact. The blood supply to these structures is left undisturbed. The entire corpus callosum is disconnected as are the white matter connections of the remaining frontal lobe and the parietal and occipital lobes. The ipsilateral cingulate gyrus is also disconnected. Complete disconnection can be technically difficult to achieve and up to a fifth of patients are subsequently found to have incomplete disconnections, many of whom continue to have seizures (84).

Peri-insular hemispherotomy and hemispheric deafferentation both emphasize disconnection. The former uses a peri-insular, suprasylvian and infrasylvian approach to a transventricular corpus callosotomy and removal of the mesial temporal structures. The latter uses a standard temporal lobectomy for ventricular access and subsequent callosotomy. Hemidecortication is an infrequently used technique where grey matter is removed or 'degloved' from underlying white matter.

The overall rates of complete or near complete seizure freedom vary between 50–94% (85–87). Seizure outcome is influenced by

Box 31.3 Candidates for hemispherectomy[a]

- Infantile spasms due to focal lesions (localization related)
- Rasmussen's encephalitis
- Sturge–Weber syndrome
- Hemispheric malformations of cortical development such as hemimegalencephaly, schizencephaly, and cortical dysplasia involving significant region of a hemisphere.
- Porencephaly syndrome
- Hemiplegia hemiconvulsion epilepsy syndrome (HHE).

[a] There may be overlap between these categories.

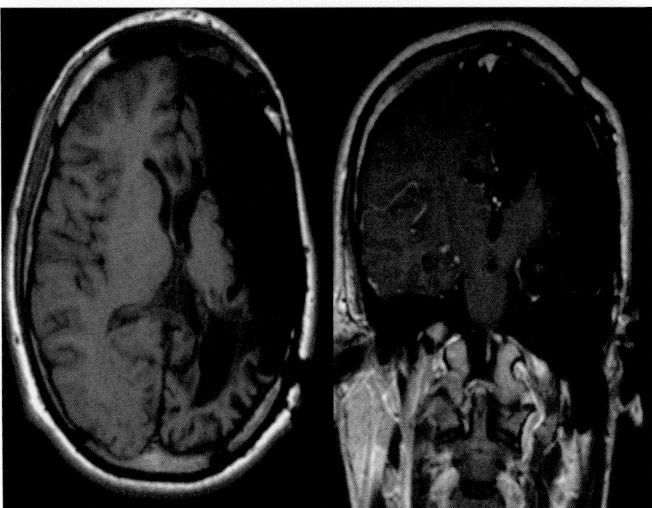

Fig. 31.5 Functional hemispherectomy in a 10-year-old patient with Rasmussen's encephalitis showing complete removal of the frontal, parietal, and temporal lobes with intact left posterior quadrant and basal ganglia structures. The resection here has been extended to include the entire frontal lobe.

brain pathology, surgical technique, the completeness of disconnection, and the extent of resection. Patients with Sturge–Weber syndrome usually have excellent results whereas patients with hemimegalencephaly frequently have poor outcomes (88). A recent study comparing peri-insular hemispherotomy and hemidecortication suggested that peri-insular hemispherotomy provided better seizure outcomes (89). Moreover, a high seizure freedom rate has been reported in patients whose deep structures were removed or disconnected (90, 91).

Although the ideal timing of hemispherectomy is unclear, key considerations are seizure-related morbidity and neuropsychological morbidity from epilepsies that are often extremely detrimental to brain development. Equally, the presence or absence of potential brain plasticity for certain brain functions is an important consideration. For example, removal or disconnection of the language areas as part of a dominant hemispherectomy in a 2-year-old child can result in reasonable relocation of language function to the contralateral, intact hemisphere. This is less likely in a 10-year-old and highly unlikely in an adult. Proximal limb power can also recover to some extent, enough to allow ambulation in many, but distal limb power and fine finger movements do not return. Studies have shown benefit in psychosocial and intellectual functions in patients who underwent surgery early (92–94). In Rasmussen's encephalitis, it is clear that a shorter period from seizure onset to surgery is associated with better seizure outcome (95). However, in some patients a longer preoperative period might enhance brain plasticity and result in better motor outcomes (96). In general, the benefits of early hemispherectomy must be weighed against postoperative deficits (97). A more recent study of hemispherectomy has demonstrated favourable outcome with low morbidity in adults as well (98).

Conclusion

Multiple subpial transection can provides a surgical option to patients with intractable focal epilepsy who are otherwise not amenable candidates for resective surgery. The application of the concept of multiple subpial transection to the hippocampus, through multiple hippocampal transection, is a potentially good alternative for high-functioning patients with mesial temporal lobe epilepsy. For devastating epilepsy, corpus callosotomy can be a good palliative option that can help improve the patient's quality of life. Hemispherectomy procedures can be extremely effective in otherwise devastating childhood epilepsies. Recent technical modifications of hemispherectomy have made the technique safer and more appealing. As experience and knowledge accrues, morbidity from these procedures will continue to lessen whilst chances of seizure freedom proportionately increase.

References

1. Morrell F, Whisler WW, Bleck TP. Multiple subpial transection: a new approach to the surgical treatment of focal epilepsy. *J Neurosurg* 1989; 70:231–9.
2. Cohen-Gadol AA, Stoffman MR, Spencer DD. Emerging surgical and radiotherapeutic techniques for treating epilepsy. *Curr Opin Neurol* 2003; 16:213–19.
3. Sawhney IM, Robertson IJ, Polkey CE, Binnie CD, Elwes RD. Multiple subpial transection: a review of 21 cases. *J Neurol Neurosurg Psychiatry* 1995; 58:344–9.
4. Rougier A, Sundstrom L, Claverie B, Saint-Hilaire JM, Labrecque R, Lurton D, *et al.* Multiple subpial transection: report of 7 cases. *Epilepsy Res* 1996; 24:57–63.
5. Hufnagel A, Zentner J, Fernandez G, Wolf HK, Schramm J, Elger CE. Multiple subpial transection for control of epileptic seizures: effectiveness and safety. *Epilepsia* 1997; 38, 678–88.
6. Mulligan LP, Spencer DD, Spencer SS. Multiple subpial transections: the Yale experience. *Epilepsia* 2001; 42:226–9.
7. Schramm J, Aliashkevich AF, Grunwald T. Multiple subpial transections: outcome and complications in 20 patients who did not undergo resection. *J Neurosurg* 2002; 97:39–47.
8. Blount JP, Langburt W, Otsubo H, Chitoku S, Ochi A, Weiss S, *et al.* Multiple subpial transections in the treatment of pediatric epilepsy. *J Neurosurg* 2004; 100:118–24.
9. Moo LR, Slotnick SD, Krauss G, Hart J. A prospective study of motor recovery following multiple subpial transections. *Neuroreport* 2002; 13:665–9.
10. Leonhardt G, Spiekermann G, Muller S, Zentner J, Hufnagel A. Cortical reorganization following multiple subpial transection in human brain—a study with positron emission tomography. *Neurosci Lett* 2000; 292:63–5.
11. Shimizu T, Maehara T, Hino T, Komori T, Shimizu H, Yagishita A, *et al.* Effect of multiple subpial transection on motor cortical excitability in cortical dysgenesis. *Brain* 2001; 124:1336–49.
12. Wyler AR, Wilkus RJ, Rostad SW, Vossler DG. Multiple subpial transections for partial seizures in sensorimotor cortex. *Neurosurgery* 1995; 37:1122–7; discussion 27–8.
13. Smith MC. Multiple subpial transection in patients with extratemporal epilepsy. *Epilepsia* 1998; 39(Suppl 4):S81–9.
14. Shimizu H, Maehara T. Neuronal disconnection for the surgical treatment of pediatric epilepsy. *Epilepsia* 2000; 41(Suppl 9):28–30.
15. Devinsky O, Romanelli P, Orbach D, Pacia S, Doyle W. Surgical treatment of multifocal epilepsy involving eloquent cortex. *Epilepsia* 2003; 44:718–23.
16. Spencer SS, Schramm J, Wyler A, O'Connor M, Orbach D, Krauss G, *et al.* Multiple subpial transection for intractable partial epilepsy: an international meta-analysis. *Epilepsia* 2002; 43:141–5.
17. Orbach D, Romanelli P, Devinsky O, Doyle W. Late seizure recurrence after multiple subpial transections. *Epilepsia* 2001; 42:1316–19.
18. Patil AA, Andrews RV, Johnson M, Rodriguez-Sierra JF. Is epilepsy surgery on both hemispheres effective? *Stereotact Funct Neurosurg* 2004; 82:214–21.
19. Desbiens R, Berkovic SF, Dubeau F, Andermann F, Laxer KD, Harvey S, *et al.* Life-threatening focal status epilepticus due to occult cortical dysplasia. *Arch Neurol* 1993; 50:695–700.
20. D'Giano CH, Del CGM, Pomata H, Rabinowicz AL. Treatment of refractory partial status epilepticus with multiple subpial transection: case report. *Seizure* 2001; 10:382–5.
21. Ma X, Liporace J, O'Connor MJ, Sperling MR. Neurosurgical treatment of medically intractable status epilepticus. *Epilepsy Res* 2001; 46:33–8.
22. Ng YT, Kim HL, Wheless JW. Successful neurosurgical treatment of childhood complex partial status epilepticus with focal resection. *Epilepsia* 2003; 44:468–71.
23. Costello DJ, Simon MV, Eskandar EN, Frosch MP, Henninger HL, Chiappa KH, *et al.* Efficacy of surgical treatment of de novo, adult-onset, cryptogenic, refractory focal status epilepticus. *Arch Neurol* 2006; 63:895–901.
24. Ng YT, Bristol RE, Schrader DV, Smith KA. The role of neurosurgery in status epilepticus. *Neurocrit Care* 2007; 7:86–91.
25. Molyneux PD, Barker RA, Thom M, van Paesschen W, Harkness WF, Duncan JS. Successful treatment of intractable epilepsia partialis continua with multiple subpial transections. *J Neurol Neurosurg Psychiatry* 1998; 65:137–8.
26. Bristol RE, Gore P, Treiman D, Smith KA. Resolution of status epilepticus after subdural grid recording and multiple subpial transections. *Barrow Quarterly* 2006; 22:8–11.
27. Morrell F, Whisler WW, Smith MC, Hoeppner TJ, de Toledo-Morrell L, Pierre-Louis SJ, *et al.* Landau–Kleffner syndrome. Treatment with subpial intracortical transection. *Brain* 1995; 118:1529–46.

28. Grote CL, Van Slyke P, Hoeppner JA. Language outcome following multiple subpial transection for Landau–Kleffner syndrome. *Brain* 1999; 122:561–6.
29. Irwin K, Birch V, Lees J, Polkey C, Alarcon G, Binnie C, *et al.* Multiple subpial transection in Landau–Kleffner syndrome. *Dev Med Child Neurol* 2001; 43:248–52.
30. Robinson RO, Baird G, Robinson G, Simonoff E. Landau–Kleffner syndrome: course and correlates with outcome. *Dev Med Child Neurol* 2001; 43:243–7.
31. Neville BG, Harkness WF, Cross JH, Cass HC, Burch VC, Lees JA, *et al.* Surgical treatment of severe autistic regression in childhood epilepsy. *Pediatr Neurol* 1997; 16:137–40.
32. Nass R, Gross A, Wisoff J, Devinsky O. Outcome of multiple subpial transections for autistic epileptiform regression. *Pediatr Neurol* 1999; 21:464–70.
33. Pondal-Sordo M, Diosy D, Tellez-Zenteno JF, Girvin JP, Wiebe S. Epilepsy surgery involving the sensory-motor cortex. *Brain* 2006; 129:3307–14.
34. Chuang MF, Harnod T, Wang PJ, Chen YH, Hsin YL. Effect of multiple subpial transection on patients with uncontrolled atypical infantile spasms. *Epilepsia* 2006; 47:659–60.
35. Sass KJ, Spencer DD, Kim JH, Westerveld M, Novelly RA, Lencz T. Verbal memory impairment correlates with hippocampal pyramidal cell density. *Neurology* 1990; 40:1694–7.
36. Rausch R, Babb TL. Hippocampal neuron loss and memory scores before and after temporal lobe surgery for epilepsy. *Arch Neurol* 1993; 50:812–17.
37. Baxendale S. Amnesia in temporal lobectomy patients: historical perspective and review. *Seizure* 1998; 7:15–24.
38. Hamberger MJ, Seidel WT, McKhann GMn, Goodman RR. Hippocampal removal affects visual but not auditory naming. *Neurology* 2010; 74:1488–93.
39. Sass KJ, Westerveld M, Buchanan CP, Spencer SS, Kim JH, Spencer DD. Degree of hippocampal neuron loss determines severity of verbal memory decrease after left anteromesiotemporal lobectomy. *Epilepsia* 1994; 35:1179–86.
40. Helmstaedter C, Petzold I, Bien CG. The cognitive consequence of resecting nonlesional tissues in epilepsy surgery-Results from MRI- and histopathology-negative patients with temporal lobe epilepsy. *Epilepsia* 2011; 52:1402–8.
41. Helmstaedter C, Roeske S, Kaaden S, Elger CE, Schramm J. Hippocampal resection length and memory outcome in selective epilepsy surgery. *J Neurol Neurosurg Psychiatry* 2011; 82:1375–81.
42. Schramm J. Temporal lobe epilepsy surgery and the quest for optimal extent of resection: a review. *Epilepsia* 2008; 49:1296–307.
43. Clusmann H, Schramm J, Kral T, Helmstaedter C, Ostertun B, Fimmers R, *et al.* Prognostic factors and outcome after different types of resection for temporal lobe epilepsy. *J Neurosurg* 2002; 97:1131–41.
44. Morino M, Uda T, Naito K, Yoshimura M, Ishibashi K, Goto T, *et al.* Comparison of neuropsychological outcomes after selective amygdalohippocampectomy versus anterior temporal lobectomy. *Epilepsy Behav* 2006; 9:95–100.
45. Helmstaedter C, Richter S, Roske S, Oltmanns F, Schramm J, Lehmann TN. Differential effects of temporal pole resection with amygdalohippocampectomy versus selective amygdalohippocampectomy on material-specific memory in patients with mesial temporal lobe epilepsy. *Epilepsia* 2008; 49:88–97.
46. Gleissner U, Helmstaedter C, Schramm J, Elger CE. Memory outcome after selective amygdalohippocampectomy: a study in 140 patients with temporal lobe epilepsy. *Epilepsia* 2002; 43:87–95.
47. Shimizu H, Kawai K, Sunaga S, Sugano H, Yamada T. Hippocampal transection for treatment of left temporal lobe epilepsy with preservation of verbal memory. *J Clin Neurosci* 2006; 13:322–8.
48. Shimizu H. Nonresective surgical procedures and electrical or magnetic stimulation for epilepsy treatment multiple hippocampal transection. In: Luders H (ed) *Textbook of Epilepsy Surgery*, pp. 1149–54. London: Informa Healthcare, 2008.
49. Patil AA, Andrews RV. Nonresective hippocampal surgery for epilepsy. *World Neurosurg* 2010; 74:645–9.
50. Van Wagenen WP, Herren RY. Surgical division of commissural pathways in the corpus callosum. *Arch Neurol Psychiatry* 1940; 44:740–59.
51. Roberts DW. The role of callosal section in surgical treatment of epilepsies. *Neurosurg Clin N Am* 1993; 4;293–300.
52. Roberts DW. Corpus callosotomy. In: Engel J, Pedley TA, eds. *Epilepsy: a comprehensive textbook*, pp. 1907–13. Philadelphia, PA: Wolters Kluwer Health/Lippincott Williams & Wilkins, 2008.
53. Spencer SS, Spencer DD, Sass K, Westerveld M, Katz A, Mattson R. Anterior, total, and two-stage corpus callosum section: differential and incremental seizure responses. *Epilepsia* 1993; 34:561–7.
54. Shim KW, Lee YM, Kim HD, Lee JS, Choi JU, Kim DS. Changing the paradigm of 1-stage total callosotomy for the treatment of pediatric generalized epilepsy. *J Neurosurg Pediatr* 2008; 2:29–36.
55. Tanriverdi T, Olivier A, Poulin N, Andermann F, Dubeau F. Long-term seizure outcome after corpus callosotomy: a retrospective analysis of 95 patients. *J Neurosurg* 2009; 110:332–42.
56. Sunaga S, Shimizu H, Sugano H. Long-term follow-up of seizure outcomes after corpus callosotomy. *Seizure* 2009; 18:124–8.
57. Jalilian L, Limbrick DD, Steger-May K, Johnston J, Powers AK, Smyth MD. Complete versus anterior two-thirds corpus callosotomy in children: analysis of outcome. *J Neurosurg Pediatr* 2010; 6:257–66.
58. Fuiks KS, Wyler AR, Hermann BP, Somes G. Seizure outcome from anterior and complete corpus callosotomy. *J Neurosurg* 1991; 74:573–8.
59. Mamelak AN, Barbaro NM, Walker JA, Laxer KD. Corpus callosotomy: a quantitative study of the extent of resection, seizure control, and neuropsychological outcome. *J Neurosurg* 1993; 79:688–95.
60. Spencer SS, Spencer DD, Williamson PD, Sass K, Novelly RA, Mattson RH. Corpus callosotomy for epilepsy. I. Seizure effects. *Neurology* 1988; 38:19–24.
61. Cukiert A, Burattini JA, Mariani PP, Yoshimura M, Ishibashi K, Goto T, *et al.* Extended, one-stage callosal section for treatment of refractory secondarily generalized epilepsy in patients with Lennox–Gastaut and Lennox-like syndromes. *Epilepsia* 2006; 47:371–4.
62. Wilson DH, Reeves AG, Gazzaniga MS. 'Central' commissurotomy for intractable generalized epilepsy: series two. *Neurology* 1982; 32:687–97.
63. Oguni H, Olivier A, Andermann F, Comair J. Anterior callosotomy in the treatment of medically intractable epilepsies: a study of 43 patients with a mean follow-up of 39 months. *Ann Neurol* 1991; 30:357–64.
64. Engel Jr J, Van Ness PC, Rasmussen TB, Ojemann LM. Outcome with respect to epileptic seizures. In: Engel Jr J (ed) *Surgical treatment of the epilepsies* (2nd edn), pp. 609–21. New York: Raven Press New York, 1993.
65. Spencer SS, Spencer DD, Glaser GH, Williamson PD, Mattson RH. More intense focal seizure types after callosal section: the role of inhibition. *Ann Neurol* 1984; 16:686–93.
66. Gates JR, Rosenfeld WE, Maxwell RE, Lyons RE. Response of multiple seizure types to corpus callosum section. *Epilepsia* 1987; 28:28–34.
67. Reutens DC, Bye AM, Hopkins IJ, Danks A, Somerville E, Walsh J, *et al.* Corpus callosotomy for intractable epilepsy: seizure outcome and prognostic factors. *Epilepsia* 1993; 34:904–9.
68. Maehara T, Shimizu H. Surgical outcome of corpus callosotomy in patients with drop attacks. *Epilepsia* 2001; 42:67–71.
69. Sass KJ, Spencer DD, Spencer SS, Novelly RA, Williamson PD, Mattson RH. Corpus callosotomy for epilepsy. II. Neurologic and neuropsychological outcome. *Neurology* 1988; 38:24–8.
70. Oguni H, Andermann F, Gotman J, Olivier A. Effect of anterior callosotomy on bilaterally synchronous spike and wave and other EEG discharges. *Epilepsia* 1994; 35:505–13.
71. Hanson RR, Risinger M, Maxwell R. The ictal EEG as a predictive factor for outcome following corpus callosum section in adults. *Epilepsy Res* 2002; 49:89–97.

72. Rathore C, Abraham M, Rao RM, George A, Sankara Sarma P, Radhakrishnan K. Outcome after corpus callosotomy in children with injurious drop attacks and severe mental retardation. *Brain Dev* 2007; 29:577–85.
73. Purves SJ, Wada JA, Woodhurst WB, Moyes PD, Strauss E, Kosaka B, *et al.* Results of anterior corpus callosum section in 24 patients with medically intractable seizures. *Neurology* 1988; 38:1194–201.
74. Fiol ME, Gates JR, Mireles R, Maxwell RE, Erickson DM. Value of intraoperative EEG changes during corpus callosotomy in predicting surgical results. *Epilepsia* 1993; 34:74–8.
75. Quattrini A, Papo I, Cesarano R, Fioravanti P, Paggi A, Ortenzi A, *et al.* EEG Patterns after callosotomy. *J Neurosurg Sci* 1997; 41:85–92.
76. McKenzie KG. The present status of a patient who had the right cerebral hemisphere removed. *JAMA* 1938; 111:168.
77. Falconer MA, Wilson PJ. Complications related to delayed hemorrhage after hemispherectomy. *J Neurosurg* 1969; 30:413–26.
78. Rasmussen T. Postoperative superficial hemosiderosis of the brain, its diagnosis, treatment and prevention. *Trans Am Neurol Assoc* 1973; 98:133–7.
79. Tuxhorn I, Holthausen H, Kotagal P, Pannek H. Hemispherectomy: post-surgical seizure frequency. In: Luders HO, ed. *Textbook of epilepsy surgery*, pp. 1249–53. London: Informa Healthcare, 2008.
80. Morino M, Shimizu H, Ohata K, Tanaka K, Hara M. Anatomical analysis of different hemispherotomy procedures based on dissection of cadaveric brains. *J Neurosurg* 2002; 97:423–31.
81. Mathern GW. Cerebral hemispherectomy: when half a brain is good enough. *Neurology* 2010; 75:1578–80.
82. Hallbook T, Ruggieri P, Adina C, Lachhwani DK, Gupta A, Kotagal P, *et al.* Contralateral MRI abnormalities in candidates for hemispherectomy for refractory epilepsy. *Epilepsia* 2010; 51:556–63.
83. Boshuisen K, van Schooneveld MM, Leijten FS, de Kort GA, van Rijen PC, Gosselaar PH, *et al.* Contralateral MRI abnormalities affect seizure and cognitive outcome after hemispherectomy. *Neurology* 2010; 75:1623–30.
84. Peacock WJ, Wehby-Grant MC, Shields WD, Shewmon DA, Chugani HT, Sankar R, *et al.* Hemispherectomy for intractable seizures in children: a report of 58 cases. *Childs Nerv Syst* 1996; 12:376–84.
85. Winston KR, Welch K, Adler JR, Erba G. Cerebral hemicorticectomy for epilepsy. *J Neurosurg* 1992; 77:889–95.
86. Davies KG, Maxwell RE, French LA. Hemispherectomy for intractable seizures: long-term results in 17 patients followed for up to 38 years. *J N*eurosurg 1993; 78:733–40.
87. Schramm J, Kral T, Clusmann H. Transsylvian keyhole functional hemispherectomy. *Neurosurgery* 2001; 49:891–900; discussion 900–1.
88. Schramm J, Clusmann H. The surgery of epilepsy. *Neurosurgery* 2008; 62(Suppl 2):463–81; discussion 81.
89. Kwan A, Ng WH, Otsubo H, Ochi A, Snead OC 3rd, Tamber MS, *et al.* Hemispherectomy for the control of intractable epilepsy in childhood: comparison of 2 surgical techniques in a single institution. *Neurosurgery* 2010; 67:429–36.
90. Shimizu H, Maehara T. Modification of peri-insular hemispherotomy and surgical results. *Neurosurgery* 2000; 47:367–72; discussion 372–3.
91. Cook SW, Nguyen ST, Hu B, Yudovin S, Shields WD, Vinters HV, *et al.* Cerebral hemispherectomy in pediatric patients with epilepsy: comparison of three techniques by pathological substrate in 115 patients. *J Neurosurg* 2004; 100:125–41.
92. Lindsay J, Ounsted C, Richards P. Hemispherectomy for childhood epilepsy: a 36-year study. *Dev Med Child Neurol* 1987; 29:592–600.
93. Wyllie E, Comair YG, Kotagal P, Raja S, Ruggieri P. Epilepsy surgery in infants. *Epilepsia* 1996; 37:625–37.
94. Basheer SN, Connolly MB, Lautzenhiser A, Sherman EM, Hendson G, Steinbok P. Hemispheric surgery in children with refractory epilepsy: seizure outcome, complications, and adaptive function. *Epilepsia* 2007; 48:133–40.
95. Villemure JG, Daniel RT. Peri-insular hemispherotomy in paediatric epilepsy. *Childs Nerv Syst* 2006; 22:967–81.
96. Graveline C, Hwang P, Bone G, Shikolka C, Wade S, Crawley A, *et al.* Evaluation of gross and fine motor functions in children with hemidecortication: predictors of outcomes and timing of surgery. *J Child Neurol* 1999; 14:304–15.
97. Ellenbogen RG, Cline MJ. Hemispherectomy: Historical perspective and current surgical overview. In: Miller JW, Silbergeld DL (eds) *Epilepsy surgery: principles and controversies*, pp. 563–76. New York: Taylor & Francis, 2005.
98. McClelland Sr, Maxwell RE. Hemispherectomy for intractable epilepsy in adults: the first reported series. *Ann Neurol* 2007; 61:372–6.

CHAPTER 32

Management of Seizures and of Epilepsy in the Emergency Department

Andrea O. Rossetti

Framing the problem: epidemiological data

Seizures represent a frequent challenge in the emergency department (ED) (1): in the US it has been estimated that yearly approximately 1 million people receive emergency treatment for seizures; of those, about 150,000 adults present with a first event, and many others with recurrent seizures; numbers in children are even higher. As a whole, this corresponds to at least 1–2% of ED admissions (2). The most common seizure type is the paediatric febrile convulsion, affecting up to 4% of children between 6 months and 6 years of age; subsequently, about 3.6% of the population will suffer from an acute symptomatic seizure (excluding febrile events), whereas 3% will be diagnosed at some point in life with epilepsy (3–5). A pre-hospital setting is frequently involved, as half of patients with seizures may arrive to the hospital by ambulance (6), and about 3% of ambulance transports are due to seizures (7), again with higher proportions (up to 9%) among the paediatric population (8, 9).

Probably reflecting underlying aetiologies, such as trauma and intoxications, males are about 1.5 times more prevalent than female subjects (2, 10); African Americans are also overrepresented as compared to Caucasians (2). Regarding age, an U-shaped curve is observed: while the yearly incidence of acute symptomatic seizures per 100,000 population in all age groups is about 40, infants show an incidence of 250, patients above 75 an incidence of 120, while middle-aged persons have an incidence of 15–40; this distribution is accounted for by febrile seizures or infections in children, and structural brain damage in elderly people (4). However, since the proportion of middle-aged persons in the population is higher than that of elderly, the absolute numbers are comparable across age strata (10).

While acute symptomatic seizures dominate the aetiological categories, about half of patients presenting with seizures to the ED have had previous episodes (2). In adults, the most common causes are related to alcohol or illicit drug intoxications (especially in the middle-aged group), trauma (younger group), cerebrovascular diseases (elderly), and previous epilepsy, including antiepileptic drug (AED) withdrawal (across all ages) (2, 10). Of note, it has been estimated that about 7% of ED seizures may represent status epilepticus (defined using a 30-minute time window) (6, 11). About one-quarter of seizure patients in the ED will be admitted to the hospital, especially if they are older and suffer from severe aetiologies or comorbidities (2). After a first ever seizure, mortality is clearly higher than in the standard population, principally owing to the underlying aetiology, with proportions around 14–18% at 6–12 months (10, 12, 13).

An American study estimated the median cost of an ED visit at 500 US$ in 2007; adding the average price of the ambulance ride (about 400 US$), the annual costs for emergency seizure care in the US may be set at around 700 million US$(1).

Facing the patient: differential diagnosis

Seizure-mimicking entities are very varied (14). Persons presenting to the ED with a suspicion of seizures fall basically into two categories: with or without loss of consciousness. In the latter setting, several other entities need to be ruled out at times. Migraine auras, which may mimic symptoms of partial seizures, last by definition more than 4 minutes, as opposed to the epileptic 'march' that develops over less than a couple of minutes. Movement disorders represent probably the most complex category from a semiological point of view (15, 16). Focal or segmental dystonias, especially if acute or paroxysmal, may be misdiagnosed as focal seizures; acute dystonias related to neuroleptic administration are usually confined to the larynx, face, and eyes; in paroxysmal disorders, the history often unravels typical triggering factors, such as movements, fasting, or exercise. Choreatic movements are usually obvious to an average experienced physician, but sometimes they may present unilaterally. Myoclonus is typically irregular, and may be accentuated by posturing or tactile stimulation, but focal seizures may be virtually identical (17). Tics are recognized by their predictable nature, and although they mostly represent a chronic condition, they may be enhanced by stress or metabolic disorders, as are abnormal startle reactions. Tremor related to Parkinsonism or other disorders may be uni- or bilateral, but often change amplitude (or disappear) after changing position. Clonus in the context of spasticity also disappears after a passive movement. Episodic ataxias are very rare, and their episodic nature (history taking!) leads to the diagnosis. Finally, "limb shaking" following transitory focal cerebrovascular involvement may also mimic focal seizures.

Facing a subject with continuing or resolved loss of consciousness, four main categories need to be considered in the differentiation

Table 32.1 Differential diagnosis between epileptic seizures and syncope

Item	Points
Lateral tongue bite	+ 2
Déjà-vu sensation	+ 1
Emotional stress	+ 1
Head turning during the spell	+ 1
Unresposive, or unusal posturing, or jerks during the spell	+ 1
Postictal confusion	+ 1
Lightheadedness	−2
Sweating	−2
Prolonged sitting or standing	−2

A score results after summing all the points. Score ≥1: the patient probably had an epileptic seizure; score <1: the patient probably had a syncope.
Adapted from Sheldon et al. (22).

from seizures: metabolic–toxic disturbances, syncope, psychogenic events, and, more rarely, sleep-related behaviours. In this context, syncope is much more frequent than seizures or other neuropsychiatic disorders: in the ED, more than 70% of patients with a history of a transitory consciousness impairment fall into this broad category, as compared to 15% with an unexplained cause, and 10% with a neurological or psychiatric origin (18–20). A careful history taking is, again, mandatory and greatly helps in the diagnosis. Syncope are typical preceded by symptoms of low brain blood perfusion, such as lightheadedness, impaired vision with a uniform grey-black character, impaired audition (such as if the patient was wearing earplugs), sweating, and nausea. Falling may be accompanied by a few uncoordinated jerks ("which are analogous to limb shaking", and whose duration may be overestimated by witnesses), and a by a pallor reflecting the preserved lung function and the impaired capillary perfusion. The duration is typically less than 30–60 seconds, and consciousness recovers rapidly, as soon as the body is in a recumbent position, unless a brain trauma has occurred (history taking with witnesses, and scalp inspection). At times, a minor anterior tongue bite may be observed, which is distinct from the often deep lateral scar seen after convulsive seizures (21). A potentially useful algorithm to differentiate seizures from syncopes has been proposed (22) (Table 32.1).

Psychogenic non-epileptic seizures (PNESs) resemble epileptic events but are not induced by neuronal hyperexcitation; although known since antiquity, they are increasingly recognized since the introduction of video-electroencephalography (EEG) some decades ago. They are reviewed in detail in Chapter 8. Their incidence is essentially unknown (23); the prevalence in the general population has been estimated at 2–33 per 100,000 (24), and up to 30–40% of patients referred to an EEG-monitoring unit for intractable seizures are diagnosed with PNES; about 10% of PNES patients also have concomitant epilepsy (25). PNES episodes, as opposed to seizures, are generally not stereotyped, suggestion-prone (in up to two-thirds of cases) (26), and may occur with or without consciousness impairment; eyes are often closed during the ictus (the specificity of this sign for PNES has been estimated at more than 90%) (27, 28); the episode may impose as uncoordinated, discontinuous, and fluctuating in intensity (29). Postictally, breathing is superficial, as opposed to the deep, slow breathing following generalized

Table 32.2 Differential diagnosis between epileptic seizures and psychogenic non-epileptic seizure (PNES)

Behavior	PNES	Epileptic seizures
Eyes	Frequently closed	Frequently open
Weeping	Possible	Exceptional ('dacrystic seizures')
Ictal movements	Multiform, uncoordinated, waxing-waning	Stereotyped, with clear start and stop
Ictal stuttering and postictal whispering	Possible	Exceptional
Ictal hyperventilation	Frequent	Exceptional
Postictal cough, nose wiping	Absent	Possible (temporal lobe seizures)
Postictal stertourous breathing	Absent	Possible (generalized convulsions)
Postictal rapid superficial breathing	Possible	Absent
Self injury	Possible	Possible
Tongue bite	Possible	Possible (generalized convulsions)
Incontinence	Possible	Possible

Adapted from LaFrance (29) and Rossetti and Kaplan (31).

epileptic convulsions (30), and during the intercritical period the patients often avoids eye contact with the examiner (31). Importantly, a physical injury may be observed in patients having PNES (32). Table 32.2 illustrates the most important discriminators between seizures and PNES. A definite PNES diagnosis can only be reached with video-EEG, and none of the mentioned clinical features is 100% specific of PNES: for example, while bilateral movements with preserved consciousness are frequently seen in PNES, these may be observed at times in generalized seizures of genetic origin (juvenile myoclonic epilepsy), or, even more rarely, during temporal lobe seizures (33). A considerable proportion of PNES patients show prolonged seizures that may be misdiagnosed as status epilepticus, leading to intensive care admission with considerable risks of overtreatment (34, 35); it is therefore paramount to suspect PNES early using the mentioned 'red flags'.

Abnormal behaviours and movements arising in sleep only, and characterized by incomplete transitions among the different states, are labelled as parasomnias (36). If related to non-rapid eye movement (REM) sleep, these are relatively frequent in childhood, where up to 20% of children may at times exhibit features of sleep-walking, nocturnal terrors, or confusional arousal, but their prevalence decreases in adulthood; there is often a family predisposition. Conversely, REM-sleep behaviour, characterized by an 'acting out' of dreams following loss of the physiological muscular atonia, is more frequent in elderly males, and may coexist with or precede neurodegenerative disorders, particularly synucleinopathies. In general, seizures tend to be briefer and present more stereotypically as compared to parasomnias (37), but without sleep video-EEG recordings diagnosis may prove difficult. An overview of useful features is given in Table 32.3.

To conclude this section, it is important to strengthen the value of a careful history taking, including interrogation of witnesses, not only to support a 'positive' diagnosis, but also to avoid

Table 32.3 Differential diagnosis between nocturnal epileptic seizures and parasomnias

Item	Nocturnal seizures	Parasomnias
Age	All ages	Children >adults
Duration	Short (<2 minutes)	May be >5 minutes
Frequency	Clusters, more on one night	Few per week
Occurrence	Stage 2 NREM-sleep	Stage 3 NREM-sleep, or REM-sleep
Symptoms	Paroxysmal arousal, focal dystonia, or (rare) complex movements	Mostly complex movements
Stereotypy	High	Low
Morning event recall	May be precise	Vague

NREM, non-rapid-eyes movement; REM, rapid-eyes movement.
Adapted from Derry et al. (37).

Table 32.4 Items to be assessed in an emergency setting facing a patient with seizures

Feature	Comment
Previous history of seizures	Orients the diagnostic work-up
Antiepileptic medication and compliance	Consider administration of the habitual medication
Use of illicit drugs/alcohol	Consider administration of thiamine
Timing (seizure start, duration)	Orients towards the presence of status epilepticus
Seizure semiology	More aggressive treatment if generalized convulsive
Concomitant health problems (diabetes!)	Consider glucose/thiamine administration
Pregnancy	Consider eclampsia and magnesium sulphate administration

Adapted from Michael and O'Connor (44).

misdiagnosis of epileptic seizures implying not only a fastidious and expensive work-up, but also a potential burden for the patient and the relatives. A minimal checklist is given in Table 32.4.

Understand what happened: diagnostic procedures

Once the diagnosis of seizure has been suspected, the diagnostic work-up has to be tailored to the situation. There are two distinctive clinical situations: first ever seizure, or recurrence in a patient already known for previous seizures. In both situations, there can be triggering factors thus generating four scenarios. In each case, the neurological examination should be considered the first 'active' test after history taking, and may orient early upon potentially life-threatening conditions (e.g. neck rigidity; stupor with risk of aspiration; petechial haemorrhages heralding a meningococcal sepsis), as well as disclose important clues regarding the seizure focus (e.g. postictal paralysis) (38). Diagnostic procedures are summarized in Table 32.5.

Table 32.5 Diagnostic procedures in patients with a suspected seizure in the emergency department

Procedure	Evidence-based	Situations when indicated
History and clinical examination	No	Always
EEG	Yes	Always in first seizures, on a patient-by-patient basis if previous seizures
CT/MRI	Yes	Always in first seizures[a], on a patient-by-patient basis if previous seizures
Laboratory (blood count, glucose, electrolytes)	No	Large panel in first seizures, on a patient-by-patient basis if previous seizures
Toxicology screen	No	Suspicion of illicit drug/medication intoxication
Lumbar puncture	No	Suspicion of meningoencephalitis
AED level	No	Suspicion of AED withdrawal or intoxication in a patient with epilepsy
Lactate	No	Suspicion of PNES vs. generalized convulsion
Prolactine	No	Suspicion of PNES vs. other loss of consciousness (seizure, syncope); repeat after 24 hours
Creatine-kinase	No	Suspicion of PNES vs. generalized convulsion
Provocative manoeuvres	No	Suspicion of PNES, under video-EEG

[a] If the EEG suggests a genetic ('idiopathic generalized') epilepsy, the test may be skipped.
AED, antiepileptic drug; PNES, psychogenic non-epileptic seizure.

The most challenging situation is the first seizure without evident provoking factors. The American Academy of Neurology (AAN) published an evidence-based practice guideline for children with non-febrile seizures; only the EEG is recommended as a standard evaluation following history taking and clinical examination, while laboratory studies, lumbar puncture, and neuroimaging are proposed only based on specific circumstances (39). More recently, this issue was also addressed for adults using the same evidence-based approach. EEG is probably helpful, with 29% of recordings unravelling 'significant abnormalities' that may predict the risk of seizure recurrence (one Class I, ten Class II studies; Level B) (40); this proportion is almost identical to a Swiss prospective survey, where 34% of EEGs after a first seizure showed epileptiform discharges, and an additional 43% unspecific abnormalities (10). Moreover, EEG results can be integrated in the classification of seizures and epilepsies. It seems advisable to perform the EEG as early as possible, since the frequency of interictal discharges tend to diminish after hours following a seizure (41). Neuroimaging studies, including computed tomography (CT) and magnetic resonance imaging (MRI), are also probably useful, with a yield of about 10%, potentially disclosing the presence of brain tumours, stroke, or other structural abnormalities (seven Class II studies, Level B) (40). An exception to the routine prescription of brain imaging may be represented by the occurrence of a first seizure in a patient with probable genetic epilepsy ('idiopathic generalized epilepsy') according to the EEG, and in absence of a head trauma.

Blood count, blood glucose, and electrolyte testing are not felt to be essential, although some abnormal results occur (two Class II and four Class III studies; Level U) (40). The use of these tests should be adapted to the specific situation; this illustrates the limits of evidence-based guidelines, and is highlighted in the aforementioned Swiss survey, where 57% of the patients with a first seizure had laboratory abnormalities potentially related to the cause or the consequence of the seizure (10). Moreover, although relatively rare, seizure generated by hypoglycaemia or non-ketotic hyperglycaemia should not be overlooked, and are readily treatable if recognized early; furthermore, metabolic disturbances may both mimic or cause seizures. Given its relatively modest cost (as compared to brain imaging and EEG), a panel including an automated blood count, glucose, sodium, calcium, albumin, C-reactive protein, creatinine, and hepatic transaminases seems reasonable in patients with first-ever seizures. Furthermore, the selective determination of serum prolactin may prove useful to differentiate a preceding loss of consciousness (due to a seizure or syncope, with raised levels) from PNES (during which the patient is not unconscious, with normal levels) (42). It is important to measure this hormone level within 20 minutes of the event, and to recheck it after 24 hours, in order to account for the circadian and cyclic (in women of childbearing age) variability of its levels. Lactic acidosis detected early after an episode is strongly suggestive of an epileptic convulsion, since during syncope and PNES the patient does breathe and muscles do not suffer from hypoxia (43). Finally, elevated creatine kinase levels can occur after epileptic convulsions, especially if prolonged, but not after PNES (34); the kinetics of this enzyme require, however, the test to be performed after at least 6–12 hours following the event. Toxicological screening and a lumbar tap are not clearly supported by evidence: studies report indeed selected populations (two Class III studies for both, Level U for both). Both should be carried out in cases where the clinician actively suspects an intoxication, or meningoencephalitis. Determination of serum AED levels may be useful in patients with epilepsy, but only if withdrawal or intoxication is suspected.

If a patient without a previous history of epilepsy presents with a seizure provoked by a potentially reversible condition, and the latter is identified (e.g. alcohol withdrawal, hypoglycaemia, acute stroke), the above-mentioned diagnostic procedures should still be applied, with more focused laboratory testing. Indeed, EEG and brain imaging can identify conditions that result in a lowered threshold for seizures: if, for example, a subject with a seizure following alcohol withdrawal has generalized spike-and-waves on the EEG, it is advisable to repeat the recording after the withdrawal in order to rule out a possible genetic epilepsy. The same patient may have an acute cerebral contusion that needs treatment in its own right.

For patients with an already established diagnosis of epilepsy, the work-up can be even more focused. A targeted approach of the underlying cause appears sufficient if this is evident (e.g. AED withdrawal, intercurrent infection), and in the absence of a head trauma or a progressive brain disorder (such as a primary tumour). If, conversely, the aetiology is obscure, the previously mentioned panel of tests should be applied. Often though brain imaging or EEG is unnecessary if the patient has completely recovered and experienced no head trauma.

Help the patient: treatment

The common practice, especially in the pre-hospital setting, of administering benzodiazepines to patients with seizures should clearly be discouraged (44), since it has no evidence base, and generates a prolonged postictal state complicating clinical assessment and having potential complications (i.e. bronchoaspiration resulting in tracheal intubation). Benzodiazepine administration should be reserved for situations of impending or manifest status epilepticus, which in adults is operationally defined as a seizure lasting for more than 5 minutes, or distinct seizures occurring without a complete recovery of the baseline state (45). This time frame is longer in children (10–5 minutes). In any case, it appears useful to obtain early an intravenous line in order to facilitate diagnostic and therapeutic steps (44). There is no need to force any object into the patient's mouth, as the tongue does not 'fall backwards' during a seizure, the force of the tonic–clonic mandibular contractions may easily put the fingers of the helper at risk, and—conversely—the teeth of the patient can be damaged from these actions (44). The seizing patient should nevertheless be protected from falling and injury, and be turned towards the recovery position as soon as the convulsion stops, for the period of the postictal state to resolve. Facing a subject experiencing a partial-complex seizure (or a confusional postictal state without deep consciousness impairment), it is helpful to bear in mind that attempts at restraint may result in an untargeted, defensive, but at time aggressive behaviour from the patient. Discussion of targeted treatment towards the aetiology of seizures in this situation is beyond the scope of this chapter, but should receive full attention as it probably represents the best prevention from seizure recurrence.

Deciding whether or not to institute AED therapy depends on the evaluation of the risk of seizure recurrence, and is guided by the diagnostic work-up. Patients with at least a putative diagnosis of epilepsy, and not only of provoked seizures, should be considered for a long-term treatment. To quantify the problem, in untreated patients at 2 years the Italian FIRST study identified a recurrence risk of 51% (46), while a more recent large European multicenter study (MESS) hold an estimate at 39% (47). Three factors appear consistently associated with a seizure relapse both in children and adults: the number of previous seizures, an abnormal EEG, especially if showing epileptiform transients (48), and a symptomatic cause (diagnosed through an abnormal neurological exam and/or brain imaging study) (49). In the MESS trial, patients with both normal EEG and neurological examination had a recurrence risk of 25% at 2 years; the relative risk increased by 1.35 if a symptomatic neurological disorder (abnormal neurological examination, brain imaging), and by 1.5 if an abnormal EEG were found (47). Patients with multiple seizures had a 1.5 higher risk of further seizures compared to patients with only one seizure (50). Other observational studies have reported similar results (51, 52). Status epilepticus at presentation bears a three times higher risk of seizure recurrence as compared to a short seizure (53). If a first seizure occurs during sleep, the recurrence risk appears greater compared to episodes arising from wakefulness (48, 54, 55), although this tendency may be in part explained by the possibility of the prior occurrence of unrecognized and undiagnosed seizures during sleep (49). Risk factors for seizure recurrence are summarized in Table 32.6.

A recent careful meta-analysis of six studies addressing the risk of seizure recurrence in patients treated versus non-treated with an AED after a first seizure showed a risk reduction of about 34% favouring the treated group. However, the MESS study clearly shows that AED treatment does not influence long-term prognosis. The study compared patients having received an early versus deferred treatment (the latter experienced thus more seizures before

Table 32.6 Risk factors associated with seizure recurrence

Feature	Comment
Abnormal EEG	Especially if showing epileptiform transients
Symptomatic cause	Summarized by abnormal neurological examination and brain imaging
Number of previous seizures	Does not influence likelihood of seizure control
Sleep-related seizures	May be a confounder number of previous seizures
Status epilepticus	High likelihood of developing epilepsy

treatment). A reduction of early seizure recurrence was observed (32% vs. 39% at 2 years), but there was no difference in terms of 2-year remission rates at 5 and 8 years (92%, 95%) (50). Due to differences inherent to the different studied populations and protocols, the FIRST study showed very similar results. While the recurrence rate at 2 years was 50% lower in the treated group (46), the chance of a 5-year remission at 10 years was identical (64% in both arms) (56). These results do not support Gower's theory that 'seizures beget seizures' (57), and suggest that epilepsy does not represent an entity progressing ominously if untreated early and that AED administration should rather not be initiated if significant doubts on an epilepsy diagnosis exist. This is highlighted in the AAN guidelines on treatment of children with first unprovoked seizures, where in view of potential side effects related to AED and the lack of evidence supporting an impact of the treatment on epilepsy development, an individualized approach is advocated (Level B) (58). Similar thoughts may apply for adults, also in view of the risk of discrimination and stigma related to epilepsy. On the other hand, regulatory implications on the quality of life, especially regarding driving, may affect the decision in this age group.

In summary, it appears reasonable to counsel a patient towards initiation of AED treatment if the diagnosis of epilepsy, intended as a first seizure together with an enduring condition implying a risk of seizure recurrence (59), is supported by complementary examinations. The choice of the AED may be made from more than 30 substances on the market, and—given major pharmacological implications—should involve, at least at the beginning, a neurologist with experience in seizure disorders. An overview of AED therapy is found in Chapter 26. As opposed to patients having seizures provoked by reversible causes, which do not need a specific treatment, those experiencing a first seizure due to an acute aetiology that may, in part, endure (e.g. brain contusion, stroke) should receive an AED for a period of weeks or months. There is, however, no evidence that continuing treatment on a long-term basis, in the absence of clear evidence of an increased risk of recurrence, is beneficial. In this context, follow-up EEGs may help in counselling the patient.

References

1. Martindale JL, Goldstein JN, Pallin DJ. Emergency department seizure epidemiology. *Emerg Med Clin North Am* 2011; 29(1):15–27.
2. Pallin DJ, Goldstein JN, Moussally JS, Pelletier AJ, Green AR, Camargo CA, Jr. Seizure visits in US emergency departments: epidemiology and potential disparities in care. *Int J Emerg Med* 2008; 1(2):97–105.
3. Febrile seizures: clinical practice guideline for the long-term management of the child with simple febrile seizures. *Pediatrics* 2008; 121(6):1281–6.
4. Annegers JF, Hauser WA, Lee JR, Rocca WA. Incidence of acute symptomatic seizures in Rochester, Minnesota, 1935–1984. *Epilepsia* 1995; 36(4):327–33.
5. Hauser WA, Annegers JF, Rocca WA. Descriptive epidemiology of epilepsy: contributions of population-based studies from Rochester, Minnesota. *Mayo Clin Proc* 1996; 71(6):576–86.
6. Krumholz A, Grufferman S, Orr ST, Stern BJ. Seizures and seizure care in an emergency department. *Epilepsia* 1989; 30(2):175–81.
7. Brokaw J, Olson L, Fullerton L, Tandberg D, Sklar D. Repeated ambulance use by patients with acute alcohol intoxication, seizure disorder, and respiratory illness. *Am J Emerg Med* 1998; 16(2):141–4.
8. Knight S, Vernon DD, Fines RJ, Dean NP. Prehospital emergency care for children at school and nonschool locations. *Pediatrics* 1999; 103(6):e81.
9. Tsai A, Kallsen G. Epidemiology of pediatric prehospital care. *Ann Emerg Med* 1987; 16(3):284–92.
10. Kawkabani A, Rossetti AO, Despland PA. Survey of management of first-ever seizures in a hospital based community. *Swiss Med Wkly* 2004; 134(39–40):586–92.
11. Huff JS, Morris DL, Kothari RU, Gibbs MA. Emergency department management of patients with seizures: a multicenter study. *Acad Emerg Med* 2001; 8(6):622–8.
12. Loiseau J, Picot MC, Loiseau P. Short-term mortality after a first epileptic seizure: a population-based study. *Epilepsia* 1999; 40(10):1388–92.
13. MacDonald BK, Johnson AL, Goodridge DM, Cockerell OC, Sander JW, Shorvon SD. Factors predicting prognosis of epilepsy after presentation with seizures. *Ann Neurol* 2000; 48(6):833–41.
14. Crompton DE, Berkovic SF. The borderland of epilepsy: clinical and molecular features of phenomena that mimic epileptic seizures. *Lancet Neurol* 2009; 8(4):370–81.
15. Onofrj M, Bonanni L, Cossu G, Manca D, Stocchi F, Thomas A. Emergencies in parkinsonism: akinetic crisis, life-threatening dyskinesias, and polyneuropathy during L-Dopa gel treatment. *Parkinsonism Relat Disord* 2009; 15(Suppl 3):S233–6.
16. Poston KL, Frucht SJ. Movement disorder emergencies. *J Neurol* 2008; 255(Suppl 4):2–13.
17. Mameniskiene R, Bast T, Bentes C, Canevini MP, Dimova P, Granata T, *et al.* Clinical course and variability of non-Rasmussen, nonstroke motor and sensory epilepsia partialis continua: A European survey and analysis of 65 cases. *Epilepsia* 2011; 52(6):1168–76.
18. Linzer M, Yang EH, Estes NA, 3rd, Wang P, Vorperian VR, Kapoor WN. Diagnosing syncope. Part 2: Unexplained syncope. Clinical Efficacy Assessment Project of the American College of Physicians. *Ann Intern Med* 1997; 127(1):76–86.
19. Linzer M, Yang EH, Estes NA, 3rd, Wang P, Vorperian VR, Kapoor WN. Diagnosing syncope. Part 1: Value of history, physical examination, and electrocardiography. Clinical Efficacy Assessment Project of the American College of Physicians. *Ann Intern Med* 1997; 126(12):989–96.
20. Sarasin FP, Louis-Simonet M, Carballo D, Slama S, Junod AF, Unger PF. Prevalence of orthostatic hypotension among patients presenting with syncope in the ED. *Am J Emerg Med* 2002; 20(6):497–501.
21. Benbadis SR, Wolgamuth BR, Goren H, Brener S, Fouad-Tarazi F. Value of tongue biting in the diagnosis of seizures. *Arch Intern Med* 1995; 155(21):2346–9.
22. Sheldon R, Rose S, Ritchie D, Connolly SJ, Koshman ML, Lee MA, *et al.* Historical criteria that distinguish syncope from seizures. *J Am Coll Cardiol* 2002; 40(1):142–8.
23. Siket MS, Merchant RC. Psychogenic seizures: A review and description of pitfalls in their acute diagnosis and management in the emergency department. *Emerg Med Clin North Am* 2011; 29(1):73–81.
24. Benbadis SR, Allen Hauser W. An estimate of the prevalence of psychogenic non-epileptic seizures. *Seizure* 2000; 9(4):280–1.

25. Benbadis SR, Agrawal V, Tatum WO. How many patients with psychogenic nonepileptic seizures also have epilepsy? *Neurology* 2001; 57(5):915–7.
26. Benbadis SR, Siegrist K, Tatum WO, Heriaud L, Anthony K. Short-term outpatient EEG video with induction in the diagnosis of psychogenic seizures. *Neurology* 2004; 63(9):1728–30.
27. Chung SS, Gerber P, Kirlin KA. Ictal eye closure is a reliable indicator for psychogenic nonepileptic seizures. *Neurology* 2006; 66(11):1730–1.
28. Syed TU, Arozullah AM, Suciu GP, Toub J, Kim H, Dougherty ML, *et al.* Do observer and self-reports of ictal eye closure predict psychogenic nonepileptic seizures? *Epilepsia* 2008; 49(5):898–904.
29. LaFrance WC, Jr. Psychogenic nonepileptic seizures. *Curr Opin Neurol* 2008; 21(2):195–201.
30. Azar NJ, Tayah TF, Wang L, Song Y, Abou-Khalil BW. Postictal breathing pattern distinguishes epileptic from nonepileptic convulsive seizures. *Epilepsia* 2008; 49(1):132–7.
31. Rossetti AO, Kaplan PW. Seizure semiology: an overview of the 'inverse problem'. *Eur Neurol* 2010; 63(1):3–10.
32. Reuber M, Pukrop R, Bauer J, Helmstaedter C, Tessendorf N, Elger CE. Outcome in psychogenic nonepileptic seizures: 1 to 10-year follow-up in 164 patients. *Ann Neurol* 2003; 53(3):305–11.
33. Nogueira RG, Sheth KN, Duffy FH, Helmers SL, Bromfield EB. Bilateral tonic-clonic seizures with temporal onset and preservation of consciousness. *Neurology* 2008; 70(22 Pt 2):2188–90.
34. Holtkamp M, Othman J, Buchheim K, Meierkord H. Diagnosis of psychogenic nonepileptic status epilepticus in the emergency setting. *Neurology* 2006; 66(11):1727–9.
35. Reuber M, Baker GA, Gill R, Smith DF, Chadwick DW. Failure to recognize psychogenic nonepileptic seizures may cause death. *Neurology* 2004; 62(5):834–5.
36. Avidan AY. Parasomnias and movement disorders of sleep. *Semin Neurol* 2009; 29(4):372–92.
37. Derry CP, Davey M, Johns M, Kron K, Glencross D, Marini C, *et al.* Distinguishing sleep disorders from seizures: diagnosing bumps in the night. *Arch Neurol* 2006; 63(5):705–9.
38. Gallmetzer P, Leutmezer F, Serles W, Assem-Hilger E, Spatt J, Baumgartner C. Postictal paresis in focal epilepsies—incidence, duration, and causes: a video-EEG monitoring study. *Neurology* 2004; 62(12):2160–4.
39. Hirtz D, Ashwal S, Berg A, Bettis D, Camfield C, Camfield P, *et al.* Practice parameter: evaluating a first nonfebrile seizure in children: report of the quality standards subcommittee of the American Academy of Neurology, The Child Neurology Society, and The American Epilepsy Society. *Neurology* 2000; 55(5):616–23.
40. Krumholz A, Wiebe S, Gronseth G, Shinnar S, Levisohn P, Ting T, *et al.* Practice Parameter: evaluating an apparent unprovoked first seizure in adults (an evidence-based review): report of the Quality Standards Subcommittee of the American Academy of Neurology and the American Epilepsy Society. *Neurology* 2007; 69(21):1996–2007.
41. Gotman J, Koffler DJ. Interictal spiking increases after seizures but does not after decrease in medication. *Electroencephalogr Clin Neurophysiol* 1989; 72(1):7–15.
42. Chen DK, So YT, Fisher RS. Use of serum prolactin in diagnosing epileptic seizures: report of the Therapeutics and Technology Assessment Subcommittee of the American Academy of Neurology. *Neurology* 2005; 65(5):668–75.
43. Lipka K, Bulow HH. Lactic acidosis following convulsions. *Acta Anaesthesiol Scand* 2003; 47(5):616–18.
44. Michael GE, O'Connor RE. The diagnosis and management of seizures and status epilepticus in the prehospital setting. *Emerg Med Clin North Am* 2011; 29(1):29–39.
45. Lowenstein DH, Bleck T, Macdonald RL. It's time to revise the definition of status epilepticus. *Epilepsia* 1999; 40(1):120–2.
46. First Seizure Trial Group (FIR.S.T. Group). Randomized clinical trial on the efficacy of antiepileptic drugs in reducing the risk of relapse after a first unprovoked tonic-clonic seizure. *Neurology* 1993; 43(3 Pt 1):478–83.
47. Kim LG, Johnson TL, Marson AG, Chadwick DW. Prediction of risk of seizure recurrence after a single seizure and early epilepsy: further results from the MESS trial. *Lancet Neurol* 2006; 5(4):317–22.
48. Hopkins A, Garman A, Clarke C. The first seizure in adult life. Value of clinical features, electroencephalography, and computerised tomographic scanning in prediction of seizure recurrence. *Lancet* 1988; 1(8588):721–6.
49. Berg AT. Risk of recurrence after a first unprovoked seizure. *Epilepsia* 2008; 49(Suppl 1):13–8.
50. Marson A, Jacoby A, Johnson A, Kim L, Gamble C, Chadwick D. Immediate versus deferred antiepileptic drug treatment for early epilepsy and single seizures: a randomised controlled trial. *Lancet* 2005; 365(9476):2007–13.
51. Berg AT, Shinnar S. The risk of seizure recurrence following a first unprovoked seizure: a quantitative review. *Neurology* 1991; 41(7):965–72.
52. Kho LK, Lawn ND, Dunne JW, Linto J. First seizure presentation: do multiple seizures within 24 hours predict recurrence? *Neurology*. 2006; 67(6):1047–9.
53. Hesdorffer DC, Logroscino G, Cascino G, Annegers JF, Hauser WA. Risk of unprovoked seizure after acute symptomatic seizure: effect of status epilepticus. *Ann Neurol* 1998; 44(6):908–12.
54. Bora I, Seckin B, Zarifoglu M, Turan F, Sadikoglu S, Ogul E. Risk of recurrence after first unprovoked tonic-clonic seizure in adults. *J Neurol* 1995; 242(3):157–63.
55. Shinnar S, Berg AT, O'Dell C, Newstein D, Moshe SL, Hauser WA. Predictors of multiple seizures in a cohort of children prospectively followed from the time of their first unprovoked seizure. *Ann Neurol* 2000; 48(2):140–7.
56. Leone MA, Solari A, Beghi E. Treatment of the first tonic-clonic seizure does not affect long-term remission of epilepsy. *Neurology* 2006; 67(12):2227–9.
57. Gowers W. *Epilepsy and other chronic convulsive disorders: their causes, symptoms and treatment.* London: J&A Churchill, 1881.
58. Hirtz D, Berg A, Bettis D, Camfield C, Camfield P, Crumrine P, *et al.* Practice parameter: treatment of the child with a first unprovoked seizure: Report of the Quality Standards Subcommittee of the American Academy of Neurology and the Practice Committee of the Child Neurology Society. *Neurology* 2003; 60(2):166–75.
59. Fisher RS, van Emde Boas W, Blume W, Elger C, Genton P, Lee P, *et al.* Epileptic seizures and epilepsy: definitions proposed by the International League Against Epilepsy (ILAE) and the International Bureau for Epilepsy (IBE). *Epilepsia* 2005; 46(4):470–2.

CHAPTER 33

Management of Status Epilepticus on the Intensive Care Unit

Erich Schmutzhard and Bettina Pfausler

Introduction

Within half an hour of generalized convulsive status epilepticus (GCSE) centrally mediated increases in adrenaline and noradrenaline lead to highly elevated blood pressure, increased cardiac output, and an increase of plasma glucose as well as cerebral blood flow. However, with progressing GCSE progressing respiratory acidosis accompanies impairment of respiration, aggravated by bronchial constriction and an increase in bronchial secretions. Beyond 60 minutes respiratory acidosis deteriorates, gas exchange being highly impaired, partial pressure of oxygen (pO_2) progressively reduced, and partial pressure of carbon dioxide (pCO_2) increased/retained. Hypotension, acidosis, hyper/hypoglycaemia, and hyperpyrexia increase acute morbidity, long-term morbidity, and mortality (1–3). Later on, GCSE may lead to rhabdomyolysis, impeding renal function and adding to acidosis, thus increasing morbidity and mortality (4). At the same time the blood–brain barrier is progressively disrupted with increased protein in the cerebrospinal fluid (3, 5, 6).

However, these metabolic derangements are not the only causes of brain injury due to GSCE; even if oxygen supply, body temperature, and all metabolic derangements are sufficiently controlled, neuronal damage still occurs and continues as a direct result of electrical seizures and neuronal depolarizations, adding to neurological long-term sequelae as cognitive impairment and memory loss (1, 6, 7). This is explained by the fact that prolonged status epilepticus (SE) results in neuronal cell loss in hippocampus pyramidal layers (2).

Intravenous anticonvulsant agents, the implementation of intensive care and neurocritical care, in particular, and increased awareness in the emergency medical community has led to decreasing morbidity and, in particular, mortality of GCSE (1, 2, 5–7). Nevertheless, any type of SE, and in particular, overt GCSE is still a major neurological emergency, and carries a mortality of up to 35% within the first 30 days (5). In most instances, mortality, being a function of age, duration, and aetiology, is mainly related to the underlying aetiology of SE (6–8). In a meta-analysis of 12 published reports (published 20–40 years ago) only 3% of the deaths could be directly linked to the GCSE itself. It might be surmised that with the advancement of neurocritical care and intensive care medicine in particular, these figures (but especially the mortality rate directly linked to the status itself/to intensive care management) will improve (9, 10).

This chapter deals with the intensive care management of patients with SE, the indication for admission to an intensive care unit (ICU)/neurocritical care unit, and stresses the complications of SE and, finally, focuses on the complications of the intensive care management steps/strategies.

Classification

Five major subtypes of SE are potential causes of intensive care management (1, 9):

1. Overt GCSE
2. Complex partial status epilepticus (CPSE)
3. Subclinical or subtle GCSE (frequently referred to as myoclonic status)
4. Partial or focal SE
5. Absence SE (petit mal status).

GCSE is the most common subtype of SE, being characterized by repetitive or continuous tonic and clonic motor activity with loss of consciousness. In the ictal electroencephalogram (EEG), bilateral epileptiform discharges are seen. If allowed to progress untreated, GCSE may evolve into 'subtle' or subclinical GCSE; in such patients minimal twitching movements of the eyelids, fingers, or in the facial muscles may be the only clinical manifestation of the SE (1, 9). However, the evolution of GCSE into subtle GCSE is associated with worsening of coma and higher morbidity and mortality (1, 9). Subtle GCSE is highly refractory to treatment carrying a higher mortality rate than overt GCSE. In a series of 94 head trauma victims, 11 had subclinical seizures, six of these 11 patients were in subtle generalized convulsive status, all of them eventually died (10). Absence SE and CPSE as well as partial/focal SE are rarely admitted to the intensive care unit, thus these conditions are not considered further here.

Box 33.1 Algorithm

- Intubation should be performed after the administration of a barbiturate bolus of 3–5 mg/kg body weight (e.g. thiopental). This dosage usually allows sufficient 'relaxation' to facilitate the placement of the endotracheal tube.
- Neuromuscular blockade should not be given in these patients; however, if absolutely necessary, vecuronium 0.1 mg/kg body weight can be considered.
- Monitor body temperature, maintain normothermia.
- Pentobarbital 5–15 mg/kg body weight over 1 hour (or thiopental 3–7 mg/kg/hour), then continue pentobarbital 0.5–5 mg/kg/hour (or continue thiopental at a rate of 1–3 mg/kg/hour) until seizures are controlled.
- Monitor with continuous EEG
- Intra-arterial line for blood gas analysis, invasive blood pressure monitoring.
- Invasive haemodynamic monitoring, e.g. PiCCO® or even more invasive monitoring.
- Titrate the dosage of barbiturates against EEG burst suppression pattern.
- Fluid management, aggressive fluid balancing, if necessary catecholamines.
- Monitoring must be on high alert to recognize any incipient nosocomial infection (regular culturing of body fluids, regular C-reactive protein, procalcitonin, white blood cell count, etc.).

Alternatives

1. Midazolam 0.2 mg/kg body weight intravenously as a bolus, followed by 1–2 mg/kg/minute for 12–24 hours.
2. Monitor with continuous EEG and blood pressure monitoring in ICU setting.
3. Propofol 1 mg/kg over 6 minutes, then 1–5 mg/kg/hour.
4. Attempt to taper after 12–24 hours.
5. Watch for hypotension and the propofol infusion syndrome.
6. Monitor with continuous EEG and blood pressure monitoring in ICU setting.

ICU management of overt GCSE

Given the risk of hypotension, respiratory depression, and metabolic acidosis, high-quality monitoring is essential in the emergency management of a patient with SE (5). If a patient with GCSE evolves into early refractory GCSE, immediate admission to a monitoring unit, even better, to an ICU (preferably a neurocritical care unit) is indicated (1, 3, 9, 10). Pulse oximetry is regularly recommended in the emergency setting as well as an oxygen supply (9, 10). However, it must be stressed that pulse oximetry can never be sufficient, and blood gas analysis must be done at the earliest possible point of time, since the increase of pCO_2 is usually not paralleled by the decrease of the pO_2. Therefore pure and only pulse oximetry is not sufficient in the emergency setting and never in the ICU setting. The immediate establishment of an intravenous line is essential, along with continuous blood pressure monitoring and ECG recording.

Treatment must never be delayed in the neurological emergency setting of a GCSE. History taking, physical examination, and primary laboratory examinations (blood gas analysis, blood glucose) must be completed rapidly (5). If in the recommended algorithm for the treatment of a generalized convulsive status the first- and second-line anticonvulsants have not terminated the GCSE, the patient needs urgent admission to an ICU, intubation, and artificial ventilation. Box 33.1 lists the recommended algorithm immediately after the admission to the neuro-ICU (1, 3, 5, 9, 10).

Adverse effects of barbiturate agents

Depending on the dosage and duration of barbiturate therapy, side effects include haemodynamic instability, leading to distributive shock, immunosuppression, and reduced gastrointestinal motility. All these side effects may limit the dose and the duration of therapy with barbiturates (2)

Patients with cardiopulmonary instability, i.e. distributive shock, need invasive blood pressure monitoring, invasive and haemodynamic monitoring, e.g. PiCCO® or even more invasive monitoring methods such as a pulmonary artery catheter (11–15). Depending on these monitoring findings, patients on barbiturate therapy need sufficient fluid management, aggressive fluid balancing, and, in most instances, catecholamines.

Haemodynamic instability potentially leading to distributive shock, reduces the cerebral perfusion and adds to injury of neuronal intracranial structures (3).

It must also be borne in mind that barbiturates lead to immunosuppression, increasing the risk of nosocomial infections, e.g. catheter-associated bloodstream infections, nosocomial ventilator-associated pneumonia, urinary tract infection, and even intestinal infection (12). Therefore careful monitoring to identify as early as possible any incipient nosocomial infection is vital. Regular culturing of body fluids, C-reactive protein, procalcitonin, white blood cell count, differential count on (at least) a daily basis are recommended (16).

Barbiturates lead to reduced gastrointestinal motility, which is particularly important in patients with haemodynamic instability, or even distributive shock, necessitating a liberal use of catecholamines. The effect of these catecholamines on the peripheral vascular system increases the blood pressure by peripheral vasoconstriction; this effect may add to the risk of nosocomial infection since the vasoconstriction may lead to (incomplete) ischaemia in the gastrointestinal wall (3). This specifically holds true in patients on therapeutic agents which reduce, per se, gastrointestinal motility. For this reason, patients on barbiturates with reduced gastrointestinal motility who require high-dose catecholamines are at high risk of experiencing transmural translocation of intestinal bacteria, e.g. Gram-negative rods (such as Enterobacteriaceae, *Escherichia coli*, or, even *Clostridia* species, etc.) (16). The intensivist must react rapidly to the clinical signs and symptoms of septic shock and/or a rapid increase of 'inflammatory parameters' (C-reactive protein, white blood cell count, procalcitonin) with the appropriate empiric antimicrobial chemotherapy. This requires best knowledge of the resistance pattern, in particular, of the Gram-negative bacteria seen in patients of the respective ICU. In the case of the occurrence of extended-spectrum beta-lactamases or carbapenemase producing Gram negatives, the empiric antimicrobial chemotherapy might even necessitate the use of polymyxin B (or E), tigecycline, or similar third-line antimicrobials (16–18).

Impaired gastrointestinal motility, in particular, of the large intestine, may be the consequence of or even be caused by antibiotic-associated ulcerative colitis due to *Clostridia* species. Constipation does not preclude the presence of a clostridial colitis, a disease with mortality rates of up to 50%, if diagnosis and appropriate management is delayed unnecessarily (3).

Adverse effects of propofol

In addition to the same problems encountered with barbiturates, propofol may, in rare instances, cause the so-called propofol infusion syndrome (PRIS) (19–22).

A propofol-related syndrome with metabolic acidosis, bradyarrhythmia, and progressive myocardial failure was first described almost 20 years and was found to carry a 30% mortality rate (22). The incidence of PRIS slightly exceeds 1% (21). Postulated risk factors include use of a high propofol dose (>83 micrograms/kg/minute), a duration of therapy of more than 48 hours, and concomitant vasopressor therapy. Patients on the ketogenic diet are possibly predisposed to develop PRIS (23). Both high-dose and concomitant vasopressor therapy are frequently necessary in patients with refractory convulsive SE. However, it needs to be stressed that PRIS can occur soon after the initiation of propofol therapy and even also at rather low dose (21). In early publications, the mortality rate was high and rhabdomyolysis was frequently seen. Although, the co-incidence of convulsive SE triggered rhabdomyolysis and PRIS has been reported only once (25), it is conceivable that patients with myoglobinuria or even frank rhabdomyolysis are at an increased risk of developing PRIS (4, 26). Therefore, careful observation is necessary when patients with refractory convulsive SE are treated with propofol.

Side effects of any type of treatment of GCSE

Hypoventilation

This should not play any role since a patient with GCSE treated at the ICU should be (must be) on an artificial ventilator. However, increased bronchial mucus production, aspirates, or bronchospasm might impair airways, ventilation, and even gas exchange. If necessary, invasive ventilation strategies must be chosen including reversal of I:E (inspiration: expiration rate), bronchoscopy, and even prone positioning (kinetic therapy) (3, 12).

Hypotension

Hypotension occurs frequently in GCSE, all treatment strategies may be associated with low blood pressure. The higher the dosage, the older the patient, and the more comorbidities, hypotension might create major intensive care problems. A central venous line is essential as is best possible fluid balancing and invasive cardiopulmonary monitoring (PiCCO®) (13–15). Pressure agents should be given liberally since hypoperfusion of the endangered brain tissue increases the risk of permanent neuronal damage, neurological sequelae, and, even more, mortality.

Cardiac arrhythmias

Phenytoin and fosphenytoin, being sodium channel blockers and class 1b antiarrhythmics, can cause ventricular arrhythmias, and changes in the PR and QRS intervals. The incidence of rhythm disturbances might be as high as 7% on phenytoin (1, 5).

Phlebitis, tissue necrosis

Extravasation of intravenous phenytoin (high pH) may cause tissue necrosis, leading finally to what is known as the 'purple glove syndrome'. Fosphenytoin carries a lower risk of phlebitis and necrosis since its pH is neutral (9, 10).

Rhabdomyolysis

Rhabdomyolysis is defined as a syndrome with myalgia and muscle weakness, caused by damage to muscle cells resulting in leakage of cellular contents, muscle enzymes, myoglobin, creatine, and electrolytes (potassium, phosphate) (26). The diagnostic main features are elevation of creatine kinase (CK) and myoglobin potentially leading to renal failure (26). It can be caused by prolonged tonic–clonic SE, the risk being higher in patients treated with propofol (2, 21, 22, 25). Deranged body-temperature regulation, notably hyperthermia, increases the risk of rhabdomyolysis (26). Furthermore, the liberal use of depolarizing muscle relaxants is a well-recognized cause of critical illness neuropathy and critical illness myopathies (26). Thus, it is conceivable that a patient with prolonged GCSE, being treated with 'immunosuppressant' dosages of thiopental and/or propofol, may develop a severe sepsis syndrome which can, in term, lead to sepsis encephalopathy, which has the potential to aggravate and propagate the SE. If this is the case and the patient continues to have a clinically overt seizure activity, the therapy of refractory GCSE itself, the ongoing systemic inflammatory response syndrome (SIRS) or sepsis syndrome and the ongoing GCSE may lead to rhabdomyolysis (26). Rhabdomyolysis may produce very high levels of CK and myoglobinaemia and myoglobinuria eventually impairing kidney function, necessitating haemofiltration or other means of extracorporeal kidney failure treatment. Continuous haemofiltration is essential to avoid acute deterioration of the cerebral function due to severe electrolyte disturbance and uraemic metabolic encephalopathy, both adding to brain oedema and cerebral metabolic disturbance (26). Finally it should be stressed that any type of haemodynamic instability or distributive shock may add to impairment of renal function, therefore kidney function must be carefully monitored from the very beginning of the treatment of a GCSE in an ICU.

Immunosuppression

This aspect has been detailed extensively earlier in the chapter. Every patient with refractory SE who needs ICU management must be intubated at the earliest point of time to avoid aspiration as a contributing factor of pneumonia in a patient who potentially develops severe infectious disease due to his/her externally caused immunosuppressive state. Any structural cause of SE, such as an intracranial space-occupying lesion or malignancy may add to the state of immunosuppression either directly or indirectly (8). Both immunosuppression due to the SE and anticonvulsive therapy such as barbiturates, increase the likelihood of developing pneumonia, especially in those patients in whom intubation was delayed and who have aspirated already.

In patients who need prolonged artificial ventilation the risk of ventilator-associated pneumonia is increased (12). Accurate knowledge of the causative agents in any particular ICU is essential to avoid unnecessary, potentially harmful antimicrobial chemotherapies and to help to choose the best possible empiric antibiotic therapy until microbiological results, obtained from blood or bronchial lavage cultures, are obtained (17, 18).

Reduced gastrointestinal motility

It is mainly the barbiturates which lead to reduced gastrointestinal motility. This is particularly important in patients with haemodynamic instability, suffering from distributive shock syndrome in which high dosages of catecholamines are needed. These catecholamines act on the peripheral vasculature, increasing the blood pressure by vasoconstriction. This vasoconstriction leads to disturbance of microcirculation in all organs, also in the entire gut. This disturbance of microcirculation together with the impairment of the gastrointestinal motility, as caused by barbiturates, increases the risk of transmural translocation of intestinal bacteria, in particular, Gram-negative rods, as Enterobacteriaceae, *Escherichia coli*, *Klebsiella* spp., but also enterococci, even *Clostridia* spp. or *Candida* spp. (17,18). Therefore, the intensivist must pay close attention to the gastrointestinal motility. One possibility is to start enteral feeding (via nasogastric tube) together with properistaltic substances as domperidone, distigminbromid, erythromycin, etc. (3).

The earliest possible recognition of an incipient Gram-negative sepsis caused by transmural location of intestinal germs is essential. A watchful and careful selection of antimicrobial chemotherapeutic agents is essential to avoid lowering of seizure thresholds by antibiotic therapy and thus aggravating and prolonging the GCSE (3). Impaired gastrointestinal motility, in particular, of the large intestine may be caused by antibiotic-associated ulcerative colitis due to *Clostridia* species. Imaging of the abdomen (abdominal computed tomography) visualizes the distended colon and helps timing of a potentially necessary colonoscopy which allows its appropriate diagnosis. Immediate and early application of oral—in case of systemic spread also additionally intravenous—metronidazole is indicated in cases where antibiotic-associated ulcerative colitis is suspected or diagnosed (17, 18).

Other complications

Rib fractures and vertebral fractures, in particular in the elderly, have been reported. Both may contribute to impairment of spontaneous ventilation adding to the risk of pneumonia (1, 3).

Unconventional therapies

Ketamine

As seizures persist, gamma-aminobutyric acid (GABA) receptors become downregulated and GABA-mediated treatments may become more and more ineffective. At this point, excitatory N-methyl-D-aspartate (NMDA) receptors and glutamate are thought to play a more important role (2). Ketamine, being a non-competitive NMDA receptor antagonist, might have a role in effectively treating prolonged electrographic seizures. Animal models have shown ketamine to be ineffective in early SE, but to be effective in reducing electrographic seizures after 1 hour or longer. There are also several case reports suggesting that this substance may have a role in the treatment of refractory SE (27). Ketamine can be used in a bolus of 2 mg/kg body weight followed by an infusion of 10–50 mg/kg/minute, a dose that does not necessarily cause respiratory depression. Unlike the earlier mentioned anaesthetic agents, in particular, barbiturates and propofol, ketamine has less haemodynamic effects being more likely to cause hypertension than hypotensive shock (27).

Lidocaine

Lidocaine is another possible alternative for the treatment of refractory SE in the ICU (28). Lidocaine functions as an antiarrhythmic, stabilizing the cardiac membrane by blocking the fast voltage-gated sodium channels. Its antiepileptic activity may also be related to sodium channel blockade. Several small case series have described rapid cessation of seizures following administration of a lidocaine bolus (2–3 mg/kg body weight given within 5 minutes); however, its effective duration is rather short. In more than half of the responders in one of the key series (28), seizures recurred within half an hour. Either a second (1–3 mg/kg) bolus or continuous infusion (0.06 mg/kg/minute—up to a maximum infusion rate of 5 mg/minute) will then need to be administered. The lidocaine infusion should not be continued for more than 12 hours. Adverse effects include paradoxical proarrhythmic and, rarely, proconvulsant effects (29). Lidocaine must be avoided in patients with significant heart disease, in particular, bradyarrhythmia or conduction block. Even worse, as lidocaine is metabolized by the liver, it should be avoided in patients with liver dysfunction (28, 29).

Isoflurane

Isoflurane is an inhalational anaesthetic. It has been given in few cases with therapy refractory GCSE. Its use is complex and cumbersome, since it needs the full-scale equipment of inhalational anaesthetic systems which usually are not available in ICUs or neuro-ICUs. Despite a successful control of GCSE, mortality remains high in those patients reported so far. Isoflurane is used in concentrations of 0.8–3%, progressively higher concentrations may be needed to control seizures; however, it may be neurotoxic when used in high doses for long time periods as evidenced by progressive T2 signal hyperintensities in thalamus and cerebellum (30).

Hypothermia

Single cases have been reported in which therapy of refractory GCSE has been contained by employing mild to moderate therapeutic hypothermia, cooling the body temperature to 32–34°C. High-quality ICU management is necessary in these patients, as hypothermia has a wide variety of potential complications, including coagulopathies, increased risk of infection, disturbance of electrolytes, cardiac arrhythmias, impairment of bowel movement, reduced intestinal absorption, etc. (31, 32).

Conclusion

All therapeutic strategies require careful monitoring of both neurological and cardiopulmonary function, as well as regular monitoring of routine laboratory parameters, including inflammatory, renal, hepatic, and coagulation parameters. In rare cases it might be advisable to supplement the electroencephalographic and cardiopulmonary monitoring by neuroimaging (magnetic resonance imaging, digital volumetric imaging) and invasive modern neuromonitoring techniques such as intracranial pressure measurement (allowing cerebral perfusion pressure management), tissue oxygen measurement, brain temperature measurement, or even microdialysis with monitoring of metabolic developments (brain tissue lactate, pyruvate/lactate ratio, glucose, glycerine, etc.). Whether the regular measurement of biomarkers of brain tissue destruction as S 100 or neuronal specific enolase add to a potential optimization of management needs to be studied.

As soon as SE is suspected, be it overt GCSE or non-convulsive status or subtle SE, continuous EEG monitoring should be initiated. All type of status epileptici need to be treated aggressively. The term subtle SE has been introduced in patients with severe structural brain damage who do not awake from coma after prolonged intensive care medicine and who do show subtle motor movement like eye lid twitching or a deviation noted only when eye lids are lifted and which frequently cannot be discovered by video-monitoring or clinical examination alone. Such status epileptici with even waxing and waning of consciousness may go unnoticed for days. Therefore, EEG monitoring in a suspected patient should be established at the earliest possible point of time.

Neurologists usually accurately diagnose convulsive SE. However, psychogenic SE can mimic the clinical manifestation of a GCSE and can even lead to intubation and use of barbiturates. It should be noted that in psychogenic SE, dysautonomia or lateral tongue biting, which are characteristic of GCSE are absent, and the periodicity of the 'tonic–clonic' movements is replaced by flailing and rocking movements. The typical lactic acidosis seen in prolonged GCSE is also absent in psychogenic SE patients. Video-EEG monitoring confirms the suspected diagnosis.

Table 33.1 Pharmaceutical agents used in intensive care units (even neurointensive care units) that may reduce seizure threshold

Antibiotics	Imipenem
	Norfloxacin
	Ciprofloxacin
	Cefepime
	Penicillin derivatives
	Betalactam antibiotics as cefepime,
Antidepressants	Amitriptyline
	Doxepin
	Nortriptyline
	Fluoxetine, sertraline
Antipsychotics	Chlorpromazine
	Haloperidol
	Thioridazine
	Perphenazine
	Trifluoperazine

Modified after Wijdicks (3).

Substances that are used regularly in any ICU, and also in neurological ICUs, that can reduce seizure threshold might be the final trigger to provoke—in an ICU—a SE. Such substances are antibiotics, antipsychotics and antidepressants, and these are listed in Table 33.1.

References

1. De Giorgio Ch, Faught E, Fujikawa DG, Vespa PM. Status epilepticus. In: Noseworthy JH (ed) *Neurological Therapeutics, Principles and Practice* (2nd edn), pp. 375–84. Oxford: Informa Healthcare, 2006.
2. Robakis TK, Hirsch LJ. Literature review, case report, and expert discussion of prolonged refractory status epilepticus. *Neurcrit Care* 2006; 4:35–46.
3. Wijdicks EFM. *The Clinical Practice of Critical Care Neurology* (2nd edn). Oxford: Oxford University Press, 2003.
4. Kreft A, Rasmussen N, Hansen LK. Refractory status epilepticus in two children with lethal rhabdomyolysis. *Ugeskr Laeger* 2008; 170:3339.
5. Wijdicks EFM. *Catastrophic Neurologic Disorders in the Emergency Department*. Oxford: Oxford University Press. 2004.
6. Neligan A, Shorvon SD. Prognostic factors, morbidity and mortality in tonic-clonic status epilepticus: a review. *Epilepsy Res* 2011; 93:1–10.
7. Neligan A, Shorvon SD. Frequency and prognosis of convulsive status epilepticus of different causes: a systematic review. *Arch Neurol* 2010; 67:931–40.
8. Tan RY, Neligan A, Shorvon SD. The uncommon causes of status epilepticus: a systematic review. *Epilepsy Res* 2010; 91:111–22.
9. Meierkord H, Boon P, Engelsen B, Göcke K, Shorvon S, Tinuper P, *et al.* European Federation of Neurological Societies. EFNS guideline on the management of status epilepticus in adults. *Eur J Neurol* 2010; 17:348–55.
10. Holtkamp M. Treatment strategies for refractory status epilepticus. *Curr Opin Crit Care* 2011; 17:94–100.
11. Belda FJ, Aguilar G, Teboul JL, Pestaña D, Redondo FJ, Malbrain M, *et al.* for the PICS Investigators' Group. Complications related to less-invasive haemodynamic monitoring. *Br J Anaesth* 2010; 106:482–6.
12. Arnold HM, Hollands JM, Skrupky LP, Mice ST. Optimizing sustained use of sedation in mechanically ventilated patients: focus on safety. *Curr Drug Saf* 2010; 5:6–12.
13. Gassanov N, Caglayan E, Nia A, Erdmann E. The PiCCO catheter. *Dtsch Med Wochenschr* 2010; 135:2311–4.
14. Hadian M, Kim HK, Severyn DA, Pinsky MR. Cross-comparison of cardiac output trending accuracy of LiDCO, PiCCO, FloTrac and pulmonary artery catheters. *Crit Care* 2010; 14(6):R212.
15. Proulx F, Lemson J, Choker G, Tibby SM (2011). Hemodynamic monitoring by transpulmonary thermodilution and pulse contour analysis in critically ill children. *Pediatr Crit Care Med* 2011; 12(4):459–66.
16. Benenson S, Temper V, Cohen MJ, Schwartz C, Hidalgo-Grass C, Block C. Imipenem disc for the detection of KPC carbapenemase-producing Enterobacteriaceae in clinical practice. *J Clin Microbiol* 2011; 49(4):1617–20.
17. Fircanis S, McKay M. Recognition and management of extended spectrum beta lactamase producing organisms (ESBL). *Med Health RI* 2010; 93 (5):161–2.
18. Oteo J, Pérez-Vázquez M, Campos J. Extended-spectrum [beta]-lactamase producing Escherichia coli: changing epidemiology and clinical impact. *Curr Opin Infect Dis* 2010; 23:320–6.
19. Fodale V, La Monaca E. Propofol infusion syndrome: An overview of a perplexing disease. *Drug Safety* 2008; 4:293–303.
20. Guitton C, Gabillet L, Latour P, Rigal JC, Boutoille D, Al Habash O, *et al.* Propofol infusion syndrome during refractory status epilepticus in a young adult: Successful ECMO Resuscitation. *Neurocrit Care* 2011; 15:139–45.

21. Roberts RJ, Barletta JF, Fong JJ, Schumaker G, Kuper PJ, Papadopoulos S, *et al.* Incidence of propofol-related infusion syndrome in critically ill adults: a prospective, multicenter study. *Crit Care* 2009; 13:R169.
22. Wong J. Propofol infusion syndrome. *Am J Therapeutics* 2010; 17:487–91.
23. Baumeister FA, Oberhoffer R, Liebhaber GM, Kunkel J, Eberhardt J, Holthausen H, *et al.* Fatal propofol infusion syndrome in association with ketogenic diet. *Neuropediatrics* 2004; 35:250–2.
24. Parke TJ, Stevens JE, Rice AS, Greenaway CL, Bray RJ, Smith PJ, *et al.* Metabolic acidosis and fatal myocardial failure after propofol infusion in children: five case reports. *BMJ* 1992; 305:613–16.
25. Zarovnaya EL, Jobst BC, Harris BT. Propofol-associated fatal myocardial failure and rhabdomyolysis in an adult with status epilepticus. *Epilepsia* 2007; 48:1002–6.
26. Renaud DL, Clarke JTR. Metabolic myopathies. In: Noseworthy JH (ed) *Neurological Therapeutics, Principles and Practice* (2nd edn), pp. 2657–68. Oxford: Informa Healthcare, 2006.
27. Prüss H, Holkamp M. Ketamine successfully terminates malignant status epilepticus. *Epilepsy Res* 2008; 82:219–22.
28. Walker IA, Slovis CM. Lidocaine in the treatment of status epilepticus. *Acad Emerg Med* 1997; 4:918–22.
29. Hattori H, Yamano T, Hayashi K, Osawa M, Kondo K, Aihara M, *et al.* Effectiveness of lidocaine infusion for status epilepticus in childhood: a retrospective multi-institutional study in Japan. *Brain Dev* 2008; 30:504–12.
30. Fugate JE, Burns JD, Wijdicks EF, Warner DO, Nakowski CJ, Rabinstein AA. Prolonged high-dose isoflurane for refractory status epilepticus: is it safe? *Anesth Analg* 2010; 111:1520–4.
31. Bleck TP. Hypothermia, hyperthermia, and other systemic factors in status epilepticus. *Epilepsia* 2009; 50(Suppl 12):10.
32. Wheless JW. Treatment of refractory convulsive status epilepticus in children: other therapies. *Semin Pediatr Neurol* 2010; 17:190–4.

CHAPTER 34

Epilepsy and Employment

Ann Jacoby

Introduction

Being employed is an important ingredient in the quality of life of people with epilepsy (1). Conversely, unemployment has been shown to be a major source of stress and increased psychopathology (2). Research into the issue of employment of people with epilepsy has generally presented a somewhat bleak account, with those affected appearing at risk in terms of both finding and maintaining employment (3), with obvious consequences for their socioeconomic status. People with epilepsy appear well aware of the risks, with employment coming near the top of the list of their concerns about the everyday implications of their condition (4). However, some brighter findings include that unemployment rates for epilepsy are lower than for other disabilities; and that among people with well-controlled seizures uncomplicated by other handicaps, employment rates may reach near-normal.

This chapter will address the objective evidence about employment rates and status in people with epilepsy; consider the employment concerns of people with epilepsy and situate the problems they face within the broader issue of epilepsy stigma; examine the evidence around internal and external factors which influence employability; and suggest what can be done to improve employment prospects people with epilepsy.

The role of employment for good quality of life

Being in employment is an important ingredient of overall quality of life, providing a sense of identity and purpose, personal status, and enhanced self-esteem (5). Conversely, unemployment has been shown to be a major source of stress, mental ill-health including depression, and physical ill-health (6, 7). Under- and unemployment represent wasted human potential and reduced societal productivity and the costs of under and unemployment in people with epilepsy have been shown to be high (8–10). It has been noted that the employment problems of people with epilepsy, 'cannot be reduced to one factor; they are, rather, the result of a bundle of adverse factors, interacting with each other in a complex fashion' (11).

Examination of the literature on employability of people with epilepsy presents a somewhat bleak picture. People with epilepsy have consistently been shown to be at risk of higher unemployment than the general population and as a direct consequence, of lower socioeconomic status (10–12); and there is evidence that in the US at least rates of employment have changed little over recent decades (9). Jennum et al. (10) examined the impact for employment and earnings of having epilepsy across almost 65,000 patients with epilepsy identified via the Danish National Patient registry and gender-matched controls. They found a greater proportion of epilepsy patients than controls were in receipt of social welfare benefits, and a lower proportion of their earned income came from employment. Interestingly, epilepsy patients were less likely to be in employment not just in the post-diagnosis period, but also prior to the diagnosis of their epilepsy.

It is also the case that some people with epilepsy are more disadvantaged in terms of employment than others—thus experiencing frequent seizures (13–16), being on multiple antiepileptic medications (16), seizure onset in childhood and adolescence (10, 16), chronological age and gender (10), having other comorbidities (17, 18) and poor self-rated health (13, 19), have all been implicated in increased disadvantage. People with epilepsy have also been shown to be at increased risk of unemployment during time periods and in geographical areas of general high unemployment (20, 21).

Of course, epilepsy is not alone among conditions of ill-health in its propensity to generate employment problems for those affected, as a recently reported study reminds us (22). Using multivariate modelling techniques, Maslow and colleagues (22) compared adult social, educational, and vocational outcomes in young adults with and without childhood-onset chronic illness (cancer, heart disease, diabetes, and epilepsy). They found that compared to controls, those with childhood-onset chronic illness had similar odds of being married or having other romantic relationships, having children, and living with their parents; but had lower odds of graduating from higher education, being employed and being higher earners and, conversely, higher odds of being in receipt of welfare benefits. These authors conclude that the contrast between social 'success' for those with chronic illness and their educational and occupational 'failure' relative to those without such illness suggests reasons for under and unemployment in this group are complex, multifactorial, and involve a range of contextual factors, all of which need to be further investigated and better understood.

Accepting the generality of the problem, it is nevertheless the case that employment status is a major concern of people with epilepsy themselves and a major contributor to their quality of life (23–25). Collings (23) identified employment (being in a secure and worthwhile job, which utilizes one's personal abilities) as the third most cited source of life fulfilment, after having a good family life and possessing self-confidence; and Bishop et al. (24) found employment status to be highly correlated with both mental well-being scores and overall quality of life. Most recently, Tlusta et al. (25) reported that employment status explained 10% of the variance in overall quality of life, as measured using the QOLIE-31, and was the strongest predictor of emotional well-being and energy/fatigue subscale scores. In the study by Gilliam et al. (26), over half of people with epilepsy interviewed identified issues around employment as a major concern for them; and Bishop (27) subsequently identified that such concerns spanned three broad areas: around applying for work and the problem of whether or not to disclose epilepsy; around maintaining employment and the possibility of covert dismissal; and around being successful in work. Bishop and Allen (28) further explored the basis for such concerns through a survey of 36 affiliate organizations of the US Epilepsy Foundation, among whom the issues most frequently raised by their members included whether or not and how best to disclose epilepsy to potential employers, violations against the American with Disabilities Act, dealing with co-workers and supervisors, the appropriateness or otherwise of particular types of employment, the implications of being in work for possible loss of health benefits, fear of having seizures in the workplace, and worries about impaired work performance. So to what extent at these concerns on the part of people with epilepsy justified?

Evidence about rates of employment, unemployment, and underemployment

Several studies have reported that rates of employment are lower and, conversely, that rates of unemployment are higher in people with epilepsy than in their comparator populations (Fig. 34.1). Thus, for example, unemployment risk was roughly doubled for men and trebled for women with epilepsy in a UK community study (21); and was approximately five times that of the general US population in the study by Fisher et al. (29)—though in contrast, in a study conducted in Sweden, Chaplin et al. (14) reported that unemployment rates among people with epilepsy were little different to those of the population as a whole, suggesting important effects of sociocultural context. However, studies which treat people with epilepsy as an undifferentiated group are misleading in as much as they fail to recognize that some people with epilepsy are at more risk than others. For example, Jacoby (13) examined employment rates in people with well-controlled epilepsy and found them to be similar to those of the general UK population; as did Ratsepp et al. (15) and Herodes et al. (30) in studies in Estonia, and Marinas et al. (16) in a study in Spain. However, in all these studies, those with continuing active epilepsy or poorly controlled seizures were, as might be expected, least likely to be employed.

The UK MESS (Multicentre Study of Early Epilepsy and Single Seizures) Study followed a cohort of individuals who had experienced only a single or a few seizures over a period of 4 years, to assess the impacts on employment status specifically (19) and quality of life more broadly (31). In those cohort members who were of working age throughout follow-up, employment rates were compared with those in the general population (19) and found to be lower, for both men and women, at all three time points for assessment (study entry and 2 and 4 years subsequently), suggesting substantial employment disadvantage from the outset. However, once again there was also clear evidence that the effects of epilepsy for employability are not uniform—thus, at all three time points, employment status was predicted by greater seizure frequency and poorer self-rated health. Of those in employment at final follow-up, three-quarters reported having had no further seizures since entry to the study. Examination of employment transitions across the course of the study revealed that there was relatively little mobility in/out of the labour market—those initially in work tended to remain so, as did those who were initially unemployed. Furthermore, those in professional or managerial posts appeared had more favourable employment trajectories than other workers, with the greatest proportion of individuals always employed and the smallest proportion never employed or losing a job after entry to the study (Table 34.1).

The finding from MESS that people with single or only a few seizures experience greater employment disadvantage than the general population from the outset of their condition is in line with the previously discussed findings reported by Jennum et al. (10). That MESS participants subsequently appear not necessarily to experience worsening employment rates over time resonates with the study in Sweden reported by Lindsten et al. (18) who also found slightly lower rates of employment following the index seizure but no evolving negative effects for employment status over a 10-year follow-up period.

Evidence of the impact of epilepsy for employability also comes from studies which have followed cohorts of patients with childhood onset epilepsy (32–34). Jalava et al. (32) reported a sevenfold risk of unemployment for those affected when compared to controls, with rates elevated even among those in long-term remission—suggesting substantial early and sustained disadvantage. In contrast, Wakamoto et al. (34) reported that though overall employment rates were lower for the group of individuals with epilepsy compared to their controls (67% compared to 97%), rates were near

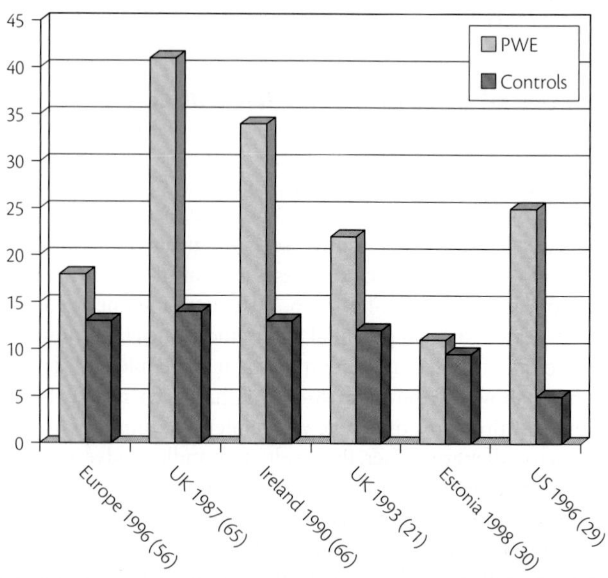

Fig. 34.1 Reported rates of unemployment of people with epilepsy (PWE).

Table 34.1 Employment trajectories between baseline and 4-year follow-up by occupational social class: men and women of working age at all time points

	Percentages in each social class			
	Professional and managerial	**Lower non-manual**	**Skilled manual**	**Semi- and unskilled manual**
Always employed during study	73.7	45.7	63.6	49.1
Never employed during study	7.9	17.1	18.2	14.6
Lost job after entry to study	7.9	22.9	9.1	12.7
Became employed after entry to study	10.5	14.3	9.1	23.6
Total	100.0	100.0	100.0	100.0

Table restricted to people with single seizures or early epilepsy who responded at all time points and supplied complete data on employment status and occupational social class. Reproduced from Holland et al. (19).

equal where the people with epilepsy were classified as 'of normal intelligence'.

Other evidence of disadvantage comes from studies by Trostle (35) in the US and Jacoby et al. (21) in the UK, both of whom reported that the proportion of people with epilepsy in managerial and non-manual positions was significantly lower than in their comparator populations; and Wadsworth (36), also in the UK, who reported that people whose epilepsy was 'uncomplicated' were nonetheless at increased risk of earning less and of experiencing reduced work opportunities than people without epilepsy.

Factors influencing employability of people with epilepsy

Craig and Oxley (37) present a four-dimensional framework of factors associated with the employment problems of people with epilepsy (Fig. 34.2). This framework suggests that both overt and covert factors and both intrinsic and extrinsic factors need to be considered. Among 'extrinsic' factors can be included the legal and statutory restrictions placed upon people with epilepsy; the lack of understanding and resultant discriminatory attitudes of employers and of fellow employees; and the low expectations for their achievement among the families and carers of people with epilepsy. Important 'intrinsic' factors could be inadequate seizure control, impaired cognitive functioning; poor self-image, and negative beliefs held by people with epilepsy in relation to their employability. Subsequent research has attempted to explore empirically the contribution these different sets of factors make to the employment difficulties faced by people with epilepsy.

Covert Extrinsic (eg. attitudes of employers, co-workers, low expectations of significant others)	Covert Intrinsic (eg. fear of discrimination, impaired self-image, low expectations, PWE beliefs re. work)
Overt extrinsic (eg. statutory limitations re. employment, driving regulations)	Overt Intrinsic (eg. Inadequate Sz control, cognitive impairment, low educational achievement)

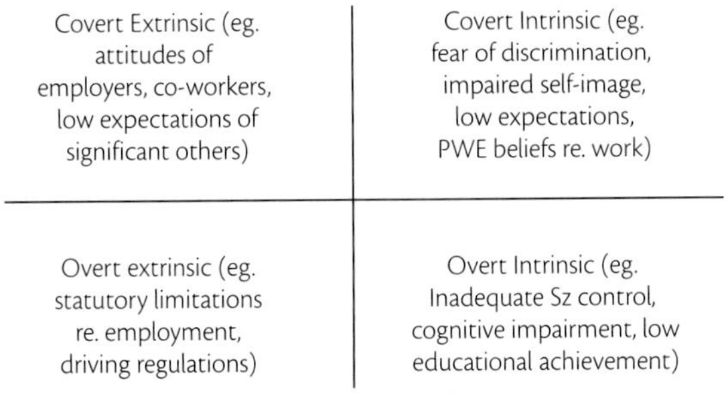

Fig. 34.2 A framework for factors associated with employability problems of people with epilepsy (PWE). Adapted from Craig and Oxley (37).

Epilepsy has a long history of associated stigma (38) which has included propositions about a link between the epileptic condition and insanity, violence, degeneracy, and inherent weaknesses of character (39). The extent to which such ideas impact on issues of employability is not necessarily easily observable, but there is nonetheless a significant body of evidence that both employers and co-workers not infrequently hold less positive attitudes than are helpful to people with epilepsy. Though the cohort studies in the US by Hicks and Hicks (40) suggest significant improvement over time in the attitudes of employers towards epilepsy, their findings are challenged by others highlighting continuing misperceptions and negative attitudes. For example, Hicks and Hicks reported that in 1986, all employers they interviewed said there were jobs in their organization fillable by people with epilepsy; whereas the proportion agreeing that this was the case was only two-thirds in a study of employers in rural areas of the US conducted at around the same time (41). Likewise, Hicks and Hicks (40) reported that 95% of their 1986 cohort of employers had knowingly employed someone with epilepsy, whereas in the study by Gade and Toutges (41), only 45% had done so. In a recent study in the UK (42), 84% of employers questioned said there were jobs in their organization fillable by people with epilepsy, but only 26% had knowingly employed someone with epilepsy. In the same study, a fifth of participating employers thought epilepsy in a prospective employee would present a major issue; and 44% thought it would cause high concern generally (Fig. 34.3) and in relation to possible absenteeism and workplace accidents (despite the lack of any substantial evidence to support these concerns). Perhaps for these reasons, 76% thought people with epilepsy should always disclose their condition to prospective employers, even when they had been seizure-free for 2 years or more.

Two interesting experiments around the issue of epilepsy and employment have been reported recently. In the first, Bishop et al. (43) set out to examine the differential effect of three different 'epilepsy labels' on employer perceptions. The labels under investigation were 'epilepsy', 'seizure disorder', and 'seizure condition'—and their relative impact was assessed by asking the research participants (employers) to rank-order the likelihood of hiring a person with each of these 'conditions' for either an assembly line position or a customer service representative position. Contrary to their expectations, the authors report that that 'epilepsy' was more favourably judged than were the terms 'seizure disorder' or 'seizure condition', perhaps, they suggest, because employers are clearer

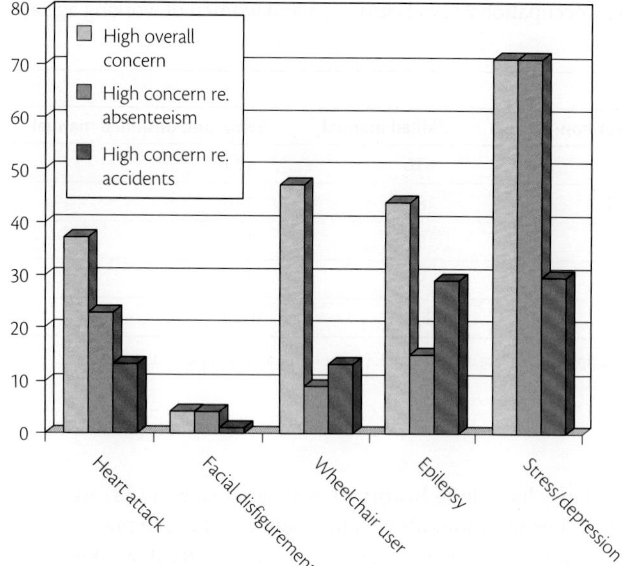

Fig. 34.3 UK employers' concerns about employing persons with health conditions. Jacoby et al. (42).

about its meaning. Whatever the reasons for this (and they undoubtedly deserve further investigation), the study confirms its authors' original hypothesis that the label used to discuss epilepsy may have a significant effect on employer perceptions.

In the second study, Parfene and colleagues (44) set out to investigate whether indirect association with epilepsy acts as a source of stigma in relation to employability, by examining workplace outcomes for hypothetical employees who did not have epilepsy themselves, but were potentially subject to stigma by association. Enlisted research participants (college enrollers) were asked to assess the likely quality of an employee's work and their own likelihood, if employing that person, of recommending them for workplace rewards or penalties, based on six different randomly allocated employee scenarios. These scenarios were identical except that the putative employee was either male or female and had either taken leave in the past year to care for a child with epilepsy or asthma or not taken any leave. Their analysis found a significant effect of leave condition, which in turn was associated with an appreciable (though non-significant) effect on work quality evaluations and a significant effect on the likelihood of work rewards and penalties—in summary, the research revealed biases against employees who took leave to care for a child with epilepsy, but not employees whose child had asthma. Their findings suggest some process of 'contamination' by association and a situation of indirect discrimination and disadvantage.

Parallel work to that involving the attitudes of employers has explored the attitudes of co-workers and supports this negative message. Harden and colleagues (45) presented a series of vignettes to US employees relating to having a co-worker with epilepsy or depression or multiple sclerosis. They found that epilepsy was least known about (perhaps because it was least disclosed by those with the condition); that employees expressed greater anxiety about interacting with a co-worker with epilepsy than one with either of the other two conditions; and expressed more anxiety about possible unpredictable behaviours on the part of a co-worker with epilepsy. They also expressed a lower level of comfort about the possibility of having to give first-aid to a co-worker with epilepsy. Harden concludes that epilepsy carries a higher risk of social avoidance than its comparator conditions of ill-health, requiring education of the public on how to manage seizures. In a UK survey (46), people with epilepsy were found to represent the second most cited health condition, after depression, as causing concern to potential co-workers.

Turning to people with epilepsy themselves, their own beliefs have also been shown to be a critical factor for their employment status (47), including beliefs about the meaning of work, concerns about safety and perceptions of workplace-related risk, and anticipation of the negative impact of seizures on work performance. In this study, informants completed a 20-item 'work beliefs' measure, scores for which were higher—in other words, more negative—for specific 'beliefs' items among those who were not in work (Table 34.2). Such negative connotations about their condition can be seen as another manifestation of 'felt' stigma (48) among people with epilepsy, which Scambler (49) suggests may be more pervasive for quality of life than any 'enacted' stigma or discrimination. Support for this proposition comes from the study by Jacoby (50), which found that whereas only 3% of people with epilepsy reported failing to get a job because of their epilepsy and only 2% could recall being treated unfairly at work because of it, around a third considered that having epilepsy made it more difficult for them than for others to secure employment.

In an analysis of internal factors influencing employability of people with epilepsy (51), being of younger age, Caucasian, with higher educational and household income levels, taking fewer antiepileptic drugs, having no other comorbidities and not being on disability benefits, having previous work experience and seeing work as personally important, and being less concerned about possible workplace discrimination were all significant predictive factors. Some of these predictor factors are almost certainly not specific to the employability of people with epilepsy and reflective of other forms of discrimination. In a multiple regression analysis, those which emerged as highly significant for people with epilepsy were belonging to a higher household income group, the perceived importance of work personally and being less concerned about possible workplace discriminations. Interestingly, clinical epilepsy

Table 34.2 Beliefs of people with epilepsy about their employability

Work belief item	Not in work (mean score[a])	In work (mean score)	P value
You have to work to be normal	2.05	3.02	0.004
I don't have enough education to work	2.73	1.48	0.0001
My family fears work injuries	3.57	1.75	0.01
I fear work injuries	2.75	1.81	0.0001
I might injure others if I have a seizure at work	3.01	2.05	0.003
Family does not want me to work	2.76	1.29	0.002
My seizures would affect my work performance	3.50	2.37	0.0001

[a] Higher scores indicate more negative responses
Adapted from Clarke et al. (47).

variables did not emerge as important in this analysis—in particular, seizure control did not emerge as a primary determinant of employability.

There is a brighter side to this somewhat bleak picture. It has been reported that employment rates in epilepsy are higher than for other disabilities (52); and, as highlighted earlier in this chapter, are near those in normal populations for people with well-controlled epilepsy (13–15, 18, 53). There is little evidence of any downward social drift following a diagnosis of epilepsy in adulthood (19, 49); and there is evidence of employment success among successful surgery patients (54, 55). Current evidence also suggests that there is little increase in risk of work absences or accidents in people with epilepsy whose seizures are satisfactorily controlled compared to the general working population. In the RESt-1 Study (56, 57), a prospective cohort study across eight countries in Europe involving around 600 people with epilepsy and matched controls, 22 people with epilepsy and nine without reported 30 and 12 accidents in the workplace, all but one of which were mild and did not require hospitalization. Though, based on these data, people with epilepsy were at roughly double the risk for work-related accidents, their accidents were minor and unrelated to seizure events; and people with epilepsy emerged as at only very slightly greater risk of having time off work. These findings support those of earlier studies such as the one by Dasgupta et al. (58) which found no evidence of increased rates of work absenteeism or work-related accidents among people with epilepsy; and by Wiebe et al. (59) who showed that though people with epilepsy reported more 'disability days', they had no higher risk of accidents than their non-epilepsy comparators.

There is also some evidence of improvements in employers' attitudes towards epilepsy. In a study conducted in 1972, Sands and Zalkind (60) reported that following an intensive educational campaign in the US, there was no discernible change in employers' attitudes to employing people with epilepsy or to the possible employment related activities of people with epilepsy; nor did employers expect to change their views. In contrast, Jacoby et al. (42) found that among UK employers questioned three decades on, the majority were willing to consider possible accommodations to conditions of work for any employees with epilepsy, including job sharing (78%), flexible working hours (72%), additional rest breaks (59%), physical modifications to the work space (54%), and alternative transport arrangements (45%). To some extent, such apparent willingness to make accommodations has almost certainly been driven by the requirements of current UK employment law, highlighting that stigma/discrimination reduction may best be attained by educational initiatives supported by statute; neither approach is, of itself, likely to be sufficient. However, measuring the real impact of legislation in protecting the employment status of people with epilepsy is difficult and the findings not always encouraging (61). For example, in a recent study by the UK Department for Work and Pensions (62), 43% of employers cited the UK Disability Discrimination Act (DDA) as a driver for making employment-related adjustments for disabled employees; but there was a decline over the previous 3-year period in the percentage actually having done so; and there was a parallel decline across the same time period in the proportion of employers reporting employing anyone with a disability. In an examination of the impact of the Americans with Disabilities Act, Roessler and Sumner (63) reported evidence of a 'catch 22' situation arising, with employers expressing concern about the productivity of employees with disabilities and chronic health conditions such as epilepsy, while at the same time being reluctant to meet the costs of now legally required job accommodations for such employees. Also somewhat worryingly, increases in the number of enquiries from people with epilepsy to the UK charity, Epilepsy Action, about the employment protection afforded by the UK DDA have been matched by a decline in those coming from employers (61).

On a more positive note, evidence of the potential for success of employment initiatives for people with epilepsy has recently been reviewed by Varekamp et al. (64). These authors identified nine studies—though none were in epilepsy—of vocational rehabilitation interventions that met specified inclusion criteria. Employment status of the discriminated group was improved in four of five studies where this was the assessed outcome; obtaining work accommodations was achieved in three of three studies; and improved psychological status of the discriminated group was achieved in two of three studies. There were some methodological weaknesses in the studies described, but nonetheless there was also some evidence of the effectiveness of the documented interventions. Work integration initiatives such as the one described by de Boer (1), that bring together government agencies, vocational consultants and people with epilepsy, offer a promising way forward; though more evidence of their success is needed to convince governments to invest meaningfully in them.

Improving employability of people with epilepsy

Given all this evidence of the continuing, if slowly lessening, employment difficulties encountered by people with epilepsy, there are some important lessons to be learnt from stigma research more broadly. First, as the empirical work reported highlights, stigma research reinforces that it is important to focus both on the targets of stigma, and on its perpetrators, the former in this instance people with epilepsy, the latter employers and co-workers. Second, stigma is a multilevel phenomenon—and stigma reduction initiatives, including those targeted at employability, need to be directed from the intrapersonal through to the social structural level. Third, stigma research shows that multistrategy initiatives are most effective—educational approaches alone are insufficient and need to be backed by other approaches such as contact between stigmatized and non-stigmatized groups; and supported by statute.

Additionally, the tendency demonstrated in studies such as those cited to consider people with epilepsy as a single, homogeneous group, needs to be challenged. Not all people with epilepsy encounter problems with employment, and employment initiatives need to target the difficult-to-employ. The evidence suggests these are most likely to be: those with uncontrolled seizures, those with additional handicaps; those with comorbidities such as depression; those from lower socioeconomic groups; those with epilepsy developing in childhood; and those with none of these problems, but fearful of workplace discrimination. The approaches taken and degree of support required will vary depending on which of these groups is being targeted.

So, what can be done to assist people with epilepsy in need to minimize the difficulties they face in the context of employment? The evidence reported here suggests the problem needs to be addressed at a number of different levels in parallel (Box 34.1).

Box 34.1 What can be done?

- At the intrapersonal level:
  - Establish the reality versus the perception of workplace discrimination.
  - Address negative beliefs about work performance and risks.
  - Provide skills-oriented support for employment.
- At the interpersonal level:
  - Address the negative beliefs and stereotypes held by others.
  - Support positive action and employment policies.
- At the community and institutional level:
  - Mount targeted educational campaigns (aimed at the general public, teachers, employers, and co-workers).
  - Invest in employment-related services and vocational rehabilitation.
- At governmental/structural level:
  - Shift power via legislation and Human Rights approaches.

At the intrapersonal level, it is important to establish the reality versus the perception of workplace discrimination; to address negative beliefs about work performance and work-related risks held by people with epilepsy; and to provide them with skills-orientated support for employment. At the interpersonal level, the negative beliefs and stereotypes held by others need to be addressed alongside initiatives that support positive action. At the community and institutional level, education campaigns targeted at the general public, teachers, employers and co-workers are required; as are employment-related and vocational rehabilitation services. At governmental level, there needs to be a continuing shift of power in favour of discriminated groups such as people with epilepsy, via legislation and Human Rights approaches.

Advocacy groups such as the epilepsy patient organizations and the International Bureau for Epilepsy Commission on Employment, statutory bodies such as the UK Disability Rights Commission and the UK Trade Union Council, and people with epilepsy themselves, informed about their rights and empowered to act for them, need to continue to challenge stigma and discrimination in the work context, so turning the question from one of 'Why employ people with epilepsy?' to that of 'Why not?'.

Conclusions

Employment status is a critical component of a person's quality of life; and initiatives aimed at improving the quality of life of people with epilepsy as a group must therefore include efforts to improve their employment status. Education of employers to allay unfounded fears and correct misperceptions about the employability of people with epilepsy is important; as is education of people with epilepsy themselves and their families, so that they can be informed and empowered potential employees. Support in law for their employability is also important. Recently, a number of programmes to reduce the barriers to employability of people with epilepsy have been instigated and shown to be potentially very effective. Learning the lessons from these programmes offers the possibility of changing a bleak employment past into a bright future for the many people with epilepsy for whom work represents an integral part of everyday life.

Acknowledgements

This chapter was originally given as a talk, 'Bleak or Bright? Changing employability of people with epilepsy', at the retirement celebration of Hanneke de Boer. I would like to thank all those people with epilepsy of the years who have contributed to the research findings reported here.

References

1. De Boer HM. Overview and perspectives of employment in people with epilepsy. *Epilepsia* 2005; 46(Suppl. 1): 52–4.
2. Hayes J, Nutman P. *Understanding the Unemployed*. London: Tavistock, 1981.
3. Smeets VMJ, van Lierop BAG, Vanhoutvin JPG, Aldenkamp AP, Nijhuis FJN. Epilepsy and employment: Literature review. *Epilepsy Behav* 2007; 10: 354–62.
4. Fisher RS, Vickrey B, Gibson P. The impact of epilepsy from the patient's perspective I. Descriptions and subjective perceptions. *Epilepsy Res* 2000; 41:39–51.
5. Jahoda M. *Employment and Unemployment: A social psychological analysis*. Cambridge: Cambridge University Press, 1982.
6. Fagin L, Little P. *The Forsaken Families*. Harmondsworth: Penguin, 1984.
7. Bartley M, Ferrie J, Montgomery SM. Living in a high-unemployment economy: understanding the health consequences. In: Marmot M, Wilkinson RG (eds) *Social Determinants of Health*, pp. 81–104. Oxford: Oxford University Press, 1999.
8. Cockerell, OC, Hart YM, Sander JWAS, Shorvon SD. The cost of epilepsy in the United Kingdom: an estimation based on the results of two population-based studies. *Epilepsy Res* 1994; 18: 249–60.
9. Begley CE, Famulari M, Annegers JF, Lairson DR. The cost of epilepsy in the United States: An estimate from population-based clinical and survey data. *Epilepsia* 2000; 41:342–51.
10. Jennum P, Gyllenborg J, Kjellberg J. The social and economic consequences of epilepsy: a controlled study. *Epilepsia* 2011; 52(5): 949–56.
11. Thorbecke R, Fraser RT. The range of needs and services in vocational employment. In: Engel J Jr, Pedley TA (eds) *Epilepsy a comprehensive textbook*, Vol 2, pp. 2211–25. Philadelphia, PA: Lippincott-Raven, 1998.
12. Collings JA, Chappell B. Correlates of employment: history and employability in a British epilepsy sample. *Seizure* 1994; 3(4):255–62.
13. Jacoby A. Impact of epilepsy on employment status: Findings from a UK study of people with well-controlled epilepsy. *Epilepsy Res* 1995; 21:125–32.
14. Chaplin JE, Wester A, Tomson T. Factors associated with the employment problems of people with established epilepsy. *Seizure* 1998; 7: 299–303.
15. Ratsepp M, Oun A, Haldre S, Kaasik AE. Felt stigma and impact of epilepsy on employment status among Estonian people: exploratory study. *Seizure* 2000; 9:394–401.
16. Marinas A, Elices E, Gil-Nagel A, Salas-Puig J, Sanchez JC, Carreño M, *et al*. Socio-occupational and employment profile of patients with epilepsy. *Epilepsy Behav* 2011; 21(3):223–7.
17. Britten N, Morgan K, Fenwick PBC, Britten H. Epilepsy and handicap from birth to age thirty-six. *Dev Med Child Neurol* 1986; 28:719–28.
18. Lindsten H, Stenlund H, Edlund C, Forsgren L. Socioeconomic prognosis after a newly diagnosed unprovoked epileptic seizure in adults: A population-based case-control study. *Epilepsia* 2002; 43(10):1239–50.

19. Holland P, Lane S, Whitehead M, Marson AG, Jacoby A. Labour market participation following onset of seizures and early epilepsy: findings from a UK cohort. *Epilepsia* 2009; 50(5):1030–39.
20. Elwes RDC, Marshall J, Beattie A, Newman PK. Epilepsy and employment: a community based survey in an area of high unemployment. *J Neurol, Neurosurg, Psychiatry* 1991; 54:200–3.
21. Jacoby A, Buck D, Baker G, McNamee P, Graham-Jones S, Chadwick D. Uptake and costs of care for epilepsy: findings from a UK regional study. *Epilepsia* 1998; 39(7):776–86.
22. Maslow GR, Haydon A, McRee AL, Ford CA, Halpern CT. Growing up with a chronic illness: social success, educational and vocational distress. *J Adolesc Health* 2011; 49(2):206–12.
23. Collings JA. Life fulfilment in an epilepsy sample from the United States. *Soc Sci Med* 1995; 40(11):1579–84.
24. Bishop M, Berven N, Hermann B. Quality of life among adults with epilepsy: An exploratory model. *Rehabil Couns Bull* 2002; 113: 87–95.
25. Tlusta E, Zarubova J, Simko J, Hojdikova H, Salek S, Vlcek J. Clinical and demographic characteristics predicting QOL in patients with epilepsy in the Czech Republic: How this can influence practice. *Seizure* 2009; 18:85–9.
26. Gilliam F, Kuzniecky R, Faught E, Black L, Carpenter G, Schrodt R. Patient-validated content of epilepsy-specific quality of life measurement. *Epilepsia* 1997; 38:233–6.
27. Bishop M. Barriers to employment among people with epilepsy: Report of a focus group. *J Vocational Rehabil* 2002; 17:281–6.
28. Bishop M, Allen C. Employment concerns of people with epilepsy and the question of disclosure: report of a survey of the epilepsy foundation. *Epilepsy Behav* 2001; 2:490–5.
29. Fisher RS. Epilepsy from the patient's perspective: Review of results of a community-based survey. *Epilepsy Behav* 2000; 1:S9–S14.
30. Herodes M, Oun A, Haldre S, Kaasik AE. Epilepsy in Estonia: A quality-of-life study. *Epilepsia* 2001; 42:1061–73.
31. Jacoby A, Lane S, Marson A, Baker GA. Relationship of clinical and quality of life trajectories following the onset of seizures: Findings from the UK MESS Study. *Epilepsia* 2011; 52(5):965–74.
32. Jalava M, Sillanpaa M, Camfield C, Camfield P. Social adjustment and competence 35 years after onset of childhood epilepsy: a prospective controlled study. *Epilepsia* 1997; 38(6):708–15.
33. Sillanpaa M, Schmidt D. Long-term employment of adults with childhood-onset epilepsy: A prospective population-based study. *Epilepsia* 2010; 51:1053–60.
34. Wakamoto H, Nagao H, Hayashi M, Morimoto T. Long-term medical, educational, and social prognoses of childhood-onset epilepsy: a population-based study in a rural district of Japan. *Brain Dev* 2000; 22:246–55.
35. Trostle JA. Managing epilepsy: a community of chronic illness in Rochester, Minnesota. PhD Thesis, University of California, 1987.
36. Wadsworth MEJ. MRC National Survey of Health & Development. Paper given at Symposium of the International Bureau for Epilepsy 2nd Commission on Epilepsy Risks and Insurability, 24th International Epilepsy Congress, Buenos Aires, 2001.
37. Craig A, Oxley J. Social aspects of epilepsy. In: Laidlaw J, Richens A, Oxley J (eds) *A Textbook of Epilepsy*, pp. 566–610. Edinburgh: Churchill Livingstone, 1993.
38. Jacoby A, Snape D, Baker GA. Epilepsy and social identity: the stigma of a chronic neurological disorder. *Lancet Neurol 2005*; 4: 171–8.
39. Temkin O. *The Falling Sickness*. Baltimore, MD: John Hopkins Press, 1971.
40. Hicks RA, Hicks MJ. Attitudes of major employers towards the employment of people with epilepsy: a 30-year study. *Epilepsia* 1991; 32:86–8.
41. Gade E, Toutges G. Employers' attitudes toward hiring epileptics: Implications for job placement. *Rehabil Counsel Bull* 1983; 26:353–6.
42. Jacoby A, Gorry J, Baker GA. Employers' attitudes to employment of people with epilepsy: Still the same old story? *Epilepsia* 2005; 46:1978–87.
43. Bishop M, Stenhoff DM, Bradley KD, Allen CA. The differential effect of epilepsy labels on employer perceptions: Report of a pilot study. *Epilepsy Behav* 2007; 11:351–6.
44. Parfene C, Stewart TL, King TZ. Epilepsy stigma and stigma by association in the workplace. *Epilepsy Behav* 2009; 15:461–6.
45. Harden CL, Kossoy A, Vera S, Nikolov B. Reaction to epilepsy in the workplace. *Epilepsia* 2004; 45:1134–40.
46. Jacoby A, Gorry J, Gamble C, Baker GA. Public knowledge, private grief: A study of public attitudes to epilepsy in the United Kingdom and implications for stigma. *Epilepsia* 2004; 45(11):1405–15.
47. Clarke BM, Upton ARM, Castellanos CM. Work beliefs and work status in epilepsy. *Epilepsy Behav* 2006; 9:119–25.
48. Scambler G, Hopkins A. Being epileptic: coming to terms with stigma. *Soc Health Illness* 1986; 8:26–43.
49. Scambler G. *Epilepsy*. London: Tavistock, 1989.
50. Jacoby A. Epilepsy and the quality of everyday life: Findings from a study of people with well-controlled epilepsy. *Soc Sci Med* 1992; 34:657–66.
51. Bautista RED, Wludyka P. Factors associated with employment in epilepsy patients. *Epilepsy Behav* 2006; 9(4):625–31.
52. Fraser RT. Epilepsy and employment: an international survey. In: Epilepsy and Employment, Proceedings of the Employment Seminar, 17th International Epilepsy Congress. Jerusalem, Israel: Heemstede IBE, 1987.
53. Hessen E, Lossius MI, Reinvang I, Gjerstad L. Predictors of neuropsychological impairment in seizure-free epilepsy patients. *Epilepsia* 2006; 47:1870–8.
54. Jones JE, Berven NL, Ramirez T, Woodard A, Hermann BP. Long-term psychosocial outcomes of anterior temporal lobectomy. *Epilepsia* 2002; 43:896–903.
55. Reid K, Herbert A, Baker GA. Epilepsy surgery: patient-perceived long-term costs and benefits. *Epilepsy Behav* 2004; 5:81–7.
56. The RESt-1 Group. Social aspects of epilepsy in the adult in seven European countries. *Epilepsia* 2000; 41(8):998–1004.
57. van den Broek M, Beghi E. Morbidity in patients with epilepsy: Type, circumstances and complications: A European cohort study. *Epilepsia* 2004; 45(6):667–72.
58. Dasgupta AK, Saunders M, Dick DJ. Epilepsy in the British Steel Corporation: an evaluation of sickness, accident and work records. *Br J Ind Med* 1982; 39:145–8.
59. Wiebe S, Bellhouse DR, Fallahay C, Eliasziw M. Burden of epilepsy: The Ontario Health Survey. *Can J Neurol Sci* 1999; 26:263–70.
60. Sands H, Zalkind SS. Effects of an educational campaign to change employer attitudes toward hiring epileptics. *Epilepsia* 1972; 13:87–96.
61. Lee P. Has disability discrimination legislation changed the legal framework for epilepsy in the United Kingdom? *Seizure* 2010; 19(10):619–22.
62. Department of Work and Pensions. *Organisations' responses to the Disability Discrimination Act: 2009 Study*. Research Report 685. London: DWP, 2009.
63. Roessler RT, Sumner G. Employer opinions about accommodating employees with chronic illness. *J Appl Rehabil Counsel* 1997; 28(3): 29–34.
64. Varekamp I, Verbeek JHAM, van Dijk FJH. How can we help employees with chronic diseases to stay at work? A review of interventions aimed at job retention and based on an empowerment perspective. *Int Arch Occup Environ Health* 2006; 80:87–97.
65. Collings JA. Psychosocial well-being and epilepsy: An empirical study. *Epilepsia* 1990; 31(4):418–26.
66. Callaghan N, Crowley M, Goggin T. Epilepsy and employment, marital, education and social status. *Ir Med J* 1992; 85:17–19.

CHAPTER 35

Sexual and Emotional Behaviour in Epilepsy

Sarah J. Wilson and Jessie Bendavid

Introduction

An intrinsic link exists between sexual and emotional functioning in humans, both of which are fundamental aspects of our behaviour. This link reflects the shared evolutionary origins of these behaviours that have arisen from common neurobiological substrates in the brain and are vital for the survival of our species (1). It is no surprise then, that disorders of one often accompany disorders of the other, as has been well described in the epilepsies. This is particularly true of certain syndromes, such as mesial temporal lobe epilepsy (MTLE), which disrupts the relevant neurobiological system (the limbic system) and thus, has a well-documented comorbidity of sexual and emotional dysfunction. In addition to the effects of recurrent seizures or a lesion, some antiepileptic drugs (AEDs) have been shown to alter sexual or emotional functioning (2) although this will not be a focus of this review. Rather, here we bring together the relatively separate research fields of sexual and emotional functioning in epilepsy, with the aim of providing a more cohesive framework for understanding relationships between the two, given their shared evolutionary and neurobiological bases. We will also consider the effects of epilepsy surgery, particularly mesial temporal lobe resection, which commonly produces changes in sexual and emotional functioning, and provides important insights into the neurobiological and psychosocial aspects of both behaviours.

The evolution of human sexuality and emotional functioning

Evolutionary theorists have proposed that the principal purpose of sexual relationships is to pass on genes to offspring, with the evolution of sexual reproduction promoting genetic diversity and increased adaptation to changing environments (3, 4). Overlaid on this is the need for an intrinsically emotional processing system that allows an organism to determine whether or not it is safe to approach another, leading to an avoidant or approach response. This includes the detection of perceived threat and the experience of fear, which is automatically processed by the amygdala in the human limbic system and leads to activation of the sympathetic nervous system and modulating systems of the hypothalamic–pituitary (HP) axis (5, 6). An approach response is also linked to the limbic system via the experience of reward, which is vital for engendering species-typical responses to important activities such as eating and mating, thereby increasing the likelihood of survival and reproduction (7, 8).

In humans, our system for approach–avoidant behaviour has evolved to incorporate more complex emotions that also promote (genetic) survival. For example, romantic love and maternal love are crucial to the perpetuation of the species by promoting reproduction and the raising of offspring, respectively. Based on this shared evolutionary purpose, it has been argued that both types of love share common neural mechanisms (9), including activation of the reward system of the brain (ventral tegmental area, ventral striatum (nucleus accumbens), and middle insula), and deactivation of regions involved in critical social judgment (such as the amygdala, mesial prefrontal cortex, and temporal poles). This implies that the apprehension with which we typically analyse faces for dangerous signs is suspended in romantic and maternal love (10), providing a means of 'overriding' our basic instinct to detect fear.

Both types of love also show unique patterns of neural activation, with romantic love selectively activating the hypothalamus, just as sexual arousal activates the hypothalamus and subcortical regions adjacent to romantic love (10). In other words, we have evolved to engage in sexual behaviour that is intrinsically linked to the experience of emotions, hence it is not surprising that both have a shared neurobiological basis in the limbic system and associated brain structures (11, 12). Since the prefrontal cortex has dense interconnections with limbic structures, particularly in the mesial prefrontal region, humans have also evolved a means of regulating their sexual behaviour and integrating their emotions with higher cognitive processes. This retains the benefits of the adaptive 'fight/flight' response while also allowing the cortical evaluation and appraisal of social situations (13).

Brain regions mediating human sexuality and emotional functioning

The results of lesion studies combined with more recent neuroimaging research have increasingly allowed us to map the networks of the brain most likely subserving human sexual and emotional functioning. The 'affective network' is now recognized to include the anterior cingulate cortex (subgenual and pregenual cingulate) and connected regions of the limbic system, such as the amygdala, entorhinal cortex, hypothalamus, and nucleus accumbens (see Fig. 35.1). This network is central to emotional processing, including vigilance, the perception and recognition of facial expressions, and fear conditioning (14). It also regulates autonomic and visceral functions, such as appetite, sleep, and sexual libido, and has been strongly implicated in depression (15–19).

As shown in Fig. 35.1, the affective network has substantial overlap with brain regions supporting sexual functioning. These include the anterior cingulate cortex and nucleus accumbens, implicated in the perceptual aspects of sexual drive, as well as the hypothalamus for mediating neuroendocrine and autonomic aspects of sexual drive and orientation (20). Also pertinent are limbic system structures, such as the amygdala, which have been implicated in sexual orientation, drive, and disorders of sexual function (11, 12, 21). The central role of the amygdala in both emotional and sexual behaviour is evident from the striking symptoms of Klüver–Bucy syndrome that can follow bilateral temporal lobectomy. Among others, these symptoms include indiscriminate sexual behaviour, hypersexuality, and unusual approach behaviours due to the absence of fear or expression of anger (the so called 'taming effect') (22).

Neocortical regions are also important in both sexual and emotional functioning. The prefrontal cortex allows us to regulate our more basic desires and instincts, including inhibition of socially inappropriate sexual behaviour or emotional responses. The orbitofrontal cortex has been particularly implicated in extinguishing conditioned fear and anticipating reward, with damage to this region typically giving rise to behavioural disinhibition (23, 24). The parietal cortex is central to somatosensory experiences including genital sensations (25, 26), and through simulation of facial expression, is considered important for the recognition of emotions (27). In other words, the complex interconnections that have formed between brain regions supporting sexual and emotional functioning in humans highlight that the determinants of sexual and emotional behaviour are multifactorial, and that the two can be influenced by similar factors given their shared evolutionary purpose.

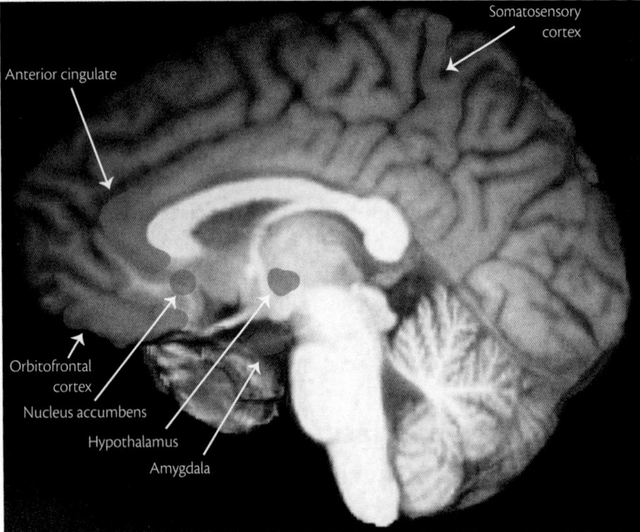

Fig. 35.1 (Also see Colour plate 19.) Sagittal view of the right hemisphere of the brain showing overlapping regions of the sexual and affective networks (approximate locations shown with shading).

Sexual and emotional functioning in epilepsy

Multiple determinants of sexual and emotional dysfunction in epilepsy

Epilepsy is becoming increasingly recognized as a disease of brain networks (28), and has well-known effects that extend beyond seizures to physical, affective, cognitive, and psychosocial domains. This is particularly the case for medically intractable seizures. For instance, long-term outcome research shows that children with medically intractable seizures are ultimately less likely to marry and have their own children, have lower socioeconomic status, poorer educational levels, and are less likely to be gainfully employed than healthy controls (29–32). These pervasive effects clearly impact upon an individual's sexual and emotional development across the lifespan, meaning that difficulties may arise at various stages that stem from different origins, but have interacting effects. Consistent with this, research to date suggests abnormally high levels of sexual, reproductive, and emotional dysfunction in epilepsy, the causes of which are likely multifactorial. Thus, research investigating the nature of sexual and emotional difficulties in epilepsy has addressed a large number of potentially causal, overlapping factors that span biological, affective, cognitive, and psychosocial domains (see Table 35.1). Currently, however, we lack a comprehensive framework that systematically accounts for the interactions between factors, within or across domains.

Within the biological domain, it has been argued that genetics plays a major role in our predisposition to episodic behavioural disturbances, with some individuals more likely to exhibit seizures or affective episodes in response to stressors (33). Dysfunction in a range of neurotransmitter systems, including serotonergic (5-HT) and noradrenergic deficits, as well as glutamate and gamma-aminobutyric acid (GABA)ergic abnormalities have been described in both affective and seizure disorders, leading to the view that they partially share pathogenic mechanisms (34, 35). For example, functional imaging studies have shown decreased binding of 5-HT_{1A} in limbic system structures and the cingulate gyrus in both epilepsy and depression (35). In addition, GABAergic interneurons form part of the core circuitry of the corticolimbic system, which regulates the release of corticotropin-releasing hormone (CRH). It has been proposed that excess secretion of CRH from the hypothalamus may trigger seizures and mood dysfunction via the HP axis. Supporting this, hyperactivity of the HP axis has been associated with seizure exacerbation (36), mood alterations (37), and reproductive and sexual dysfunction (38).

The HP axis stimulates hormonal secretion from regions such as the gonads and adrenal glands, which the liver and kidneys ultimately metabolize. Epileptiform discharges, particularly those arising in the temporolimbic circuit, have been associated with abnormal hormone secretion and higher rates of sexual reproduction disorders in women with epilepsy, such as polycystic ovarian syndrome and menstrual dysfunction (38–41). Similarly in men with epilepsy, reduced potency, abnormal semen analysis, and hypogonadotropic hypogonadism have been reported (42, 43). Higher rates of sexual dysfunction, such as erectile dysfunction in

Table 35.1 Overlapping factors that may be associated with sexual and emotional dysfunction in epilepsy

Domain	Sexual dysfunction	Emotional dysfunction
Biological	Limbic system dysfunction: ◆ Amygdala abnormalities	Limbic system dysfunction: ◆ Amygdala and hippocampal abnormalities
	HP axis dysfunction: ◆ Altered secretion of sex hormones ◆ Sexual and reproductive dysfunction	HP axis dysfunction: ◆ Excess secretion of cortisol ◆ mood disturbance
Treatment effects	Antiepileptic drugs: ◆ Altered sex hormone binding proteins ◆ Decreased testosterone, sexual libido	Antiepileptic drugs: ◆ Altered inhibitory neurotransmitter release ◆ Lowered mood
	Selective serotonin reuptake inhibitors (for mood disturbance) ◆ Reduced sexual libido, delayed orgasm	
Affective	Impaired emotional recognition: ◆ Altered close relationships and sexual functioning	Impaired emotional recognition: ◆ Mood disturbance
Cognitive	Autobiographical memory impairment: ◆ Altered sense of self, sexual confidence	Autobiographical memory impairment: ◆ Risk factor for depression
	Impaired social cognition: ◆ Sexual anxiety	Impaired social cognition: ◆ Lowered mood, heightened anxiety
Psychological	Low self-esteem and internal locus of control: ◆ Reduced sense of sexual attractiveness ◆ Reduced libido, sexual dysfunction	Low self-esteem and internal locus of control: ◆ Risk factor for mood disturbance
Psychosocial	Relationship difficulties	Relationship difficulties
	Reduced social activities	Reduced social activities
	Reduced quality of life	Reduced quality of life

men (44) and vaginismus and dyspareunia in women (45) have also been noted, with bioactive available testosterone levels related to the level of sexual dysfunction in both men and women with TLE (41). AEDs may also alter concentrations of sex steroid hormones leading to sexual and reproductive dysfunction (46). For example, enzyme-inducing AEDs have been shown to lower serum levels of sex hormones and have been linked to a range of reproductive disorders (47). AEDs have also been associated with arousal difficulties, decreased libido, anorgasmia, and sexual anxiety, with dysfunction particularly evident in individuals with higher depression scores (48, 49). Related to this, known anticonvulsant mechanisms of action, such as the potentiation of GABAergic neurotransmitter release, have been related to lowered mood (50).

The HP axis has direct projections from the hippocampus and amygdala, allowing their function to influence hormone release. In turn, high cortisol levels, reflecting a hyperactive HP axis, have been detected in individuals with epilepsy (51) or depression (52), and have been suggested to result in hippocampal atrophy (52). Abnormalities of the hippocampus or amygdala commonly give rise to seizures in MTLE (53), and volumetric changes in the hippocampus and amygdala have been related to mood disturbance (depression and anxiety) and sexual functioning (21, 54–56). In the literature, TLE has a long-standing association with hyposexuality (57) and heightened mood disturbance, particularly a high comorbidity of anxiety and depression (58). This is not surprising given the typical seizure network in TLE, as revealed by measures of regional cerebral blood flow (59), overlaps with the affective and sexual networks of the brain, likely altering HP axis function and accounting for the heightened comorbidity of emotional, sexual and reproductive dysfunction.

In addition to heightened sexual and mood comorbidities, habitual activity in the TLE seizure network or the presence of a limbic system lesion could be expected to disrupt basic emotional processes mediated by the affective network, such as emotional recognition (60). In support of this, over the last 10 years an increasing number of studies have reported emotion recognition deficits and impairments in social cognition in people with epilepsy, particularly MTLE. Given the relatively recent emergence of this intriguing research field, it will be reviewed in greater detail later (see 'Emotional processing and social cognition in epilepsy' section). The point here, however, is that impairments in emotional recognition and social cognition may directly contribute to mood disturbance, and lead to difficulties with close relationships and sexual intimacy. Arguably, they may also contribute to the report of reduced libido and sexual dysfunction in depressed individuals.

Within the cognitive domain, memory dysfunction has long been regarded as the chief neuropsychological concern in TLE (61, 62). Some degree of memory impairment can be documented in almost all cases, with ongoing seizure activity deepening and extending memory impairments in the long term (63). The learning of new, arbitrarily-related events and information has been ascribed to the mesial temporal region, particularly the entorhinal–hippocampal interface (64). Within this declarative memory system, autobiographic memory binds events and people encountered in space and time with accompanying emotional experiences to create self-narrative (65). This is reflected in the well-established behavioural overlap between autobiographic memory and mood. For instance, impoverished autobiographic memory is considered a trait-like vulnerability factor for developing depression as well as a maintaining factor, leading to poor prognosis and long-term adjustment difficulties (66). A strong neurobiological overlap between autobiographic memory and mood has also been demonstrated (67), with the mesial temporal region independently implicated in autobiographic memory dysfunction (68) and depressive symptomatology in TLE (54, 69).

Conceivably, the effects of habitual seizures on autobiographic memory functioning and the ability to construct a coherent self-narrative may ultimately lead to the development of an altered sense of self. Consistent with this, the psychological effects of seizures have been shown to include a reduced sense of personal autonomy, lowered self-esteem, and perceived loss of self-control (70–72). The unpredictable nature of seizures may particularly impact upon the attribution of an internal locus of control, presumably via mechanisms of learned helplessness (73). Such mechanisms have been strongly implicated in treatment adherence, adjustment to illness, and the experience of mood disturbance, particularly depression (74). Loss of an internal locus of control may also undermine an individual's sexual identity and sense of sexual attractiveness, thereby contributing to lowered libido and sexual dysfunction (75).

Combined, the biological, affective, cognitive, and psychological factors canvassed above contribute to the well-recognized deleterious psychosocial effects of epilepsy, particularly in medically intractable epilepsy. These include impaired physical functioning, reduced vocational and community integration, disrupted family functioning and carer burden, decreased marriage rates, social stigma and isolation, and reduced quality of life (71, 76, 77). Fig. 35.2 provides a possible framework for understanding the complex interactions between biological, cognitive, and psychosocial factors, both within and across domains, in terms of their impact upon sexual and emotional functioning. In this figure, two key pathways are highlighted that recognize the proposed role of HP axis dysfunction and emotional processing deficits in sexual, reproductive, and emotional difficulties.

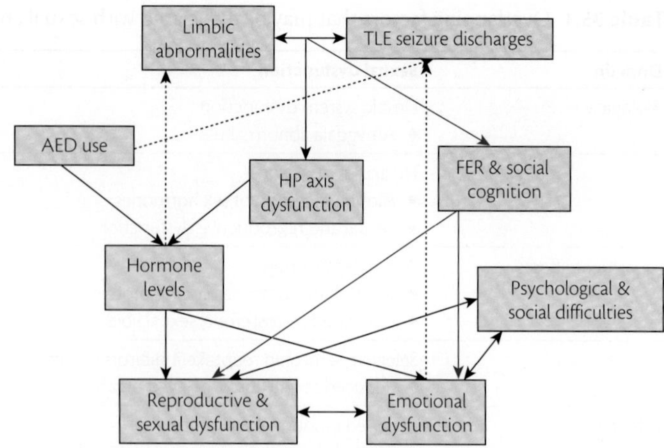

Fig. 35.2 A preliminary framework highlighting the complexity of interactions between factors impacting upon sexual and emotional functioning in epilepsy. Within this framework, two key pathways are shown. First, seizure discharges and limbic abnormalities may cause HP axis dysfunction, resulting in altered hormone release and reproductive, sexual and emotional dysfunction (black arrows). Second, seizure discharges and limbic abnormalities may produce deficits in facial emotional recognition (FER) and social cognition that contribute to mood disturbance and impair sexual functioning (dashed black arrows).

Emotional processing and social cognition in epilepsy

Recognition of facial emotions

Human facial expressions provide vital information for engaging in effective social interactions and intimate relationships, which are central to our emotional well-being and perceived quality of life (78). The ability to recognize emotions is typically assessed in terms of the six basic emotions of fear, anger, sadness, disgust, happiness, and surprise (79). In epilepsy, studies investigating facial emotion recognition (FER) have revealed significant impairment in people with generalized epilepsy, frontal lobe epilepsy, and most notably MTLE (see Table 35.2). This impairment is suspected to result from the effects of epileptiform discharges or a lesion in limbic system structures, such as the hippocampus or amygdala. Other epilepsy-related factors have also been consistently identified, such as an early age of first or habitual seizure onset, and right-sided laterality of the seizure focus (see Table 35.2).

Various methods have been used to assess FER abilities. Typically, an individual is required to name one of the basic emotions depicted in a photograph, or to match the photo with a verbal label or target photo. Evidence from these tasks suggests that patients with right TLE are more likely to experience emotional processing difficulties than those with left TLE (80–83), although left TLE patients may still show impairment relative to controls (83, 84). Notably, the importance of an intact right amygdala has been highlighted, particularly for the recognition of 'withdrawal' emotions, such as fear (80–90), sadness (80, 82, 83, 86, 90), and disgust (82–84, 86, 90).

Several studies have found that early onset of habitual seizures, especially before a proposed critical age of approximately 5 years, is common in patients with FER impairment (81–84, 88). This is particularly the case for fear recognition deficits (81, 82, 84, 88). For example, individuals with right MTLE and early seizure onset showed impaired fear recognition that was associated with decreased activation of the limbic network during an FER task compared to controls (81). In addition, those with early onset but not late onset MTLE had impaired fear recognition compared to controls (81, 84, 87, 88), with younger age at first seizure and epilepsy onset correlated with greater levels of FER impairment (83). Febrile convulsions have also been correlated with FER impairment in right TLE (81, 82), and specifically linked to impaired fear recognition in TLE (84). These findings lend support to the proposed 'early-onset' hypothesis that epileptiform discharges may alter plasticity in regions pertinent to FER, leading to impaired neural development and life-long FER difficulties (88).

Researchers have noted that the early-onset hypothesis is supported by the observation that anterior temporal lobectomy (ATL) and accompanying seizure freedom rarely lead to improved FER, particularly post-right ATL (85–88, 90). For example, Shaw and colleagues prospectively assessed FER in patients undergoing ATL and found some improvement in fear recognition after left ATL but no change after right ATL. Other studies have suggested that right ATL may impair FER, including recognition of fear, sadness, and disgust compared to controls (85–88, 90). These studies, however, did not always account for preoperative FER performance, or

Table 35.2 Studies examining emotional processing and social cognition in epilepsy

Authors (reference)	Sample	Task	Results
Facial emotion recognition (FER)			
Batut et al. 2006 (80)	12 MTLE 15 controls	Implicit and explicit processing of positive and negative facial emotions	Right MTLE were impaired at FER, especially fear Implicit: MTLE made more errors in FER than controls Explicit: MTLE were impaired in fear and sadness recognition
Benuzzi et al. 2004 (81)	8 right MTLE 5 left MTLE 14 controls	Emotion recognition in morphed faces Viewing fearful versus neutral faces (fMRI)	Right MTLE were impaired for fear, with early onset most impaired Impaired fear processing was associated with reduced limbic activation, particularly in right MTLE
Golouboff et al. 2008 (84)	Children: 29 TLE (13 right, 16 left) 8 frontocentral epilepsy 37 controls	Match facial expression with an emotion	All fear impaired individuals had TLE, with early onset TLE significantly impaired Left TLE impaired for fear and neutrality, right TLE for disgust, frontocentral epilepsy for happiness
Meletti et al. 2003 (82)	33 TLE (MTS) 30 TLE (lesion) 33 extratemporal 50 controls	Match facial expression with an emotion	Right MTS were impaired at FER, particularly for fear, sadness and disgust recognition. In right TLE, the degree of FER impairment correlated with age at first seizure and age at epilepsy onset
Meletti et al. 2009 (83)	140 MTLE 36 lateral TLE 50 controls	Match facial expression with an emotion	Bilateral, right, and left MTLE were impaired for all emotions except happiness. Early onset MTLE correlated with FER dysfunction
Anterior temporal lobectomy (ATL) studies			
Adolphs et al. 2001 (85)	11 right ATL 15 left ATL 50 brain-injured controls	Rate facial expressions against a basic emotion	Right ATL were significantly impaired for fear compared to controls Age at seizure onset correlated with recognition of fearful faces
Anderson et al. 2000 (86)	12 right ATL 11 left ATL 23 controls	Evaluation of facial expression against an emotional term	Right ATL most impaired for fear, disgust, and sadness compared to other groups
Hlobil et al. 2008 (87)	76 MTLE: 36 pre-ATL 40 post-ATL 45 right, 31 left 39 early onset 37 late onset 28 controls	Choose photo of facial expression among photos of distractor emotions	Early onset right MTLE were impaired for fear compared to all other groups Post-ATL: happiness recognition was improved compared to pre-ATL
McClelland et al. 2006 (88)	Right ATL 7 early onset 5 late onset 10 controls	Match facial expression with an emotion	Post-ATL: early onset less accurate at matching fearful faces compared to controls and late onset despite seizure freedom
Social cognition			
Farrant et al. 2005 (96)	14 FLE 14 controls	Happe's strange stories Faux pas task Humour appreciation Inferring mental states from eye gaze Match facial expression with an emotion	FLE showed a trend for impairment on the faux pas task and no impairment on the story task FLE were impaired on the humour and eye gaze tasks FLE were impaired in facial emotion recognition, especially fear, anger, and sadness
Reynders et al. 2005 (89)	37 TLE_{IF} 14 $TLE_{no\ IF}$ 10 IGE 12 controls	Match facial expression with an emotion Social judgement of approachability and trustworthiness	All epilepsy groups were impaired for fear detection TLE_{IF} were significantly impaired compared to $TLE_{no\ IF}$ and IGE Fear recognition deficits were associated with impaired judgments of trustworthiness
Schachter et al. 2006 (95)	27 MTLE: 14 right, 13 left 16 pre-surgery 11 post-surgery 27 extramesial 12 controls	Faux pas task	MTLE were significantly impaired at detecting faux pas pre- and postsurgery Right MTLE worse than left MTLE

(Continued)

Table 35.2 *(Continued)*

Authors (reference)	Sample	Task	Results
Schilbach et al. 2007 (94)	10 female left TLE 10 female controls	Virtual character's direction of gaze and type of facial expression	Left TLE group showed an 'egocentric bias' where they perceived all communication toward them as socially relevant
Shaw et al. 2007 (90)	19 TLE: pre- & post-ATL 10 right TLE 9 left TLE	Happe's strange stories Faux pas task Intensity ratings of facial emotions	No significant effects for theory of mind tasks. Pre-ATL, patients gave higher incongruent ratings for facial expressions compared to control data. Post-ATL, left TLE evaluated fearful faces in a more normative way
Walpole et al. 2008 (93)	16 TLE 14 controls	Match facial expression with an emotion Emotional intelligence (EQ-i)	TLE group impaired on both tasks

ATL, anterior temporal lobectomy; FLE, frontal lobe epilepsy; IGE, idiopathic generalized epilepsy; MTLE, mesial temporal lobe epilepsy; MTS, mesial temporal sclerosis; TLE, temporal lobe epilepsy; TLE_{IF}, TLE with ictal fear.

age of habitual seizure onset. In the latter case, McClelland and colleagues (88) found that early-onset MTLE patients showed fear recognition impairments after surgery, while later onset patients showed comparable performance to controls.

Considered overall, the studies reported in the field to date (Table 35.2) generally indicate that right ATL may impair FER, likely reflecting the fundamental role of the right amygdala in emotional processing. Conversely, FER functioning following left ATL is comparable to controls, and improvements may be evident relative to preoperative performance. The findings should be considered relative to the age of onset of habitual seizures, with early onset showing minimal change in FER after ATL, while later onset may show signs of improvement. Patients at particular disadvantage are those with early onset right TLE, who may show life-long difficulties recognizing withdrawal emotions. Such difficulties are likely to impact upon social cognition generally, and sexual functioning in particular, and are consistent with the report of increased sexual changes following right versus left ATL (91) reviewed in greater detail below (see 'Interictal sexual behaviour and behavioural change after epilepsy surgery' section).

Social cognition

Few studies have examined social cognition in epilepsy, despite its importance for perceiving social signals and interpreting the actions of others, as well as guiding our own social behaviour. Some studies have employed both FER and social cognition tasks (see Table 35.2) given the importance of accurately recognizing emotions for social cognition, and thus the likely effects of epileptiform discharges on the neural circuitry relevant to both (60, 92). The most common paradigm used to assess social cognition in epilepsy has involved inferring the mental states of others (so called 'theory of mind'), typically using stories that contain social faux pas or require a non-literal interpretation. This ability is pertinent to cognitive and emotional empathy and is fundamental to effective social functioning. Emotional intelligence, social judgments of trustworthiness and approachability, and interpreting eye gaze have also been examined (Table 2).

Given the small number of studies performed to date, only preliminary conclusions can be drawn. However, these generally support impaired social cognition in epilepsy that may relate to the degree of FER impairment. In particular, social cognition deficits have been observed in most (89, 93, 94), but not all samples with TLE (90), despite the use of different measures of social cognition. Patients with MTLE have especially poor performance compared to non-mesial patients, with a right-sided laterality effect reported by Schachter and colleagues (95) on a social faux pas task. Considering the role of the prefrontal cortex in social behaviour, it is not surprising that frontal lobe epilepsy has also been associated with deficits on some social cognition tasks (96). These include impaired recognition of humour and the use of eye gaze to infer mental states in others, as well as mild difficulties recognizing social faux pas (96). Epilepsy variables, such as the age of onset of habitual seizures, their duration, frequency, or laterality of focus have not shown consistent positive effects, although considerably more research is required to investigate this important domain of cognitive functioning, with preliminary studies clearly highlighting its relevance in people with TLE.

Interictal sexual behaviour and behavioural change after epilepsy surgery

Similar to research investigating emotional processing and social cognition, there is a paucity of studies examining sexual behaviour in people with epilepsy. There are even fewer studies assessing change in sexual behaviour following epilepsy surgery, although existing research again provides an important foundation on which to build (see Table 35.3). Reports of ictal sexual phenomenon in the literature are quite rare, and include sexual auras, genital sensations during seizures, and genital and sexual automatisms (97, 98). These have been found to occur in individuals with frontal lobe epilepsy, idiopathic generalized epilepsy, and TLE, with the mesial temporal region implicated in their origin (98–100). As already noted, interictal changes in sexual behaviour have also been reported, most commonly hyposexuality in TLE (41, 44, 45, 101–104). This has typically been defined as sexual activity less than once per month (57, 105–109), comprising a decrease in sexual desire and/or arousal, and more frequently reported in patients with right compared to left TLE (41, 101).

A key challenge for investigating change in interictal sexual functioning is defining what might constitute 'normal' sexual behaviour, given its significant variability in the general population (110). One approach to addressing this issue involves obtaining an individual's subjective view of what constitutes 'normal', and then measuring change relative to this baseline. Using this approach,

Table 35.3 Studies examining sexual functioning in epilepsy

Authors (reference)	Sample	Task	Results
Daniele et al. 1997 (101)	22 male TLE 23 female TLE 30 controls	Sexual Interest and Sexual Performance Questionnaire	Right TLE showed reduced sexual interest compared to left TLE in men and women when implicitly explored
Duncan et al. 2009 (44)	69 men with epilepsy 50 male controls	Sexual Desire Inventory Sexual Response Inventory Sexual Self-Efficacy Scale—Erectile Function	Patients had lower scores on the Sexual Desire Inventory and the Sexual Self-Efficacy Scale compared to controls
Herzog et al. 2003 (41)	36 females: 16 right TLE 20 left TLE 9 TLE (treated) 12 controls	Arizona Sexual Experience Scale	TLE had significantly higher scores than controls 5 treated left TLE had scores in the normal range Right TLE had abnormally high scores compared to controls
Jensen et al. 1990 (113)	86 people with epilepsy	Interview	Frequency of sexual dysfunction in epilepsy did not differ from data acquired in a previous study with diabetic patients and controls
Morrell and Guldner 1996 (45)	99 focal epilepsy 17 primary generalized epilepsy	Sexual Arousability Inventory—Expanded Sexual Behaviour Inventory Sexual Functioning Inventory	Patients reported altered sexual function compared to control data Focal epilepsy patients were more sexually anxious than control data
Saunders and Rawson 1970 (102)	100 males: 65 idiopathic epilepsy 33 TLE 2 cortical seizures	Interview	TLE had disrupted sexual behaviour
Shukla et al. 1979 (104)	44 TLE: 30 male, 14 female 47 generalized epilepsy: 34 male, 13 female	Interview	In each gender, hyposexuality was more common in TLE compared to generalized epilepsy
Silveira et al. 2001 (103)	39 people with epilepsy 39 controls	Interview Follow-up interview at 2 years	Hyposexuality was more frequent among people with epilepsy, particularly TLE. Follow-up: sexual function improved in patients with good seizure control
Temporal lobe resection studies			
Baird et al. 2002 (112)	7 TLR with hypersexuality	Case series	5 patients had bilateral temporal lobe abnormalities. All patients had psychosocial adjustment issues that preceded hypersexuality
Baird et al. 2003 (91)	58 TLR 16 ETR	Interview & questionnaire	Postoperative sexual change: more likely in TLR than ETR, right than left TLR, and in females
Baird et al. 2004 (21)	45 TLR 46 controls	Interview & questionnaire T1-weighted MRI	Postoperative sexual increase was associated with a larger contralateral amygdalar volume. Volume was positively correlated with maximum degree of sexual change postsurgery

ETR, extratemporal resection; TLE, temporal lobe epilepsy; TLR, temporal lobe resection.

patients with focal seizures typically regarded a 'normal' sex drive as wanting to have sex once to a few times per week, and similarly, a 'normal' sex life as having sex once to a few times per week (91). Following epilepsy surgery, those undergoing temporal lobe resection for TLE were significantly more likely to report a sexual increase to 'normal' levels, compared to those undergoing extratemporal resections. This was particularly evident following right-sided resections in the first 3 months after surgery, and was more commonly reported by females (91).

An interesting parallel can be drawn between this profile and the evolution of mood change, specifically depression, after surgery. It is also more common in the first 3 months and more likely to present *de novo* following mesial temporal lobe resection, compared to non-mesial resection (111). In both profiles the change is heralded by psychosocial disruption, most notably altered family functioning and relationship dynamics that likely exacerbate the appearance of the change (111, 112). Anxiety and depression may accompany more extreme changes in sexual behaviour after surgery, such as hypersexuality (112). This is not surprising given that both have been linked to the preoperative integrity of limbic system structures. In the case of sexual change, a positive correlation has been reported between contralateral amygdala volume and sexual drive, and in the case of mood change, a negative association has been reported between contralateral hippocampal volume and the experience of depression after surgery (21, 54).

Conclusions

For most people, a meaningful life includes intimate emotional and sexual relationships and reproduction. There is an intrinsic link between emotional and sexual functioning that is evident from their shared evolutionary purpose and their interconnected brain circuitry. From this, behaviours such as monogamy and face-to-face copulation have developed to promote bonding and sexual reproduction, and facilitate feelings of love and intimacy. In other words, emotional and sexual behaviour constitute core aspects of our social relationships and psychological functioning, and are central to our perceived quality of life.

In this chapter, we have deliberately juxtaposed research on emotional and sexual functioning in epilepsy, to allow links between these research fields to emerge that might support a more cohesive framework. This research indicates that people with epilepsy, particularly MTLE, are more likely to experience emotional and sexual dysfunction and reproductive disorders. Biologically, this is thought to reflect disruption to limbic system structures and associated brain regions common to their neural networks. The cause of the dysfunction may also include psychological, cognitive, and social factors; however, within this multifactorial framework, two key mechanisms have gained increasing research support. The first proposes that a hyperactive HP axis leads to excess hormone secretion and subsequent emotional and sexual dysfunction. The second relates to a basic impairment in facial emotion recognition that is a core skill on which our emotional regulation depends, and on which we base a range of complex behaviours including social and sexual relationships. Of note, this research has pointed to the fundamental role of the right amygdala in impaired recognition of withdrawal emotions, particularly in patients with TLE onset early in development.

The comorbidity of emotional and sexual dysfunction in epilepsy has also been found to vary with the medical treatment undertaken, with AEDs and temporal lobe resection having differential but well-documented effects. Although not the focus of this review, AEDs can alter sex hormone concentrations and neurotransmitter release that may have detrimental effects on sexual and reproductive function, and sedating effects on mood. Disruption of limbic system function via temporal lobe resection has also been associated with lowered mood, but increased sex drive, both of which are typically accompanied by impaired psychosocial functioning. These findings highlight the complexity of interactions underpinning emotional and sexual change in epilepsy and the need to consider individual differences in clinical presentation. Greater understanding of this complexity promises improved treatments that may ultimately benefit both the emotional and sexual functioning of people with epilepsy. At present, mood disorders remain underdiagnosed and sexual functioning is often not discussed in clinical practice. Likewise in research, few studies have examined the links between emotional and sexual functioning in pre- or postoperative samples. As a first step, addressing these challenges will move us towards identifying appropriate interventions that can better preserve sexual and emotional functioning, thereby enhancing quality of life for people with epilepsy.

References

1. Darwin C. *The expression of emotion in man and animals*. London: HarperCollins, 1872.
2. Hamed SA. Neuroendocrine hormonal conditions in epilepsy: relationship to reproductive and sexual functions. *Neurologist* 2008; 14(3):157–69.
3. Fisher RA. *The genetical theory of natural selection* (2nd edn). New York: Dover, 1958.
4. Muller HJ. The relation of recombination to mutational advance. *Mutat Res* 1964; 106:2–9.
5. LeDoux JE. Emotional memory systems in the brain. *Behav Brain Res* 1993; 58(1–2):69–79.
6. Adolphs R, Tranel D, Damasio H, Damasio A. Impaired recognition of emotion in facial expressions following bilateral damage to the human amygdala. *Nature* 1994; 372(6507):669–72.
7. Glickman SE, Schiff BB. A biological theory of reinforcement. *Psychol Rev* 1967; 74(2):81–109.
8. Olds J, Milner P. Positive reinforcement produced by electrical stimulation of septal area and other regions of rat brain. *J Comp Physiol Psychol* 1954; 47(6):419–27.
9. Bartels A, Zeki S. The neural correlates of maternal and romantic love. *Neuroimage* 2004; 21(3):1155–66.
10. Zeki S. The neurobiology of love. *FEBS Lett* 2007; 581:2575–9.
11. Baird AD, Wilson SJ, Bladin PF, Saling MM, Reutens DC. Neurological control of human sexual behaviour: insights from lesion studies. *J Neurol Neurosurg Psychiatry* 2007; 78(10):1042–9.
12. Rees PM, Fowler CJ, Maas CP. Sexual function in men and women with neurological disorders. *Lancet* 2007; 369(9560):512–25.
13. Barbas H. Connections underlying the synthesis of cognition, memory, and emotion in primate prefrontal cortices. *Brain Res Bull* 2000; 52(5):319–30.
14. Adolphs R. Recognizing emotion from facial expressions: psychological and neurological mechanisms. *Behav Cogn Neurosci Rev* 2002; 1(1):21–62.
15. Sheline YI, Price JL, Yan Z, Mintun MA. Resting-state functional MRI in depression unmasks increased connectivity between networks via the dorsal nexus. *Proc Natl Acad Sci U S A* 2010; 107(24):11020–5.
16. Mayberg HS, Liotti M, Brannan SK, McGinnis S, Mahurin RK, Jerabek PA, *et al.* Reciprocal limbic-cortical function and negative mood: converging PET findings in depression and normal sadness. *Am J Psychiatry* 1999; 156(5):675–82.
17. Johansen-Berg H, Gutman DA, Behrens TE, Matthews PM, Rushworth MF, Katz E, *et al.* Anatomical connectivity of the subgenual cingulate region targeted with deep brain stimulation for treatment-resistant depression. *Cereb Cortex* 2008; 18(6):1374–83.
18. Phillips ML, Drevets WC, Rauch SL, Lane R. Neurobiology of emotion perception II: Implications for major psychiatric disorders. *Biol Psychiatry* 2003; 54(5):515–28.
19. Kennedy SH, Evans KR, Krüger S, Mayberg HS, Meyer JH, McCann S, *et al.* Changes in regional brain glucose metabolism measured with positron emission tomography after paroxetine treatment of major depression. *Am J Psychiatry* 2001; 158(6):899–905.
20. Pfaus JG, Damsma G, Wenkstern D, Fibiger HC. Sexual activity increases dopamine transmission in the nucleus accumbens and striatum of female rats. *Brain Res* 1995; 693(1–2):21–30.
21. Baird AD, Wilson SJ, Bladin PB, Saling MM, Reutens DC. The amygdala and sexual drive: Insights from temporal lobe resection in intractable epilepsy. *Ann Neurol* 2004; 55(1):87–96.
22. Klüver H, Bucy PC. Preliminary analysis of functions of the temporal lobes in monkeys. *Arch Neurol Psychiatry* 1939; 42:979–1000.
23. Kahnt T, Heinzle J, Park SQ, Haynes JD. The neural code of reward anticipation in human orbitofrontal cortex. *Proc Natl Acad* Sci U S A 2010; 107(13):6010–15.
24. Peters F, Perani D, Herholz K, Holthoff V, Beuthien-Baumann B, Sorbi S, *et al.* Orbitofrontal dysfunction related to both apathy and disinhibition in frontotemporal dementia. *Dement Geriatr Cogn Disord* 2006; 21(5–6):373–9.
25. Toone B. Sex, sexual seizures and the female with epilepsy. In: Trimble MR (eds) *Women and epilepsy*, pp. 201–6. West Sussex: John Wiley & Sons, 1991.

26. Toone B. Epilepsy and sexual life. In: Hopkins A, Shorvon S, Cascino G (eds) *Epilepsy* (2nd edn), pp. 557–64. London: Chapman & Hall, 1995.
27. Adolphs R, Damasio H, Tranel D, Cooper G, Damasio AR. A role for somatosensory cortices in the visual recognition of emotion as revealed by 3-D lesion mapping. *J Neurosci* 2000; 20:2683–90.
28. Carney PW, Masterton RAJ, Harvey AS, Scheffer IE, Berkovic SF, Jackson GD. The core network in absence epilepsy. *Neurology* 2010; 75:904–11.
29. Ounsted CJ, Richards P. *Temporal lobe epilepsy: a biographical study 1948–1986*. Oxford: Mac Keith Press, Blackwell Scientific Publications, 1987.
30. Shackleton DP, Trenité K-N, de Craen AJM, Vandenbroucke JP, Westendorp RGJ. Living with epilepsy: long-term prognosis and psychosocial outcomes. *Neurology* 2003; 61(1):64–70.
31. Sillanpää M. Children with epilepsy as adults: Outcome after 30 years of follow-up. *Acta Paediatr Scand* 1990; 368:1–78.
32. Sillanpää M, Haataja L, Shinnar S. Perceived impact of childhood-onset epilepsy on quality of life as an adult. *Epilepsia* 2004; 45(8): 971–7.
33. Jobe PC. Common pathogenic mechanisms between depression and epilepsy: an experimental perspective. *Epilepsy Behav* 2003; 4(Suppl. 3):S14–24.
34. Jobe PC, Dailey JW, Wernicke JF. A noradrenergic and serotonergic hypothesis of the linkage between epilepsy and affective disorders. *Crit Rev Neurobiol*. 1999; 13(4):317–56.
35. Kanner AM. Depression and epilepsy: A bidirectional relation? *Epilepsia* 2011; 52(Suppl. 1):21–7.
36. Kumar A, Jin Z, Bilker W, Udupa J, Gottlieb G. Late-onset minor and major depression: early evidence for common neuroanatomical substrates detected by using MRI. *Proc Natl Acad Sci U S A* 1998; 95(13):7654–8.
37. Appelhof bc, Huyser J, Verweij M, Brouwer JP, van Dyck R, Fliers E, *et al*. Glucocorticoids and relapse of major depression (dexamethasone/corticotropin-releasing hormone test in relation to relapse of major depression). *Biol Psychiatry* 2006; 59(8):696–701.
38. Morris GL 3rd, Vanderkolk C. Human sexuality, sex hormones, and epilepsy. *Epilepsy Behav* 2005; 7(Suppl. 2):S22–8.
39. Herzog AG, Coleman AE, Jacobs AR, Klein P, Friedman MN, Drislane FW, *et al*. Interictal EEG discharges, reproductive hormones and menstrual disorders in epilepsy. *Ann Neurol* 2003; 54(5):625–37.
40. Klein P, Serje A, Pezzullo JC. Premature ovarian failure in women with epilepsy. *Epilepsia* 2001; 42:1584–9.
41. Herzog AG, Coleman AE, Jacobs AR, Klein P, Friedman MN, Drislane FW, *et al*. Relationship of sexual dysfunction to epilepsy laterality and reproductive hormone levels in women. *Epilepsy Behav* 2003; 4(4):407–13.
42. Isojärvi JI, Taubøll E, Herzog AG. Effects of antiepileptic drugs on reproductive endocrine function in individuals with epilepsy—a review. *CNS Drugs* 2005; 19(3):207–23.
43. Taneja N, Kucheria K, Jain S, Maheshwari MC. Effect of phenytoin on semen. *Epilepsia* 1994; 35(1):136–40.
44. Duncan S, Talbot A, Sheldrick R, Caswell H. Erectile function, sexual desire, and psychological well-being in men with epilepsy. *Epilepsy Behav* 2009; 15(3):351–7.
45. Morrell MJ, Guldner GT. Self-reported sexual function and sexual arousability in women with epilepsy. *Epilepsia* 1996; 37(12):1204–10.
46. Stoffel-Wagner B, Bauer J, Flügel D, Brennemann W, Klingmüller D, Elger CE. Serum sex hormones are altered in patients with chronic temporal lobe epilepsy receiving anticonvulsant medication. *Epilepsia* 1998; 39(11):1164–73.
47. Morrell MJ, Flynn KL, Seale CG, Done S, Paulson AJ, Flaster ER, *et al*. Reproductive dysfunction in women with epilepsy: antiepileptic drug effects on sex-steroid hormones. *CNS Spectr* 2001; 6(9):771–2, 83–6.
48. Morrell MJ, Flynn KL, Doñe S, Flaster E, Kalayjian L, Pack AM. Sexual dysfunction, sex steroid hormone abnormalities, and depression in women with epilepsy treated with antiepileptic drugs. *Epilepsy Behav* 2005; 6(3):360–5.
49. Zelená V, Kuba R, Soška V, Rektor I. Depression as a prominent cause of sexual dysfunction in women with epilepsy. *Epilepsy Behav* 2011; 20(3):539–44.
50. Reijs R, Aldenkamp AP, De Krom M. Mood effects of antiepileptic drugs. *Epilepsy Behav* 2004; 5(Suppl. 1):S66–76.
51. Zobel A, Wellmer J, Schulze-Rauschenbach S, Pfeiffer U, Schnell S, Elger C, *et al*. Impairment of inhibitory control of the hypothalamic pituitary adrenocortical system in epilepsy. *Eur Arch Psychiatry Clin Neurosci* 2004; 254(5):303–11.
52. Sapolsky RM. The possibility of neurotoxicity in the hippocampus in major depression: a primer on neuron death. *Biol Psychiatry* 2000; 48(8):755–65.
53. Kondziella D, Alvestad S, Vaaler A, Sonnewald U. Which clinical and experimental data link temporal lobe epilepsy with depression? *J Neurochem* 2007; 103(6):2136–52.
54. Wrench J, Wilson SJ, Bladin PF, Reutens DC. Hippocampal volume and major depression: Insights from epilepsy surgery. *J Neurol Neurosurg Psychiatry* 2009; 80(5):539–44.
55. Halley SA, Wrench JM, Reutens DC, Wilson SJ. (2010). The amygdala and anxiety after epilepsy surgery. *Epilepsy Behav* 2010; 18(4):431–6.
56. Bremner JD, Narayan M, Anderson ER, Staib LH, Miller HL, Charney DS. Hippocampal volume reduction in major depression. *Am J Psychiatry* 2000; 157(1):115–18.
57. Blumer D, Walker AE. Sexual behavior in temporal lobe epilepsy. A study of the effects of temporal lobectomy on sexual behavior. *Arch Neurol* 1967; 16(1):37–43.
58. Kimiskidis VK, Triantafyllou NI, Kararizou E, Gatzonis SS, Fountoulakis KN, Siatouni A, *et al*. Depression and anxiety in epilepsy: the association with demographic and seizure-related variables. *Ann Gen Psychiatry* 2007; 6:28.
59. Blumenfeld H, McNally KA, Vanderhill SD, Paige AL, Chung R, Davis K, *et al*. Positive and negative network correlations in temporal lobe epilepsy. *Cereb Cortex* 2004; 14(8):892–902.
60. Adolphs R. Neural systems for recognizing emotion. *Curr Opin Neurobiol* 2002; 12(2):169–77.
61. Alessio A, Bonilha L, Rorden C, Kobayashi E, Min LL, Damasceno BP, *et al*. Memory and language impairments and their relationships to hippocampal and perirhinal cortex damage in patients with medial temporal lobe epilepsy. *Epilepsy Behav* 2006; 8(3):593–600.
62. Wilson SJ, Engel J Jr. Diverse perspectives on developments in epilepsy surgery. *Seizure* 2010; 19(10):659–68.
63. Helmstaedter C, Sonntag-Dillender M, Hoppe C, Elger CE. Depressed mood and memory impairment in temporal lobe epilepsy as a function of focus lateralization and localization. *Epilepsy Behav* 2004; 5(5):696–701.
64. Saling MM. Verbal memory in mesial temporal lobe epilepsy: beyond material specificity. *Brain* 2009; 132:570–82.
65. Baddeley A. The concept of episodic memory. *Philos Trans R Soc Lond B Biol Sci* 2001; 356(1413):1345–50.
66. Gibbs BR, Rude SS. Overgeneral autobiographical memory as depression vulnerability. *Cognit Ther Res* 2004; 28(4):511–26.
67. Naylor E, Clare L. Awareness of memory functioning, autobiographical memory and identity in early stage dementia. *Neuropsychol Rehabil* 2008; 18(5–6):590–606.
68. St-Laurent M, Moscovitch M, Levine B, McAndrews MP. Determinants of autobiographical memory in patients with unilateral TLE or excisions. *Neuropsychologia* 2009; 47:2211–21.
69. Briellmann RS, Hopwood MJ, Jackson GD. Major depression in TLE with hippocampal sclerosis: clinical and imaging correlates. *J Neurol Neurosurg* Psychiatry 2007; 78(11):1226–30.
70. Baker GA, Hargis E, Hsih MM, Mounfield H, Arzimanoglou A, Glauser T, *et al*. Perceived impact of epilepsy in teenagers and young adults: an international survey. *Epilepsy Behav* 2008; 12(3):395–401.

71. Jacoby A, Baker GA, Steen N, Potts P, Chadwick DW. The clinical course of epilepsy and its psychosocial correlates: findings from a U.K. Community study. *Epilepsia.* 1996; 37(2):148–61.
72. Asadi-Pooya AA, Schilling CA, Glosser D, Tracy JI, Sperling MR. Health locus of control in patients with epilepsy and its relationship to anxiety, depression, and seizure control. *Epilepsy Behav* 2007; 11(3):347–50.
73. De Vellis RF, De Vellis BM, Wallston BS, Wallston KA. Epilepsy and learned helplessness. *Basic Appl Soc Psych* 1980; 1:241–53.
74. Affleck G, Tennen H, Pfeiffer C, Fifield J. Appraisals of control and predictability in adapting to a chronic disease. *J Pers Soc Psychol* 1987; 53(2):273–9.
75. Monga U, Tan G, Ostermann HJ, Monga TN. Sexuality in head and neck cancer patients. *Arch Phys Med Rehabil* 1997; 78(3):298–304.
76. Smeets VM, van Lierop BA, Vanhoutvin JP, Aldenkamp AP, Nijhuis FJ. Epilepsy and employment: literature review. *Epilepsy Behav* 2007; 10(3):354–62.
77. Austin JK, deBoer H. Disruptions in social functioning and services facilitating adjustment for the child and adult. In: Engel J Jr, Pedley TA (eds) *Epilepsy: A comprehensive textbook*, pp. 2191–201. Philadelphia, PA: Lippincott-Raven, 1997.
78. Headey B, Wearing A. *Understanding happiness: a theory of subjective well*-being. Melbourne: Longman Cheshire, 1992.
79. Ekman P, Friesen WV. Constants across cultures in the face and emotion. *J Pers Soc Psychol* 1971; 17(2):124–9.
80. Batut AC, Gounot D, Namer IJ, Hirsch E, Kehrli P, Metz-Lutz MN. Neural responses associated with positive and negative emotion processing in patients with left versus right temporal lobe epilepsy. *Epilepsy Behav* 2006; 9(3):415–23.
81. Benuzzi F, Meletti S, Zamboni G, Calandra-Buonaura G, Serafini M, Lui F, *et al.* Impaired fear processing in right mesial temporal sclerosis: a fMRI study. *Brain Res Bull* 2004; 63(4):269–81.
82. Meletti S, Benuzzi F, Rubboli G, Cantalupo G, Stanzani Maserati M, Nichelli P, *et al.* Impaired facial emotion recognition in early-onset right mesial temporal lobe epilepsy. *Neurology* 2003; 60(3):426–31.
83. Meletti S, Benuzzi F, Cantalupo G, Rubboli G, Tassinari CA, Nichelli P. Facial emotion recognition impairment in chronic temporal lobe epilepsy. *Epilepsia* 2009; 50(6):1547–59.
84. Golouboff N, Fiori N, Delalande O, Fohlen M, Dellatolas G, Jambaqué I. Impaired facial expression recognition in children with temporal lobe epilepsy: impact of early seizure onset on fear recognition. *Neuropsychologia* 2008; 46(5):1415–28.
85. Adolphs R, Tranel D, Damasio H. Emotion recognition from faces and prosody following temporal lobectomy. *Neuropsychology* 2001; 15(3):396–404.
86. Anderson AK, Spencer DD, Fulbright RK, Phelps EA. Contribution of the anteromedial temporal lobes to the evaluation of facial emotion. *Neuropsychology* 2000; 14(4):526–36.
87. Hlobil U, Rathore C, Alexander A, Sarma S, Radhakrishnan K. Impaired facial emotion recognition in patients with mesial temporal lobe epilepsy associated with hippocampal sclerosis (MTLE-HS): Side and age at onset matters. *Epilepsy Res* 2008; 80(2–3):150–7.
88. McClelland S 3rd, Garcia RE, Peraza DM, Shih TT, Hirsch LJ, Hirsch J, *et al.* Facial emotion recognition after curative nondominant temporal lobectomy in patients with mesial temporal sclerosis. *Epilepsia* 2006; 47(8):1337–42.
89. Reynders HJ, Broks P, Dickson JM, Lee CE, Turpin G. Investigation of social and emotion information processing in temporal lobe epilepsy with ictal fear. *Epilepsy Behav* 2005; 7(3):419–29.
90. Shaw P, Lawrence E, Bramham J, Brierley B, Radbourne C, David AS. A prospective study of the effects of anterior temporal lobectomy on emotion recognition and theory of mind. *Neuropsychologia* 2007; 45(12):2783–90.
91. Baird AD, Wilson SJ, Bladin PF, Saling MM, Reutens DC. Sexual outcome after epilepsy surgery. *Epilepsy Behav* 2003; 4(3):268–78.
92. Adolphs R. The neurobiology of social cognition. *Curr Opin Neurobiol* 2001; 11(2):231–9.
93. Walpole P, Isaac CL, Reynders HJ. A comparison of emotional and cognitive intelligence in people with and without temporal lobe epilepsy. *Epilepsia* 2008; 49(8):1470–4.
94. Schilbach L, Koubeissi MZ, David N, Vogeley K, Ritzl EK. Being with virtual others: studying social cognition in temporal lobe epilepsy. *Epilepsy Behav* 2007; 11(3):316–23.
95. Schachter M, Winkler R, Grunwald T, Kraemer G, Kurthen M, Reed V, *et al.* Mesial temporal lobe epilepsy impairs advanced social cognition. *Epilepsia* 2006; 47(12):2141–6.
96. Farrant A, Morris RG, Russell T, Elwes R, Akanuma N, Alarcón G, *et al.* Social cognition in frontal lobe epilepsy. *Epilepsy Behav* 2005; 7(3):506–16.
97. Aull-Watschinger S, Pataraia E, Baumgartner C. Sexual auras: predominance of epileptic activity within the mesial temporal lobe. *Epilepsy Behav* 2008; 12(1):124–7.
98. Leutmezer F, Serles W, Bacher J, Gröppel G, Pataraia E, Aull S, *et al.* Genital automatisms in complex partial seizures. *Neurology* 1999; 52(6):1188–91.
99. Dobesberger J, Walser G, Unterberger I, Embacher N, Luef G, Bauer G, *et al.* Genital automatisms: a video-EEG study in patients with medically refractory seizures. *Epilepsia* 2004; 45(7):777–80.
100. Mascia A, Di Gennaro G, Esposito V, Grammaldo LG, Meldolesi GN, Giampà T, *et al.* Genital and sexual manifestations in drug-resistant partial epilepsy. *Seizure* 2005; 14(2):133–8.
101. Daniele A, Azzoni A, Bizzi A, Rossi A, Gainotti G, Mazza S. Sexual behavior and hemispheric laterality of the focus in patients with temporal lobe epilepsy. *Biol Psychiatry* 1997; 42(7):617–24.
102. Saunders M, Rawson M. Sexuality in male epileptics. *J Neurol Sci* 1970; 10(6):577–83.
103. Silveira DC, Souza EA, Carvalho JF, Guerreiro CA. Interictal hyposexuality in male patients with epilepsy. *Arq Neuropsiquiatr* 2001; 59(1):23–8.
104. Shukla GD, Srivastava ON, Katiyar bc. Sexual disturbances in temporal lobe epilepsy: a controlled study. *Br J Psychiatry* 1979; 134:288–92.
105. Kolárský A, Freund K, Machek J, Polák O. Male sexual deviation. Association with early temporal lobe damage. *Arch Gen Psychiatry* 1967; 17(6):735–43.
106. Gastaut H, Collomb H. Etude du comportment sexuel chez les epileptiques psychomoteurs. *Ann Med Psychol* 1954; 11:657–96.
107. Blumer D. Hypersexual episodes in temporal lobe epilepsy. *Am J Psychiatry* 1970; 126:1099–106.
108. Herzog AG, Seibel MM, Schomer DL, Vaitukaitis JL, Geschwind N. Reproductive endocrine disorders in women with partial seizures of temporal lobe origin. *Arch Neurol* 1986; 43(4):341–6.
109. Herzog AG, Seibel MM, Schomer DL, Vaitukaitis JL, Geschwind N. Reproductive endocrine disorders in men with partial seizures of temporal lobe origin. *Arch Neurol* 1986; 43(4):347–50.
110. Jayne C, Gago BA. Diagnosis and treatment of female sexual arousal disorder. *Clin Obstet Gynecol* 2009; 52(4):675–81.
111. Wrench JM, Rayner G, Wilson SJ. Profiling the evolution of depression after epilepsy surgery. *Epilepsia* 2011; 52(5):900–8.
112. Baird AD, Wilson SJ, Bladin PF, Saling MM, Reutens DC. Hypersexuality after temporal lobe resection. *Epilepsy Behav* 2002; 3(2):173–81.
113. Jensen P, Jensen SB, Sørensen PS, Bjerre BD, Rizzi DA, Sørensen AS. Sexual dysfunction in male and female patients with epilepsy: a study of 86 outpatients. *Arch Sex Behav* 1990; 19(1):1–14.

CHAPTER 36

Epilepsy: Cognition and Memory in Adults

Sallie Baxendale

Introduction

Epilepsy may be a condition defined by seizures, but seizures remain rare events for the majority of people with the diagnosis. Whilst up to two-thirds may become seizure free on antiepileptic medications, difficulties in memory and other cognitive problems associated with the condition (and its treatment) are encountered on a daily basis by many people with epilepsy. As the likelihood and concomitant fear of a seizure recedes following the instigation of an optimal antiepileptic treatment regimen, it is often the underlying cognitive difficulties that become distressing daily reminders of the diagnosis.

The extent of the problem

It is important to make a distinction between subjective complaints and objective measures of cognitive impairment in epilepsy, particularly in the memory domain. There is a poor correlation between scores on standardized neuropsychological tests of memory function and scores on self-report measures of everyday memory problems. However, patient ratings of memory complaints are closely related to measures of anxiety and depression (1–3) and some have argued that memory complaints in epilepsy are a reflection of difficulties adjusting to, or coping with, the condition (4). Others argue that the poor correlations reflect the artificial nature of standardized memory tests and the fact that they bear little relation to either the demands placed on memory in everyday situations or the specific nature of the memory complaints of some patients. The poor ecological validity of pencil and paper memory tests is particularly relevant for patients who complain of a loss of autobiographical memory (5). Amnesia for past events, such as holidays or weddings, can be a particular feature of patients with frontal lobe epilepsy and is also commonly reported interictally by patients with transient epileptic amnesia (5, 6). Hermann and Langfitt (7) point out that 'memory' is often employed as a catchall phrase that patients use as a shorthand to describe a broad spectrum of cognitive difficulties. These can range from word-finding difficulties to difficulties in recognizing faces; route finding to remembering why you have come into the kitchen. From a neuropsychological perspective, different processes and substrates may underpin each of these functions, but from a patient's perspective they all represent examples of 'a dreadful memory'.

Thus, estimates of the prevalence of memory difficulties in epilepsy based on self-report measures from patient samples may represent a wide range of cognitive difficulties and other factors associated with mood and psychological adjustment. Estimates based on clinical studies using formal neuropsychological measures may also overestimate the extent of the problem, as patients who undertake a formal assessment normally only do so following concerns about their memory or a deterioration in other cognitive domains. Notwithstanding these caveats, there is a general consensus that the prevalence of memory and other cognitive problems within the epilepsy population as a whole is high.

Epilepsy is over-represented in people with a low intelligence quotient (IQ), often due to the extensive underlying cerebral abnormalities that lead to both limited cognitive abilities and recurrent seizures (8). However, when people with an IQ of 70 or below are discounted, the mean IQ of people with epilepsy falls slightly below, but within the average range of normative healthy samples and is distributed across a normal bell curve.

Factors affecting cognition and memory

There are many factors that contribute to cognitive dysfunction in epilepsy. Some of these factors may be fixed (e.g. the underlying pathology) while others may be more fluid or transient (e.g. mood, side effects of antiepileptic medications). Other factors may represent the course of the disease (e.g. episodes of status epilepticus, the effects of aging). These factors all interact to shape the nature and extent of the cognitive deficits in each individual with epilepsy. See Table 36.1.

Fixed factors

Although a seizure is often the first overt sign of neurological dysfunction, there is increasing evidence that many people eventually diagnosed with epilepsy have pre-existing signs of cerebral dysfunction. Epilepsy has long been associated with depression and this has traditionally been understood as a response to the significant personal and practical changes a diagnosis of epilepsy brings. However, in a series of population studies, Dale Hesdorffer and her colleagues from Columbia University, New York have demonstrated that depression is a risk factor for developing epilepsy and that mood disturbance often predates the first seizure (9–11).

Table 36.1 Fixed, fluid, and cumulative factors that influence neuropsychological function in epilepsy

Fixed factors	Variable factors	History of the disease
Nature of underlying pathology	Medication	Episodes of status epilepticus
Laterality of pathology	Interictal/subclinical EEG abnormalities	Repeated generalized seizures
Locality of pathology	Seizure control	Head injuries
Age onset of pathology/ seizures	Mood	
	Motivation	
Age onset of treatment	Quality of sleep	
Impact on education	Proximity of last seizure to assessment	
Gender		
Intellectual capacity		

Adapted from Baxendale and Thompson (15).

In the Standard And New Antiepileptic Drugs (SANAD) study, researchers in Liverpool, UK examined the neuropsychological profiles of 155 newly diagnosed people with epilepsy, before they had started any treatments (12). They found that newly diagnosed patients with epilepsy performed more poorly than healthy controls on six of 14 cognitive measures, with memory functions and psychomotor speed particularly affected. Cognitive performance was not related to the type of epilepsy diagnosed or measures of low mood. The researchers concluded that many newly diagnosed, untreated patients with epilepsy are cognitively compromised before they start taking antiepileptic drugs. This is unsurprising given that the location, type, and extent of brain pathology are all significant factors in determining the associated cognitive difficulties.

Temporal lobe pathology

The mesial temporal structures play a critical role in the learning and consolidation of new material. In patients with hippocampal sclerosis (one of the most common pathologies seen in focal temporal lobe epilepsies) the extent of hippocampal volume loss in the dominant hemisphere, quantified using magnetic resonance imaging volumetry, correlates with scores on tests of verbal learning and recall. These correlations have been corroborated with postoperative cell counting studies that have found significant correlations between the neuronal densities in resected hippocampal specimens and preoperative scores on verbal memory tests. See Baxendale for a review (13). Whilst the role of the hippocampi in memory function has long been recognized, Saling has recently presented a persuasive argument that the perirhinal cortex is also a key node in a more extensive memory network (14).

The material-specific model of memory function has been a dominant concept in the neuropsychological understanding of memory function for over 50 years (15). Based on postoperative studies of early epilepsy surgery patients, this model postulates that verbal memory functions are associated with the dominant medial structures whilst non-verbal memory functions are associated with non-dominant mesial structures. However, this model has recently been challenged on both theoretical and clinical grounds following critical re-evaluations of the classic literature often cited in support of the model (14, 15). The verbal versus non-verbal specialisms of the mesial temporal structures where they do exist, are just that—specialisms, they do not represent exclusive functions. Thus is it common for people with pathology in the right temporal lobe to have some degree of verbal memory impairment; similarly people with left temporal lobe pathology may demonstrate impairments on memory tests involving both verbal and non-verbal material. Fig. 36.1 represents the mean scores of 417 adult patients with medically intractable epilepsy and unilateral hippocampal sclerosis on a range of cognitive tasks including measures of intellectual function, verbal and visual learning, and expressive language function. This figure graphically illustrates the range and extent of cognitive deficits associated with an apparently discreet localized underlying lesion. On the memory tasks, the mean performance of the epilepsy groups falls at about the 10th percentile of that of the normal population. Thus whilst some patients with temporal lobe epilepsy (TLE) may have normal memory function, they will be in the minority.

Hermann et al. (16) examined the neuropsychological profiles of 96 patients with epilepsy and compared them with matched healthy controls to determine whether distinct cognitive phenotypes could be identified in TLE. They identified three distinct types of cognitive profile. Almost half of the sample (47%) were minimally impaired. A second group (24%) were impaired on memory measures whilst the remainder (29%) were impaired on a much broader range of tasks including measures of memory, executive function, and processing speed. Differences in brain structure are associated with each profile, with increasing abnormalities in temporal and extratemporal cortical thickness and decreasing volumes of the subcortical structures (hippocampus, thalamus, basal ganglia) distinguishing the cognitive phenotypes in a broadly step-wise fashion, according to the extent of the neuropsychological deficits (17).

Although it is in its infancy at present, this phenotypical approach may have important implications for the counselling of TLE patients regarding changes in cognition over time and also for the interpretation of the global declines in function often seen clinically in patients who have been followed for many years.

Frontal lobe pathology

Whilst people with frontal lobe epilepsy (FLE) may achieve comparable scores on formal tests of learning and recall to their counterparts with a temporal focus, their performance is often qualitatively very different. Frontal lesions are associated with difficulties in placing past events in order, or within the correct time frame. Confabulation and intrusions may be prominent, when recall of the original material is weak. Thus the FLE patient may be able to provide a fulsome (albeit inaccurate) recount of a story they have just heard, in stark contrast to TLE patients, who are often unable to provide much detail and who are generally very aware of their poor recall. Recall is not always disrupted in FLE. In some cases, recognition memory can be impaired in the context of intact recall abilities. This may be due to interference from distraction items in recognition memory tests. Difficulties in recalling the source of new information (the where, when, and how you learnt something new) are also associated with frontal lobe disturbance.

Cahn-Weiner et al. (18) compared the memory and executive functions of FLE and TLE patients on cognitively-based daily living tasks. They expected the TLE patients to be more impaired on memory tasks, whilst the FLE patients would be more impaired on tests that employed executive function. However, they did not find this double dissociation, but rather both groups were significantly

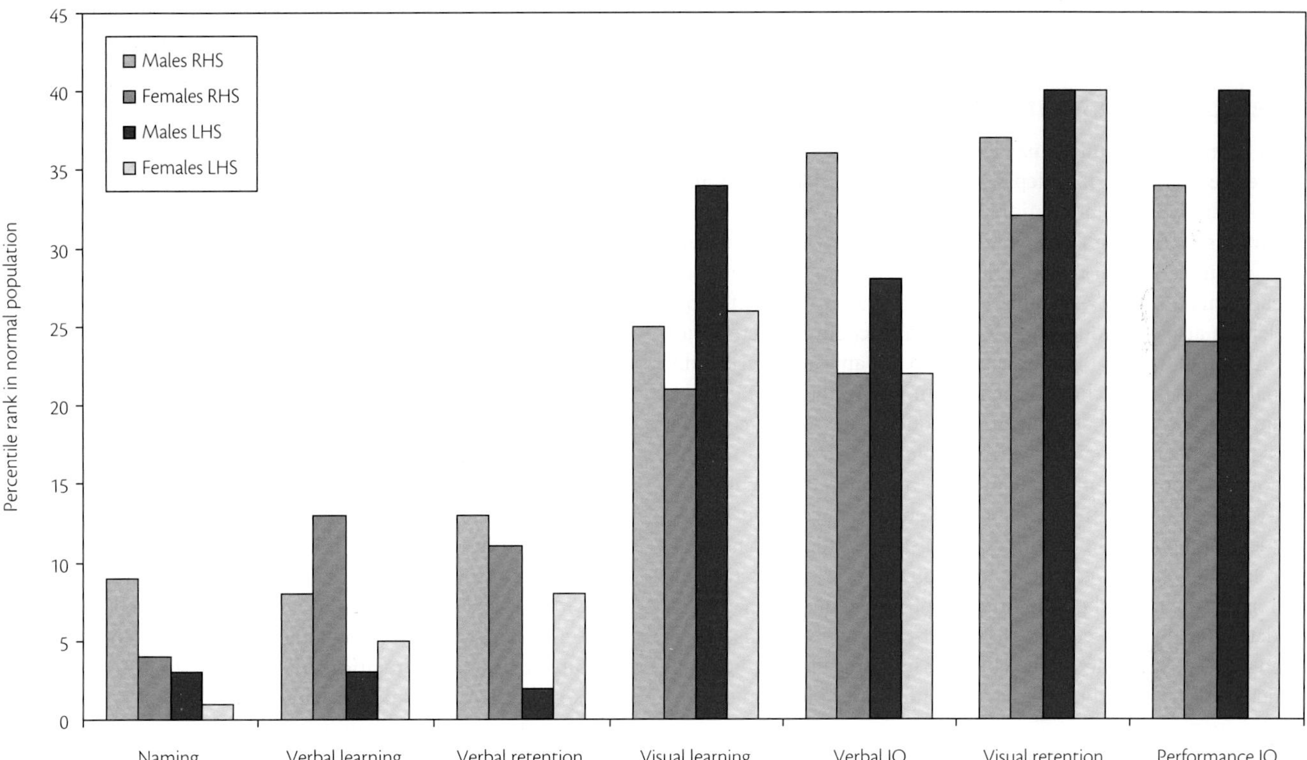

Fig. 36.1 Mean scores of patients with unilateral hippocampal sclerosis (n = 417) on standardized neuropsychological tests of intellect, learning, memory, and language, plotted against the percentile rank of healthy controls. Adapted from Baxendale et al. (20).

impaired on the memory tasks whilst their executive function scores fell within normal limits. Language problems were also found in both groups. The authors concluded that a wide range of cognitive problems were found in both groups, despite the apparent focal nature of their pathology.

Aetiology

Whilst the focus of much early research was on the effects of the location of the underlying lesion in epilepsy, clinicians and researchers have recently begun to appreciate that the nature of the lesion may play just as important a role in shaping the characteristics and extent of any associated neuropsychological deficit. Very early developmental lesions, such as dysembroplastic neuroepithelial tumours (DNET), and other forms of cortical dysplasia may be associated with relatively little cognitive disturbance as cognitive functions are reorganized during subsequent cognitive development. However, fast-growing tumours that occur in an adult brain that has developed normally can have a devastating impact on neighbouring cortical functions. Thus similar-sized lesions, in the same location, can have a very different impact on cognitive function in different patients dependent on the aetiology of the pathology.

In the general population, women generally have better verbal abilities than men and this pattern appears to hold for women with epilepsy, whose verbal memory deficits may not be as marked as those observed in matched male groups. Female epilepsy patients also have a gender advantage over males in delayed facial recognition (19). However, gender may play a role in mediating the effects of underlying pathology on cognitive function, and females with left-sided hippocampal sclerosis may be particularly vulnerable to more widespread cognitive dysfunction beyond the memory domain (20).

Fluid factors

Seizure control can have a significant impact on cognitive function. Clusters of seizures may lead to temporarily reduced memory function and a reduced attention span. The proximity of a seizure to a neuropsychological assessment may have a significant impact on the results.

Nocturnal seizures disrupt sleep patterns, which can decrease cognitive efficiency the following day. Interictal subclinical electroencephalogram (EEG) disturbances can significantly interfere with normal brain function. Disruptions in cognitive processing consequent on these otherwise subclinical abnormalities are sometimes detected when neuropsychological testing is conducted during a routine EEG recording.

Low mood and anxiety (common comorbidities in epilepsy) are associated with reduced learning capacity and increased difficulties in recall. Mood disturbance is also a significant factor in self-reported memory function. Salas-Puig et al. (1) examined the contribution of clinical and demographic factors to scores on a memory complaint questionnaire. They found that measures of anxiety and depression explained over a third of the variance in the self-perception of memory disturbance. Independent of formal neuropsychological test results, patients' perceptions of cognitive difficulties are also significantly correlated with measures of quality of life in epilepsy (21).

Developmental course of epilepsy

Whilst cognitive difficulties may be present early on and may even predate the diagnosis of epilepsy (22), repeated seizures can also lead to a stepwise deterioration in memory function for some patients across the adult lifespan. Cell death following status epilepticus can lead to an irrevocable decline in cognitive function. Repeated head injuries sustained as the result of frequent drop attacks can also lead to a stepwise pattern of cognitive deterioration. Although frequent partial seizures do not appear to accelerate normal age-related decline in memory function, the same cannot be said for generalized convulsions. Frequent generalized convulsions have been associated with accelerated deterioration in memory function in some patients (23). Helmsteadter et al. (24) report that memory functions may never fully develop in adults who develop epilepsy in childhood. Whilst the gradient of normal age-related decline in cognitive function may be similar to that observed in the normal population, people with epilepsy may start this decline from a lower level than their healthy peers This lower starting level means that they will become impaired at an earlier age. Gender and side of pathology may also influence long-term trajectories of cognitive decline (20).

Treatments

Many of the treatments that are effective in controlling seizures also have side effects that affect cognition. Different cognitive profiles are associated with each antiepileptic medication. Most GABA (gamma-aminobutyric acid) inhibitory agents are associated with mental slowing (25). As a general rule of thumb, cognitive problems usually increase with the dose and number of different medications taken. Antiepileptic drug toxicity can result in very marked cognitive decline in a poorly monitored patient. Although cognitive side effects are generally thought to be less pronounced with the newer antiepileptic medications, caution should be exercised in the introduction of some of these. Topiramate can result in markedly reduced verbal fluency and processing (26, 27). Although some have found that the cognitive side effects can be reduced following gradual titration (28), others have suggested that the presence of word finding difficulties appears to be a phenomenon independent from titration schedule and is a side effect that occurs in a subgroup of patients with a specific biological vulnerability (29). Fortunately, the cognitive difficulties associated with topiramate appear to be reversed following discontinuation of the drug (30).

Although epilepsy surgery can be associated with postoperative decline in memory function, individual postoperative trajectories can differ significantly. Whilst approximately one-third of patients may experience a significant decline in memory function following a unilateral temporal lobe resection, memory functions for the majority may remain unchanged and can actually improve in approximately 20% of some surgical series (31). Postoperative change is governed by a variety of pre-, peri-, and postoperative factors. Preoperative risk factors for postoperative decline in memory function include good preoperative function and surgery on the language dominant hemisphere. Although the role of postoperative seizures on memory function is complex following surgery (32–36), there are some patients who suffer the 'double whammy' of a significant postoperative deterioration of memory functions and ongoing seizures following surgery. The lifetime risk of developing an amnesic syndrome is increased following surgery if the contralateral hippocampal structures become damaged following an episode of status or a severe cluster of seizures. This is not just a theoretical risk; a number of such case studies have been reported in the literature (37–39).

Social and psychological impact

Cognitive difficulties in epilepsy can have a significant impact on the quality of life of those affected. It can be difficult for friends, family, and colleagues to understand the nature of a poor memory and this can lead to frustration and interpersonal conflict. In the workplace, cognitive failures can be mistaken for carelessness or a lack of ability. This can limit the economic opportunities open to people with epilepsy. Baxendale et al. (40) found that it was the extent of memory difficulties, rather than a diagnosis of epilepsy or overall level of intellectual function, that had the greatest association with low socioeconomic status in people with epilepsy.

The embarrassment of being unable to recall a friend's name can be acute. In personal relationships, failure to recall important events or facts can be misinterpreted as disinterest. As a result, many people with memory difficulties find their social circle gradually shrinking over the years. Within the family, familiarity with an individual's memory difficulties can lead to gradual exclusion from joint decisions as relatives become impatient with the need for constant repetition.

Neuropsychological rehabilitation

A neuropsychological assessment forms the basis for all rehabilitation efforts for cognitive problems in epilepsy. Approaches to cognitive rehabilitation fall into three main categories. The first are strategy based. For memory difficulties these may include teaching the patient strategies that help them to process new information in greater depth, in a variety of ways. Mnemonic strategies may be useful for people with epilepsy but generalization of this technique to everyday situations outside the clinic is usually modest or even absent. Success is largely dependent on small, individualized, concrete goals (41). Another common strategy is the method of loci, where lists of items are recalled via visual imagery, the more bizarre imagery the better. Schefft et al. (42) reported some improvements in formal memory test scores in patients with epilepsy who were taught to use a self-generated encoding procedure. The patients with a left temporal seizure onset (who had the poorest memory performance in a didactic control condition) benefited the most from the self-generation condition. It remains unknown whether these improvements last. In postoperative patients it appears that patients who have undergone a left temporal lobectomy and who are in the greatest need of rehabilitation benefit less from rehabilitation strategies than those with more residual function remaining following surgery (43). Memory strategies can be very time consuming to master and require a high level of motivation from the patient for any real level of success. Wider cognitive deficits may mean it is not easy for some to employ visual imagery. As a result, many patients find these methods difficult to adopt and apply effectively in their everyday lives.

The second rehabilitation approach involves environmental adaptations. These can range from simple techniques to ease the nuisance of everyday memory difficulties to more complex interventions to reduce the impact of impulsive or disinhibited behaviours associated with frontal lobe dysfunction. These adaptations range from the use of diaries, calendars, 'Post-it' notes, and telephone pads to structural changes within the workplace to allow behavioural prompts from handheld devices, computer systems, and even colleagues, where appropriate. These environmental adaptations often involve the development of routines that need to become second nature to ensure success.

The planning of these strategies relies heavily on finding the appropriate external prompt to shore up the failing internal cognitive functions. Each neuropsychological rehabilitation package will be unique to the individual and will be drawn up on the basis of the results from a detailed clinical interview and a formal neuropsychological assessment. Relatives and work colleagues may also need to be actively involved in some rehabilitation strategies, particularly where frontal lobe functions are compromised.

Acceptance of cognitive difficulties as an integral part of having epilepsy is a fundamental adjustment that many patients with epilepsy must make. Many have never been explicitly told this and they continue to strive for a remedy many years after diagnosis. Many of the factors that underpin cognitive difficulties in epilepsy are fixed and cannot be changed. Memory functions will not get better, although neuropsychological rehabilitation can help to develop ways around the nuisance of frequent memory failures. An early explanation that cognitive difficulties are an integral part of the condition can help the long-term adjustment to living with epilepsy. The third approach to neuropsychological rehabilitation may employ a cognitive behavioural or psychotherapeutic approach to help the patient work through the issues of loss that are inevitably associated with the development of this acceptance.

References

1. Salas-Puig J, Gil-Nagel A, Serratosa JM, Sanchez-Alvarez JC, Elices E, Villanueva V, *et al.* Self-reported memory problems in everyday activities in patients with epilepsy treated with antiepileptic drugs. *Epilepsy Behav* 2009; 14(4):622–7.
2. Baxendale S, Thompson P. Defining meaningful postoperative change in epilepsy surgery patients: measuring the unmeasurable? *Epilepsy Behav* 2005; 6(2):207–11.
3. Rayner G, Wrench JM, Wilson SJ. Differential contributions of objective memory and mood to subjective memory complaints in refractory focal epilepsy. *Epilepsy Behav* 2010; 19(3):359–64.
4. Hall KE, Isaac CL, Harris P. Memory complaints in epilepsy: an accurate reflection of memory impairment or an indicator of poor adjustment? A review of the literature. *Clin Psychol Rev* 2009; 29(4):354–67.
5. Zeman A, Butler C. Transient epileptic amnesia. *Curr Opin Neurol* 2010; 23(6):610–16.
6. Butler CR, Zeman AZ. Recent insights into the impairment of memory in epilepsy: transient epileptic amnesia, accelerated long-term forgetting and remote memory impairment. *Brain* 2008; 13(Pt 9): 2243–63.
7. Hermann B, Langfitt J. Forgetting to remember in epilepsy: a family affair? *Neurology* 2010; 75(24):2144–55.
8. Davies R, Baxendale S, Thompson P, Duncan JS. Epilepsy surgery for people with a low IQ. *Seizure* 2009; 18(2):150–2.
9. Hesdorffer DC, Hauser WA, Annegers JF, Cascino G. Major depression is a risk factor for seizures in older adults. *Ann Neurol* 2000; 47(2):246–9.
10. Hesdorffer DC, Hauser WA, Olafsson E, Ludvigsson P, Kjartansson O. Depression and suicide attempt as risk factors for incident unprovoked seizures. *Ann Neurol* 2006; 59(1):35–41.
11. Hesdorffer DC, Ludvigsson P, Hauser WA, Olafsson E, Kjartansson O. Co-occurrence of major depression or suicide attempt with migraine with aura and risk for unprovoked seizure. *Epilepsy Res* 2007; 75(2–3):220–3.
12. Taylor J, Kolamunnage-Dona R, Marson AG, Smith PE, Aldenkamp AP, Baker GA. Patients with epilepsy: cognitively compromised before the start of antiepileptic drug treatment? *Epilepsia* 2010; 51(1):48–56.
13. Baxendale SA. The hippocampus: functional and structural correlations. *Seizure* 1995; 4(2):105–17.
14. Saling MM. Verbal memory in mesial temporal lobe epilepsy: beyond material specificity. *Brain* 2009; 132(Pt 3):570–82.
15. Baxendale S, Thompson P. Beyond localization: the role of traditional neuropsychological tests in an age of imaging. *Epilepsia* 2010; 51(11):2225–30.
16. Hermann B, Seidenberg M, Lee EJ, Chan F, Rutecki P. Cognitive phenotypes in temporal lobe epilepsy. *J Int Neuropsychol Soc* 2007; 13(1):12–20.
17. Dabbs K, Jones J, Seidenberg M, Hermann B. Neuroanatomical correlates of cognitive phenotypes in temporal lobe epilepsy. *Epilepsy Behav* 2009; 15(4):445–51.
18. Cahn-Weiner DA, Wittenberg D, McDonald C. Everyday cognition in temporal lobe and frontal lobe epilepsy. *Epileptic Disord* 2009; 11(3):222–7.
19. Bengner T, Fortmeier C, Malina T, Lindenau M, Voges B, Goebell E, *et al.* Sex differences in face recognition memory in patients with temporal lobe epilepsy, patients with generalized epilepsy, and healthy controls. *Epilepsy Behav* 2006; 9(4):593–600.
20. Baxendale S, Heaney D, Thompson PJ, Duncan JS. Cognitive consequences of childhood-onset temporal lobe epilepsy across the adult lifespan. *Neurology* 2010; 75(8):705–11.
21. Baker GA, Taylor J, Hermann B. How can cognitive status predispose to psychological impairment? *Epilepsy Behav* 2009; 15(Suppl 1): S31–S35.
22. Baker GA, Taylor J, Aldenkamp AP. Newly diagnosed epilepsy: Cognitive outcome after 12 months. *Epilepsia* 2011; 52(6):1084–91.
23. Thompson PJ, Duncan JS. Cognitive decline in severe intractable epilepsy. *Epilepsia* 2005; 46(11):1780–7.
24. Helmstaedter C, Elger CE. Chronic temporal lobe epilepsy: a neurodevelopmental or progressively dementing disease? *Brain* 2009; 132(Pt 10):2822–30.
25. Cavanna AE, Ali F, Rickards HE, McCorry D. Behavioral and cognitive effects of anti-epileptic drugs. *Discov Med* 2010; 9(45):138–44.
26. Gomer B, Wagner K, Frings L, Saar J, Carius A, Harle M, *et al.* The influence of antiepileptic drugs on cognition: a comparison of levetiracetam with topiramate. *Epilepsy Behav* 2007; 10(3):486–94.
27. Blum D, Meador K, Biton V, Fakhoury T, Shneker B, Chung S, *et al.* Cognitive effects of lamotrigine compared with topiramate in patients with epilepsy. *Neurology* 2006; 67(3):400–6.
28. Aldenkamp AP, De KM, Reijs R. Newer antiepileptic drugs and cognitive issues. *Epilepsia* 2003; 44(Suppl 4):21–9.
29. Mula M, Trimble MR, Thompson P, Sander JW. Topiramate and word-finding difficulties in patients with epilepsy. *Neurology* 2003; 60(7):1104–7.
30. Kockelmann E, Elger CE, Helmstaedter C. Significant improvement in frontal lobe associated neuropsychological functions after withdrawal of topiramate in epilepsy patients. *Epilepsy Res* 2003; 54(2–3):171–8.
31. Baxendale S, Thompson PJ, Duncan JS. Improvements in memory function following anterior temporal lobe resection for epilepsy. *Neurology* 2008; 71(17):1319–25.
32. Alpherts WC, Vermeulen J, van Rijen PC, da Silva FH, van Veelen CW. Verbal memory decline after temporal epilepsy surgery?: A 6-year multiple assessments follow-up study. *Neurology* 2006; 67(4):626–31.

33. Alpherts WC, Vermeulen J, Hendriks MP, Franken ML, van Rijen PC, Lopes da Silva FH, *et al.* Long-term effects of temporal lobectomy on intelligence. *Neurology* 2004; 62(4):607–11.
34. Andersson-Roswall L, Engman E, Samuelsson H, Malmgren K. Cognitive outcome 10 years after temporal lobe epilepsy surgery: a prospective controlled study. *Neurology* 2010; 74(24):1977–85.
35. Engman E, Andersson-Roswall L, Samuelsson H, Malmgren K. Serial cognitive change patterns across time after temporal lobe resection for epilepsy. *Epilepsy Behav* 2006; 8(4):765–72.
36. Helmstaedter C, Kurthen M, Lux S, Reuber M, Elger CE. Chronic epilepsy and cognition: a longitudinal study in temporal lobe epilepsy. *Ann Neurol* 2003; 54(4):425–32.
37. Dietl T, Urbach H, Helmstaedter C, Staedtgen M, Szentkuti A, Grunwald T, *et al.* Persistent severe amnesia due to seizure recurrence after unilateral temporal lobectomy. *Epilepsy Behav* 2004; 5(3): 394–400.
38. Oxbury S, Oxbury J, Renowden S, Squier W, Carpenter K. Severe amnesia: an usual late complication after temporal lobectomy. *Neuropsychologia* 1997; 35(7):975–88.
39. Loring DW, Hermann BP, Meador KJ, Lee GP, Gallagher BB, King DW, *et al.* Amnesia after unilateral temporal lobectomy: a case report. *Epilepsia* 1994; 35(4):757–63.
40. Baxendale S, Heaney D. Socioeconomic status, cognition, and hippocampal sclerosis. *Epilepsy Behav* 2011; 20(1):64–7.
41. Ponds RW, Hendriks M. Cognitive rehabilitation of memory problems in patients with epilepsy. *Seizure* 2006; 15(4):267–73.
42. Schefft BK, Dulay MF, Fargo JD, Szaflarski JP, Yeh HS, Privitera MD. The use of self-generation procedures facilitates verbal memory in individuals with seizure disorders. *Epilepsy Behav* 2008; 13(1):162–8.
43. Helmstaedter C, Loer B, Wohlfahrt R, Hammen A, Saar J, Steinhoff BJ, *et al.* The effects of cognitive rehabilitation on memory outcome after temporal lobe epilepsy surgery. *Epilepsy Behav* 2008; 12(3):402–9.

CHAPTER 37

Legal Aspects of Epilepsy and Epilepsy and Driving

Morris Odell

Legal aspects of epilepsy

Epilepsy has always occupied a distinctive place among the various medical conditions that come to medico-legal attention, possibly because of its sometimes spectacular manifestations of paroxysmal disability, and misconceptions regarding automatic or violent behaviour occurring during or after a seizure. Automatism is sometimes claimed as a defence for criminal actions occurring while a person is suffering a seizure. The word 'automatism' has a particular meaning in law, which is not necessarily the same as its pure clinical usage to describe unconscious behaviour; however, a detailed discussion of the resulting legal issues is beyond the scope of this chapter (1, 2). Potentially dangerous or criminal behaviour may be exhibited by patients with epilepsy but may not necessarily be associated with epilepsy per se. Violent and aggressive behaviour may be interictal and unrelated to a seizure although underlying psychiatric conditions or brain injury may be common to both. True ictal violence may be attributed to automatisms associated with complex partial seizures, myoclonic seizures, and similar types of epilepsy but this occurs without purpose or conscious control. Actions may appear to be destructive, violent, or aggressive but they are not directed and are not modified to suit the circumstances. In the postictal state a person may be psychotic, delirious, disorientated, and confused. Actions may seem purposeful but they are based on an altered sensorium with impaired cognition and decision-making ability. An example of this might be resisting or lashing out at someone trying to restrain or assist the delirious person.

In cases where epileptic automatism is claimed as a defence it is necessary to prove the person was actually having a seizure and was ictal or postictal at the time of the incident. The seizure must occur suddenly and there must be demonstrable impaired consciousness. Alternatively it should be demonstrated that the behaviour in question was characteristic of a typical seizure for that person. Video electroencephalogram (EEG) monitoring may be required and detailed neurological and forensic psychiatric assessment is always advisable (3). It is uncommon for criminal activity to be caused by epileptic seizures. In one British study, epilepsy was cited in only 7.3% of criminal cases found 'not guilty by reason of insanity' between 1975 and 2001. In the majority of these cases there were associated factors such as intoxications and psychiatric comorbidities that could not be excluded as contributing factors (4).

Epilepsy and driving

Epilepsy is probably the most common neurological disorder seen in the general community and all general practitioners and neurologists will have patients with a history of seizures and who are taking anticonvulsant medication. Epilepsy has the potential to cause a wide range of episodic disability from minor disturbances of perception or movement to complete loss of consciousness and this may result in adverse events associated with complex or dangerous activities including driving. Behaviour and events associated with seizures or postictal states may be of major medico-legal significance. Even though drug treatment of epilepsy has the potential to produce side effects that affect behaviour or driving ability, in practice it is the risk of a seizure that is the defining criterion for holding a licence (5). Despite this, the relative risk of crashes attributed to fitting drivers is low (6), possibly because of medical management of epileptic patients and consequent advice regarding licensing. However, one study in a country with no regulations regarding fitness to drive of epilepsy patients but a low population density found similar low risk, with the overall relative risk for 'traffic violations' being only 1.95 (6, 7). The relative risk of a crash in drivers with known epilepsy is usually quoted as less than 2 which must be put into the context of, for instance, the much higher relative risk associated with alcohol and drug use, and the increased crash risk of healthy drivers between the ages of 18 and 25 compared to middle-aged experienced drivers. Many other medical conditions are related to similar degrees of crash risk as epilepsy, but this is not always recognized in a consistent manner in various fitness to drive regulations. There are also significant differences in crash risk between drivers with epilepsy under treatment or advice (who have a very low relative risk) and the epilepsy population as a whole where the risk of a crash is increased by 40–100% (8). This probably represents the difference in severity of the condition between epilepsy patients who can obtain a licence and those who cannot satisfy the authorities that they are fit to drive (9). As epilepsy is a condition that relies on historical details for clinical decision-making, it is perhaps not surprising that there is a perception that many drivers with epilepsy do not tell their doctors the truth (10). Social and work pressures are often cited as reasons why poorly controlled patients continue to drive (11, 12).

Sudden loss of consciousness during an epileptic fit is obviously incompatible with maintaining control of a motor vehicle although a more or less universal finding is that *crash* frequency in drivers with epilepsy is only 50–60% of *seizure* frequency while driving. This probably reflects the inclusion of seizures without loss of consciousness in studies, or the perception of an imminent seizure allowing the driver to pull over. It may also represent interictal events which have a minor and subtle effect on consciousness and performance (13). However, it may also be a fortuitous finding due more to luck and the real risk is potentially much higher (14). The types of crashes have also been reported to be different from 'general' crashes in being more commonly in open areas rather than built-up areas, against an immovable object rather than a vehicle, and causing less severe injuries (15).

There are many different types of epilepsies which may differ in some respects in their potential effect on licensing policy although they have a common thread of paroxysmal gross impairment separated by periods of relative normality. Complex partial and generalized tonic–clonic seizures (primary or secondary) are the types most commonly associated with crashes (14). These are completely incapacitating during the ictal phase and are associated with a variable postictal period where the driver may remain incapacitated despite a partial return of consciousness. Involuntary motor movements during partial seizures have also been noted to contribute to crashes. Other forms are less commonly causes of crashes, with simple partial or uncomplicated myoclonic seizures where consciousness is preserved being rarely involved. Psychogenic pseudoseizures rarely occur in dangerous situations and should not affect driving; however, it is not always possible to be sure whether the events really are psychogenic unless they can be captured during EEG monitoring (16). Licensing guidelines for patients with epilepsy therefore may require identification of a specific epilepsy syndrome and monitoring of treatment. Because the oversight of epilepsy by clinicians rests largely on evidence from the patient regarding the frequency of seizures, it is important for doctors to assess the reliability of the history. Information from family members can be helpful in this regard. It is important to differentiate between the risk of having a seizure (whether behind the wheel or not) and the risk of having a crash. This is especially problematic as most licensing guidelines specify a fixed fit-free period and recording of this historical data is likely to be adversely affected by bias in histories given to clinicians (17). Objective evidence of seizure frequency and type may come from police reports, hospital records, or observations made during admissions for monitoring. Clinical evidence of brain imaging or EEG may be helpful in establishing a diagnosis and serum drug levels may be helpful in monitoring treatment. Video EEG monitoring extended over a period of a day or more is a useful aid to assessment in cases where the extent of seizure control is doubtful (18).

When a person is actually suffering a seizure, they are unconscious and technically incapable of controlling a motor vehicle. This has implications for criminal proceedings where it is necessary to prove intent or negligence for certain acts such as culpable driving, vehicular homicide, or similar offences. If a person is incapacitated by a seizure or a postictal state it can be argued that they were not actually in control of the vehicle or responsible for their actions. The question of automatism may also arise. Arguments can be made that negligence extends to driving with untreated or inadequately treated epilepsy or after a negligent decision not to inform a doctor or to drive against medical advice. A number of legal cases have explored this issue with varying outcomes, not always consistent with each other (19).

Another important medico-legal issue is the estimation of risk of seizure recurrence in patients who have ceased anticonvulsant medication. There are many variables here, including the type of epilepsy and the indications for ceasing treatment (20). Patients with generalized tonic–clonic seizures and those on multiple drug therapy present the greatest risk of seizure recurrence. Studies have shown variable periods of increased risk in patients withdrawn from medication with increased risk in some cases persisting for long periods. Patients recommenced on treatment after a recurrent seizure have an increased risk over the next 12 months compared to patients started on treatment, probably reflecting the increased severity of epilepsy which has recurred after treatment withdrawal (21). However, there are unpredictable variables introduced because of uncertainties in following-up patients remaining on treatment. The most significant factor in assessing risk is the time since the last seizure rather than the time off medication.

Therapeutic measures in epilepsy cases may also have a bearing on fitness to drive even though seizures are controlled. Visual field defects resulting from epilepsy surgery or treatment with certain drugs such as vigabatrin may be severe enough to render a person unfit to drive (22). Many anticonvulsant drugs have undesirable side effects such as sedation, confusion, incoordination, or other psychomotor effects that can affect driving ability. In most cases these are either transient, due to wrong dosing or may be avoided with a change of medication. It is important to keep these effects in mind when treating patients with epilepsy.

Reporting of drivers with epilepsy or any other medical condition to the driver licensing authority (Driver and Vehicle Licensing Agency in the UK) is a source of anxiety for many doctors. In some jurisdictions reporting is compulsory, which makes the decision easy, but there may be an adverse impact on the doctor–patient relationship and the reliability of the history of seizure control. This aspect of licensing policy involves a breach of confidentiality and raises ethical and medico-legal questions which have been debated vociferously in the literature (23–25). In some jurisdictions doctors are protected from litigation by the driver if it can be shown that they acted in good faith when reporting. Regardless of whether reporting is compulsory, it is always good practice to discuss the situation fully with the patient and attempt to explain the reasons why they should not be driving. Doctors who deal with epileptic patients need to be familiar with local fitness to drive requirements (26) and should be proactive in counselling the patient regarding driving (27). Medical notes are documents which may be examined in court and therefore all aspects of these discussions and decisions should be meticulously recorded.

Medical standards for drivers with epilepsy are concerned with the following aspects:

- The existence of a prescribed seizure-free period. Periods vary with different jurisdictions and the evidence base for them may not be strong (28); however, as a general rule, the risk of a recurrence is reduced as the seizure-free period increases (29).
- The type of seizures being experienced. In some jurisdictions a distinction is made regarding 'safe' seizures such as purely sensory phenomena or those occurring in or from sleep which by their nature are not likely to disturb driving. The recurrence rate

Table 37.1 Private licensing guidelines for drivers with epilepsy (31)

Disorder	Canada	Australia	UK	USA	New Zealand	Sweden
	CMA (2006)	**Austroads (2006 and 2012)**	**Drivers Medical Group, Swansea (2008)**	**Utah Driver License Division (2006)**	**Land Transport Safety Authority (2002)**	**Swedish National Road Administration (1999)**
Auras and minor epilepsy (absences)	May drive if: ◆ seizure pattern has been stable for at least 12 months ◆ no generalized seizures ◆ neurologist gives approval ◆ no impairment of cognition or consciousness ◆ no head or eye deviation with seizures	Not addressed	If patient suffered an attack whilst awake—must desist from driving for minimum 1 year from date of attack before licence may be issued. 3-year licence issue is dependent on patient being treatment compliant and if driving is unlikely to cause danger to the public. 70 licence restored if seizure free for minimum 7 years (with medication if necessary)	An unrestricted licence may be issued if seizure or episode free for 5 years, without medication. OR seizure free for 3–12 months without medication or with medication but no side effects. Reviews are required 6-monthly, yearly, or 2-yearly. Speed, area, and time of day restriction apply, depending on the length of time without seizures. 6-monthly review required	Regarded as a partial epilepsy attack and treat as uncontrolled epilepsy. May resume driving after 1 year free of any epileptic seizures. Upon specialist advice this period may be reduced if further seizures are unlikely	Not addressed
First, isolated epileptic seizure (prior to epilepsy diagnosis)	Desist from driving for 3 months. Neurological assessment including EEG (awake and asleep) and appropriate imaging preferable	Desist from driving for 6 months. This may be reduced on medical advice	May resume driving until the age of 70 after 1 year free of any epileptic seizures. Medical opinion required before driving again. Special consideration may be given if a non-recurring cause of the seizure is clearly identified	Whilst under evaluation, a restricted licence may be issued subject to medical advice	May resume driving after 1 year free of any epileptic seizures. Upon specialist advice this period may be reduced if further seizures are unlikely	Licence denied due to any of the following: ◆ seizure in the last 2 years ◆ EEG test and medical history show high risk of loss of consciousness ◆ no evidence of epileptiform activity on EEG. Exceptions may be made if a favourable prognosis is made, e.g. seizures are unlikely to reoccur
Epilepsy diagnosis	May resume driving after 6 months free of seizures and on medication. 12 months if seizures associated with altered awareness have occurred in last 2 years. GP conversant with participant compliance. Person to be warned about the effects of fatigue and alcohol	Conditional licence granted if seizure free for 6 months. Annual review required	If patient suffered an attack whilst awake—must desist from driving for minimum 1 year from date of attack before licence may be issued. 3-year licence will be issued until the age of 70 if the driver is seizure free for at least 7 years since the last attack with medication, if required. Exceptions can be made if the seizure occurs during an acute head injury or intracranial surgery	An unrestricted licence may be issued if seizure or episode free for 5 years, without medication. OR seizure free for 3–12 months without medication or with medication but no side effects. Reviews are required 6-monthly, yearly, or 2-yearly. Speed, area, and time of day restriction apply, depending on the length of time without seizures. 6-monthly review required	May resume driving after 1 year free of any epileptic seizures. Upon specialist advice this period may be reduced if further seizures are unlikely.	Licence denied due to any of the following: ◆ seizure in the last 2 years ◆ EEG test and medical history show high risk of loss of consciousness ◆ no evidence of epileptiform activity on EEG. Exceptions may be made if a favourable prognosis is made, e.g. seizures are unlikely to reoccur

Continued

Table 37.1 (*Continued*)

Disorder	Canada	Australia	UK	USA	New Zealand	Sweden
	CMA (2006)	**Austroads (2006 and 2012)**	**Drivers Medical Group, Swansea (2008)**	**Utah Driver License Division (2006 and 2012)**	**Land Transport Safety Authority (2002)**	**Swedish National Road Administration (1999)**
Seizures while sleeping	Drive after 1 year from initial seizure if drug levels are therapeutic	Conditional licence may be issued after 1 year seizure-free period since last seizure whilst awake	If attack occurred whilst asleep, must desist from driving for minimum 1 year. If attacks occur for 3 years whilst asleep, and no attacks when awake then patient may be licensed. If attack when awake occurs, then as above. 3-year licence issue is dependent on patient's being treatment compliant and if driving is unlikely to cause danger to the public	If seizures have occurred only whilst asleep over a period of 3 years or more and confirmed by a medical report, the person may be issued with a licence after a 'suitable interval'	May resume driving after 1 year if no seizures whilst awake and seizure pattern upon waking or during sleep remains unchanged	Licence denied due to any of the following: 1. Seizure in the last 2 years. 2. EEG test and medical history show high risk of loss of consciousness. 3. No evidence of epileptiform activity on EEG
Withdrawal of medication	Desist from driving for 3 months after withdrawal or change of medication *If seizures recur:* can resume driving on resumption of previously effective medications. Resume driving after 3 months if seizure free *Long-term withdrawal:* patients can drive any class of vehicle after being seizure free for 5 years and if no epileptiform activity is recorded during a waking and sleep EEG obtained in the 6 months prior to driving	Desist from driving during withdrawal period and for 3 months after this. On medical advice and with low risk of seizure, may not need to curtail driving	Desist from driving during withdrawal period and for 6 months after this. Exceptions can be made depending on the physician's advice	Person may qualify for a licence, subject to medical report and after a corrective adjustment to medication has been made and a 'suitable interval' has elapsed	A reduction in the requirement for a person to be seizure-free for 1 year prior to resuming driving may be considered if the seizure occurred whilst medication was being withdrawn or modified under medical direction	Exceptions to the requirement for a person to be seizure free in the previous 2 years may be made if the seizures resulted from attempted withdrawal of medication on medical advice. The length of any post-seizure observation period may be specified on a case-by-case basis
Epilepsy treated by surgery	May resume driving after 1-year seizure-free period after surgery. May be reduced to 6 months on neurologist advice	Conditional licence may be issued after 1 year seizure-free period after surgery	Not addressed	Not addressed	Not addressed	Not specifically addressed

of awake seizures after some sleep-related seizures is usually low enough to allow licensing in many jurisdictions (30).

- Compliance with prescribed medication.
- Compliance with behavioural measures. These may include restrictions on driving when tired or sleep deprived, or restrictions to driving at certain times.
- Abstention from other drugs or alcohol which may precipitate seizures or affect control of the condition.
- A much more stringent criterion is applied to commercial or heavy vehicle drivers with epilepsy. This is intended to ensure (within the limits of knowledge of the condition) that drivers have a risk of a seizure no greater than that of the general population.

As Table 37.1 illustrates, a variety of approaches is taken by different licensing authorities and the specifics of licensing guidelines vary between different jurisdictions.

References

1. Fenwick P. Automatism, medicine and the law. *Psychol Med Monogr Suppl* 1990; 17:1–27.
2. Beran RG. Automatism: comparison of common law and civil law approaches—a search for the optimal. *J Law Med* 2002; 10(1):61–8.
3. Marsh L, Krauss GL. Aggression and violence in patients with epilepsy. *Epilepsy Behav* 2000; 1(3):160–8.
4. Reuber M, Mackay RD. Epileptic automatisms in the criminal courts: 13 cases tried in England and Wales between 1975 and 2001. *Epilepsia* 2008; 49(1):138–45.
5. Somerville ER, Black AB, Dunne JW. Driving to distraction—certification of fitness to drive with epilepsy. *Med J Aust* 2010; 192(6):342–4.
6. Hansotia P, Broste SK. The effect of epilepsy or diabetes mellitus on the risk of automobile accidents. *N Engl J Med* 1991; 324(1):22–6.
7. Bener A, Murdoch JC, Achan NV, Karama AH, Sztriha L. The effect of epilepsy on road traffic accidents and casualties. *Seizure* 1996; 5(3):215–19.
8. Taylor J, Chadwick D, Johnson T. Risk of accidents in drivers with epilepsy. *J Neurol Neurosurg Psychiatry* 1996; 60(6):621–7.
9. Sillanpaa M, Shinnar S. Obtaining a driver's license and seizure relapse in patients with childhood-onset epilepsy. *Neurology* 2005; 64(4):680–6.
10. Elliott JO, Long L. Perceived risk, resources, and perceptions concerning driving and epilepsy: A patient perspective. *Epilepsy Behav* 2008; 13(2):381–6.
11. Bautista RE, Wludyka P. Driving prevalence and factors associated with driving among patients with epilepsy. *Epilepsy Behav* 2006; 9(4):625–31.
12. Polychronopoulos P, Argyriou AA, Huliara V, Sirrou V, Gourzis P, Chroni E. Factors associated with poor compliance of patients with epilepsy driving restrictions. *Neurology* 2006; 67(5):869–71.
13. Berkovic SF. Epilepsy syndromes: effects on cognition, performance and driving ability. *Med Law* 2001; 20(4):547–51.
14. Gastaut H, Zifkin BG. The risk of automobile accidents with seizures occurring while driving: relation to seizure type. *Neurology* 1987; 37(10):1613–16.
15. Hasegawa S, Kumagai K, Kaji S. Epilepsy and driving: a survey of automobile accidents attributed to seizure. *Jpn J Psychiatry Neurol* 1991; 45(2):327–31.
16. Specht U, Thorbecke R. Should patients with psychogenic nonepileptic seizures be allowed to drive? Recommendations of German experts. *Epilepsy Behav* 2009; 16(3):547–50.
17. Beaussart M, Beaussart-Defaye J, Lamiaux JM, Grubar JC. Epileptic drivers—a study of 1,089 patients. *Med Law* 1997; 16(2):295–306.
18. Kamel JT, Christensen B, Odell MS, D'Souza WJ, Cook MJ. Evaluating the use of prolonged video-EEG monitoring to assess future seizure risk and fitness to drive. *Epilepsy & Behavior* 2010; 19(4):608–11.
19. McSherry B. Epilepsy, automatism and culpable driving. *Med Law* 2002; 21(1):133–53.
20. Medical Research Council. Randomised study of antiepileptic drug withdrawal in patients in remission. *Lancet* 1991; 337(8751):1175–80.
21. Bonnett LJ, Shukralla A, Tudur-Smith C, Williamson PR, Marson AG. Seizure recurrence after antiepileptic drug withdrawal and the implications for driving: further results from the MRC Antiepileptic Drug Withdrawal Study and a systematic review. *J Neurol Neurosurg Psychiatry* 2011; 82:1328–33.
22. Ray A, Pathak-Ray V, Walters R, Hatfield R. Driving after epilepsy surgery: effects of visual field defects and epilepsy control: British Journal of Neurosurgery. *Br J Neurosurg* 2002; 16(5):456–60.
23. Black AB, Lai NY. Epilepsy and driving in South Australia—an assessment of compulsory notification. *Med Law* 1997; 16(2):253–67.
24. Black AB. Confidentiality and driver licensing authorities. *Med Law* 2003; 22(2):333–43.
25. Remillard GM, Zifkin BG, Andermann F. Epilepsy and motor vehicle driving—a symposium held in Quebec City, November 1998. *Can J Neurol Sci* 2002; 29(4):315–25.
26. Vogtle LK, Martin R, Russell Foushee H, Edward Faught R. A comparison of physicians' attitudes and beliefs regarding driving for persons with epilepsy. *Epilepsy Behav* 2007; 10(1):55–62.
27. Shareef YS, McKinnon JH, Gauthier SM, Noe KH, Sirven JI, Drazkowski JF. Counseling for driving restrictions in epilepsy and other causes of temporary impairment of consciousness: How are we doing? *Epilepsy Behav* 2009; 14(3):550–2.
28. Drazkowski JF, Fisher RS, Sirven JI, Demaerschalk BM, Uber-Zak L, Hentz JG, *et al.* Seizure-related motor vehicle crashes in Arizona before and after reducing the driving restriction from 12 to 3 months. *Mayo Clin Proc* 2003; 78(7):819–25.
29. Krauss GL, Krumholz A, Carter RC, Li G, Kaplan P. Risk factors for seizure-related motor vehicle crashes in patients with epilepsy. *Neurology* 1999; 52(7):1324–9.
30. Thomas RH, King WH, Johnston JA, Smith PE. Awake seizures after pure sleep-related epilepsy: a systematic review and implications for driving law. *J Neurol Neurosurg Psychiatry* 2010; 81(2):130–5.
31. Charlton JL, Koppel S, Odell MS, Devlin A, Langford J, O'Hare M, *et al.* Influence of chronic illness on crash involvement of motor vehicle drivers Report #300. Influence of chronic illness on crash involvement of motor vehicle drivers Report #300. Victoria: Monash University Accident Research Centre, 2010.

of awake seizures after some sleep-related seizures, is usually low enough to allow licensing in many jurisdictions (30).

- Compliance with prescribed medication.
- Compliance with behavioural measures. These may include restrictions on driving when tired or sleep deprived or restrictions to driving in certain times.
- Abstention from other drugs or alcohol which may precipitate seizures or affect control of the condition.
- A much more stringent criterion is applied to commercial or heavy vehicle drivers with epilepsy. This is intended to ensure (within the limits of knowledge of the condition) that drivers have a risk of a seizure no greater than that of the general population.

As Table 37.1 illustrates, a variety of approaches is taken by different licensing authorities and the specifics of licensing guidelines vary between different jurisdictions.

References

1. Fenwick P. Automatism, medicine and the law. Psychol Med Monogr Suppl 1990; 17:1–27.
2. Beran RG. Automatism: commentary on common law and enabling approaches—a search for the optimal. J Law Med 2002; 10(1):61–8.
3. Marsh L, Krauss GL. Aggression and violence in patients with epilepsy. Epilepsy Behav 2000; 1(3):160–8.
4. Reuber M, Mackay RD. Epileptic automatisms in the criminal courts: 13 cases tried in England and Wales between 1975 and 2001. Epilepsia 2008; 49(1):138–45.
5. Somerville ER, Black AB, Dunne JW. Driving to distraction—certification of fitness to drive with epilepsy. Med J Aust 2010; 192(6):342–4.
6. Hansotia P, Broste SK. The effect of epilepsy or diabetes mellitus on the risk of automobile accidents. N Engl J Med 1991; 324(1):22–6.
7. Beran A, Murdoch JC, Avrahami M, Karkaus MS, Szmuk L. The effect of epilepsy on road traffic accidents and casualties. Seizure 1992; 1(1):7–19.
8. Taylor J, Chadwick D, Johnson T. Risk of accidents in drivers with epilepsy. J Neurol Neurosurg Psychiatry 1996; 60(6):621–7.
9. Sillanpää M, Shinnar S. Obtaining a driver's license and seizure relapse in patients with childhood-onset epilepsy. Neurology 2005; 64(4):680–6.
10. Elliott JO, Long L. Perceived risk, resources, and perceptions concerning driving and epilepsy: A patient's perspective. Epilepsy Behav 2008; 13(2):381–6.
11. Sundelin HE, Chang Z. Driving prevalence and factors associated with driving among patients with epilepsy. Epilepsy Behav 2016; [illegible]
12. Pitts [illegible] S, Haigh AA, Haitlan T, Shroff V, [illegible] Elabeiri T. Patients' notification about the compliance of a clinic with epilepsy driving guidelines. Neurology 2012; [illegible]
13. Krauss GL. The law standards for seizure and epilepsy and driving. Epilepsy Behav 2011; [illegible]
14. Gastaut H, Zifkin BG. The risk of automobile accidents with seizures occurring while driving: relation to seizure type. Neurology 1987; 37(10):1613–16.
15. Hasegawa S, Kumagai K, Kaji S. Epilepsy and driving: a survey of automobile accidents attributed to seizure. Jpn J Psychiatry Neurol 1991; 45(2):327–31.
16. Specht U, Thorbecke R. Should patients with psychogenic nonepileptic seizures be allowed to drive? Recommendations of German experts. Epilepsy Behav 2009; 16(4):547–50.
17. Benbadis M, Beaussart-Defaye J, Lamiaux JM, Lopes JL. Epileptic drivers—a study of 1,089 patients. Med Law 1991; 10(3):295–306.
18. Kanaan JE, Christensen J, O'Dell MP, [illegible] W, Cook MJ. Evaluating the use of prolonged video-EEG monitoring to assess future seizure risk and fitness to drive. Epilepsy & Behavior 2016; [illegible]
19. Shorvon SD. Epilepsy, automatism and culpable driving. Med Law 2012; 21(1):133–56.
20. Medical Research Council Randomised study of antiepileptic drug withdrawal in patients in remission. Lancet 1991; 337(8751):1175–80.
21. Bonnett LJ, Shukralla A, Tudur-Smith C, Williamson PR, Marson AG. Seizure recurrence after antiepileptic drug withdrawal and the implications for driving: further results from the MRC Antiepileptic Drug Withdrawal Study and a systematic review. J Neurol Neurosurg Psychiatry 2011; 82(12):1328–33.
22. Ray A, Pathak-Ray V, Walters R, Hatfield R. Driving after epilepsy surgery: effects of visual field defects and epilepsy control. British Journal of Neurosurgery. Br J Neurosurg 2002; 16(5):496–501.
23. Black AB, Lai NY. Epilepsy and driving in South Australia—an assessment of compulsory notification. Med Law 1997; 16(2):253–67.
24. Black AB. Confidentiality and driver licensing authorities. Vic Law 2006; 2(1):1–45.
25. Remillard GM, Zifkin BG, Andermann F. Epilepsy and motor vehicle driving—a symposium held in Quebec City, November 1998. Can J Neurol Sci 2002; 29(4):315–25.
26. Vogtle LK, Martin R, Faught E, Foushee HR, Edward Faught R. A comparison of physicians' attitudes and beliefs regarding driving for persons with epilepsy. Epilepsy Behav 2007; 10(1):95–8.
27. Shareef YS, McKinnon JH, Gauthier SM, Noe KH, Sirven JI, Drazkowski JF. Counseling for driving restrictions in epilepsy and other causes of temporary impairment of consciousness: How are we doing? Epilepsy Behav 2009; 14(3):550–2.
28. Drazkowski JF, Fisher RS, Sirven JI, Demaerschalk BM, Uber-Zak L, Hentz JG, et al. Seizure-related motor vehicle crashes in Arizona before and after reducing the driving restriction from 12 to 3 months. Mayo Clin Proc 2003; 78(7):819–25.
29. Krauss GL, Krumholz A, Carter RC, Li G, Kaplan P. Risk factors for seizure-related motor vehicle crashes in patients with epilepsy. Neurology 1999; 52(7):1324–9.
30. Gastaut H, King WH, Johnston IG, Zifkin BG. Awake seizures after pure sleep-related epilepsy: a systematic review and implications for driving law. J Neurol Neurosurg Psychiatry 2016; 85(12):1320–5.
31. Charlton JL, Koppel S, Odell M, Devlin A, Langford J, O'Hare M, et al. Influence of chronic illness on crash involvement of motor vehicle drivers: 2nd edition. Influence of chronic illness on crash involvement of motor vehicle drivers (report 300). Monash University Accident Research Centre, 2010.

Index